ERRATA

The National Diet and Nutrition Survey: adults aged 19 to 64 years.
Volume 1: Types and quantities of foods consumed.
Henderson L, Gregory J, Swan G. TSO (London, 2002).

ISBN   0 11 621566 6

Since its publication in December 2002, an error has come to light in the derivation of consumption data for the following food types:

>Other cereals
>Cream
>Other milk
>Beef, veal & dishes
>Table sugar
>Fruit juice
>Concentrated soft drinks - not low calorie, as consumed
>Concentrated soft drinks - low calorie, as consumed
>Coffee, as consumed
>Tea, as consumed
>Other beverages, dry weight
>Soup

The following tables have been revised to show correct consumption figures and are available at www.food.gov.uk/science/:

>Tables 2.10(a) and 2.10(b); Tables 2.11(a), 2.11(b) and 2.11(c)
>Tables 2.12(a) and 2.12(b); Tables 2.13(a) and 2.13(b)
>Table 2.14; Table 2.16(b); Table 2.17(b)
>Tables A2(a), A3(a), A4(a), A5(a), A6(a), A7(a) and A8.

Data on nutrient intakes are not affected by this error.

The National Diet and Nutrition Survey: young people aged 4 to 18 years.
Volume 1: Report of the diet and nutrition survey.
Gregory JR, Lowe S, Bates CJ, Prentice A, Jackson LV, Smithers G, Wenlock R, Farron M. TSO (London, 2000).

ISBN   0 11 621265 9

The error noted above affects the consumption data for the following food types for the NDNS of young people aged 4 to 18 years:
>Whole milk
>Cream
>Other milk
>Concentrated soft drinks - not low calorie, as consumed
>Concentrated soft drinks - low calorie, as consumed
>Coffee, as consumed
>Tea, as consumed
>Other beverages, dry weight

Revised consumption figures for these food types are available at www.food.gov.uk/science/.

continued over

The National Diet and Nutrition Survey: adults aged 19 to 64 years.
Volume 2: Energy, protein, carbohydrate, fat and alcohol intake.
Henderson L, Gregory J, Irving K, Swan G. TSO (London, 2003).

ISBN   0 11 621567 4

CORRECTIONS

Page 9, section 2.2, para 1, second and third sentences to read:
'The mean daily total energy intake for men was 9.72MJ (2313kcal) and for women, 6.87MJ (1632kcal) ($p < 0.01$). Mean intake for men was significantly higher than for women in all age groups ($p < 0.01$).

Page 9, section 2.2, para 3, second and third sentences to read:
'The mean daily food energy intake for men was 8.88MJ (2110kcal) and for women, 6.54MJ (1554kcal) ($p < 0.01$). Mean intake for men was significantly higher than for women in all age groups ($p < 0.01$).

The National Diet and Nutrition Survey: adults aged 19 to 64 years.
Volume 3: Vitamin and mineral intake and urinary analytes.
Henderson L, Irving K, Gregory J, Bates CJ, Prentice A, Perks J, Swan G, Farron M. TSO (London, 2003).

ISBN   0 11 621568 2

CORRECTIONS

Page 12, section 2.2.1 Pre-formed retinol
For 'mg' read 'µg'.

Page 17, section 2.3.7, para 2, first sentence:
For '41mg for men' read '41µg for men'.

Page 17, section 2.3.7, para 6, second sentence:
For 'within the range 10mg to 200mg' read 'within the range 10µg to 200µg'.

Office for National Statistics
January 2004

Volume 4

The National Diet & Nutrition Survey: adults aged 19 to 64 years

Nutritional status (anthropometry and blood analytes), blood pressure and physical activity

Dave Ruston
Jacqueline Hoare
Lynne Henderson
Jan Gregory
Office for National Statistics

with **Christopher J Bates**
Ann Prentice
Maureen Birch
Medical Research Council Human Nutrition Research

Gillian Swan
Melanie Farron
Food Standards Agency

A survey carried out in Great Britain on behalf of the Food Standards Agency and the Departments of Health by the Office for National Statistics and Medical Research Council Human Nutrition Research

London: TSO

ISBN 0 11 621569 0

Contact points

For enquiries about this publication, contact
Lynne Henderson
Tel: **020 7533 5385**
E-mail: **lynne.henderson@ons.gov.uk**

To order this publication, call TSO
on **0870 600 5522**. See also inside back cover.

For general enquiries, contact the National Statistics
Customer Enquiry Centre on **0845 601 3034**
(minicom: 01633 812399)
E-mail: **info@statistics.gov.uk**
Fax: 01633 652747
Letters: Room D.115, Government Buildings,
Cardiff Road, Newport NP10 8XG

You can also find National Statistics on the Internet
at **www.statistics.gov.uk**

About the Office for National Statistics

The Office for National Statistics (ONS) is the government
agency responsible for compiling, analysing and disseminating
many of the United Kingdom's economic, social and
demographic statistics, including the retail prices index, trade
figures and labour market data, as well as the periodic census of
the population and health statistics. The Director of ONS is also
the National Statistician and the Registrar General for England
and Wales, and the agency administers the statutory registration
of births, marriages and deaths there.

This report has been produced by the Office for National
Statistics in accordance with the Official Statistics Code of
Practice.

Contents

		Page
Foreword		**vi**
Authors' acknowledgements		**vii**
Notes to the tables		**viii**
1	**Background, research design and response**	**1**
1.1	The National Diet and Nutrition Survey Programme	1
1.2	The sample design and selection	2
1.3	The components of the survey	3
	1.3.1 The dietary and post-dietary record interview	3
	1.3.2 The dietary record	3
	1.3.3 Anthropometry	4
	1.3.4 Blood pressure	5
	1.3.5 24-hour urine collection	6
	1.3.6 Blood analysis	7
	1.3.7 Physical activity	8
1.4	Response and weighting	9
2	**Anthropometry**	**15**
2.1	Introduction	15
2.2	Height	16
2.3	Weight	16
2.4	Body mass index	16
2.5	Waist and hip circumferences	17
2.6	Variations in measurements	18
	2.6.1 Variation in height	18
	2.6.2 Variation in weight	19
	2.6.3 Variation in BMI	19
	2.6.4 Variation in waist to hip ratio	19
2.7	Characteristics found to be independently associated with anthropometric measurements	19
	2.7.1 Findings	19
2.8	Comparison with 1986/87 Adults Survey	20
2.9	Comparison with Health Survey for England 2001	20

3	**Blood pressure**	**33**
	3.1 Introduction	33
	3.1.1 Blood pressure measurements used in the analyses	33
	3.1.2 Interpretation of blood pressure levels	34
	3.2 Systolic and diastolic blood pressure	34
	3.2.1 Systolic blood pressure	34
	3.2.2 Diastolic blood pressure	35
	3.3 Variation in blood pressure	35
	3.3.1 Region and household receipt of benefits	36
	3.3.2 Correlation of systolic blood pressure with urinary sodium excretion	36
	3.4 Characteristics found to be independently associated with variation in blood pressure	36
	3.4.1 Findings	36
	3.5 Comparison with Health Survey for England 2001	37
4	**Blood analytes**	**47**
	4.1 Introduction	47
	4.1.1 Obtaining the blood sample	47
	4.1.2 Analysis of the blood samples	47
	4.2 Haematology, including measures of iron status	48
	4.2.1 The analytes and results	48
	4.2.2 Correlation with dietary intakes and other blood analytes	50
	4.2.3 Variation in the concentrations of haematology analytes and measures of iron status	50
	4.3 Water soluble vitamins and plasma total homocysteine	50
	4.3.1 The analytes and results	50
	4.3.2 Correlation with dietary intakes	53
	4.3.3 Variation in the levels of water soluble vitamins and plasma total homocysteine	53
	4.4 Fat soluble vitamins and carotenoids	54
	4.4.1 The analytes and results	54
	4.4.2 Correlation with dietary intakes	56
	4.4.3 Variation in the concentrations of fat soluble vitamins and carotenoids	56
	4.5 Blood lipids	57
	4.5.1 The analytes and results	57
	4.5.2 Variation in the concentrations of plasma total, plasma HDL and plasma LDL cholesterol	58
	4.6 Other analytes	58
	4.6.1 The analytes and results	58
	4.6.2 Variation in the concentrations and levels of other analytes	59

5   Physical activity   101

5.1   Introduction   101

5.2   Findings   102

        5.2.1   Measures of physical activity   102

        5.2.2   Self-reported levels of physical activity   102

        5.2.3   Time spent in activities of at least moderate
                intensity and vigorous/very vigorous intensity   102

5.3   Variation in physical activity   103

        5.3.1   Region and household receipt of benefits   103

        5.3.2   Correlation with energy and macronutrient
                intakes, anthropometric measurements and
                blood pressure   104

5.4   Characteristics found to be independently associated
        with measures of physical activity   104

        5.4.1   Findings   104

5.5   Comparison with Health Survey for England 1998   104

        5.5.1   Findings   105

Appendices

        A   Sampling errors and statistical methods   115

        B   Unweighted base numbers   133

        C   Weights for results from analysis of blood samples   137

        D   Physical activity   139

        E   Glossary of abbreviations, terms and survey definitions   145

        F   List of tables   151

Foreword

This survey, of a national sample of adults aged 19 to 64 years, is one of a programme of national surveys with the aim of gathering information about the dietary habits and nutritional status of the British population. The results of the survey will be used to develop nutrition policy and to contribute to the evidence base for Government advice on healthy eating.

This report covers physical measurements, blood pressure, physical activity levels and a range of biochemical indices of nutritional status derived from analysis of blood samples. It is the fourth in a series on the findings of this survey. The first report, covering foods consumed, was published in December 2002. The second report, covering intakes of energy and macronutrients, and the third, covering vitamin and mineral intakes and urinary analytes, were published in July 2003. A summary report will complete the series later in 2004.

The work described in this series of reports results from a successful collaboration between the Food Standards Agency and the Department of Health, who jointly funded the collection of the survey data, with the Office for National Statistics and the Medical Research Council Human Nutrition Research.

We warmly welcome this fourth report of the latest survey in the National Diet and Nutrition Survey programme and express our thanks to all the respondents who took part.

Sir John Krebs
Chairman
Food Standards Agency

Melanie Johnson
Minister for Public Health
Department of Health

Authors' acknowledgements

We would like to thank everyone who contributed to the survey and the production of this report:

- the respondents without whose co-operation the survey would not have been possible;

- the ONS interviewers who recruited the respondents and carried out all the fieldwork stages of the survey;

- ONS colleagues in the Sampling Implementation Unit, Field Branch, Business Solutions, Methodology Unit and Project Support Branch, in particular, Amanda Wilmot, Jo Bacon, Bev Botting, Goli Lashkari, Ann Whitby, Michaela Pink, Karen Irving, Caroline Ojemuyiwa, Michael Staley, Glenn Edy, Andrew Tollington, Dave Elliot, Jeremy Barton and Tracie Goodfellow;

- the ONS nutritionists, namely Debbie Hartwell, Michaela Davies, Sui Yip, Laura Hopkins, Jessica Ive, Sarah Oyston, Claire Jaggers and Robert Anderson;

- the ONS editors, namely Angela Harris, Carole Austen, Mike Donovan, Nina Hall, Sue Heneghan, Sarah Kelly, Dave Philpot, Colin Wakeley, Carol Willis and Heather Yates;

- staff of the Medical Research Council Human Nutrition Research (HNR), particularly Steve Austin, Dr Jayne Perks and Dr Andy Coward;

- the phlebotomists and local laboratory personnel who were recruited by HNR to take the blood samples, and process and store the blood specimens;

- Professor Elaine Gunter, Chief, National Health and Nutrition Examination Survey (NHANES) Laboratory, Centres for Disease Control and Prevention, Atlanta, USA, for an independent review of the methodology for the blood and urine collection and laboratory analyses;

- Professor Angus Walls for his contribution to the oral health component and briefing the interviewers on the procedures for the self-tooth and amalgam-filling count;

- Professor Chris Skinner and Dr David Holmes at the University of Southampton for an independent review of response to this NDNS and an assessment of non-response bias;

- David Marker at Westat for an independent review of NDNS methodology and procedures;

- the professional staff at the Food Standards Agency and the Department of Health, in particular Jamie Blackshaw, Susan Church, Michael Day, Miguel Goncalves, Hannah Green, Tom Murray, John Pascoe, Rebecca Preston, Dr Roger Skinner and Alette Weaver of the Food Standards Agency; Richard Bond, Tony Boucher, Ian Cooper, Dr Sheela Reddy and Robert Wenlock of the Department of Health.

Notes to the tables

Tables showing percentages

In general, percentages are shown if the base is 30 or more. Where a base number is less than 30, actual numbers are shown within square brackets.

The row or column percentages may add to 99% or 101% because of rounding and weighting.

The varying positions of the bases in the tables denote the presentation of different types of information. Where the base is at the foot of the table, the whole distribution is presented and the individual percentages add to between 99% and 101%. Where the base is given in a column, the figures refer to the proportion of respondents who had the attribute being discussed, and the complementary proportion, to add to 100%, is not shown in the table.

In tables showing cumulative percentages the row labelled 'All' is always shown as 100%. The proportion of cases falling above the upper limit of the previous band can be calculated by subtracting from 100 the proportion in the previous band. Actual maximum values are not shown in tables of cumulative percentages, since they could vary for different subgroups being considered within the same tables.

Unless shown as a separate group, or stated in the text or a footnote to a table, estimates have been calculated for the total number of respondents in the subgroup, excluding those not answering. Base numbers shown in the tables are the total number of respondents in the subgroup, including those not answering.

The total column may include cases from small subgroups not shown separately elsewhere on the tables, therefore the individual column bases may not add to the base in the total column.

Conventions

The following conventions have been used in the tables:

..	data not available
-	category not applicable; no cases
0	values less than 0.5%
[ ]	numbers inside square brackets are the actual numbers of cases, when the base is fewer than 30.

Tables showing descriptive statistics – mean, percentiles, standard deviation

These are shown in tables to an appropriate number of decimal places.

Significant differences

Differences commented on in the text are shown as being significant at the 95% or 99% confidence levels (p<0.05 and p<0.01). Throughout this volume, the terms 'significant' and 'statistically significant' are used interchangeably. Where differences are shown or described as being 'not statistically significant' or 'ns' this indicates p>0.05. The formulae used to test for significant differences are given in Appendix A, pages 115-131.

As a general indication of those groups showing the largest differences, the differences between all pairs of groups were tested for statistical significance. Because of this 'trawling' approach, real statistical significance levels are lower than indicated here and some of the reported significant differences are likely to be spurious. However, these significance tests can still be validly used for testing hypotheses suggested by earlier work.

Where differences between subgroups are compared for a number of variables, for example differences between respondents in different age groups in mean systolic blood pressure, the significance level shown ($p < 0.05$ or $p < 0.01$) applies to all comparisons, unless otherwise stated.

Standard deviations

Standard deviations for estimates of mean values are shown in the tables and have been calculated for a simple random sample design. In testing for the significant difference between two sample estimates, proportions or means, the sampling error calculated as for a simple random design was multiplied by an assumed design factor of 1.5, to allow for the complex sample design. The reader is referred to Appendix A for an account of the method of calculating true standard errors and for tables of design factors for the main variables and subgroups used throughout this volume. In general, design factors were below 1.5. Therefore although not commented on in the text, there will be some differences in sample proportions and means, that are significantly different, at least at the $p < 0.05$ level.

Weighting

Unless otherwise stated, all proportions and means presented in the tables in the substantive chapters in this volume are taken from data weighted to compensate for the differential probabilities of selection and non-response. Base numbers are presented weighted. All base numbers are given in italics. *See* Appendix B for unweighted base numbers, and Appendix D of the Technical Report online for more details on the weighting: accessible at http://www.food.gov.uk/science.

1 Background, research design and response

This volume presents findings on physical measurements, blood pressure, blood samples, analysed for a range of biochemical indices of nutritional status, and physical activity, from a survey of the diet and nutrition of adults aged 19 to 64 years living in private households in Great Britain, carried out between July 2000 and June 2001. It is the fourth volume in a series that also covers food and nutrient intake data derived from the analyses of dietary records and the analyses of urine samples[1]. This first chapter of this volume describes the background to the National Diet and Nutrition Survey (NDNS) of adults aged 19 to 64 years, its main aims, research designs and methodologies and response. Chapter 2 reports on the anthropometric data – the measurements of height, weight, waist and hip circumferences, and derived indices. Chapter 3 reports on the results of the blood pressure measurements. The results from the analyses of the samples of blood are presented in Chapter 4. Where relevant, the associations between dietary intakes and blood levels are examined. The final substantive chapter reports on the physical activity information collected in the physical activity diaries. Differences are considered by age, sex, region and household receipt of benefits. Where appropriate, comparisons are made between this survey and the Dietary and Nutritional Survey of British Adults aged 16 to 64 years carried out in 1986/87[2].

A Technical Report containing the methodological chapters and appendices is available online[3]. Like previous surveys in the NDNS programme, following publication of the final summary volume, a copy of the survey database, containing the full data set will be deposited with The Data Archive at the University of Essex. Independent researchers who wish to carry out their own analyses should apply to the Archive for access[4].

1.1 The National Diet and Nutrition Survey Programme

The survey forms part of the National Diet and Nutrition Survey (NDNS) programme, which was set up jointly by the Ministry of Agriculture, Fisheries and Food (MAFF)[5] and the Department of Health in 1992 following the successful Dietary and Nutritional Survey of British Adults aged 16 to 64 years carried out in 1986/87 (1986/87 Adults Survey)[2]. MAFF's responsibility for the NDNS programme has now transferred to the Food Standards Agency.

The NDNS programme aims to provide comprehensive, cross-sectional information on the dietary habits and nutritional status of the population of Great Britain. The results of the surveys within the programme are used to develop nutrition policy at a national and local level, and to contribute to the evidence base for Government advice on healthy eating.

The NDNS programme is intended to:

- provide detailed quantitative information on the food and nutrient intakes, sources of nutrients and nutritional status of the population under study as a basis for Government policy;

- describe the characteristics of individuals with intakes of specific nutrients that are above and below the national average;

- provide a database to enable the calculation of likely dietary intakes of natural toxicants, contaminants, additives and other food chemicals for risk assessment;

- measure blood and urine indices that give evidence of nutritional status or dietary biomarkers and to relate these to dietary, physiological and social data;

- provide height, weight and other measurements of body size on a representative sample of individuals and examine their relationship to social, dietary, health and anthropometric data as well as data from blood analyses;

- monitor the diet of the population under study to establish the extent to which it is adequately nutritious and varied;

- monitor the extent of deviation of the diet of specified groups of the population from that recommended by independent experts as optimum for health, in order to act as a basis for policy development;

- help determine possible relationships between diet and nutritional status and risk factors in later life;

- assess physical activity levels of the population under study; and

- provide information on oral health in relation to dietary intake and nutritional status.

The NDNS programme consists of a planned programme of cross-sectional surveys of representative samples of defined age groups of the population. The surveys of older adults, pre-school children, and young people have been published[6,7,8]. The last national survey of diet and nutrition in adults was the 1986/87 Adults Survey[2].

1.2 The sample design and selection

A nationally representative sample of adults aged 19 to 64 years living in private households was required. The sample was selected using a multi-stage random probability design with postal sectors as first stage units. The sampling frame included all postal sectors within mainland Great Britain; selections were made from the small users' Postcode Address File. The frame was stratified by 1991 Census variables. A total of 152 postal sectors was selected as first stage units, with probability proportional to the number of postal delivery points, and 38 sectors were allocated to each of four fieldwork waves. The allocation took account of the need to have approximately equal numbers of households in each wave of fieldwork and for each wave to be nationally representative.

From each postal sector 40 addresses were randomly selected[9].

Eligibility was defined as being aged between 19 and 64 and not pregnant or breastfeeding at the time of the doorstep sift[10]. Where there was more than one adult between the ages of 19 and 64 years living in the same household, only one was selected at random to take part in the survey[11]. A more detailed account of the sample design is given in Appendix D of the Technical Report[3]. In keeping with the ONS normal fieldwork procedures, a letter was sent to each household in the sample in advance of the interviewer calling, telling them briefly about the survey (*see* Appendix A of the Technical Report[3]).

As in previous surveys in the NDNS series, fieldwork covered a 12-month period, to cover any seasonality in eating behaviour, for example, potential reduction in the consumption of salad vegetables during the winter months, and seasonality in the nutrient content of foods, for example, in the vitamin A content of whole milk. The 12-month fieldwork period was divided into four fieldwork waves, each of three months duration[12]. The fieldwork waves were:

Wave 1: July to September 2000

Wave 2: October to December 2000

Wave 3: January to March 2001

Wave 4: April to June 2001

Feasibility work carried out between September and December 1999 by the ONS and the Medical Research Council Human Nutrition Research (HNR) tested all the components of the survey and made recommendations for revisions for the mainstage. For a subgroup of the feasibility study sample, the validity of the dietary recording methodology was tested using the doubly labelled water methodology to compare energy expenditure against reported energy intake. Further details of the design and results of the feasibility study are summarised in Appendix C of the Technical Report[3].

Because this survey, in common with other surveys in the NDNS series, includes invasive procedures such as venepuncture to take a blood sample, and measurements with possible clinical significance (that is the results of the blood analysis and measurement of blood pressure) it was necessary to obtain approval for the survey protocol from a Multi-centre Research Ethics Committee (MREC), and the National Health Service Local Research Ethics Committees covering each of the 152 sampled areas. Further details of the ethics approval process are given in Appendix N of the Technical Report[3].

1.3 The components of the survey

The survey design included: an interview to provide information about the socio-demographic circumstances of the respondent and their household, their medication and eating and drinking habits; a weighed dietary record of all food and drink consumed over seven consecutive days; a record of bowel movements and a record of physical activity for the same seven days; physical measurements of the respondent (height, weight, waist and hip circumferences); blood pressure measurements; and a request for a sample of blood and a 24-hour urine collection. Respondents were also asked to do a self-count of the number of teeth and amalgam fillings they had, and provide a sample of tap water from their home for analysis of fluoride.

1.3.1 The dietary and post-dietary record interview

The interview comprised two parts. An initial face-to-face interview using computer-assisted personal interviewing methods (CAPI) to collect information about the respondent's household, their usual dietary behaviour, consumption of artificial sweeteners, herbal teas and other drinks; any foods that were avoided and the reasons for doing so, including vegetarianism and dieting behaviours; the use of salt at the table and in cooking; and the use of fluoride preparations and dietary supplements. Information was also collected on: the respondent's health status; their smoking and drinking habits; socio-economic characteristics; and, for women in defined age groups, the use of the contraceptive pill, menopausal state and use of hormone replacement therapy.

There was also a short interview, using CAPI, conducted at the end of the seven dietary recording days (post-dietary record interview). Respondents were asked about any problems they experienced in keeping the diary, whether their consumption of specific foods had changed during the seven days and whether they had been unwell at all during the recording period. Respondents were also asked to complete an eating restraint questionnaire, using computer assisted self-interviewing (CASI) or on paper. Information was also collected on prescribed medications taken during the seven days and levels of physical activity.

The interview questionnaire is reproduced in Appendix A of the Technical Report[3].

1.3.2 The dietary record

The survey used a weighed intake methodology since its main aims were to provide detailed quantitative information on the range and distribution of intakes of foods and nutrients for respondents aged 19 to 64 years in Great Britain, and to investigate relationships between nutrient intakes, physical activity levels and various nutritional status and health measures. The advantages and disadvantages of this method and the factors affecting the choice are discussed in Appendix F of the Technical Report[3]. Appendix F also gives further details on the dietary methodology and the recording and coding procedures.

A feasibility study concluded that it was possible to collect dietary information for a seven-day period from respondents and that the quality of information would be acceptable (*see* Appendix C of the Technical Report[3]). Respondents were asked to keep a weighed record of all food and drink they consumed, both in and out of the home, over seven consecutive days. Each respondent was issued with a set of accurately calibrated Soehnle Quanta digital food scales and two recording diaries; the 'Home Record' diary for use when it was possible for foods to be weighed, generally foods eaten in the home; and a smaller 'Eating and Drinking Away From Home' diary (the 'Eating Out' diary) for use when foods could not be weighed, generally foods eaten away from home. The respondent was also issued with a pocket-sized notebook for recording any of this information in circumstances where they were reluctant or it was inappropriate to carry the 'Eating Out' diary. The instruction and recording pages from these documents relating to the dietary information are included in Appendix A of the Technical Report[3].

The 'Home Record' diary was the main recording and coding document. For each item consumed over the seven days a description of the item was recorded, including the brand name of the product and, where appropriate, the method of preparation. Also recorded was the weight served and the weight of any leftovers, the time food was eaten, whether it was eaten at home or elsewhere, and whether fruit and vegetables were home grown, defined as being grown in the household's own garden or allotment.

Everything consumed by the respondent had to be recorded, including medicines taken by mouth, vitamin and mineral supplements, and drinks of water. Respondents were encouraged to weigh everything they could and where a served item could not be weighed, respondents were asked to record a description of the portion size, or to describe the size of the item in some other way. Each separate item of food in a served portion needed to be weighed separately in order that the nutrient composition of each food item could be calculated. In addition, recipes for all home-made dishes were collected.

A large amount of detail needed to be recorded in the dietary record to enable similar foods prepared and cooked by different methods to be coded correctly, as such foods will have different nutrient compositions.

The 'Eating Out' diary was intended to be used only when it was not possible to weigh the food items. In such cases, respondents were asked to write down as much information as possible about each food item consumed, particularly the portion size and an estimate of the amount of any left over.

Where the respondent consumed food or drink items provided by their workplace or college, the interviewer was required to visit the workplace/college canteen to collect further information from the catering manager about, for example, cooking methods, portion sizes and types of fats used (see Appendix A of the Technical Report[3]).

A food code list, giving code numbers for about 3,500 items and a full description of each item, was prepared by nutritionists at the Food Standards Agency and the ONS, for use by the interviewers. As fieldwork progressed, further codes were added to the food code list for home-made recipe dishes and new products found in the dietary record. A page from the food code list is reproduced in Appendix A of the Technical Report[3].

After the interviewers had coded the entries in the dietary records, ONS headquarters coding and editing staff checked the documents. ONS nutritionists carried out initial checks for completeness of the dietary records, dealt with specific queries from interviewers and coding staff, and advised on and checked the quality of coding, with advice from the Food Standards Agency nutritionists. Computer checks for completeness and consistency of information were run on the dietary and questionnaire data. Information from the dietary record was linked to the nutrient databank and nutrient intakes were calculated from quantities of food consumed. This nutrient databank, which was compiled by the Food Standards Agency, holds information on 56 nutrients for each of the 6,000 food codes. Further details of the nutrient databank are provided in Appendix H of the Technical Report[3]. Each food

code used was also allocated to one of 115 subsidiary food groups; these were aggregated into 57 main food groups and further aggregated into 11 food types (see Appendix G of the Technical Report[3]).

1.3.3 Anthropometry

One of the main aims of this survey is to provide anthropometric data on a representative sample of adults, which can be related to socio-demographic and dietary data. Anthropometry, the measurement of body size, weight and proportions, is an intrinsic part of any nutritional survey and can be an indicator of health, development and growth. Derived indices, for instance to assess the ratio of waist to hip circumferences, provide additional information.

In deciding which measurements should be taken a number of factors were considered. These included the acceptability of the measurement to the respondent, whether there was equipment suitable for use in the home and whether interviewers could be trained to take the measurements accurately.

All respondents were eligible to have measurements of standing height, weight and waist and hip circumferences taken. Height and weight can also be used to calculate the Quetelet or Body Mass Index (weight[kg]/height[m]^2) or other indices which control for variations in body weight associated with height. The ratio of waist to hip circumference gives indirect information on the distribution of body fat stores. Several studies in adults have shown that the location of body fat is associated with health risks, in particular cardio-vascular disease[13].

ONS interviewers have taken measurements of height, weight and waist and hip circumferences on surveys of adults and young people[2,7,8,14,15]. All interviewers were trained in accurate measurement techniques at personal briefings. Once trained, any interviewer working on a subsequent, non-consecutive wave of fieldwork attended a one-day refresher briefing where they were retrained in these techniques. Interviewers were able to practise the measurement techniques at the briefings.

Interviewers were allowed to take the measurements at any point after the dietary interview had been completed; it was thought that specifying a particular time to take the measurements could affect response.

Interviewers recorded the measurement, the date on which it was taken, and if there were any special circumstances which might have affected the accuracy of the measurement (*see* M1, Appendix A of the Technical Report[3]). The Department of Health advised on circumstances that were likely to affect the accuracy to such an extent that the measurement should be excluded from the analysis. This included, for example, the respondent being unable to keep the correct posture when standing height was being measured, or their hair being arranged in a 'permanent' style which affected the measurement of standing height. Each measurement was made twice, repeating the same protocol. For further details of the measurement techniques, *see* Appendix J of the Technical Report[3].

Standing height

Height was measured using the Leicester Height Measure[16]. This was the instrument of choice for the NDNS of young people aged 4 to 18 years[8]. The Measure consists of a base plate, four measuring rods, which slot together, two stabilising bars and a head plate, which slides up and down the vertical measuring rods. Measurements were made in centimetres and millimetres.

The respondent was asked to remove their shoes and socks and to wear as few clothes as possible. The respondent was positioned with their feet together and flat on the base plate of the Measure, their arms loosely at their side, and with their head and back straight and against the vertical measuring rods. The respondent's head was correctly positioned in the Frankfort plane[17] by the interviewer and the alignment checked using a card. Once the correct position was achieved the interviewer lowered the head plate until it just touched the top of the respondent's head. The interviewer then asked the respondent to take a breath and stand as tall as possible, without lifting their heels off the base plate.

Weight

Weight was taken using Soehnle Quantratronic scales, Models 7300 and 7306, calibrated in 100 gram units. The scales were checked for accuracy and calibrated by a specialist contractor prior to the start of fieldwork[18]. During the fieldwork period the batteries were regularly changed.

The scale was placed on a hard, level surface. If only a carpeted surface was available then the interviewer noted this. The time of day for taking the measurement was not standardised.

The respondent was asked to wear only light clothing while being weighed; heavy items of clothing, including shoes, trainers and jackets and any heavy jewellery, keys and money were removed where possible. A record was made of which items of clothing the respondent was wearing while being weighed.

Waist and hip circumferences

The waist is defined as the midway point between the iliac crest and the lower rib. The hip circumference is defined as being the maximum circumference over the buttocks and below the iliac crest.

In preparation for these measurements the respondent was asked to wear only light clothing and to have recently emptied their bladder. In particular they were asked to remove any belts or items in pockets that might affect only one of the circumferences and therefore change the ratio between the waist and hip measurements. Respondents were also asked to adjust the position of their clothing to try to achieve a similar thickness at both measurement positions.

An insertion tape was passed around the circumference, adjusted and checked for horizontal alignment[19]. Having achieved satisfactory positioning of the tape the interviewer then asked the respondent to continue breathing normally, that is, not to hold in the breath, and the measurement was made at the end of a normal expiration. Measurements were made and recorded to the nearest millimetre.

Each respondent was given a record card with his or her measurements.

1.3.4 Blood pressure

High blood pressure is an important and known risk factor for cardiovascular disease in adults[20]. Blood pressure could only be taken if written consent from the respondent to take the measurement was obtained[21]. Consent to notify the respondent's GP of their participation in the survey and signed consent to send a record of the blood pressure measurements to the respondent's GP was also sought, but if not obtained, or the respondent was not registered with a GP, the blood pressure measurement was taken and duty of care passed to the survey doctor. If the respondent did not consent to informing their GP or the survey doctor then a blood pressure measurement was not taken.

Blood pressure was measured using the Dinamap 8100 oscillometric monitor[22]. This device was previously used to measure blood pressure on the NDNS of young people aged 4 to 18 years[8] and the Health Survey for England[23], and was the instrument of choice principally for reasons of methodological comparability between all these surveys, instrument reliability and ease of use. A summary review of studies comparing the Dinamap with other devices, including the standard mercury syphgmomanometer, was reported in the NDNS of young people aged 4 to 18 years[8]. Although the mercury sphygmomanometer is relatively cheap, it requires more training to use correctly than an automated device. For epidemiological purposes, automated devices have the advantage that observers need not be highly trained medical or nursing personnel. ONS interviewers are easily able to learn the technique and the risk of inter-observer bias is reduced.

Measurements were made on the respondent's right arm. Three different size cuffs were available and each had markings to indicate, whether, after wrapping the cuff around the upper arm, the cuff selected was the appropriate size[24]. The respondent was asked to remove any jacket, jumper or cardigan they were wearing, and if they were wearing a garment with sleeves, to remove their right arm from the sleeve. If they were unwilling to comply with this, and provided their circulation was not impeded, they were asked to roll the sleeve so that it would be above the top edge of the cuff.

The time of day when the measurements were taken was not standardised but when arranging an appointment interviewers asked the respondent not to eat, drink, smoke or exercise in the 30 minutes prior to the measurement being made. Interviewers subsequently checked whether these instructions had been carried out, and if not and they were unable to reschedule the visit they recorded the relevant details on the measurement schedule.

The respondent was seated so that they were relaxed and had their feet flat on the floor. The right arm was rested on a support at a height that brought the antecubital fossa to approximately heart level. The lower edge of the cuff was placed about 2cm above the elbow crease and the arrow marked on the cuff placed over the brachial artery. The cuff was wrapped to a tightness that allowed two fingers to be inserted between it and the respondent's arm at the top and bottom edges of the cuff.

The respondent was then asked to sit quietly for about 5 minutes before the measurements were taken while the interviewer explained what would happen when the Dinamap was switched on. Three measurements were then taken at one-minute intervals, recording diastolic, systolic and mean arterial blood pressure and pulse rate.

The measurements were recorded on the measurement schedule, with details of any difficulties that might have affected the readings.

For further details of the procedures for taking blood pressure measurements see Appendix J of the Technical Report[3].

Reporting blood pressure

Immediately after the blood pressure measurements were taken, the interviewer sent a copy of the readings to HNR where they were scrutinised by the survey doctor and then sent with an appropriate covering letter to the respondent's GP (see Appendix L of the Technical Report[3]). If the respondent did not have a GP or had not consented to their notification the survey doctor would feed the results back to the respondent. Where the readings obtained by the interviewer were unusually high, defined as all three readings being equal to or above 160mmHg systolic pressure and/or equal to or above 90mmHg diastolic pressure, the interviewer immediately delivered a copy of the results with a standard accompanying letter to the respondent's GP. The interviewer also contacted the survey doctor by telephone, to ensure that the survey doctor was sufficiently informed to discuss the readings with the GP should the need arise, and provided respondent details, including age and weight. If the respondent did not have a GP or had not consented to their GP being informed of their participation, then in the case of high blood pressure readings the interviewer would inform the survey doctor immediately and the survey doctor would contact the respondent to discuss and advise him/her on what further action to take.

1.3.5 24-hour urine collection

The relationship between dietary intakes of sodium, present in salt (sodium chloride), and other dietary components and blood pressure has been investigated in relation to the established association between hypertension and cardiovascular disease. The Scientific Advisory Committee on Nutrition in its recent report on salt and health concluded that reducing the average population salt intake would proportionally lower population average blood pressure levels and confer significant public health benfits by contributing to a reduction in the burden of cardiovascular disease[25]. It was considered important therefore that this survey obtained information on both sodium intakes and blood pressure .

It is not possible to obtain accurate estimates of dietary intake of sodium from weighed food intake information, mainly because it is not possible to assess accurately the amount of salt added to food in cooking or at the table. Estimates of sodium and potassium intakes can be obtained by measuring their urinary excretion, assuming the body is in balance for these minerals.

Since the rate of excretion of both sodium and potassium varies with intake, the best estimate of intake is obtained from the analysis of a urine sample taken from a complete 24-hour collection, which allows for the fluctuations in intake over the collection period. A spot urine sample is not sufficiently representative to provide a valid long-term estimate of intakes, and hence excretion, of sodium and potassium. There were some concerns about the acceptability of a 24-hour collection among this population following the response in the feasibility study for the NDNS of adults aged 65 or over[6]. However, the feasibility study for this NDNS found the 24-hour collection method to be acceptable to respondents (see Appendix C of the Technical Report[3]).

The aim was to have a complete collection of urine over a 24-hour period from as many of the respondents as possible, and to analyse a sample from the complete collection for sodium, potassium, creatinine, urea and fluoride.

The collection of a complete 24-hour urine sample is a demanding task, and previous experience has shown that samples are frequently incomplete. Therefore, an additional procedure, 'PABA-check', has been devised. This is designed to monitor the completeness of the collection by asking respondents to take three 80mg tablets of para-aminobenzoic acid (PABA) at intervals during the 24-hour collection period. Measurement of the PABA concentration and total volume of the collected sample permits the calculation of the percentage recovery of the administered PABA, which in turn is a measure of completeness of the 24-hour urine collection. The taking of PABA required signed consent from the respondents.

The use of this procedure in this survey was approved by the Multi-centre and Local Research Ethics Committees and was successfully piloted in the feasibility study. It was included in part of Wave 1 of the mainstage survey. One respondent in Wave 1 exhibited an acute allergic reaction with generalised urticaria and periorbital oedema soon after taking the three PABA doses. Although this occurrence may have been a chance association, the survey doctor decided, after seeking external advice, to recommend the discontinuation of the PABA-check procedure as a precaution[26]. From part-way through Wave 1 until the end of the survey, all subsequent 24-hour urine collections were made without PABA-check[27].

Respondents were provided with an explanation of the procedures for making the 24-hour urine collection and the purpose of this (see L2 and L5, Appendix K of the Technical Report[3]). They were also provided with instructions (W3) on how to take the subsamples of the urine, under supervision by the interviewer, and a form (M3A) on which to record the date of collection, times of taking the PABA tablets and any problems with the urine collection or PABA procedures. The procedure without PABA was essentially the same, except that all of the equipment, forms and procedural elements that were specific to the PABA-check procedure, were omitted. More detailed information was collected on M3A about missed collections. On the day after starting the collection the interviewer paid another visit to the respondent to weigh the collection and take the sub-samples. For further details on the procedure and equipment provided to respondents and interviewers see Appendix P of the Technical Report[3].

Once the 24-hour collection was completed, the urine collection was thoroughly mixed. The interviewer weighed the total collection twice and recorded both measurements on form M3B (see Appendix K of the Technical Report[3]). The respondent was then asked to take four aliquots, each 10ml, from the total collection using Sarstedt syringes. If the respondent was unable, or unwilling, to take the aliquots themselves, the interviewers were asked to take the subsamples if they were happy to do so. If the collection was tainted with blood no subsamples were taken. The interviewer added pre-printed cryo-labels to the aliquots, added the date to these, and then transferred all four to the postal plastic containers. These were then placed in the cardboard box and then in the Jiffy bag along with completed forms M3A and M3B. The Jiffy bag was sealed with parcel tape and posted to HNR.

Samples were sent by first class post to HNR where they were analysed. On arrival at HNR the samples were stored at −40°C or lower.

If the respondent failed to make a full 24-hour collection ethics approval did not allow for a second attempt. Aliquots were still taken, from the incomplete collection, and a note made of the reasons why a full collection had not been made.

1.3.6 Blood analysis

A further aim of the NDNS programme is to measure haematological and other blood indices that give evidence of nutritional status and to relate these to dietary and social data.

All procedures associated with obtaining and analysing the blood samples were contracted to HNR whose staff worked closely with the ONS throughout all stages of the survey. All procedures were tested in the feasibility study to ensure that they were safe and acceptable to respondents, those taking the blood samples and to the medical profession (*see* Appendix C of the Technical Report[3]). Details of the recruitment and training of the blood takers, and of the recruitment of local laboratories are provided in Appendix N of the Technical Report[3].

Explicit formal consent was required for taking the blood sample from respondents. Interviewers were required to tell the respondent at the time they conducted the dietary interview that their consent to a blood sample being taken would be sought. This was to avoid the possibility that having built a rapport with the interviewer, respondents might have felt obliged to consent to the venepuncture procedure against their true wishes. Respondents were given time to consider whether they wished to participate in this component or not. Written consent for the procedure was sought, as well as consent for HNR to inform the respondent's GP of the results for the clinically significant analytes. If the respondent was not registered with a GP, or consent to pass information to the GP was not given, a blood sample could still be taken provided the respondent provided written consent. In these circumstances the duty of care passed to the survey doctor.

Agreement to this aspect of the survey was independent of agreement to other components in the survey, and was not associated with the £10 gift voucher given to the respondent for completing the full seven-day dietary record. Respondents were told that they were free to withdraw their consent to any procedure at any point, even after the consent form had been signed. Further details of the consent procedures are given in Appendix N of the Technical Report[3].

Blood was taken by the phlebotomist in the respondent's home with the ONS interviewer present. Screening questions were asked by the phlebotomists before attempting to obtain the sample. Questions were asked to ensure exclusion of any respondents with known clotting or bleeding disorders or those taking anticoagulant drugs. If the respondent volunteered that they were HIV or hepatitis B positive, blood was not taken.

The blood samples were collected by the phlebotomist using the Sarstedt Monovette blood-collection system with butterfly or fixed needle, according to their preference. The Monovette system of blood collection is an enclosed system which allows the safe, spill-free collection of blood which is critical in the home environment. It can also offer trace element contamination control and is manufactured from plastic which allows the safe transport of the sample, inside an outer rigid plastic container, through the postal system. Ethics approval allowed for a maximum of two attempts to obtain the blood sample (maximum 30ml).

Details of the procedures for taking blood samples and the processing and storage procedures are described in Appendix O of the Technical Report[3].

Reporting procedures

Respondents and their GPs, if consent to inform the GP was given, were informed by letter of the results of a selected number of analytes which were of clinical significance (*see* Appendix L of Technical Report[3]). This letter also reported the blood pressure measurements for the respondent where these had been taken. Letters to GPs and respondents contained identical results sheets together with information on normal ranges. On request, the survey doctor provided advice to GPs about the need for follow-up tests.

Results for the following assays were reported:

- full blood count (including haemoglobin concentration) and differential blood count

- plasma cholesterol concentration and total cholesterol/HDL ratio

- serum and red cell folate concentration

- serum vitamin B_{12} concentration

- plasma homocysteine concentration if abnormal

- measures of iron status concentration

- plasma 25-hydroxyvitamin D concentration (a measure of vitamin D status)

- blood mercury concentration

Any abnormality of potential clinical significance in any of the unreported analytes, for example, a toxic selenium concentration, was also reported to the respondent and to their GP if consent was obtained.

1.3.7 Physical activity

The main purpose in collecting information on levels of physical activity was to allow an investigation of the relationships between dietary intakes, particularly energy intake, body composition, that is body mass index, and physical activity levels.

If the body does not use all the energy it takes in as food for activity, growth, thermogenesis, for example then it will be stored. Over time, this will lead to an increase in body weight, which if it continues leads to an increased risk of obesity. The risk of cardio-vascular disease increases with obesity and many other illnesses and conditions are related to being overweight[29]. This survey provided the opportunity to relate activity levels to energy intake and body size.

Respondents were asked to record their physical activity over the same seven days as the dietary recording period. The feasibility study showed that the seven-day diary method was appropriate for the collection of data for respondents in this survey.

The recording pages for physical activity were included in the 'Diary of Activities and Eating and Drinking Away from Home' (see Appendix A of the Technical Report[3]). It was felt inappropriate within the context of an already onerous survey to ask respondents to provide detailed information on how all their time was spent, for example, by obtaining a 'time-use' diary. It was considered sufficient to collect information which would allow adults to be classified into broad bands of activity level, for example, very inactive, inactive or active. The diary asked for details of time spent on a list of specified activities. Information was collected on duration and intensity of activity.

Information was collected for each of the seven days on the time spent:

- asleep, including napping;

- at work;

- at college;

- walking briskly or at an average pace;

- in a range of listed household or similar activities – light and heavy housework, gardening, DIY jobs and active caring;

- in a range of listed sports and leisure activities or similar activities, including whether the respondent got 'out of breath and sweaty' doing the activity.

For respondents in employment their hours worked were recorded and they were asked to provide details of what they did in their job so it could be categorised as being of either light, moderate or hard intensity.

Each of the prompted activities has an associated metabolic equivalent value (MET), for example volleyball has a MET value of 4.0[30]. This was used to group activities into different levels of intensity: sleep, very light/light, moderate or hard/very hard. The total time spent in activities of different levels of intensity was calculated for each diary day. Time spent in very/light or light activities was calculated by subtracting the time spent sleeping and in activities of moderate and hard/very hard intensity from 24 hours. This meant that very light/light activities did not have to be recorded separately.

Multiplying the time spent in an activity by its MET value produces a calculated activity score, representing the level of energy expenditure for that respondent. Further details on the calculated activity score and other derived measures of physical activity are given in Appendix D.

1.4 Response and weighting

Table 1.1 shows response to the dietary interview (the responding sample) and dietary record (the diary sample) overall and by fieldwork wave[12]. Of the 5,673 addresses issued[31] to the interviewers, 35% were ineligible for the survey (see Chapter 2 of the Technical Report[3]). This high rate of ineligibility is mainly due to the exclusion of those aged under 19 years and those aged 65 or over. Just over one-third of the eligible sample, 37%, refused outright to take part in the survey. Only 2% of the eligible sample were not contacted. Overall, 61% of the eligible sample completed the dietary interview, including 47% who completed a full seven-day dietary record. Overall, 77% of those who completed the dietary interview completed a full seven-day dietary record.

Table 1.2 shows response to the anthropometric measurements and blood pressure by fieldwork wave[12], sex and age of respondent and the social class of the household reference person[32]. For each of the measurements, at least 77% of the responding sample and 93% of the diary sample had the measurement taken. Table 1.3 shows the proportion of respondents who consented to having a blood sample taken and the proportion of cases where a sample was obtained. Overall, 63% of the responding sample and 78% of the diary sample consented to having a blood sample taken. A blood sample was obtained for 95% of those who consented (60% of the responding sample and 74% of the diary sample).

While there has been a general fall in response to government social surveys over the last decade[32], the level of refusal to this NDNS was higher than expected. Steps were taken at an early stage to improve response, and included reissuing non-productive cases[33], developing the interviewer training to address further response issues, this included providing general guidance on approaching and explaining the survey to respondents, and increased support to the interviewers and their managers. This met with some success so that in Wave 4 a higher proportion of the eligible sample, 67%, completed the dietary interview compared with previous waves, 56% to 60%.

Those who completed the dietary record had a similar demographic profile, by sex, age and social class of the Household Reference Person to those who completed the dietary interview (*see* also Chapter 2 of the Technical Report[3]). There were no significant differences by sex and age or by social class of the Household Reference Person in co-operation rates for the anthropometric and blood pressure measurements or in the proportions consenting to a blood sample, where venepuncture was attempted and where a blood sample was obtained.

The potential for bias in any dataset increases as the level of non-response increases. Assessing bias is particularly difficult when there is little or no information on particular subgroups within the study population. An independent evaluation of the potential impact of non-response bias was undertaken by the University of Southampton[34]. The authors concluded that there was no evidence to suggest serious non-response bias, although this should be interpreted with caution as bias estimates were based upon assumptions about the total refusals and non-contacts for whom there was very little information. The authors recommended population-based weighting by sex, age and region. Indeed, without weighting for the differential response effect, estimates for different groups would be biased estimates because, in particular, they under-represent men and the youngest age group. To correct for this, the data presented in this volume and the other volumes of this survey have been weighted using a combined weight, based on differential sampling probabilities and differential non-response. Bases in tables are weighted bases scaled back to the number of cases in the appropriate sample. Unweighted bases are given in Appendix B on pages 133-135. Further details of the weighting procedures are given in Appendix D of the Technical Report[3].

In summary, the estimates presented in this report result from weighting the data as effectively as possible using the available information. However, results should be interpreted with caution, particularly where the sample sizes are low. The reader should note that the sample size in Scotland is particularly low and therefore standard errors may be large (see Appendix A, pages 115-131, for further details on standard errors).

(Tables 1.1 to 1.3)

References and endnotes

[1] The other volumes in this series are:

(i) Henderson L, Gregory J, Swan G. *National Diet and Nutrition Survey: adults aged 19 to 64 years. Volume 1: Types and quantities of foods consumed.* TSO (London, 2002);

(ii) Henderson L, Gregory J, Irving K, Swan G. *National Diet and Nutrition Survey: adults aged 19 to 64 years. Volume 2: Energy, protein, carbohydrate, fat and alcohol intake.* TSO (London, 2003);

(iii) Henderson L, Irving K, Gregory J, Bates CJ, Prentice A, Perks J, Swan G, Farron M. *National Diet and Nutrition Survey: adults aged 19 to 64 years. Volume 3: Vitamin and mineral intake and urinary analytes.* TSO (London, 2003);

(iv) Summary report, providing a summary of the key findings from the four volumes, to be published in spring 2004.

[2] Gregory J, Foster K, Tyler H, Wiseman M. *The Dietary and Nutritional Survey of British Adults.* HMSO (London, 1990).

[3] The Technical Report is available online at http://www.food.gov.uk/science.

[4] For further information about the archived data contact:

The Data Archive
University of Essex
Wivenhoe Park
Colchester
Essex CO4 3SQ
United Kingdom
Tel: (UK) 01206 872001
Fax: (UK) 01206 872003
E-mail: archive@essex.ac.uk
Website: www.data-archive.ac.uk

[5] Responsibility for this survey and the National Diet and Nutrition Survey programme transferred from the Ministry of Agriculture, Fisheries and Food to the Food Standards Agency on its establishment in April 2000.

[6] Finch S, Doyle W, Lowe C, Bates CJ, Prentice A, Smithers G, Clarke PC. *National Diet and Nutrition Survey: people aged 65 years and over. Volume 1: Report of the diet and nutrition survey.* TSO (London, 1998).

[7] Gregory JR, Collins DL, Davies PSW, Hughes JM, Clarke PC. *National Diet and Nutrition Survey: children aged 1$\frac{1}{2}$ to 4$\frac{1}{2}$ years. Volume 1: Report of the diet and nutrition survey.* HMSO (London, 1995).

[8] Gregory JR, Lowe S, Bates CJ, Prentice A, Jackson LV, Smithers G, Wenlock R, Farron M. *National Diet and Nutrition Survey: young people aged 4 to 18 years. Volume 1: Report of the diet and nutrition survey.* TSO (London, 2000).

[9] Initially 30 addresses were selected within each postal sector. Results from Wave 1 indicated a higher level of age-related ineligibles than expected and a much lower response rate. In order to increase the actual number of diaries completed and to give interviewers enough work an extra 10 addresses, in each sector, were selected for Waves 2, 3 and 4.

[10] The diet and physiology of pregnant or breastfeeding women is likely to be so different from those of other

similarly aged women as possibly to distort the results. Further, as the number of pregnant or breastfeeding women identified within the overall sample of 2000 would not be adequate for analysis as a single group, it was decided that they should be regarded as ineligible for interview.

11 Selecting only one eligible adult per household reduces the burden of the survey on the household and therefore reduces possible detrimental effects on co-operation and data quality. It also reduces the clustering of the sample associated with similar dietary behaviour within the same household and improves the precision of the estimates.

12 As in some cases fieldwork extended beyond the end of the three-month fieldwork wave, or cases were re-allocated to another fieldwork wave, cases have been allocated to a wave for analysis purposes as follows. Any case started more than four weeks after the end of the official fieldwork wave has been allocated to the actual quarter in which it started. For example, all cases allocated to Wave 1 and started July to October 2000 appear as Wave 1 cases. Any case allocated to Wave 1 and started in November 2000 or later appears in a subsequent wave; for example a case allocated to Wave 1 which started in November 2000 is counted as Wave 2. All cases in Wave 4 (April to June 2001) had been started by the end of July 2001.

13 International Obesity Task Force. Obesity: preventing and managing the global epidemic. Report of WHO consultation on obesity, Geneva, 3–5 June 1998. WHO (Geneva, 1998).

14 White A, Nicolaas G, Foster K, Browne F, Carey S. *Health Survey for England 1991*. HMSO (London, 1993).

Breeze E, Maidment A, Bennett N, Flatley J, Carey S. *Health Survey for England 1992*. HMSO (London, 1994).

Bennett N, Dodd T, Flatley J, Freeth S, Bolling K. *Health Survey for England 1993*. HMSO (London, 1995).

15 Knight I. *The Heights and Weights of Adults in Great Britain*. HMSO (London, 1984).

16 The Leicester Height Measure is available from the Child Growth Foundation, 2 Mayfield Avenue, Chiswick, London W4 1PW, UK.

17 To achieve the correct Frankfort position, the bottom of the orbital socket should be in a horizontal line with the external auditory meatus.

18 Scales were checked and calibrated by CHASMOR, 18 Camden High Street, London NW1 6JH, UK.

19 Insertion tapes, fitted with a metal buckle and calibrated in centimetres and millimetres, were supplied by CHASMOR, 18 Camden High Street, London NW1 6JH, UK.

20 Prospective Studies Collaboration. Age specific relevance of usual blood pressure to vascular mortality: a meta-analysis of individual data for one million adults in 61 prospective studies. *Lancet* 2002; **360**: 1903–13.

21 Details of the consent procedures are given in Appendix N of the Technical Report (*see* Note 3).

22 Dinamap monitors were supplied by GE Medical Systems, DINAMAP Centre of Excellence, Monitor House, Unit 3 Cherrywood, Chineham Business Park, Basingstoke, Hampshire, RG24 8WKF and maintained by Marquette Hellige, Montagu Court, Kettering Parkway, Kettering, Northamptonshire NN15 6XR, UK.

23 Erens B, Primatesta P, Prior G (Eds) *Health Survey for England The Health of Minority Ethnic Groups 1999: Volume 2: Methodology and Documentation*. TSO (London, 2001).

24 Small adult cuff: 17–25cm; standard adult cuff: 23–33cm; large adult cuff; 31–40cm.

25 Scientific Advisory Committee on Nutrition. Salt and Health. TSO (London, 2003).

26 The respondent was offered the opportunity of a additional test under medical supervision to ascertain any allergic reaction. This challenge test was performed in July 2001 and concluded that PABA was not the cause of the respondent's allergic symptoms.

27 Subsequent to the removal of the PABA check a decision was made to use plasma creatinine as an indicator of the completeness of the 24-hour urine collection. Further details on this and results from the PABA-check and plasma creatinine are given in Volume 3, Chapter 4, sections 4.1.1 and 4.1.2.

28 National Audit Office. *Tackling obesity in England*. TSO (London, 2001).

29 A MET is a multiple of the resting rate of oxygen consumption, or the ratio of working metabolic rate to resting metabolic rate (WMR/RMR). One MET represents the resting metabolic rate, approximately equal to an energy expenditure of one kilocalorie (kcal) per kilogram body weight per hour (kcal/kg/hour). An individual participating in physical activity at 2 METs is consuming oxygen at twice the resting rate. A list of activities with associated MET values can be found in: Ainsworth BE et al. Compendium of Physical Activities: classification of energy costs of human physical activities. *Med. Sci. Sports Exerc.* 1993; **25(1)**: 71–80.

30 Initially 1,140 addresses were issued per wave. This was increased in Wave 2 to 1,520 addresses, 40 in each quota of work. In Wave 3, 27 addresses were withdrawn. These were unapproachable due to access restrictions in place because of the foot-and-mouth disease outbreak.

31 This is the member of the household in whose name the accommodation is owned or rented, or is otherwise responsible for the accommodation (*see* Appendix E – Glossary).

32 Martin J and Matheson J. Responses to declining response rates on government surveys. *Survey Methodology Bulletin* 1999; **45**: 33–37.

33 Non-productive cases are those where the interviewer was unable to make contact with the selected household or respondent (non-contacts) and where the household or selected respondent refused to take part in the survey (refusals). Addresses that were returned to the office coded as refusals or non-contacts were considered for reissue. Where it was thought that a non-productive case might result in at least a dietary interview (for example, where the selected respondent had said they were too busy at the time of the original call but would be available at a later date) these addresses were issued to interviewers working in subsequent waves of fieldwork.

34 Skinner CJ and Holmes D (2001) *The 2000–01 National Diet and Nutrition Survey of Adults Aged 19–64 years: The Impact of Non-response*. University of Southampton. Reproduced as Appendix E of the Technical Report (*see* Note 3).

Table 1.1

Response to the dietary interview and seven-day dietary record by wave of fieldwork*

Unweighted data

Numbers and percentages

| | Wave of fieldwork | | | | | | | | All | |
| | Wave 1: July–September | | Wave 2: October–December | | Wave 3: January–March | | Wave 4: April–June | | | |
	No.	%	No.	%	No.	%	No.	%	No.	%
Set sample = 100%	1098	100	1397	100	1450	100	1728	100	5673	100
Ineligible	382	35	514	37	515	36	558	32	1969	35
Eligible sample = 100%	716	100	883	100	935	100	1170	100	3704	100
Non-contacts	12	2	24	3	23	2	30	3	89	2
Refusals	271	38	369	42	364	39	360	31	1364	37
Co-operation with:										
dietary interview	433	60	490	56	548	59	780	67	2251	61
seven-day dietary record	325	45	385	44	429	46	585	50	1724	47

Note: * For productive cases, fieldwork wave is defined as the wave (quarter) in which the dietary interview took place; for unproductive cases, fieldwork wave is the wave in which the case was issued (or reissued) (see note 12).

Table 1.2

Co–operation with anthropometric measurements and blood pressure by wave of fieldwork, sex and age of respondent and social class of household reference person

Unweighted data   Numbers and percentages

Wave of fieldwork, sex and age of respondent and social class of household reference person	Height			Weight			Waist and hip circumference			Blood pressure		
	No.	as percentage of:		No.	as percentage of:		No.	percentage of:		No.	as percentage of:	
		responding sample	diary sample		responding sample	diary sample		responding sample	diary sample		responding sample	diary sample
Fieldwork wave:												
Wave 1	356	82	97	356	82	97	354	82	97	347	80	98
Wave 2	402	82	96	405	83	96	402	82	96	395	81	95
Wave 3	433	79	92	432	79	92	426	78	91	408	74	88
Wave 4	609	78	94	608	78	94	601	77	93	589	76	91
Men aged (years):												
19-24	65	76	93	65	76	93	64	74	93	62	72	90
25-34	172	78	94	171	78	94	170	78	94	169	77	94
35-49	328	83	96	329	84	97	328	83	96	323	82	96
50-64	249	81	94	250	81	94	246	80	93	244	79	93
All	814	81	95	815	81	95	808	80	94	798	79	94
Women aged (years):												
19-24	83	76	87	83	76	87	82	75	87	81	74	87
25-34	216	78	95	213	77	94	213	77	94	209	75	92
35-49	393	81	96	396	81	96	387	80	94	374	77	92
50-64	294	80	94	294	80	94	293	79	94	277	75	91
All	986	79	94	986	79	94	975	78	94	941	76	91
Social class of household reference person:												
Non-manual	1024	82	96	1026	82	96	1018	82	95	992	80	94
Manual	738	78	94	738	78	94	729	77	94	712	75	92
All	**1800**	**80**	**95**	**1801**	**80**	**95**	**1783**	**79**	**94**	**1739**	**77**	**93**

Table 1.3

Co–operation with blood sample by wave of fieldwork, sex and age of respondent and social class of household reference person

Unweighted data

Numbers and percentages

	Consent obtained:			Venepuncture attempted:				Blood sample obtained:			
	No.	as percentage of:		No.	as percentage of:			No.	as percentage of:		
		responding sample	diary sample		responding sample	diary sample	consenting sample		responding sample	diary sample	consenting sample
Fieldwork wave:											
Wave 1	290	67	83	284	66	82	98	278	64	80	96
Wave 2	328	67	81	320	65	79	98	313	64	78	95
Wave 3	326	59	73	316	58	71	97	315	57	70	97
Wave 4	475	61	76	459	59	75	97	441	57	71	93
Men aged (years):											
19–24	49	57	74	48	56	72	98	47	55	70	96
25–34	125	57	72	121	55	70	97	120	55	69	96
35–49	262	66	82	256	65	80	98	254	64	79	97
50–64	205	66	81	197	64	78	96	194	63	77	95
All	641	64	79	622	62	77	97	615	61	76	96
Women aged (years):											
19–24	61	56	72	58	53	70	95	53	49	64	87
25–34	163	59	74	161	58	73	99	159	57	72	98
35–49	319	66	79	313	64	77	98	306	63	75	96
50–64	235	64	79	225	61	76	96	214	58	72	91
All	778	63	77	757	61	75	98	732	59	73	94
Social class of household reference person:											
Non–manual	809	65	79	785	63	77	97	771	62	76	95
Manual	579	61	77	764	60	75	132	548	58	73	95
All	**1419**	**63**	**78**	**1379**	**61**	**76**	**97**	**1347**	**60**	**74**	**95**

2 Anthropometry

2.1 Introduction

This chapter presents anthropometric data on the height, weight and waist and hip circumferences of adults aged 19 to 64 years. Data are also presented on the derived measures of body mass index (BMI) and waist to hip ratio. Descriptive statistics are presented for men and women separately by age group. Both bivariate and multivariate analyses are presented showing the relationship between variations in the anthropometric measurements and various socio-demographic, behavioural and dietary factors. The rationale for each of the anthropometric measurements and the protocol, equipment and methodologies used are described in Chapter 1 of this report and in Appendix J of the Technical Report[1].

Data from the Dietary and Nutritional Survey of British Adults aged 16 to 64 years carried out in 1986/87 (1986/87 Adults Survey)[2] and the Health Survey for England 2001 (HSfE)[3] are presented for comparison. Data from the 1986/87 Adults Survey are available for height, weight and BMI. Data from the HSfE are available for height, weight, BMI and waist to hip ratio for adults aged 16 to 64 years.

All 2,251 respondents were eligible for measurements, but not all of the respondents co-operated with every measurement. The response rate for each measurement is given in Chapter 1 of this report. The bases shown in the tables within this chapter therefore vary between measurements. The number of cases for which individual measurements were missing was small enough that it was possible to use a single set of weights for all of the measurements[4]. Unweighted bases are presented in Appendix B.

Data are presented for men and women in four age groups. For the purpose of these analyses age was calculated by subtracting the respondent's date of birth from the date when each measurement was made. There was no requirement for all of the anthropometric measurements to be made at the same visit. It is possible that some respondents may be classified in different age groups for the anthropometric measurements than for other components of the survey.

The interviewers were asked to attempt each measurement twice. In the analyses, the mean of the two recorded measurements was taken. Agreement between the two measurements was checked and cases were included where the percentage difference was less than 15%. Not all participants co-operated with both measurements. In the small number of cases where only one measurement was taken, this measurement was used in the analyses.

The interviewers were asked to record if measurements were taken under any special circumstances, for example if the person was unable to stand fully upright while the height measurement was made. In addition, consistency checks were made within the data for each measurement. Where a measurement lay at either extreme of the distribution, all of the anthropometric measurements were scrutinised for inconsistency for that individual. Measurements that were considered unreliable were excluded from the analyses.

2.2 Height

Height measurements were achieved for a total of 1,800 respondents (unweighted). The measurements for one respondent were excluded due to unreliability, as the respondent was unable to stand upright due to an injured back. For another respondent one measurement was taken in an incorrect standing position and therefore was excluded. In this case the other measurement was used.

Table 2.1 shows descriptive statistics for height for men and women by age group. Acceptable measures of height were obtained for 814 men and 985 women (unweighted). Generally, for men and women within each age group, the mean values were close to median values. This indicates that the distribution of data is normal[5].

The mean height for men was 176cm and the mean height for women was significantly lower at 162cm (p<0.01). Men were significantly taller than women in each age group (p<0.01).

Men aged 25 to 34 years, with a mean height of 177cm, were significantly taller than men aged 50 to 64 years, 175cm (p<0.05). Women aged 19 to 49 years were significantly taller than women aged 50 to 64 years (19 to 24 years: p<0.01; 25 to 49 years: p<0.05). The lower height of men and women in the oldest group compared with younger groups may reflect either a true loss of height with age as a result of spinal compression, or a shorter adult stature as a result of differences in growth during childhood (see Section 2.8).

(Table 2.1)

2.3 Weight

Weight is a useful measure for inter-group comparisons, but there are a number of difficulties associated with the measurement. The weight of an individual can vary from day to day and at different times of the day for the same individual. There are also problems with the interpretation of the measurement as weight is highly correlated with height. Also, weight alone is not a measure of body fat, since the measurement includes the weights of non-fat tissue, bone and body fluids.

Measurements were achieved for 1,801 respondents, representing 815 men and 986 women (unweighted). None of the measurements taken were considered unreliable and so no exclusions were made. There were no cases where only one measurement was recorded. The weights shown here have not been adjusted to take account of the weight of clothing although a

Clothing Record in the Measurements Schedule was kept to report the items of clothing that were worn while the weight measurement was taken (see Appendix A of the Technical Report[1]).

Table 2.2 shows descriptive statistics for weight for men and women by age group. Generally, the mean values were slightly higher than the median values for both men and women within each age group. This indicates that there were a small number of cases within each age group with relatively large weight measurements[5].

The mean weight for men was 84kg, significantly higher than the mean weight for women, 69kg (p<0.01). Men were significantly heavier than women in each age group (p<0.01).

Men aged 19 to 24 years were significantly lighter, 79kg, than men aged 50 to 64 years, 87kg (p<0.05). Women aged 25 to 34 years were significantly lighter than women aged 50 to 64 years, 67kg compared with 71kg (p<0.05).

(Table 2.2)

2.4 Body mass index

Body weight alone is not a good indicator of obesity, or a useful predictor of morbidity or mortality as it is strongly correlated with height. However, weight can be adjusted for height to give an indicator of body shape that is independent of height and provides a measure of 'fatness'.

Of the various indices that standardise weight by height, the most widely used is the Quetelet or Body Mass Index (BMI). To be a useful measure of obesity, BMI should be uncorrelated with height, but there is a low correlation between BMI and height in adults. BMI does have the disadvantage, because it is solely based on measurements of height and weight, of giving a potentially misleading level of fatness in lean individuals with muscular physiques. BMI is calculated as weight (kg) / height (m^2) and in adults is customarily grouped as follows[6]:

Descriptor	Index
Underweight	20 or less
Average	over 20 to 25
Overweight	over 25 to 30
Obese	over 30

The data presented here are based on 1,788 respondents who recorded a measurement of both height and weight as previously described. BMI was calculated for 810 men and 978 women (unweighted).

Table 2.3 shows descriptive statistics for BMI for men and women by age group. Generally, for men and women and within each age group, the mean values were higher than the median values[5]. This shows that there were a small number of cases within each age group with a relatively high BMI.

Mean BMI for men was 27.2 and for women was 26.4 (p<0.05). For both men and women BMI increased with age. Men and women aged 19 to 34 years had significantly lower BMI than those aged 50 to 64 years (women aged 19 to 24 years: p<0.05; all others: p<0.01). For example, for men aged 19 to 24 years, the mean BMI was 25.1 compared with 28.4 for men aged 50 to 64 years (p<0.01). For women aged 19 to 24 years, the mean BMI was 24.8 compared with 27.4 for those women aged 50 to 64 years (p<0.05).

The data show that men were significantly more likely than women to be overweight or obese, that is having a BMI of over 25.0, 66% of men and 53% of women (p<0.01). Forty-two per cent of men and 32% of women were classified as overweight (p<0.01) and one in four men, 25%, and one in five women, 20%, were classified as obese, that is having a BMI of over 30.0 (ns).

A significantly lower proportion of men and women aged 19 to 34 years were classified as overweight or obese than the oldest group of men and women (men aged 25 to 34 years: p<0.05; all others: p<0.01). For example, 43% of men and 39% of women aged 19 to 24 years were classified as overweight or obese compared with 78% and 64% of the oldest group of men and women respectively. In addition, a significantly lower proportion of the youngest group of men were classified as at least overweight, 43%, compared with men aged 35 to 49 years, 70% (p<0.01).

A significantly higher proportion of women were classified as underweight compared with men. Seven per cent of women and 3% of men were classified as underweight, that is having a BMI of 20 or less (p<0.05). The proportion of women aged 19 to 24 years classified as underweight, 19%, was significantly higher than for women aged 35 to 64 years, 4% (p<0.05).

(Table 2.3)

2.5 Waist and hip circumferences

There has been increasing interest in the distribution of body fat as an important indicator of increased risk of cardiovascular disease[6]. The potential health risks associated with being overweight vary depending on where the body fat is distributed. Where fat is deposited centrally around the abdominal region (indicated by a high waist-to-hip ratio) rather than peripherally, around the hip, there is an increased risk of suffering heart disease, diabetes, gallstones, varicose veins and other diseases[6].

Waist and hip measurements were taken from a total of 1,783 respondents, 808 men and 975 women (unweighted). One respondent admitted to breathing in during the first measurement so this was excluded from the analysis. The second measurement was reliable and therefore included. One female respondent had both hip measurements excluded, as they were estimated values that could not be validated without height and weight data. As a result, waist to hip ratios were calculated for a total of 1,782 respondents, 808 men and 974 women.

Waist circumference

Table 2.4 shows descriptive statistics for waist circumference for men and women by age group. For both men and women in each age group, the mean values were slightly higher than median values for waist circumference[5]. This indicates that there were a small number of cases within each age group with relatively large waist circumferences.

The mean waist circumference for men was 95cm and was significantly smaller for women, 82cm (p<0.01). For all age groups men had a significantly greater waist circumference than women (p<0.01).

For both men and women, waist circumference increased with age. Men and women aged 19 to 49 years had significantly smaller waist circumferences than those aged 50 to 64 years (p<0.01). For example, men and women aged 19 to 24 years had mean waist circumferences of 89cm and 78cm respectively, compared with 100cm and 86cm for men and women aged 50 to 64 years (p<0.01). In addition, both men and women aged 19 to 34 years had significantly smaller waist circumferences than those aged 35 to 49 years (men: p<0.01; women: p<0.05).

The waist circumference can be used as a measure of increased risk of metabolic complications of obesity. Guidelines suggest that for men a waist circumference greater than 102cm, and for women greater than 88cm, indicates a substantially increased risk of metabolic complications of obesity[7].

Overall, 29% of men had a waist circumference greater than 102cm and 26% of women had a waist circumference greater than 88cm.

Compared with men aged 19 to 49 years, a significantly higher proportion of men in the oldest age group had a waist circumference of greater than 102cm (19 to 24 years: p<0.05; all others: p<0.01).

A significantly higher proportion of women aged 35 to 64 years compared with women aged 19 to 34 years had a waist circumference of greater than 88cm (35 to 49 years: p<0.05; 50 to 64 years: p<0.01).

(Table 2.4)

Hip circumference

Table 2.5 shows descriptive statistics for hip circumference for men and women by age group. Generally, within each sex and age group, mean values were higher than median values[5]. This indicates that within each age group there were some respondents with relatively large hip circumferences.

There were no significant sex or age differences in mean hip circumference for men or women.

(Table 2.5)

Waist to hip ratio

The waist to hip ratio is a measure of distribution of body fat (both subcutaneous and intra-abdominal). The ratio is calculated as waist circumference (cm) / hip circumference (cm). Guidelines suggest that for men a waist to hip ratio of 0.95 or greater, and for women 0.85 or greater, indicate a potential health risk[8].

Table 2.6 shows descriptive statistics for waist to hip ratio for men and women by age group. The distribution of waist to hip ratio was close to a normal distribution for men and women[5].

Men had a significantly greater mean waist to hip ratio, 0.90, than women, 0.79 (p<0.01). This was true for all age groups (p<0.01).

Waist to hip ratio increased with increasing age for both men and women. For men and women, all age groups had a significantly greater mean waist to hip ratio than the age group below them, except for those aged 25 to 34 years compared with those aged 19 to 24 years (women aged 35 to 49 years compared with 25 to 34 years: p<0.05; all others: p<0.01). For example, men and women aged 50 to

64 years had a mean waist to hip ratio of 0.94 and 0.81 respectively, compared with 0.91 and 0.79 respectively for those aged 35 to 49 years (p<0.01).

Overall, 23% of men had a waist to hip ratio that was 0.95 or greater and 15% of women had a waist to hip ratio of 0.85 or greater.

A significantly higher proportion of men in the two oldest age groups had a waist to hip ratio that was 0.95 or greater than men in the two youngest age groups (19 to 24 years compared with 35 to 49 years: p<0.05; all others: p<0.01). For example, 37% of men aged 50 to 64 years had a waist to hip ratio of 0.95 or greater, compared with 12% of men aged 19 to 24 years (p<0.01).

A significantly higher proportion of women in the oldest age group, 26%, had a waist to hip ratio that was 0.85 or greater than women aged 19 to 49 years (p<0.01).

(Table 2.6)

2.6 Variations in measurements

Table 2.7 shows the relationship between anthropometric measurements and region[9] for men and women. Table 2.8 shows the relationship between measurements and whether someone in the respondent's household was in receipt of certain state benefits[10] for men and women.

As shown in previous tables (see Tables 2.1 to 2.6), anthropometric measures vary by age and sex. When interpreting data on variation by region or household benefit status, it is important to bear in mind that any significant associations between anthropometric measurements and these variables may be a result of the variation in age distributions.

For further analysis of the association between socio-demographic characteristics and anthropometric measurements see Section 2.7 where the technique of multiple regression was used to identify factors independently associated with BMI and waist to hip ratio.

2.6.1 Variation in height

There were no significant differences in the mean height of men or women according to the region in which they lived.

Men living in households not in receipt of benefits were significantly taller, 176cm, than men living in benefit households, 174cm (p<0.05). There was no significant difference in mean height by household benefit status for women.

(Tables 2.7 and 2.8)

2.6.2 Variation in weight

There were no significant differences in mean weight for men or women according to the region in which they lived or household benefit status.

(Tables 2.7 and 2.8)

2.6.3 Variation in BMI

There were no significant regional differences in mean BMI for men. Women in Scotland had a significantly lower mean BMI, 24.9, than women in Central and South West regions of England and in Wales, 27.0 (p<0.05).

There were no statistically significant differences in BMI for men or women according to whether they lived in households in receipt of benefits or not.

(Tables 2.7 and 2.8)

2.6.4 Variation in waist to hip ratio

Men living in Scotland had a significantly greater waist to hip ratio, 0.92, than men living in London and the South East, 0.89 (p<0.05).

Women living in the Northern region had a significantly greater waist to hip ratio than women in any other region (Scotland and Central and South West of England and in Wales: p<0.05; London and the South East: p<0.01).

For men there was no significant difference in waist to hip ratio according to household benefit status. Women in benefit households had a significantly greater waist to hip ratio, 0.80 than women in non-benefit households, 0.78 (p<0.01).

(Tables 2.7 and 2.8)

2.7 Characteristics found to be independently associated with anthropometric measurements

Previous research has shown that various socio-demographic, dietary and physiological factors are associated with variations in body size, and some of these factors are known to be inter-related[2,3,11]. This section considers the combined effect of various socio-demographic, dietary and physiological characteristics on BMI and waist to hip ratio. The technique of multiple regression is used to build a model from those characteristics which most explain the anthropometric measurements.

As shown in previous tables (see Tables 2.3 and 2.6), there is a strong association between sex and BMI and waist to hip ratios, so each multiple regression analysis is presented separately for men and women. To control for the effects of age, this variable was included in each regression analysis.

Tables 2.9 and 2.10 show the socio-demographic, dietary and physiological factors which were significantly associated with BMI and waist to hip ratio when bivariate analyses were carried out, in addition to the previously shown relationships with region and household benefit status[12]. Those independent variables that were found to be significantly associated with the measurements in a bivariate relationship were then included in the multiple regression model[13].

(Tables 2.9 and 2.10)

Tables 2.11 to 2.14 give standardised regression coefficients for a number of characteristics, the independent variables, associated with variation in the anthropometric measurements, the dependent variable, produced using the technique of multiple regression. The tables of results identify those characteristics which are related to the measurements after controlling for the effects of the other characteristics included in the analysis. All regression models are only deemed meaningful when a high percentage of the variance in the dependent variable is explained. The technique of multiple regression calculates coefficients based on the number of cases for which there are valid values for all the variables included in the analysis. Further information on the statistical method and interpretation of output from multiple regression analysis is given in Appendix A[14].

(Tables 2.11 to 2.14)

2.7.1 Findings

Characteristics independently associated with BMI

Tables 2.11 and 2.12 show that the best multiple regression models that could be developed using the most relevant independent variables for the dependent variable BMI were able to explain 41% of the variance for men and 33% of the variance for women.

(Tables 2.11 and 2.12)

Characteristics independently associated with waist to hip ratio

Tables 2.13 and 2.14 show that the best multiple regression models that could be developed using the most relevant independent variables for the dependent variable waist to hip ratio were able to explain 48% of the variance for men and 29% of the variance for women.

(Tables 2.13 and 2.14)

2.8 Comparison with 1986/87 Adults Survey

Table 2.15 compares data from this present survey of adults with data on anthropometric measurements from the Dietary and Nutritional Survey of British Adults aged 16 to 64 years carried out in 1986/87 (1986/87 Adults Survey)[2]. Data are presented for men and women by age for height, body weight and body mass index (BMI). Comparisons are made between comparable age groups in the two surveys; no attempt is made to use the data to undertake cohort analysis. It should be noted that in the 1986/87 Adults Survey the youngest age group was aged 16 to 24 years, while in the current NDNS the youngest age group was adults aged 19 to 24 years. This should be borne in mind where there are differences between these groups. A summary of the methodology and findings from the 1986/87 Adults Survey is given in Appendix S of the Technical Report[1].

Table 2.15 shows that the mean height of men overall was higher in the present NDNS, 176cm, than in the 1986/87 Adults Survey, 174cm (p<0.01). Men aged 35 to 49 years and 50 to 64 years were significantly taller in the present study, 176cm and 175cm respectively, than in the 1986/87 Adults Survey, 174cm and 173cm respectively (p<0.05). There were no significant differences in mean height for women overall or in any age group between this survey and the 1986/87 Adults Survey.

For both men and women, mean weight was significantly higher in the present NDNS, 84kg and 69kg respectively, than in the 1986/87 Adults Survey, 76kg for men and 64kg for women respectively (p<0.01). This was true for men in all age groups (p<0.01). For example, in this survey the mean weight of men aged 50 to 64 years was 87kg and in the 1986/87 Adults Survey was 78kg (p<0.01). Only women in the two older age groups (35 to 64 years) had greater mean weight in the present survey than in the 1986/87 Adults Survey (35 to 49 years: p<0.01; 50 to 64 years: p<0.05).

Mean BMI was significantly higher in this survey for both men and women, 27.2 and 26.4 respectively, than in the 1986/87 Adults Survey, 24.9 and 24.6 respectively (p<0.01). This was true for men in all age groups (16/19 to 24 years: p<0.05; all others: p<0.01) and for women aged 25 to 49 years (25 to 34 years: p<0.05; 35 to 49 years: p<0.01). For example, the mean BMI of men and women aged 35 to 49 years in this survey was 27.4 and 26.7 respectively, compared with 25.6 and 24.8 respectively in the 1986/87 Adults Survey (p<0.01).

(Table 2.15)

2.9 Comparison with Health Survey for England 2001

Table 2.16 compares data from this survey for respondents in England only with data on anthropometric measurements from the Health Survey for England 2001 (HSfE)[3]. The HSfE was based on a multi-stage probability sample of addresses drawn from the Postcode Address File. 15,647 adults aged 16 and over were interviewed. The measurement procedures were similar to the present NDNS, except nurses took the anthropometric measurements in the HSfE whereas trained interviewers took anthropometric measurements on the NDNS. Summaries of the key findings and methodology from the Health Survey for England 2001 are provided in two reports[15,16].

Data are presented for men and women by age for height, body weight, body mass index (BMI) and waist to hip ratio. It should be noted that in the HSfE the youngest age group was aged 16 to 24 years, while in the current NDNS the youngest age group was adults aged 19 to 24 years. This should be borne in mind where there are differences between these groups. Age groups for this survey were redefined to match those of the HSfE so that better comparisons could be made: 16/19 to 24 years, 25 to 34 years, 35 to 44 years, 45 to 54 years, 55 to 64 years. It should also be noted that weight measurements from the HSfE shown here have not been adjusted to take account of the weight of clothing. The NDNS follows the same protocol and has not made adjustments to take account of the weight of clothing.

There were no significant differences between the two surveys in mean height or in mean weight by age group for men or women.

There were no significant differences between the two surveys in BMI for men or women overall or by age, or in the proportion of respondents classified as overweight (BMI over 25.0 to 30.0) or obese (BMI over 30.0).

Men aged 45 to 64 years and women aged 25 to 54 years had a lower mean waist to hip ratio in this survey than in the HSfE (women aged 25 to 44 years: p<0.05; all others: p<0.01).

(Table 2.16)

References and endnotes

1   The Technical Report is available online at http://www.food.gov.uk/science.

2   Gregory J, Foster K, Tyler H, Wiseman M. *The Dietary and Nutritional Survey of British Adults*. HMSO (London, 1990).

3   Bajekal M, Primatesta P and Prior G. Eds. *Health Survey for England 2001*. TSO (London, 2003).

4   Weighting was needed to compensate for unequal probabilities of selection because only one household was selected at multi-household addresses and only one adult was selected for interview from households containing more than one eligible adult (*see* Appendix D of the Technical Report, *see* Note 1). Weighting factors were derived to compensate for differential non-response by comparing the proportions of respondents consenting to height measurements by sex, age and region, with the corresponding proportion in the population using population estimates (*see* Appendix D of the Technical Report). Where other anthropometric measurements were achieved but not height, the weighting factors were calculated using the data for height.

5   Distribution of data was evaluated using the skewness statistic in SPSS. If the skewness statistic was less than twice the standard error of the statistic then data were considered to be normally distributed.

6   International Obesity Task Force. Obesity: preventing and managing the global epidemic. *Report of WHO consultation on obesity, Geneva, 3-5 June 1998*. WHO (Geneva, 1998).

7   Garrow JS, James WPT and Ralph A. *Human Nutrition and Dietetics* (10th Edition). Churchill Livingstone (UK, 2000).

8   Although there is no consensus on cut off points for waist to hip ratio, previous health research in England (including Health Survey for England 2001, *see* Note 3) has used ratios >=0.95 for men and >=0.85 for women based on US/Canadian guidelines (US Department of Agriculture. *Report of the dietary guidelines advisory committee on the dietary guidelines for Americans*. Washington: 1990).

9   The areas included in each of the four analysis 'regions' are given in the response chapter, Chapter 2 of the Technical Report (*see* Note 1). Definitions of 'regions' are given in the Glossary (*see* Appendix E).

10   Households receiving certain benefits are those where someone in the respondent's household was currently receiving Working Families Tax Credit or had, in the previous 14 days, drawn Income Support or (Income-related) Job Seeker's Allowance. Definitions of 'household' and 'benefits (receiving)' are given in the Glossary (*see* Appendix E).

11   Gregory J, Lowe S, Bates CJ, Prentice A, Jackson LV, Smithers G, Wenlock, R, Farron M. *National Diet and Nutrition Survey: young people aged 4 to 18 years. Volume 1: Report of the diet and nutrition survey*. TSO (London, 2000).

12   Bivariate analyses of continuous variables were carried out using the Pearson correlation coefficient and analyses of categorical variables tested the difference between means. It should be noted that where correlations are statistically significant the relationship between the two variables may not necessarily be causal; other factors may have affected the size of the correlation.

13   The regression models are constructed by carrying out bivariate analyses and incorporating variables with significant associations. It should be noted that this method of selection can lead to important variables being left out as additive or interactive effects can only be identified using multiple regression.

14   The model is tested by an ANOVA (*see* Appendix E - Glossary) to determine whether all the regression coefficients are zero in the population, and shows that there are significant linear relationships between the independent variables and the dependent variable.

15   Health Survey for England 2001 – Summary of key findings is available online at http://www.official-documents.co.uk/document/deps/doh/survey01/skf/skf.htm.

16   Health Survey for England 2001 – Methodology and documentation is available online at http://www.official-documents.co.uk/document/deps/doh/survey01/md/md.htm.

Table 2.1

Percentage distribution of height by sex and age of respondent

Cumulative percentages

Height (cm)	Men aged (years):				All men	Women aged (years):				All women
	19–24	25–34	35–49	50–64		19–24	25–34	35–49	50–64	
	cum %	cum %	cum %	cum %	cum %	cum %	cum %	cum %	cum %	cum %
Less than 150	-	-	-	-	-	2	4	1	5	3
Less than 155	-	-	-	0	0	7	11	10	17	12
Less than 160	1	-	1	1	1	30	36	40	46	40
Less than 165	4	3	4	9	5	64	67	72	75	71
Less than 170	12	13	20	25	19	84	90	91	95	91
Less than 175	31	34	46	49	42	98	98	97	99	98
Less than 180	68	69	72	77	72	100	100	100	100	100
Less than 185	92	87	92	94	92					
Less than 190	97	99	98	99	98					
All	100	100	100	100	100					
Base	112	229	263	264	869	110	220	331	270	930
Mean (average value)	177	177	176	175	176	163	162	162	160	162
Median	178	178	176	176	177	163	163	162	161	162
Lower 2.5 percentile	163	165	161	162	162	150	148	151	148	150
Upper 2.5 percentile	190	188	190	188	188	175	173	175	173	174
Standard deviation	6.6	6.1	6.8	6.9	6.7	5.9	6.3	5.8	6.3	6.1

Table 2.2

Percentage distribution of body weight by sex and age of respondent

Cumulative percentages

Body weight (kg)	Men aged (years):				All men	Women aged (years):				All women
	19–24	25–34	35–49	50–64		19–24	25–34	35–49	50–64	
	cum %	cum %	cum %	cum %	cum %	cum %	cum %	cum %	cum %	cum %
Less than 45	-	-	-	-	-	1	1	0	2	1
Less than 50	3	-	-	-	0	12	6	1	4	4
Less than 55	3	1	0	-	1	21	16	12	9	13
Less than 60	8	2	1	1	2	40	34	27	20	28
Less than 65	24	7	5	3	7	61	51	45	35	45
Less than 70	35	12	16	10	16	70	65	58	55	60
Less than 75	46	32	26	23	29	77	77	70	70	72
Less than 80	60	49	38	36	43	84	87	79	81	82
Less than 85	66	63	55	49	57	90	91	85	85	87
Less than 90	74	71	66	63	67	90	94	91	90	91
Less than 100	87	88	87	83	86	94	97	97	97	97
Less than 110	97	99	94	94	96	98	98	99	99	99
All	100	100	100	100	100	100	100	100	100	100
Base	111	228	265	265	870	110	215	334	270	928
Mean (average value)	79	83	85	87	84	66	67	70	71	69
Median	77	81	83	85	82	62	65	67	69	66
Lower 2.5 percentile	50	61	62	65	61	46	47	51	46	47
Upper 2.5 percentile	115	109	119	117	115	112	104	103	106	104
Standard deviation	17.1	13.1	14.4	14.9	14.8	16.3	13.3	15.7	14.0	14.8

Table 2.3

Percentage distribution of body mass index by sex and age of respondent

Cumulative percentages

Body mass index (kg/m²)	Men aged (years):				All men	Women aged (years):				All women
	19–24	25–34	35–49	50–64		19–24	25–34	35–49	50–64	
	cum %	cum %	cum %	cum %	cum %	cum %	cum %	cum %	cum %	cum %
18.5 or less	7	1	0	-	1	7	4	1	3	3
20.0 or less	9	5	2	1	3	19	9	4	4	7
22.5 or less	38	15	9	6	14	39	30	23	17	25
25.0 or less	57	40	30	22	34	61	56	46	36	47
30.0 or less	82	82	75	68	75	86	84	77	78	80
35.0 or less	97	97	94	92	94	94	95	93	90	93
All	100	100	100	100	100	100	100	100	100	100
Base	110	227	263	264	864	110	213	331	269	922
Mean (average value)	25.1	26.4	27.4	28.4	27.2	24.8	25.4	26.7	27.4	26.4
Median	24.1	26.0	26.8	27.5	26.5	23.7	24.0	25.4	26.9	25.4
Lower 2.5 percentile	17.0	19.1	20.9	21.3	19.3	18.1	18.2	19.6	17.3	18.3
Upper 2.5 percentile	41.1	35.3	37.2	37.8	37.3	42.9	37.6	41.2	40.9	40.8
Standard deviation	5.22	4.06	4.23	4.83	4.63	5.74	5.00	5.75	5.50	5.58

Table 2.4

Percentage distribution of waist circumference by sex and age of respondent

Cumulative percentages

Waist circumference (cm)	Men aged (years):				All men	Women aged (years):				All women
	19–24	25–34	35–49	50–64		19–24	25–34	35–49	50–64	
	cum %	cum %	cum %	cum %	cum %	cum %	cum %	cum %	cum %	cum %
65 or less	-	-	-	-	-	4	5	2	2	3
70 or less	3	1	1	-	1	26	13	13	5	12
75 or less	13	3	2	0	3	53	37	29	14	29
80 or less	26	12	6	1	9	68	57	46	33	48
85 or less	49	27	14	5	19	77	78	64	56	66
88 or less	54	36	23	9	26	80	84	71	66	74
90 or less	63	42	30	15	33	83	85	75	72	78
95 or less	74	65	53	33	53	91	93	86	80	86
100 or less	78	78	65	52	66	95	95	93	88	92
102 or less	78	82	73	57	71	95	96	95	89	93
110 or less	92	96	89	83	89	99	97	97	94	96
120 or less	99	99	96	95	97	100	100	100	98	99
130 or less	100	100	100	100	100				99	100
All									100	
Base	111	228	263	261	862	110	214	329	269	922
Mean (average value)	89	92	96	100	95	78	80	82	86	82
Median	86	92	94	99	94	74	77	81	84	81
Lower 2.5 percentile	68	74	76	83	74	62	62	65	66	64
Upper 2.5 percentile	120	111	122	124	121	106	111	112	118	112
Standard deviation	13.4	10.3	11.2	10.2	11.7	11.0	10.8	11.6	12.9	12.1

23

Table 2.5

Percentage distribution of hip circumference by sex and age of respondent

Cumulative percentages

Hip circumference (cm)	Men aged (years):				All men	Women aged (years):				All women
	19–24	25–34	35–49	50–64		19–24	25–34	35–49	50–64	
	cum %	cum %	cum %	cum %	cum %	cum %	cum %	cum %	cum %	cum %
Less than 90	2	2	2	-	1	9	5	3	6	5
Less than 95	26	9	9	2	9	27	17	16	12	16
Less than 100	42	30	26	15	26	47	39	37	27	36
Less than 105	67	55	54	43	52	72	64	57	51	59
Less than 110	70	76	77	71	74	82	80	73	73	76
Less than 115	87	90	90	85	88	88	91	86	84	87
Less than 120	94	96	97	97	96	91	94	93	89	92
All	100	100	100	100	100	100	100	100	100	100
Base	111	228	263	261	862	110	214	329	269	922
Mean (average value)	103	105	105	107	105	102	103	104	106	104
Median	102	104	104	106	104	100	102	103	104	103
Lower 2.5 percentile	90	91	90	95	91	85	87	88	87	87
Upper 2.5 percentile	126	121	122	124	123	130	131	129	134	130
Standard deviation	9.8	8.1	8.2	7.4	8.3	11.6	10.1	10.2	11.4	10.8

Table 2.6

Percentage distribution of waist to hip ratio by sex and age of respondent

Cumulative percentages

Waist to hip ratio	Men aged (years):				All men	Women aged (years):				All women
	19–24	25–34	35–49	50–64		19–24	25–34	35–49	50–64	
	cum %	cum %	cum %	cum %	cum %	cum %	cum %	cum %	cum %	cum %
Less than 0.70	-	1	1	-	0	12	6	4	2	5
Less than 0.75	2	1	1	-	1	46	38	26	17	29
Less than 0.80	15	8	3	1	5	77	73	60	49	62
Less than 0.85	56	29	14	4	20	95	91	87	74	85
Less than 0.90	74	66	45	23	47	100	99	96	90	95
Less than 0.95	88	90	74	63	77		100	99	97	99
Less than 1.00	100	98	93	90	95			100	99	100
All		100	100	100	100				100	
Base	111	228	263	261	862	110	214	329	268	921
Mean (average value)	0.86	0.88	0.91	0.94	0.90	0.76	0.77	0.79	0.81	0.79
Median	0.85	0.88	0.91	0.94	0.90	0.76	0.77	0.78	0.80	0.78
Lower 2.5 percentile	0.75	0.76	0.80	0.83	0.78	0.67	0.66	0.69	0.71	0.68
Upper 2.5 percentile	0.99	0.99	1.05	1.04	1.02	0.87	0.88	0.92	0.96	0.93
Standard deviation	0.062	0.060	0.062	0.050	0.064	0.049	0.056	0.059	0.066	0.062

Table 2.7

Anthropometric measurements by sex of respondent and region

Measurement	Region															
	Scotland				Northern				Central, South West and Wales				London and the South East			
	Mean	Median	sd	Base	Mean	Median	sd	Base	Mean	Median	sd	Base	Mean	Median	sd	Base
Men																
Height (cm)	174	175	6.4	63	176	175	6.5	252	176	177	6.9	306	177	178	6.6	247
Body weight (kg)	86	84	15.5	63	84	82	15.0	251	84	84	14.5	308	83	81	14.8	248
BMI (kg/m²)	28.3	27.9	4.90	63	27.4	26.7	4.67	249	27.1	26.5	4.42	306	26.7	26.1	4.73	246
Waist circumference (cm)	98	97	11.6	63	96	94	11.4	250	95	94	11.2	303	94	94	12.4	246
Hip circumference (cm)	107	106	8.8	63	105	104	8.8	250	105	104	7.6	303	105	104	8.3	246
Waist to hip ratio	0.92	0.92	0.061	63	0.91	0.90	0.064	250	0.91	0.91	0.064	303	0.89	0.90	0.065	246
Women																
Height (cm)	162	162	5.7	71	162	162	6.4	241	161	161	5.9	338	162	162	6.3	281
Body weight (kg)	65	64	14.4	68	70	66	14.6	241	70	68	15.3	336	68	66	14.5	283
BMI (kg/m²)	24.9	24.2	5.18	68	26.6	25.4	5.52	240	27.0	26.4	5.88	333	25.8	24.7	5.25	281
Waist circumference (cm)	80	77	11.8	66	84	82	11.6	239	83	81	12.9	335	81	79	11.4	282
Hip circumference (cm)	102	101	10.3	66	104	103	10.5	239	105	103	11.9	335	104	102	9.7	282
Waist to hip ratio	0.78	0.77	0.058	66	0.80	0.80	0.061	239	0.79	0.78	0.063	335	0.78	0.77	0.060	282

Table 2.8

Anthropometric measurements by sex of respondent and whether someone in the respondent's household was receiving certain benefits

Measurement	Whether receiving benefits							
	Receiving benefits				Not receiving benefits			
	Mean	Median	sd	Base	Mean	Median	sd	Base
Men								
Height (cm)	174	174	6.3	118	176	177	6.7	751
Body weight (kg)	84	82	16.6	121	84	83	14.5	749
BMI (kg/m²)	27.7	27.1	5.35	118	27.1	26.5	4.50	746
Waist circumference (cm)	96	94	13.5	119	95	94	11.3	744
Hip circumference (cm)	105	104	10.0	119	105	105	7.9	744
Waist to hip ratio	0.91	0.91	0.067	119	0.90	0.90	0.064	744
Women								
Height (cm)	161	161	6.1	167	162	162	6.1	764
Body weight (kg)	68	65	15.9	165	69	67	14.6	763
BMI (kg/m²)	26.3	25.7	6.14	164	26.4	25.4	5.45	758
Waist circumference (cm)	84	83	13.9	164	82	80	11.6	758
Hip circumference (cm)	104	102	13.2	164	104	103	10.2	758
Waist to hip ratio	0.80	0.80	0.061	164	0.78	0.78	0.062	758

Table 2.9

Socio-demographic, dietary and physiological factors associated with BMI in bivariate analysis

Men	Women
Age at measurement (years)**	Age at measurement (years)**
Average calculated activity score	Average calculated activity score
Average daily alcohol intake (g)	Average daily alcohol intake (g)
Average daily total energy intake (MJ)	Average daily total energy intake (MJ)
Current smoking**	Current smoking*
Ethnicity of respondent	Ethnicity of respondent
Gross weekly household income	Gross weekly household income**
Grouped Standard Region	Grouped Standard Region*
Household benefit status	Household benefit status
Household composition*	Household composition
Limited activity due to illness or disability	Limited activity due to illness or disability**
Mean diastolic pressure (mmHg)**	Mean diastolic pressure (mmHg)**
Mean systolic pressure (mmHg)**	Mean systolic pressure (mmHg)**
Percentage food energy from protein**	Percentage food energy from protein**
Percentage food energy from saturated fatty acids	Percentage food energy from saturated fatty acids*
Percentage food energy from total carbohydrate**	Percentage food energy from total carbohydrate
Percentage food energy from total fat	Percentage food energy from total fat*
Percentage total energy from protein**	Percentage total energy from protein**
Percentage total energy from saturated fatty acids	Percentage total energy from saturated fatty acids
Percentage total energy from starch	Percentage total energy from starch**
Percentage total energy from total carbohydrate**	Percentage total energy from total carbohydrate
Percentage total energy from total sugars**	Percentage total energy from total sugars**
Reported dieting to lose weight**	Reported dieting to lose weight**
Self-reported alcohol consumption	Self-reported alcohol consumption
Self-reported physical activity level	Self-reported physical activity level**
Social class of household reference person	Social class of household reference person**
Vegetarian or vegan	Vegetarian or vegan
Waist to hip ratio**	Waist to hip ratio**
Wave of interview	Wave of interview

Note: * p<0.05; ** p<0.01

Table 2.10

Socio-demographic, dietary and physiological factors associated with waist to hip ratio in bivariate analysis

Men	Women
Age at measurement (years)**	Age at measurement (years)**
Average calculated activity score	Average calculated activity score
Average daily alcohol intake (g)	Average daily alcohol intake (g)
Average daily total energy intake (MJ)	Average daily total energy intake (MJ)
BMI (kg/m²)**	BMI (kg/m²)**
Current smoking	Current smoking*
Ethnicity of respondent	Ethnicity of respondent
Gross weekly household income	Gross weekly household income**
Grouped Standard Region*	Grouped Standard Region**
Household benefit status	Household benefit status*
Household composition**	Household composition*
Limited activity due to illness or disability	Limited activity due to illness or disability**
Mean systolic pressure (mmHg)**	Mean systolic pressure (mmHg)**
Mean diastolic pressure (mmHg)**	Mean diastolic pressure (mmHg)**
Percentage food energy from total carbohydrate**	Percentage food energy from total carbohydrate
Percentage food energy from total fat	Percentage food energy from total fat**
Percentage food energy from protein**	Percentage food energy from protein
Percentage food energy from saturated fatty acids	Percentage food energy from saturated fatty acids*
Percentage total energy from total carbohydrate**	Percentage total energy from total carbohydrate*
Percentage total energy from protein**	Percentage total energy from protein
Percentage total energy from saturated fatty acids	Percentage total energy from saturated fatty acids
Percentage total energy from starch	Percentage total energy from starch
Percentage total energy from total sugars**	Percentage total energy from total sugars
Reported dieting to lose weight**	Reported dieting to lose weight*
Self-reported alcohol consumption	Self-reported alcohol consumption**
Self-reported physical activity level*	Self-reported physical activity level
Social class of household reference person*	Social class of household reference person**
Vegetarian or vegan	Vegetarian or vegan
Wave of interview	Wave of interview

Note: * p<0.05; ** p<0.01

Table 2.11

Linear regression model for BMI: men

Characteristic	Unstandardised coefficient (B)	Standard error of B	Standardised regression coefficient (β)	T-value
Constant	−14.031	2.487		−5.642***
Waist to hip ratio	39.319	2.335	0.551	16.836***
Age at measurement (years)	−0.054	0.014	−0.153	−3.876***
Current smoking	−1.249	0.287	−0.127	−4.357***
Percentage total energy from protein†	0.188	0.048	0.119	3.910***
Reported dieting to lose weight	1.425	0.426	0.098	3.345**
Systolic blood pressure (mmHg)	0.029	0.012	0.092	2.337*
Diastolic blood pressure (mmHg)	0.023	0.017	0.056	1.313
Household composition				
Living alone	−0.146	0.302	−0.020	−0.484
Living with spouse or partner, no dependent children	0.169	0.228	0.031	0.743
Living with other adults, no spouse or dependent children	−0.346	0.297	−0.051	−1.165
Living with dependent children, with or without spouse	0.322	0.224	0.044	1.439
Percentage total energy from total sugars	−0.016	0.028	−0.022	−0.583
Percentage total energy from total carbohydrate†	−0.001	0.025	−0.002	−0.049
Percentage of variance explained		41%		
Number of respondents		765		

Note: * p<0.05; ** p<0.01; *** p<0.001

† For men, percentage food energy from protein and carbohydrate were significantly correlated with BMI in bivariate analysis, but these variables were not included in the multiple regression models. This is because alcohol intake was not found to be significantly associated with BMI, so percentage of total energy from protein and total carbohydrate, which includes alcohol intake, were chosen preferentially.

Table 2.12

Linear regression model for BMI: women

Characteristic	Unstandardised coefficient (B)	Standard error of B	Standardised regression coefficient (β)	T–value
Constant	−12.194	3.815		−3.196 **
Waist to hip ratio	27.769	2.974	0.311	9.337 ***
Systolic blood pressure (mmHg)	0.078	0.015	0.234	5.243 ***
Diastolic blood pressure (mmHg)	−0.005	0.021	−0.010	−0.245
Reported dieting to lose weight	2.936	0.405	0.230	7.255 ***
Self-reported physical activity level				
Very physically active	−1.401	0.353	−0.122	−3.965 ***
Fairly physically active	−0.144	0.271	−0.016	−0.530
Not very physically active	0.950	0.323	0.090	2.943 **
Not at all physically active	0.595	0.536	0.052	1.109
Region				
Scotland	−0.645	0.460	−0.068	−1.401
Northern	−0.581	0.304	−0.080	−1.910
Central, South West and Wales	0.733	0.270	0.111	2.716 **
London and the South East	0.492	0.290	0.052	1.696
Percentage total energy from protein[†,††]	0.184	0.062	0.110	2.944 **
Current smoking	−1.067	0.368	−0.092	−2.898 **
Gross weekly household income				
Less than £160	−0.880	0.353	−0.114	−2.495 *
£160 - less than £400	0.705	0.263	0.082	2.681 **
£400 & over	0.175	0.255	0.023	0.689
Percentage total energy from starch[†]	0.098	0.039	0.107	2.490 *
Percentage food energy from saturated fatty acids	0.002	0.001	0.093	2.093 *
Limited activity due to illness or disability	0.611	0.261	0.071	2.337 *
Social class of household reference person				
Non-manual	−0.473	0.375	−0.048	−1.262
Manual	0.636	0.380	0.064	1.674
Unclassified	−0.164	0.668	−0.017	−0.245
Age at measurement (years)	−0.020	0.016	−0.045	−1.209
Percentage total energy from total sugars[†]	0.002	0.036	0.002	0.044
Percentage of variance explained		33%		
Number of respondents		780		

Note: * $p<0.05$; ** $p<0.01$; *** $p<0.001$

[†] Percentage food energy from total fat and total carbohydrate were highly correlated with percentage total energy from total sugars, protein and starch (variance inflation factor >10). It is difficult to distinguish the effects in a multiple regression of highly correlated characteristics if they are all included and the results may be unreliable, so percentage food energy from total fat and total carbohydrate were dropped from the regression.

[††] For women, percentage food energy from protein was significantly correlated with BMI in bivariate analysis, but this variable was not included in the multiple regression model. This is because alcohol intake was not found to be significantly associated with BMI, so percentage of total energy from protein, which includes alcohol intake, was chosen preferentially.

Table 2.13

Linear regression model for waist to hip ratio: men

Characteristic	Unstandardised coefficient (B)	Standard error of B	Standardised regression coefficient (β)	T–value
Constant	0.665	0.024		28.048***
Body mass index (kg/m²)	0.007	0.000	0.467	16.033***
Age at measurement (years)	0.002	0.000	0.320	9.111***
Social class of household reference person				
Non-manual	0.008	0.005	0.067	1.690
Manual	0.020	0.005	0.160	4.034***
Unclassified	−0.028	0.009	−0.230	−3.084 **
Percentage total energy from protein†	−0.002	0.001	−0.073	−2.537 *
Self-reported physical activity				
Very physically active	−0.009	0.004	−0.065	−2.445 *
Fairly physically active	−0.000	0.003	−0.004	−0.158
Not very physically active	0.009	0.004	0.071	2.618 **
Not at all physically active	0.000	0.006	0.000	0.004
Reported dieting to lose weight	0.011	0.006	0.054	1.960 *
Percentage total energy from total sugars	−0.001	0.000	−0.056	−1.621
Percentage total energy from total carbohydrate†	0.000	0.000	−0.123	−0.367
Systolic blood pressure (mmHg)	0.000	0.000	−0.004	−0.100
Diastolic blood pressure (mmHg)	0.000	0.000	0.065	1.605
Region				
Scotland	0.005	0.005	0.045	1.059
Northern	−0.001	0.003	−0.011	−0.316
Central, South West and Wales	0.002	0.003	0.020	0.556
London and the South East	−0.006	0.003	−0.050	−1.867
Household composition				
Living alone	−0.002	0.004	−0.019	−0.507
Living with spouse or partner, no dependent children	0.000	0.003	0.004	0.112
Living with other adults, no spouse or dependent children	−0.003	0.004	0.026	0.646
Living with dependent children, with or without spouse	0.004	0.003	0.041	1.423
Percentage of variance explained		48%		
Number of respondents		764		

Note: * $p<0.05$; ** $p<0.01$; *** $p<0.001$

† For men, percentage food energy from protein and total carbohydrate were significantly correlated with waist to hip ratio in bivariate analysis, but these variables were not included in the multiple regression model. This is because alcohol intake was not found to be significantly associated with waist to hip ratio, so percentage of total energy from protein and total carbohydrate, which includes alcohol intake, were chosen preferentially.

Table 2.14

Linear regression model for waist to hip ratio: women

Characteristic	Unstandardised coefficient (B)	Standard error of B	Standardised regression coefficient (β)	T–value
Constant	0.576	0.045		12.944***
Body mass index (kg/m²)	0.004	0.000	0.326	9.444***
Age at measurement (years)	0.001	0.000	0.240	5.945***
Gross weekly household income				
Less than £160	0.017	0.005	0.201	3.446***
£160 - less than £400	−0.003	0.003	−0.036	−1.111
£400 & over	−0.014	0.004	−0.161	−3.719***
Current smoking	0.017	0.004	0.134	4.064***
Self-reported alcohol consumption				
Non/light drinker	0.005	0.004	0.056	1.466
Within weekly guidelines[†]	−0.007	0.003	−0.090	−2.651 **
Above weekly guidelines[†]	0.002	0.004	0.017	0.439
Region				
Scotland	−0.003	0.005	−0.028	−0.566
Northern	0.008	0.003	0.099	2.293 *
Central, South West and Wales	−0.004	0.003	−0.053	−1.246
London and the South East	−0.001	0.003	−0.010	−0.323
Systolic blood pressure (mmHg)	0.000	0.000	0.035	0.745
Diastolic blood pressure (mmHg)	0.000	0.000	0.085	1.990
Reported dieting to lose weight	0.000	0.005	0.001	0.035
Percentage food energy from total fat	0.000	0.000	0.065	0.871
Percentage food energy from saturated fatty acids	0.000	0.000	−0.066	−1.159
Percentage total energy from total carbohydrate	0.000	0.000	0.043	0.747
Social class of household reference person				
Non-manual	0.003	0.004	−0.026	−0.639
Manual	−0.001	0.005	−0.013	−0.309
Unclassified	0.004	0.008	0.039	0.532
Household composition				
Living alone	0.000	0.005	0.000	0.000
Living with spouse or partner, no dependent children	−0.004	0.004	−0.042	−1.080
Living with other adults, no spouse or dependent children	0.009	0.006	0.061	1.549
Living with dependent children, with spouse	0.000	0.004	−0.001	−0.021
Living with dependent children, without spouse	−0.004	0.006	−0.032	−0.697
Household receiving benefits	0.000	0.007	0.001	0.013
Limited activity due to illness or disability	0.002	0.003	0.023	0.734
Percentage of variance explained		29%		
Number of respondents		*778*		

Note: * $p<0.05$; ** $p<0.01$; *** $p<0.001$

   [†] *Weekly guidelines were set at a maximum number of 21 units of alcohol a week for men, and 14 units a week for women. Current guidelines are a maximum daily amount of 4 units for men and 3 units for women.*

Table 2.15

Comparison of anthropometric measurements with the 1986/87 Adults Survey*

Measurement	Age of respondent (years):									
	1986/87 Adults Survey*				All	2000/01 NDNS				All
	16–24	25–34	35–49	50–64	16–64	19–24	25–34	35–49	50–64	19–64
Men										
Height (cm)										
mean	175	176	174	173	174	177	177	176	175	176
median	175	176	174	172	174	178	178	176	176	177
se/sd**	0.5	0.4	0.3	0.4	0.2	6.6	6.1	6.8	6.9	6.7
Base	223	269	370	298	1160	112	229	263	264	869
Body weight (kg)										
mean	70	76	78	78	76	79	83	85	87	84
median	70	75	77	77	75	77	81	83	85	82
se/sd**	0.7	0.7	0.6	0.6	0.3	17.1	13.1	14.4	14.9	14.8
Base	225	279	379	311	1194	111	228	265	265	870
BMI (kg/m²)										
mean	22.9	24.6	25.6	25.9	24.9	25.1	26.4	27.4	28.4	27.2
median	22.4	24.4	25.1	25.8	24.6	24.1	26.0	26.8	27.5	26.5
se/sd**	0.22	0.20	0.19	0.19	0.11	5.22	4.06	4.23	4.83	4.63
Base	222	269	369	298	1158	110	227	263	264	864
Women										
Height (cm)										
mean	163	163	162	160	162	163	162	162	160	162
median	163	163	162	159	162	163	163	162	161	162
se/sd**	0.5	0.4	0.3	0.3	0.2	5.9	6.3	5.8	6.3	6.1
Base	194	261	402	306	1163	110	220	331	270	930
Body weight (kg)										
mean	61	63	65	66	64	66	67	70	71	69
median	58	60	63	63	62	62	65	67	69	67
se/sd**	1.0	0.9	0.6	0.8	0.4	16.3	13.3	15.7	14.0	14.8
Base	196	267	411	315	1189	110	215	334	270	928
BMI (kg/m²)										
mean	22.9	23.9	24.8	26.2	24.6	24.8	25.4	26.7	27.4	26.4
median	21.9	22.5	24.1	24.7	23.6	23.7	24.0	25.4	26.9	25.4
se/sd**	0.35	0.33	0.21	0.33	0.15	5.74	5.00	5.75	5.50	5.58
Base	193	261	402	305	1161	110	213	331	269	922

Note: * Gregory JR et al. The Dietary and Nutritional Survey of British Adults. HMSO (London, 1990).

** The 1986/87 survey reported standard errors; the present survey reports standard deviations.

Table 2.16

Comparison of anthropometric measurements with the Health Survey for England 2001*

Measurement	Age of respondent (years):									
	2001 Health Survey for England*					2000/01 NDNS - England only				
	16–24	25–34	35–44	45–54	55–64	19–24	25–34	35–44	45–54	55–64
Men										
Height (cm)										
mean	177	177	176	175	173	177	177	176	176	174
se/sd**	0.3	0.2	0.2	0.2	0.2	6.8	6.1	6.8	6.5	7.1
Base	774	1071	1244	1145	980	105	211	167	155	134
Body weight (kg)										
mean	76	83	86	85	84	78	83	86	86	86
se/sd**	0.5	0.5	0.4	0.4	0.4	16.1	13.0	15.0	13.5	15.7
Base	758	1060	1232	1124	973	104	210	169	155	134
BMI (kg/m^2)										
mean	24.1	26.4	27.4	27.9	27.9	24.9	26.5	27.7	27.5	28.1
se/sd**	0.16	0.13	0.13	0.13	0.13	4.98	4.11	4.53	4.02	5.13
Base	757	1051	1220	1112	958	102	209	167	155	134
Waist to hip ratio										
mean	0.84	0.89	0.91	0.94	0.95	0.86	0.88	0.91	0.92	0.93
se/sd**	0.002	0.002	0.002	0.002	0.002	0.061	0.061	0.060	0.063	0.046
Base	599	863	1055	1005	879	103	209	167	153	134
Women										
Height (cm)										
mean	163	163	162	161	161	164	162	162	161	161
se/sd**	0.2	0.2	0.2	0.2	0.2	5.6	6.3	5.7	6.5	6.3
Base	915	1365	1613	1396	1073	93	192	202	198	133
Body weight (kg)										
mean	65	69	70	72	73	67	66	69	72	70
se/sd**	0.5	0.4	0.4	0.4	0.4	16.4	12.9	15.1	16.0	12.2
Base	863	1227	1524	1342	1056	93	190	203	198	134
BMI (kg/m^2)										
mean	24.1	25.8	26.6	27.6	28.1	25.1	25.3	26.5	27.6	27.1
se/sd**	0.17	0.15	0.14	0.15	0.16	5.79	4.82	5.69	5.88	4.84
Base	856	1221	1513	1331	1038	93	188	202	198	132
Waist to hip ratio										
mean	0.77	0.78	0.80	0.82	0.83	0.77	0.77	0.79	0.80	0.82
se/sd**	0.002	0.002	0.002	0.002	0.002	0.051	0.057	0.059	0.059	0.069
Base	678	1031	1309	1204	950	93	193	200	197	133

Note: *   Bajekal M, Primatesta P and Prior G. Eds. Health Survey for England 2001. TSO (London, 2003).
       ** The 2001 Health Survey for England reported standard errors; the present survey reports standard deviations.

3 Blood pressure

3.1 Introduction

This chapter presents descriptive data on blood pressure for adults aged 19 to 64 years. Both bivariate and multivariate analyses are presented showing the relationship between blood pressure and various socio-demographic and dietary factors.

All 2,251 respondents were eligible for blood pressure measurements, but not all of the respondents co-operated with this component of the survey. The rationale for making blood pressure measurements and the protocol, equipment and methodologies used are described in Chapter 1 of this report and in Appendix J of the Technical Report[1]. Information on response is also included in Chapter 1 of this report. Data are presented weighted[2]; unweighted bases are presented in Appendix B.

3.1.1 Blood pressure measurements used in the analyses

Blood pressure measurements were only made if signed consent had been obtained both to taking the measurements and to passing the readings to the respondent's General Practitioner and/or the survey doctor[3]. If both these consents were obtained then three measurements of blood pressure were made at pre-set intervals of one minute (*see* Chapter 1 and Appendix J of the Technical Report[1]).

Since the first measurement might have been artificially high, particularly if the respondent was anxious, the first reading from each set of three measurements was excluded and the mean of the subsequent two readings calculated. It is this average value that has been used for analyses and is presented in the tables in this chapter. For two respondents, only the first measurement was successfully achieved and these cases have been excluded from the analysis.

Where it was only possible to make two blood pressure measurements for a respondent, the second reading alone has been used in the analysis. Seven cases had just one measurement included in the analysis. None of the measurements was considered unreliable and so no exclusions were made for this reason[4].

This method of treating and presenting the data has been used in previous NDNS and other surveys, including major national surveys where blood pressure measurements have been made[5,6,7]. It is believed to be more likely to approximate to the respondent's usual blood pressure, which in turn is more likely to predict adverse cardiovascular events[8].

Interviewers were encouraged to report any difficulties they had in making the blood pressure measurements or any unusual circumstances; these were recorded on the measurement schedule M1 (*see* Appendix A of the Technical Report[1]). Difficulty in wrapping the blood pressure cuff, either because the respondent had a conical-shaped upper arm or the circumference of their arm was larger than a cuff of the appropriate width, was reported in about 2% of cases. Where at least two successful measurements were made they have been included in the analyses, even if difficulties were reported.

Of all the respondents who consented to blood pressure measurements, 119 (7%) were taking prescribed anti-hypertensive medication at the time of measurement. Of these, 58 were men, of whom, one was aged 25 to 34 years, 12 were aged 35 to 49 years and 45 were aged 50 to 64 years. For women, a total of 61 were taking anti-hypertensive medication, of whom, four were aged 25 to 34 years, 11 were aged 35 to 49 years and 46 were aged 50 to 64 years. Mean values for all respondents were compared to mean values for respondents excluding those taking prescribed anti-hypertensive medication and little difference was noted[9]. Therefore all respondents have been included in the analyses in this Chapter.

3.1.2 Interpretation of blood pressure levels

As described in Chapter 1 and Appendix J of the Technical Report[1], the Dinamap 8100 automatic monitor used in this survey has been validated in several studies, but compared with measurements made using a mercury sphygmomanometer, the Dinamap has been shown to produce higher systolic and lower diastolic blood pressure levels in adults[10,11]. The Dinamap 8100 is no longer recommended by the European Society of Hypertension due to its inaccuracies for clinical uses, particularly for diastolic blood pressures[12]. It has been used in this survey to allow for comparisons with other health surveys and also to maintain continuity within the National Diet and Nutrition Survey programme.

The differences between blood pressure measurements made using the Dinamap monitor and those which have been made using a different instrument, in particular those using an ausculatory method, mean that direct comparison between measurements are inadvisable. Since the previous Dietary and Nutritional Survey of British Adults aged 16 to 64 years carried out in 1986/87 (1986/87 Adults Survey)[5] used Accutorr sphygmomanometers, which detect pressures by means of oscillometry, results from this present study and the 1986/87 Adults Survey are not compared. However, the Dinamap 8100 was used to measure blood pressure in the Health Survey for England 2001 (HSfE)[7] and therefore results from the HSfE are presented for comparison with data for England from the present NDNS in Section 3.5.

In interpreting the blood pressure results for the respondents in this survey, it should be remembered that these are cross-sectional data, in that blood pressure was measured at a single point in time, and blood pressure is likely to vary over time.

There has been much debate on the relative importance of systolic and diastolic blood pressure, and in general, systolic and diastolic blood pressure correlate highly. In epidemiological studies both are important risk factors for cardiovascular disease[13], but in practice systolic blood pressure should be regarded as the most important[14].

The latest guidelines on the management of hypertension issued by the World Health Organization (WHO)[15] indicate that both hypertension (defined as 140/90mmHg or above) and 'high normal' blood pressure (between 130/85mmHg and 140/90mmHg) pose a threat to health[16]. These guidelines classify optimal blood pressure as less than 120/80mmHg while normal blood pressure is classified as less than 130/85mmHg.

It should be noted that there may be inconsistencies in the data when making comparisons against the WHO guidelines since these were based on mercury sphygmomanometer measurements and are being compared with measurements from the Dinamap 8100 (which can provide inaccurate diastolic blood pressure measurements as described above). This may therefore explain in part why some respondents have optimal systolic and not optimal diastolic blood pressures, and vice versa.

3.2 Systolic and diastolic blood pressure

Blood pressure measurements are presented for 797 men and 939 women (unweighted). Distributions and descriptive statistics are given for measurements of systolic and diastolic pressures by sex and age group. Comparisons with the WHO guidelines are made for each sex and age group. For the purpose of these analyses age was calculated by subtracting the respondent's date of birth from the date when the blood pressure measurement was made.

3.2.1 Systolic blood pressure[17]

Table 3.1 shows descriptive statistics for systolic blood pressure for men and women by age group. Generally, the mean values were slightly higher than the median values for both men and women within each age group. This indicates that there were a small number of cases within each age group with relatively high systolic blood pressure measurements[18].

Mean systolic blood pressure for men, 130mmHg, was significantly higher than for women, 122mmHg (p<0.01). Men aged 19 to 49 years had significantly higher systolic blood pressure than women of the same age (p<0.01).

Both men and women in the oldest age group had significantly higher mean systolic blood pressure than those aged 19 to 49 years (p<0.01). In addition, women aged 35 to 49 years had a significantly higher mean systolic blood pressure of 120mmHg, compared with 114mmHg for those aged 19 to 24 and 25 to 34 years (p<0.01).

Overall, 22% of men and 13% of women had systolic blood pressure that is considered hypertensive and 24% of men and 13% of women had systolic blood pressure that is considered 'high normal' based on the WHO guidelines[15] (p<0.01). Twenty-four per cent of men and 51% of women had systolic blood pressure that is considered optimal (less than 120mmHg) (p<0.01).

Using the guidelines on hypertension issued by the WHO[15], the proportion of both men and women who had systolic blood pressure classified as either hypertensive or 'high normal' increased with age. Conversely, the proportion of both men and women who had mean systolic blood pressure classified as optimal generally decreased with age.

A significantly higher proportion of men and women aged 50 to 64 years had systolic blood pressure that is classified as hypertensive than all younger men and women (p<0.01). In addition, a higher proportion of women aged 35 to 49 years than women aged 19 to 24 years had systolic blood pressure that is classified as hypertensive, 7% and 1% respectively (p<0.05).

A significantly higher proportion of men aged 25 to 34 years, 33%, had systolic blood pressure that is classified as optimal compared with the oldest group of men, 16% (p<0.05). Women aged 50 to 64 years and those aged 35 to 49 years were less likely than women in younger age groups to have optimal systolic blood pressure (p<0.01).

(Table 3.1)

3.2.2 Diastolic blood pressure[17]

Table 3.2 shows descriptive statistics for diastolic blood pressure for men and women by age group. Generally, for men and women within each age group, the mean values were close to median values. This indicates that the distribution of data is normal[18].

Mean diastolic blood pressure for men, 73mmHg, was significantly higher than for women, 68mmHg (p<0.01). Men aged 35 to 64 years had significantly higher mean diastolic blood pressures than women of the same age (p<0.01).

Generally, mean diastolic blood pressure increased with age for both men and women; those aged 35 to 64 years had significantly higher mean diastolic blood pressure than those aged 19 to 34 years (p<0.01). In addition, women aged 25 to 34 years had significantly higher diastolic blood pressure than women aged 19 to 24 years, 65mmHg and 62mmHg respectively (p<0.05), and women aged 50 to 64 years had significantly higher diastolic blood pressure, 72mmHg, than women aged 35 to 49 years, 69mmHg (p<0.01).

Overall, 7% of men and 3% of women had diastolic blood pressure that is considered hypertensive, that is at or above 90mmHg, based on the guidelines issued by the WHO[15] (p<0.05). Seventy-one per cent of men and 86% of women had diastolic blood pressure that is considered optimal (less than 80mmHg) (p<0.01).

Using the guidelines on hypertension issued by the WHO[15], the proportion of both men and women who had mean diastolic blood pressure classified as either hypertensive or 'high normal' increased with age. Conversely, the proportion of both men and women who had mean diastolic blood pressure classified as optimal decreased with age.

A higher proportion of men aged 35 to 64 years compared with men aged 25 to 34 years had diastolic blood pressure classified as hypertensive (50 to 64 years: p<0.01; 35 to 49 years: p<0.05).

All men and women aged 19 to 24 years had diastolic blood pressure that is classified as optimal; a significantly higher proportion than men and women aged 25 to 64 years (p<0.01). In addition, a significantly higher proportion of men aged 25 to 34 years compared with men 35 to 64 years had diastolic blood pressure that is classified as optimal (p<0.01). For women, a higher proportion of those aged 25 to 34 years than women in the oldest age group had diastolic blood pressure classified as optimal (p<0.01).

(Table 3.2)

3.3 Variation in blood pressure

In this section, variation in the average blood pressure measurements is considered in relation to socio-demographic and dietary factors. Table 3.3 shows the relationship between blood pressure and region[19], Table 3.4 between blood pressure and whether someone in the respondent's household was in receipt of certain state benefits[20] and Table 3.5 shows the relationship between systolic blood pressure and urinary sodium excretion. All three tables present data separately for men and women.

As shown in previous tables (*see* Tables 3.1 and 3.2), blood pressure varies by sex and age. When interpreting data on variation by region or household benefit status, it is important to bear in mind that any significant associations between blood pressure measurements and these variables may be a result of the variation in age distributions.

For further analysis of the association between socio-demographic and dietary characteristics and blood pressure measurements *see* Section 3.4 where the technique of multiple regression was used to identify factors independently associated with blood pressure level.

3.3.1 Region and household receipt of benefits

There were no statistically significant differences in mean systolic or diastolic blood pressures for men or women according to the region in which they lived or household benefit status.

(Tables 3.3 and 3.4)

3.3.2 Correlation of systolic blood pressure with urinary sodium excretion

Table 3.5 shows that the correlation coefficients between systolic blood pressure and urinary sodium excretion are generally low for all groups. This indicates that, based on the data from this survey, there was no correlation between systolic blood pressure and urinary sodium.

(Table 3.5)

3.4 Characteristics found to be independently associated with variation in blood pressure

Previous research has shown that various socio-demographic and dietary factors are associated with variations in blood pressure, and some of these factors are known to be inter-related[5,13,21]. This section considers the combined effect of these variables on blood pressure, using the technique of multiple regression to build a model from those characteristics which most explain the blood pressure measurements.

As shown in previous tables, there is a strong association between sex and blood pressure measurements, so each multiple regression analysis is presented separately for men and women. To control for the effects of age, this variable was included in each regression analysis.

Tables 3.6 and 3.7 show the socio-demographic and dietary factors that were significantly associated with blood pressure when bivariate analyses were carried out[22]. Independent variables that were found to be significantly associated with the measurements in a bivariate relationship were included in the multiple regression model[23].

(Tables 3.6 and 3.7)

Tables 3.8 to 3.11 give standardised regression coefficients for a number of characteristics, the independent variables, associated with variation in the blood pressure measurements, the dependent variable, produced using the technique of multiple regression. The tables of results identify those characteristics which are related to the measurements after controlling for the effects of the other characteristics included in the analysis. All regression models are only deemed meaningful when a high percentage of the variance in the dependent variable is explained. The technique of multiple regression calculates coefficients based on the number of cases for which there are valid values for all the variables included in the analysis. Further information on the statistical method and interpretation of output from multiple regression analysis is given in Appendix A[24].

(Tables 3.8 to 3.11)

3.4.1 Findings

Characteristics independently associated with systolic blood pressure

Tables 3.8 and 3.9 show that the best multiple regression models that could be developed using the most relevant independent variables for the dependent variable, systolic blood pressure, explained 50% and 59% of the variance for men and women respectively, which still leaves a substantial proportion of variance to be explained. As expected, the variable that contributed most to the estimate of systolic blood pressure in the regression models was diastolic blood pressure, as these variables are known to be highly correlated.

(Tables 3.8 and 3.9)

Characteristics independently associated with diastolic blood pressure

Tables 3.10 and 3.11 show that the best multiple regression models that could be developed using the most relevant independent variables for the dependent variable, diastolic blood pressure, explained 59% and 50% of the variance for men and women respectively, which still leaves a substantial proportion of variance to be explained. As expected, the variable that contributed most to the estimate of systolic blood pressure in the regression models was diastolic blood pressure, as these variables are known to be highly correlated.

(Tables 3.10 and 3.11)

3.5 Comparison with Health Survey for England 2001

Table 3.12 compares data from the present NDNS for respondents in England only with blood pressure data from the Health Survey for England 2001 (HSfE)[7]. The HSfE was based on a multi-stage probability sample of addresses drawn from the Postcode Address File. 15,647 adults aged 16 and over were interviewed. A summary of the key findings and methodology from the Health Survey for England 2001 are provided in two reports[25, 26].

The blood pressure measurement procedures used in the present NDNS were similar in the HSfE, but measurements in the NDNS were made by a trained interviewer whereas a nurse made the measurements in the HSfE. Differences in measurement procedures, such as non-standardised time of day for measurement, instrument calibration and choices of cuff sizes, in addition to modest inter-survey differences may result in measurement differences that are of methodological origin.

Data are presented for men and women by age for both systolic and diastolic blood pressure. It should be noted that in the HSfE the youngest age group was aged 16 to 24 years, while in the present NDNS the youngest age group was adults aged 19 to 24 years. This should be borne in mind where there are differences between these groups. Age groups for the present NDNS were redefined to match those of the HSfE so that meaningful comparisons could be made: 16/19 to 24 years, 25 to 34 years, 35 to 44 years, 45 to 54 years, 55 to 64 years.

Mean systolic blood pressure was generally lower in the present NDNS than in the HSfE for each sex/age group. For men aged 25 to 34 years and 45 to 54 years, mean systolic blood pressure was significantly lower in the present NDNS than in the HSfE (p<0.01). For women aged 16/19 to 54 years, mean systolic blood pressure was significantly lower in the present NDNS than in the HSfE (16/19 to 24 years: p<0.05; all others: p<0.01).

Mean diastolic blood pressure was generally lower in the present NDNS than in the HSfE for each sex/age group. For men aged 25 to 34 years and 45 to 64 years, mean diastolic blood pressure was significantly lower in the present survey than in the HSfE (p<0.05). For example, mean diastolic blood pressure for men aged 25 to 34 years in the present NDNS was 68mmHg compared with 71mmHg for men of the same age in the HSfE (p<0.05).

For women aged 25 to 54 years mean diastolic blood pressure was significantly lower in the present survey than in the HSfE (35 to 44 years: p<0.05; all others: p<0.01). For example, women aged 45 to 54 years had mean diastolic blood pressure of 70mmHg in the present NDNS compared with 74mmHg in the HSfE (p<0.01).

Given that the same equipment was used to make the blood pressure measurements, it may be possible that the data from the different surveys illustrate what is frequently referred to as 'the white coat effect', that is a tendency for blood pressure to rise when it is measured by a doctor or nurse[27, 28].

(Table 3.12)

References and endnotes

1   The Technical Report is available online at http://www.food.gov.uk/science.

2   Weighting was needed to compensate for unequal probabilities of selection because only one household was selected at multi-household addresses and only one adult was selected for interview from households containing more than one eligible adult (*see* Appendix D of the Technical Report, *see* Note 1). Weighting factors were derived to compensate for differential non-response by comparing the proportions, by sex, age and region, of respondents consenting to blood pressure measurements with the corresponding proportion in the population using population estimates (*see* Appendix D of the Technical Report).

3   If the respondent was not registered with a General Practitioner the duty of care passed to the survey doctor and blood pressure measurements could still be taken.

4   Where systolic or diastolic pressures varied between readings by more than 20%, potential data entry errors were checked by using the recorded Mean Arterial Pressure (MAP) from the M1 (*see* Appendix A of the Technical Report, *see* Note 1) with a derived value for MAP which was calculated by adding the level of the diastolic pressure to one third of the difference between the systolic and diastolic pressures.

5   Gregory J, Foster K, Tyler H, Wiseman M. *The Dietary and Nutritional Survey of British Adults.* HMSO (London, 1990).

6   Finch S, Doyle W, Lowe C, Bates CJ, Prentice A, Smithers G, Clarke PC. *National Diet and Nutrition Survey: people aged 65 years and over. Volume 1: Report of the diet and nutrition survey.* TSO (London, 1998).

7   Bajekal M, Primatesta P and Prior G. Eds. *Health Survey for England 2001.* TSO (London, 2003).

8   Petrie JC, O'Brien ET, Littler WA, de Swiet M. Recommendations on blood pressure measurement. *BMJ* 1986; **293**: 611–615.

9   For both systolic and diastolic blood pressure, there was less than one per cent difference for men and women in all age groups when comparing mean values for all respondents with mean values for respondents excluding those taking prescribed anti-hypertensive medication.

10   Bolling K. *The Dinamap Calibration Study.* HMSO (London, 1994).

11   O'Brien E, Atkins N. Accuracy of the Dinamap portable monitor, model 8100; a review of the evidence for accuracy. *Blood Pressure Monitoring* 1997; **2**: 31–33.

12 O'Brien E, Waeber B, Parati G, Staessen J, Myers MG. BP Measuring Devices: recommendations of the European Society of Hypertension. *BMJ* 2001; **322**: 531–536.

13 Stamler J, Stamler R, Neaton JD. Blood pressure, systolic and diastolic, and cardiovascular risks. US population data. *Arch Intern Med* 1993; **153**: 598–615.

14 Ramsay LE, Williams B, Johnston DG, MacGregor GA, Poston L, Potter JF *et al.* Guidelines for management of hypertension: report of the third working party of the British Hypertension Society, 1999: summary. *J Hum Hypertens* 1999; **13**: 569–592.

15 Chalmers J et al. WHO-ISH Hypertension Guidelines Committee. 1999 World Health Organization – International Society of Hypertension Guidelines for the management of hypertension. *Journal of Hypertension* 1999; **17**: 151–183.

16 Thresholds for treatment intervention can be evaluated independently for systolic and diastolic blood pressure when considering elevated blood pressure levels.

17 Values for systolic and diastolic pressures are *average* values, derived as described in Section 3.1.1 of this chapter. Mean values refer to the mean of the average systolic or diastolic pressures as appropriate.

18 Distribution of data was evaluated using the skewness statistic in SPSS. If the skewness statistic was less than twice the standard error of this statistic then data were considered to be normally distributed.

19 The areas included in each of the four analysis 'regions' are given in the response chapter, Chapter 2 of the Technical Report (*see* Note 1). Definitions of 'regions' are given in the Glossary (*see* Appendix E).

20 Households receiving certain benefits are those where someone in the respondent's household was currently receiving Working Families Tax Credit or had, in the previous 14 days, drawn Income Support or (Income-related) Job Seeker's Allowance. Definitions of 'household' and 'benefits (receiving)' are given in the Glossary (*see* Appendix E).

21 Gregory J, Lowe S, Bates CJ, Prentice A, Jackson LV, Smithers G, Wenlock, R, Farron M. *National Diet and Nutrition Survey: young people aged 4 to 18 years. Volume 1: Report of the diet and nutrition survey.* TSO (London, 2000).

22 Bivariate analyses of continuous variables were carried out using the Pearson correlation coefficient and analyses of categorical variables tested the difference between means. It should be noted that where correlations are statistically significant the relationship between the two variables may not necessarily be causal; other factors may have affected the size of the correlation.

23 The regression models are constructed by carrying out bivariate analyses and incorporating variables with significant associations. It should be noted that this method of selection can lead to important variables being left out as additive or interactive effects can only be identified using multiple regression.

24 The model is tested by an ANOVA (*see* Appendix E - Glossary) to determine whether all the regression coefficients are zero in the population, and shows that there are significant linear relationships between the independent variables and the dependent variable.

25 Health Survey for England 2001 – Summary of key findings is available online at http://www.official-documents.co.uk/document/deps/doh/survey01/skf/skf.htm.

26 Health Survey for England 2001 – Methodology and documentation is available online at http://www.official-documents.co.uk/document/deps/doh/survey01/md/md.htm.

27 Tsai P-S. White coat hypertension: understanding the concept and examining the significance. *Journal of Clinical Nursing* 2002; **11(6)**: 715–722.

28 Verdecchia P, O'Brien E, Pickering T, Staessen JA, Parati G, Myers M, Palatini P. When can the practising physician suspect white coat hypertension? Statement from the Working Group on Blood Pressure Monitoring of the European Society of Hypertension. *American Journal of Hypertension* 2003; **16(1)**: 87–91.

Table 3.1

Percentage distribution of systolic blood pressure by sex and age of respondent

Cumulative percentages

Systolic blood pressure (mmHg)	Men aged (years):				All men	Women aged (years):				All women
	19–24	25–34	35–49	50–64		19–24	25–34	35–49	50–64	
	cum %	cum %	cum %	cum %	cum %	cum %	cum %	cum %	cum %	cum %
Less than 100	-	2	1	0	1	2	7	5	1	4
Less than 105	-	5	2	2	2	12	25	10	6	13
Less than 110	1	10	4	4	5	36	42	24	8	25
Less than 115	11	18	13	7	12	53	58	39	16	39
Less than 120	28	33	24	16	24	74	69	52	24	51
Less than 125	51	50	41	24	40	85	83	67	34	63
Less than 130	67	62	59	36	54	94	93	79	43	74
Less than 140	88	86	82	63	78	99	97	93	67	87
Less than 150	96	98	93	80	91	100	99	98	86	95
Less than 160	100	100	97	92	97		100	99	93	98
All			100	100	100			100	100	100
Base	109	221	255	255	839	105	212	320	260	897
Mean (average value)	127	125	129	136	130	114	114	120	133	122
Median	124	124	128	134	128	114	112	119	132	120
Lower 5.0 percentile	112	104	111	112	109	100	98	100	104	100
Upper 5.0 percentile	148	146	153	166	155	134	136	142	164	149
Standard deviation	10.7	13.0	13.4	16.7	14.7	9.6	11.4	13.8	18.2	16.2

Table 3.2

Percentage distribution of diastolic blood pressure by sex and age of respondent

Cumulative percentages

Diastolic blood pressure (mmHg)	Men aged (years):				All men	Women aged (years):				All women
	19–24	25–34	35–49	50–64		19–24	25–34	35–49	50–64	
	cum %	cum %	cum %	cum %	cum %	cum %	cum %	cum %	cum %	cum %
Less than 50	1	2	0	-	1	5	5	2	2	3
Less than 55	9	10	2	2	5	17	13	6	3	8
Less than 60	24	22	7	3	12	42	31	20	13	23
Less than 65	53	43	16	7	25	66	53	36	27	41
Less than 70	80	58	28	15	39	87	71	53	42	58
Less than 75	96	77	44	35	57	95	84	72	60	74
Less than 80	100	88	62	55	71	100	91	85	76	86
Less than 85		96	79	75	85		97	93	88	93
Less than 90		98	91	88	93		98	97	94	97
Less than 95		100	96	95	97		99	99	98	99
All			100	100	100		100	100	100	100
Base	109	221	255	255	839	105	212	320	260	897
Mean (average value)	64	68	76	79	73	62	65	69	72	68
Median	64	67	77	78	73	61	64	68	72	68
Lower 5.0 percentile	53	52	58	63	54	50	50	54	56	52
Upper 5.0 percentile	74	84	94	96	92	76	82	87	90	87
Standard deviation	6.5	10.0	11.4	9.6	11.4	7.6	9.9	10.2	10.7	10.6

Table 3.3

Blood pressure by sex of respondent and region

Blood pressure (mmHg)	Sex of respondent and region							
	Men				Women			
	Scotland	Northern	Central, South West and Wales	London and the South East	Scotland	Northern	Central, South West and Wales	London and the South East
Systolic pressure								
Mean	127	131	131	129	121	123	122	120
Median	127	129	128	129	119	120	120	118
5th percentile	102	108	112	108	100	102	101	100
10th percentile	108	113	115	112	106	106	104	102
90th percentile	143	152	149	145	138	146	144	141
95th percentile	144	163	154	151	144	156	151	146
Standard deviation	12.9	16.7	14.1	13.5	13.9	16.7	17.0	15.4
Diastolic pressure								
Mean	72	74	74	72	69	69	68	67
Median	71	74	74	72	69	69	67	67
5th percentile	54	54	56	53	52	50	53	53
10th percentile	57	60	59	57	55	56	56	56
90th percentile	86	88	88	86	86	82	82	82
95th percentile	89	93	94	89	88	87	86	88
Standard deviation	10.9	11.9	11.4	10.9	11.0	10.8	10.4	10.6
Base	*62*	*242*	*299*	*237*	*67*	*233*	*330*	*266*

Table 3.4

Blood pressure by sex of respondent and whether someone in the respondent's household was receiving certain benefits

Blood pressure (mmHg)	Sex of respondent and whether receiving benefits			
	Men		Women	
	Receiving benefits	Not receiving benefits	Receiving benefits	Not receiving benefits
Systolic pressure				
Mean	130	130	120	122
Median	129	128	119	120
5th percentile	108	109	102	100
10th percentile	112	113	103	104
90th percentile	152	148	140	144
95th percentile	156	155	145	151
Standard deviation	15.2	14.6	15.2	16.4
Diastolic pressure				
Mean	72	73	68	68
Median	73	73	68	68
5th percentile	53	55	51	53
10th percentile	56	59	55	56
90th percentile	88	87	80	82
95th percentile	94	92	90	87
Standard deviation	12.2	11.2	10.8	10.6
Base	*119*	*720*	*163*	*734*

Table 3.5

Pearson correlation coefficients for systolic blood pressure with urinary sodium excretion

Sex and age of respondent	Correlation of systolic blood pressure with:	
	urinary sodium (mmol/24h)*	*Base*
Men aged (years):		
19–24	0.00	*53*
25–34	0.13	*137*
35–49	0.08	*174*
50–64	−0.16**	*189*
All men	−0.02	*553*
Women aged (years):		
19–24	0.23	*51*
25–34	0.08	*128*
35–49	0.02	*210*
50–64	0.12	*193*
All women	0.01	*582*

Note: * *Only includes samples where a full 24 hour collection was achieved.*
    ** *$p<0.05$*

Table 3.6

Socio-demographic, dietary and physiological factors associated with systolic blood pressure in bivariate analysis

Men	Women
Age at measurement (years)**	Age at measurement (years)**
Average calculated activity score	Average calculated activity score*
Average daily alcohol intake (g)**	Average daily alcohol intake (g)
Average daily intake of total cholesterol (mg)	Average daily intake of total cholesterol (mg)**
Current smoking	Current smoking
Eating affected by being unwell	Eating affected by being unwell
Ethnicity of respondent	Ethnicity of respondent
Gross weekly household income	Gross weekly household income*
Grouped Standard Region	Grouped Standard Region
Household benefit status	Household benefit status
Household composition**	Household composition**
Limited activity due to illness or disability	Limited activity due to illness or disability*
Mean diastolic pressure (mmHg)**	Mean diastolic pressure (mmHg)**
Mean body weight (kg)**	Mean body weight (kg)**
Reported dieting to lose weight*	Reported dieting to lose weight
Self-reported physical activity level	Self-reported physical activity level
Social class of household reference person	Social class of household reference person
Urinary potassium: urinary creatinine ratio (mol/mol)	Urinary potassium: urinary creatinine ratio (mol/mol)*
Urinary sodium: urinary creatinine ratio (mol/mol)	Urinary sodium: urinary creatinine ratio (mol/mol)
Urinary sodium excretion (mmol/24h)	Urinary sodium excretion (mmol/24h)
Vegetarian or vegan	Vegetarian or vegan
Wave of interview	Wave of interview
Whether adds salt to cooking	Whether adds salt to cooking
Whether adds salt to food at the table	Whether adds salt to food at the table

Note: * p<0.05; ** p<0.01

Table 3.7

Socio-demographic, dietary and physiological factors associated with diastolic blood pressure in bivariate analysis

Men	Women
Age at measurement (years)**	Age at measurement (years)**
Average calculated activity score*	Average calculated activity score*
Average daily alcohol intake (g)**	Average daily alcohol intake (g)*
Average daily intake of total cholesterol (mg)	Average daily intake of total cholesterol (mg)
Current smoking	Current smoking
Eating affected by being unwell	Eating affected by being unwell
Ethnicity of respondent	Ethnicity of respondent
Gross weekly household income	Gross weekly household income
Grouped Standard Region	Grouped Standard Region
Household benefit status	Household benefit status
Household composition**	Household composition**
Limited activity due to illness or disability	Limited activity due to illness or disability
Mean systolic pressure (mmHg)**	Mean systolic pressure (mmHg)**
Mean body weight (kg)**	Mean body weight (kg)**
Reported dieting to lose weight	Reported dieting to lose weight
Self-reported physical activity level	Self-reported physical activity level
Social class of household reference person	Social class of household reference person*
Urinary potassium: urinary creatinine ratio (mol/mol)*	Urinary potassium: urinary creatinine ratio (mol/mol)**
Urinary sodium: urinary creatinine ratio (mol/mol)	Urinary sodium: urinary creatinine ratio (mol/mol)
Urinary sodium excretion (mmol/24h)	Urinary sodium excretion (mmol/24h)
Vegetarian or vegan	Vegetarian or vegan
Wave of interview	Wave of interview
Whether adds salt to cooking	Whether adds salt to cooking
Whether adds salt to food at the table	Whether adds salt to food at the table

Note: * p<0.05; ** p<0.01

Table 3.8

Linear regression model for systolic blood pressure: men

Characteristic	Unstandardised coefficient (B)	Standard error of B	Standardised regression coefficient (β)	T–value
Constant	59.695	3.115		19.161 ***
Diastolic blood pressure (mmHg)	0.881	0.039	0.692	22.658 ***
Household composition				
Living alone	0.412	0.884	0.018	0.466
Living with spouse or partner, no dependent children	0.973	0.667	0.056	1.458
Living with other adults, no spouse or dependent children	1.262	0.866	0.059	1.458
Living with dependent children, with or without spouse	−2.647	0.647	−0.113	−4.088 ***
Body weight (kg)	0.092	0.027	0.093	3.381 ***
Reported dieting to lose weight	1.935	1.223	0.042	1.583
Age at measurement (years)	−0.055	0.038	−0.049	−1.450
Average daily alcohol intake (g)	−0.002	0.015	−0.003	−0.102
Percentage of variance explained		50%		
Number of respondents		*758*		

Note: * p<0.05; ** p<0.01; *** p<0.001

Table 3.9

Linear regression model for systolic blood pressure: women

Characteristic	Unstandardised coefficient (B)	Standard error of B	Standardised regression coefficient (β)	T–value
Constant	41.019	5.510		7.444 ***
Diastolic blood pressure (mmHg)	0.877	0.039	0.584	22.221 ***
Age at measurement (years)	0.352	0.041	0.265	8.674 ***
Gross weekly household income				
Less than £160	3.394	0.940	0.147	3.609 ***
£160 to less than £400	−0.783	0.652	−0.030	−1.202
£400 & over	−2.611	0.669	−0.113	−3.903 ***
Household composition				
Living alone	−1.157	1.130	−0.031	−1.023
Living with spouse or partner, no dependent children	1.745	0.811	0.066	2.151 *
Living with other adults, no spouse or dependent children	5.735	1.168	0.146	4.911 ***
Living with dependent children, with spouse	−2.104	0.801	−0.075	−2.627 **
Living with dependent children, without spouse	−4.220	1.310	−0.113	−3.222 **
Body weight (kg)	0.145	0.028	0.133	5.194 ***
Calculated physical activity score[†]	−0.028	0.102	−0.007	−0.276
Limited activity due to illness	−1.895	1.037	−0.047	−1.828
Average daily cholesterol intake (mg)	0.000	0.004	0.000	−0.018
Urinary potassium: urinary creatinine ratio	−0.128	0.190	−0.018	−0.675
Percentage of variance explained		59%		
Number of respondents		*705*		

Note: * p<0.05; ** p<0.01; *** p<0.001

   † The calculated physical activity score ranges from 32 to 78, with an overall mean of 42 for women. The higher the score, the more physically active a respondent is. For more information see Appendix D.

Table 3.10

Linear regression model for diastolic blood pressure: men

Characteristic	Unstandardised coefficient (B)	Standard error of B	Standardised regression coefficient (β)	T–value
Constant	0.466	3.465		0.135
Systolic blood pressure (mmHg)	0.477	0.022	0.613	22.097 ***
Age at measurement (years)	0.226	0.029	0.257	7.911 ***
Household composition				
Living alone	−0.320	0.701	−0.017	−0.457
Living with spouse or partner, no dependent children	0.226	0.522	0.016	0.432
Living with other adults, no spouse or dependent children	−1.659	0.702	−0.095	−2.363 *
Living with dependent children, with or without spouse	1.754	0.515	0.094	3.407 ***
Average daily alcohol intake (g)	0.039	0.012	0.084	3.259 **
Calculated physical activity score[†]	−0.040	0.029	−0.035	−1.367
Urinary potassium: urinary creatinine ratio	0.210	0.192	0.029	1.094
Body weight (kg)	0.015	0.021	0.019	0.716
Percentage of variance explained		59%		
Number of respondents		630		

Note: * p<0.05; ** p<0.01; *** p<0.001

[†] *The calculated physical activity score ranges from 36 to 100, with an overall mean of 46 for men. The higher the score, the more physically active a respondent is. For more information see Appendix D.*

Table 3.11

Linear regression model for diastolic blood pressure: women

Characteristic	Unstandardised coefficient (B)	Standard error of B	Standardised regression coefficient (β)	T–value
Constant	10.216	4.175		2.447 *
Systolic blood pressure (mmHg)	0.475	0.021	0.717	22.453 ***
Social class of household reference person				
Non–manual	2.382	0.662	0.122	3.596 ***
Manual	1.108	0.687	0.056	1.613
Unclassified	−3.490	1.204	−0.179	−2.899 **
Household composition				
Living alone	−0.330	0.802	−0.013	−0.411
Living with spouse or partner, no dependent children	−0.414	0.539	−0.024	−0.768
Living with other adults, no spouse or dependent children	−2.919	0.854	−0.112	−3.419 ***
Living with dependent children, with spouse	1.379	0.560	0.073	2.463 *
Living with dependent children, without spouse	2.283	0.901	0.090	2.535 *
Average daily alcohol intake (g)	0.056	0.025	0.062	2.277 *
Urinary potassium: urinary creatinine ratio	0.131	0.135	0.027	0.967
Calculated physical activity score[†]	−0.056	0.025	0.062	−0.740
Age at measurement (years)	−0.020	0.031	−0.023	−0.645
Body weight (kg)	0.003	0.021	0.004	0.134
Percentage of variance explained		50%		
Number of respondents		696		

Note: * p<0.05; ** p<0.01; *** p<0.001

[†] *The calculated physical activity score ranges from 32 to 78, with an overall mean of 42 for women. The higher the score, the more physically active a respondent is. For more information see Appendix D.*

Table 3.12

Comparison of blood pressure measurements with the Health Survey for England 2001*

Measurement	Age of respondent (years):									
	2001 Health Survey for England*					2000/01 NDNS - England only				
	16–24	25–34	35–44	45–54	55–64	19–24	25–34	35–44	45–54	55–64
Men										
Systolic pressure (mmHg)										
mean	130	130	130	136	142	127	126	130	130	138
se/sd**	0.5	0.4	0.4	0.5	0.6	10.9	13.1	12.6	14.7	18.1
Diastolic pressure (mmHg)										
mean	64	71	76	81	82	64	68	76	78	79
se/sd**	0.4	0.4	0.3	0.4	0.4	6.7	10.0	11.5	10.6	9.4
Base	*516*	*711*	*917*	*877*	*786*	*101*	*203*	*161*	*147*	*131*
Women										
Systolic pressure (mmHg)										
mean	120	120	123	132	140	115	114	118	126	137
se/sd**	0.5	0.4	0.4	0.5	0.7	9.8	11.5	13.2	16.2	18.3
Diastolic pressure (mmHg)										
mean	63	68	71	74	75	62	65	69	70	72
se/sd**	0.4	0.3	0.3	0.4	0.4	7.9	9.8	9.8	11.0	10.5
Base	*582*	*896*	*1144*	*1056*	*866*	*92*	*190*	*196*	*188*	*130*

Note: * Bajekal M, Primatesta P and Prior G. Eds. Health Survey for England 2001. TSO (London, 2003).

   ** The 2001 Health Survey for England reported standard errors; the present survey reports standard deviations.

4 Blood analytes

4.1 Introduction

This chapter reports on the results from the analysis of the blood samples. Chapter 1 of this report describes the purpose, methodologies and other procedures associated with obtaining venous blood samples from respondents in this survey and response rates. The Technical Report[1] details the procedures for obtaining and processing the samples (Appendix N) and describes the assay techniques and quality assurance data (Appendix O). Appendix M of the Technical Report lists the analytes in priority order for analysis.

4.1.1 Obtaining the blood sample

All 2,251 respondents were asked to consent to give a blood sample. Respondents who consented to giving a blood sample were visited by a phlebotomist to attempt venepuncture, accompanied by an interviewer. In this survey, unlike in some of the previous NDNS surveys[2,3], respondents were not asked to provide a fasting blood sample nor was the blood sample necessarily collected in the early morning.

A total of 1,419 respondents consented to having a blood sample taken. Venepuncture was attempted for 1,379 of those who consented to the procedure. Samples were obtained from a total of 1,347 respondents (60% of the responding sample). Reasons for a sample not being obtained, when prior consent had been given, included not being able to find a suitable vein or a vein collapsing during the procedure.

4.1.2 Analysis of the blood samples

Some of the posted blood samples reached the laboratory several days after posting due to delays at sorting centres[4]. The effect of postal delays and subsequent haemolysis of some samples was addressed by applying a correction factor[5]. Appendix O of the Technical Report[1] describes how samples were handled.

As described and shown in Appendix M of the Technical Report[1], the analytes were priority ordered to take account of technical constraints and clinical and policy relevance. Where it was not possible to obtain a sufficient volume of blood for the full range of analytes, the assays were carried out in the order of priority, and thus not all the assays were carried out on all the samples. The base numbers in the tables of results therefore vary for different analytes. The results for some analytes were routinely reported to the respondent and their GP (Appendix N of the Technical Report[1]).

As with data presented elsewhere in this report, the results for each of the blood analytes have been weighted at case level for both differential non-response and differential sampling probabilities and the tables present weighted data. The weights were derived for three groups of blood analytes (*see* Appendix C). Unweighted base numbers are shown in Appendix B.

Data are presented giving distributions and descriptive statistics for the blood analytes by sex and age. For the purpose of these analyses age was calculated by subtracting the respondent's date of birth from the date when the blood sample was obtained. For selected analytes, tables are given showing the variation in analyte concentration between various subgroups in the sample based on region and whether someone in the respondent's household was receiving certain benefits. Again for selected analytes, tables are also given showing correlation coefficients between the analyte and dietary intake of the relevant nutrient[6] and other blood analytes. Correlations were run on weighted data, within age groups[7].

It should be noted that for certain analytes, the mean value was considerably different from the median value for all or some sex/age groups. This indicates that there were a small number of respondents within each age/sex group who had extreme values in relation to the overall distribution[8].

For convenience of presentation and discussion the analytes are divided into the following main groups:

- haematology, including measures of iron status

- water soluble vitamins and plasma total homocysteine

- fat soluble vitamins and carotenoids

- blood lipids

- other analytes.

No comparison with blood analytes data from the Dietary and Nutritional Survey of British Adults aged 16 to 64 years carried out in 1986/87 (1986/87 Adults Survey)[9] has been undertaken because differences in the analytical methods used mean that the data from the two surveys are generally not comparable.

4.2 Haematology, including measures of iron status

4.2.1 The analytes and results

Tables 4.1 to 4.7 show the results for haematology analytes, including serum ferritin, for respondents by sex and age.

Haemoglobin concentration (grams /decilitre)

Haemoglobin is the oxygen-carrying, iron-containing molecule in red blood cells. Circulating levels of haemoglobin are indicative of the oxygen-carrying capacity of the blood. A low haemoglobin concentration can indicate iron deficiency. The World Health Organization's (WHO) lower limits for haemoglobin concentration are 13.0g/dl for men and 12.0g/dl for women[10]. Concentrations lower than these are indicative of anaemia. The haemoglobin concentrations of women of childbearing age tend to be lower because of menstrual loss. Upper limits of haemoglobin have been set at 18g/dl for men and 16.5g/dl for women[11].

Mean haemoglobin concentration was 15.1g/dl for men and significantly lower, 13.4g/dl, for women (p<0.01). This difference between men and women was observed within each age group.

For both men and women there were no significant differences in mean haemoglobin concentration by age.

Three per cent of men had a haemoglobin concentration below the WHO lower limit for adult men (13.0g/dl) and 8% of women had a concentration below the WHO lower limit for adult women (12.0g/dl) (p<0.01). There were no significant age differences for men or women.

(Table 4.1)

Mean corpuscular volume (MCV) (femtolitres)

The MCV is a measure of the average size of the red blood cells, and for adults is usually between 83fl and 101fl[11]. A low MCV (microcytosis) is usually an indication of iron deficiency. High MCV (macrocytosis) may be due to alcohol abuse, liver disease, hypothyroidism and folate or vitamin B_{12} deficiency.

The mean MCV was 92.9fl for men and 93.4fl for women (ns). The two youngest groups of men had a significantly lower mean MCV, 91.0fl and 90.9fl respectively, than the oldest group of men, 95.0fl (p<0.01). There were no significant age differences for women.

Three per cent of men and 4% of women had an MCV below 83.0fl, the lower end of the normal range for adults, suggesting iron deficiency. For men and women there were no significant age differences in the proportion with mean MCV below 83.0fl. Seven per cent of men and 11% of women had an MCV at or above 101.0fl (ns).

(Table 4.2)

Haematocrit (packed cell volume – PCV) (litres/litre fractional volume)

The haematocrit is the proportion of the blood volume taken up by the red cells, and is determined by the cell size and number. A lower concentration may indicate abnormal cell development, as shown by abnormally small red blood cells (microcytosis). Cells containing less haemoglobin may also be abnormally pale (hypochromic). Typically, iron deficiency produces a microcytic, hypochromic picture. In men haematocrit is usually between 0.40l/l and 0.50l/l and in women between 0.36l/l and 0.46l/l[11].

Overall, and within each age group, men had a significantly higher haematocrit than women, 0.459l/l and 0.413l/l respectively (p<0.01). There were no significant age differences for men or women.

Overall, four per cent of men and 5% of women (ns) had a haematocrit concentration below the lower limit of the usual range, 0.40l/l for men and 0.36l/l for women. There were no significant differences by age in the proportions of men and women who had a haematocrit concentration below the lower limit.

(Table 4.3)

Plasma iron (micromoles/litre)

Although it is normal for plasma iron concentration for an individual to vary throughout the day and between days, a low concentration, below 13µmol/l in adults, is indicative of iron-deficiency, inflammation, infection, surgery and/or chronic disease. High concentrations are indicative of liver disease, hypoplastic anaemia, ineffective erthyropoiesis and/or iron overload. For men and women the normal range is between 13µmol/l and 32µmol/l[11].

Mean plasma iron concentration for men was 17.0µmol/l and for women 16.1µmol/l (ns). There were no significant differences by age for either men or women.

Overall, 26% of men and 33% of women (ns) had a plasma iron concentration below 13.0µmol/l, the lower limit of the normal range. There were no significant age differences in the proportion below this value for either men or women. One per cent of men and 2% of women had a mean concentration of 32µmol/l or above, the upper limit of the normal range (ns).

(Table 4.4)

Total iron-binding capacity (TIBC) (micromoles/litre)

Extracellular iron in the blood is bound to the protein, transferrin. The total iron-binding capacity (TIBC) reflects the amount of transferrin that is available to bind iron. The laboratory method measures the amount of iron required to achieve complete saturation of the transferrin. TIBC is raised in iron-deficiency anaemia, but is lowered with infections, malignant disease, renal disease and iron overload[12]. For adults the normal range is 45µmol/l to 70µmol/l[11].

The mean TIBC for men in the survey was 61.5µmol/l, significantly lower than the mean value for women, 63.8µmol/l (p<0.01). Women in the youngest age group had a significantly higher mean TIBC, 66.1µmol/l, than those aged 50 to 64 years, 61.7µmol/l (p<0.05). There were no significant age differences for men.

One per cent of men and 2% of women had a TIBC below 45.0µmol/l, the lower limit of the normal adult range (ns). There were no significant age differences for men or women.

A lower proportion of men, 14%, than women, 24%, had a TIBC at or above 70.0µmol/l, the upper limit of the normal range (p<0.01). The proportion of women with levels at or above the upper limit decreased significantly with age, from 32% of those aged 25 to 34 years to 16% of those aged 50 to 64 years (p<0.05). There were no significant age differences for men.

(Table 4.5)

Percentage saturation of plasma iron (%)

Transferrin is the circulating transport protein for iron. The percentage of transferrin that is saturated with iron is derived from plasma iron and total iron-binding capacity (TIBC). A decrease in percentage saturation is an indicator of a progressive iron deficiency state with depleted iron stores. When the percentage transferrin saturation drops to a certain level haemoglobin formation is likely to be impaired. For adults this level is usually considered to be 15%[13].

Overall mean plasma iron percentage saturation was 28.1% for men and 26.0% for women (p<0.05). There were no significant differences by age for either men or women.

A significantly higher proportion of women, 16%, than men, 7%, had low plasma iron percentage saturation, that is less than 15% (p<0.01). There were no significant differences by age for men or women.

(Table 4.6)

Serum ferritin (micrograms/litre)

Serum ferritin gives an indication of the level of iron stores as well as being an acute phase reactant that is raised in response to infection or inflammation.

The normal range for serum ferritin is generally taken to be 20µg/l to 300µg/l for men and 15µg/l to 150µg/l for women[11]. Raised serum ferritin concentrations should be interpreted with care as they can result from inflammatory conditions, liver disease or other chronic disorders. Low concentrations indicate low iron stores.

Mean serum ferritin was 120μg/l for men and significantly lower, 53μg/l, for women (p<0.01).

Men and women in the youngest age group had significantly lower mean concentrations of serum ferritin than those in the oldest age group. Mean serum ferritin for those aged 19 to 24 years was 78μg/l for men and 41μg/l for women compared with 145μg/l and 71μg/l respectively for men and women aged 50 to 64 years (p<0.01).

Four per cent of men and 11% of women had a mean serum ferritin concentration below the lower limit of the normal range (p<0.01).

(Table 4.7)

4.2.2 Correlation with dietary intakes and other blood analytes

Table 4.8 gives correlation coefficients for haemoglobin and serum ferritin concentrations with dietary intakes of haem, non-haem and total iron from all sources, including supplements. In addition, Tables 4.9 and 4.10 give correlation coefficients for haemoglobin and serum ferritin concentrations with plasma iron percentage saturation and α_1-antichymotrypsin.

It should be noted that where correlations are statistically significant the relationship between the analyte and intake may not necessarily be causal; other factors, in particular the respondent's health at the time, may have affected the size of the correlation. Further, multiple tests for significance can suggest associations or differences that may have arisen by chance.

Table 4.8 shows that the correlation coefficients between serum ferritin and dietary intakes of haem, non-haem and total iron, and between haemoglobin and dietary intakes of haem, non-haem and total iron, were very low for all groups. This indicates that, based on the data from this survey, there were no correlations between these measures.

(Table 4.8)

Table 4.9 shows correlation coefficients for serum ferritin and haemoglobin with plasma iron percentage saturation. The correlation coefficients were generally very low in all groups indicating that, based in the data from this survey, there were no correlations between these measures.

(Table 4.9)

Plasma α_1-antichymotrypsin (α_1-ACT) is a positive acute phase reactant and is discussed later in this chapter (*see* Section 4.6.1). The correlation coefficients between serum ferritin and α_1-ACT, and between haemoglobin and α_1-ACT, were very low in all groups indicating that, based on the data from this survey, there were no correlations between these measures.

(Table 4.10)

4.2.3 Variation in the concentrations of haematology analytes and measures of iron status

Results for the main haematology analytes and measures of iron status were examined in relation to the region[14] in which the respondent lived and whether someone in the respondent's household was receiving certain state benefits[15].

There were no significant regional differences or differences by household benefit status for men or women in mean concentrations of any of the haematology analytes or measures of iron status.

(Tables 4.11 and 4.12)

4.3 Water soluble vitamins and plasma total homocysteine

4.3.1 The analytes and results

Plasma vitamin C (micromoles/litre)

Plasma vitamin C concentrations reflect recent dietary intakes of vitamin C, with values of less than 11μmol/l indicative of biochemical depletion[16].

Mean plasma vitamin C concentration was significantly higher for women than for men, 60.9μmol/l and 52.2μmol/l respectively (p<0.01). There were no significant differences by age for men or women.

Overall 5% of men and 3% of women had a plasma vitamin C concentration below 11μmol/l (ns). There were no significant differences by age for men or women.

(Table 4.13)

Red cell folate and serum folate (nanomoles/litre)

The term folate includes several derivatives of the parent molecule folic acid (pteroyl monoglutamic acid). Red cell folate is usually a better measure of long-term status than plasma folate because it reflects body stores at the time of red cell synthesis. The folate status of women of childbearing age is a particular public health issue due to the risk of having babies with neural tube defects[17].

Folate values and normal ranges are assay-method dependent, which makes it difficult to compare values directly between different studies and surveys. The following interpretation of ranges have been suggested[18]:

for red cell folate:

deficient	less than 337nmol/l
intermediate	337nmol/l to < 422nmol/l
normal	422nmol/l to 1463nmol/l

for serum folate:

deficient	less than 6.3nmol/l
intermediate	6.3nmol/l to < 7.0nmol/l
normal	7.0nmol/l to 28.1nmol/l

In adults, a red cell folate concentration below 230nmol/l is considered to be severely deficient, while concentrations between 230nmol/l and 345nmol/l indicate marginal status[19]. Based on an older assay, the normal range for serum folate concentration in adults is usually considered to be between 7nmol/l and 46nmol/l[11]. Statistically defined upper limits for nutrients such as folate do not have any well-established or nutritional significance.

The mean concentration of *red cell folate* in the samples provided by men in this survey was 694nmol/l and for women 685nmol/l (ns). For both men and women, mean concentration for those in the oldest group was significantly higher than for those in the youngest group. For example, for the youngest group of men and women mean red cell folate was 561nmol/l and 576nmol/l, respectively, compared with 773nmol/l for men and 768nmol/l for women aged 50 to 64 years (p<0.01).

Concentrations of red cell folate less than 350nmol/l were found in 5% of the samples from both men and women. For women, 8% of those in the youngest age group, 4% of those aged 25 to 34 years and 5% of those aged 35 to 49 years had red cell folate concentrations below 350nmol/l (ns). No more than 1% of any age/sex group had a red cell folate concentration of less than 230nmol/l, indicating that severe red cell folate deficiency is negligible in this sample.

Mean *serum folate* concentration was similar for men and women, 20.8nmol/l and 22.1nmol/l respectively (ns). For men, mean concentration increased significantly from 17.4nmol/l for those aged 19 to 24 years to 22.9nmol/l for those aged 50 to 64 years (p<0.01). There were no significant age differences for women.

One per cent of men and less than 0.5% of women had a serum folate concentration below 7.0nmol/l, the lower level of the normal range.

(Tables 4.14 and 4.15)

Serum vitamin B_{12} (picomoles/litre)

Serum concentration of vitamin B_{12} is a good indicator of vitamin B_{12} status. Vitamin B_{12}, with folate, is required for methyl group transfer during protein metabolism and DNA synthesis. Vitamin B_{12} is also required to maintain the integrity of the nervous system. Poor vitamin B_{12} status may be due to low dietary intake, malabsorption or pernicious anaemia. For adults, the lower level of normality for serum vitamin B_{12} concentration is usually taken as 118pmol/l[11].

There was no significant difference between men and women in mean concentration of serum vitamin B_{12}, 298pmol/l and 288pmol/l respectively. For men, there were no significant differences in mean concentration of serum vitamin B_{12} by age. For women, however, mean concentration increased with age from 247pmol/l for those aged 19 to 24 years and 259pmol/l for those aged 25 to 34 years, to 329pmol/l for those aged 50 to 64 years (p<0.05).

There were no men in the two youngest age groups with a serum vitamin B_{12} concentration below 118pmol/l, but 2% and 3% of men in the two older groups had concentrations below this, the lower level of normality for adults. Overall, 4% of women had a serum vitamin B_{12} concentration below 118pmol/l. There were no significant age differences for men or women.

(Table 4.16)

Erythrocyte Transketolase Activation Coefficient (ETKAC)

As with most water-soluble vitamins, there is virtually no recognisable store of non-functional thiamin in the body and the only reserve is that which is functionally bound to enzymes within the tissues. The *Erythrocyte Transketolase Activation Coefficient (ETKAC)* depends on the reactivation of the cofactor-depleted red cell enzyme transketolase *in vitro*. This index is sensitive to the lower to moderate range of intakes of thiamin. For adults, values above 1.25 are indicative of biochemical thiamin deficiency[13].

Table 4.17 shows that mean ETKAC for men, 1.15, was significantly higher than the mean ratio for women, 1.14 (p<0.01). For both men and women there were no significant age differences.

EGRAC than those living in non-benefit households (p<0.05).

There were no significant differences associated with household benefit status for either men or women for mean serum folate, serum vitamin B_{12}, ETKAC, ETK-B, EAATAC or plasma total homocysteine.

(Table 4.25)

4.4 Fat soluble vitamins and carotenoids

4.4.1 The analytes and results

Plasma retinol (vitamin A) (micromoles/litre)

Plasma retinol is related to long-term dietary intake of vitamin A. The plasma concentration is homeostatically controlled with little variation either within or between subjects. For adults, concentrations below 0.35µmol/l are considered to be severely deficient and concentrations between 0.35µmol/l and 0.70µmol/l indicate marginal status[13].

Mean plasma retinol concentration was significantly higher for men, 2.02µmol/l, than for women, 1.82µmol/l (p<0.01). Except for those aged 50 to 64 years, this difference was true within all age groups (25 to 34 years: p<0.05; all others: p<0.01).

Mean plasma retinol concentration increased significantly with age. For men in the youngest age group the mean concentration was 1.81µmol/l and increased to 2.08µmol/l for those aged 35 to 49 years, and 2.13µmol/l for those aged 50 to 64 years (35 to 49 years: p<0.05; 50 to 64 years: p<0.01). For women, the mean concentration for those aged 19 to 49 years was 1.75µmol/l in each group compared with 1.99µmol/l for those aged 50 to 64 years (19 to 24 years: p<0.05; all others: p<0.01).

There were no men or women with plasma retinol values of less than 0.35µmol/l. The only group to have concentrations between 0.35µmol/l and 0.70µmol/l, indicating marginal status, were men aged 50 to 64 years, 1% of whom had a concentration between these values.

(Table 4.26)

Plasma α- and β-carotene and α- and β-cryptoxanthin (micromoles/litre)

These are all carotenoids with vitamin A activity and reflect short to medium term intakes over a wide range. Concentration of carotenoids may be influenced by conversion to vitamin A, the

conversion being dependent on vitamin A status and requirements. This may confound comparisons between dietary intakes and blood concentrations.

For both α- and β-carotene, mean concentrations were significantly higher for women than men. The mean α-carotene concentration was 0.064µmol/l for men and 0.081µmol/l for women and the mean β-carotene concentration was 0.216µmol/l and 0.304µmol/l for men and women respectively (p<0.01).

Mean α-carotene concentrations were significantly lower in the youngest group of men and women, 0.039µmol/l and 0.048µmol/l respectively, than in the oldest groups, 0.074µmol/l and 0.101µmol/l (p<0.01).

The mean β-carotene concentration for men increased significantly from 0.143µmol/l for those aged 19 to 24 years to 0.221µmol/l for those aged 35 to 49 years and 0.248µmol/l for those aged 50 to 64 years (35 to 49 years: p<0.05; 50 to 64 years: p<0.01). The only significant age difference for women was between those aged 25 to 34 years and the oldest age group, 0.245µmol/l and 0.384µmol/l respectively (p<0.05).

(Tables 4.27 and 4.28)

The mean concentration of α-cryptoxanthin was 0.041µmol/l for men and 0.035µmol/l for women (ns). There were no significant age differences in mean α-cryptoxanthin concentrations for either men or women.

Overall, mean β-cryptoxanthin concentration was significantly lower for men than for women, 0.118µmol/l and 0.148µmol/l respectively (p<0.01).

Mean β-cryptoxanthin concentration was 0.123µmol/l for women aged 19 to 24 years and increased to 0.181µmol/l for those women aged 50 to 64 years (p<0.05). For men there were no significant age differences in mean β-cryptoxanthin concentrations.

(Tables 4.29 and 4.30)

Plasma lycopene and plasma lutein and zeaxanthin (micromoles/litre)

Lycopene, lutein and zeaxanthin are also carotenoids but with no provitamin A activity. The main sources of dietary lycopene are tomatoes and processed tomato products. Plasma lutein and zeaxanthin may be a useful marker of green vegetable intake.

Mean plasma lycopene concentration for men was 0.467µmol/l and for women, 0.463µmol/l (ns). For both men and women there were no significant age differences in mean concentration.

Mean concentration of plasma lutein and zeaxanthin was 0.27µmol/l for men and 0.29µmol/l for women (ns). Men in the youngest age group had a significantly lower mean concentration than men in all other age groups. Mean plasma lutein and zeaxanthin was 0.20µmol/l for men aged 19 to 24 years compared with 0.26µmol/l for men aged 25 to 34 years, 0.28µmol/l for men aged 35 to 49 years and 0.30µmol/l for those aged 50 to 64 years (25 to 34 years: p<0.05; 35 to 64 years: p<0.01). There were no significant age differences for women.

(Tables 4.31 and 4.32)

Plasma 25-hydroxyvitamin D (nanomoles/litre)

Plasma 25-hydroxyvitamin D (25-OHD) is derived from ergocalciferol and cholecalciferol which is obtained from the diet and from synthesis in the skin of cholecalciferol during ultraviolet irradiation from sunlight. It is a measure of vitamin D status and reflects the availability of vitamin D in the body from both dietary and endogenous sources. Factors influencing exposure to sunlight, such as the time of year, habit of dress and time spent outdoors should therefore be considered when interpreting 25-OHD results. Vitamin D is required for calcium absorption from the intestine as well as for a range of other metabolic processes. Traditionally 25nmol/l has been used as the lower threshold for plasma 25-OHD[26] but this has been questioned recently and there is currently no consensus[27].

Mean concentration of plasma 25-OHD for men was 48.3nmol/l and for women 49.6nmol/l (ns). Men in the youngest age group had a significantly lower mean plasma 25-OHD concentration, 40.6nmol/l, than those in the oldest age group, 51.6nmol/l (p<0.05). There were no significant age differences for women. Overall, 14% of men and 15% of women had a plasma 25-OHD concentration lower than 25nmol/l.

(Table 4.33)

Seasonal variation in concentration of plasma 25-OHD

Vitamin D synthesised by the skin in the presence of sunlight is an important source and plasma concentrations of 25-OHD are likely to be higher during the summer months. Plasma 25-OHD concentration was therefore tabulated by the month when the blood sample was taken[28].

Table 4.34 and Figure 4.1 illustrate the variation in mean plasma 25-OHD concentration for men and women by when the blood sample was taken. The mean plasma 25-OHD concentration for both men and women was higher for respondents who provided a sample in the summer months, July to September, than for those who gave a sample at other times of the year (both sexes: p<0.01). Mean concentrations were also significantly higher in samples obtained between October and December than in those obtained between January and March (men: p<0.01; women: p<0.05) and for men, but not women, between samples obtained in October to December compared with those obtained between April and June (p<0.05).

Men who provided a sample of blood during July to September were significantly less likely to have a 25-OHD concentration below 25nmol/l than those who gave a sample at other times of the year (October to December: p<0.05; all others: p<0.01). This was also true for women providing a sample in July to September compared with those providing a sample in January to March or April to June (April to June: p<0.05; January to March: p<0.01). Nearly one quarter of men and women, 24% and 23% respectively, who provided a sample in the months January to March had a 25-OHD concentration below 25nmol/l.

(Table 4.34 and Figure 4.1)

Plasma α- and γ-tocopherol (micromoles/litre)

Plasma tocopherol concentration can be used as a measure of vitamin E status. α-tocopherol is the predominant form in human tissues. It has the highest biological activity and is the most resistant to oxidation. Increased concentration of plasma lipids appears to cause tocopherols to partition out of cellular membranes, thus increasing concentrations of tocopherol and resulting in a correlation between tocopherol and total lipid in the blood, particularly with the cholesterol fraction. For this reason plasma tocopherol can be usefully expressed as a ratio of tocopherol to cholesterol (µmol/mmol)[29], enabling comparisons to be made between age groups with different plasma lipid levels.

For adults plasma tocopherols below 11.6µmol/l, or a tocopherol to cholesterol ratio of below 2.25µmol/mmol, tend to cause red blood cells to haemolyse after exposure to oxidising agents. This is sometimes considered to be an indicator of biochemical deficiency but is not indicative of a clinical deficiency of vitamin E. The Committee on Medical Aspects of Food and Nutrition Policy (COMA) Panel on Dietary Reference Values considered a tocopherol to cholesterol ratio of 2.25µmol/mmol to be the lowest satisfactory value for adults[30].

Mean α-tocopherol concentration was 21.1μmol/l for men and 20.6μmol/l for women (ns). Men in the youngest age group had a significantly lower mean α-tocopherol concentration than men in all other age groups. Mean α-tocopherol was 16.6μmol/l for men aged 19 to 24 years compared with 19.7μmol/l for men aged 25 to 34 years, 22.0μmol/l for men aged 35 to 49 years and 23.3μmol/l for those aged 50 to 64 years (25 to 34 years: p<0.05; 35 to 64 years: p<0.01). Similarly, mean α-tocopherol concentration was lower for women in the youngest group, 16.6μmol/l, compared with 20.3μmol/l for those aged 35 to 49 and 24.7μmol/l for those in the oldest age group (both: p<0.01).

Overall, 4% of men and women had a mean α-tocopherol concentration below 11.6μmol/l, the lower limit of the normal range for adults. There were no significant age differences in the proportions below the normal range.

Mean concentration of γ-tocopherol was 1.26μmol/l for men and 1.21μmol/l for women (ns). The mean γ-tocopherol concentration for men aged 19 to 24 years, 1.09μmol/l, was significantly lower than for men aged 35 to 49 years, 1.29μmol/l, and men aged 50 to 64 years, 1.31μmol/l (all: p<0.05). There were no significant age differences for women.

(Tables 4.35 and 4.36)

The mean tocopherol to cholesterol ratio was 4.06μmol/mmol for men and 3.96μmol/mmol for women (ns). For men, the ratio increased from 3.76μmol/mmol for those aged 19 to 24 years to 4.22μmol/mmol for those aged 50 to 64 years (p<0.05). For women the mean ratio increased from 3.71μmol/mmol for those aged 25 to 34 years to 4.03μmol/mmol for those aged 35 to 49 years and 4.17μmol/mmol for 50 to 64 year olds (35 to 49 years: p<0.05; 50 to 64 years: p<0.01).

One per cent of men and 2% of women had a tocopherol to cholesterol ratio below 2.25μmol/mmol, the lowest satisfactory value for adults. There were no significant age differences for men or women in the proportion below this value.

(Table 4.37)

4.4.2 Correlation with dietary intakes

The correlation coefficients between plasma retinol and dietary intakes of α-carotene, β-carotene and vitamin A (expressed as retinol equivalents) were extremely low for all groups. This indicates that, based on the data from this survey, there were no correlations between these measures.

(Table 4.38)

The correlation coefficients between plasma α-carotene and dietary intake of α-carotene were generally low for all groups, indicating that these measures were poorly correlated in this dataset.

The correlation coefficients between plasma β-carotene and dietary intake of β-carotene were generally low for all groups, except for women aged 19 to 24 years, where there was a high positive correlation.

(Tables 4.39 and 4.40)

Tables 4.41 and 4.42 show correlation coefficients between plasma 25-OHD and dietary intake of vitamin D by, respectively, sex and age of the respondent and time of year when the blood sample was taken. The correlation coefficients in both tables were generally low for all groups. This indicates that, based on the data from this survey, there was no correlation between these measures.

(Table 4.41 and 4.42)

The correlation coefficients between the tocopherol to cholesterol ratio and dietary intake of vitamin E were generally low for all groups, indicating that these measures were poorly correlated in this dataset.

(Table 4.43)

4.4.3 Variation in the concentrations of fat soluble vitamins and carotenoids

Tables 4.44 and 4.45 show variations in mean concentrations of fat soluble vitamins and carotenoids according to the region in which the respondent lived[14] and whether someone in the respondent's household was receiving certain state benefits[15].

There were no consistent patterns of differences in mean concentrations of fat soluble vitamins and carotenoids associated with region.

Women living in London and the South East had a higher mean concentration of plasma β-carotene than women in any other region. Mean plasma β-carotene concentration for women in London and the South East was 0.404μmol/l compared with 0.255μmol/l for those in Scotland, 0.231μmol/l in the Northern region and 0.288μmol/l in Central and South West regions of England and in Wales (Northern: p<0.01; all others: p<0.05). In addition, women living in London and the South East had a significantly higher mean α-carotene concentration, 0.101μmol/l, than those in the Northern region, 0.072μmol/l (p<0.05).

Women in Scotland, along with both men and women in London and the South East, had a significantly higher mean concentration of plasma β-cryptoxanthin than those in the Northern region and Central and South West regions of England and in Wales (Central and South West regions of England and Wales compared with London and the South East: p<0.01; all others: p<0.05).

Men in Scotland and both men and women in the Northern region had a significantly lower mean concentration of plasma lutein and zeaxanthin than those in London and the South East (men: p<0.05; women: p<0.01).

The mean plasma tocopherol to cholesterol ratio was significantly lower for women in Scotland, 3.54μmol/mmol, than for women living in Central and South West regions of England and in Wales, 4.04μmol/mmol, and London and the South East, 4.02μmol/mmol (p<0.05).

There were no significant regional differences for men or women for plasma retinol, plasma α-cryptoxanthin, plasma lycopene, plasma 25-OHD, plasma α- or γ-tocopherol.

(Table 4.44)

For women, mean concentrations of α- and β-carotene, α- and β-cryptoxanthin, lycopene, lutein and zeaxanthin, and plasma 25-hydroxyvitamin D were significantly lower for those in benefit households than for those living in non-benefit households (α-cryptoxanthin and plasma 25-hydroxyvitamin D: p<0.05; all others: p<0.01). For example, mean α-carotene concentration for women living in benefit households was 0.054μmol/l compared with 0.087μmol/l for those in non-benefit households. For these analytes, there were no significant differences for men associated with household benefit status.

For both men and women, mean α-tocopherol concentration was lower in benefit households than non-benefit households (men: p<0.05; women: p<0.01). There were no significant differences for men or women for mean concentrations of plasma retinol, γ-tocopherol or tocopherol to cholesterol ratio by household benefit status.

(Table 4.45)

4.5 Blood lipids

4.5.1 The analytes and results

In adults, circulating levels of plasma total cholesterol and its subfractions are among the predictors of coronary heart disease (CHD)[31]. They vary with age, genetic and environmental influences, including dietary factors, notably the amount of saturated fatty acids in the diet. The absolute risk of CHD increases with age but the interactions of risk factors, including plasma cholesterol, cigarette smoking, high blood pressure and body weight obscure individual relationships with CHD. High levels of total cholesterol occur in some diseases, for example kidney, liver and thyroid disorders or in diabetes.

Cholesterol circulates in the body bound to a variety of proteins, namely the lipoproteins. Cholesterol bound to low density lipoproteins *(LDL cholesterol)* is the major proportion of total circulating cholesterol. In adults, the risk of CHD is positively correlated with concentrations of both total cholesterol and LDL cholesterol. Cholesterol bound to high density lipoproteins *(HDL cholesterol)* is a smaller proportion of the total and may be inversely related to the development of CHD.

It is generally accepted that a plasma total cholesterol concentration below 5.2mmol/l represents an optimal level, 5.2mmol/l to 6.4mmol/l mildly elevated, 6.5mmol/l to 7.8mmol/l moderately elevated and above 7.8mmol/l a severely elevated level[32].

In this survey LDL cholesterol was not directly measured but is calculated by subtraction of HDL cholesterol from total cholesterol, uncorrected for plasma triglycerides; for brevity the term *LDL cholesterol* has been used for *non-HDL cholesterol*. Measurement of triglycerides concentration was not attempted in this survey because a fasting blood sample is required for this analyte and results from non-fasting samples would not have been interpretable.

Plasma cholesterol (millimoles/litre)

Table 4.46 shows that mean *plasma total cholesterol* concentration was 5.21mmol/l for men and 5.25mmol/l for women (ns). There were no significant age differences for men or women.

Over half, 52%, of men and women had plasma total cholesterol concentrations below 5.20mmol/l, the optimal level for total cholesterol. Over a third, 34%, of men and women had concentrations between 5.20mmol/l and 6.50mmol/l, which indicates mildly elevated cholesterol levels. Twelve per cent of men and 11% of women had moderately elevated cholesterol levels, at 6.50mmol/l to 7.80mmol/l. Two per cent of men and 3% of women had a mean concentration of 7.80mmol/l or above, which indicates a severely elevated level of total cholesterol.

For both men and women the proportion with plasma total cholesterol concentration below 5.20mmol/l decreased with age. For example, for the youngest group of men and women 84% and 83%, respectively, had concentrations below 5.20mmol/l compared with 41% of men and 25% of women in the oldest age group (both sexes: p<0.01).

In contrast, no men or women in the 19 to 24 age group had a mean concentration of 7.80mmol/l or above, indicating a severely elevated level of total cholesterol. The proportion of women with a mean plasma total cholesterol concentration of 7.80mmol/l or above increased from 1% of those aged 25 to 34 years to 9% of those aged 50 to 64 years (p<0.01). There were no significant age differences for men.

Table 4.47 shows mean *HDL cholesterol* concentration by age and sex. There was no significant difference in mean concentration between men and women, 1.07mmol/l and 1.28mmol/l respectively. For both sexes there were no significant differences by age.

Overall, men and women had a similar mean LDL cholesterol concentration, 4.15mmol/l and 3.97mmol/l respectively (ns). However, men aged 25 to 34 years and 35 to 49 years had a significantly higher mean concentration than women of the same age. Mean LDL concentration for men aged 25 to 34 years and 35 to 49 years was 4.00mmol/l and 4.34mmol/l respectively, and for women in the same age groups, 3.57mmol/l and 3.85mmol/l (25 to 34 years: p<0.05; 35 to 49 years: p<0.01). There were no significant differences by age for men or women.

(Tables 4.46 to 4.48)

4.5.2 Variation in the concentrations of plasma total, plasma HDL and plasma LDL cholesterol

Tables 4.49 and 4.50 show variations in mean concentrations of plasma total, plasma HDL and plasma LDL cholesterol according to the region in which the respondent lived[14] and whether someone in the respondent's household was receiving certain state benefits[15].

There were no significant regional differences in mean cholesterol concentrations for men and few for women. However, mean HDL cholesterol concentration was significantly higher for women in Scotland, 1.46mmol/l, than for those in the Northern region, 1.24mmol/l, and in Central and South West regions of England and in Wales, 1.23mmol/l (p<0.05). In addition, women in London and the South East had a higher mean HDL

cholesterol concentration than those living in Central and South West regions of England and in Wales (p<0.05).

(Table 4.49)

There were no significant differences in the mean concentration of the blood lipids by household benefit status.

(Table 4.50)

4.6 Other analytes

4.6.1 The analytes and results

Plasma selenium (micromoles/litre), red cell selenium (micromoles/litre) and erythrocyte glutathione peroxidase activity (GSH-Px) (nanomoles/milligram haemoglobin/minute)

Selenium is an essential trace element[33]. It forms part of the structure of certain proteins, and plays a key role in a number of metabolic processes including antioxidant systems and thyroid hormone metabolism.

There are well-confirmed pathological syndromes associated with selenium deficiency as well as selenium toxicity. However, there is increasing evidence that relatively high intakes, within the safe range, may have a protective action against some kinds of cancer[34], and other studies have explored the relationships between selenium status or indicators and functional indicators such as immune cell function[35] or risk of vascular disease[36].

Most studies have reported either plasma, serum or red blood cell selenium concentration levels, the latter being considered a longer term indicator of variations in dietary selenium intake[37]. The largest fraction of selenium, among all components of blood, is in the erythrocytes[38]. As it has been claimed that plasma selenium may be an acute phase reactant[39,40], red cell selenium may be a better measure of selenium status because red cell nutrient levels are less affected by acute phase status than plasma nutrient levels. However, red blood selenium may be influenced by disease states, as well as age[41]. Another favoured measure is blood glutathione peroxidase (GSH-Px) (functional index)[42], a selenoenzyme which can be measured in either blood cells or plasma.

As shown in Table 4.51, mean *plasma selenium* concentration for men and women was 1.11µmol/l and 1.10µmol/l respectively (ns). For both men and women mean concentration increased significantly with age. For example, for the youngest age group the mean concentration was 1.03µmol/l for both men and women compared with 1.15µmol/l for men and 1.17µmol/l for women in the oldest age group (p<0.01).

Mean concentration of *red cell selenium* for men was 1.60µmol/l and significantly higher, 1.80µmol/l, for women (p<0.01). This difference was observed for all age groups except for those aged 50 to 64 years (p<0.01).

For men, mean concentration of red cell selenium was significantly lower for those aged 19 to 24 years than for men in any other age group. The mean concentration for men aged 19 to 24 years was 1.42µmol/l compared with 1.60µmol/l for those aged 25 to 34 years and 1.64µmol/l for those aged 35 to 64 years (19 to 24 years: p<0.05; all others: p<0.01). For women there were no significant age differences.

Mean *GSH-Px* for men was 121.9nmol/mg Hb/min and for women, 127.2nmol/mg Hb/min (p<0.05). There were no significant age differences for men or women.

(Tables 4.51 to 4.53)

Plasma α_1-antichymotrypsin concentration (grams/litre)

α_1-antichymotrypsin (α_1-ACT) is known as a positive acute phase reactant. It is produced in the liver in response to inflammation. Ferritin is also an acute phase reactant and blood α_1-ACT and ferritin concentrations may be raised in response to infection or inflammation (*see* Section 4.2.1). The measurement of α_1-ACT can provide independent evidence of infection or inflammation that can assist in the interpretation of haematology and plasma nutrient index assays, especially plasma ferritin. For adults, the normal upper limit for α_1-ACT is usually considered to be 0.65g/l[43].

Overall, mean α_1-ACT was significantly lower for men, 0.30g/l, than for women, 0.31g/l (p<0.01). Women aged 19 to 49 years had significantly lower mean concentrations than those in the oldest group. Mean α_1-ACT was 0.29g/l for women aged 19 to 24 years, 0.30g/l for those aged 25 to 34 years and 0.31g/l for those aged 35 to 49 years compared with 0.34g/l for those aged 50 to 64 years (p<0.01). There were no significant age differences for men.

One per cent of women aged 50 to 64 years had a mean concentration at 0.65g/l or above, the upper α_1-ACT limit of normality. None of the other age groups had a α_1-ACT concentration above the upper limit.

(Table 4.54)

Blood mercury (nanomoles/litre)

Whole blood mercury reflects total exposure to mercury. The main source of mercury exposure is methylmercury found in contaminated fish. Mercury vapour from amalgam tooth fillings and ethylmercury in the form of thiomerosal added as an antiseptic to widely used vaccines both contribute smaller amounts[44]. Mercury has no known function in humans and is a toxin[45].

Current knowledge of normal mercury concentration in blood and plasma is incomplete[46] and a review of all published data on mercury concentration concluded that only tentative values could be established[47]. Expert opinion suggests that levels above 16nmol/l for non-occupationally exposed individuals are unusual and indicate increased uptake[48]. Opinions differ as to what level suggests excessive exposure or abnormal uptake.

Mean blood mercury concentration was 7.5nmol/l for men and 8.6nmol/l for women (ns). Generally for men, mean blood mercury concentrations appeared to increase with age. The mean concentration for men aged 19 to 24 years, 3.8nmol/l, was significantly lower than for those aged 25 to 34 years, 6.3nmol/l, those aged 35 to 49 years, 8.7nmol/l and those aged 50 to 64 years, 9.0nmol/l (25 to 34 years: p<0.05; others: p<0.01). The only significant age difference for women was between the youngest age group and the oldest age group, where mean concentration increased from 6.1nmol/l to 10.6nmol/l (p<0.05).

Overall, 9% of men and 10% of women had a mercury concentration at or above 16.0nmol/l. The proportion of men with concentrations at 16.0nmol/l or above increased significantly with age, from 1% of those aged 19 to 24 years to 14% of those aged 50 to 64 years (p<0.01). For women there were no significant differences in the proportion with concentrations at 16.0nmol/l or above by age.

(Table 4.55)

4.6.2 Variation in the concentrations and levels of other analytes

Table 4.56 shows the variation in concentrations and levels of other analytes for men and women associated with the region in which the respondent lived[14]. There were no consistent patterns of differences in mean concentrations or levels associated with region.

Both mean concentrations of plasma selenium and red cell selenium were significantly higher for women living in London and the South East than for those in the Northern region and in Central and

South West regions of England and in Wales (red cell selenium in Central and South West regions of England and in Wales: $p<0.01$; others: $p<0.05$).

The mean GSH-Px was significantly lower for men living in Scotland compared with those living in all other regions (Northern region: $p<0.05$; others: $p<0.01$). For women, those living in Scotland had lower mean GSH-Px than women living in London and the South East ($p<0.01$).

Men living in London and the South East had a significantly higher mean blood mercury concentration, 9.4nmol/l, than those in Central and South West regions of England and in Wales, 6.7nmol/l ($p<0.05$).

There were no significant differences for men or women in mean α_1-ACT concentrations associated with region.

(Table 4.56)

Table 4.57 shows the variation in levels of other analytes according to whether the respondent lived in a household which was receiving certain state benefits or not[15].

Men and women living in benefit households had a significantly lower mean plasma selenium concentration and a lower mean blood mercury concentration than those in non-benefit households (plasma selenium and men: $p<0.05$; blood mercury and women: $p<0.05$; others: $p<0.01$). In addition, women in benefit households had a significantly lower mean concentration of red cell selenium, 1.65µmol/l, than those in non-benefit households, 1.84µmol/l ($p<0.01$).

There were no significant differences for men or women in mean α_1-ACT concentrations or mean GSH-Px by household benefit status.

(Table 4.57)

References and endnotes

[1] The Technical Report is available online at http://www.food.gov.uk/science.

[2] Gregory J, Lowe S, Bates CJ, Prentice A, Jackson LV, Smithers G, Wenlock, R, Farron M. *National Diet and Nutrition Survey: young people aged 4 to 18 years. Volume 1: Report of the diet and nutrition survey.* TSO (London, 2000).

[3] Finch S, Doyle W, Lowe C, Bates CJ, Prentice A, Smithers G, Clarke PC. *National Diet and Nutrition Survey: people aged 65 years and over. Volume 1: Report of the diet and nutrition survey.* TSO (London,1998).

[4] Some of the posted blood samples reached Great Ormond Street Haematology Laboratory several days after posting. About 60% of all samples were delayed by 24 hrs or more and about 30% were delayed by 48 hrs or more. Different analytes have different sensitivities to the effects of delay.

[5] For some of the analytes measured in samples that had been sent through the post there was a significant linear correlation between the assay values and the magnitude of the delay time, and in some there was also a small but significant difference in values obtained from the small number of slightly haemolysed samples. In order to correct for these two potential errors, the following mathematical corrections were employed. For each analyte where there was a significant correlation with delay time, each result was corrected (up or down) by the product of number of hours delay and the slope of the overall rate of change per hour. For each analyte where there was a significant effect of haemolysis, the results from the haemolysed samples were multiplied by a correction factor (between 0.969 and 1.023) which represented the ratio of the overall mean values of the haemolysed and non-haemolysed samples.

[6] When interpreting results, it should be noted that there was a time lag between the blood sample being obtained and the original dietary recording period (mean 14 days). It should also be noted that the results of the blood sample analyses measure nutritional status in the longer term which may not necessarily be reflected by dietary intake over the relatively short period of seven days.

[7] Pearson correlation coefficients were calculated in SPSS. Weighting factors, for non-response and sampling probability, were scaled (normalised) to the original, unweighted sample size before running the SPSS procedure on weighted data. Pearson correlation coefficients are robust to departures from normally distributed data, that is skewed data, provided the value of the population coefficient is low, which it is for these data. See:

Gayen AK. The distribution of Student's t in random samples of any size drawn from non-normal universes. *Biometrica* 1949; **36**: 353.

Gayen AK. The distribution of the variance ratio in random samples of any size drawn for non-normal universes. *Biometrica* 1950; **37**: 236.

Gayen AK. Significance of difference between the means of two non-random samples. *Biometrica* 1950; **37**: 399.

Gayen AK. The frequency distribution of the product-moment correlation coefficient in random samples of any size drawn for non-normal universes. *Biometrica* 1951; **38**: 219.

[8] Distribution of data was evaluated using the skewness statistic in SPSS. If the skewness statistic is less than twice the standard error of the statistic then data were considered to be normally distributed.

For all age/sex groups, plasma vitamin C was found to be normally distributed. All other blood analytes were found to be not normally distributed for at least one age/sex group. For all age/sex groups, the following analytes were found to be skewed: Red cell folate, serum vitamin B_{12}, erythrocyte glutathione peroxidase, blood mercury, total iron-binding capacity, plasma total homocysteine, plasma 25-hydroxyvitamin D, plasma α-tocopherol to total cholesterol ratio, plasma α_1-antichymotrypsin, plasma β-carotene, plasma β-cryptoxanthin, plasma lycopene, and plasma lutein and zeaxanthin.

[9] Gregory J, Foster K, Tyler H, Wiseman M. *The Dietary and Nutritional Survey of British Adults.* HMSO (London, 1990).

[10] World Health Organization. *Nutritional Anaemias.* Technical Report Series: 503. WHO (Geneva, 1972).

[11] Dacie JV, Lewis SM. *Practical Haematology.* 9th Edition. Churchill Livingstone (Edinburgh, 2001).

12 Worwood M. Iron deficiency anaemias. In: *Practical Haematology*. Eds. Dacie JV, Lewis SM. 9th Edition. Churchill Livingstone (Edinburgh, 2001).

13 Bates CJ, Thurnham DI, Bingham SA, Margetts BM, Nelson M. Biochemical Markers of Nutrient Intake. In: *Design Concepts in Nutritional Epidemiology*. 2nd Edition. OUP (Oxford, 1997) pp 170–240.

14 The areas included in each of the four analysis 'regions' are given in the response chapter, Chapter 2 of the Technical Report (*see* Note 1). Definitions of 'regions' are given in the glossary (*see* Appendix E).

15 Households receiving certain benefits are those where someone in the respondent's household was currently receiving Working Families Tax Credit or had, in the previous 14 days, drawn Income Support or (Income-related) Job Seeker's Allowance. Definitions of 'household' and 'benefits (receiving)' are given in the Glossary (*see* Appendix E).

16 Sauberlich HE. Vitamin C status: methods and findings. *Ann N Y Acad Sci* 1971; **24**: 444–454.

17 Cziezel AE, Dudas I. Prevention of the first occurrence of neural tube defects by periconceptional vitamin supplementation. *N Engl J Med* 1992; **327**: 1832–35.

18 Based on an analysis of 170 serum samples and 140 whole blood samples. Abbott Laboratories, Diagnostics Division, IMx system: Folate, Technical Information Leaflet, 1997.

19 Sauberlich HE, Skala JH, Dowdy RP. *Laboratory tests for the assessment of nutritional status*. CRC Press (Cleveland, Ohio, 1974).

20 Gregory J, Collins DL, Davies PSW, Hughes JM, Clarke PC. *National Diet and Nutrition Survey: children aged 1½ to 4½ years. Volume 1: Report of the diet and nutrition survey*. HMSO (London, 1995).

21 Boushey C, Beresford SAA, Omenn GS, Motulsky AG. A quantitative assessment of plasma homocysteine as a risk factor for vascular disease: probable benefits of increasing folic acid intakes. *JAMA* 1995; **274**: 1049–57.

22 Wald DS, Law M, Morris JK, Homocysteine and Cardiovascular Disease: Evidence on Causality from a Meta-Analysis. *BMJ* 2002; **325**: 1202–9.

23 Bates CJ, Mansoor MA, Gregory J, Pentieva K, Prentice A. Correlates of plasma homocysteine, cysteine and cysteinyl-glycine in respondents in the British National Diet and Nutrition Survey of Young People Aged 4-18 Years, and a comparison with the Survey of People Aged 65 Years and Over. *Br J Nut* 2002; **87**: 71–79.

24 Malinow MR, Bostom AG, Krauss RM. Homocyst(e)ine, diet, and cardiovascular diseases: a statement for healthcare professionals from the Nutrition Committee, American Heart Association. *Circulation* 1999; **99**: 178–182.

25 See also http://www.homocysteine.net/pages/guidelines/1/overview.html.

26 Department of Health Report on Health and Social Subjects, No. 49. *Nutrition and bone health with particular reference to calcium and vitamin D*. TSO (London, 1998).

27 Bates CJ, Carter GD, Mishra GD, O'Shea D, Jones J, Prentice A. In a population study, can parathyroid hormone aid the definition of adequate vitamin D status? A study of people aged 65 years and over from the British National Diet and Nutrition Survey. *Osteoporos Internat* 2003 (in press).

28 A two-way ANOVA test was used to determine that plasma 25-hydroxyvitamin D was significantly related to the date of blood sample being taken whilst controlling for sex of the respondent.

29 Calculated as the ratio of plasma α-tocopherol to plasma total cholesterol.

30 Department of Health. Report on Health and Social Subjects: 41. *Dietary Reference Values for Food Energy and Nutrients for the United Kingdom*. HMSO (London, 1991).

31 Department of Health. Report on Health and Social Subjects: 46. *Nutritional Aspects of Cardiovascular Disease*. HMSO (London, 1994).

32 The British Cardiac Society, British Hyperlipidaemia Association, British Hypertension Society, endorsed by the British Diabetic Association, have issued guidance published in the article 'Joint British recommendations on prevention of coronary heart disease in clinical practice' *Heart* 1998; **80**: 1–29.

33 Rayman MP. The importance of selenium to human health. *Lancet* 2000; **356**: 233–41.

34 Combs GF. Impact of selenium and cancer-prevention findings on the nutrition-health paradigm. *Nutrition and Cancer* 2001; **40**: 6–11.

35 Beck MA, Nelson HK, Shi Q et al. Selenium deficiency increases the pathology of an influenza virus infection. *FASEB J* 2001; **15**: 1481–83.

36 Salonen JT, Huttunen JK. Se in cardiovascular diseases. *Ann Clin Res* 1986; **18**: 30–35.

37 Bates CJ, Thane CW, Prentice A, Delves HT, Gregory J. Selenium status and associated factors in a British National Diet and Nutrition Survey: young people aged 4–18. *Eur J Clin Nutr* 2002; **56**: 873–881.

38 Rukgauer M, Zeyfang A, Uhland K , Kruse-Jarres JD. Isolation of corpuscular components of whole blood for the determination of selenium in red cells. *J Trace Elem Med Biol* 1995; **9**: 130–35.

39 Sattar N, Eatock F, Fell GS, O'Reilly D. Selenium: an acute phase reactant. *Ann Clin Biochem* 1997; **34**: 437–9.

40 Galloway P, McMillan DC, Sattar N. Effect of the inflammatory response on trace element and vitamin status. *Ann Clin Biochem* 2000; **37**: 289–97.

41 Miller L, Mills BJ, Blotcky AJ, Lindeman RD. Red blood cell and serum selenium concentrations as influenced by age and selected diseases. *J Amer Coll Nutr* 1983; **4**: 331–41.

42 Neve J. Methods in determination of selenium status. *J Trace Elem Electrolytes Health Dis* 1991; **5**: 1–17.

43 Calvin J, Price CP. Measurement of serum α_1-antichymotrypsin by immunoturbidimetry. *Ann Clin Biochem* 1986; **213**: 206–209.

44 Clarkson TW. The three modern faces of mercury. *Environ Health Perspect* 2002; **110**:11–23.

45 Bakir F, Damlugi SF, Amin-Zaki L, Murtadha M, Khalidi A, Al-Rawi NY, Tikriti S, Dhahir HI, Clarkson TW, Smith JC, Doherty RA. Methylmercury poisoning in Iraq. *Science* 1973; **181**: 230–241.

46 'Dental Amalgam' A report with reference to the Medical Devices Directive 93/42/EEC from an Ad Hoc Working Group mandated by DG111 of the European Commission, 1998.

47 Brune D, Nordberg GF, Vesterberg O, Gerhardsson L, Wester PO. A Review of Normal Concentrations of Mercury in Human Blood. *Sci Total Environ* 1991; **100**: 235–282.

48 Work was conducted by Human Nutrition Research and reported to the Food Standards Agency Committee on Toxicity *see* report no. 21 (2002). The reference levels quoted are from the HSE Guidance Booklet, 6th Edition (1993).

Table 4.1

Percentage distribution of haemoglobin concentration by sex and age of respondent

Cumulative percentages

Haemoglobin concentration (g/dl)	Men aged (years):				All men	Women aged (years):				All women
	19–24	25–34	35–49	50–64		19–24	25–34	35–49	50–64	
	cum %	cum %	cum %	cum %	cum %	cum %	cum %	cum %	cum %	cum %
Less than 11.0	-	1	0	0	0	3	-	2	2	2
Less than 12.0	-	1	1	0	1	7	8	10	7	8
Less than 12.5	-	1	1	0	1	16	14	18	16	16
Less than 13.0	-	2	4	3	3	32	34	35	31	33
Less than 13.5	6	6	5	9	6	45	61	54	51	54
Less than 14.0	8	10	9	15	11	58	78	74	67	71
Less than 14.5	17	24	22	29	24	84	88	90	80	86
Less than 15.0	36	41	43	49	43	96	95	97	89	94
Less than 16.0	83	78	77	86	81	100	100	100	99	100
Less than 17.0	97	99	97	98	98				100	
All	100	100	100	100	100					
Base	83	170	191	194	638	81	162	243	196	683
Mean (average value)	15.2	15.1	15.1	14.9	15.1	13.5	13.3	13.3	13.5	13.4
Median	15.3	15.2	15.2	15.0	15.2	13.7	13.2	13.3	13.4	13.4
Lower 2.5 percentile	13.0	13.0	12.7	12.8	12.9	10.8	11.5	10.9	11.2	11.1
Upper 2.5 percentile	17.2	16.9	17.0	16.8	16.9	15.0	15.1	15.1	15.7	15.3
Standard deviation	0.96	1.04	1.05	1.04	1.04	1.05	0.91	1.03	1.14	1.04

Table 4.2

Percentage distribution of mean corpuscular volume by sex and age of respondent

Cumulative percentages

Mean corpuscular volume (fl)	Men aged (years):				All men	Women aged (years):				All women
	19–24	25–34	35–49	50–64		19–24	25–34	35–49	50–64	
	cum %	cum %	cum %	cum %	cum %	cum %	cum %	cum %	cum %	cum %
Less than 79.0	2	2	1	0	1	3	3	1	2	2
Less than 83.0	7	4	3	0	3	4	5	4	4	4
Less than 86.0	15	13	9	5	10	9	9	12	8	9
Less than 89.0	31	29	22	14	23	27	22	22	18	22
Less than 92.0	63	57	40	28	44	41	48	38	36	40
Less than 95.0	79	81	64	51	67	67	71	59	60	63
Less than 99.0	94	95	84	78	87	88	84	80	83	83
Less than 101.0	97	98	92	87	93	88	92	87	90	89
All	100	100	100	100	100	100	100	100	100	100
Base	83	170	191	194	638	81	162	243	196	683
Mean (average value)	91.0	90.9	93.3	95.0	92.9	92.8	92.7	93.9	93.7	93.4
Median	90.5	91.3	93.4	94.9	92.7	93.3	92.1	93.7	93.8	93.4
Lower 2.5 percentile	80.8	74.1	80.9	85.4	82.4	71.9	78.8	81.6	80.4	80.4
Upper 2.5 percentile	102.1	100.0	106.1	106.6	103.8	106.3	107.3	106.5	104.8	106.3
Standard deviation	5.11	5.15	6.01	5.58	5.79	6.77	6.07	6.55	5.95	6.30

Table 4.3

Percentage distribution of haematocrit by sex and age of respondent

Cumulative percentages

Haematocrit (l/l)	Men aged (years):				All men	Women aged (years):				All women
	19–24	25–34	35–49	50–64		19–24	25–34	35–49	50–64	
	cum %	cum %	cum %	cum %	cum %	cum %	cum %	cum %	cum %	cum %
Less than 0.360	-	2	1	-	1	10	5	4	3	5
Less than 0.375	-	3	1	0	1	13	12	12	8	11
Less than 0.400	4	4	4	4	4	24	31	29	26	28
Less than 0.425	13	11	14	14	13	64	68	67	63	65
Less than 0.450	45	44	47	44	45	87	90	93	85	89
Less than 0.475	69	70	67	71	69	95	98	98	94	97
Less than 0.500	86	91	85	85	87	96	100	100	98	99
All	100	100	100	100	100	100			100	100
Base	83	170	191	194	638	81	162	243	196	683
Mean (average value)	0.460	0.457	0.460	0.460	0.459	0.416	0.411	0.411	0.417	0.413
Median	0.460	0.460	0.460	0.460	0.460	0.420	0.410	0.410	0.410	0.410
Lower 2.5 percentile	0.380	0.356	0.380	0.390	0.380	0.340	0.350	0.340	0.350	0.340
Upper 2.5 percentile	0.511	0.520	0.534	0.520	0.520	0.501	0.470	0.470	0.480	0.480
Standard deviation	0.0308	0.0333	0.0363	0.0341	0.0341	0.0372	0.0316	0.0314	0.0352	0.0334

Table 4.4

Percentage distribution of plasma iron by sex and age of respondent

Cumulative percentages

Plasma iron (μmol/l)	Men aged (years):				All men	Women aged (years):				All women
	19–24	25–34	35–49	50–64		19–24	25–34	35–49	50–64	
	cum %	cum %	cum %	cum %	cum %	cum %	cum %	cum %	cum %	cum %
Less than 8.0	-	6	2	3	3	10	9	10	5	8
Less than 10.0	2	15	5	9	9	33	16	19	10	17
Less than 13.0	27	33	21	26	26	41	36	34	25	33
Less than 16.0	50	54	48	50	50	47	49	55	49	51
Less than 20.0	68	74	74	71	72	76	73	79	81	78
Less than 25.0	83	93	91	89	90	91	88	90	93	91
Less than 30.0	92	98	98	99	97	98	95	97	97	97
Less than 32.0	97	100	99	99	99	100	96	98	99	98
All	100		100	100	100		100	100	100	100
Base	81	165	190	190	627	77	158	238	194	668
Mean (average value)	17.8	16.2	17.3	17.1	17.0	15.6	16.5	15.9	16.3	16.1
Median	16.1	15.6	16.2	16.1	16.0	17.0	16.2	15.2	16.0	15.9
Lower 2.5 percentile	10.0	6.7	8.6	6.2	7.6	4.0	4.6	5.7	7.2	5.6
Upper 2.5 percentile	33.8	30.5	29.7	28.7	30.5	28.9	33.4	30.5	31.4	30.9
Standard deviation	6.69	5.80	5.54	6.53	6.08	6.60	7.17	6.60	5.54	6.45

Table 4.5

Percentage distribution of total iron–binding capacity by sex and age of respondent

Cumulative percentages

Total iron–binding capacity (μmol/l)	Men aged (years):				All men	Women aged (years):				All women
	19–24	25–34	35–49	50–64		19–24	25–34	35–49	50–64	
	cum %	cum %	cum %	cum %	cum %	cum %	cum %	cum %	cum %	cum %
Less than 45.0	–	2	2	1	1	–	1	4	2	2
Less than 50.0	12	9	5	6	8	3	3	8	7	6
Less than 55.0	17	21	16	23	20	5	12	19	22	16
Less than 60.0	44	49	42	46	45	20	27	41	49	37
Less than 65.0	70	67	71	68	69	57	49	61	68	60
Less than 70.0	83	83	88	88	86	67	68	79	84	76
Less than 75.0	93	91	96	94	94	86	80	89	94	88
Less than 80.0	97	96	99	97	97	92	91	94	96	93
All	100	100	100	100	100	100	100	100	100	100
Base	81	165	188	189	624	77	158	238	193	666
Mean (average value)	61.8	61.8	61.2	61.5	61.5	66.1	66.8	62.8	61.7	63.8
Median	61.2	60.1	61.0	61.1	61.0	63.0	65.2	61.9	60.2	62.8
Lower 2.5 percentile	47.5	46.1	45.1	47.3	46.9	49.3	48.9	43.8	44.8	45.1
Upper 2.5 percentile	81.3	81.3	75.9	82.1	80.9	86.8	90.3	84.7	82.9	86.2
Standard deviation	8.39	9.38	8.00	9.01	8.72	8.82	11.36	10.14	9.75	10.38

Table 4.6

Percentage distribution of plasma iron % saturation by sex and age of respondent

Cumulative percentages

Plasma iron % saturation (%)	Men aged (years):				All men	Women aged (years):				All women
	19–24	25–34	35–49	50–64		19–24	25–34	35–49	50–64	
	cum %	cum %	cum %	cum %	cum %	cum %	cum %	cum %	cum %	cum %
Less than 10.0	-	1	0	3	1	8	7	7	3	6
Less than 15.0	6	13	3	6	7	27	17	18	8	16
Less than 20.0	17	25	17	22	20	42	36	32	22	31
Less than 25.0	47	47	40	41	43	51	56	47	44	49
Less than 30.0	66	69	62	60	64	61	70	66	67	67
Less than 35.0	71	81	77	77	77	85	83	78	83	82
Less than 40.0	82	92	89	87	88	92	89	88	92	90
Less than 45.0	87	94	94	93	93	96	94	96	95	95
All	100	100	100	100	100	100	100	100	100	100
Base	81	165	188	189	624	77	158	238	192	665
Mean (average value)	29.7	26.6	28.5	28.2	28.1	24.3	25.3	26.1	27.1	26.0
Median	25.1	26.3	27.1	27.3	26.7	24.4	22.6	25.5	27.1	25.3
Lower 2.5 percentile	12.7	10.8	13.7	9.0	12.1	5.4	6.3	7.9	9.1	7.8
Upper 2.5 percentile	64.1	50.3	50.8	51.3	52.0	46.6	50.2	50.3	52.3	50.2
Standard deviation	13.17	9.77	9.29	10.02	10.24	11.20	11.47	11.15	9.82	10.88

Table 4.7

Percentage distribution of serum ferritin by sex and age of respondent

Cumulative percentages

Serum ferritin (μg/l)	Men aged (years):				All men	Women aged (years):				All women
	19–24	25–34	35–49	50–64		19–24	25–34	35–49	50–64	
	cum %	cum %	cum %	cum %	cum %	cum %	cum %	cum %	cum %	cum %
Less than 15	-	-	2	2	1	16	8	12	8	11
Less than 20	4	0	6	5	4	30	18	24	15	21
Less than 25	7	1	7	8	6	33	27	32	18	27
Less than 40	15	10	11	14	12	59	59	57	32	51
Less than 50	18	18	18	19	18	70	73	67	42	62
Less than 60	30	24	23	23	24	78	77	76	50	69
Less than 75	42	36	33	32	35	88	89	84	63	79
Less than 100	77	57	52	45	55	97	94	91	79	89
Less than 150	96	78	73	65	75	100	99	97	91	96
All	100	100	100	100	100		100	100	100	100
Base	85	169	186	194	633	80	156	238	195	670
Mean (average value)	78	101	129	145	120	41	43	49	71	53
Median	78	89	96	109	92	34	34	37	60	40
Lower 2.5 percentile	18	26	14	17	18	10	9	6	4	7
Upper 2.5 percentile	177	201	512	505	371	102	144	170	232	163
Standard deviation	34.2	52.2	109.7	157.9	112.1	26.2	30.8	46.7	54.4	45.6

Table 4.8

Pearson correlation coefficients for serum ferritin and haemoglobin with dietary intake of iron

	Men aged (years):				All men	Women aged (years):				All women
	19–24	25–34	35–49	50–64		19–24	25–34	35–49	50–64	
Serum ferritin with dietary intakes of:										
Haem iron	0.28*	0.11	0.24**	0.09	0.16**	−0.11	0.05	0.08	0.21**	0.15**
Non–haem iron	0.08	−0.08	0.01	0.02	0.03	0.00	−0.02	−0.05	−0.03	−0.03
Total iron	0.11	−0.07	0.04	0.02	0.05	−0.01	−0.02	−0.05	−0.02	−0.03
Base	80	154	177	190	600	74	150	224	191	639
Haemoglobin with dietary intakes of:										
Haem iron	−0.07	−0.10	−0.02	0.12	0.00	0.21	0.12	−0.02	0.13	0.10*
Non–haem iron	−0.27*	0.25**	−0.08	0.04	0.02	0.10	−0.11	−0.13	0.05	−0.07
Total iron	−0.28*	0.24**	−0.08	0.05	0.02	0.11	−0.10	−0.13	0.06	−0.06
Base	78	155	181	190	604	76	155	229	192	652

Note: * p<0.05; ** p<0.01

Table 4.9

Pearson correlation coefficients for serum ferritin and haemoglobin with plasma iron % saturation

	Men aged (years):				All men	Women aged (years):				All women
	19–24	25–34	35–49	50–64		19–24	25–34	35–49	50–64	
Serum ferritin with:										
Plasma iron % saturation	0.06	0.15	0.19*	0.38**	0.23**	0.43**	0.22**	0.25**	0.13	0.22**
Base	*83*	*164*	*179*	*189*	*614*	*71*	*154*	*234*	*187*	*646*
Haemoglobin with:										
Plasma iron % saturation	0.24*	0.21**	0.16*	0.26**	0.21**	0.15	0.28**	0.37**	0.28**	0.30**
Base	*81*	*165*	*183*	*189*	*619*	*73*	*159*	*238*	*189*	*658*

Note: * $p<0.05$; ** $p<0.01$

Table 4.10

Pearson correlation coefficients for serum ferritin and haemoglobin with plasma α_1–antichymotrypsin

	Men aged (years):				All men	Women aged (years):				All women
	19–24	25–34	35–49	50–64		19–24	25–34	35–49	50–64	
Serum ferritin with:										
Plasma α_1–antichymotrypsin	–0.12	0.14	–0.05	–0.13	–0.03	0.11	–0.12	–0.01	0.06	0.08*
Base	*83*	*161*	*171*	*180*	*595*	*71*	*151*	*229*	*185*	*636*
Haemoglobin with:										
Plasma α_1–antichymotrypsin	–0.12	–0.21**	0.10	–0.18*	–0.12**	0.05	0.21**	0.12	0.05	0.12**
Base	*81*	*162*	*174*	*181*	*599*	*73*	*156*	*233*	*187*	*648*

Note: * $p<0.05$; ** $p<0.01$

Table 4.11

Haematology analytes by sex of respondent and region

Sex of respondent and analytes	Units	Region							
		Scotland				Northern			
		Mean	Median	sd	Base	Mean	Median	sd	Base
Men									
Haemoglobin concentration	g/dl	15.1	15.1	0.85	53	15.1	15.1	0.99	178
Mean corpuscular volume	fl	93.5	92.5	6.26	53	92.7	92.7	5.80	178
Haematocrit	l/l	0.455	0.460	0.0325	53	0.460	0.460	0.0354	178
Plasma iron	μmol/l	17.5	16.8	5.59	54	17.5	15.8	6.15	169
Total iron-binding capacity	μmol/l	62.9	60.4	8.86	54	62.4	61.1	8.30	168
Iron % saturation	%	28.6	28.1	10.62	54	28.4	26.6	10.07	168
Serum ferritin	μg/l	139	103	108.1	53	111	86	93.6	176
Women									
Haemoglobin concentration	g/dl	13.6	13.8	0.98	53	13.4	13.5	1.01	178
Mean corpuscular volume	fl	94	93	4.9	53	94	94	5.8	178
Haematocrit	l/l	0.415	0.420	0.0303	53	0.416	0.411	0.0336	178
Plasma iron	μmol/l	17.4	15.5	7.12	50	16.2	15.5	6.38	175
Total iron-binding capacity	μmol/l	64.6	62.7	11.18	50	63.5	62.8	9.16	175
Iron % saturation	%	28.4	28.6	13.33	50	26.1	24.9	10.70	174
Serum ferritin	μg/l	51	28	58.5	51	58	44	47.0	175

Central, South West and Wales				London and the South East				Sex of respondent and analytes	Units
Mean	Median	sd	Base	Mean	Median	sd	Base		
								Men	
15.1	15.1	0.94	226	15.0	15.2	1.23	181	Haemoglobin concentration	g/dl
92.9	92.4	5.08	226	92.8	92.8	6.48	181	Mean corpuscular volume	fl
0.458	0.460	0.0316	226	0.460	0.460	0.0364	181	Haematocrit	l/l
16.7	15.8	6.37	227	16.7	15.7	5.78	176	Plasma iron	µmol/l
60.7	61.2	8.33	226	61.3	60.5	9.49	176	Total iron-binding capacity	µmol/l
28.0	27.0	10.69	226	27.6	26.3	9.73	176	Iron % saturation	%
115	92	100.3	225	128	99	140.1	179	Serum ferritin	µg/l
								Women	
13.4	13.3	1.06	258	13.2	13.2	1.05	194	Haemoglobin concentration	g/dl
94	94	6.7	258	93	93	6.5	194	Mean corpuscular volume	fl
0.414	0.410	0.0343	258	0.410	0.410	0.0326	194	Haematocrit	l/l
16.3	16.2	6.67	250	15.5	15.7	6.01	192	Plasma iron	µmol/l
63.6	62.1	10.98	250	64.3	63.3	10.48	191	Total iron-binding capacity	µmol/l
26.4	26.2	11.05	250	24.7	23.9	10.02	191	Iron % saturation	%
52	41	41.7	249	50	37	45.4	194	Serum ferritin	µg/l

Table 4.12

Haematology analytes by sex of respondent and whether someone in the respondent's household was receiving certain benefits

Sex of respondent and analytes	Units	Whether receiving benefits								
		Receiving benefits				Not receiving benefits			
		Mean	Median	sd	Base	Mean	Median	sd	Base
Men									
Haemoglobin concentration	g/dl	15.0	15.0	1.23	86	15.1	15.2	1.00	552
Mean corpuscular volume	fl	92.5	92.6	7.22	86	92.9	92.7	5.54	552
Haematocrit	l/l	0.457	0.460	0.0352	86	0.459	0.460	0.0340	552
Plasma iron	μmol/l	16.9	16.3	5.95	85	17.0	15.9	6.11	542
Total iron-binding capacity	μmol/l	61.3	61.6	7.79	85	61.5	60.9	8.87	539
Iron % saturation	%	28.3	26.9	10.98	85	28.0	26.7	10.12	539
Serum ferritin	μg/l	97	78	76.7	84	123	94	116.2	549
Women									
Haemoglobin concentration	g/dl	13.4	13.4	1.20	131	13.4	13.3	1.00	552
Mean corpuscular volume	fl	93.5	92.9	7.14	131	93.4	93.4	6.09	552
Haematocrit	l/l	0.416	0.410	0.0393	131	0.413	0.410	0.0318	552
Plasma iron	μmol/l	15.9	15.0	7.69	129	16.2	15.9	6.12	538
Total iron-binding capacity	μmol/l	65.2	64.4	10.76	129	63.5	62.5	10.28	537
Iron % saturation	%	25.4	23.5	13.41	129	26.1	25.8	10.19	536
Serum ferritin	μg/l	47	33	41.2	126	55	42	46.5	543

Table 4.13

Percentage distribution of plasma vitamin C by sex and age of respondent

Cumulative percentages

Plasma vitamin C (μmol/l)	Men aged (years):				All men	Women aged (years):				All women
	19–24	25–34	35–49	50–64		19–24	25–34	35–49	50–64	
	cum %	cum %	cum %	cum %	cum %	cum %	cum %	cum %	cum %	cum %
Less than 11.0	7	5	4	5	5	4	3	4	3	3
Less than 30.0	12	20	22	25	21	9	14	15	15	14
Less than 50.0	39	42	50	48	46	26	37	36	30	33
Less than 60.0	57	57	66	63	62	46	44	47	44	45
Less than 70.0	81	72	79	73	76	73	59	65	60	63
Less than 80.0	84	88	91	85	88	84	75	78	78	78
Less than 90.0	89	93	97	91	93	91	84	91	89	89
Less than 100.0	95	97	99	96	97	92	90	95	92	93
All	100	100	100	100	100	100	100	100	100	100
Base	79	156	180	178	593	72	151	234	188	644
Mean (average value)	54.6	54.2	50.0	51.6	52.2	60.1	62.9	58.8	62.2	60.9
Median	59.0	56.6	49.8	50.8	52.6	62.1	63.5	61.0	63.6	63.0
Lower 2.5 percentile	6.8	8.1	7.2	6.6	7.0	5.2	9.1	8.5	9.9	9.5
Upper 2.5 percentile	101.9	109.2	98.1	108.4	103.1	109.1	119.2	108.5	109.4	109.9
Standard deviation	24.42	25.81	22.79	27.85	25.40	23.54	30.00	26.49	27.15	27.24

Table 4.14

Percentage distribution of red cell folate by sex and age of respondent

Cumulative percentages

Red cell folate (nmol/l)	Men aged (years):				All men	Women aged (years):				All women
	19–24	25–34	35–49	50–64		19–24	25–34	35–49	50–64	
	cum %	cum %	cum %	cum %	cum %	cum %	cum %	cum %	cum %	cum %
Less than 230	-	1	1	-	1	-	-	-	0	0
Less than 350	13	4	5	2	5	8	4	5	6	5
Less than 425	19	20	12	10	14	22	14	15	10	14
Less than 500	50	29	21	20	27	31	34	28	20	28
Less than 600	73	46	38	37	44	61	56	49	35	48
Less than 800	89	70	76	64	73	85	84	72	58	72
Less than 1000	93	86	93	78	86	97	94	85	81	87
Less than 1200	95	91	96	88	92	100	97	93	91	94
All	100	100	100	100	100		100	100	100	100
Base	83	170	189	194	636	81	161	243	197	683
Mean (average value)	561	688	677	773	694	576	630	691	768	685
Median	492	629	644	688	633	526	562	612	696	610
Lower 2.5 percentile	231	319	278	360	287	283	332	319	317	320
Upper 2.5 percentile	1338	1319	1245	1531	1426	1016	1255	1448	1651	1392
Standard deviation	261.6	281.4	244.8	319.7	288.2	194.4	274.6	293.4	317.4	293.0

Table 4.15

Percentage distribution of serum folate by sex and age of respondent

Cumulative percentages

Serum folate (nmol/l)	Men aged (years):				All men	Women aged (years):				All women
	19–24	25–34	35–49	50–64		19–24	25–34	35–49	50–64	
	cum %	cum %	cum %	cum %	cum %	cum %	cum %	cum %	cum %	cum %
Less than 6.3	-	1	1	1	1	-	-	0	-	0
Less than 7.0	-	1	1	1	1	-	-	1	-	0
Less than 10.0	12	7	3	6	6	6	7	5	5	6
Less than 15.0	42	30	27	21	28	32	30	27	21	27
Less than 20.0	68	60	56	47	56	53	52	48	38	47
Less than 25.0	82	74	72	62	71	75	71	63	58	65
Less than 28.1	92	83	80	67	78	79	83	72	65	73
Less than 30.0	93	87	84	73	83	83	86	78	70	78
Less than 35.0	100	94	93	88	93	94	93	91	87	90
Less than 40.0		99	99	96	98	100	99	98	99	99
All		100	100	100	100		100	100	100	100
Base	83	169	188	196	636	81	159	240	197	678
Mean (average value)	17.4	20.1	20.9	22.9	20.8	20.6	21.2	21.9	23.7	22.1
Median	16.4	18.8	19.0	21.4	18.8	19.7	19.5	20.6	22.6	21.0
Lower 2.5 percentile	7.2	8.8	9.4	7.8	8.1	9.2	8.4	8.6	9.3	8.9
Upper 2.5 percentile	32.9	38.5	37.6	40.3	39.4	35.6	38.3	38.9	39.6	39.2
Standard deviation	7.07	8.16	8.02	9.40	8.55	8.03	11.13	8.95	9.00	9.46

Table 4.16

Percentage distribution of serum vitamin B$_{12}$ by sex and age of respondent

Cumulative percentages

Serum vitamin B$_{12}$ (pmol/l)	Men aged (years):				All men	Women aged (years):				All women
	19–24	25–34	35–49	50–64		19–24	25–34	35–49	50–64	
	cum %	cum %	cum %	cum %	cum %	cum %	cum %	cum %	cum %	cum %
Less than 118	-	-	2	3	2	5	5	4	3	4
Less than 150	3	2	8	8	6	17	14	8	7	10
Less than 200	27	16	21	19	20	31	34	29	19	27
Less than 250	44	33	40	37	38	57	54	47	36	47
Less than 300	62	60	55	59	59	73	75	61	57	65
Less than 350	78	73	72	71	73	87	85	74	72	78
Less than 450	90	95	94	87	92	96	93	91	85	91
Less than 550	96	97	97	94	96	100	97	97	95	97
All	100	100	100	100	100		100	100	100	100
Base	84	168	187	193	632	79	158	239	191	667
Mean (average value)	286	298	294	308	298	247	259	288	329	288
Median	261	279	281	276	276	233	237	255	285	263
Lower 2.5 percentile	138	139	121	95	128	111	85	99	110	104
Upper 2.5 percentile	614	581	575	665	614	525	590	613	691	573
Standard deviation	111.2	101.8	108.1	155.1	123.2	91.3	121.9	145.4	273.9	185.3

Table 4.17

Percentage distribution of erythrocyte transketolase activation coefficient (ETKAC) by sex and age of respondent

Cumulative percentages

ETKAC (ratio)	Men aged (years):				All men	Women aged (years):				All women
	19–24	25–34	35–49	50–64		19–24	25–34	35–49	50–64	
	cum %	cum %	cum %	cum %	cum %	cum %	cum %	cum %	cum %	cum %
Greater than 1.25	-	3	2	5	3	-	1	2	1	1
Greater than 1.20	18	23	14	19	19	7	8	14	9	10
Greater than 1.18	21	28	22	23	24	10	14	17	13	14
Greater than 1.15	58	45	43	45	46	36	40	33	29	34
Greater than 1.13	80	71	64	59	66	52	58	55	45	53
Greater than 1.10	96	92	91	89	91	88	86	86	79	84
Greater than 1.05	100	99	97	97	98	100	98	97	99	98
All		100	100	100	100		100	100	100	100
Base	83	164	189	192	628	74	162	241	195	672
Mean (average value)	1.16	1.16	1.15	1.15	1.15	1.14	1.15	1.14	1.13	1.14
Median	1.16	1.15	1.15	1.15	1.15	1.14	1.14	1.14	1.13	1.14
Lower 2.5 percentile	1.09	1.06	1.05	1.04	1.06	1.07	1.06	1.04	1.06	1.06
Upper 2.5 percentile	1.24	1.26	1.25	1.27	1.26	1.22	1.25	1.25	1.23	1.24
Standard deviation	0.040	0.047	0.049	0.064	0.053	0.036	0.060	0.057	0.049	0.054

Table 4.18

Percentage distribution of erythrocyte transketolase basal activity (ETK-B) by sex and age of respondent

Cumulative percentages

ETK-B (μmol/g Hb/min)	Men aged (years):				All men	Women aged (years):				All women
	19–24	25–34	35–49	50–64		19–24	25–34	35–49	50–64	
	cum %	cum %	cum %	cum %	cum %	cum %	cum %	cum %	cum %	cum %
Less than 0.50	2	2	2	4	2	-	-	3	1	1
Less than 0.60	14	15	12	10	12	3	9	11	7	9
Less than 0.65	36	28	29	25	28	12	20	24	16	19
Less than 0.70	57	44	44	39	44	18	28	39	31	32
Less than 0.75	69	55	60	55	58	30	42	50	49	46
Less than 0.80	83	74	80	74	77	50	62	69	62	63
Less than 0.90	95	90	95	96	94	86	88	91	86	88
Less than 1.00	100	97	99	100	99	95	97	98	96	97
All		100	100		100	100	100	100	100	100
Base	83	167	191	192	633	74	162	242	195	673
Mean (average value)	0.70	0.73	0.71	0.73	0.72	0.79	0.76	0.74	0.77	0.76
Median	0.69	0.71	0.72	0.73	0.72	0.80	0.76	0.75	0.75	0.76
Lower 2.5 percentile	0.51	0.51	0.48	0.48	0.49	0.57	0.50	0.47	0.55	0.51
Upper 2.5 percentile	0.95	1.16	0.96	0.92	0.95	1.03	1.00	1.00	1.05	1.02
Standard deviation	0.107	0.151	0.124	0.104	0.125	0.110	0.124	0.128	0.128	0.126

Table 4.19

Percentage distribution of erythrocyte glutathione reductase activation coefficient (EGRAC) by sex and age of respondent

Cumulative percentages

EGRAC (ratio)	Men aged (years):				All men	Women aged (years):				All women
	19–24	25–34	35–49	50–64		19–24	25–34	35–49	50–64	
	cum %	cum %	cum %	cum %	cum %	cum %	cum %	cum %	cum %	cum %
Greater than 1.70	6	5	2	3	4	10	8	6	4	6
Greater than 1.60	17	12	9	9	11	19	19	11	10	13
Greater than 1.50	25	20	16	15	18	35	35	20	16	24
Greater than 1.40	59	40	37	30	38	66	53	40	33	44
Greater than 1.30	82	70	67	54	66	77	78	69	50	66
Greater than 1.20	100	96	86	84	90	91	95	91	82	90
All		100	100	100	100	100	100	100	100	100
Base	83	167	191	192	633	74	162	242	195	673
Mean (average value)	1.45	1.40	1.37	1.35	1.38	1.45	1.44	1.40	1.34	1.40
Median	1.44	1.37	1.36	1.32	1.36	1.47	1.41	1.36	1.31	1.38
Lower 2.5 percentile	1.22	1.16	1.10	1.12	1.12	1.08	1.12	1.09	1.08	1.09
Upper 2.5 percentile	1.77	1.88	1.69	1.78	1.77	1.98	1.89	1.88	1.79	1.85
Standard deviation	0.132	0.163	0.176	0.171	0.169	0.194	0.179	0.206	0.179	0.194

Table 4.20

Percentage distribution of erythrocyte aspartate aminotransferase activation coefficient (EAATAC) by sex and age of respondent

Cumulative percentages

EAATAC (ratio)	Men aged (years):				All men	Women aged (years):				All women
	19–24	25–34	35–49	50–64		19–24	25–34	35–49	50–64	
	cum %	cum %	cum %	cum %	cum %	cum %	cum %	cum %	cum %	cum %
Greater than 2.10	1	4	6	5	5	3	5	6	5	5
Greater than 2.00	4	10	13	11	10	12	8	12	13	11
Greater than 1.90	29	23	25	22	24	20	23	22	27	24
Greater than 1.80	55	48	45	39	45	29	39	39	43	39
Greater than 1.70	77	78	70	61	70	51	66	58	66	61
Greater than 1.60	95	97	89	86	91	78	88	81	83	83
Greater than 1.50	99	98	95	95	96	98	97	94	91	94
All	100	100	100	100	100	100	100	100	100	100
Base	83	167	191	192	633	74	162	242	195	673
Mean (average value)	1.81	1.81	1.80	1.77	1.79	1.74	1.78	1.77	1.79	1.77
Median	1.84	1.78	1.79	1.74	1.78	1.71	1.75	1.75	1.76	1.75
Lower 2.5 percentile	1.56	1.53	1.45	1.38	1.46	1.47	1.48	1.28	1.41	1.41
Upper 2.5 percentile	2.07	2.19	2.21	2.31	2.19	2.23	2.27	2.20	2.17	2.22
Standard deviation	0.134	0.156	0.195	0.204	0.182	0.183	0.177	0.232	0.241	0.218

Table 4.21

Percentage distribution of plasma total homocysteine by sex and age of respondent

Cumulative percentages

Plasma total homocysteine (µmol/l)	Men aged (years):				All men	Women aged (years):				All women
	19–24	25–34	35–49	50–64		19–24	25–34	35–49	50–64	
	cum %	cum %	cum %	cum %	cum %	cum %	cum %	cum %	cum %	cum %
Greater than 18.0	13	6	5	6	7	3	1	3	5	3
Greater than 14.0	23	14	16	19	17	12	5	10	12	10
Greater than 12.0	41	26	31	37	33	16	20	20	29	22
Greater than 10.0	66	57	56	70	62	34	39	38	49	41
Greater than 9.0	77	74	74	83	77	42	54	54	65	56
Greater than 8.0	85	87	88	94	89	53	69	74	79	72
Greater than 6.0	100	100	100	99	100	79	94	96	94	93
All				100		100	100	100	100	100
Base	81	162	179	181	603	77	154	233	190	654
Mean (average value)	12.5	11.1	11.1	12.4	11.7	9.3	9.6	10.4	10.6	10.1
Median	11.1	10.2	10.5	11.4	10.6	8.6	9.2	9.2	9.9	9.4
Lower 2.5 percentile	6.5	6.9	6.8	6.9	6.8	5.2	4.4	5.8	5.1	5.2
Upper 2.5 percentile	26.5	19.9	19.7	25.9	22.3	21.9	15.8	20.6	19.2	19.2
Standard deviation	5.37	4.00	3.21	5.52	4.55	3.86	2.93	6.56	3.40	4.76

Table 4.22

Pearson correlation coefficients for plasma vitamin C with dietary intake of vitamin C and fruit and vegetable intake[†]

Sex and age of respondent	Correlation of plasma vitamin C with:		
	Dietary intake of vitamin C	Fruit and vegetable consumption	Base
Men aged (years):			
19–24	0.36**	0.39**	75
25–34	0.36**	0.34**	141
35–49	0.16*	0.25**	171
50–64	0.48**	0.41**	174
All men	0.25**	0.29**	560
Women aged (years):			
19–24	0.17	0.08	66
25–34	0.41**	0.32**	144
35–49	0.42**	0.44**	221
50–64	0.55**	0.33**	184
All women	0.41**	0.33**	615

Note: * p<0.05; ** p<0.01

[†] Average daily consumption of fruit and vegetables (grams) including composite dishes (all fruit juice counted as one portion; all baked beans and other pulses counted as one portion). See Volume 1, Chapter 2, Section 2.4 for methodology for deriving fruit and vegetable consumption (Henderson L, Gregory J, Swan G. National Diet and Nutrition survey: adults aged 19 to 64 years. Volume 1: Types and quantities of foods consumed. TSO (London, 2002)).

Table 4.23

Pearson correlation coefficients for dietary intakes of folate with red cell folate and serum folate

Sex and age of respondent	Correlation of dietary intakes of folate with:			
	Red cell folate	Base	Serum folate	Base
Men aged (years):				
19–24	0.37**	78	0.28 *	78
25–34	0.30**	155	0.30 **	154
35–49	0.26**	179	0.29 **	178
50–64	0.36**	190	0.40 **	192
All men	0.32**	603	0.33 **	602
Women aged (years):				
19–24	0.39**	76	0.35 **	76
25–34	0.42**	154	0.33 **	153
35–49	0.53**	229	0.46 **	227
50–64	0.22**	192	0.21 **	192
All women	0.33**	651	0.28 **	648

Note: * p<0.05; ** p<0.01

Table 4.24

Water soluble vitamins and plasma total homocysteine by sex of respondent and region

Sex of respondent and analytes	Units	Region							
		Scotland				Northern			
		Mean	Median	sd	Base	Mean	Median	sd	Base
Men									
Plasma vitamin C	µmol/l	42.0	42.8	23.48	48	50.7	51.1	25.45	155
Red cell folate	nmol/l	719	646	327.1	53	698	644	288.2	177
Serum folate	nmol/l	19.0	16.5	8.61	53	21.3	19.9	7.86	176
Serum vitamin B_{12}	pmol/l	304	305	85.4	51	302	278	116.7	175
ETKAC*	ratio	1.14	1.14	0.053	54	1.15	1.15	0.053	171
ETK-B**	µmol/g Hb/min	0.78	0.78	0.102	54	0.72	0.72	0.104	171
EGRAC***	ratio	1.40	1.38	0.165	54	1.37	1.35	0.177	171
EAATAC****	ratio	1.69	1.67	0.142	54	1.81	1.79	0.195	171
Plasma total homocysteine	µmol/l	12.8	10.4	8.31	53	11.2	10.1	3.68	167
Women									
Plasma vitamin C	µmol/l	62.9	66.6	28.07	54	57.6	62.5	25.08	170
Red cell folate	nmol/l	684	574	351.6	53	705	632	281.0	179
Serum folate	nmol/l	18.4	18.1	6.62	54	22.7	19.9	11.33	179
Serum vitamin B_{12}	pmol/l	279	273	95.3	53	281	265	134.9	173
ETKAC*	ratio	1.14	1.13	0.038	54	1.14	1.14	0.052	177
ETK-B**	µmol/g Hb/min	0.78	0.77	0.085	54	0.76	0.75	0.124	177
EGRAC***	ratio	1.46	1.46	0.202	54	1.37	1.35	0.173	177
EAATAC****	ratio	1.71	1.72	0.153	54	1.79	1.76	0.267	177
Plasma total homocysteine	µmol/l	10.4	9.2	4.14	50	9.9	9.3	3.17	174

Note: *   erythrocyte transketolase activation coefficient.
      **   erythrocyte transketolase basal activity.
      ***   erythrocyte glutathione reductase activation coefficient.
      **** erythrocyte aspartate aminotransferase activation coefficient.

Central, South West and Wales				London and the South East				Sex of respondent and analytes	Units
Mean	Median	sd	Base	Mean	Median	sd	Base		
								Men	
51.9	51.5	26.25	220	56.8	57.2	23.88	169	Plasma vitamin C	μmol/l
678	629	292.0	226	704	626	272.2	181	Red cell folate	nmol/l
20.1	18.6	8.72	226	21.8	19.3	8.87	181	Serum folate	nmol/l
280	264	111.9	227	316	290	147.7	179	Serum vitamin B_{12}	pmol/l
1.16	1.16	0.045	228	1.16	1.15	0.061	175	ETKAC*	ratio
0.72	0.71	0.127	229	0.72	0.72	0.141	179	ETK-B**	μmol/g Hb/min
1.38	1.36	0.169	229	1.38	1.37	0.163	179	EGRAC***	ratio
1.79	1.79	1.790	229	1.80	1.79	0.177	179	EAATAC****	ratio
11.9	11.0	4.53	218	11.5	10.9	3.52	166	Plasma total homocysteine	μmol/l
								Women	
62.5	64.1	29.09	243	61.2	60.6	26.28	178	Plasma vitamin C	μmol/l
668	605	272.1	256	690	614	313.3	194	Red cell folate	nmol/l
22.1	22.2	8.73	253	22.6	21.4	8.97	191	Serum folate	nmol/l
277	245	126.7	249	311	265	281.6	192	Serum vitamin B_{12}	pmol/l
1.14	1.14	0.047	250	1.15	1.14	0.065	192	ETKAC*	ratio
0.77	0.78	0.121	250	0.73	0.73	0.139	192	ETK-B**	μmol/g Hb/min
1.39	1.37	0.173	250	1.42	1.39	0.229	192	EGRAC***	ratio
1.76	1.74	0.202	250	1.79	1.78	0.200	192	EAATAC****	ratio
10.6	9.4	6.24	244	9.8	9.2	3.78	186	Plasma total homocysteine	μmol/l

Table 4.25

Water soluble vitamins and plasma total homocysteine by sex of respondent and whether someone in the the respondent's household was receiving certain benefits

Sex of respondent and analytes	Units	Whether receiving benefits							
		Receiving benefits				Not receiving benefits			
		Mean	Median	sd	Base	Mean	Median	sd	Base
Men									
Plasma vitamin C	μmol/l	43.1	41.9	24.70	82	53.6	54.8	25.23	510
Red cell folate	nmol/l	617	544	245.7	85	706	643	292.6	551
Serum folate	nmol/l	19.1	17.7	8.04	85	21.1	19.0	8.61	551
Serum vitamin B$_{12}$	pmol/l	275	257	99.9	85	302	279	126.2	547
ETKAC*	ratio	1.17	1.16	0.044	85	1.15	1.15	0.054	543
ETK-B**	μmol/g Hb/min	0.71	0.70	0.110	85	0.73	0.72	0.127	548
EGRAC***	ratio	1.43	1.38	0.164	85	1.37	1.36	0.169	548
EAATAC****	ratio	1.82	1.79	0.206	85	1.79	1.78	0.178	548
Plasma total homocysteine	μmol/l	12.4	11.0	5.37	81	11.6	10.6	4.40	523
Women									
Plasma vitamin C	μmol/l	49.4	48.2	28.33	126	63.7	65.5	26.23	518
Red cell folate	nmol/l	616	563	249.8	130	701	623	300.1	552
Serum folate	nmol/l	20.7	19.0	8.79	129	22.4	21.4	9.59	548
Serum vitamin B$_{12}$	pmol/l	262	258	100.0	128	294	265	199.9	539
ETKAC*	ratio	1.14	1.14	0.051	129	1.14	1.14	0.054	542
ETK-B**	μmol/g Hb/min	0.75	0.75	0.124	129	0.76	0.76	0.127	543
EGRAC***	ratio	1.42	1.41	0.191	129	1.39	1.37	0.195	543
EAATAC****	ratio	1.76	1.73	0.216	129	1.78	1.75	0.218	543
Plasma total homocysteine	μmol/l	10.7	9.9	3.96	127	10.0	9.2	4.93	527

Note: * erythrocyte transketolase activation coefficient.
** erythrocyte transketolase basal activity.
*** erythrocyte glutathione reductase activation coefficient.
**** erythrocyte aspartate aminotransferase activation coefficient.

Table 4.26

Percentage distribution of plasma retinol by sex and age of respondent

Cumulative percentages

Plasma retinol (μmol/l)	Men aged (years):				All men	Women aged (years):				All women
	19–24	25–34	35–49	50–64		19–24	25–34	35–49	50–64	
	cum %	cum %	cum %	cum %	cum %	cum %	cum %	cum %	cum %	cum %
Less than 0.70	-	-	-	1	0	-	-	-	-	-
Less than 1.00	1	2	2	2	2	2	3	1	1	2
Less than 1.20	6	4	4	3	4	15	10	6	5	8
Less than 1.50	22	14	13	9	13	29	30	28	20	26
Less than 1.83	63	42	35	32	40	59	63	61	44	57
Less than 2.00	75	59	47	45	53	65	71	76	59	68
Less than 2.15	78	72	59	52	63	74	80	83	66	77
Less than 2.50	87	90	79	75	82	99	92	95	84	92
Less than 3.00	100	98	95	92	96	100	100	100	93	98
All		100	100	100	100				100	100
Base	75	152	175	175	576	72	146	219	179	616
Mean (average value)	1.81	1.94	2.08	2.13	2.02	1.75	1.75	1.75	1.99	1.82
Median	1.71	1.88	2.04	2.12	1.96	1.68	1.71	1.72	1.88	1.76
Lower 2.5 percentile	1.03	1.01	1.14	1.15	1.04	1.00	0.94	1.07	1.08	1.01
Upper 2.5 percentile	2.82	2.92	3.22	3.37	3.19	2.45	2.65	2.68	3.85	2.89
Standard deviation	0.451	0.456	0.549	0.565	0.529	0.426	0.456	0.404	0.630	0.505

Table 4.27

Percentage distribution of plasma α–carotene by sex and age of respondent

Cumulative percentages

Plasma α–carotene (μmol/l)	Men aged (years):				All men	Women aged (years):				All women
	19–24	25–34	35–49	50–64		19–24	25–34	35–49	50–64	
	cum %	cum %	cum %	cum %	cum %	cum %	cum %	cum %	cum %	cum %
Less than 0.010	6	2	4	2	3	-	2	3	2	2
Less than 0.020	24	12	12	8	12	17	10	9	4	9
Less than 0.030	46	21	25	20	25	33	20	14	13	17
Less than 0.040	66	37	40	29	39	50	34	25	22	29
Less than 0.060	96	68	62	51	65	80	60	52	52	57
Less than 0.080	100	82	79	66	79	90	75	65	59	69
Less than 0.100		87	84	74	84	97	80	70	61	73
Less than 0.120		97	93	86	93	100	90	84	76	85
All		100	100	100	100		100	100	100	100
Base	75	152	175	175	576	72	146	219	179	616
Mean (average value)	0.039	0.059	0.067	0.074	0.064	0.048	0.075	0.080	0.101	0.081
Median	0.040	0.050	0.050	0.060	0.050	0.045	0.060	0.060	0.060	0.060
Lower 2.5 percentile	0.010	0.011	0.010	0.020	0.010	0.020	0.016	0.010	0.020	0.020
Upper 2.5 percentile	0.080	0.160	0.159	0.180	0.160	0.100	0.180	0.190	0.320	0.230
Standard deviation	0.0170	0.0322	0.0913	0.0458	0.0599	0.0200	0.0914	0.0582	0.1028	0.0808

Table 4.28

Percentage distribution of plasma β–carotene by sex and age of respondent

Cumulative percentages

Plasma β-carotene (μmol/l)	Men aged (years):				All men	Women aged (years):				All women
	19–24	25–34	35–49	50–64		19–24	25–34	35–49	50–64	
	cum %	cum %	cum %	cum %	cum %	cum %	cum %	cum %	cum %	cum %
Less than 0.050	12	6	6	4	6	8	6	3	2	4
Less than 0.100	37	27	25	20	26	41	25	17	11	20
Less than 0.150	62	47	46	42	47	58	40	29	26	34
Less than 0.250	86	64	72	66	70	80	67	55	45	58
Less than 0.350	97	84	83	77	83	90	84	69	61	73
Less than 0.450	98	92	91	85	90	94	91	81	71	82
Less than 0.550	98	96	93	90	94	94	95	87	76	86
All	100	100	100	100	100	100	100	100	100	100
Base	75	152	175	175	576	72	146	219	179	616
Mean (average value)	0.143	0.209	0.221	0.248	0.216	0.233	0.245	0.301	0.384	0.304
Median	0.120	0.160	0.150	0.180	0.160	0.125	0.180	0.230	0.281	0.210
Lower 2.5 percentile	0.030	0.040	0.030	0.033	0.030	0.030	0.036	0.040	0.050	0.040
Upper 2.5 percentile	0.485	0.590	0.787	0.830	0.690	2.502	0.751	1.010	1.410	1.118
Standard deviation	0.1340	0.1532	0.2408	0.2149	0.2024	0.4795	0.3417	0.2653	0.3396	0.3401

Table 4.29

Percentage distribution of plasma α–cryptoxanthin by sex and age of respondent

Cumulative percentages

Plasma α–cryptoxanthin (μmol/l)	Men aged (years):				All men	Women aged (years):				All women
	19–24	25–34	35–49	50–64		19–24	25–34	35–49	50–64	
	cum %	cum %	cum %	cum %	cum %	cum %	cum %	cum %	cum %	cum %
Less than 0.008	2	-	3	2	2	-	-	1	2	1
Less than 0.014	11	7	10	25	14	14	12	16	24	17
Less than 0.020	45	29	33	46	38	28	38	43	55	43
Less than 0.030	67	54	58	69	62	58	65	72	73	69
Less than 0.040	80	73	79	82	78	77	78	82	83	81
Less than 0.060	93	86	93	91	91	95	91	93	93	93
Less than 0.080	94	92	97	95	95	100	95	94	95	96
Less than 0.100	94	93	97	96	95		95	95	96	96
All	100	100	100	100	100		100	100	100	100
Base	75	152	175	175	576	72	146	219	179	616
Mean (average value)	0.052	0.047	0.039	0.035	0.041	0.034	0.039	0.037	0.032	0.035
Median	0.030	0.030	0.030	0.030	0.030	0.030	0.030	0.030	0.020	0.030
Lower 2.5 percentile	0.009	0.010	0.000	0.010	0.010	0.010	0.010	0.010	0.010	0.010
Upper 2.5 percentile	0.434	0.200	0.146	0.190	0.203	0.077	0.194	0.170	0.130	0.167
Standard deviation	0.0947	0.0570	0.0420	0.0375	0.0547	0.0166	0.0387	0.0415	0.0315	0.0359

Table 4.30

Percentage distribution of plasma β–cryptoxanthin by sex and age of respondent

Cumulative percentages

Plasma β–cryptoxanthin (μmol/l)	Men aged (years):				All men	Women aged (years):				All women
	19–24	25–34	35–49	50–64		19–24	25–34	35–49	50–64	
	cum %	cum %	cum %	cum %	cum %	cum %	cum %	cum %	cum %	cum %
Less than 0.030	6	1	4	10	6	2	3	6	5	4
Less than 0.040	17	4	11	15	11	5	7	10	11	9
Less than 0.080	41	30	35	38	35	37	37	33	31	34
Less than 0.120	65	71	65	66	67	76	57	59	50	58
Less than 0.160	86	84	83	79	82	83	71	73	65	71
Less than 0.220	96	91	92	89	91	93	86	85	77	84
Less than 0.280	100	95	95	94	95	93	91	93	82	90
All		100	100	100	100	100	100	100	100	100
Base	75	152	175	175	576	72	146	219	179	616
Mean (average value)	0.103	0.122	0.119	0.119	0.118	0.123	0.141	0.134	0.181	0.148
Median	0.090	0.100	0.100	0.100	0.100	0.100	0.110	0.110	0.130	0.110
Lower 2.5 percentile	0.020	0.040	0.030	0.020	0.020	0.033	0.030	0.030	0.020	0.030
Upper 2.5 percentile	0.233	0.420	0.382	0.340	0.350	0.430	0.488	0.370	0.670	0.530
Standard deviation	0.0540	0.0818	0.0818	0.0837	0.0794	0.0859	0.1063	0.0957	0.1779	0.1281

Table 4.31

Percentage distribution of plasma lycopene by sex and age of respondent

Cumulative percentages

Plasma lycopene (µmol/l)	Men aged (years):				All men	Women aged (years):				All women
	19–24	25–34	35–49	50–64		19–24	25–34	35–49	50–64	
	cum %	cum %	cum %	cum %	cum %	cum %	cum %	cum %	cum %	cum %
Less than 0.125	5	4	7	9	7	5	6	4	5	5
Less than 0.250	30	25	25	29	27	22	29	20	26	24
Less than 0.375	50	41	46	57	49	48	56	44	45	48
Less than 0.500	64	57	61	72	64	65	68	61	62	63
Less than 0.625	73	66	69	81	72	79	80	73	79	77
Less than 0.750	92	74	77	87	81	90	88	85	85	86
Less than 0.875	93	87	88	92	90	90	92	93	88	91
All	100	100	100	100	100	100	100	100	100	100
Base	75	152	175	175	576	72	146	219	179	616
Mean (average value)	0.442	0.514	0.487	0.416	0.467	0.452	0.426	0.474	0.484	0.463
Median	0.360	0.410	0.400	0.340	0.380	0.395	0.330	0.420	0.410	0.390
Lower 2.5 percentile	0.087	0.120	0.100	0.080	0.090	0.100	0.106	0.110	0.092	0.100
Upper 2.5 percentile	1.260	1.200	1.247	1.260	1.211	1.360	1.202	1.150	1.467	1.276
Standard deviation	0.2798	0.3098	0.3092	0.2794	0.2988	0.2878	0.2769	0.2662	0.3309	0.2914

Table 4.32

Percentage distribution of plasma lutein and zeaxanthin by sex and age of respondent

Cumulative percentages

Plasma lutein and zeaxanthin (µmol/l)	Men aged (years):				All men	Women aged (years):				All women
	19–24	25–34	35–49	50–64		19–24	25–34	35–49	50–64	
	cum %	cum %	cum %	cum %	cum %	cum %	cum %	cum %	cum %	cum %
Less than 0.10	9	0	2	3	3	2	3	2	1	2
Less than 0.15	29	13	14	12	15	14	15	13	7	12
Less than 0.20	49	37	30	25	33	30	27	32	14	25
Less than 0.25	76	60	52	44	55	63	53	56	32	49
Less than 0.30	84	69	66	55	66	78	72	67	41	62
Less than 0.35	92	81	77	71	78	86	89	79	56	75
Less than 0.40	100	86	84	80	85	91	93	85	68	83
Less than 0.45		92	89	86	91	93	94	90	80	88
All		100	100	100	100	100	100	100	100	100
Base	75	152	175	175	576	72	146	219	179	616
Mean (average value)	0.20	0.26	0.28	0.30	0.27	0.26	0.25	0.27	0.37	0.29
Median	0.20	0.23	0.25	0.27	0.24	0.23	0.25	0.24	0.33	0.26
Lower 2.5 percentile	0.07	0.10	0.11	0.08	0.09	0.09	0.08	0.09	0.11	0.10
Upper 2.5 percentile	0.37	0.68	0.65	0.69	0.65	0.66	0.53	0.56	0.85	0.71
Standard deviation	0.082	0.134	0.145	0.156	0.142	0.126	0.116	0.125	0.854	0.164

Table 4.33

Percentage distribution of plasma 25-hydroxyvitamin D by sex and age of respondent

Cumulative percentages

Plasma 25-hydroxyvitamin D (nmol/l)	Men aged (years):				All men	Women aged (years):				All women
	19–24	25–34	35–49	50–64		19–24	25–34	35–49	50–64	
	cum %	cum %	cum %	cum %	cum %	cum %	cum %	cum %	cum %	cum %
Less than 12.0	-	1	1	0	1	-	2	1	1	1
Less than 20.0	15	7	7	5	8	15	9	8	4	8
Less than 25.0	24	16	12	9	14	28	13	15	11	15
Less than 30.0	35	25	19	15	22	28	24	26	22	25
Less than 40.0	61	40	41	32	41	54	40	43	35	41
Less than 50.0	70	57	58	49	57	67	50	57	49	54
Less than 60.0	83	72	73	68	72	78	66	72	64	69
Less than 70.0	90	80	85	85	84	83	76	84	78	80
Less than 80.0	95	86	93	91	91	93	85	89	88	88
Less than 100.0	98	98	99	97	98	96	95	98	98	97
All	100	100	100	100	100	100	100	100	100	100
Base	81	165	190	190	627	78	158	239	194	670
Mean (average value)	40.6	48.8	47.8	51.6	48.3	44.5	51.9	47.9	51.8	49.6
Median	34.1	44.9	44.8	50.7	45.5	39.3	49.8	43.6	51.5	46.5
Lower 2.5 percentile	13.5	17.7	13.5	16.1	14.6	12.8	12.6	13.5	14.4	13.3
Upper 2.5 percentile	89.0	96.4	88.7	105.5	97.1	103.9	113.4	96.6	99.8	102.6
Standard deviation	21.93	23.33	21.03	21.16	22.02	23.77	26.94	22.75	22.55	23.96

Table 4.34

Percentage distribution of plasma 25-hydroxyvitamin D by date blood sample taken and sex of respondent

Cumulative percentages

Plasma 25-hydroxyvitamin D (nmol/l)	Wave 1: July-September		Wave 2: October-December		Wave 3: January-March		Wave 4: April-June		All	
	Men	Women	Men	Women	Men	Women	Men	Women	Men	Women
	cum %	cum %	cum %	cum %	cum %	cum %	cum %	cum %	cum%	cum%
Less than 12.0	-	0	1	1	1	3	0	1	1	1
Less than 20.0	1	4	6	3	12	16	10	8	8	8
Less than 25.0	1	6	12	13	24	23	16	17	14	15
Less than 30.0	2	11	22	22	37	36	24	29	22	25
Less than 40.0	13	19	38	42	63	55	45	47	41	41
Less than 50.0	25	29	57	55	75	70	67	61	57	54
Less than 60.0	44	41	70	73	88	81	83	78	72	69
Less than 70.0	61	59	88	84	93	92	93	85	84	80
Less than 80.0	75	72	92	90	97	95	97	93	91	88
Less than 100.0	95	92	97	98	99	100	100	98	98	97
All	100	100	100	100	100			100	100	100
Base	153	161	120	140	168	152	186	218	627	670
Mean (average value)	64.9	64.5	48.4	48.4	38.7	40.8	43.3	45.5	48.3	49.6
Median	64.2	65.6	45.7	43.2	33.9	36.7	41.3	41.2	45.5	46.5
Lower 2.5 percentile	30.0	18.4	15.8	18.5	13.2	9.5	16.2	15.5	14.6	13.3
Upper 2.5 percentile	114.6	121.3	107.3	99.4	85.6	93.1	82.3	96.4	97.1	102.6
Standard deviation	21.59	25.37	21.31	21.02	18.70	20.78	17.70	21.84	22.02	23.96

Table 4.35

Percentage distribution of plasma α–tocopherol by sex and age of respondent

Cumulative percentages

Plasma α–tocopherol (μmol/l)	Men aged (years):				All men	Women aged (years):				All women
	19–24	25–34	35–49	50–64		19–24	25–34	35–49	50–64	
	cum %	cum %	cum %	cum %	cum %	cum %	cum %	cum %	cum %	cum %
Less than 11.6	8	3	3	4	4	9	10	2	1	4
Less than 15.0	38	20	16	10	18	44	27	12	5	17
Less than 18.0	67	42	33	20	36	65	57	36	14	38
Less than 21.0	91	60	52	40	56	84	75	61	29	58
Less than 25.0	95	80	68	64	74	97	90	86	58	80
Less than 30.0	96	98	88	88	92	100	99	93	82	92
Less than 35.0	96	100	95	92	95		100	97	92	97
All	100		100	100	100			100	100	100
Base	75	152	175	175	576	72	146	219	179	616
Mean (average value)	16.6	19.7	22.0	23.3	21.1	16.6	17.8	20.3	24.7	20.6
Median	15.7	19.0	20.3	22.4	20.2	16.3	17.2	20.3	24.0	19.7
Lower 2.5 percentile	9.6	10.5	11.3	10.6	10.7	7.6	9.7	12.0	13.9	10.6
Upper 2.5 percentile	39.2	31.2	38.7	43.8	38.0	28.6	28.6	35.4	41.7	36.0
Standard deviation	5.62	5.30	7.53	7.34	7.05	4.53	4.67	5.54	6.70	6.32

Table 4.36

Percentage distribution of plasma γ–tocopherol by sex and age of respondent

Cumulative percentages

Plasma γ–tocopherol (μmol/l)	Men aged (years):				All men	Women aged (years):				All women
	19–24	25–34	35–49	50–64		19–24	25–34	35–49	50–64	
	cum %	cum %	cum %	cum %	cum %	cum %	cum %	cum %	cum %	cum %
Less than 0.75	10	2	1	2	3	5	5	6	5	5
Less than 1.00	35	27	20	15	22	44	32	26	31	31
Less than 1.15	70	48	43	37	46	73	59	48	49	54
Less than 1.25	80	61	53	47	57	78	68	61	55	63
Less than 1.50	92	83	76	79	81	92	88	80	78	83
Less than 2.00	96	94	96	96	95	97	99	95	97	97
All	100	100	100	100	100	100	100	100	100	100
Base	75	152	175	175	576	72	146	219	179	616
Mean (average value)	1.09	1.25	1.29	1.31	1.26	1.16	1.14	1.24	1.24	1.21
Median	1.04	1.17	1.22	1.26	1.19	1.01	1.11	1.18	1.17	1.14
Lower 2.5 percentile	0.43	0.73	0.81	0.79	0.71	0.73	0.45	0.55	0.72	0.59
Upper 2.5 percentile	2.58	2.33	2.35	2.12	2.25	3.96	1.91	2.23	2.01	2.06
Standard deviation	0.389	0.378	0.367	0.362	0.377	0.591	0.310	0.403	0.394	0.410

Table 4.37

Percentage distribution of tocopherol to cholesterol ratio* by sex and age of respondent

Cumulative percentages

Tocopherol to cholesterol ratio (μmol/mmol)	Men aged (years):				All men	Women aged (years):				All women
	19–24	25–34	35–49	50–64		19–24	25–34	35–49	50–64	
	cum %	cum %	cum %	cum %	cum %	cum %	cum %	cum %	cum %	cum %
Less than 2.25	1	1	1	1	1	-	2	1	3	2
Less than 3.25	24	22	25	19	22	27	33	21	14	22
Less than 3.75	58	53	44	36	46	56	58	42	40	47
Less than 4.25	75	67	64	58	64	79	79	67	63	70
Less than 4.75	88	82	79	77	80	93	90	82	80	85
Less than 5.25	92	90	86	82	87	97	94	91	87	91
Less than 6.25	99	98	95	95	96	100	99	97	95	97
All	100	100	100	100	100		100	100	100	100
Base	81	156	170	173	580	72	149	222	183	626
Mean (average value)	3.76	3.97	4.11	4.22	4.06	3.69	3.71	4.03	4.17	3.96
Median	3.55	3.75	3.94	4.06	3.85	3.70	3.63	3.92	3.95	3.81
Lower 2.5 percentile	2.74	2.48	2.44	2.50	2.48	2.38	2.28	2.52	2.11	2.38
Upper 2.5 percentile	6.21	7.38	7.41	7.01	7.06	6.15	6.01	6.35	8.46	6.35
Standard deviation	0.851	1.022	1.292	1.115	1.122	0.787	0.872	1.025	1.243	1.054

Note: * α–tocopherol to total cholesterol ratio.

Table 4.38

Pearson correlation coefficients for plasma retinol with dietary intake of α–carotene, β–carotene and vitamin A (retinol equivalents)

Sex and age of respondent	Correlation of plasma retinol with dietary intake of:			Base
	α–carotene	β–carotene	vitamin A (retinol equivalents)	
Men aged (years):				
19–24	0.17	0.09	−0.01	70
25–34	−0.01	0.11	−0.07	139
35–49	−0.08	−0.03	0.10	166
50–64	−0.18*	−0.11	0.03	171
All men	−0.05	0.02	0.08*	546
Women aged (years):				
19–24	0.11	−0.10	−0.09	68
25–34	0.06	0.10	0.17*	138
35–49	−0.05	0.01	−0.01	207
50–64	−0.03	0.01	0.06	176
All women	0.02	0.03	0.08*	590

Note: * p<0.05

Table 4.39

Pearson correlation coefficients for plasma α–carotene with dietary intake of α–carotene

Sex and age of respondent	Correlation of plasma α–carotene with:	
	Dietary intake of α–carotene	*Base*
Men aged (years):		
19–24	0.24*	*70*
25–34	0.20*	*139*
35–49	0.06	*166*
50–64	0.26**	*171*
All men	0.16**	*546*
Women aged (years):		
19–24	0.11	*68*
25–34	0.52**	*138*
35–49	0.32**	*207*
50–64	0.49**	*176*
All women	0.44**	*590*

*Note: * p<0.05; ** p<0.01*

Table 4.40

Pearson correlation coefficients for plasma β–carotene with dietary intake of β–carotene

Sex and age of respondent	Correlation of plasma β–carotene with:	
	Dietary intake of β–carotene	*Base*
Men aged (years):		
19–24	–0.04	*70*
25–34	0.13	*139*
35–49	0.11	*166*
50–64	0.29**	*171*
All men	0.20**	*546*
Women aged (years):		
19–24	0.91**	*68*
25–34	0.45**	*138*
35–49	0.44**	*207*
50–64	0.38**	*176*
All women	0.54**	*590*

*Note: ** p<0.01*

Table 4.41

Pearson correlation coefficients for plasma 25-hydroxyvitamin D with dietary intake of vitamin D

Sex and age of respondent	Correlation of plasma 25-hydroxyvitamin D with:	
	Dietary intake of vitamin D	Base
Men aged (years):		
19–24	0.59**	77
25–34	0.14	150
35–49	0.16*	181
50–64	0.17*	186
All men	0.21**	594
Women aged (years):		
19–24	0.12	73
25–34	0.25**	151
35–49	0.23**	225
50–64	0.33**	191
All women	0.24**	640

Note: * $p<0.05$; ** $p<0.01$

Table 4.42

Pearson correlation coefficients for plasma 25-hydroxyvitamin D with dietary intake of vitamin D by date blood sample taken

Date blood sample taken	Correlation of plasma 25-hydroxyvitamin D with:	
	Dietary intake of vitamin D	Base
July to September		
Men	0.16	153
Women	0.29**	147
October to December		
Men	0.29**	116
Women	0.24**	132
January to March		
Men	0.34**	160
Women	0.34**	148
April to June		
Men	0.26**	173
Women	0.18**	212

Note: ** $p<0.01$

Table 4.43

Pearson correlation coefficients for tocopherol to cholesterol ratio[†] with dietary intake of vitamin E

Sex and age of respondent	Correlation of tocopherol to cholesterol ratio with:	
	Dietary intake of vitamin E	Base
Men aged (years):		
19–24	0.17	77
25–34	0.25**	142
35–49	0.11	162
50–64	0.17*	168
All men	0.15**	549
Women aged (years):		
19–24	0.02	68
25–34	0.17*	141
35–49	0.41**	210
50–64	0.41**	181
All women	0.38**	600

Note: * p<0.05; ** p<0.01

[†] α–tocopherol to total cholesterol ratio.

Table 4.44

Fat soluble vitamins and carotenoids by sex of respondent and region

Sex of respondent and analytes	Units	Region							
		Scotland				Northern			
		Mean	Median	sd	Base	Mean	Median	sd	Base
Men									
Plasma retinol	μmol/l	2.09	2.06	0.446	51	1.99	1.95	0.516	155
Plasma α-carotene	μmol/l	0.063	0.056	0.0504	51	0.059	0.05	0.0371	155
Plasma β-carotene	μmol/l	0.177	0.13	0.1631	51	0.221	0.16	0.1925	155
Plasma α-cryptoxanthin	μmol/l	0.054	0.03	0.0741	51	0.035	0.03	0.0505	155
Plasma β-cryptoxanthin	μmol/l	0.128	0.1	0.0999	51	0.114	0.1	0.085	155
Plasma lycopene	μmol/l	0.469	0.368	0.3351	51	0.527	0.47	0.3297	155
Plasma lutein and zeaxanthin	μmol/l	0.23	0.21	0.114	51	0.25	0.23	0.111	155
Plasma 25-hydroxyvitamin D	nmol/l	43.7	44	20.58	54	50.9	47.5	24.76	169
Plasma α-tocopherol	μmol/l	20.4	19.1	6.27	51	21.4	20.5	7.39	155
Plasma γ-tocopherol	μmol/l	1.27	1.21	0.411	51	1.27	1.21	0.381	155
Plasma α-tocopherol to total cholesterol ratio	μmol/mmol	3.87	3.58	0.932	53	4.09	3.84	1.086	162
Women									
Plasma retinol	μmol/l	1.86	1.81	0.46	47	1.82	1.78	0.534	161
Plasma α-carotene	μmol/l	0.075	0.06	0.0471	47	0.072	0.06	0.0515	161
Plasma β-carotene	μmol/l	0.255	0.19	0.2176	47	0.231	0.19	0.1732	161
Plasma α-cryptoxanthin	μmol/l	0.047	0.03	0.0466	47	0.037	0.02	0.0448	161
Plasma β-cryptoxanthin	μmol/l	0.194	0.17	0.1151	47	0.131	0.1	0.1039	161
Plasma lycopene	μmol/l	0.431	0.32	0.2961	47	0.44	0.36	0.2736	161
Plasma lutein and zeaxanthin	μmol/l	0.3	0.28	0.158	47	0.26	0.23	0.121	161
Plasma 25-hydroxyvitamin D	nmol/l	42.5	35.3	20.62	52	52.4	48.2	24.36	176
Plasma α-tocopherol	μmol/l	19.5	19	5.97	47	20.7	19.7	6.22	161
Plasma γ-tocopherol	μmol/l	1.17	1.11	0.389	47	1.17	1.11	0.392	161
Plasma α-tocopherol to total cholesterol ratio	μmol/mmol	3.54	3.66	0.746	48	3.89	3.8	0.949	165

Central, South West and Wales				London and the South East				Sex of respondent and analytes	Units
Mean	Median	sd	Base	Mean	Median	sd	Base		
								Men	
2.05	1.95	0.545	212	1.99	1.94	0.545	159	Plasma retinol	μmol/l
0.061	0.05	0.0361	212	0.071	0.06	0.0954	159	Plasma α-carotene	μmol/l
0.203	0.15	0.1762	212	0.24	0.18	0.249	159	Plasma β-carotene	μmol/l
0.042	0.03	0.0503	212	0.044	0.03	0.0569	159	Plasma α-cryptoxanthin	μmol/l
0.107	0.09	0.0647	212	0.133	0.12	0.0822	159	Plasma β-cryptoxanthin	μmol/l
0.444	0.359	0.2908	212	0.437	0.36	0.2569	159	Plasma lycopene	μmol/l
								Plasma lutein and	
0.28	0.23	0.154	212	0.3	0.27	0.154	159	zeaxanthin	μmol/l
48.6	45.7	20.84	227	46.7	44.8	20.93	159	Plasma 25-hydroxyvitamin D	nmol/l
21.2	20.5	6.93	212	20.8	19.6	7.12	159	Plasma α-tocopherol	μmol/l
1.25	1.18	0.373	212	1.25	1.18	0.369	159	Plasma γ-tocopherol	μmol/l
								Plasma α-tocopherol to	
4.12	3.86	1.223	210	4	3.9	1.076	155	total cholesterol ratio	μmol/mmol
								Women	
1.84	1.75	0.534	230	1.78	1.74	0.448	178	Plasma retinol	μmol/l
0.073	0.06	0.0578	230	0.101	0.06	0.1216	178	Plasma α-carotene	μmol/l
0.288	0.2	0.35	230	0.404	0.264	0.4332	178	Plasma β-carotene	μmol/l
0.033	0.03	0.0302	230	0.034	0.03	0.0297	178	Plasma α-cryptoxanthin	μmol/l
0.126	0.1	0.0984	230	0.18	0.13	0.1694	178	Plasma β-cryptoxanthin	μmol/l
0.45	0.37	0.3004	230	0.509	0.46	0.2911	178	Plasma lycopene	μmol/l
								Plasma lutein and	
0.29	0.26	0.181	230	0.33	0.29	0.17	178	zeaxanthin	μmol/l
51.1	49.5	25.05	250	46.9	44.8	22.43	192	Plasma 25-hydroxyvitamin D	nmol/l
20.6	19.6	6.22	230	20.8	19.7	6.64	178	Plasma α-tocopherol	μmol/l
1.24	1.14	0.467	230	1.21	1.17	0.347	178	Plasma γ-tocopherol	μmol/l
								Plasma α-tocopherol to	
4.04	3.85	1.165	233	4.02	3.89	1.043	181	total cholesterol ratio	μmol/mmol

Table 4.45

Fat soluble vitamins and carotenoids by sex of respondent and whether someone in the respondent's household was receiving certain benefits

Sex of respondent and analytes	Units	Whether receiving benefits							
		Receiving benefits				Not receiving benefits			
		Mean	Median	sd	Base	Mean	Median	sd	Base
Men									
Plasma retinol	µmol/l	1.94	1.96	0.525	76	2.03	1.96	0.529	500
Plasma α-carotene	µmol/l	0.054	0.040	0.0347	76	0.065	0.050	0.0627	500
Plasma ß-carotene	µmol/l	0.199	0.130	0.1686	76	0.218	0.160	0.2071	500
Plasma α-cryptoxanthin	µmol/l	0.046	0.030	0.0838	76	0.041	0.030	0.0489	500
Plasma ß-cryptoxanthin	µmol/l	0.111	0.090	0.0893	76	0.119	0.100	0.0778	500
Plasma lycopene	µmol/l	0.409	0.366	0.2831	76	0.475	0.390	0.3004	500
Plasma lutein and zeaxanthin	µmol/l	0.24	0.20	0.140	76	0.28	0.25	0.142	500
Plasma 25-hydroxyvitamin D	nmol/l	42.3	36.4	21.79	85	49.2	46.9	21.92	542
Plasma α-tocopherol	µmol/l	18.8	18.1	6.02	76	21.4	20.4	7.13	500
Plasma γ-tocopherol	µmol/l	1.20	1.15	0.356	76	1.27	1.21	0.379	500
Plasma α-tocopherol to total cholesterol ratio	µmol/mmol	3.84	3.59	1.014	77	4.09	3.88	1.135	504
Women									
Plasma retinol	µmol/l	1.82	1.79	0.494	120	1.82	1.74	0.508	496
Plasma α-carotene	µmol/l	0.054	0.050	0.0363	120	0.087	0.060	0.0871	496
Plasma ß-carotene	µmol/l	0.189	0.150	0.1593	120	0.332	0.230	0.3655	496
Plasma α-cryptoxanthin	µmol/l	0.028	0.020	0.0271	120	0.037	0.030	0.0375	496
Plasma ß-cryptoxanthin	µmol/l	0.114	0.090	0.0920	120	0.156	0.120	0.1341	496
Plasma lycopene	µmol/l	0.364	0.310	0.2254	120	0.487	0.420	0.3005	496
Plasma lutein and zeaxanthin	µmol/l	0.25	0.22	0.139	120	0.30	0.27	0.168	496
Plasma 25-hydroxyvitamin D	nmol/l	43.5	35.3	23.94	129	51.1	48.7	23.75	541
Plasma α-tocopherol	µmol/l	18.8	18.2	5.52	120	21.0	19.9	6.43	496
Plasma γ-tocopherol	µmol/l	1.14	1.10	0.336	120	1.22	1.15	0.424	496
Plasma α-tocopherol to total cholesterol ratio	µmol/mmol	3.77	3.72	0.895	121	4.00	3.85	1.085	505

Table 4.46

Percentage distribution of plasma total cholesterol by sex and age of respondent

Cumulative percentages

Plasma total cholesterol (mmol/l)	Men aged (years):				All men	Women aged (years):				All women
	19–24	25–34	35–49	50–64		19–24	25–34	35–49	50–64	
	cum %	cum %	cum %	cum %	cum %	cum %	cum %	cum %	cum %	cum %
Less than 3.00	-	2	2	1	1	4	1	0	1	1
Less than 3.50	10	7	4	3	5	11	5	3	1	4
Less than 4.00	32	18	12	8	15	33	17	12	2	13
Less than 4.50	69	35	19	19	30	47	38	25	7	25
Less than 5.20	84	59	44	41	52	83	68	52	25	52
Less than 5.80	90	78	64	60	70	93	87	78	41	71
Less than 6.50	100	90	85	78	86	100	94	92	67	86
Less than 7.80		98	98	98	98		99	99	91	97
All		100	100	100	100		100	100	100	100
Base	*81*	*164*	*186*	*187*	*618*	*77*	*157*	*234*	*192*	*659*
Mean (average value)	4.40	5.04	5.38	5.56	5.21	4.46	4.84	5.13	6.06	5.25
Median	4.29	4.93	5.41	5.56	5.14	4.55	4.69	5.16	6.05	5.18
Lower 2.5 percentile	3.20	2.99	3.06	3.35	3.20	2.83	3.01	3.44	4.16	3.31
Upper 2.5 percentile	6.33	7.80	7.47	7.76	7.64	6.04	6.92	7.17	8.69	8.02
Standard deviation	0.839	1.139	1.124	1.126	1.155	0.800	0.970	0.995	1.225	1.180

Table 4.47

Percentage distribution of plasma high density lipoprotein cholesterol by sex and age of respondent

Cumulative percentages

Plasma high density lipoprotein cholesterol (mmol/l)	Men aged (years):				All men	Women aged (years):				All women
	19–24	25–34	35–49	50–64		19–24	25–34	35–49	50–64	
	cum %	cum %	cum %	cum %	cum %	cum %	cum %	cum %	cum %	cum %
Less than 0.70	7	6	9	8	8	-	3	3	2	2
Less than 0.80	15	17	19	16	17	5	3	5	5	5
Less than 1.00	43	44	46	42	44	24	20	22	18	21
Less than 1.20	77	77	77	69	74	52	42	45	38	43
Less than 1.40	92	91	89	84	89	76	68	71	64	69
Less than 1.60	100	98	95	92	96	90	86	84	79	84
All		100	100	100	100	100	100	100	100	100
Base	81	164	186	186	617	77	157	234	192	659
Mean (average value)	1.06	1.04	1.04	1.12	1.07	1.21	1.26	1.27	1.34	1.28
Median	1.07	1.02	1.01	1.04	1.02	1.18	1.24	1.24	1.31	1.25
Lower 2.5 percentile	0.68	0.61	0.56	0.64	0.64	0.75	0.66	0.70	0.69	0.73
Upper 2.5 percentile	1.49	1.58	1.87	1.85	1.74	1.71	1.97	2.34	2.36	2.28
Standard deviation	0.219	0.244	0.295	0.411	0.316	0.264	0.322	0.391	0.400	0.367

Table 4.48

Percentage distribution of plasma low density lipoprotein cholesterol* by sex and age of respondent

Cumulative percentages

Plasma low density lipoprotein cholesterol (mmol/l)	Men aged (years):				All men	Women aged (years):				All women
	19–24	25–34	35–49	50–64		19–24	25–34	35–49	50–64	
	cum %	cum %	cum %	cum %	cum %	cum %	cum %	cum %	cum %	cum %
Less than 2.00	3	2	2	-	2	3	3	1	1	2
Less than 2.70	22	10	7	7	10	23	16	12	2	11
Less than 3.00	40	20	14	10	18	26	21	19	7	17
Less than 3.40	60	30	23	18	28	57	49	35	13	34
Less than 4.10	81	61	42	39	51	86	77	63	31	60
Less than 4.80	89	78	65	61	71	96	90	83	57	79
Less than 5.50	100	90	85	81	87	100	96	94	80	91
Less than 6.20		94	96	94	96		98	98	88	95
All		100	100	100	100		100	100	100	100
Base	81	164	186	187	618	77	157	234	192	659
Mean (average value)	3.35	4.00	4.34	4.44	4.15	3.26	3.57	3.85	4.72	3.97
Median	3.18	3.84	4.39	4.37	4.09	3.24	3.43	3.79	4.59	3.82
Lower 2.5 percentile	1.84	1.86	2.00	2.25	2.10	1.86	1.94	2.20	2.71	2.09
Upper 2.5 percentile	5.37	6.77	6.78	6.64	6.62	4.98	5.84	6.00	7.22	6.84
Standard deviation	0.880	1.171	1.166	1.140	1.179	0.750	0.980	0.998	1.229	1.162

Note: * Calculated as non-high density lipoprotein cholesterol (non-HDL).

Table 4.49

Blood lipids by sex of respondent and region

Sex of respondent and analytes	Units	Region							
		Scotland				Northern			
		Mean	Median	sd	Base	Mean	Median	sd	Base
Men									
Plasma total cholesterol	mmol/l	5.27	5.20	0.872	54	5.24	5.26	1.261	169
Plasma high density lipoprotein cholesterol	mmol/l	1.10	1.01	0.355	54	1.05	1.05	0.266	169
Plasma low density lipoprotein cholesterol*	mmol/l	4.17	4.09	0.948	54	4.19	4.29	1.322	169
Women									
Plasma total cholesterol	mmol/l	5.50	5.44	1.108	50	5.34	5.20	1.108	175
Plasma high density lipoprotein cholesterol	mmol/l	1.46	1.38	0.382	50	1.24	1.21	0.370	175
Plasma low density lipoprotein cholesterol*	mmol/l	4.04	3.94	1.136	50	4.10	3.89	1.131	175

*Note: * Calculated as non-high density lipoprotein cholesterol (non-HDL).*

Central, South West and Wales				London and the South East				Sex of respondent and analytes	Units
Mean	Median	sd	Base	Mean	Median	sd	Base		
								Men	
5.18	4.97	1.097	222	5.21	5.20	1.203	172	Plasma total cholesterol	mmol/l
1.07	1.02	0.376	222	1.07	1.04	0.262	172	Plasma high density lipoprotein cholesterol	mmol/l
4.11	3.91	1.081	222	4.15	4.07	1.222	172	Plasma low density lipoprotein cholesterol*	mmol/l
								Women	
5.18	5.15	1.206	246	5.20	4.96	1.223	188	Plasma total cholesterol	mmol/l
1.23	1.19	0.346	246	1.34	1.31	0.366	188	Plasma high density lipoprotein cholesterol	mmol/l
3.95	3.84	1.182	246	3.86	3.63	1.166	188	Plasma low density lipoprotein cholesterol*	mmol/l

Table 4.50

Blood lipids by sex of respondent and whether someone in the respondent's household was receiving certain benefits

| Sex of respondent and analytes | Units | Whether receiving benefits | | | | | | | |
| | | Receiving benefits | | | | Not receiving benefits | | | |
		Mean	Median	sd	Base	Mean	Median	sd	Base
Men									
Plasma total cholesterol	mmol/l	4.97	5.02	1.184	82	5.25	5.15	1.147	535
Plasma high density lipoprotein cholesterol	mmol/l	1.03	0.96	0.308	82	1.07	1.04	0.317	535
Plasma low density lipoprotein cholesterol*	mmol/l	3.94	4.04	1.282	82	4.18	4.09	1.160	535
Women									
Plasma total cholesterol	mmol/l	5.07	4.98	1.259	129	5.30	5.20	1.156	530
Plasma high density lipoprotein cholesterol	mmol/l	1.22	1.20	0.370	129	1.30	1.25	0.365	530
Plasma low density lipoprotein cholesterol*	mmol/l	3.85	3.80	1.209	129	4.00	3.83	1.149	530

Note: * Calculated as non-high density lipoprotein cholesterol (non-HDL).

Table 4.51

Percentage distribution of plasma selenium by sex and age of respondent

Cumulative percentages

| Plasma selenium (μmol/l) | Men aged (years): | | | | All men | Women aged (years): | | | | All women |
	19–24	25–34	35–49	50–64		19–24	25–34	35–49	50–64	
	cum %	cum %	cum %	cum %	cum %	cum %	cum %	cum %	cum %	cum %
Less than 0.60	-	-	-	-	-	-	-	-	-	-
Less than 0.70	3	0	0	1	1	2	1	1	-	1
Less than 0.80	6	2	3	3	3	4	5	4	2	4
Less than 0.90	15	8	10	8	9	21	17	12	8	13
Less than 1.00	38	24	24	19	24	42	38	29	21	30
Less than 1.10	74	57	44	39	50	65	65	56	45	56
Less than 1.20	91	81	65	62	72	88	78	78	68	76
Less than 1.30	95	89	87	82	87	97	90	90	84	89
Less than 1.40	95	93	93	93	93	100	95	94	91	94
All	100	100	100	100	100		100	100	100	100
Base	83	169	190	195	636	76	159	244	195	674
Mean (average value)	1.03	1.10	1.13	1.15	1.11	1.03	1.07	1.09	1.17	1.10
Median	1.04	1.07	1.11	1.14	1.10	1.04	1.05	1.07	1.11	1.07
Lower 2.5 percentile	0.65	0.84	0.78	0.79	0.79	0.72	0.74	0.75	0.82	0.77
Upper 2.5 percentile	1.46	1.47	1.58	1.50	1.49	1.32	1.46	1.52	1.84	1.53
Standard deviation	0.150	0.160	0.182	0.199	0.182	0.151	0.205	0.176	0.332	0.240

Table 4.52

Percentage distribution of red cell selenium by sex and age of respondent

Cumulative percentages

Red cell selenium (µmol/l)	Men aged (years):				All men	Women aged (years):				All women
	19–24	25–34	35–49	50–64		19–24	25–34	35–49	50–64	
	cum %	cum %	cum %	cum %	cum %	cum %	cum %	cum %	cum %	cum %
Less than 1.00	8	-	2	1	2	1	-	1	-	0
Less than 1.25	25	9	11	14	13	2	7	8	11	8
Less than 1.40	50	36	25	29	32	14	15	21	23	19
Less than 1.50	63	49	37	41	45	27	24	29	32	29
Less than 1.75	86	67	67	67	70	47	48	49	59	52
Less than 2.00	96	89	85	84	87	87	71	70	75	74
Less than 2.50	100	99	97	97	98	100	92	93	92	93
All		100	100	100	100		100	100	100	100
Base	81	163	182	191	617	74	158	237	189	658
Mean (average value)	1.42	1.60	1.64	1.64	1.60	1.73	1.83	1.80	1.82	1.80
Median	1.40	1.51	1.60	1.59	1.55	1.75	1.76	1.76	1.68	1.73
Lower 2.5 percentile	0.82	1.11	1.03	1.03	1.03	1.26	1.05	1.08	1.08	1.08
Upper 2.5 percentile	2.11	2.40	2.53	2.50	2.46	2.31	3.05	2.79	3.46	3.04
Standard deviation	0.286	0.328	0.356	0.422	0.369	0.276	0.453	0.457	0.816	0.569

Table 4.53

Percentage distribution of blood glutathione peroxidase (GSH-Px) by sex and age of respondent

Cumulative percentages

Blood glutathione peroxidase (nmol/mg Hb/min)	Men aged (years):				All men	Women aged (years):				All women
	19–24	25–34	35–49	50–64		19–24	25–34	35–49	50–64	
	cum %	cum %	cum %	cum %	cum %	cum %	cum %	cum %	cum %	cum %
Less than 60.0	-	-	-	-	-	-	1	-	-	0
Less than 70.0	-	1	1	-	1	-	1	-	-	0
Less than 80.0	4	6	3	4	4	-	3	1	1	2
Less than 90.0	11	12	10	10	11	9	12	8	3	8
Less than 100.0	24	26	25	24	25	14	23	19	11	17
Less than 110.0	39	40	40	36	39	30	32	37	25	32
Less than 120.0	55	56	53	45	52	37	52	46	42	45
Less than 130.0	69	67	62	60	64	45	65	60	54	58
Less than 140.0	83	76	71	70	74	57	76	70	66	69
Less than 160.0	97	90	88	88	90	82	90	87	87	87
Less than 180.0	97	97	94	97	96	93	97	94	97	96
All	100	100	100	100	100	100	100	100	100	100
Base	81	163	184	187	615	74	161	237	188	661
Mean (average value)	118.5	119.5	123.4	124.1	121.9	134.0	122.5	126.8	129.2	127.2
Median	116.0	114.0	116.0	123.0	117.0	132.0	119.0	121.0	124.0	121.0
Lower 2.5 percentile	73.0	75.8	78.0	77.5	77.0	84.0	76.0	81.1	83.7	81.0
Upper 2.5 percentile	183.6	184.0	198.2	184.0	190.0	264.0	185.9	200.0	189.0	193.2
Standard deviation	24.20	27.45	31.06	29.36	28.79	36.39	30.49	31.93	27.85	31.14

Table 4.54

Percentage distribution of plasma α_1– antichymotrypsin by sex and age of respondent

Cumulative percentages

Plasma α_1–antichymotrypsin (g/l)	Men aged (years):				All men	Women aged (years):				All women
	19–24	25–34	35–49	50–64		19–24	25–34	35–49	50–64	
	cum %	cum %	cum %	cum %	cum %	cum %	cum %	cum %	cum %	cum %
Less than 0.18	1	3	3	2	2	-	-	0	-	0
Less than 0.22	23	11	15	11	14	17	10	6	3	7
Less than 0.25	32	26	23	17	23	34	18	15	6	16
Less than 0.30	73	62	52	44	55	52	51	45	28	42
Less than 0.35	92	89	86	81	86	86	83	82	67	78
Less than 0.45	98	96	99	95	97	93	99	98	95	97
Less than 0.65	100	100	100	100	100	100	100	100	99	100
All									100	
Base	81	162	179	181	603	77	154	233	190	654
Mean (average value)	0.28	0.29	0.29	0.31	0.30	0.29	0.30	0.31	0.34	0.31
Median	0.28	0.28	0.29	0.31	0.29	0.28	0.29	0.30	0.33	0.31
Lower 2.5 percentile	0.20	0.17	0.17	0.16	0.18	0.18	0.20	0.20	0.22	0.20
Upper 2.5 percentile	0.39	0.50	0.43	0.53	0.49	0.51	0.41	0.45	0.50	0.47
Standard deviation	0.065	0.073	0.066	0.079	0.072	0.074	0.058	0.061	0.073	0.068

Table 4.55

Percentage distribution of blood mercury by sex and age of respondent

Cumulative percentages

Blood mercury (nmol/l)	Men aged (years):				All men	Women aged (years):				All women
	19–24	25–34	35–49	50–64		19–24	25–34	35–49	50–64	
	cum %	cum %	cum %	cum %	cum %	cum %	cum %	cum %	cum %	cum %
Less than 0.5	6	4	-	1	2	8	5	1	1	3
Less than 1.0	19	4	1	2	4	8	7	2	2	4
Less than 2.5	55	18	14	11	20	31	23	10	9	15
Less than 4.0	72	43	28	26	37	49	40	25	21	30
Less than 7.0	84	67	53	55	61	64	66	50	56	57
Less than 10.0	89	77	69	70	74	84	78	71	70	74
Less than 13.0	97	91	84	81	87	91	87	82	82	84
Less than 16.0	99	96	90	86	91	91	92	90	88	90
All	100	100	100	100	100	100	100	100	100	100
Base	81	169	190	195	636	80	160	246	198	683
Mean (average value)	3.8	6.3	8.7	9.0	7.5	6.1	7.2	8.6	10.6	8.6
Median	2.3	4.8	6.6	6.3	5.5	4.3	4.7	7.0	6.6	6.2
Lower 2.5 percentile	0.2	0.4	1.0	1.0	0.5	0.1	0.1	0.9	1.3	0.4
Upper 2.5 percentile	14.4	23.9	33.7	32.6	27.1	22.6	33.8	28.9	57.4	33.4
Standard deviation	4.28	5.09	8.66	8.37	7.50	6.05	7.41	7.06	15.99	10.53

Table 4.56

Other analytes by sex of respondent and region

Sex of respondent and analytes	Units	Region							
		Scotland				Northern			
		Mean	Median	sd	Base	Mean	Median	sd	Base
Men									
Plasma selenium	μmol/l	1.09	1.10	0.184	54	1.12	1.10	0.215	176
Red cell selenium	μmol/l	1.65	1.69	0.316	53	1.59	1.56	0.322	171
Erythrocyte glutathione peroxidase activity	nmol/mg Hb/min	104.0	99.0	25.54	51	120.3	115.0	26.69	171
Plasma α_1–antichymotrypsin	g/l	0.29	0.29	0.053	53	0.30	0.29	0.062	167
Blood mercury	nmol/l	7.4	5.9	5.52	54	6.8	4.9	6.43	176
Women									
Plasma selenium	μmol/l	1.07	1.08	0.150	52	1.08	1.07	0.160	178
Red cell selenium	μmol/l	1.87	1.85	0.488	50	1.76	1.71	0.367	175
Erythrocyte glutathione peroxidase activity	nmol/mg Hb/min	115.3	107.0	27.63	52	125.8	120.0	32.55	174
Plasma α_1–antichymotrypsin	g/l	0.30	0.30	0.061	50	0.32	0.31	0.076	174
Blood mercury	nmol/l	7.4	6.5	5.52	52	7.5	5.6	7.64	179

NDNS adults aged 19 to 64, Volume 4 2004

Central, South West and Wales				London and the South East				Sex of respondent and analytes	Units
Mean	Median	sd	*Base*	Mean	Median	sd	*Base*		
								Men	
1.10	1.08	0.162	*226*	1.13	1.12	0.168	*179*	Plasma selenium	μmol/l
1.56	1.48	0.410	*218*	1.65	1.60	0.369	*175*	Red cell selenium	μmol/l
126.7	127.0	26.91	*222*	122.7	117.0	31.88	*172*	Erythrocyte glutathione peroxidase activity	nmol/mg Hb/min
0.29	0.29	0.076	*218*	0.30	0.29	0.082	*166*	Plasma α_1–antichymotrypsin	g/l
6.7	4.9	6.29	*228*	9.4	6.5	9.80	*178*	Blood mercury	nmol/l
								Women	
1.07	1.05	0.200	*252*	1.16	1.09	0.340	*192*	Plasma selenium	μmol/l
1.70	1.62	0.439	*244*	1.96	1.87	0.809	*190*	Red cell selenium	μmol/l
124.5	120.0	28.27	*245*	135.3	133.0	32.57	*190*	Erythrocyte glutathione peroxidase activity	nmol/mg Hb/min
0.31	0.31	0.067	*244*	0.31	0.30	0.063	*186*	Plasma α_1–antichymotrypsin	g/l
8.2	6.2	11.46	*259*	10.3	6.6	12.26	*194*	Blood mercury	nmol/l

Table 4.57

Other analytes by sex of respondent and whether someone in the respondent's household was receiving certain benefits

Sex of respondent and analytes	Units	Whether receiving benefits							
		Receiving benefits				Not receiving benefits			
		Mean	Median	sd	Base	Mean	Median	sd	Base
Men									
Plasma selenium	µmol/l	1.05	1.02	0.193	86	1.12	1.10	0.178	550
Red cell selenium	µmol/l	1.54	1.44	0.347	81	1.61	1.57	0.372	536
Erythrocyte glutathione peroxidase activity	nmol/mg Hb/min	119.8	117.0	25.78	84	122.3	117.0	29.24	531
Plasma α_1-antichymotrypsin	g/l	0.31	0.30	0.071	81	0.29	0.29	0.072	523
Blood mercury	nmol/l	5.3	3.5	4.95	86	7.9	5.7	7.77	550
Women									
Plasma selenium	µmol/l	1.01	0.98	0.171	131	1.12	1.08	0.249	543
Red cell selenium	µmol/l	1.65	1.61	0.362	130	1.84	1.77	0.603	528
Erythrocyte glutathione peroxidase activity	nmol/mg Hb/min	123.3	119.0	32.26	129	128.2	122.0	30.82	532
Plasma α_1-antichymotrypsin	g/l	0.32	0.31	0.079	127	0.31	0.30	0.065	527
Blood mercury	nmol/l	6.4	4.2	7.25	131	9.1	6.6	11.11	552

Figure 4.1

Comparison of mean plasma 25-OHD levels by date of blood sample taken by sex of respondent

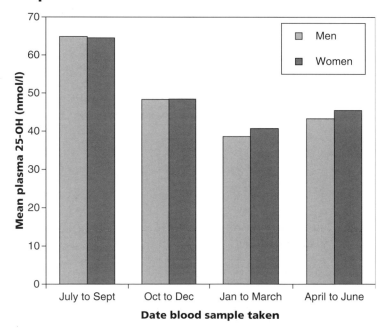

5 Physical activity

5.1 Introduction

This chapter reports on the results from the analysis of the physical activity data. All respondents were asked to record detailed information on their daily activities over the same seven-day period as the dietary record. This was recorded in the 'Diary of Activities and Eating and Drinking Away from Home' (*see* Appendix A of the Technical Report[1]). Chapter 1 of this report gives further details of the methodology. Appendix D gives further details of the data editing process, data quality and the derivation of different measures of physical activity.

The Health Development Agency and Health Survey for England give the following definitions of physical activity[2,3].

Physical activity

Any force exerted by skeletal muscle that results in energy expenditure above resting level.

Exercise

A subset of physical activity, which is volitional, planned, structured, repetitive and aimed at improvement or maintenance of any aspect of fitness or health.

Moderate intensity physical activity

Activities with an energy cost of at least 5 kcal/min but less than 7.5 kcal/min, usually equivalent to brisk walking, which might be expected to leave the participant feeling warm or slightly out of breath.

Vigorous intensity physical activity

Activities with an energy cost of at least 7.5 kcal/min, usually equivalent to at least slow jogging, which might be expected to leave the participant feeling out of breath and sweaty.

The main purpose in collecting physical activity information was to allow an investigation of the relationships between physical activity levels and dietary intakes, particularly energy intake and body composition. If the body does not use all the energy it takes in as food for activity, growth and thermogenesis, for example, then it will be stored. Over time this will lead to an increase in body weight, which if it continues leads to an increased risk of obesity. Obesity can increase the risk of chronic diseases in later life including coronary heart disease and diabetes[4,5].

There is a wealth of data on the health benefits of physical activity, including the prevention or delay of high blood pressure, reduction in the risk of some cancers and maintenance of bone density, therefore helping prevent osteoporosis[6]. There is general consensus on the amount and type of physical activity that is beneficial to health[7]. The Department of Health (DH) recommendation for adults is[2,3]:

> At least 30 minutes of physical activity on five or more days of the week. This physical activity should be of at least moderate intensity – similar to brisk walking. Activity can be taken in bouts of 10 to 15 minutes, allowing for accumulation of activity throughout the day.

Data from this survey on energy intake show that mean daily total energy intakes were below Estimated Average Requirements (EARs)[8] for each sex and age group (see Volume 2, Chapter 2[9]). It has been suggested that this disparity could arise from an inadequate energy intake, a biased low estimate of intake due to respondents mis-reporting their actual intake or modifying their diet during the recording period, or an overestimate of energy requirements[10,11]. This survey provided the opportunity to estimate energy expenditure from records of physical activity and relate this to energy intake and body size (BMI and waist to hip ratio).

5.2 Findings

5.2.1 Measures of physical activity

Self-reported levels of physical activity were asked in the dietary interview. All respondents were asked whether they considered themselves to be very physically active, fairly physically active, not very physically active or not at all physically active.

Complete seven-day physical activity diaries were obtained from 1,658 respondents, 741 men and 917 women. From these diaries, the duration of participation in different activities of varying intensity can be estimated. The time spent in activities of moderate and vigorous/very vigorous intensity during the seven-day recording period were calculated, and added together to give the total time spent in activities of 'at least moderate intensity'. Data are presented on the various measures derived from the physical activity data, including mean hours spent in activities of at least moderate intensity per day and mean hours spent in activities of vigorous/very vigorous intensity per day.

Data for these measures are presented for both men and women separately by age group. Tables are also presented showing the breakdown between physical activity and the region in which the respondent lived and whether someone in the respondent's household was in receipt of certain benefits. In addition, bivariate[12] and multivariate analyses are presented showing the relationship between the measures of physical activity and key socio-demographic, physiological and behavioural factors. Data on the number of days per week on which respondents spent 30 minutes or more in activities of at least moderate intensity are given for the NDNS and the Health Survey for England (HSfE)[13] and discussed in relation to the DH recommendation noted above.

5.2.2 Self-reported levels of physical activity

Table 5.1 gives the distributions for self-reported levels of physical activity from the dietary interview. Over half of men and women in the responding sample, 51% and 52% respectively, reported that they were fairly physically active, and around a fifth of men and women, 21% and 17% respectively, reported that they were very physically active. Just under a quarter of men and women reported that they were not very physically active, 23% and 24% respectively, and 5% of men and 6% of women reported being not at all physically active. There were no significant sex or age differences in the proportion of respondents who reported each level of physical activity.

(Table 5.1)

5.2.3 Time spent in activities of at least moderate intensity and vigorous/very vigorous intensity

Table 5.2 shows that, overall, 17% of men and 16% of women did not record spending any time in activities of at least moderate intensity during the seven-day recording period (ns). Men and women aged 50 to 64 years were significantly more likely to have not recorded any time in activities of at least moderate intensity, 24% and 20% respectively, than those aged 25 to 34 years, 9% and 10% respectively (men: p<0.01; women: p<0.05).

Table 5.2 also shows the mean hours spent in activities of at least moderate intensity. On average, men spent 2.2 hours per day and women 1.2 hours per day in activities of at least moderate intensity (medians 0.6 hours and 0.5 hours) (p<0.01). Within each age group, men spent significantly more time than women in activities of at least moderate intensity (19 to 24 years: p<0.05; all others: p<0.01).

Generally, for men, mean hours spent in activities of at least moderate intensity decreased with age. Men aged 19 to 34 years spent significantly more time in activities of at least moderate intensity than the oldest group of men (19 to 24: p<0.05; 25 to 34: p<0.01). Men aged 19 to 24 years spent, on average, 2.9 hours per day and those aged 25 to 34 years spent 2.7 hours per day in activities of at least moderate intensity compared with 1.5 hours for those aged 50 to 64 years. There were no significant age differences for women.

For all sex/age groups, the mean time spent in activities of at least moderate intensity was considerably higher than the median value. This indicates that there were a small number of respondents within each sex/age group who recorded spending relatively long periods of time in activities of at least moderate intensity[14]. For instance, at the upper 2.5 percentile, the time spent in activities of at least moderate intensity recorded by men was more than 8.0 hours and by women more than 6.0 hours. It is likely that the large amounts of time spent in activities of at least moderate intensity at the upper end of the distribution are due to the respondent working in occupations categorised as moderate or hard/very hard work (see Appendix D).

(Table 5.2)

Table 5.3 shows that 39% of men and 28% of women recorded spending some time in activities of vigorous/very vigorous intensity over the seven-day recording period (p<0.01). Generally, the proportion of men and women who recorded spending time in activities of vigorous/very vigorous intensity decreased with age. For men, 53% of those aged 25 to 34 years recorded spending time in activities of vigorous/very vigorous intensity compared with 22% of those aged 50 to 64 years (p<0.01). Similarly, the youngest group of women were significantly more likely than the oldest group of women to have recorded taking part in vigorous/very vigorous activity during the seven-day recording period, 41% compared with 18% (p<0.05).

Overall, men spent significantly more time, on average, in activities of vigorous/very vigorous intensity than women, 0.5 hours and 0.1 hours respectively (medians 0.0 hours for both sexes) (p<0.01). This difference between men and women was true for age groups 25 to 34 years and 35 to 49 years (p<0.01).

Men aged 25 to 34 years, and women aged 19 to 24 years, spent significantly longer in activities of vigorous/very vigorous intensity, 0.8 hours and 0.2 hours respectively, than men and women aged 50 to 64 years, 0.3 hours and 0.1 hours respectively (p<0.05).

For all sex/age groups, the mean time spent in activities of vigorous/very vigorous intensity was higher than the median value. This indicates that there were a small number of respondents within each sex/age group who recorded spending a lot of time in activities of vigorous/very vigorous intensity[14]. For instance, at the upper 2.5 percentile the amount of time spent in activities of vigorous/very vigorous intensity ranged from 4.4 hours for the oldest group of men to 8.6 hours for those

aged 25 to 34 years. As for time spent in activities of at least moderate intensity, it is likely that the large amount of time spent in activities of vigorous/very vigorous intensity at the upper end of the distribution is due to the respondent working in occupations categorised as hard/very hard work, for example hard physical labour (see Appendix D).

(Table 5.3)

The DH recommendation for adults is that they should participate in at least 30 minutes of at least moderate activity on at least five days of the week[2,3]. Table 5.4 shows data on the number of days per week respondents spent 30 minutes or more in activities of at least moderate intensity.

Overall, 36% of men and 26% of women spent 30 minutes or more per day in activities of at least moderate intensity on five or more days (p<0.01). For men, the proportion who spent 30 minutes or more in activities of at least moderate intensity on five or more days was 49% of the youngest age group and 46% of those aged 25 to 34 years compared with 24% of those aged 50 to 64 years (19 to 24 years: p<0.05; 25 to 34 years: p<0.01). There were no significant age differences for women.

(Table 5.4)

5.3 Variation in physical activity

In this section, variation in measures of physical activity is considered in relation to socio-demographic and dietary factors, and anthropometric and blood pressure measurements.

5.3.1 Region and household receipt of benefits

Table 5.5 shows the mean number of hours spent in activities of at least moderate intensity per day in relation to the region in which the respondent lived[15].

For women, there were no significant regional differences in the mean hours spent in activities of at least moderate intensity. The only significant difference for men was for those living in Central and South West regions of England and in Wales who spent longer in activities of at least moderate intensity than those in London and the South East, 2.6 hours compared with 1.7 hours (p<0.05).

(Table 5.5)

Table 5.6 shows mean hours spent in activities of at least moderate intensity per day according to whether someone in the respondent's household was receiving certain state benefits[16]. There were no significant differences by household benefit status for men or women.

(Table 5.6)

5.3.2 Correlations with energy and macronutrient intakes, anthropometric measurements and blood pressure

Table 5.7 gives correlation coefficients for the relationships between the time spent in activities of at least moderate intensity and dietary intake, as measured by average daily total energy intake, percentage food energy from total fat, protein, total carbohydrate and non-milk extrinsic sugars and percentage total energy from alcohol. The tables are restricted to those respondents who completed a seven-day dietary and physical activity diary. Tables 5.8 and 5.9 give correlation coefficients for the relationships between the time spent in activities of at least moderate intensity per day and, respectively, anthropometric measurements indicating body size[17] and blood pressure.

It should be noted that where correlations are statistically significant the relationship between the two variables may not necessarily be causal; other factors, for example, the respondent's health at the time, may have affected the size of the correlation.

Tables 5.7, 5.8 and 5.9 show that the correlation coefficients between time spent in activities of at least moderate intensity and these variables are extremely low for all groups. This indicates that, based on the data from this survey, there was no correlation between the time spent in activities of at least moderate intensity and the measures of average intake of energy and macronutrients, anthropometric measurements and blood pressure.

(Tables 5.7 to 5.9)

5.4 Characteristics found to be independently associated with measures of physical activity

Various socio-demographic, physiological and behavioural factors have been shown to be associated with physical activity, defined as time spent in activities of at least moderate intensity (see Sections 5.2 and 5.3) but some of these factors are known to be inter-related. This section considers the combined effect of these variables on time spent in activities of at least moderate intensity. The technique of multiple regression is used to build a model from those characteristics which most explain the physical activity measurements.

As noted above (see Section 5.2.3), there is a strong association between sex and physical activity, so each multiple regression analysis is presented separately for men and women. To control for the effects of age, this variable was included in each regression analysis.

Table 5.10 shows the socio-demographic, dietary and physiological factors which were significantly associated with time spent in activities of at least moderate intensity when bivariate analyses were carried out, in addition to the previously shown relationships with region and household benefit status[18]. Those independent variables that were found to be significantly associated with the measurements in a bivariate relationship were then included in the multiple regression model[19].

(Table 5.10)

Tables 5.11 and 5.12 give standardised regression coefficients for a number of characteristics, the independent variables, associated with variation in the physical activity measure, the dependent variable, produced using the technique of multiple regression. The tables of results identify those characteristics which are related to the measurements after controlling for the effects of the other characteristics included in the analysis. All regression models are deemed meaningful when a high percentage of the variance is explained. The technique of multiple regression calculates coefficients based on the number of cases for which there are valid values for all the variables included in the analysis. Further information on the statistical method and interpretation of output from multiple regression analysis is given in Appendix A[20].

5.4.1 Findings

Tables 5.11 and 5.12 show that the best multiple regression models that could be developed using the most relevant independent variables for the dependent variable, time spent in activities of at least moderate intensity, were able to explain 23% and 5% of the variance for men and women respectively.

(Tables 5.11 and 5.12)

5.5 Comparison with Health Survey for England 1998

Table 5.13 compares data from the present NDNS for respondents in England only with physical activity data from the Health Survey for England 1998 (HSfE)[3]. The HSfE was based on a multi-stage probability sample of addresses drawn from the Postcode Address File. 15,908 adults aged 16 and over were interviewed. A summary of the key findings and methodology from the Health Survey for England 1998 is provided in two volumes[21].

There are several important differences between the HSfE and the NDNS in terms of the data collection method for physical activity; these are described in Appendix I of the Technical Report[1]. In particular it should be noted that the HSfE used a seven-day recall compared with the NDNS which used a seven-day diary. In addition, for the HSfE activities lasting less than 15 minutes were excluded whereas activities in the NDNS lasting less than 10 minutes were excluded.

Data are presented for men and women by age. It should be noted that in the HSfE the youngest age group was aged 16 to 24 years, while in the present NDNS the youngest age group was adults aged 19 to 24 years. This should be borne in mind where there are differences between these groups. Age groups for the present NDNS were redefined to match those of the HSfE so that meaningful comparisons could be made: 16/19 to 24 years, 25 to 34 years, 35 to 44 years, 45 to 54 years, 55 to 64 years.

5.5.1 Findings

The following discussion focuses on differences between the two surveys in relation to the DH recommendation for adults discussed in Section 5.2.3.

Table 5.13 shows that for men aged 35 to 44 and 55 to 64 years the proportion who recorded spending at least 30 minutes in activities of at least moderate intensity on five days a week or more was significantly lower in the NDNS than in the HSfE, 32% and 21% compared with 43% and 32% ($p < 0.01$). For women, there were no significant age differences between the NDNS and HSfE.

For both men and women there were no significant differences by age between the NDNS and the HSfE in the proportion reporting participating in activities of at least moderate intensity for 30 minutes or more on at least one day during the reference period.

(Table 5.13)

References and endnotes

1   The Technical Report is available online at http://www.food.gov.uk/science.

2   Health Development Agency. *Physical Activity*. Online: http://www.hda-online.org.uk/html/research/physicalactivity.html.

3   Prior G. 'Physical Activity' In: *Health Survey for England: Cardiovascular Disease*. TSO (London, 1998).

4   National Audit Office. *Tackling obesity in England*. TSO (London, 2001).

5   National Heart Forum. *Physical activity and coronary heart disease*. Online: http://www.heartforum.org.uk/physicalactivity.html.

6   Health Development Agency. *Physical activity: health benefits*. Online: http://www.hda-online.org.uk/html/research/pa_healthbenefits.html.

7   U.S. Department of Health and Human Services. *Physical activity and health: A report of the Surgeon General*. National Centre for Chronic Disease Prevention and Health Promotion (Atlanta, GA: U.S. 1994).

8   Estimates of energy requirements of different population groups are termed 'Estimated Average Requirements' (EARs) and are defined as the energy intake estimated to meet the average requirements of the population group.

    Department of Health. Report on Health and Social Subjects: 41. *Dietary Reference Values for Food Energy and Nutrients for the United Kingdom*. HMSO (London, 1991).

9   Henderson L, Gregory J, Irving K, Swan G. *The National Diet and Nutrition Survey: adults aged 19 to 64 years. Volume 2: Energy, protein, carbohydrate, fat and alcohol intake*. TSO (London, 2003).

10 Finch S, Doyle W, Lowe C, Bates CJ, Prentice A, Smithers G, Clarke PC. *National Diet and Nutrition Survey: people aged 65 years and over. Volume 1: Report of the diet and nutrition survey*. TSO (London, 1998).

11 Gregory J, Lowe S, Bates CJ, Prentice A, Jackson LV, Smithers G, Wenlock R, Farron M. *National Diet and Nutrition Survey: young people aged 4 to 18 years. Volume 1: Report of the diet and nutrition survey*. TSO (London, 2000).

12 It should be noted that statistically significant correlation results do not necessarily indicate any direct health or clinical meaning.

13 *See* Note 3. This was the most recent year that physical activity data were available for the general population.

14 Distribution of data was evaluated using the skewness statistic in SPSS. If the skewness statistic was less than twice the standard error of this statistic then data were considered to be normally distributed.

15 The areas included in each of the four analysis 'regions' are given in the response chapter, Chapter 2 of the Technical Report (*see* Note 1). Definitions of 'regions' are given in the Glossary (*see* Appendix E).

16 Households receiving certain benefits are those where someone in the respondent's household was currently receiving Working Families Tax Credit or had, in the previous 14 days, drawn Income Support or (Income-related) Job Seeker's Allowance. Definitions of 'household' and 'benefits (receiving)' are given in the Glossary (*see* Appendix E).

17 It should be noted that anthropometric measurements used are reflections of body composition in the longer term which may not necessarily be reflected by self-reported physical activity levels over a short term period.

[18] Bivariate analyses of continuous variables were carried out using the Pearson correlation coefficient and analyses of categorical variables tested the difference between means. It should be noted that where correlations are statistically significant the relationship between the two variables may not necessarily be causal; other factors may have affected the size of the correlation.

[19] The regression models are constructed by carrying out bivariate analyses and incorporating variables with significant associations. It should be noted that this method of selection can lead to important variables being left out as additive or interactive effects can only be identified using multiple regression.

[20] The model is tested by an ANOVA (*see* Appendix E - Glossary) to determine whether all the regression coefficients are zero in the population, and shows that there are significant linear relationships between the independent variables and the dependent variable.

[21] Health Survey for England 1998 - Volume 1 provides a summary of key findings and Volume 2 details the methodology. Both are available online at http://www.archive.official-documents.co.uk//document/doh/survey98/hse98.htm.

Table 5.1

Percentage distribution of self–reported levels of physical activity by sex and age of respondent

Responding sample   Percentages

Reported level of activity at dietary interview	Men aged (years):				All men	Women aged (years):				All women
	19–24	25–34	35–49	50–64		19–24	25–34	35–49	50–64	
	%	%	%	%	%	%	%	%	%	%
Not at all physically active	7	4	5	5	5	8	6	5	8	6
Not very physically active	24	23	25	20	23	27	23	26	22	24
Fairly physically active	43	53	52	53	51	53	57	48	52	52
Very physically active	26	21	18	21	21	12	15	20	18	17
Base	142	284	329	330	1085	136	275	415	336	1162

Table 5.2

Percentage distribution of mean hours spent in activity of at least moderate intensity* per day by sex and age of respondent

Respondents who completed physical activity diary   Cumulative percentages

Hours spent in activity of at least moderate intensity per day during the 7-day recording period	Men aged (years):				All men	Women aged (years):				All women
	19–24	25–34	35–49	50–64		19–24	25–34	35–49	50–64	
	cum %	cum %	cum %	cum %	cum %	cum %	cum %	cum %	cum %	cum %
None**	20	9	16	24	17	19	10	16	20	16
Less than quarter of an hour	25	19	33	39	30	31	30	31	42	34
Less than half an hour	38	35	45	54	44	54	46	50	56	51
Less than one hour	43	49	63	69	58	67	64	68	73	68
Less than an hour and a half	51	58	69	74	66	74	74	78	81	77
Less than two hours	54	62	73	79	70	78	77	82	84	81
Less than three hours	64	66	75	85	74	85	85	87	91	87
Less than four hours	64	70	77	86	76	91	92	90	94	92
Less than six hours	72	81	87	88	84	96	96	95	97	96
Less than eight hours	96	91	96	96	95	99	98	99	100	99
All	100	100	100	100	100	100	100	100		100
Base	104	211	243	243	801	100	202	305	249	857
Mean (average value)	2.9	2.7	2.0	1.5	2.2	1.3	1.3	1.2	1.0	1.2
Median	1.4	1.1	0.6	0.4	0.6	0.4	0.6	0.5	0.4	0.5
Lower 2.5 percentile	0.0	0.0	0.0	0.0	0.0	0.0	0.0	0.0	0.0	0.0
Upper 2.5 percentile	8.3	9.6	9.4	8.4	9.0	6.3	7.4	7.0	6.2	6.4
Standard deviation	3.00	3.10	2.81	2.45	2.86	1.77	1.92	1.87	1.52	1.78

Note: * Includes moderate, vigorous and very vigorous activity .

** This category includes respondents who did not participate in any moderate, vigorous or very vigorous activity during the recording period.

Table 5.3

Percentage distribution of mean hours spent in vigorous or very vigorous activity per day by sex and age of respondent

Respondents who completed physical activity diary

Cumulative percentages

Hours spent in vigorous or very vigorous activity per day during the 7-day recording period	Men aged (years):				All men	Women aged (years):				All women
	19–24	25–34	35–49	50–64		19–24	25–34	35–49	50–64	
	cum %	cum %	cum %	cum %	cum %	cum %	cum %	cum %	cum %	cum %
None*	56	47	60	78	61	59	65	74	82	72
Less than quarter of an hour	64	64	75	85	74	74	85	86	91	86
Less than half an hour	75	76	84	93	84	90	95	95	97	95
Less than one hour	88	88	92	97	92	98	99	99	100	99
Less than an hour and a half	91	91	93	97	93	98	99	100		100
All	100	100	100	100	100	100	100			
Base	104	211	243	243	801	100	202	305	249	857
Mean (average value)	0.7	0.8	0.6	0.3	0.5	0.2	0.1	0.1	0.1	0.1
Median	0.0	0.1	0.0	0.0	0.0	0.0	0.0	0.0	0.0	0.0
Lower 2.5 percentile	0.0	0.0	0.0	0.0	0.0	0.0	0.0	0.0	0.0	0.0
Upper 2.5 percentile	7.2	8.6	6.5	4.4	7.1	1.0	0.7	0.6	0.6	0.6
Standard deviation	1.66	2.11	1.69	1.11	1.67	0.29	0.24	0.32	0.15	0.26

Note: * This category includes respondents who did not participate in any vigorous or very vigorous activity during the recording period. Respondents in this category may still have taken part in moderate intensity activity.

Table 5.4

Participation in at least 30 minutes of activity of at least moderate intensity* per day by sex and age of respondent

Respondents who completed physical activity diary

Percentages

Number of days per week that 30 minutes or more per day spent in activity of at least moderate intensity	Men aged (years):				All men	Women aged (years):				All women
	19–24	25–34	35–49	50–64		19–24	25–34	35–49	50–64	
	%	%	%	%	%	%	%	%	%	%
None	21	12	20	30	21	20	14	21	24	20
One or two days a week	14	21	27	28	24	36	29	29	34	31
Three or four days a week	17	21	19	18	19	15	26	24	21	23
Five or more days a week	49	46	34	24	36	29	30	25	22	26
Base	104	211	243	243	801	100	202	305	249	857

Note: * Includes moderate, vigorous and very vigorous activity.

Table 5.5

Mean hours spent in activities of at least moderate intensity* per day by sex of respondent and region

Region	Sex of respondent							
	Men				Women			
	Mean	Median	sd	Base	Mean	Median	sd	Base
Scotland	2.1	0.4	2.98	59	1.3	0.4	1.93	65
Northern	2.0	0.6	2.76	229	1.0	0.4	1.58	218
Central, South West and Wales	2.6	1.0	3.08	279	1.3	0.6	1.88	313
London and the South East	1.7	0.6	2.56	234	1.1	0.4	1.77	261

Note: * Includes moderate, vigorous and very vigorous activity.

Table 5.6

Mean hours spent in activities of at least moderate intensity* per day by sex of respondent and whether someone in the respondent's household was receiving certain benefits

Sex of respondent	Whether receiving benefits							
	Receiving benefits				Not receiving benefits			
	Mean	Median	sd	Base	Mean	Median	sd	Base
Men	2.0	0.5	2.76	105	2.2	0.6	2.87	696
Women	1.2	0.7	1.48	147	1.2	0.5	1.84	710

Note: * Includes moderate, vigorous and very vigorous activity.

Table 5.7

Pearson correlation coefficients for hours spent in activities of at least moderate intensity[†] per day with energy and macronutrient intakes

Sex and age of respondent	Correlation of hours spent in activities of at least moderate intensity with:						
	Average daily total energy intake (MJ)	Percentage of total energy from alcohol	Percentage food energy from:				Base
			Total fat	Protein	Total carbohydrate	Non-milk extrinsic sugars	
Men aged (years):							
19–24	0.14	0.04	0.25 *	−0.16	−0.17	−0.13	102
25–34	0.20 **	−0.16 *	0.06	−0.04	−0.02	−0.06	207
35–49	0.19 **	−0.03	0.03	−0.11	0.03	−0.02	235
50–64	0.24 **	−0.02	0.08	−0.06	−0.04	−0.09	240
All men	0.19 **	−0.05	0.09 *	−0.09 **	−0.02	−0.03	784
Women aged (years):							
19–24	−0.05	−0.03	−0.12	−0.02	0.11	0.08	98
25–34	−0.09	−0.10	0.02	0.00	−0.02	−0.02	201
35–49	0.04	−0.15 *	0.02	0.03	−0.03	−0.08	299
50–64	0.14 *	−0.06	0.01	−0.10	0.04	0.05	248
All women	0.02	−0.10 **	0.00	−0.03	0.01	−0.01	847

Note: * $p<0.05$; ** $p<0.01$

† Includes moderate, vigorous and very vigorous activity.

Table 5.8

Pearson correlation coefficients for hours spent in activities of at least moderate intensity[†] per day with anthropometric measurements

Sex and age of respondent	Correlation of hours spent in activities of at least moderate intensity with:			
	Body mass index (kg/m²)	Base	Waist to hip ratio	Base
Men aged (years):				
19–24	0.10	95	0.21*	97
25–34	0.21**	199	0.14*	199
35–49	−0.04	236	0.01	236
50–64	0.04	233	0.06	230
All men	0.02	762	0.00	763
Women aged (years):				
19–24	0.07	93	0.14	93
25–34	0.13	190	0.01	190
35–49	0.04	294	−0.01	293
50–64	−0.07	231	−0.03	232
All women	0.03	807	−0.02	808

Note: * p<0.05; ** p<0.01

[†] Includes moderate, vigorous and very vigorous activity .

Table 5.9

Pearson correlation coefficients for hours spent in activities of at least moderate intensity[†] per day with blood pressure

Sex and age of respondent	Correlation of hours spent in activities of at least moderate intensity with:		
	Systolic blood pressure (mmHg)	Diastolic blood pressure (mmHg)	Base
Men aged (years):			
19–24	0.15	0.04	93
25–34	0.11	−0.01	201
35–49	−0.14 *	−0.08	235
50–64	0.02	0.02	226
All men	−0.04	−0.11 **	754
Women aged (years):			
19–24	−0.01	0.03	93
25–34	0.00	−0.04	185
35–49	−0.03	−0.07	284
50–64	−0.15 *	−0.10	223
All women	−0.08 *	−0.07 *	786

Note: * p<0.05; ** p<0.01

[†] Includes moderate, vigorous and very vigorous activity .

Table 5.10

Socio-demographic, dietary and physiological factors associated with hours spent in activities of at least moderate intensity[†] in bivariate analysis

Men	Women
Age (years)**	Age (years)*
Average daily alcohol intake (g)	Average daily alcohol intake (g)
Average daily total energy intake (MJ)**	Average daily total energy intake (MJ)
BMI (kg/m²)	BMI (kg/m²)
Current smoking	Current smoking
Employment status**	Employment status**
Ethnicity of respondent	Ethnicity of respondent
Gross weekly household income**	Gross weekly household income*
Grouped Standard Region*	Grouped Standard Region
Household benefit status	Household benefit status
Household composition*	Household composition
Limited activity due to illness or disability*	Limited activity due to illness or disability*
Mean diastolic pressure (mmHg)**	Mean diastolic pressure (mmHg)*
Mean systolic pressure (mmHg)	Mean systolic pressure (mmHg)*
Percentage food energy from protein**	Percentage food energy from protein
Percentage food energy from total carbohydrate	Percentage food energy from total carbohydrate
Percentage food energy from total fat*	Percentage food energy from total fat
Percentage total energy from alcohol	Percentage total energy from alcohol**
Percentage total energy from protein*	Percentage total energy from protein
Percentage total energy from total carbohydrate	Percentage total energy from total carbohydrate
Percentage total energy from total fat*	Percentage total energy from total fat
Percentage total energy from total sugars	Percentage total energy from total sugars
Reported dieting to lose weight	Reported dieting to lose weight
Self-reported alcohol consumption	Self-reported alcohol consumption
Self-reported physical activity level**	Self-reported physical activity level**
Social class of household reference person**	Social class of household reference person*
Vegetarian or vegan	Vegetarian or vegan
Waist to hip ratio	Waist to hip ratio
Wave of interview	Wave of interview

Note: * p<0.05; ** p<0.01

[†] Includes moderate, vigorous and very vigorous activity.

Table 5.11

Linear regression model for time spent in activities of at least moderate intensity per day: men

Characteristic	Unstandardised coefficient (B)	Standard error of B	Standardised regression coefficient (β)	T-value
Constant	0.463	1.098		0.422
Social class of household reference person				
Non-manual	−0.284	0.269	−0.053	−1.053
Manual	1.466	0.264	0.266	5.557 ***
Unclassified	−1.182	0.485	−0.219	−2.437 *
Age (years)	−0.039	0.010	−0.177	−3.972 ***
Self-reported physical activity level				
Very physically active	0.880	0.200	0.148	4.400 ***
Fairly physically active	−0.083	0.167	−0.017	−0.500
Not very physically active	−0.807	0.195	−0.139	−4.143 ***
Not at all physically active	0.011	0.342	0.002	0.032
Gross weekly household income				
Less than £160	−0.816	0.281	−0.187	−2.906 **
£160 - less than £400	0.534	0.186	0.104	2.864 **
£400 & over	0.282	0.197	0.065	1.432
Employment status				
In employment	0.689	0.253	0.162	2.727 **
Unemployed	−0.487	0.354	−0.067	−1.375
Economically inactive	−0.202	0.257	−0.048	−0.785
Average daily total energy intake (MJ)	0.152	0.042	0.129	3.655 ***
Household composition				
Living alone	−0.276	0.224	−0.060	−1.229
Living with spouse or partner, no dependent children	0.232	0.172	0.067	1.350
Living with other adults, no spouse or dependent children	−0.160	0.218	−0.037	−0.734
Living with dependent children, with or without spouse	0.204	0.164	0.044	1.246
Region				
Scotland	0.281	0.278	0.055	1.014
Northern	−0.164	0.175	−0.043	−0.940
Central, South West and Wales	0.193	0.165	0.054	1.173
London and the South East	−0.311	0.172	−0.061	−1.802
Percentage total energy from total fat[†]	0.024	0.017	0.048	1.436
Limited activity due to illness or disability	−0.126	0.259	−0.017	−0.485
Diastolic blood pressure (mmHg)	−0.004	0.009	−0.016	−0.435
Percentage total energy from protein[†]	0.010	0.035	0.010	0.284
Percentage of variance explained		23%		
Number of respondents		*732*		

Note: * $p<0.05$; ** $p<0.01$; *** $p<0.001$

[†] *For men, percentage food energy from protein and percentage food energy from total fat were significantly correlated with average time spent in activities of at least moderate intensity at the bivariate stage but these variables were not included in the multiple regression model. This is because alcohol intake was not found to be significantly associated with time spent in activities of at least moderate intensity, therefore percentage of total energy from protein and percentage of total energy from total fat, which includes alcohol intake, were chosen preferentially.*

Table 5.12

Linear regression model for time spent in activities of at least moderate intensity per day: women

Characteristic	Unstandardised coefficient (B)	Standard error of B	Standardised regression coefficient (β)	T-value
Constant	1.938	0.530		3.658 ***
Self-reported physical activity level				
Very physically active	0.327	0.137	0.090	2.395 *
Fairly physically active	0.180	0.104	0.063	1.729
Not very physically active	0.136	0.124	0.040	1.102
Not at all physically active	−0.644	0.203	−0.176	−3.172 **
Social class of household reference person				
Non-manual	−0.436	0.141	−0.140	−3.092 **
Manual	−0.099	0.143	−0.031	−0.693
Unclassified	0.535	0.250	0.172	2.140 *
Percentage total energy from alcohol	−0.027	0.012	−0.080	−2.176 *
Limited activity due to illness or disability	−0.321	0.162	−0.074	−1.979 *
Employment status				
In employment	0.173	0.164	0.088	1.055
Unemployed	0.005	0.287	0.001	0.017
Economically inactive	−0.177	0.168	−0.090	−1.055
Gross weekly household income				
Less than £160	−0.111	0.145	−0.045	−0.768
£160 - less than £400	0.132	0.104	0.069	1.271
£400 & over	−0.021	0.103	−0.009	−0.206
Age (years)	−0.005	0.006	−0.036	−0.819
Diastolic blood pressure (mmHg)	0.001	0.008	0.004	0.079
Systolic blood pressure (mmHg)	−0.003	0.006	−0.030	−0.556
Percentage of variance explained		5%		
Number of respondents		*749*		

Note: * p<0.05; ** p<0.01; *** p<0.001

Table 5.13

Participation in at least 30 minutes of activity of at least moderate intensity* per day by sex and age of respondent compared with the Health Survey for England 1998**

Percentages

Number of days per week that 30 minutes or more per day spent in activity of at least moderate intensity*	Men aged (years):					Women aged (years):				
	16/19–24***	25–34	35–44	45–54	55–64	16/19–24***	25–34	35–44	45–54	55–64
	%	%	%	%	%	%	%	%	%	%
2000/01 NDNS – England only†										
None	20	14	20	25	27	23	15	21	24	29
One or two days a week	13	21	28	27	30	36	28	30	27	31
Three or four days a week	17	22	21	18	23	15	29	23	27	18
Five or more days a week	50	44	32	30	21	26	29	26	22	22
Base	*96*	*191*	*150*	*143*	*126*	*88*	*177*	*185*	*179*	*125*
1998 Health Survey for England††										
None	10	11	15	22	34	20	15	16	21	29
Less than one day a week****	6	11	12	11	10	13	13	14	13	13
One or two days a week	15	19	20	21	17	22	26	25	23	26
Three or four days a week	11	11	9	10	7	13	15	14	13	12
Five or more days a week	58	48	43	36	32	32	31	32	30	21
Base	*875*	*1338*	*1305*	*1289*	*987*	*1006*	*1630*	*1573*	*1484*	*1148*

Note: * Includes moderate, vigorous and very vigorous activity.

** Erens B, Primatesta P. Eds. Health Survey for England: Cardovascular Disease 1998. TSO (London, 1999).

*** Health Survey for England figures include respondents aged 16 to 24.

**** The total number of activity days each respondent reported in the past four weeks was divided by four to produce a weekly figure. A comparable category for the present NDNS is not meaningful.

† Figures based on participation for at least 10 minutes.

†† Figures based on participation for at least 15 minutes.

Appendix A   Sampling errors and statistical methods

1   Sampling errors

This section examines the sources of error associated with survey estimates and presents sampling errors of survey estimates, referred to as standard errors, and design factors for a number of key variables shown in this volume. It should be noted that tables showing standard errors in the main part of this volume have assumed a simple random sample design. In testing for the significance of the differences between two survey estimates, proportions or means, the standard error calculated as for a simple random sample design was multiplied by an assumed, conservative, design factor of 1.5 to allow for the complex sample design.

The estimates presented in the main part of this volume are based on data weighted to correct both for differential sampling probability and for differential non-response. The sampling errors presented in this appendix were calculated after applying a weight to compensate for differential sampling probability and differential non-response. The sample was also post-stratified, so that it matched the population distribution in terms of age, sex and region[1].

1.1   The accuracy of survey results

Survey results are subject to various sources of error. The total error in a survey estimate is the difference between the estimate derived from the data collected and the true value for the population. It can be thought of as being comprised of random and systematic errors, and each of these two main types of error can be subdivided into error from a number of different sources.

1.1.1 Random error

Random error is the part of the total error which would be expected to average zero if a number of repeats of the same survey were carried out based on different samples from the same population.

An important component of random error is sampling error, which arises because the estimate is based on a survey rather than a census of the population. The results of this or any other survey would be expected to vary from the true population values. The amount of variation depends on both the size of the sample and the sample design.

Random error may also arise from other sources such as the respondent's interpretation of the questions. As with all surveys carried out by the ONS, considerable efforts were made on this survey to minimise these effects through interviewer training and through feasibility work; however it is likely some will remain that are not possible to quantify.

1.1.2 Systematic error

Systematic error, or bias, applies to those sources of error that will not average to zero over a number of repeats of the survey. The category includes, for example, bias due to omission of certain parts of the population from the sampling frame, or bias due to interviewer or coder variation. A substantial effort is put into avoiding systematic errors but it is likely that some will remain.

Non-response bias is a systematic error that is of particular concern. It occurs if non-respondents to the survey, or to particular components of the survey, differ significantly in some respect from respondents, so that the responding sample is not representative of the total population. Non-response can be minimised by training interviewers in how to deal with potential refusals and with strategies to minimise non-contacts. However, a certain level of non-response is inevitable in any voluntary survey. The resulting bias is, however, dependent not only on the absolute level of non-response, but on the extent to which non-respondents differ from respondents in terms of the measures that the survey aims to estimate.

Although respondents were encouraged to take part in all components of the survey, some refused certain components. Chapter 2 of the Technical Report[2] examines the characteristics of groups responding to the different parts of the survey package. The analysis of the region, sex and age profile of respondents compared with population estimates showed evidence of some response bias. In particular, there was an under representation of men, and of people aged 19 to 24 years. The data for the main part of this volume (and all volumes in the series) were therefore weighted for differential non-response by sex, age and region.

1.2   Standard errors for estimates for the NDNS of adults aged 19 to 64 years

As described in Chapter 1 and Appendix D of the Technical Report[2], this survey used a complex sample design, which involved both clustering and stratification. In considering the accuracy of estimates, standard errors calculated on the basis of a simple random sample design will be incorrect because of the complex sample design.

The sample for this survey was clustered using postcode sectors as primary sampling units (PSUs). Clustering can increase standard errors if there is a lot of variation in characteristics between the PSUs, but little variation within them. By contrast, stratification tends to reduce standard errors especially where the stratification factors are correlated to the survey estimate. Stratifying the sample ensures that certain sections of the population are represented in the sample. The main stratifier used on this survey was Standard Statistical Region (SSR). The PSUs were further stratified by population density, socio-economic group and car ownership (*see* Appendix D of the Technical Report[2]).

In a complex sample design, the size of the standard error of any estimate depends on how the characteristic of interest is spread within and between PSUs and strata: this is taken into account by pairing adjacent PSUs from the same strata. The squared differences in the estimates between successive PSUs from the same strata are calculated and summed to produce the standard error.

The majority of estimates in this survey take the form of ratio estimates, either means or proportions. The formula to calculate the standard error of these is:

$$se\ (r)= \frac{1}{x}\ [var(y) + r^2\ var\ (x) - 2r\ cov(y,x)]^{1/2}$$

where the ratio $r = y/x$.

The method explicitly allows for the fact that the percentages and means are actually ratios of two survey estimates, both of which are subject to random error. The value *se (r)* is the estimate of the standard error of the ratio, *r*, expressed in terms of *se(y)* and *se(x)* which are the estimated standard errors of *y* and *x*, and *cov(y,x)* which is their estimated covariance. The resulting estimate is slightly biased and only valid if the denominator is not too variable[3]. The ratio means for age groups have standard errors equal to zero for the full sample because both the numerator and the denominator have been set to equal the population totals and thus cannot vary for any selected sample.

The method of standard error estimation compares the successive differences between totals of the characteristic of interest for adjacent PSUs (postal sectors)[4]. The characteristic is the numerator, for example body mass index, and the sample size is the denominator in the ratio estimate[5]. The ordering of PSUs reflects the ranking of postal sectors on the stratifiers used in the sample design.

Tables A1 to A4 give standard errors, taking account of the complex sample design used on this survey, for the key variables presented in this volume. Standard errors for estimates by household benefit status and region, are shown separately for men and women to reflect the way they are presented in the main part of the volume.

1.3   Estimating standard errors for other survey estimates

Although standard errors can be calculated readily by computer, there are practical problems in presenting a large number of survey estimates. One solution is to calculate standard errors for selected variables and, from these, identify design factors appropriate for the specific survey design and for different types of survey variable. The standard error of other survey measures can then be estimated using an appropriate design factor, together with the sampling error assuming a simple random sample.

1.3.1 The Design Factor (deft)

The effect of a complex sample design can be quantified by comparing the observed variability in the sample with the expected variability had the survey used a simple random sample. The most commonly used statistic is the design factor *(deft)*, which is calculated as a ratio of the standard error for a survey estimate allowing for the full complexity of the sample design (including weighting), to the standard error assuming that the result has come from a simple random sample. The deft can be used as a multiplier to the standard error based on a simple random sample, $se(p)_{srs}$, to give the standard error of the complex design, $se(p)$, by using the following formula:

$$se(p) = deft \times se(p)_{srs}$$

Tables A1 to A4 show deft values for certain measures for respondents who completed that component of the survey. The deft value varies between survey variables, reflecting the degree to which the characteristic is clustered within PSUs or is distributed between strata. Variables which are highly correlated to the post-strata should also have reduced deft values. For a single variable, the deft value can also vary according to the size of the subgroup on which the estimate is based because smaller subgroups can be less affected by clustering.

Table A1 shows deft values for age group, region and household benefit status for the diary sample, Table A2 for physiological measurements, Tables A3(a) and (b) for blood analytes and Table A4 for measures of physical activity. For age group, region and household benefit status, where geographic clustering would be expected, six out of ten of the deft values for men and eight out of ten for women are less than 1.2. Deft values of this order are considered to be small and they indicate that, in this survey, the characteristic is not markedly clustered geographically. Two of these deft values are above 1.5 for both sexes.

For women, 61% of the deft values presented in Tables A2 to A4 are less than 1.2, while for men 43% are less than 1.2. For women, 2% of the deft

values are greater than 1.5, while for men, 6% are greater than 1.5.

(Tables A1 to A4)

1.3.2 Testing differences between means and proportions

Standard errors can be used to test whether an observed difference between two proportions or means in the sample is likely to be due to sampling error. An estimate for the standard error of a difference between percentages, from the same sample, assuming a simple random sample is:

$$se_1(p_1 \text{-} p_2) = \sqrt{[(p_1 q_1 / n_1) + (p_2 q_2 / n_2)]}$$

where p_1 and p_2 are the observed percentages for the two subsamples, q_1 and q_2 are respectively *(100–p_1)* and *(100–p_2)*, and n_1 and n_2 are the subsample sizes.

The equivalent formula for the standard error of the difference between the means for subsamples 1 and 2 is:

$$se_2 (diff) = \sqrt{(se_1^2 + se_2^2)}$$

Allowance for the complex sample design is then made by multiplying the standard errors se_1 and se_2 from the above formula by the appropriate deft values.

In this volume the calculation of the difference between proportions and means assumed a deft of 1.5 across all survey estimates. The calculation of complex sampling errors and design factors for key characteristics show that this was a conservative estimate for some characteristics for some age and sex groups, but was an optimistic estimate for other characteristics. Therefore there will be some differences in sample proportions and means which are not commented on in the text, but that are significantly different, at least at the p<0.05 level. Equally, there will be some differences that are described as significant in the text, but that are not significantly different when the complex sampling design is taken into account. An indication of the characteristics for which significance tests are likely to provide false-positives or false-negatives can be gained by looking at the size of the deft values in the tables in this appendix.

Confidence intervals can be calculated around a survey estimate using the standard error for that estimate. For example, the 95% confidence interval is calculated as 1.96 times the standard error on either side of the estimated proportion or mean value. At the 95% confidence level, over many repeats of the survey under the same conditions, 95% of these confidence intervals would contain the population estimate. However, when assessing the results of a survey, it is usual to assume that there is only a 5% chance that the true population value will fall outside the 95% confidence interval calculated for the survey estimate.

2   Multiple Regression

The substantive chapters of this volume present results from multiple regression analyses. These analyses were carried out in SPSS version 10.1 using the 'enter' method.

In each analysis age was always included as an independent variable and the regression analyses were run separately for men and women. For each regression the procedure was first run to identify any collinear variables. After excluding one from the pair of any collinear variables the procedure was run again. All the regression analyses were carried out using weights for the dependent variable in the analysis[6].

2.1   The multiple regression analysis method[7]

Most of the tables shown in this volume are based on bivariate analysis. These tables show the relationship between two reported or measured variables, for example, the proportion of respondents living in different regions with different mean body weight. What these tables do not show, however, is how other factors may interrelate with the independent variable; for example, how age, sex and household composition interrelate to explain variations in diastolic blood pressure.

Figure A1 shows how each of the variables, x_1 and x_2, make an independent contribution to the dependent variable, y, but that there is an area of x_1 that overlaps with x_2. By carrying out a multiple regression analysis the overlap between x_1 and x_2 is eliminated, so that the contribution x_1 makes to y can be measured after controlling for (eliminating) the overlapping contribution of x_2.

Figure A1

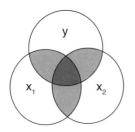

Multiple regression is a multivariate statistical technique that describes the relationship between one survey variable, the dependent variable, for example the diastolic blood pressure of the respondent and several other variables, the independent variables, for example, age, sex and household composition. For example, Table 3.10 of this volume shows the results of regression where the dependent variable is the diastolic blood pressure for a man aged between 19 and 64 years. The regression calculates a coefficient for each independent variable which quantifies the effect that a change in that variable will have on the predicted diastolic blood pressure, leaving all other variables in the regression unchanged (*see* Section 2.3 below).

When running regression the interest is in testing whether, for a given model, there is a relationship between the dependent variable and the independent variables in the population. This is done by testing whether the coefficient for the independent variable is equal to zero. A variable is judged to be statistically different from zero if it is significant at the 95% level or above. This means that if there were no relationship in the population between the dependent and the independent variable, there would be a probability of 5% or less that the regression would have estimated a coefficient that was different from zero.

2.1.1   Assumptions for multiple regression analysis

The technique of multiple regression requires a number of conditions of the data to be met or assumed; some are appropriate only to the analysis of particular types of dataset, for example time series, and are not presented here. The assumptions made in respect of the NDNS data for multiple regression analysis were as follows:

- *Linearity and normal distribution*

  The technique of multiple regression calculates coefficients that describe linear relationships between variables and assume that the residuals (the difference between the actual value of the dependent variable and that predicted by the model) are normally distributed. If the residuals are not normally distributed, the significance tests will not be valid. In order to facilitate normally distributed residuals, where the NDNS data for any of the dependent variables included in the analysis were strongly skewed[8] they were transformed by taking the natural log (ln) before being added to the analysis model.

- *Values for the independent variables in repeated samples are fixed*

  The assumption is that if multiple samples are drawn, an independent variable will take the same value in each sample. Chapter 2 of the Technical Report[2] shows that for several of the socio-demographic variables used in the multiple regression analysis, the NDNS sample gave comparable results to those found in other surveys.

- *Collinearity (or multicollinearity)*

  The assumption is that no two independent variables are close or exact linear combinations of one another. When two variables are strongly positively correlated (collinear), the standard errors will be inflated, making the significance tests misleading. In SPSS, the multiple regression analysis produces a Pearson correlation matrix and two 'collinearity statistics': the *tolerance* and the *variance inflation factor* (VIF). The *tolerance* of a variable is $1-R_i^2$ where R_i is the multiple correlation coefficient when the *i*th independent variable is predicted from the other independent variables. The *VIF* is *1/tolerance*. A value of 10 or more for the *VIF* indicates the presence of significant collinearity between the independent variable against which it appears and one or more of the other independent variables included in the model. The Pearson correlation coefficient matrix gives correlation coefficients for the relationship between each of the independent variables and is used to identify which are strongly correlated.

For each multiple regression analysis carried out, all of the independent variables considered important in explaining the dependent variable were included in an initial regression analysis. The output from this initial analysis identified independent variables with a *VIF* value of greater than 10, and the Pearson correlation matrix was used to show which variables were strongly correlated so that one or more could be excluded from the analysis. The decision about which variable(s) to exclude from the regression analysis was made with reference to which might be the more important factor, either in terms of predictive value or in terms of policy relevance.

2.1.2 Preparing variables for multiple regression analysis

In a multiple regression analysis the dependent variable must be continuous and the independent variables either continuous or dichotomous. Independent categorical variables with more than two categories must be transformed into dichotomous ('dummy') variables before being included in the analysis.

For categorical variables with two categories, the two possible 'dummy' variables are complementary. For example, for whether the respondent 'smoked cigarettes at all nowadays' the two possible 'dummy' variables are:

smoke cigarettes at all nowadays? yes = 1, no = 0
smoke cigarettes at all nowadays? yes = 0, no = 1

The SPSS multiple regression program tests the independent variables for multicollinearity, as described above. Where there is a strong correlation between two variables, the statistics produced by the analysis are not valid and one of the collinear variables must be excluded. However, where there is an exact correlation between two variables, for example where two 'dummy' variables are complementary parts of the same variable, SPSS automatically excludes one from the analysis and uses it as the 'reference category'. For a dichotomous variable the regression coefficient gives the expected difference of being in one category (the category that takes the value 1) rather than the other (the category that takes the value 0).

For categorical variables with more than two categories, dichotomous 'dummy' variables need to be created. For example, for region with four categories, four 'dummy' variables need to be created to indicate whether or not the respondent lived in each region. Thus the first 'dummy' variable would be categorised 'Living in Scotland' and 'Not living in Scotland', the second 'Living in Northern region' and 'Not living in Northern region' and so on. If all four 'dummy' variables for regions are included in the analysis, one is automatically treated as the reference category and the unstandardised coefficients are interpreted with reference to that category. However, to provide correlation coefficients that can be interpreted as deviations from the average effect of all categories, it is necessary to use the 'enter' method for the procedure and to run two versions of each regression analysis.

For example for 'region' in the NDNS dataset two sets of 'dummy' variables were created with one (reference) category coded as −1 and one category excluded:

Set 1:

'Dummy' 1 = (Scotland = 1) (Northern = 0) (Central and South West of England and Wales = 0) (London and South East = −1)

'Dummy' 2 = (Scotland = 0) (Northern = 1) (Central and South West of England and Wales = 0) (London and South East = −1)

'Dummy' 3 = (Scotland = 0) (Northern = 0) (Central and South West of England and Wales = 1) (London and South East = −1)

Set 2:

'Dummy' A = (Scotland = −1) (Northern = 1) (Central and South West of England and Wales = 0) (London and South East = 0)

'Dummy' B = (Scotland = −1) (Northern = 0) (Central and South West of England and Wales = 1) (London and South East = 0)

'Dummy' C = (Scotland = −1) (Northern = 0) (Central and South West of England and Wales = 0) (London and South East = 1)

Note that for the first set the London and the South East category is set to −1 and there is no 'dummy' variable for London and the South East. In the second set, Scotland is set to −1 and there is no 'dummy' variable for Scotland. Any two categories could have been excluded.

The same procedure was used for all categorical variables for which there were more than two categories, producing two sets of 'dummy' variables that were run in two versions of the same multiple regression analysis. It is only necessary to run the regressions twice, no matter how many categorical variables are included. Where a 'dummy' variable appears in both versions of the analysis, the coefficients and standard errors are the same and the constant term has increased by the same amount. Having run both versions of the regression analysis, the results can be summarised in a single table.

2.2   The interpretation of statistics produced by multiple regression analysis

The **constant** is the predicted value of the dependent variable when all of the independent variables are held at zero.

The **unstandardised coefficient (B)** quantifies the *effect* that a change in the independent variable will have on the dependent variable, *holding all other variables in the regression analysis constant*.

This coefficient should not be used to indicate which independent variable is the best predictor of the dependent variable as the magnitude of the coefficients depends on the units in which the variables are measured.

The **adjusted R^2** is an assessment of the overall fit of the model and is interpreted as the percentage of the variance in the dependent variable that is explained by all of the independent variables included in the regression model. The adjusted R^2 is used in place of the R^2 value because the number of variables in the model does not affect it.

The **standardised coefficient (Beta, β)** is standardised for the units of measurement of the independent variable. It shows what the relative effect of each independent variable would be if they were all measured using the same scale. It indicates which independent variable is the best predictor of the dependent variable, with the highest value being the best predictor.

SPSS also gives **t values** and **significance levels** identifying those variables where the regression coefficients are significantly related to the dependent variable after controlling the effects of the other variables included in the analysis. The tables given in this volume show the significance level for each coefficient ($p<0.05$, $p<0.01$ or $p<0.001$[9]). Unstandardised and standardised regression coefficients are only shown in the tables in this volume for variables significantly related to the dependent variable.

2.3   Predicting values from a multiple regression analysis

For categorical variables the coefficients quantify the effect that having a particular characteristic will have on the dependent variable. For a dichotomous variable, the regression coefficient gives the expected difference of being in one category (the category that takes the value 1) rather than the other (the one that takes the value 0). For categorical variables with more than two categories the constant plus the value of the unstandardised coefficient for the independent variable gives the predicted value of the dependent variable for someone with that characteristic, when the values of all the other independent variables in the regression analysis are set to zero.

For continuous variables the value of the coefficient represents the contribution to the dependent variable per unit of the independent variable. For example, for 'body weight' this would be per kilogram if the unit for the variable was kilograms, or per gram if the unit for the variable was grams. The coefficient is multiplied by the value of the continuous variable for which the prediction is being made before being added to the constant. For example, if body weight = 50kg and the value of the unstandardised coefficient B = 0.45, then a value of 22.5 (equal to 0.45 * 50) is added to the constant.

A worked example is given below to show how systolic blood pressure can be predicted from a multiple regression analysis where diastolic blood pressure, household composition and body weight were all found to be statistically independently related to systolic blood pressure.

For example, from Table 3.8, a man who had a diastolic blood pressure of 82mmHg and weighed 91.5kg who lived with dependent children and his spouse/partner would have a predicted systolic blood pressure of:

56.70 + (0.88 x 82) − 2.65 + (0.09 x 91.5) = 134mmHg

where 56.70 (constant)

+0.88(per mmHg diastolic blood pressure)
−2.65(living with dependent children and spouse)
+0.09(per kg body weight).

As explained previously, the adjusted R^2 is used as an assessment of the overall fit of the model and is interpreted as the percentage of the variance in the dependent variable that is explained by all of the independent variables included in the regression model. It is generally expected that the amount of variance in the dependent variable which can be explained by a model will be low when analysing 'real-life' health data.

References and endnotes

[1]   Weighting for different sampling probabilities results in larger sampling errors than for an equal-probability sample without weights. However, using population totals to control for differential non-response tends to lead to a reduction in the errors. The method used to calculate the sampling errors identifies the weighting for unequal sampling probabilities and to the population separately and adjusts the sampling errors accordingly.

[2]   The Technical Report is available online at http://www.food.gov.uk/science.

[3]   This variability of the denominator can be measured by the coefficient of variation of x, denoted by $cv(x)$, which is the standard error of x expressed as a proportion of x.

$$cv(x) = \frac{se(x)}{x}$$

It has been suggested that the ratio estimator should not be used if $cv(x)$ is greater than 0.2. For the standard errors produced here, the denominators for the ratios were number of men and number of women. Both of these totals were constant, determined by the post-stratification and, therefore, there is no variation in these denominators and hence the cv of the denominator will be zero.

[4]   The calculation of standard errors and design factors for this survey used the package STATA. For further details of the method of calculation see: Elliot D. A comparison of software for producing sampling errors on social surveys. *Survey Methodology Bulletin* 1999; **44**: 27–36.

[5]   For a survey of this kind the sample size is subject to random fluctuation, both within each PSU and overall. This is because the number of adults identified in each PSU is dependent on which households are sampled and there will be differing amounts of non-response. There is more control in the (weighted) sample sizes of subgroups such as age and sex since these variables were used as post-stratifiers.

[6]   These weights adjusted for differential sampling probability and differential non-response.

[7]   For a more detailed description of multiple regression analysis using *SPSS, see Chapter 18, SPSS for Windows. Base Systems User's Guide*. SPSS Inc. (Chicago, 1993).

[8]   A skewness value of +1.0 represents extreme positive skewness and a value of -1.0 extreme negative skewness. Loether HJ, McTavish DG. *Descriptive and inferential statistics: an introduction*. 2nd edition. Allyn and Bacon (Massachusetts, 1980).

[9]   In the tables presenting results from multiple regression, variables that are significantly different at the 95%, 99% and 99.9% levels are indicated by one, two and three asterisks respectively.

Table A1

True standard errors and design factors for socio-demographic characteristics of the diary sample by sex of respondent

Diary sample   Numbers

	Men			Women		
	% (p)	Standard error of p*	Design factor	% (p)	Standard error of p*	Design factor
Age group						
19–24 years	13	0.00	0.00	12	0.00	0.00
25–34 years	26	0.00	0.00	24	0.00	0.00
35–49 years	30	0.00	0.00	36	0.00	0.00
50–64 years	30	0.00	0.00	29	0.00	0.00
Region						
Scotland	8	0.92	0.98	7	0.86	0.98
Northern	28	1.14	0.73	26	0.96	0.65
Central, South West and Wales	35	2.54	1.54	37	2.62	1.62
London and the South East	29	2.48	1.58	30	2.57	1.67
Household receipt of benefits						
Receiving benefits	13	1.47	1.25	17	1.47	1.17
Not receiving benefits	87	1.47	1.25	83	1.47	1.17
Sample size		*833*			*891*	

Note: * The ratio means for age groups for the diary sample have standard errors equal to zero because both the numerator and the denominator have been set to equal the population totals and thus cannot vary for any selected sample.

Table A2

True standard errors and design factors for physiological measurements by sex and age of respondent

| Physiological measurements | Age (years): | | | | | | | | | | | |
| | 19–24 | | | | 25–34 | | | | 35–49 | | | |
	Mean r	Standard error of r	Design factor	Base	Mean r	Standard error of r	Design factor	Base	Mean r	Standard error of r	Design factor	Base
Men												
Anthropometric measurements												
Height (cm)	177	0.9	1.45	112	177	0.5	1.18	229	176	0.4	0.98	263
Body weight (kg)	79	2.2	1.35	111	83	0.8	1.28	228	85	0.8	0.87	265
Waist circumference (cm)	89	1.8	1.42	111	92	0.8	1.18	228	96	0.6	0.82	263
Hip circumference (cm)	103	1.3	1.38	111	105	0.7	1.25	228	105	0.5	0.90	263
BMI (kg/m²)	25.1	0.64	1.29	110	26.4	0.35	1.32	227	27.4	0.21	0.81	263
Waist to hip ratio	0.86	0.009	1.50	111	0.88	0.005	1.31	228	0.91	0.004	0.92	263
Blood pressure												
Systolic blood pressure (mmHg)	127	1.6	1.59	109	125	1.0	1.12	221	129	0.9	1.03	255
Diastolic blood pressure (mmHg)	64	0.9	1.38	109	68	0.8	1.21	221	76	0.7	0.97	255
Women												
Anthropometric measurements												
Height (cm)	163	0.7	1.27	110	162	0.5	1.10	220	162	0.3	1.05	331
Body weight (kg)	66	2.1	1.35	110	67	1.0	1.05	215	70	0.8	0.95	334
Waist circumference (cm)	78	1.4	1.35	110	80	0.7	0.99	214	82	0.6	1.00	329
Hip circumference (cm)	102	1.4	1.29	110	103	0.7	1.07	214	104	0.5	0.98	329
BMI (kg/m²)	24.8	0.71	1.30	110	25.4	0.38	1.11	213	26.7	0.30	0.95	331
Waist to hip ratio	0.76	0.006	1.34	110	0.77	0.004	0.98	214	0.79	0.003	1.07	329
Blood pressure												
Systolic blood pressure (mmHg)	114	1.3	1.43	105	114	1.0	1.28	212	120	0.8	1.08	320
Diastolic blood pressure (mmHg)	62	1.0	1.38	105	65	0.8	1.21	212	69	0.5	0.95	320

Numbers

Physiological measurements

50-64				All				
Mean r	Standard error of r	Design factor	Base	Mean r	Standard error of r	Design factor	Base	
								Men
								Anthropometric measurements
175	0.5	1.11	264	176	0.3	1.26	869	Height (cm)
87	1.1	1.17	265	84	0.6	1.18	870	Body weight (kg)
100	0.6	0.97	261	95	0.4	1.11	862	Waist circumference (cm)
107	0.5	1.05	261	105	0.3	1.13	862	Hip circumference (cm)
28.4	0.32	1.08	264	27.2	0.17	1.09	864	BMI (kg/m^2)
0.94	0.003	0.99	261	0.90	0.002	1.13	862	Waist to hip ratio
								Blood pressure
136	1.3	1.25	255	130	0.6	1.21	839	Systolic blood pressure (mmHg)
79	0.7	1.15	255	73	0.4	1.06	839	Diastolic blood pressure (mmHg)
								Women
								Anthropometric measurements
160	0.4	1.10	270	162	0.2	1.14	930	Height (cm)
71	1.0	1.13	270	69	0.6	1.19	928	Body weight (kg)
86	0.9	1.09	269	82	0.4	1.10	922	Waist circumference (cm)
106	0.7	1.14	269	104	0.4	1.13	922	Hip circumference (cm)
27.4	0.41	1.23	269	26.4	0.22	1.21	922	BMI (kg/m^2)
0.81	0.004	1.06	268	0.79	0.002	1.10	921	Waist to hip ratio
								Blood pressure
133	1.3	1.12	260	122	0.6	1.15	897	Systolic blood pressure (mmHg)
72	0.6	0.98	260	68	0.4	1.05	897	Diastolic blood pressure (mmHg)

Table A3(a)

True standard errors and design factors for selected blood analytes by age of respondent: men

Blood analytes	Men aged (years):											
	19–24				25–34				35–49			
	Mean r	Standard error of r	Design factor	Base	Mean r	Standard error of r	Design factor	Base	Mean r	Standard error of r	Design factor	Base
Haemoglobin concentration (g/dl)	15.2	0.14	1.39	83	15.1	0.10	1.21	170	15.1	0.07	0.99	191
Mean cell volume (fl)	91.0	0.74	1.34	83	90.9	0.40	1.02	170	93.3	0.54	1.24	191
Haematocrit (l/l)	0.460	0.0047	1.39	83	0.457	0.0032	1.25	170	0.460	0.0031	1.19	191
Plasma iron (μmol/l)	17.8	1.03	1.39	81	16.2	0.55	1.22	165	17.3	0.35	0.88	190
Total iron-binding capacity (μmol/l)	61.8	1.33	1.44	81	61.8	0.93	1.28	165	61.2	0.52	0.90	188
Iron % saturation (%)	29.7	2.09	1.44	81	26.6	0.89	1.17	165	28.5	0.64	0.94	188
Serum ferritin (μg/l)	78	5.2	1.39	85	101	5.6	1.41	169	129	7.9	0.99	186
Plasma vitamin C (μmol/l)	54.6	4.22	1.54	79	54.2	2.79	1.35	156	50.0	1.47	0.87	180
Red cell folate (nmol/l)	561	37.9	1.33	83	688	28.6	1.33	170	677	16.8	0.95	189
Serum folate (nmol/l)	17.4	1.05	1.36	83	20.1	0.81	1.29	169	20.9	0.51	0.88	188
Serum vitamin B$_{12}$ (pmol/l)	286	17.0	1.41	84	298	10.6	1.35	168	294	8.4	1.07	187
ETKAC(ratio)*	1.16	0.007	1.59	83	1.16	0.004	1.16	164	1.15	0.003	0.92	189
ETK-B (μmol/g Hb/min)**	0.70	0.019	1.66	83	0.73	0.017	1.48	167	0.71	0.008	0.91	191
EGRAC(ratio)***	1.45	0.020	1.39	83	1.40	0.018	1.40	167	1.37	0.012	0.98	191
EAATAC(ratio)****	1.81	0.023	1.58	83	1.81	0.014	1.16	167	1.80	0.013	0.90	191
Plasma total homocysteine (μmol/l)	12.5	0.86	1.46	81	11.1	0.38	1.23	162	11.1	0.19	0.77	179
Plasma retinol (μmol/l)	1.81	0.078	1.51	75	1.94	0.052	1.41	152	2.08	0.047	1.13	175
Plasma α-carotene (μmol/l)	0.039	0.0027	1.39	75	0.059	0.0036	1.36	152	0.067	0.0074	1.08	175
Plasma β-carotene (μmol/l)	0.143	0.0206	1.34	75	0.209	0.0171	1.38	152	0.221	0.0211	1.16	175
Plasma α-cryptoxanthin (μmol/l)	0.052	0.0129	1.18	75	0.047	0.0060	1.31	152	0.039	0.0033	1.05	175
Plasma β-cryptoxanthin (μmol/l)	0.103	0.0092	1.48	75	0.122	0.0080	1.20	152	0.119	0.0056	0.91	175
Plasma lycopene (μmol/l)	0.442	0.0467	1.45	75	0.514	0.0372	1.48	152	0.487	0.0302	1.29	175
Plasma lutein and zeaxanthin (μmol/l)	0.20	0.013	1.39	75	0.26	0.013	1.24	152	0.28	0.011	0.98	175
Plasma 25-hydroxyvitamin D (nmol/l)	40.6	3.77	1.56	81	48.8	2.57	1.42	165	47.8	1.83	1.21	190
Plasma α-tocopherol (μmol/l)	16.6	0.91	1.42	75	19.7	0.54	1.27	152	22.0	0.54	0.95	175
Plasma γ-tocopherol (μmol/l)	1.09	0.065	1.45	75	1.25	0.040	1.32	152	1.29	0.027	0.96	175
Plasma α-tocopherol to total cholesterol ratio (μmol/mmol)	3.76	0.131	1.40	81	3.97	0.112	1.37	156	4.11	0.107	1.08	170
Plasma total cholesterol (mmol/l)	4.40	0.134	1.45	81	5.04	0.112	1.26	164	5.38	0.070	0.84	186
Plasma high density lipoprotein cholesterol (mmol/l)	1.06	0.036	1.48	81	1.04	0.024	1.25	164	1.04	0.022	1.01	186
Plasma low density lipoprotein cholesterol (mmol/l)*****	3.35	0.140	1.44	81	4.00	0.117	1.28	164	4.34	0.069	0.81	186
Plasma selenium (μmol/l)	1.03	0.027	1.66	83	1.10	0.016	1.27	169	1.13	0.014	1.05	190
Red cell selenium (μmol/l)	1.39	0.055	1.50	83	1.57	0.030	1.10	169	1.62	0.029	0.97	190
Blood glutathione peroxidase (nmol/mg Hb/min)	118.5	3.97	1.49	81	119.5	2.78	1.30	163	123.4	3.70	1.62	184
Plasma α$_1$-antichymotrypsin (g/l)	0.28	0.011	1.47	81	0.29	0.006	1.08	162	0.29	0.004	0.79	179
Blood mercury (nmol/l)	3.8	0.58	1.24	81	6.3	0.48	1.23	169	8.7	0.74	1.18	190

Note: *   erythrocyte transketolase activation coefficient.

   **   erythrocyte transketolase basal activity.

   ***   erythrocyte glutathione reductase activation coefficient.

   ****   erythrocyte aspartate aminotransferase activation coefficient.

   ***** calculated as non-high density lipoprotein cholesterol (non-HDL).

Numbers

Blood analytes

50–64				All men				
Mean r	Standard error of r	Design factor	Base	Mean r	Standard error of r	Design factor	Base	
14.9	0.09	1.23	194	15.1	0.05	1.26	638	Haemoglobin concentration (g/dl)
95.0	0.46	1.16	194	92.9	0.29	1.26	638	Mean cell volume (fl)
0.460	0.0032	1.31	194	0.459	0.0020	1.47	638	Haematocrit (l/l)
17.1	0.53	1.11	190	17.0	0.30	1.26	627	Plasma iron (μmol/l)
61.5	0.65	1.00	189	61.5	0.37	1.07	624	Total iron-binding capacity (μmol/l)
28.2	0.79	1.09	189	28.1	0.53	1.28	624	Iron % saturation (%)
145	12.2	1.08	194	120	5.6	1.25	633	Serum ferritin (μg/l)
51.6	2.14	1.03	178	52.2	1.18	1.13	593	Plasma vitamin C (μmol/l)
773	28.9	1.26	194	694	12.1	1.06	636	Red cell folate (nmol/l)
22.9	0.79	1.19	196	20.8	0.39	1.16	636	Serum folate (nmol/l)
308	11.7	1.05	193	298	6.3	1.28	632	Serum vitamin B$_{12}$ (pmol/l)
1.15	0.005	1.01	192	1.15	0.003	1.26	628	ETKAC(ratio)*
0.73	0.009	1.23	192	0.72	0.007	1.47	633	ETK-B (μmol/g Hb/min)**
1.35	0.014	1.17	192	1.38	0.008	1.19	633	EGRAC(ratio)***
1.77	0.015	0.99	192	1.79	0.007	1.04	633	EAATAC(ratio)****
12.4	0.42	1.03	181	11.7	0.20	1.06	603	Plasma total homocysteine (μmol/l)
2.13	0.049	1.14	175	2.02	0.031	1.41	576	Plasma retinol (μmol/l)
0.074	0.0041	1.18	175	0.064	0.003	1.20	576	Plasma α-carotene (μmol/l)
0.248	0.0187	1.15	175	0.216	0.0124	1.47	576	Plasma β-carotene (μmol/l)
0.035	0.0036	1.28	175	0.041	0.0033	1.44	576	Plasma α-cryptoxanthin (μmol/l)
0.119	0.0073	1.15	175	0.118	0.0043	1.31	576	Plasma β-cryptoxanthin (μmol/l)
0.416	0.0264	1.25	175	0.467	0.0225	1.81	576	Plasma lycopene (μmol/l)
0.30	0.013	1.08	175	0.27	0.007	1.22	576	Plasma lutein and zeaxanthin (μmol/l)
51.6	1.70	1.11	190	48.3	1.35	1.54	627	Plasma 25-hydroxyvitamin D (nmol/l)
23.3	0.62	1.12	175	21.1	0.38	1.29	576	Plasma α-tocopherol (μmol/l)
1.31	0.030	1.10	175	1.26	0.021	1.32	576	Plasma γ-tocopherol (μmol/l)
4.22	0.102	1.21	173	4.06	0.071	1.53	580	Plasma α-tocopherol to total cholesterol ratio (μmol/mmol)
5.56	0.099	1.21	187	5.21	0.053	1.14	618	Plasma total cholesterol (mmol/l)
1.12	0.038	1.28	186	1.07	0.015	1.19	617	Plasma high density lipoprotein cholesterol (mmol/l)
4.44	0.101	1.21	187	4.15	0.052	1.11	618	Plasma low density lipoprotein cholesterol (mmol/l)*****
1.15	0.013	0.92	195	1.11	0.008	1.15	636	Plasma selenium (μmol/l)
1.61	0.038	1.20	195	1.57	0.020	1.24	638	Red cell selenium (μmol/l)
124.1	2.57	1.20	187	121.9	2.26	1.95	615	Blood glutathione peroxidase (nmol/mg Hb/min)
0.31	0.006	0.96	181	0.30	0.003	1.13	603	Plasma α$_1$-antichymotrypsin (g/l)
9.0	0.71	1.19	195	7.5	0.34	1.14	636	Blood mercury (nmol/l)

Table A3(b)

True standard errors and design factors for selected blood analytes by age of respondent: women

Blood analytes	Women aged (years):											
	19–24				25–34				35–49			
	Mean r	Standard error of r	Design factor	Base	Mean r	Standard error of r	Design factor	Base	Mean r	Standard error of r	Design factor	Base
Haemoglobin concentration (g/dl)	13.5	0.16	1.38	81	13.3	0.08	1.15	162	13.3	0.07	1.08	243
Mean cell volume (fl)	92.8	1.10	1.48	81	92.7	0.65	1.37	162	93.9	0.45	1.07	243
Haematocrit (l/l)	0.416	0.0056	1.36	81	0.411	0.0032	1.30	162	0.411	0.0022	1.10	243
Plasma iron (μmol/l)	15.6	1.02	1.37	77	16.5	0.58	1.02	158	15.9	0.41	0.96	238
Total iron-binding capacity (μmol/l)	66.1	1.44	1.44	77	66.8	0.92	1.02	158	62.8	0.7	1.07	238
Iron % saturation (%)	24.3	1.79	1.41	77	25.3	0.93	1.02	158	26.1	0.77	1.06	238
Serum ferritin (μg/l)	41	4.0	1.36	80	43	2.9	1.19	156	49	2.8	0.92	238
Plasma vitamin C (μmol/l)	60.1	3.25	1.18	72	62.9	2.82	1.16	151	58.8	2.13	1.23	234
Red cell folate (nmol/l)	576	33.4	1.56	81	630	24.7	1.14	161	691	19.6	1.04	243
Serum folate (nmol/l)	20.6	1.23	1.39	81	21.2	0.97	1.11	159	21.9	0.6	1.04	240
Serum vitamin B$_{12}$ (pmol/l)	247	13.6	1.33	79	259	11.6	1.20	158	288	8.6	0.91	239
ETKAC (ratio)*	1.14	0.005	1.26	74	1.15	0.004	0.96	162	1.14	0.004	1.04	241
ETK-B (μmol/g Hb/min)**	0.79	0.017	1.35	74	0.76	0.014	1.40	162	0.74	0.01	1.18	242
EGRAC (ratio)***	1.45	0.029	1.28	74	1.44	0.016	1.12	162	1.40	0.015	1.15	242
EAATAC (ratio)****	1.74	0.031	1.46	74	1.78	0.016	1.18	162	1.77	0.017	1.14	242
Plasma total homocysteine (μmol/l)	9.3	0.57	1.30	77	9.6	0.29	1.24	154	10.4	0.37	0.86	233
Plasma retinol (μmol/l)	1.75	0.070	1.41	72	1.75	0.044	1.17	146	1.75	0.026	0.97	219
Plasma α-carotene (μmol/l)	0.048	0.0039	1.48	72	0.075	0.0082	1.09	146	0.080	0.0045	1.16	219
Plasma β-carotene (μmol/l)	0.233	0.0737	1.31	72	0.245	0.0304	1.08	146	0.301	0.0216	1.21	219
Plasma α-cryptoxanthin (μmol/l)	0.034	0.0026	1.32	72	0.039	0.0041	1.30	146	0.037	0.0031	1.10	219
Plasma β-cryptoxanthin (μmol/l)	0.123	0.0170	1.69	72	0.141	0.0096	1.10	146	0.134	0.0062	0.96	219
Plasma lycopene (μmol/l)	0.452	0.0504	1.50	72	0.426	0.0252	1.10	146	0.474	0.0204	1.14	219
Plasma lutein and zeaxanthin (μmol/l)	0.26	0.022	1.49	72	0.25	0.010	1.08	146	0.27	0.01	1.17	219
Plasma 25-hydroxyvitamin D (nmol/l)	44.5	3.85	1.44	78	51.9	2.80	1.31	158	47.9	1.62	1.10	239
Plasma α-tocopherol (μmol/l)	16.6	0.73	1.37	72	17.8	0.38	0.98	146	20.3	0.34	0.91	219
Plasma γ-tocopherol (μmol/l)	1.16	0.109	1.58	72	1.14	0.032	1.27	146	1.24	0.028	1.01	219
Plasma α-tocopherol to total cholesterol ratio (μmol/mmol)	3.69	0.132	1.43	72	3.71	0.078	1.09	149	4.03	0.067	0.98	222
Plasma total cholesterol (mmol/l)	4.46	0.122	1.35	77	4.84	0.076	0.99	157	5.13	0.059	0.91	234
Plasma high density lipoprotein cholesterol (mmol/l)	1.21	0.042	1.41	77	1.26	0.028	1.11	157	1.27	0.03	1.16	234
Plasma low density lipoprotein cholesterol (mmol/l)*****	3.26	0.110	1.29	77	3.57	0.080	1.02	157	3.85	0.065	0.99	234
Plasma selenium (μmol/l)	1.03	0.024	1.40	76	1.07	0.018	1.11	159	1.09	0.013	1.16	244
Red cell selenium (μmol/l)	1.76	0.053	1.34	78	1.80	0.043	1.17	160	1.76	0.032	0.99	246
Blood glutathione peroxidase (nmol/mg Hb/min)	134.0	6.27	1.49	74	122.5	2.98	1.25	161	126.8	3.02	1.46	237
Plasma α$_1$-antichymotrypsin (g/l)	0.29	0.011	1.36	77	0.30	0.006	1.22	154	0.31	0.004	0.97	233
Blood mercury (nmol/l)	6.1	0.85	1.27	80	7.2	0.75	1.28	160	8.6	0.44	0.97	246

Note: *   erythrocyte transketolase activation coefficient.

      **   erythrocyte transketolase basal activity.

      ***   erythrocyte glutathione reductase activation coefficient.

      ****   erythrocyte aspartate aminotransferase activation coefficient.

      ***** calculated as non-high density lipoprotein cholesterol (non-HDL).

Numbers

Blood analytes

50–64				All women				
Mean r	Standard error of r	Design factor	Base	Mean r	Standard error of r	Design factor	Base	
13.5	0.09	1.10	196	13.4	0.05	1.21	683	Haemoglobin concentration (g/dl)
93.7	0.47	1.11	196	93.4	0.31	1.27	683	Mean cell volume (fl)
0.417	0.0029	1.14	196	0.413	0.0017	1.36	683	Haematocrit (l/l)
16.3	0.46	1.16	194	16.1	0.29	1.17	668	Plasma iron (μmol/l)
61.7	0.90	1.29	193	63.8	0.42	1.06	666	Total iron-binding capacity (μmol/l)
27.1	0.86	1.22	192	26.0	0.49	1.17	665	Iron % saturation (%)
71	4.2	1.08	195	53	1.7	0.95	670	Serum ferritin (μg/l)
62.2	2.18	1.10	188	60.9	1.33	1.24	644	Plasma vitamin C (μmol/l)
768	24.1	1.07	197	685	12.4	1.11	683	Red cell folate (nmol/l)
23.7	0.62	0.96	197	22.1	0.44	1.20	678	Serum folate (nmol/l)
329	25.4	1.28	191	288	9.2	1.28	667	Serum vitamin B$_{12}$ (pmol/l)
1.13	0.003	0.81	195	1.14	0.002	0.89	672	ETKAC (ratio)*
0.77	0.010	1.11	195	0.76	0.007	1.46	673	ETK-B (μmol/g Hb/min)**
1.34	0.013	1.02	195	1.40	0.009	1.21	673	EGRAC (ratio)***
1.79	0.023	1.32	195	1.77	0.012	1.45	673	EAATAC (ratio)****
10.6	0.27	1.11	190	10.1	0.18	0.97	654	Plasma total homocysteine (μmol/l)
1.99	0.050	1.07	179	1.82	0.026	1.29	616	Plasma retinol (μmol/l)
0.101	0.0069	0.90	179	0.081	0.0028	0.85	616	Plasma α-carotene (μmol/l)
0.384	0.0247	0.98	179	0.304	0.0179	1.31	616	Plasma β-carotene (μmol/l)
0.032	0.0026	1.10	179	0.035	0.0021	1.46	616	Plasma α-cryptoxanthin (μmol/l)
0.181	0.0149	1.12	179	0.148	0.0062	1.20	616	Plasma β-cryptoxanthin (μmol/l)
0.484	0.0269	1.09	179	0.463	0.0170	1.45	616	Plasma lycopene (μmol/l)
0.37	0.019	1.17	179	0.29	0.008	1.24	616	Plasma lutein and zeaxanthin (μmol/l)
51.8	1.94	1.20	194	49.6	1.34	1.44	670	Plasma 25-hydroxyvitamin D (nmol/l)
24.7	0.49	0.99	179	20.6	0.26	1.01	616	Plasma α-tocopherol (μmol/l)
1.24	0.032	1.10	179	1.21	0.021	1.30	616	Plasma γ-tocopherol (μmol/l)
4.17	0.101	1.11	183	3.96	0.054	1.28	626	Plasma α-tocopherol to total cholesterol ratio (μmol/mmol)
6.06	0.086	0.98	192	5.25	0.038	0.83	659	Plasma total cholesterol (mmol/l)
1.34	0.029	1.00	192	1.28	0.015	1.06	659	Plasma high density lipoprotein cholesterol (mmol/l)
4.72	0.086	0.97	192	3.97	0.041	0.90	659	Plasma low density lipoprotein cholesterol (mmol/l)*****
1.17	0.029	1.21	195	1.10	0.011	1.17	674	Plasma selenium (μmol/l)
1.79	0.070	1.15	198	1.78	0.026	1.12	681	Red cell selenium (μmol/l)
129.2	2.45	1.21	188	127.2	2.12	1.75	661	Blood glutathione peroxidase (nmol/mg Hb/min)
0.34	0.006	1.08	190	0.31	0.003	1.18	654	Plasma α$_1$-antichymotrypsin (g/l)
10.6	1.49	1.31	198	8.6	0.54	1.34	683	Blood mercury (nmol/l)

Table A4

True standard errors and design factors for measures of physical activity by sex and age of respondent

Physical activity diary sample

Measures of physical activity	Age (years):											
	19–24				25–34				35–49			
	Mean r	Standard error of r	Design factor	*Base*	Mean r	Standard error of r	Design factor	*Base*	Mean r	Standard error of r	Design factor	*Base*
Men												
Hours spent in activities of at least moderate intensity per day	2.86	0.401	1.37	*104*	2.69	0.267	1.25	*211*	2.01	0.198	1.10	*243*
Hours spent in activities of vigorous intensity per day	0.67	0.215	1.33	*104*	0.82	0.191	1.32	*211*	0.55	0.114	1.05	*243*
Women												
Hours spent in activities of at least moderate intensity per day	1.27	0.188	1.07	*100*	1.34	0.14	1.04	*202*	1.24	0.121	1.13	*305*
Hours spent in activities of vigorous intensity per day	0.17	0.04	1.31	*100*	0.10	0.02	1.00	*202*	0.09	0.02	0.82	*305*

Numbers

Measures of physical activity

50–64				All				
Mean r	Standard error or r	Design factor	*Base*	Mean r	Standard error of r	Design factor	*Base*	
								Men
								Hours spent in activities of at least
1.52	0.201	1.28	*243*	2.15	0.127	1.26	*801*	moderate intensity per day
								Hours spent in activities of vigorous
0.25	0.090	1.27	*243*	0.55	0.077	1.30	*801*	intensity per day
								Women
								Hours spent in activities of at least
0.97	0.113	1.17	*249*	1.19	0.072	1.18	*857*	moderate intensity per day
								Hours spent in activities of vigorous
0.05	0.010	1.12	*249*	0.09	0.008	0.85	*857*	intensity per day

Appendix B   Unweighted base numbers

Table B1

Unweighted base numbers: dietary interview, seven–day dietary record and physical activity record by sex of respondent

	Dietary interview	Seven–day weighed dietary record	Seven–day physical activity record
Age			
Men aged (years):			
19–24	86	61	61
25–34	219	160	155
35–49	394	303	296
50–64	309	242	229
All men	1008	766	741
Women aged (years):			
19–24	109	78	75
25–34	277	211	206
35–49	487	379	358
50–64	370	290	278
All women	1243	958	917
Region			
Men			
Scotland	80	53	47
Northern	267	195	191
Central, South West and Wales	337	274	262
London and the South East	324	244	241
Women			
Scotland	111	70	69
Northern	341	256	248
Central, South West and Wales	436	350	330
London and the South East	355	282	270
Household receipt of benefits*			
Men			
Receiving benefits	145	106	102
Not receiving benefits	863	660	639
Women			
Receiving benefits	283	199	193
Not receiving benefits	960	759	724
All	**2251**	**1724**	**1658**

Note: * Receipt of benefits was asked of the respondent about themselves, their partner or anyone else in the household. Benefits asked about were Working Families Tax Credit, Income Support and (Income–related) Job Seeker's Allowance.

Table B2

Unweighted base numbers: anthropometry and blood pressure by sex of respondent

	Height	Weight	BMI	Waist circumference	Hip circumference and waist to hip ratio	Blood pressure
Age						
Men aged (years):						
19–24	65	65	64	64	64	62
25–34	171	170	169	170	170	168
35–49	329	330	328	328	328	324
50–64	249	250	249	246	246	243
All men	814	815	810	808	808	797
Women aged (years):						
19–24	82	82	82	82	82	80
25–34	217	214	212	213	213	210
35–49	391	395	391	387	387	373
50–64	295	295	293	293	292	276
All women	985	986	978	975	974	939
Region						
Men						
Scotland	52	52	52	52	52	51
Northern	212	212	210	210	210	207
Central, South West and Wales	290	291	290	287	287	286
London and the South East	260	260	258	259	259	253
Women						
Scotland	75	73	73	71	71	70
Northern	268	268	267	264	264	254
Central, South West and Wales	353	352	349	349	348	342
London and the South East	289	293	289	291	291	273
Household receipt of benefits*						
Men						
Receiving benefits	115	117	115	115	115	116
Not receiving benefits	699	698	695	693	693	681
Women						
Receiving benefits	214	214	211	211	210	208
Not receiving benefits	771	772	767	764	764	731
All	**1799**	**1801**	**1788**	**1783**	**1782**	**1736**

Note: * Receipt of benefits was asked of the respondent about themselves, their partner or anyone else in the household. Benefits asked about were Working Families Tax Credit, Income Support and (Income–related) Job Seeker's Allowance.

Table B3

Unweighted base numbers: blood analytes by sex of respondent

	Blood sample*		
	Plasma retinol	Haemoglobin	Plasma iron
Age			
Men aged (years):			
19–24	45	45	45
25–34	107	119	115
35–49	213	245	243
50–64	168	191	189
All men	533	600	592
Women aged (years):			
19–24	44	53	47
25–34	146	157	154
35–49	278	298	296
50–64	191	210	206
All women	659	718	703
Region			
Men			
Scotland	45	45	46
Northern	140	155	148
Central, South West and Wales	191	211	214
London and the South East	157	189	184
Women			
Scotland	46	50	48
Northern	177	191	189
Central, South West and Wales	245	272	263
London and the South East	191	157	203
Household receipt of benefits**			
Men			
Receiving benefits	76	85	84
Not receiving benefits	457	515	508
Women			
Receiving benefits	149	162	159
Not receiving benefits	510	556	544
All	**1192**	**1318**	**1295**

Note:*   Blood analytes shown are those used to derive weighting factors for groups of analytes with similar numbers of reported results.
** Receipt of benefits was asked of the respondent about themselves, their partner or anyone else in the household. Benefits asked about were Working Families Tax Credit, Income Support and (Income–related) Job Seeker's Allowance.

Appendix C Weights for results from analysis of blood samples

Weights were derived for results from the analysis of blood samples. Three weighting factors were calculated based on similar numbers of reported results for different analytes and similarity of socio-demographic characteristics.

The three groups were as follows:

Group 1: Non-response weight based on the number of haemoglobin results

Applies to:

> Haemoglobin
> Mean corpuscular volume (MCV)
> Haematocrit
> Serum ferritin
> Plasma vitamin C
> Red cell folate
> Serum folate
> Serum vitamin B_{12}
> Erythrocyte Transketolase Activation Coefficient (ETKAC)
> Erythrocyte Transketolase Basal Activity (ETK-B)
> Erythrocyte Glutathione Reductase Activation Coefficient (EGRAC)
> Erythrocyte Aspartate Aminotransferase Activation Coefficient (EAATAC)
> Plasma selenium
> Red cell selenium
> Erythrocyte glutathione peroxidase
> Blood mercury

Group 2: Non-response weight based on the number of results for plasma iron

Applies to:

> Plasma iron
> Plasma total iron-binding capacity (TIBC)
> Plasma iron % saturation
> Plasma total homocysteine
> Plasma 25-hydroxyvitamin D (25-OHD)
> Plasma α-tocopherol to total cholesterol ratio
> Plasma total cholesterol
> HDL cholesterol
> LDL cholesterol
> Plasma α_1-antichymotrypsin (α_1 - ACT)

Group 3: Non-response weight based on the number of plasma retinol results

Applies to:

Plasma retinol
Plasma α-carotene
Plasma β-carotene
Plasma α-cryptoxanthin
Plasma β-cryptoxanthin
Plasma lycopene
Plasma lutein and zeaxanthin
Plasma α-tocopherol
Plasma γ-tocopherol

Appendix D   Physical activity

1   Introduction

This appendix describes the editing of the physical activity data, data quality and provides additional information on the derived measures of physical activity. Details of the methodology for collecting information on physical activity are given in Chapter 1 of this report and in Appendix I of the Technical Report[1].

2   Editing the data on physical activities

Interviewers entered the physical activity diary data into their laptop computer and internal consistency checks were applied to avoid mis-keying, for example to check that the time spent in all activities did not add up to more than 24 hours. Data were subsequently assessed at HQ on a number of criteria.

The following checks were carried out on all physical activity diaries.

- Coding of occupation activity level.

- Time went to bed and got up on any diary day.

- Correct use of 24-hour clock, particularly in recording time went to bed/ got up on any diary day.

- If less than one hour or more than 12 hours of sleep were recorded on any diary day.

- If less than 60 minutes of very light/light activity was calculated on any diary day.

- If the time spent in any 'other' activity was greater than 3 hours.

- Any recorded activities less than 10 minutes.

Respondents were asked during the post-dietary recording period interview whether they had done any paid or voluntary work during the recording period and, if so, what tasks were involved in this work. The activity level was then coded according to whether it involved very light/light work, e.g. mainly sitting, standing or walking, the use of light tools, light assembly or repair, but no heavy lifting or carrying; moderate work, e.g. mainly walking, lifting or carrying light loads; or hard/very hard work, e.g. mainly hard physical labour. All occupations that were coded as moderate or hard/very hard were checked for accuracy of coding against the Physical Activity Diary Coding Guide for Occupations (*see* Appendix I of the Technical Report[1]). This led to a downward revision of the activity code for main occupation in 184 of 812 cases (23%) and for the second occupation in 15 of 54 cases (28%). If the respondent did not complete the post-dietary interview or did not answer the questions on occupation activity level, their occupation activity level was coded at HQ using information on industry and occupation collected during the dietary interview, in line with the Physical Activity Diary Coding Guide for Occupations.

The time the respondent went to bed and got up each day is required in order to calculate time spent sleeping. All cases were checked for completeness of this information. If time went to bed and/or time got up was missing an estimate was made based on the time recorded for other days in the diary. In total, 12 cases were missing this information on at least one day. Where information about sleep was missing for more than two days of the seven-day recording period, this case was checked for completeness of other information, for example, whether the respondent went to work, how long they spent at work, participation in activities. In two cases, there appeared to be no data recorded and the case was removed from analysis of physical activity data. In seven cases, the time went to bed on one of the diary days was equal to the time recorded for getting up. In five of the seven cases, this was due to a data keying error. In the other two cases the respondent was working shifts and as they had slept during the day had recorded their time sleeping under the question 'spent any other time asleep today' and then recorded the same time for going to bed and getting up. In 495 cases the time the respondent went to bed on the last day of the recording period was not recorded on the diary. Values were imputed based on the time the respondent recorded going to bed over the preceding seven days.

All cases were checked for appropriate use of the 24-hour clock. In 30 cases, the data entered for the time the respondent went to bed and got up, along with other information on activity, suggested that the 24-hour clock had not been used. For example, where the time went to bed last night was entered as 11:30, but the time he/she got up was entered as 7:00. In such cases the time went to bed was changed to reflect the 24-hour clock.

If the time recorded participating in any activity on any day of the diary was less than 10 minutes then this was checked for accuracy of keying[2]. If the figure had been keyed correctly then this entry was deleted.

The time spent in very light/light activities is calculated as the time leftover from 24 hours after time spent sleeping and time spent in moderate and vigorous/very vigorous activities is deducted. In 25 cases the derived time spent in very light/light activities was less than 60 minutes. In the majority of these cases, this was due to errors in data keying, for example, 600 minutes brisk walking entered instead of 60 minutes, or to duplication in recorded activities, for example, someone who worked as a childminder recording eight hours at work and also eight hours active childcare for the same day. Duplication errors were most frequent where time spent at work was entered both for work and either a prompted activity or an 'other' activity, or where time spent in an activity was recorded both for a prompted

activity and an 'other' activity. Entries were only edited where duplication was clear and in deciding which entry to delete priority was given firstly to time at work and then to activities which were on the prompted list.

All 'other' household and sports activities were checked. Where possible, 'other' activities were recoded into the prompted list of activities. 'Other' activities that were coded to the wrong intensity level were recoded to the correct level and those that were not of at least moderate intensity were deleted. Most wrongly categorised activities over-estimated the intensity level, for example, including time spent shopping as a moderate or vigorous activity when it should have been coded as a light activity.

After editing, 'other' activities that remained, included:

- less common sports activities, for example, canoeing, horse riding;

- playing with or exercising pets, in particular dogs;

- active hobbies, for example, woodwork, bell ringing.

3   Data quality

After editing, some preliminary analysis was carried out to investigate the quality of the final information on activities. Figures D1 and D2 show the mean number of different activities of at least moderate intensity participated in by diary day and day of the week respectively. Figure D1 shows that the mean number of activities recorded decreased over the seven days of record keeping, with the greatest mean number of activities recorded on Day 1 and the fewest recorded on Day 5. This suggests possible over-reporting of physical activity in the first few days of recording. Figure D2 shows that on average more activities of at least moderate intensity were recorded on Tuesdays, Wednesdays and Fridays than were recorded on other days of the week. The lowest mean number of activities was recorded on Sundays.

Although there was no strict protocol for which days the diaries were started, practical fieldwork reasons meant that diaries were less likely to be started on weekend days than on weekdays. Analysis showed that Day 1 of record keeping was most frequently a Tuesday (22%), Wednesday (21%) or Thursday (20%) and least frequently a Monday (7%) or Sunday (3%) (table not shown).

Figures D1 and D2 therefore suggest either that respondents were more active mid-week compared with the weekend or that as the seven-day recording period progressed they tended to omit to record all their activities.

4   Derived measures of physical activity

Two measures of level of physical activity were derived from the available data; the mean hours spent in activities of at least moderate intensity per day and the calculated activity score. These measures are derived in part from information on duration of activity. Any upward rounding of activity time will therefore result in an overestimate of energy expenditure as represented by the calculated activity score. However, this may in part be offset by any under-recording of the number of activities participated in.

4.1   Calculating time spent in activities of moderate and vigorous/very vigorous intensity

In order to collect data on activities of moderate and vigorous/very vigorous intensity, the diary page provided a list of common activities against which the respondent could record any time spent that day. Activities were grouped according to whether they were household activities (including walking) or sports activities. Respondents were able to record activities participated in that were not already listed, prompts were provided to establish the intensity level involved.

On each diary day respondents were asked if they had gone to work and the hours worked per day were recorded. The activity level of the respondent's occupation was recorded during the post-dietary recording period interview.

To allow comparisons between the activity of respondents in the present NDNS, the Department of Health recommendations and data from the Health Survey for England, the time spent in all activities of moderate, vigorous and very vigorous intensity was combined to give the category 'at least moderate intensity'.

4.2   Calculating the activity score

For all respondents for whom physical activity data were available, a physical activity score was calculated using data on intensity and duration of activity following the procedure proposed by Blair (1984) for the 7-Day Recall Physical Activity Questionnaire[3]. These data were added to the database but the results are not presented in Chapter 5. This is because the results suggest

that when compared to the physical activity data derived from the mean hours spent in activities of at least moderate intensity per day, the activity score overestimates the level of physical activity for this dataset.

The advantage of the calculated activity score method is that since very light/light activity is obtained by subtraction from 24 hours, most individuals have to account only for time spent asleep and for relatively brief periods of time engaged in moderate and vigorous/very vigorous activities. The assumption underlying the calculation of the activity score is that most adults spend most of their waking hours in light activity.

Activities can be classified by their 'energy cost' measured in metabolic equivalents (METs[4]) into the following intensity levels:

Sleep	= average 1.0 MET
Very light/light activity	= average 2.0 METs (e.g. sitting, watching television, light household chores)
Moderate activity	= average 4.0 METs (e.g. heavy household chores, badminton, swimming)
Vigorous/very vigorous	= average 7.5 METs (e.g. basketball, athletics)

Resting metabolism, defined as 1 MET, is approximately equal to an energy expenditure of one kilocalorie (kcal) per kilogram per hour (kcal/kg/hour). For adults an average body weight of 60kg is assumed and therefore for an average adult 1 MET is equal to 60kcal/hour or 1kcal/min. For adults METs are therefore taken as numerically equivalent to energy expenditure. An example of how the calculated activity score is derived for one day is given in table D1.

The score is derived by multiplying the duration of each activity (hours) by the average MET score for the intensity of the activity. The total for each day is taken and the average daily total energy expenditure calculated.

As with the previous NDNS survey of younger people[5], the categories 'very light' and 'light' have been combined into a single 'very light/light'

Table D1   Example of calculated activity score for one day:

Type of activity	Total time spent (hours)	MET value for the type of activity	Activity score
Sleep	9.0	1.0	9.00
Very light/light activities	13.5	2.0	27.00
Moderate activities	1.0	4.0	4.00
Vigorous/very vigorous activities	0.5	7.5	3.75
Total	24.0		43.75

category. In the current survey, the categories vigorous and very vigorous have also been combined into a 'vigorous/very vigorous' category. This approach is suggested by Blair (1984) for simplified self-administered physical activity instruments[3]. The MET values for the categories are calculated as an average for the activities corresponding to that category. For example, vigorous/very vigorous activities have MET values ranging from 6.0 to 10.0. An average of 7.5 was taken based on the type of activities that could be coded as vigorous/very vigorous.

For adults, calculated activity scores of 40 or above indicate a relatively active lifestyle, scores in the mid to high 30s indicate an inactive lifestyle and those in the low 30s indicate a very inactive lifestyle[3]. Overall, 84% of men and 74% of women in this NDNS had a calculated activity score indicative of a relatively active lifestyle, and no men and less than 0.5% of women an inactive lifestyle (data not shown).

References and endnotes

[1]   The Technical Report is available online at http://www.food.gov.uk/science.

[2]   Respondents were asked to record only activities they had done for at least 10 minutes. Time was recorded to the nearest 10 minutes.

[3]   Blair SN. How to assess exercise habits and physical fitness. In: Matarazzo JD et al. Eds. *Behavioural Health: A Handbook of Health Enhancement and Disease Prevention.* Wiley & Sons (New York, 1984).

[4]   A MET is a multiple of the resting rate of oxygen consumption, or the ratio of working metabolic rate to resting metabolic rate (WMR/RMR). One MET represents the resting metabolic rate, so that an individual participating in physical activity at 2 METs is consuming oxygen at twice the resting rate.

[5]   Gregory J, Lowe S, Bates CJ, Prentice A, Jackson LV, Smithers G, Wenlock R, Farron M. *National Diet and Nutrition Survey: young people aged 4 to 18 years. Volume 1: Report of the diet and nutrition survey.* TSO (London, 2000).

Figure D1

The mean number of activities of at least moderate intensity in which respondents participated by diary day

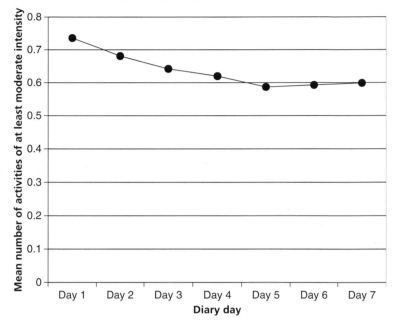

Figure D2

The mean number of activities of at least moderate intensity in which respondents participated by the day of the week

Appendix E   Glossary of abbreviations, terms and survey definitions

ANOVA	Analysis of variance. This identifies those factors which are independently associated with the variable of interest by allowing the effect on the variable of a number of characteristics to be considered simultaneously. It identifies those characteristics and factors which explain a significant amount of the total variation in the variable of interest after allowing for the other variables.
Benefits (receiving)	Receipt of Working Families Tax Credit by the respondent or anyone in their household at the time of the interview, or receipt of Income Support, or (Income-related) Job Seeker's Allowance by the respondent or anyone in their household in the 14 days prior to the date of interview.
BMI	*See* Body Mass Index
Body Mass Index	A measure of body 'fatness' which standardises weight for height: calculated as [weight(kg)/ height(m^2)]. Also known as the Quetelet Index.
COMA	The Committee on Medical Aspects of Food and Nutrition Policy.
CAPI	Computer assisted personal interviewing.
CASI	Computer assisted self-interviewing. The respondent is given the opportunity to enter their responses directly onto the laptop. This technique is used to collect data of a sensitive or personal nature, for example, information on contraception.
Cum %	Cumulative percentage (of a distribution).
Deft	Design factor; *see* Notes to Tables and Appendix A.
DH	The Department of Health.
Diary sample	Respondents for whom a seven-day dietary record was obtained.
Doubly labelled water method (DLW)	A method for assessing total energy expenditure, used to validate dietary assessment methods by comparison with estimated energy intake. The respondent drinks a measured dose of water labelled with the stable isotopes $^2H_2$ and ^{18}O and collects urine samples over the next 10 to 15 days. Energy expenditure is calculated from the excretion rates of the isotopes.

Dna	Does not apply.
EAATAC	The erythrocyte aspartate aminotransferase activation coefficient, an index of vitamin B_6 status.
EGRAC	The erythrocyte glutathione reductase activation coefficient, an index of riboflavin status.
ETKAC	The erythrocyte transketolase activation coefficient, an index of thiamin status.
ETK-B	The erythrocyte transketolase basal activity.
GSH-Px	The erythrocyte glutathione peroxidase activity.
HDL cholesterol	High density lipoprotein cholesterol.
HNR	Medical Research Council Human Nutrition Research, Cambridge.
Household	The standard definition used in most surveys carried out by the ONS and comparable with the 1991 Census definition of a household was used in this survey. A household is defined as a single person or group of people who have the accommodation as their only or main residence and who either share one main meal a day or share the living accommodation. (*See* McCrossan E. *A Handbook for interviewers.* HMSO: London 1991.)
HRP	Household Reference Person. This is the member of the household in whose name the accommodation is owned or rented, or is otherwise responsible for the accommodation. In households with a sole householder that person is the household reference person, in households with *joint* householders the person with the *highest income* is taken as the household reference person, if both householders have exactly the same income, the *older* is taken as the household reference person. This differs from Head of Household in that female householders with the highest income are now taken as the HRP, and in the case of joint householders, income then age, rather than sex then age is used to define the HRP.
HSfE	Health Survey for England.
LDL (-calc) cholesterol	Low density lipoprotein cholesterol. LDL cholesterol was not measured in this survey. Total serum cholesterol minus *HDL cholesterol* is taken as an approximation of LDL cholesterol, uncorrected for triglycerides. For brevity the term LDL (-calc) cholesterol is used for non-HDL cholesterol.

MAFF	The Ministry of Agriculture, Fisheries and Food.
Manual social class	Respondents living in households where the household reference person was in an occupation ascribed to *Social Classes III manual, IV or V.*
MAP	Mean arterial pressure.
Mean	The average value.
Median	*See* Percentiles.
MET	Metabolic equivalent. For adults, metabolic equivalents are taken as numerically equivalent to energy expenditure. For an average adult, 1 MET is equal to 60kcal/hour or 1 kcal/min.
MCV	Mean corpuscular volume.
MRC	The Medical Research Council.
na	Not available, not applicable.
NDNS	The National Diet and Nutrition Survey.
No.	Number (of cases).
Non-manual social class	Respondents living in households where the household reference person was in an occupation ascribed to *Social Class I, II or III non-manual.*
ns	Not statistically significant.
ONS	Office for National Statistics.
PAF	Postcode Address File; the sampling frame for the survey.
Percentiles	The percentiles of a distribution divide it into equal parts. The median of a distribution divides it into two equal parts, such that half the cases in the distribution fall, or have a value, above the median, and the other half fall, or have a value below the median.
Physical activity sample	Those respondents for whom a seven-day physical activity diary was obtained.
Plasma 25-hydroxyvitamin D; plasma 25-OHD	The biochemical index of vitamin D.
Plasma ascorbate	The biochemical index of vitamin C.
PSU	Primary Sampling Unit; for this survey, postcode sectors.
Quetelet index	*See* Body Mass Index.

Region	Based on the Standard regions and grouped as follows:

Scotland

Northern
North
Yorkshire and Humberside
North West

Central, South West and Wales
East Midlands
West Midlands
East Anglia
South West
Wales

London and the South East
London
South East

The regions of England are as constituted after local government reorganisation on 1 April 1974. The regions as defined in terms of counties are listed in Chapter 2 of the Technical report (*see* www.food.gov.uk/science).

Responding sample	Respondents who completed the dietary interview and may/may not have co-operated with other components of the survey.
sd/Std Dev	Standard deviation. An index of variability which is calculated as the square root of the variance and is expressed in the same units used to calculate the *mean*.
se	Standard error. An indication of the reliability of an estimate of a population parameter, which is calculated by dividing the *standard deviation* of the estimate by the square root of the sample size.
Social class	Based on the Registrar General's Standard Occupational Classification, Volume 4, TSO (2001). Social class was ascribed on the basis of the occupation of the household reference person. The classification used in the tables is as follows:

	Description	Social Class
	Non-manual	
	Professional and intermediate	I and II
	Skilled occupations,	III non-manual
	non-manual	
	Manual	
	Skilled occupations, manual	III manual
	Partly-skilled and unskilled	IV and V
	occupations	
TIBC	Total iron-binding capacity.	
Wave; Fieldwork wave	The 3-month period in which fieldwork was carried out.	
	Wave 1: July to September 2000	
	Wave 2: October to December 2000	
	Wave 3: January to March 2001	
	Wave 4: April to June 2001	
WHO	World Health Organization.	

Appendix F   List of tables

1: Background, research design and response

Tables

1.1   Response to the dietary interview and seven-day dietary record by wave of fieldwork

1.2   Co-operation with anthropometric measurements and blood pressure by wave of fieldwork, sex and age of respondent and social class of household reference person

1.3   Co-operation with blood sample by wave of fieldwork, sex and age of respondent and social class of household reference person

2: Anthropometry

Tables

2.1   Percentage distribution of height by sex and age of respondent

2.2   Percentage distribution of body weight by sex and age of respondent

2.3   Percentage distribution of body mass index by sex and age of respondent

2.4   Percentage distribution of waist circumference by sex and age of respondent

2.5   Percentage distribution of hip circumference by sex and age of respondent

2.6   Percentage distribution of waist to hip ratio by sex and age of respondent

2.7   Anthropometric measurements by sex of respondent and region

2.8   Anthropometric measurements by sex of respondent and whether someone in the respondent's household was receiving certain benefits

2.9   Socio-demographic, dietary and physiological factors associated with BMI in bivariate analysis

2.10   Socio-demographic, dietary and physiological factors associated with waist to hip ratio in bivariate analysis

2.11   Linear regression model for BMI: men

2.12   Linear regression model for BMI: women

2.13   Linear regression model for waist to hip ratio: men

2.14   Linear regression model for waist to hip ratio: women

2.15   Comparison of anthropometric measurements with the 1986/87 Adults Survey

2.16   Comparison of anthropometric measurements with the Health Survey for England 2001

3: Blood pressure

Tables

3.1   Percentage distribution of systolic blood pressure by sex and age of respondent

3.2   Percentage distribution of diastolic blood pressure by sex and age of respondent

3.3   Blood pressure by sex of respondent and region

3.4   Blood pressure by sex of respondent and whether someone in the respondent's household was receiving certain benefits

3.5   Pearson correlation coefficients for systolic blood pressure with urinary sodium excretion

3.6   Socio-demographic, dietary and physiological factors associated with systolic blood pressure in bivariate analysis

3.7   Socio-demographic, dietary and physiological factors associated with diastolic blood pressure in bivariate analysis

3.8   Linear regression model for systolic blood pressure: men

3.9   Linear regression model for systolic blood pressure: women

3.10   Linear regression model for diastolic blood pressure: men

3.11   Linear regression model for diastolic blood pressure: women

3.12   Comparison of blood pressure measurements with the Health Survey for England 2001

4: Blood analytes

Tables

4.1   Percentage distribution of haemoglobin concentration by sex and age of respondent

4.2   Percentage distribution of mean corpuscular volume by sex and age of respondent

4.3   Percentage distribution of haematocrit by sex and age of respondent

4.4   Percentage distribution of plasma iron by sex and age of respondent

4.5   Percentage distribution of total iron-binding capacity by sex and age of respondent

4.6   Percentage distribution of plasma iron % saturation by sex and age of respondent

4.7   Percentage distribution of serum ferritin by sex and age of respondent

4.8   Pearson correlation coefficients for serum ferritin and haemoglobin with dietary intake of iron

4.9   Pearson correlation coefficients for serum ferritin and haemoglobin with plasma iron % saturation

4.10   Pearson correlation coefficients for serum ferritin and haemoglobin with plasma α_1 - antichymotrypsin

4.11   Haematology analytes by sex of respondent and region

4.12   Haematology analytes by sex of respondent and whether someone in the respondent's household was receiving certain benefits

4.13   Percentage distribution of plasma vitamin C by sex and age of respondent

4.14   Percentage distribution of red cell folate by sex and age of respondent

4.15   Percentage distribution of serum folate by sex and age of respondent

4.16   Percentage distribution of serum vitamin B_{12} by sex and age of respondent

4.17   Percentage distribution of erythrocyte transketolase activation coefficient (ETKAC) by sex and age of respondent

4.18   Percentage distribution of erythrocyte transketolase basal activity (ETK-B) by sex and age of respondent

4.19   Percentage distribution of erythrocyte glutathione reductase activation coefficient (EGRAC) by sex and age of respondent

4.20   Percentage distribution of erythrocyte aspartate aminotransferase activation coefficient (EAATAC) by sex and age of respondent

4.21   Percentage distribution of plasma total homocysteine by sex and age of respondent

4.22   Pearson correlation coefficients for plasma vitamin C with dietary intake of vitamin C and fruit and vegetable intake

4.23   Pearson correlation coefficients for dietary intakes of folate with red cell folate and serum folate

4.24   Water soluble vitamins and plasma total homocysteine by sex of respondent and region

4.25   Water soluble vitamins and plasma total homocysteine by sex of respondent and whether someone in the respondent's household was receiving certain benefits

4.26   Percentage distribution of plasma retinol by sex and age of respondent

4.27   Percentage distribution of plasma α-carotene by sex and age of respondent

4.28   Percentage distribution of plasma β-carotene by sex and age of respondent

4.29   Percentage distribution of plasma α-cryptoxanthin by sex and age of respondent

4.30   Percentage distribution of plasma β-cryptoxanthin by sex and age of respondent

4.31   Percentage distribution of plasma lycopene by sex and age of respondent

4.32   Percentage distribution of plasma lutein and zeaxanthin by sex and age of respondent

4.33   Percentage distribution of plasma 25-hydroxyvitamin D by sex and age of respondent

4.34   Percentage distribution of plasma 25-hydroxyvitamin D by date blood sample taken and sex of respondent

4.35   Percentage distribution of plasma α-tocopherol by sex and age of respondent

4.36   Percentage distribution of plasma γ-tocopherol by sex and age of respondent

4.37   Percentage distribution of tocopherol to cholesterol ratio by sex and age of respondent

4.38   Pearson correlation coefficients for plasma retinol with dietary intake of α-carotene, β-carotene and vitamin A (retinol equivalents)

4.39   Pearson correlation coefficients for plasma α-carotene with dietary intake of α-carotene

4.40   Pearson correlation coefficients for plasma β-carotene with dietary intake of β-carotene

4.41   Pearson correlation coefficients for plasma 25-hydroxyvitamin D with dietary intake of vitamin D

4.42   Pearson correlation coefficients for plasma 25-hydroxyvitamin D with dietary intake of vitamin D by date blood sample taken

4.43   Pearson correlation coefficients for tocopherol to cholesterol ratio with dietary intake of vitamin E

4.44   Fat soluble vitamins and carotenoids by sex of respondent and region

4.45   Fat soluble vitamins and carotenoids by sex of respondent and whether someone in the respondent's household was receiving certain benefits

4.46   Percentage distribution of plasma total cholesterol by sex and age of respondent

4.47   Percentage distribution of plasma high density lipoprotein cholesterol by sex and age of respondent

4.48   Percentage distribution of plasma low density lipoprotein cholesterol by sex and age of respondent

4.49   Blood lipids by sex of respondent and region

4.50   Blood lipids by sex of respondent and whether someone in the respondent's household was receiving certain benefits

4.51   Percentage distribution of plasma selenium by sex and age of respondent

4.52   Percentage distribution of red cell selenium by sex and age of respondent

4.53   Percentage distribution of blood glutathione peroxidase (GSH-Px) by sex and age of respondent

4.54   Percentage distribution of plasma α_1-antichymotrypsin by sex and age of respondent

4.55   Percentage distribution of blood mercury by sex and age of respondent

4.56   Other analytes by sex of respondent and region

4.57   Other analytes by sex of respondent and whether someone in the respondent's household was receiving certain benefits

Figures

4.1   Comparison of mean plasma 25-OHD levels by date of blood sample taken by sex of respondent

5: Physical activity

Tables

5.1   Percentage distribution of self-reported levels of physical activity by sex and age of respondent

5.2   Percentage distribution of mean hours spent in activity of at least moderate intensity per day by sex and age of respondent

5.3   Percentage distribution of mean hours spent in vigorous or very vigorous activity per day by sex and age of respondent

5.4   Participation in at least 30 minutes of activity of at least moderate intensity per day by sex and age of respondent

5.5   Mean hours spent in activities of at least moderate intensity per day by sex of respondent and region

5.6   Mean hours spent in activities of at least moderate intensity per day by sex of respondent and whether someone in the respondent's household was receiving certain benefits

5.7   Pearson correlation coefficients for hours spent in activities of at least moderate intensity per day with energy and macronutrient intakes

5.8   Pearson correlation coefficients for hours spent in activities of at least moderate intensity per day with anthropometric measurements

5.9   Pearson correlation coefficients for hours spent in activities of at least moderate intensity per day with blood pressure

5.10   Socio-demographic, dietary and physiological factors associated with hours spent in activities of at least moderate intensity in bivariate analysis

5.11   Linear regression model for time spent in activities of at least moderate intensity per day: men

5.12   Linear regression model for time spent in activities of at least moderate intensity per day: women

5.13   Participation in at least 30 minutes of activity of at least moderate intensity per day by sex and age of respondent compared with the Health Survey for England 1998

Appendix A: Sampling errors and statistical methods

Tables

A1   True standard errors and design factors for socio-demographic characteristics of the diary sample by sex of respondent

A2   True standard errors and design factors for physiological measurements by sex and age of respondent

A3   True standard errors and design factors for selected blood analytes by sex and age of respondent

A4   True standard errors and design factors for measures of physical activity by sex and age of respondent

Figures

A1   Multiple regression analysis method

Appendix B: Unweighted base numbers

Tables

B1   Unweighted base numbers: dietary interview, seven-day dietary record and physical activity record by sex of respondent

B2   Unweighted base numbers: anthropometry and blood pressure by sex of respondent

B3   Unweighted base numbers: blood analytes by sex of respondent

Appendix D: Physical activity

Figures

D1   The mean number of activities of at least moderate intensity in which respondents participated by diary day

D2   The mean number of activities of at least moderate intensity in which respondents participated by the day of the week

Physiology of Exercise

McGraw Hill **Higher Education**

EXERCISE PHYSIOLOGY: THEORY AND APPLICATION TO FITNESS AND
PERFORMANCE, SIXTH EDITION

ISBN-13: 978-0-07-110726-6
ISBN-10: 0-07-110726-6

www.mhhe.com

dedicated to LOU and ANN
for their love, patience, and support

Brief Contents

SECTION 1

Physiology of Exercise   1

1 Physiology of Exercise in the United States—Its Past, Its Future   2

2 Control of the Internal Environment   14

3 Bioenergetics   23

4 Exercise Metabolism   52

5 Hormonal Responses to Exercise   73

6 Measurement of Work, Power, and Energy Expenditure   106

7 The Nervous System: Structure and Control of Movement   120

8 Skeletal Muscle: Structure and Function   140

9 Circulatory Responses to Exercise   169

10 Respiration During Exercise   200

11 Acid-Base Balance During Exercise   230

12 Temperature Regulation   241

13 The Physiology of Training: Effect on $\dot{V}O_2$ Max, Performance, Homeostasis, and Strength   260

SECTION 2

Physiology of Health and Fitness   278

14 Patterns in Health and Disease: Epidemiology and Physiology   288

15 Work Tests to Evaluate Cardiorespiratory Fitness   299

16 Exercise Prescriptions for Health and Fitness   320

17 Exercise for Special Populations   337

18 Body Composition and Nutrition for Health   359

SECTION 3

Physiology of Performance   407

19 Factors Affecting Performance   408

20 Laboratory Assessment of Human Performance   421

21 Training for Performance   441

22 Training for the Female Athlete, Children, and Special Populations   463

23 Nutrition, Body Composition, and Performance   477

24 Exercise and the Environment   499

25 Ergogenic Aids   522

Contents

Preface   xi

SECTION 1

Physiology of Exercise   1

Chapter 1 Physiology of Exercise in the United States—Its Past, Its Future   2
European Heritage   3
Harvard Fatigue Laboratory   4
Physical Fitness   5
Physical Education to Exercise Science   7
Graduate Study and Research in the Physiology of Exercise   8
Professional Societies and Research Journals   10
Translation of Exercise Physiology to the Consumer   11

Chapter 2 Control of the Internal Environment   14
Homeostasis: Dynamic Constancy   15
Control Systems of the Body   16
Nature of the Control Systems   17
Negative Feedback   18
Gain of a Control System   18
Examples of Homeostatic Control   18
Regulation of Arterial Blood Pressure   18
Regulation of Blood Glucose   19
Stress Proteins Assist in the Regulation of Cellular Homeostasis   19
Exercise: A Test of Homeostatic Control   21

Chapter 3 Bioenergetics   23
Cell Structure   24
Biological Energy Transformation   25
Cellular Chemical Reactions   25
Oxidation-Reduction Reactions   27
Enzymes   28

Fuels for Exercise   31
Carbohydrates   31
Fats   32
Proteins   32
High-Energy Phosphates   33
Bioenergetics   33
Anaerobic ATP Production   33
Aerobic ATP Production   38
Aerobic ATP Tally   46
Efficiency of Oxidative Phosphorylation   46
Control of Bioenergetics   46
Control of ATP-PC System   47
Control of Glycolysis   47
Control of Krebs Cycle and Electron Transport Chain   48
Interaction Between Aerobic/Anaerobic ATP Production   48

Chapter 4 Exercise Metabolism   52
Energy Requirements at Rest   53
Rest-to-Exercise Transitions   53
Recovery from Exercise: Metabolic Responses   54
Metabolic Responses to Exercise: Influence of Duration and Intensity   57
Short-Term, Intense Exercise   57
Prolonged Exercise   58
Incremental Exercise   58
Estimation of Fuel Utilization During Exercise   61
Factors Governing Fuel Selection   62
Exercise Intensity and Fuel Selection   62
Exercise Duration and Fuel Selection   63
Interaction of Fat/Carbohydrate Metabolism   64
Body Fuel Sources   65

Chapter 5 Hormonal Responses to Exercise   73
Neuroendocrinology   74
Blood Hormone Concentration   75
Hormone-Receptor Interaction   76

Hormones: Regulation and Action 78
  Hypothalamus and the Pituitary Gland 79
  Thyroid Gland 81
  Parathyroid Gland 82
  Adrenal Gland 82
  Pancreas 85
  Testes and Ovaries 86
Hormonal Control of Substrate Mobilization
  During Exercise 92
  Muscle-Glycogen Utilization 92
  Blood Glucose Homeostasis During Exercise 93
  Hormone-Substrate Interaction 100

**Chapter 6 Measurement of Work, Power,
and Energy Expenditure 106**
Units of Measure 107
  Metric System 107
  SI Units 107
Work and Power Defined 107
  Work 107
  Power 108
Measurement of Work and Power 109
  Bench Step 109
  Cycle Ergometer 110
  Treadmill 110
Measurement of Energy Expenditure 111
  Direct Calorimetry 111
  Indirect Calorimetry 112
Estimation of Energy Expenditure 112
Calculation of Exercise Efficiency 115
  Factors That Influence Exercise Efficiency 115
Running Economy 117

**Chapter 7 The Nervous System: Structure
and Control of Movement 120**
General Nervous System Functions 121
Organization of the Nervous System 121
  Structure of the Neuron 122
  Electrical Activity in Neurons 122
Sensory Information and Reflexes 129
  Proprioceptors 129
  Muscle Chemoreceptors 130
  Reflexes 130
Somatic Motor Function 131
Vestibular Apparatus and Equilibrium 132
Motor Control Functions of the Brain 132
  Brain Stem 133
  Cerebrum 133
  Cerebellum 134
Motor Functions of the Spinal Cord 134
Control of Motor Functions 135
Autonomic Nervous System 136
Exercise Enhances Brain Health 137

**Chapter 8 Skeletal Muscle: Structure
and Function 140**
Structure of Skeletal Muscle 141
Neuromuscular Junction 143

Muscular Contraction 144
  Overview of the Sliding Filament Model 144
  Energy for Contraction 145
  Regulation of Excitation-Contraction Coupling 145
Fiber Types 149
  Biochemical and Contractile Characteristics of
  Skeletal Muscle 149
  Characteristics of Individual Fiber Types 152
  Fiber Types and Performance 154
Alterations in Skeletal Muscle Due to Exercise,
  Inactivity, and Aging 155
  Exercise-Induced Changes in Skeletal Muscles 155
  Muscle Atrophy Due to Inactivity 155
  Age-Related Changes in Skeletal Muscle 157
Muscle Actions 158
Speed of Muscle Action and Relaxation 159
Force Regulation in Muscle 160
Force-Velocity/Power-Velocity
  Relationships 161
Receptors in Muscle 163
  Muscle Spindle 163
  Golgi Tendon Organs 164

**Chapter 9 Circulatory Responses
to Exercise 169**
Organization of the Circulatory System 170
  Structure of the Heart 170
  Pulmonary and Systemic Circuits 171
Heart: Myocardium and Cardiac Cycle 171
  Myocardium 171
  Cardiac Cycle 174
  Arterial Blood Pressure 176
  Factors That Influence Arterial Blood Pressure 177
  Electrical Activity of the Heart 178
Cardiac Output 181
  Regulation of the Heart Rate 182
  Regulation of Stroke Volume 183
Hemodynamics 186
  Physical Characteristics of Blood 186
  Relationships Among Pressure, Resistance,
  and Flow 186
  Sources of Vascular Resistance 187
Changes in Oxygen Delivery to Muscle During
  Exercise 188
  Changes in Cardiac Output During Exercise 188
  Changes in Arterial-Mixed Venous O_2 Content
  During Exercise 189
  Redistribution of Blood Flow During Exercise 189
  Regulation of Local Blood Flow During Exercise 190
Circulatory Responses to Exercise 192
  Emotional Influence 192
  Transition from Rest to Exercise 192
  Recovery from Exercise 192
  Incremental Exercise 192
  Arm versus Leg Exercise 193
  Intermittent Exercise 194
  Prolonged Exercise 194
Regulation of Cardiovascular Adjustments to
  Exercise 195

Chapter 10 Respiration During Exercise 200
  Function of the Lung 201
  Structure of the Respiratory System 201
    Conducting Zone 202
    Respiratory Zone 204
  Mechanics of Breathing 204
    Inspiration 204
    Expiration 204
    Airway Resistance 206
  Pulmonary Ventilation 207
  Pulmonary Volumes and Capacities 208
  Diffusion of Gases 210
  Blood Flow to the Lung 211
  Ventilation-Perfusion Relationships 212
  O_2 and CO_2 Transport in Blood 213
    Hemoglobin and O_2 Transport 213
    Oxyhemoglobin Dissociation Curve 213
    O_2 Transport in Muscle 215
    CO_2 Transport in Blood 215
  Ventilation and Acid-Base Balance 217
  Ventilatory and Blood-Gas Responses to Exercise 217
    Rest-to-Work Transitions 217
    Prolonged Exercise in a Hot Environment 217
    Incremental Exercise 218
  Control of Ventilation 219
    Ventilatory Regulation at Rest 219
    Ventilatory Control During Submaximal Exercise 222
    Ventilatory Control During Heavy Exercise 222
  Do the Lungs Adapt to Exercise Training? 224
  Does the Pulmonary System Limit Maximal Exercise Performance? 224

Chapter 11 Acid-Base Balance During Exercise 230
  Acids, Bases, and pH 231
  Hydrogen Ion Production During Exercise 232
  Importance of Acid-Base Regulation During Exercise 234
  Acid-Base Buffer Systems 234
    Intracellular Buffers 234
    Extracellular Buffers 235
  Respiratory Influence on Acid-Base Balance 236
  Regulation of Acid-Base Balance via the Kidneys 236
  Regulation of Acid-Base Balance During Exercise 237

Chapter 12 Temperature Regulation 241
  Overview of Heat Balance During Exercise 242
  Temperature Measurement During Exercise 243
  Overview of Heat Production/Heat Loss 243
    Heat Production 243

    Heat Loss 244
    Heat Storage in the Body During Exercise 245
  Body's Thermostat—Hypothalamus 247
    Shift in the Hypothalamic Thermostat Set Point Due to Fever 248
  Thermal Events During Exercise 249
  Exercise in the Heat 250
    Sweat Rates During Exercise 251
    Exercise Performance in a Hot Environment 252
    Gender and Age Differences in Thermoregulation 253
    Heat Acclimatization 254
    Loss of Acclimatization 256
  Exercise in a Cold Environment 256
    Cold Acclimatization 256

Chapter 13 The Physiology of Training: Effect on $\dot{V}O_2$ Max, Performance, Homeostasis, and Strength 260
  Principles of Training 261
    Overload 261
    Specificity 262
  Research Designs to Study Training 262
  Endurance Training and $\dot{V}O_2$ Max 262
    Training Programs and Changes in $\dot{V}O_2$ Max 263
  $\dot{V}O_2$ Max: Cardiac Output and the Arteriovenous O_2 Difference 264
    Stroke Volume 265
    Arteriovenous O_2 Difference 267
  Detraining and $\dot{V}O_2$ Max 268
  Endurance Training. Effects on Performance and Homeostasis 269
    Biochemical Adaptations and the Oxygen Deficit 271
    Biochemical Adaptations and the Plasma Glucose Concentration 271
    Biochemical Adaptations and Blood pH 273
    Biochemical Adaptations and Lactate Removal 274
  Endurance Training: Links Between Muscle and Systemic Physiology 275
    Peripheral Feedback 277
    Central Command 277
  Physiological Effects of Strength Training 278
  Physiological Mechanisms Causing Increased Strength 279
    Neural Factors 279
    Muscular Enlargement 280
    Concurrent Strength and Endurance Training 281

SECTION 2

Physiology of Health and Fitness 287

Chapter 14 Patterns in Health and Disease: Epidemiology and Physiology 288
  Epidemiology 289

Coronary Heart Disease 291
  Physical Inactivity as a Risk Factor 292
Physiology 294
Synthesis 296

Chapter 15 Work Tests to Evaluate Cardiorespiratory Fitness 299

Testing Procedures 300
  Screening 300
  Resting and Exercise Measures 302
Field Tests for Estimating CRF 302
  Maximal Run Tests 302
  Walk Tests 304
  Canadian Home Fitness Test 304
Graded Exercise Tests: Measurements 305
  Heart Rate 305
  Blood Pressure 305
  ECG 306
  Rating of Perceived Exertion 306
  Termination Criteria 307
$\dot{V}O_2$ Max 308
  Estimation of $\dot{V}O_2$ Max from Last Work Rate 309
  Estimation of $\dot{V}O_2$ Max from Submaximal HR Response 309
Graded Exercise Test: Protocols 311
  Treadmill 312
  Cycle Ergometer 313
  Step Test 314

Chapter 16 Exercise Prescriptions for Health and Fitness 320

Prescription of Exercise 321
  Dose-Response 322
  Physical Activity and Health 323
General Guidelines for Improving Fitness 325
  Screening 325
  Progression 325
  Warm-Up, Stretch, and Cool-Down, Stretch 325
Exercise Prescription for CRF 325
  Frequency 326
  Duration 326
  Intensity 326
Sequence of Physical Activity 329
  Walking 329
  Jogging 329
  Games and Sports 330
Strength and Flexibility Training 331
Environmental Concerns 332

Chapter 17 Exercise for Special Populations 337

Diabetes 338
  Exercise and the Diabetic 339
Asthma 342
  Diagnosis and Causes 342
  Prevention/Relief of Asthma 343
  Exercise-Induced Asthma 343

Chronic Obstructive Pulmonary Disease 345
  Testing and Training 345
Hypertension 346
Cardiac Rehabilitation 347
  Population 347
  Testing 348
  Exercise Programs 348
Exercise for Older Adults 349
Exercise During Pregnancy 352

Chapter 18 Body Composition and Nutrition for Health 359

Nutritional Goals 360
Standards of Nutrition 362
Classes of Nutrients 363
  Water 363
  Vitamins 364
  Minerals 364
  Carbohydrates 368
  Fats 372
  Protein 373
Meeting the Guidelines and Achieving the Goals 374
  Food Group Plans 374
  Evaluating the Diet 375
Body Composition 376
  Methods of Assessing Overweight and Obesity 377
  Methods of Measuring Body Composition 378
  Two-Component System of Body Composition 380
  Body Fatness for Health and Fitness 383
Obesity and Weight Control 384
  Obesity 384
Diet, Exercise, and Weight Control 388
  Energy and Nutrient Balance 389
  Diet and Weight Control 390
  Energy Expenditure and Weight Control 391

SECTION 3

Physiology of Performance 407

Chapter 19 Factors Affecting Performance 408

Sites of Fatigue 409
  Central Fatigue 409
  Peripheral Fatigue 410
Factors Limiting All-Out Anaerobic Performances 413
  Ultra Short-Term Performances (Less than Ten Seconds) 413
  Short-Term Performances (10 to 180 Seconds) 415
Factors Limiting All-Out Aerobic Performances 415
  Moderate-Length Performances (Three to Twenty Minutes) 415

Intermediate-Length Performances (Twenty-One to Sixty Minutes) 416
Long-Term Performances (One to Four Hours) 417
Athlete as Machine 418

Chapter 20 Laboratory Assessment of Human Performance 421

Laboratory Assessment of Physical Performance 422
Physiological Testing: Theory and Ethics 422
What the Athlete Gains by Physiological Testing 422
What Physiological Testing Will Not Do 423
Components of Effective Physiological Testing 423
Direct Testing of Maximal Aerobic Power 424
Specificity of Testing 424
Exercise Test Protocol 425
Determination of Peak $\dot{V}O_2$ in Paraplegic Athletes 425
Laboratory Tests to Predict Endurance Performance 426
Use of the Lactate Threshold to Evaluate Performance 426
Measurement of Critical Power 428
Tests to Determine Exercise Economy 429
Estimating Success in Distance Running Using the Lactate Threshold and Running Economy 429
Determination of Anaerobic Power 430
Tests of Ultra Short-Term Maximal Anaerobic Power 431
Tests of Short-Term Anaerobic Power 433
Evaluation of Muscular Strength 434
Criteria for Selection of a Strength-Testing Method 434
Isometric Measurement of Strength 435
Free-Weight Testing of Strength 435
Isokinetic Assessment of Strength 436
Variable-Resistance Measurement of Strength 437

Chapter 21 Training for Performance 441

Training Principles 442
Overload, Specificity, and Reversibility 442
Influence of Gender, Initial Fitness Level, and Genetics 443
Components of a Training Session: Warm-Up, Workout, and Cool Down 444
Training to Improve Aerobic Power 444
Interval Training 445
Long, Slow-Distance Exercise 446
High-Intensity, Continuous Exercise 446
Injuries and Endurance Training 447
Training for Improved Anaerobic Power 447
Training to Improve the ATP-PC System 448
Training to Improve the Glycolytic System 448

Training to Improve Muscular Strength 448
Progressive Resistance Exercise 450
General Strength-Training Principles 450
Free Weights versus Machines 451
Combined Strength- and Endurance-Training Programs 451
Gender Differences in Response to Strength Training 451
Muscle Soreness 453
Training for Improved Flexibility 456
Year-Round Conditioning for Athletes 457
Off-Season Conditioning 457
Preseason Conditioning 457
In-Season Conditioning 457
Common Training Mistakes 458

Chapter 22 Training for the Female Athlete, Children, and Special Populations 463

Factors Important to Women Involved in Vigorous Training 464
Exercise and Menstrual Disorders 464
Training and Menstruation 465
The Female Athlete and Eating Disorders 465
Bone Mineral Disorders and the Female Athlete 466
Training During Pregnancy 466
Risk of Knee Injury in Female Athletes 466
Sports Conditioning for Children 469
Training and the Cardiopulmonary System 469
Training and the Musculoskeletal System 469
Competitive Training for Diabetics 470
Training for Asthmatics 472
Epilepsy and Physical Training 472
Does Exercise Promote Seizures? 473
Risk of Injury Due to Seizures 473

Chapter 23 Nutrition, Body Composition, and Performance 477

Nutrition and Performance 478
Carbohydrate 478
Protein 482
Water and Electrolytes 486
Minerals 489
Vitamins 490
Precompetition Diet 491
Body Composition and Performance 492
Somatotype 492
Body Fatness and Performance 492

Chapter 24 Exercise and the Environment 499

Altitude 500
Atmospheric Pressure 500
Short-Term Anaerobic Performance 500
Long-Term Aerobic Performance 501
Maximal Aerobic Power and Altitude 501
Adaptation to High Altitude 503
Training for Competition at Altitude 504
The Quest for Everest 506

Heat   509
  Hyperthermia   509
Cold   512
  Environmental Factors   512
  Insulating Factors   513
  Energy Production   515
  Dealing with Hypothermia   516
Air Pollution   516
  Particulate Matter   517
  Ozone   517
  Sulfur Dioxide   517
  Carbon Monoxide   517

Chapter 25 Ergogenic Aids   522
Research Design Concerns   523
Dietary Supplements   524
Aerobic Performance   524
  Oxygen   524
  Blood Doping   527
Anaerobic Performance   529
  Blood Buffers   529
Drugs   530
  Amphetamines   530
  Caffeine   531
  Cocaine   534
  Nicotine   535
Physical Warm-Up   536

Appendixes

Appendix A   Calculation of Oxygen Uptake and Carbon Dioxide Production   A-1
Appendix B   Estimated Energy Expenditure during Selected Activities   A-5
Appendix C   PARmed-X Physical Activity Readiness Medical Examination   A-17
Appendix D   Dietary Reference Intakes: Macronutrients   A-18
Appendix E   Dietary Reference Intakes: Vitamins and Minerals   A-20
Appendix F   Dietary Reference Intakes: Estimated Energy Requirements   A-24
Appendix G   Percent Fat Estimate for Men: Sum of Triceps, Chest, and Subscapula Skinfolds   A-25
Appendix H   Percent Fat Estimate for Women: Sum of Triceps, Abdomen, and Suprailium Skinfolds   A-26

Glossary   G-1
Credits   C-1
Index   I-1

Preface

Similar to previous editions, the sixth edition of *Exercise Physiology: Theory and Application to Fitness and Performance* is intended for students of exercise science, clinical exercise physiology, physical education, sport physiology, athletic training and sports medicine, and physical therapy. The goal of this text is to provide the student with an up-to-date understanding of the physiology of exercise. In addition, the book contains extensive practical and clinical applications, including work tests to evaluate cardiorespiratory fitness and information on exercise training for improvements in health-related fitness and sports performance.

This book is intended for a one-semester, upper-level undergraduate or beginning graduate exercise physiology course. Clearly, the text contains more material than can be covered during a typical fifteen-week semester. This is by design. The book was written to be comprehensive in order to afford instructors a great deal of freedom to select the material that they consider most important for the makeup of their class.

NEW TO THIS EDITION

Updated Content and New Research

As always, the sixth edition highlights the latest research in exercise physiology. This focus is reflected throughout the book—in expanded text discussions, new and revised box features, new figures and references, and new suggested readings. In this new edition, students will learn new information about the negative health consequences of hypertension, up-to-date information about the impact of exercise on the lungs, the latest research on creatine supplementation, new clinical applications of exercise physiology, an expanded treatment of exercise prescription for different populations, and up-to-date information on nutrition based on current dietary guidelines.

New Illustrations

Many illustrations have been updated, and numerous new illustrations have been added to complement the text discussions. Besides enhancing the book's visual appeal, these illustrations make the content easier for students to understand and reinforce their learning.

New or Expanded Topics

The content of this new edition has been updated overall, including the references and readings. The following list includes examples of changes that have made the sixth edition more complete and up to date:

Chapter 1 Physiology of Exercise in the United States—Its Past, Its Future
- New highlight on Dr. Brenda Bigland-Richie
- Updated ACSM certification categories
- Updated professional societies and research journals

Chapter 2 Control of the Internal Environment
- Revised Figure 2.1
- Updated references and readings

Chapter 3 Bioenergetics
- New A Closer Look box explaining nomenclature for lactic acid and lactate
- Expanded discussion of factors affecting enzyme activity; includes two new illustrations
- New Clinical Applications box explaining diagnostic use of enzyme activity in blood
- New section discussing the nomenclature and six classes of enzymes; includes new table
- Several new and improved illustrations
- Updated Winning Edge box with latest new information on creatine supplementation

Chapter 4 Exercise Metabolism
- New section on energy requirement at rest
- Expanded discussion of the concept of onset of blood lactate accumulation (OBLA)

- Updated and revised information on protein metabolism during exercise

Chapter 5 Hormonal Responses to Exercise
- Update on anabolic steroids, highlighting major league baseball's dilemma
- Updated information on each of the major hormones as they respond to or influence exercise

Chapter 6 Measurement of Work, Power, and Energy Expenditure
- Updated references and readings

Chapter 7 The Nervous System: Structure and Control of Movement
- Expanded discussion of resting membrane potential and ion channel function
- New illustrations present ion exchange across neuron membrane

Chapter 8 Skeletal Muscle: Structure and Function
- New sections on skeletal muscle plasticity and exercise
- Updated and expanded information on muscle fatigue during exercise
- New section on disuse muscle atrophy
- New information related to aging and skeletal muscle
- Several new illustrations

Chapter 9 Circulatory Responses to Exercise
- Updated information on comparison between skeletal muscle myocytes and cardiac myocytes
- New information on the negative health consequences of hypertension
- Expanded discussion of the regulation of blood pressure
- Revised and updated discussion of regulation of stroke volume
- Updated and revised section on regulation of local blood flow
- New and updated illustrations

Chapter 10 Respiration During Exercise
- New and updated illustrations
- Updated information on the effect of exercise training on the lung
- New discussion of the use of pulmonary function testing to diagnose COPD

Chapter 11 Acid-Base Balance During Exercise
- New A Closer Look box on exercise-induced acidosis
- Revised and updated Winning Edge box on ingestion of bicarbonate buffers and human performance

Chapter 12 Temperature Regulation
- New material on heat storage in the body during exercise

- New A Closer Look box on calculation of body temperature increase during exercise
- Updated information on measurement of core temperature, muscle fatigue during exercise in hot environments, and prevention of dehydration during exercise

Chapter 13 The Physiology of Training: Effect on $\dot{V}O_2$ Max, Performance, Homeostasis, and Strength
- Expanded discussion of immune function and exercise
- Expanded treatment of resistance training

Chapter 14 Patterns in Health and Disease: Epidemiology and Physiology
- New A Closer Look box on leading vs. actual causes of death
- New A Closer Look box featuring Harvard Alumni Study and Aerobic Center Longitudinal Study

Chapter 15 Work Tests to Evaluate Cardiorespiratory Fitness
- New A Closer Look box on Progressive Aerobic Cardiovascular Endurance Run (PACER test)

Chapter 16 Exercise Prescriptions for Health and Fitness
- Overall content updated based on new ACSM and other exercise guidelines
- Updated references and readings

Chapter 17 Exercise for Special Populations
- Extensive chapter revision based on new exercise guidelines
- Updated section on diabetes
- Revised and updated section on asthma
- Updated section on hypertension
- Revised and updated section on pregnancy

Chapter 18 Body Composition and Nutrition for Health
- Extensive revision of all dietary information
- New Ask the Expert feature on tracking obesity-related risks
- Revised dietary standards based on 2005 Dietary Guidelines for Americans
- Updated vitamin and mineral tables
- New Clinical Applications box on glycemic index
- Presentation and discussion of MyPyramid
- Updated discussion of body composition with addition of air displacement plethysmography
- Updated section on physical activity and obesity (weight control)

Chapter 19 Factors Affecting Performance
- Miscellaneous updates to content
- Updated references and readings

Chapter 20 Laboratory Assessment of Human
Performance
- New material on jumping tests to determine
  anaerobic power
- Revised and updated information regarding
  isometric measurement of strength
- Several new illustrations

Chapter 21 Training for Performance
- Updated information on single vs. multiple
  sets for strength-training
- Revised and updated discussion of strength-
  training principles
- Updated material on exercise-induced muscle
  soreness
- Revised and updated information on flexibility

Chapter 22 Training for the Female Athlete, Children,
and Special Populations
- Updated information on female athlete triad;
  includes new illustration
- Revised and updated illustrations
- New section on risk of knee injury in female
  athletes

Chapter 23 Nutrition, Body Composition, and
Performance
- New Winning Edge box on hyponatremia
- Miscellaneous updates to other sections to
  add new information

Chapter 24 Exercise and the Environment
- Expanded treatment of lactate paradox in
  A Closer Look box
- More information on acclimatization to
  prevent heat-related deaths
- Expanded discussion of pollution and exercise

Chapter 25 Ergogenic Aids
- New information to update various topics
- Expanded discussion of caffeine
- Extensive revision of section on warm-up
- New section on stretching as part of warm-up
  discussion

SUCCESSFUL FEATURES

Contents and Organization

All topics in exercise physiology addressed in this
text are presented in a contemporary fashion and
supported by up-to-date references. The text is divided into three sections: (1) Physiology of Exercise,
(2) Physiology of Health and Fitness, and (3) Physiology of Performance. Section One (Physiology of Exercise) contains 13 chapters that provide the necessary
background for the beginning student of exercise
physiology to understand the role of the major organ
systems of the body in maintaining homeostasis during exercise. In fact, a major theme of this section is

that almost all organ systems work to help maintain a
relatively stable internal environment during exercise.
Also included are chapters that present an overview
of biological control systems; bioenergetics; exercise
metabolism; endocrine function during exercise; techniques for measurement of work, power, and energy
expenditure; neuromuscular function during exercise; cardiopulmonary responses to exercise; acid-
base regulation during exercise; temperature regulation; and the effects of endurance training on various
organ systems.

Sections Two and Three are designed to show
how the information presented in Section One is
applied to fitness and performance. These two sections distinguish between exercise programs that are
appropriate for attainment of health-related fitness
goals and those needed to realize world-class or individual maximal performance goals. Section Two
(Physiology of Health and Fitness) contains five chapters dealing with health-related fitness: (1) factors
that limit health and fitness; (2) work tests used to
evaluate cardiorespiratory fitness; (3) training methods for fitness; (4) exercise concerns for special populations; and (5) body composition and nutritional
concerns for health.

Section Three (Physiology of Performance) includes seven chapters dealing with the physiology
of performance: (1) factors affecting performance;
(2) work tests to evaluate performance; (3) training
techniques for improvement of performance; (4) training concerns for special populations; (5) nutrition,
body composition, performance; (6) environmental
influences on performance; and (7) ergogenic aids. A
unique aspect of Sections Two and Three is that they
include two chapters on exercise training for special
populations. These chapters feature discussions of
exercise for women, asthmatics, diabetics, and the
elderly.

Writing Style and Presentation

The concepts in this text are presented in a simple
and straightforward way. The writing style is key to
making the content understandable to all students.
Illustrations and examples are commonly used to
clarify or further explain a concept. Key terms are
shown in bold type, defined as they are presented,
and organized in a glossary at the end of the book.

Pedagogical Aids

The following teaching aids have proved to be successful in earlier editions and so have been included
in this new edition.

Objectives The list of objectives at the beginning of
each chapter presents the key concepts that students
will need to understand. This tool helps students

focus their attention so that they will be well prepared for participating in class discussions and for taking examinations.

Outlines Each chapter includes an outline of topics that shows how the chapter is organized. With major headings and their page numbers listed, students can find key topics quickly as they prepare for class and review for examinations.

Key Terms The most important terms for learning are presented on the first page of each chapter. These terms are shown in bold type in the text, where they are explained and discussed. This visual emphasis makes it easy for students to locate the key terms and reinforce their learning.

In Summary The short summaries presented at the end of each major discussion prompt students to review what they have just learned. This helps them retain key concepts and be well prepared for the upcoming discussions.

A Closer Look This feature offers an in-depth view of topics of special interest to students. By encouraging students to think further about what they have just read, these boxes reinforce the text discussion and enhance student learning. Topics include anabolic steroids and performance, calculation of body temperature increase during exercise, and low-intensity exercise as a way of burning fat.

Research Focus No matter what their career direction is, students in exercise physiology need to be informed about the latest research in the field. The research boxes will keep them up to date on issues such as the repeated bout effect related to muscle soreness and the importance of nitric oxide as a vasodilator.

Clinical Applications How is knowledge in exercise physiology used in clinical settings? This feature shows students how their learning can be applied to health care, sports medicine, and physical therapy. For example, it demonstrates how beta-blockers affect exercise heart rate and how exercise and weight control are related.

The Winning Edge These boxes focus on how athletes find the "extra edge" that can make the difference between victory and defeat. Is maximum oxygen uptake important in distance running performance? What is the best way to use sets in strength training? What are the implications of the female athlete triad?

Ask the Expert This feature offers students a question-and-answer look at what leading scientists have to say about important issues in exercise physiology. What are the issues involved in tracking obesity-related risk? What special considerations are associated with children and exercise? How does exercise affect bone health?

Study Questions A set of study questions appears at the end of each chapter. This study tool helps students analyze the chapter content and prepare for exams.

Suggested Readings Students who want to learn more about topics presented in the text can refer to this chapter list for specific books and articles of interest.

Appendixes *Exercise Physiology* includes eight appendixes that are valuable resources for the student. New appendixes for this edition include the PARmed-X Physical Activity Readiness Medical Examination (Appendix C), Dietary Reference Intakes: Macronutrients (Appendix D), Dietary Reference Intakes: Vitamins and Minerals (Appendix E), and Dietary Reference Intakes: Estimated Energy Requirements (Appendix F).

Glossary The glossary that appears at the end of this book provides quick and easy access to definitions for all the key terms.

SUPPLEMENTS

Instructor's Resource CD-ROM (ISBN 0-07-302865-7)

This CD-ROM includes all the resources you need to help teach your course: It works in both Windows and Macintosh environments and includes the following teaching tools:

Instructor's Manual This manual includes key concepts, lecture outlines, suggested activities, and readings.

Test Bank The electronic Test Bank (Microsoft Word files), which includes the same questions presented in the Computerized Test Bank, is offered as an alternative version.

Computerized Test Bank The Test Bank is available with the EZ Test computerized testing software, which provides a powerful, easy-to-use way to create printed quizzes and exams. EZ Test runs on both Windows and Macintosh systems. For secure online testing, exams created in EZ Test can be exported to WebCT, Blackboard, PageOut, and EZ Test Online. EZ Test is packaged with a Quick Start Guide. Once the program is installed, you have access to the complete

User's Manual, including Flash tutorials. Additional help is available at www.mhhe.com/eztest.

PowerPoint slides A comprehensive set of Power-Point lecture slides for your course completes this package of tools. The slides correspond to the content in each chapter of *Exercise Physiology*, making it easier for you to teach and ensuring that your students will be able to follow your lectures point by point. You can modify the presentation as much as you like to meet the needs of your course.

Image Library This collection contains all the illustrations presented in the text. Images can be selected for use in conjunction with lectures, classroom discussions, and PowerPoint slides.

Online Learning Center
www.mhhe.com/powers6e

The Online Learning Center to accompany *Exercise Physiology* offers a number of special resources for instructors and students:

For the instructor:
- Downloadable PowerPoint presentations
- Instructor's Manual
- Image Library

For the student:
- Practice quizzes
- Glossary and flashcards
- Animations
- Learning objectives
- Chapter outlines
- Suggested readings
- Links to professional organizations
- Career information

Anatomy & Physiology Revealed
CD-ROM Series

This amazing multimedia tool is designed to help students learn and review human anatomy using cadaver specimens. Detailed cadaver photos blended together with a state-of-the-art layering technique provide a uniquely interactive dissection experience.
CD #1: Skeletal/Muscular Systems
(ISBN 0-07-312323-4)
CD #2: Nervous System
(ISBN 0-07-312321-8)
CD #3: Cardiovascular, Respiratory, and Lymphatic Systems
(ISBN 0-07-321550-3)

CD #4: Digestive, Endocrine, Urinary, and Reproductive Systems
(ISBN 0-07-321551-1)

NutriCalc Plus

This dietary analysis program features an easy-to-use interface that allows users to track their nutrient and food group intakes, energy expenditures, and weight control goals. NutriCalc Plus is available on CD-ROM (ISBN 0-07-319532-4) or as an online version (ISBN 0-07-292127-7).

Primis Online
www.mhhe.com/primis/online

Primis Online is a database-driven publishing system that allows you to create customized textbooks, lab manuals, or readers for your courses directly from the Primis Web site. The custom text can be delivered in print or electronic (eBook) form. A Primis eBook is a digital version of the customized text sold directly to students as a file downloadable to their computer or accessed online by password. Motor Learning and Control can be customized using Primis Online.

PageOut
www.pageout.net

PageOut is a free, easy-to-use program that lets you quickly develop Web sites for your courses. With PageOut, you can create a course home page, an instructor home page, an interactive syllabus that can be linked to elements in the Online Learning Center, Web links, online discussion areas, an online gradebook, and much more. Contact your local sales representative to obtain a password.

Course Management Systems
www.mhhe.com/solutions

The McGraw-Hill Instructor Advantage program offers access to a complete online teaching Web site called the Knowledge Gateway, toll-free phone support, and unlimited e-mail support directly from WebCT and Blackboard. Instructors who use 500 or more copies of a text can enroll in the Instructor Advantage Plus program, which provides on-campus, hands-on training from a certified platform specialist.

A Guided Tour of *Exercise Physiology*

What are the latest research findings in exercise physiology? Want to understand how this information applies to exercise science, sports, athletic training, or physical therapy? Trying to improve your grade? The special features in *Exercise Physiology: Theory and Application to Fitness and Performance* will help you do all this and more! Let's take a look inside this book . . .

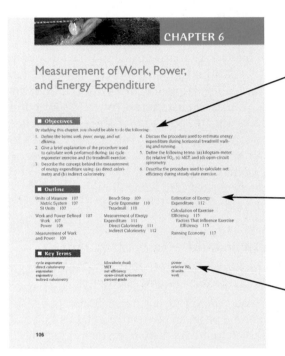

Learning Objectives

The objectives at the beginning of each chapter help you focus on the key points for learning. Use this tool to prepare for class discussions and exams.

Outline of Topic

How is each chapter organized? The outline shows you at a glance—page numbers will help you locate key topics quickly as you study.

Key Terms

The key terms are highlighted when they are introduced and defined in the text. This visual emphasis makes the terms easy to locate and remember.

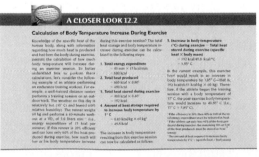

In Summary

Each major section is followed by a summary of its main ideas. Take a few minutes to review those key concepts before starting the next section.

Ask the Expert

This question-and-answer feature lets you find out what leading scientists have to say about topics such as obesity-related risks and the effect of exercise on bone health.

A Closer Look

These boxes offer an in-depth view of chapter topics. Examples include how to calculate body temperature increase during exercise and the PACER test.

Research Focus

Can exercise prevent or delay the onset of type 2 diabetes? Why is nitric oxide an important vasodilator? Look here for the latest findings on such topics.

Clinical Applications

Learn how exercise physiology is used in the clinical setting. How can enzyme activity in the blood be used to diagnose certain diseases? What does the glycemic index tell us?

The Winning Edge

What new information about the female athlete triad is available? How does hyponatremia affect performance? Check these boxes to see how scientific findings can be used in sports.

Study Questions

Check how well you understand the chapter content with these questions. Use them to prepare for exams.

Suggested Readings

Want to know more about a topic in this book? Look here for a list of readings available for further exploration.

Up-to-Date References

Each chapter includes a comprehensive reference list of journal articles and texts that reflect the up-to-date content in this book.

REFERENCES

1. Abernethy, P., R. Thayer, and A. Taylor. 1990. Acute and chronic responses of skeletal muscle to endurance and sprint exercise: A review. *Sports Medicine* 10:365–89.
2. Adams, G. et al. 1993. Skeletal muscle myosin heavy chain composition and resistance training. *Journal of Applied Physiology* 74:911–15.
3. Alway, S. et al. 1990. Muscle cross-sectional area and torque in resistance trained subjects. *European Journal of Applied Physiology* 60:86–90.
4. Appell, H. 1990. Muscular atrophy following immobilization. A review. *Sports Medicine* 10:42–58.
5. Armstrong, R. et al. 1983. Differential inter- and intra-muscular responses to exercise. Considerations in use of the biopsy technique. In *Biochemistry of Exercise*, eds. H. Knuttgen, J. Vogel, and J. Poortmans, 775–80. Champaign, IL: Human Kinetics.
6. Armstrong, R., and H. Laughlin. 1985. Muscle function during locomotion in mammals. In *Circulation, Respiration, and Metabolism*, ed. R. Giles, 56–63. New York: Springer-Verlag.
7. Bagby, G., W. Sembrowich, and P. Gollnick. 1972. Myosin ATPase and fiber type composition from trained and untrained rat skeletal muscle. *Journal of Applied Physiology* 223:1415–17.
8. Baldwin, K. et al. 1972. Respiratory capacity of white, red, and intermediate muscle: Adaptive response to exercise. *Journal of Applied Physiology* 222:373–78.
9. Bar, A., and D. Pette. 1988. Three fast myosin heavy chains in adult rat skeletal muscle. *FEBS Letters* 235:153–54.
10. Barton-Davis, E. et al. 1998. Viral mediated expression of insulin-like growth factor I blocks the age-related loss of skeletal muscle function. *Proceedings of the National Academy of Sciences* 95:15603–7.
11. Billeter, R., and H. Hoppeler. 1992. Muscular basis of strength. In *Strength and Power in Sport*, ed. P. Komi, 39–63. Oxford: Blackwell Scientific Publishing.
12. Black, R. 1991. Muscle strength as an indicator of the habitual level of physical activity. *Medicine and Science in Sports and Exercise* 23:1375–81.
13. Bobbert, M., G. Ettema, and P. Huijing. 1990. The force-length relationship of a muscle-tendon complex. Experimental results and model calculations. *European Journal of Applied Physiology* 61:323–29.
14. Booth, F., and D. Thomason. 1991. Molecular and cellular adaptation of muscle in response to exercise: Perspectives of various models. *Physiological Reviews* 71:541–85.
15. Booth, F. and S. Weeden. 1993. Structural aspects of aging human skeletal muscle. In *Musculoskeletal Soft-tissue Aging: Impact on Mobility*, ed. J. Buckwalter, V. Goldberg, and S. Woo. Rosemont, IL: American Academy of Orthopaedic Surgeons.
16. Booth, F.W. and D. S. Criswell. 1997. Molecular events underlying skeletal muscle atrophy and the development of effective countermeasures. *International Journal of Sports Medicine* 18 (Suppl. 4): S265–69.
17. Bottinelli, R., M. Canepari, C. Reggiani, and G. Stienen. 1994. Myofibrillar ATPase activity during isometric contractions and isomyosin composition in rat single skinned muscle fibres. *Journal of Physiology (London)* 481:663–75.
18. Brooks, G., T. Fahey, T. White, and K. Baldwin. 2000. *Exercise Physiology: Human Bioenergetics and Its Applications*. New York: McGraw-Hill Companies.
19. ———. 1957. *Fundamentals of Human Performance*. New York: Macmillan.
20. Buchthal, F., and H. Schmalbruch. 1970. Contraction times and fiber types in intact human muscle. *Acta Physiologica Scandanavica* 79:435–45.
21. Burke, R. 1986. The control of muscle force: Motor unit recruitment and firing pattern. In *Human Muscle Power*, ed. N. Jones, N. McCartney, and A. McComas, 97–109. Champaign, IL: Human Kinetics.
22. Caiozzo, V. et al. 1997. Single fiber analyses of Type IIa myosin heavy chain distribution in hyper- and hypothyroid soleus. *American Journal of Physiology* 265:C842–49.
23. Cairns, S., A. Knicker, M. Thompson, and D. Sjogaard. 2005. Evaluation of models used to study neuromuscular fatigue. *Exercise and Sport Science Review* 33:9–16.
24. Carlson, F., and D. Wilkie. 1974. *Muscle Physiology*. Englewood Cliffs, NJ: Prentice-Hall.
25. Carmeli, E., R. Coleman, and A. Z. Reznick. 2002. The biochemistry of aging muscle. *Experimental Gerontology* 37:477–89.
26. Conley, K. 1994. Cellular energetics during exercise. *Advances in Veterinary Science and Comparative Medicine* 38A:1–39.
27. Costill, D., W. Fink, and M. Pollock. 1976. Muscle fiber composition and enzyme activities of elite distance runners. *Medicine and Science in Sports* 8:96.
28. Demirel, H., S. Powers, H. Naito, M. Hughes, and J. Coombes. 1999. Exercise-induced alterations in skeletal muscle myosin heavy chain phenotype: dose-response relationship. *Journal of Applied Physiology* 86:1002–8.
29. Deliabourenza, K., Kawano, M. Deering, D. Falk, D. Van Gammeren, T. Yimlamai, G. Ordway, and S. Powers. 2005. Mechanical ventilation induces alterations of the ubiscuitin-proteasome pathway in the diaphragm. *Journal of Applied Physiology* 95:1314–21.
30. Devor, S. and T. White. 1995. Myosin heavy chain phenotype in regenerating skeletal muscle is affected by thyroid hormone. *Medicine and Science in Sports and Exercise* 27:674–61.
31. Ebashi, S. 1976. Excitation-contraction coupling. *Annual Review of Physiology* 38:293–309.
32. ———. 1991. Excitation-contraction coupling. *Annual Review of Physiology* 53:1–16.
33. Edgerton, V. et al. 1983. Muscle fiber activation and recruitment. In *Biochemistry of Exercise*, ed. H. Knuttgen, J. Vogel, and J. Poortmans, 31–49. Champaign, IL: Human Kinetics.
34. Edgerton, V. et al. 1986. Morphological basis of skeletal muscle power output. In *Human Muscle Power*, ed. N. Jones, N. McCartney, and A. McComas, 43–58. Champaign, IL: Human Kinetics.
35. Edman, K. 1992. Contractile performance of skeletal muscle fibers. In *Strength and Power in Sport*, ed. P. Komi, 96–114. Oxford: Blackwell Scientific Publishing.
36. Edstrom, L., and L. Grimby. 1986. Effect of exercise on the motor unit. *Muscle and Nerve* 9:104–26.
37. Faulkner, J., D. Claflin, and K. McCully. 1986. Power output of fast and slow fibers from human skeletal muscles. In *Human Muscle Power*, ed. N. Jones, N. McCartney, and A. McComas, 81–90. Champaign, IL: Human Kinetics.
38. Fauteck, S., and S. Kandarian. 1995. Sensitive detection of myosin heavy chain composition in skeletal muscle under different loading conditions. *American Journal of Physiology* 37:C419–C424.

166 Section One Physiology of Exercise

Online Learning Center
www.mhhe.com/powers6e

Visit the Online Learning Center for all the resources you need to get the most out of this text. There you'll find:

- Practice quizzes
- Flashcards for key terms
- Animations
- Learning objectives
- Chapter outlines
- Suggested readings
- Links to professional organizations
- Career information

Acknowledgments

A text like Exercise Physiology: Theory and Application to Fitness and Performance is not the effort of two authors, but represents the contributions of hundreds of scientists throughout the world. While it is not possible to acknowledge every contributor to this work, we would like to recognize the following scientists who have greatly influenced our thinking, careers, and lives in general: Drs. Bruno Balke, Ralph Beadle, Ronald Byrd, Jerome Dempsey, Stephen Dodd, H. V. Forster, B. D. Franks, Steven Horvath, Henry Montoye, Francis Nagle, Michael Pollock, and Hugh G. Welch.

In addition, we would like to thank the following reviewers, who provided helpful comments about the fifth edition of Exercise Physiology:

William Beam
California State University, Fullerton

Frank Bosso
Youngstown State University

Joseph Chromiak
Mississippi State University

Lisa Colvin
University of Louisiana at Monroe

Glen Fincher II
Ashland University

Guy Leadbetter III
Mesa State College

Allen Parcell
Brigham Young University

Linda Tecklenburg
Wilmington College

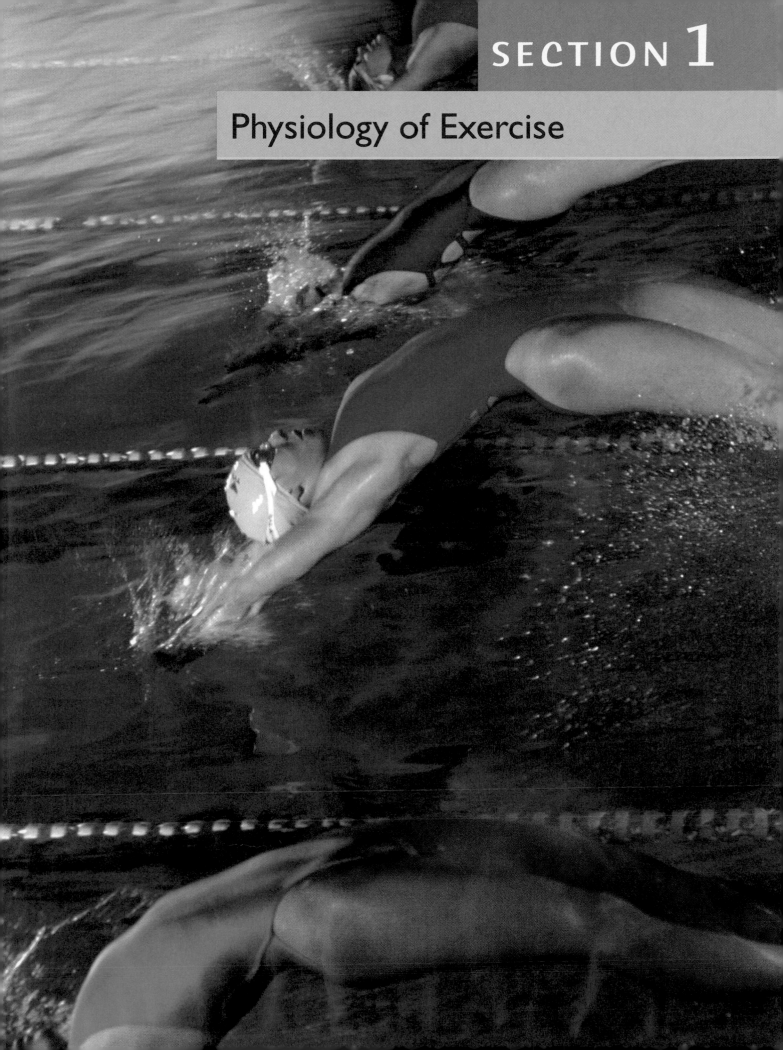

SECTION 1

Physiology of Exercise

Physiology of Exercise in the United States—Its Past, Its Future

■ Objectives

By studying this chapter, you should be able to do the following:

1. Name the three Nobel Prize winners whose research work involved muscle or muscular exercise.

2. Describe the role of the Harvard Fatigue Laboratory in the history of exercise physiology in the United States.

3. Describe factors influencing physical fitness in the United States over the past century.

■ Outline

European Heritage   3

Harvard Fatigue Laboratory   4

Physical Fitness   5

Physical Education to Exercise Science   7

Graduate Study and Research in the Physiology of Exercise   8

Professional Societies and Research Journals   10

Translation of Exercise Physiology to the Consumer   11

Does one have to have a "genetic gift" of speed to be a world-class runner, or is it all due to training? What happens to your heart rate when you take a fitness test that increases in intensity each minute? What changes occur in your muscles as a result of an endurance training program that allows you to run at faster speeds over longer distances? The answers to these and other questions are provided throughout this text. However, we go beyond simple statements of fact to show how information about the physiology of exercise is applied to the prevention of and rehabilitation from coronary heart disease, the performances of elite athletes, and the ability of a person to work in adverse environments such as high altitudes. The acceptance of terms such as *sports physiology*, *sports nutrition*, and *sports medicine* is evidence of the growth of interest in the application of physiology of exercise to real-world problems. Before we take you on this journey, we need to take a brief look at the history of exercise physiology to understand where we are and where we are going.

EUROPEAN HERITAGE

A good starting place to discuss the history of exercise physiology in the United States is in Europe. Three scientists, A. V. Hill of Britain, August Krogh of Denmark, and Otto Meyerhof of Germany, received Nobel Prizes for research on muscle or muscular exercise (9). Hill and Meyerhof shared the Nobel Prize in Physiology or

Medicine in 1922. Hill was recognized for his precise measurements of heat production during muscle contraction and recovery, and Meyerhof for his discovery of the relationship between the consumption of oxygen and the measurement of lactic acid in muscle. Hill was trained as a mathematician before becoming interested in physiology. In addition to his work cited for the Nobel Prize, his studies on humans led to the development of a framework around which we understand the physiological factors related to distance running performance (4) (see A Closer Look 1.1).

Although Krogh received his Nobel Prize for his research on the function of the capillary circulation, he is also known for designing a considerable amount of instrumentation used in exercise physiology research. A precise gas analyzer to measure CO_2 within 0.001%, an accurate mechanically braked cycle ergometer, and a precision balance to weigh exercising human subjects within a few grams (13) are but three examples of Krogh's resourcefulness. The August Krogh Institute in Denmark contains some of the most prominent exercise physiology laboratories in the world. Marie Krogh, his wife, was a noted scientist in her own right and was recognized for her innovative work on measuring the diffusing capacity of the lung. We recommend the biography of the Kroghs written by their daughter, Bodil Schmit-Nielsen (see Suggested Readings), for those interested in the history of the physiology of exercise.

There are several other European scientists who must be mentioned, not only because of their

A CLOSER LOOK 1.1

In the years following the awarding of the Nobel Prize to Hill and Meyerhof in 1922, Hill carried out experiments on exercising humans and established classical concepts in exercise physiology that are with us today. Hill had subjects, including himself, run around an 85-meter grass track while wearing a mouthpiece, a gas collection (Douglas) bag, and a three-way valve to start and stop gas collection. Numerous measurements of oxygen uptake, made at both submaximal and maximal sustainable speeds, provided data that allowed Hill and his colleagues to characterize how humans respond to such exercise. The following terms, assigned to some of the responses, are "classics" in exercise physiology:

- *steady-state oxygen uptake*: After an initial increase in oxygen uptake at the onset of exercise, the oxygen uptake stabilizes at a value proportional to submaximal speed, and remains at that level as long as the speed remains constant.
- *maximal oxygen uptake*: The upper limit in the body's ability to consume oxygen, which Hill believed was linked to the body's capacity for oxygen transport (see chapter 13).

Hill also measured oxygen uptake in recovery from exercise and named the elevated oxygen uptake the *oxygen debt*. He surmised that the body was able to use energy at a high rate during exercise—beyond what could be provided by oxygen consumption—and the body had to "repay" that energy credit in recovery (chapter 4 will have more on that). Lastly, Hill also predicted that superior running performance was linked to a high maximal oxygen uptake and a low oxygen requirement for running (good running economy). See chapter 19 for more on the factors affecting performance.

Hill made enormous contributions to the field of exercise physiology. For an interesting history of Hill that goes beyond his scientific accomplishments, read Bassett's review in the Suggested Readings. A Closer Look 1.2 describes the work of a scientist who was influenced and encouraged by Hill.

A CLOSER LOOK 1.2

One scientist whose roots can be traced to A. V. Hill is Dr. Brenda Bigland-Ritchie. As a graduate student, she was encouraged by Hill to examine the oxygen cost of doing positive and negative work, to parallel the experiments he had done in shortening and lengthening contractions in isolated muscle. In a very clever design, Brenda Bigland, Murdoch Ritchie (her future husband), and Bud Abbott arranged two bicycles back to back such that one rider pedaled forward and one pedaled backward—the same muscles were involved, but one muscle group was being lengthened while the other was being shortened. Positive work (shortening) required much more energy than negative work at the same power output. In 1953, Bigland-Ritchie stepped away from science while she raised her family, and it wasn't until 1969 that she completed her Ph.D. She then took a teaching position at Quinnipiac College in Connecticut and restarted her scientific studies in collaboration with another new Ph.D., Joseph J. Woods. Dr. Bigland-Ritchie's research focused on skeletal muscle physiology with specific interest in the relationship between muscle force and the electrical activity of the muscle. However, it is her work on the causes of neuromuscular fatigue for which she is internationally known (33). We refer the interested reader to an autobiographical piece by Dr. Bigland-Ritchie in a book dedicated to her (see Gandevia et al. in the Suggested Readings).

contributions to the physiology of exercise, but because their names are commonly used in a discussion of exercise physiology. J. S. Haldane did some of the original work on the role of CO_2 in the control of breathing. Haldane also developed the respiratory gas analyzer that bears his name (13). C. G. Douglas did pioneering work with Haldane in the role of O_2 and lactic acid in the control of breathing during exercise, including some work conducted at various altitudes. The canvas-and-rubber gas collection bag used for many years in exercise physiology laboratories around the world carries Douglas's name. A contemporary of Douglas, Christian Bohr of Denmark, did the classic work on how O_2 binds to hemoglobin. The "shift" in the oxygen-hemoglobin dissociation curve due to the addition of CO_2 bears his name. It was in Bohr's lab that Krogh got his start on a career studying respiration and exercise in humans (13).

IN SUMMARY

- Three physiologists, A. V. Hill, August Krogh, and Otto Meyerhof, received the Nobel Prize for work related to muscle or muscular exercise.

HARVARD FATIGUE LABORATORY

A focal point in the history of exercise physiology in the United States is the Harvard Fatigue Laboratory. Professor L. J. Henderson organized the laboratory within the Business School to conduct physiological research on industrial hazards. Dr. David Bruce Dill was the research director from the time the laboratory opened in 1927 until it closed in 1947 (16). Table 1-1

TABLE 1.1	Active Research Areas in the Harvard Fatigue Laboratory

Metabolism
    Maximal oxygen uptake
    Oxygen debt
    Carbohydrate and fat metabolism during
       long-term work
Environmental physiology
    Altitude
    Dry and moist heat
    Cold
Clinical physiology
    Gout
    Schizophrenia
    Diabetes
Aging
    Basal metabolic rate
    Maximal oxygen uptake
    Maximal heart rate
Blood
    Acid-base balance
    O_2 saturation: role of PO_2, PCO_2, and carbon
       monoxide
Nutrition
    Nutritional assessment techniques
    Vitamins
    Foods
Physical fitness
    Harvard Step Test

shows that the laboratory conducted research in numerous areas, in the laboratory and in the field, and the results of those early studies have been supported by recent investigations. Dill's classic text, *Life, Heat, and Altitude* (12), is recommended reading for any stu-

FIGURE 1.1 Comparison of old and new technology used to measure oxygen consumption and carbon dioxide production during exercise. (*Left:* The Carnegie Institute of Washington, D.C.; *Right:* Quinton Instrument Co.)

dent of exercise and environmental physiology. Much of the careful and precise work of the laboratory was conducted using the now-classic Haldane analyzer for respiratory gas analysis and the van Slyke apparatus for blood-gas analysis. The advent of computer-controlled equipment in the 1980s has made data collection easier, but has not improved on the accuracy of measurement (see figure 1.1).

The Harvard Fatigue Laboratory attracted doctoral students as well as scientists from other countries. Many of the alumni from the laboratory are recognized in their own right for excellence in research in the physiology of exercise. Two doctoral students, Steven Horvath and Sid Robinson, went on to distinguished careers at the Institute of Environmental Stress in Santa Barbara and Indiana University, respectively. Foreign "Fellows" included E. Asmussen, E. H. Christensen, M. Nielsen, and the Nobel Prize winner August Krogh from Denmark. These scientists brought new ideas and technology to the lab, participated in laboratory and field studies with other staff members, and published some of the most important work in the physiology of exercise between 1930 and 1980. Rudolpho Margaria, from Italy, went on to extend his classic work on oxygen debt and described the energetics of locomotion. Peter F. Scholander, from Norway, gave us his chemical gas analyzer that is a primary method of calibrating tank gas used to standardize electronic gas analyzers (16).

In summary, under the leadership of Dr. D. B. Dill, the Harvard Fatigue Laboratory became a model for research investigations into exercise and environmental physiology, especially as it relates to humans. When the laboratory closed and the staff dispersed, the ideas, techniques, and approaches to scientific inquiry were distributed throughout the world, and with them, Dill's influence in the area of environmental and exercise physiology. Dr. Dill continued his research outside Boulder City, Nevada, into the 1980s. He died at the age of 93 in 1986.

Progress toward understanding any issue in exercise physiology transcends time, national origin, and scientific training. Solutions to difficult questions require the interaction of scientists from diverse disciplines and professions such as physiology, biochemistry, molecular biology, and medicine. We will highlight several scientists with our Ask the Expert boxes throughout the text, both to introduce them to you and for them to share their current ideas. However, we would like to recommend a recently published text, *Exercise Physiology—People and Ideas* (see the Suggested Readings) to further your understanding of important historical connections. In this book, internationally known scientists provide an historical treatment of a number of important issues in exercise physiology with an emphasis on the cross-continent flow of energy and ideas. It is in this context that you will get to know those who have gone before and those who are currently leading the charge.

IN SUMMARY

■ The Harvard Fatigue Laboratory was a focal point in the development of exercise physiology in the United States. Dr. D. B. Dill directed the laboratory from its opening in 1927 until its closing in 1947. The body of research in exercise and environmental physiology produced by that laboratory forms the basis of much of what we know today.

PHYSICAL FITNESS

Physical fitness is a popular topic today, and its popularity has been a major factor in motivating college students to pursue careers in physical education, physiology of exercise, health education, nutrition, physical therapy, and medicine. In 1980, the Public Health Service listed "physical fitness and exercise" as one of fifteen areas of concern related to improving the country's overall health (28). While this might appear to be an unprecedented event, similar interests and concerns about physical fitness existed in this country over one hundred years ago. Between the Civil War and the First World War (WW I), physical education was primarily concerned with the development and maintenance of fitness, and many of the leaders in physical education were trained in medicine (10, p. 5). For example, Dr. Dudley Sargent, hired by Harvard University in 1879, set up a physical training program with individual exercise prescriptions to improve a person's structure and function to achieve "that prime physical condition called fitness—fitness for work, fitness for play, fitness for anything a man may be called upon to do" (31, p. 297).

Sargent was clearly ahead of his time in promoting health-related fitness. Later, war became a primary force driving this country's interest in physical fitness. Concerns about health and fitness were raised during WW I and WW II when large numbers of draftees failed the induction exams due to mental and physical defects (15, p. 407). These concerns influenced the type of physical education programs in the schools during these years, making them resemble premilitary training programs (37, p. 484).

The present interest in physical activity and health was stimulated in the early 1950s by two major findings: (1) autopsies of young soldiers killed during the Korean War showed that significant coronary artery disease had already developed, and (2) Hans Kraus showed that American children performed poorly on a minimal muscular fitness test compared to European children (37, p. 516). Due to the latter finding, President Eisenhower initiated a conference in 1955 that resulted in the formation of the President's Council on Youth Fitness. The American Association for Health, Physical Education, and Recreation (AAHPER) supported these activities and in 1957 developed the AAHPER Youth Fitness Test with national norms to be used in physical education programs throughout the country. Before he was inaugurated, President Kennedy expressed his concerns about the nation's fitness in an article published in *Sports Illustrated*, called "The Soft American" (21):

> For the physical vigor of our citizens is one of America's most precious resources. If we waste and neglect this resource, if we allow it to dwindle and grow soft, then we will destroy much of our ability to meet the great and vital challenges which confront our people. We will be unable to realize our full potential as a nation.

During Kennedy's term the council's name was changed to the "President's Council on Physical Fit-

ness" to highlight the concern for fitness. The name was changed again in the Nixon administration to the current "President's Council on Physical Fitness and Sports," which supports fitness not only in schools but in business and industry. Items in the Youth Fitness Test were changed over the years, and in 1980 the American Alliance for Health, Physical Education, Recreation, and Dance (AAHPERD) published a separate *Health-Related Physical Fitness Test Manual* (1) to distinguish between "performance testing" (e.g., 50-yard dash) and "fitness testing" (e.g., skinfold thickness). This health-related test battery is consistent with the direction of lifetime fitness programs, being concerned with obesity, cardiorespiratory fitness, and low-back function. For those readers interested in the history of fitness testing in schools, we recommend Park's monograph in the Suggested Readings.

Paralleling this interest in the physical fitness of youth was the rising concern about the death rate from coronary heart disease in the middle-aged American male population. Epidemiological studies of the health status of the population underscored the fact that degenerative diseases related to poor health habits (e.g., high-fat diet, smoking, inactivity) were responsible for more deaths than the classic infectious and contagious diseases. In 1966, a major symposium highlighted the need for more research in the area of physical activity and health (29). In the 1970s, there was an increase in the use of exercise tests to diagnose heart disease and to aid in the prescription of exercise programs to improve cardiovascular health. Large corporations developed "executive" fitness programs to improve the health status of that high-risk group. While most Americans are now familiar with such programs, and some students of exercise physiology seek careers in "Corporate Fitness," such programs are not new. The photos in figures 1.2 and

FIGURE 1.2 A group of businessmen in a dancing class under the direction of Oliver E. Hebbert.

FIGURE 1.3 Roof of the former John Wanamaker store, Philadelphia, showing running track, basketball, and tennis courts.

IN SUMMARY

- Fitness has been an issue in this country from the latter part of the nineteenth century until the present. War or the threat of war exerted a strong influence on fitness programs in the public schools.
- Recent interest in fitness is related to the growing concern over the high death rates from disease processes that are attributable to preventable factors, such as poor diet, lack of exercise, and smoking. The government and professional organizations have responded to this need by educating the public about these problems.
- Schools are now using health-related fitness tests such as the skinfold estimation of body fatness, rather than the more traditional performance tests, to evaluate a child's physical fitness.

1.3, taken from the 1923 edition of McKenzie's *Exercise in Education and Medicine* (24), show a group of businessmen in costume doing dance exercises (figure 1.2), and fitness facilities on the roof of a large inner-city department store (figure 1.3). In short, the idea that regular physical activity is an important part of a healthy lifestyle was "rediscovered." If any questions remained about the importance of physical activity to health, the publication of the Surgeon General's report put them to rest (see A Closer Look 1.3).

PHYSICAL EDUCATION TO EXERCISE SCIENCE

Undergraduate academic preparation in physical education has changed over the past four decades to reflect the explosion in the knowledge base related to the physiology of exercise, biomechanics, and exercise prescription. This occurred at a time of a reduced

A CLOSER LOOK 1.3

By the early to mid 1980s, it had become clear that physical inactivity was a major public health concern (28). In 1992, the American Heart Association made physical inactivity a major risk factor for cardiovascular diseases, just like smoking, high blood pressure, and high serum cholesterol (3). In 1995, the Centers for Disease Control and Prevention (CDC) and the American College of Sports Medicine published a public health physical activity recommendation that "Every U.S. adult should accumulate 30 minutes or more of moderate-intensity physical activity on most, preferably all, days of the week" (27). A year later, the *Surgeon General's Report on Physical Activity and Health* was published (35). This report

highlighted the fact that physical inactivity was killing U.S. adults, and the problem was a big one—60% of U.S. adults did not engage in the recommended amount of physical activity, and 25% were not active at all. This report was based on the large body of evidence available from epidemiological studies, small-group training studies, and clinical investigations showing the positive effects of an active lifestyle. For example, physical activity was shown to:

- lower the risk of dying prematurely and from heart disease
- reduce the risk of developing diabetes and high blood pressure

- help maintain weight and healthy bones, muscles, and joints
- help lower blood pressure in those with high blood pressure
- promote psychological well-being

Since the publication of the *Surgeon General's Report*, the obesity epidemic has focused special attention on the amount of physical activity needed to achieve and maintain a healthy weight. The *Dietary Guidelines for Americans 2005* (36) provides guidance for both caloric intake and physical activity related to this issue. We will present more on this in later chapters.

need for school-based physical education teachers and an increased need for exercise professionals in the preventive and clinical settings. These factors, as well as others, led some college and university departments to change their names from Physical Education to Exercise Science. This trend is likely to continue as programs move further away from traditional roots in education and become integrated within colleges of Arts and Sciences or Allied Health Professions (34). There has been an increase in the number of programs requiring undergraduates to take one year of calculus, chemistry, and physics, and courses in organic chemistry, biochemistry, anatomy, physiology, and nutrition. In many colleges and universities, there is now little difference between the first two years of requirements in a pre-physical therapy or pre-medical track and the track associated with fitness professions. The differences among these tracks lie in the "application" courses that follow. Biomechanics, physiology of exercise, fitness assessment, exercise prescription, exercise leadership, and so on belong to the physical education/exercise science track. However, it must again be pointed out that this new trend is but another example of a rediscovery of old roots rather than a revolutionary change. Kroll describes two four-year professional physical education programs in the 1890s, one at Stanford and the other at Harvard, that were the forerunners of today's programs (22, pp. 51–64). They included the detailed scientific work and application courses with clear prerequisites cited. Finally, considerable time was allotted for laboratory work. No doubt, Lagrange's 1890 text, *Physiology of Bodily Exercise* (23), served as an important reference source for these students. The expectations and goals of those programs were almost identical to those specified for current exercise physiology undergraduate tracks. In fact, one of the aims of the Harvard program was to allow a student to pursue the study of medicine after completing two years of study (22, p. 61).

GRADUATE STUDY AND RESEARCH IN THE PHYSIOLOGY OF EXERCISE

While the Harvard Fatigue Laboratory was closing in 1947, the country was on the verge of a tremendous expansion in the number of universities offering graduate study and research opportunities in exercise physiology. A 1950 survey showed that only 16 colleges or universities had research laboratories in departments of physical education (17). By 1966, 151 institutions had research facilities, 58 of them in exercise physiology (37, p. 526). This expansion was due to

the availability of more scientists trained in the research methodology of exercise physiology, the increased number of students attending college due to the GI Bill and student loans, and the increase in federal dollars to improve the research capabilities of universities (8, 34).

"The scholar's work will be multiplied many fold through the contribution of his students." This quote, taken from Montoye and Washburn (25), expresses a view that has helped attract researchers and scholars to universities. Evidence to support this quote was presented in the form of genealogical charts of contributors to the *Research Quarterly* (26). These charts showed the tremendous influence a few people had through their students in the expansion of research in physical education. Probably the best example of this is Thomas K. Cureton, Jr., of the University of Illinois, a central figure in the training of productive researchers in exercise physiology and fitness. The Illinois Research Laboratory dates from 1944 (22, pp. 177–83), and it focused attention on the physiology of fitness. The *Proceedings* of a symposium honoring Cureton in 1969 listed the sixty-eight Ph.D. students who completed their work under his direction (14). While Cureton's scholarly record includes hundreds of research articles and dozens of books dealing with physical fitness, the publications of his students in the areas of epidemiology, fitness, cardiac rehabilitation, and exercise physiology represent the "multiplying effect" that students have on a scholar's productivity (see A Closer Look 1.4).

An example of a major university program that can trace its lineage to the Harvard Fatigue Laboratory is found at Pennsylvania State University. Dr. Ancel Keys, a staff member at the Harvard Fatigue Laboratory, brought Henry Longstreet Taylor back to the Laboratory for Physiological Hygiene at the University of Minnesota, where he received his Ph.D. in 1941 (7). Taylor subsequently advised the research work of Elsworth R. Buskirk, who designed and directed the Laboratory for Human Performance Research (Noll Laboratory) at Pennsylvania State University. Noll Laboratory continues in the tradition of the Harvard Fatigue Laboratory with a comprehensive research program of laboratory and field research into basic exercise, environmental, and industrial research questions (6). However, it is clear that excellent research in exercise and environmental physiology is conducted in laboratories other than those that have a tie to the Harvard Fatigue Lab. Laboratories are found in physical education departments, physiology departments in medical schools, clinical medicine programs at hospitals, and in independent facilities like the Cooper Institute for Aerobics Research. The proliferation and specialization of research involving exercise is discussed in the next section.

A CLOSER LOOK 1.4

Bruno Balke

Given the introduction to this chapter, it should be no surprise that some scientists who have had an impact on the present state of exercise physiology, fitness, and cardiac rehabilitation in the United States received their training in Europe. Dr. Bruno Balke received his training in medicine and physical education in Germany and was invited to this country by Dr. Ulrich Luft in 1950. During the 1950s, he did research on high-altitude tolerance and high-speed flight for the Civil Aeromedical Research Institute and the United States Air Force. His research on work-capacity testing on the treadmill led to the development of the exercise test protocols that bear his name. In addition, his distance-run field test to eval-

uate cardiovascular fitness (maximal aerobic power) was modified by Ken Cooper for use in the well-known *Aerobics* book (11).

Balke was active in the early days of the American College of Sports Medicine (ACSM), serving as its president in 1966. He was a prime mover in the development of the ACSM certifications for exercise leaders of fitness and cardiac rehabilitation programs (see later discussion in the Translation of Exercise Physiology to the Consumer section) and was actively involved in the teaching and practical examinations associated with those certification workshops.

Balke left government service in 1963 to create the Biodynamics Labo-

ratory at the University of Wisconsin, Madison. Francis J. Nagle followed in 1964, and both had joint appointments with the physical education and physiology departments. Balke's quantitative approach to human physiological questions, especially as they related to fitness and performance, set the standard for other graduate exercise physiology programs. Balke enjoyed teaching others how to do things, and he viewed as his greatest accomplishment the graduation of the Ph.D. students from his lab who would now teach others (20). This is another example of how a scholar's work is multiplied by that of his or her students. Balke died in 1999 at the age of 92.

TABLE 1.2	**Significant Exercise Physiology Subject Matter Areas that Were Investigated Between 1954 and 1994**

A. Basic Exercise Physiology
- Exercise Specificity
- Exercise Prescription
- Central and Peripheral Responses and Adaptations
- Responses of Diseased Populations
- Action of Transmitters
- Regulation of Receptors
- Cardiovascular and Metabolic Feed Forward and Feedback Mechanisms
- Substrate Utilization Profiles
- Matching Mechanisms for Oxygen Delivery and Demand
- Mechanisms of Signal Transduction
- Intracellular Lactate Mechanisms

- Plasticity of Muscle Fibers
- Motor Functions of the Spinal Cord
- Hormonal Responses
- The Hypoxemia of Severe Exercise
- Cellular and Molecular Adaptive Responses

B. Applied Exercise Physiology
- Performance of Elite Athletes
- Performance and Heat Stress
- Exercise at Altitude
- Nutritional Aspects of Exercise
- Fluid Balance During Exercise
- Performance and Ergogenic Aids
- Training for Physical Fitness

From: C. M. Tipton, Contemporary exercise physiology: Fifty years after the closure of Harvard Fatigue Laboratory. In *Exercise and Sport Sciences Reviews*, vol. 26, pp. 315–39. Edited by J. O. Holloszy. Baltimore: Williams & Wilkins.

Table 1.2, from Tipton's look at the fifty years following the closing of the Harvard Fatigue Lab, shows the subject matter areas that were studied in considerable detail between 1954 and 1994 (34). A great number of these topics fit into the broad area of systemic physiology or were truly applied physiology issues. In the future, Tipton believes that many of the most important questions in the physiology of exer-

cise will be answered by those with special training in molecular biology. In fact, as biology and physiology programs shift their emphasis to the molecular approach, exercise science programs may be the primary academic department in which whole-body studies in exercise physiology will take place. We recommend the chapters by Tipton (34) and Buskirk and Tipton (8) for those interested in a detailed look at the development of exercise physiology in the United States.

IN SUMMARY

- The increase in research in exercise physiology was a catalyst that propelled the transformation of physical education departments into exercise science departments. The number of exercise physiology laboratories increased dramatically between the 1950s and 1970s, with many dealing with problems requiring specialized training in human physiology. That emphasis has been replaced with a focus on molecular biology as an essential ingredient to solving basic science issues related to physical activity and health.

PROFESSIONAL SOCIETIES AND RESEARCH JOURNALS

The expansion of interest in exercise physiology and its application to fitness and rehabilitation resulted in an increase in the number of professional societies in which scientists and clinicians could present their work. Prior to 1950, the two major societies concerned with physiology of exercise and its application were the American Physiological Society (APS) and the American Association of Health, Physical Education, and Recreation (AAHPER). The need to bring together physicians, physical educators, and physiologists interested in physical activity and health into one professional society resulted in the founding of the American College of Sports Medicine (ACSM) in 1954 (see Berryman's history of the ACSM in the Suggested Readings). The ACSM now has more than 20,000 members with twelve regional chapters throughout the country, each holding its own annual meeting to present research, sponsor symposiums, and promote sports medicine.

The growth of research journals has paralleled the increased number of professional societies. During the time of the Harvard Fatigue Laboratory, much of the research was published in the following journals: *Journal of Biological Chemistry, American Journal of Physiology, Arbeitsphysiologie* (*European Journal of Occupational and Applied Physiology*), *Journal of Clinical Investigation, Journal of Aviation Medicine, Journal of Nutrition,* and *Journal of Physiology.* In 1948, the American Physiological Society published the *Journal of Applied Physiology* to bring together the research work in exercise and environmen-

tal physiology. In 1969, the American College of Sports Medicine published the research journal *Medicine and Science in Sports* to support the growing productivity of its members. More recently, the *International Journal of Sports Medicine, Sports Medicine, Journal of Cardiopulmonary Rehabilitation,* and *Journal of Strength and Conditioning Research* have been introduced to report and review research. The latter two journals are linked to the American Association of Cardiovascular and Pulmonary Rehabilitation and the National Strength and Conditioning Association, respectively.

One of the clear consequences of this increase in research activity is the degree to which scientists must specialize in order to compete for research grants and to manage the research literature. Laboratories may focus on neuromuscular physiology, cardiac rehabilitation, or the influence of exercise on bone structure. Graduate students need to specialize earlier in their careers as researchers, and undergraduates must investigate graduate programs very carefully to make sure they meet their career goals (19).

This specialization in research has generated comments about the need to emphasize "basic" research examining the mechanisms underlying a physiological issue rather than "applied" research, which might describe responses of persons to exercise, environmental, or nutritional factors. It would appear that both types of research are needed and, to some extent, such a separation is arbitrary. For example, one scientist might study the interaction of exercise intensity and diet on muscle hypertrophy, another may characterize the changes in muscle cell size and contractile protein, a third might study changes in the energetics of muscle contraction relative to cytoplasmic enzyme activities, and a fourth might study the gene expression needed to synthesize that contractile protein. Where does "applied" research begin and "basic" research end? In the introduction to his text *Human Circulation* (30), Loring Rowell provided a quote from T. H. Huxley that bears on this issue:

> I often wish that this phrase "applied science," had never been invented. For it suggests that there is a sort of scientific knowledge of direct practical use, which can be studied apart from another sort of scientific knowledge, which is of no practical utility, and which is termed "pure science." But there is no more complete fallacy than this. What people call applied science is nothing but the application of pure science to particular classes of problems. It consists of deductions from those principles, established by reasoning and observation, which constitute pure science. No one can safely make these

deductions until he has a firm grasp of the principles; and he can obtain that grasp only by personal experience of the operations of observation and of reasoning on which they are found (18).

Solutions to chronic disease problems related to physical inactivity (e.g., type 2 diabetes, obesity) will come from a range of scientific disciplines—from epidemiologists on the one hand (35) to cell biologists on the other (5). We hope that all forms of inquiry are supported by fellow scientists such that present theories related to exercise physiology are continually questioned and modified. Lastly, we completely agree with the sentiments expressed in a statement ascribed to Arthur B. Otis: "Physiology is a good way to make a living and still have fun" (32).

IN SUMMARY

- The growth and development of exercise physiology laboratories in the 1950s and 1960s increased the opportunities for graduate study and research.
- Graduates from these laboratories contributed to the increase in research productivity and the number of research journals and professional societies.

TRANSLATION OF EXERCISE PHYSIOLOGY TO THE CONSUMER

The practical implications of the "fitness boom" include an increase in the number of "health spas" offering fitness or weight-control programs, and an explosion in the number of diet and exercise books selling easy ways to shed pounds and inches. It is clear that there has been and continues to be a need to provide correct information to the consumer about the "facts" related to exercise and weight control, and to provide some guidelines about the qualities to look for in an instructor associated with health and fitness programs. Most readers are familiar with the videotapes, DVDs, and books based on the fitness programs of movie stars, and they are also aware that some of what is offered may not be very sound. Fortunately, there are a number of well-known scientists and scholars in the area of exercise physiology and fitness who are now writing "popular" books related to fitness issues.

Concern over the qualifications of fitness instructors has been addressed by professional societies that offer "certification programs" for those interested in a career in fitness programming. The American College of Sports Medicine (ACSM) provided leadership in this area by initiating certification programs in 1975 for those involved in cardiac rehabilitation programs. Current certifications include ACSM Certified Personal Trainer, ACSM Health/Fitness Instructor, ACSM Exercise Specialist, and ACSM Registered Clinical Exercise Physiologist (2). In like manner, increased recognition of the importance of muscular strength in health and fitness led to the development of the Strength and Conditioning Specialist certification by the National Strength and Conditioning Association. The certifications are recognized by those involved in fitness programs as imparting a high standard of professional achievement.

Colleges and universities responded to this need for qualified personnel to direct exercise and weight-control programs. Many exercise science departments offer undergraduate and graduate courses to train students for a career in fitness and cardiac rehabilitation programs, or for advanced graduate study leading to a career in research and teaching at the university level. The growth in these programs occurred at the same time that there was a glut in the job market for physical education positions in the public schools. The colleges and universities had simply overproduced physical education teachers at a time when teaching positions were decreasing. One can only hope that as more and more colleges and universities develop these undergraduate fitness tracks, the quality of the graduate will be maintained and the market will not be saturated. On the other hand, the increase in the number of well-educated people who can provide quality programming for the apparently healthy individual might be properly timed for the current teacher shortage in the school systems.

IN SUMMARY

- To meet the needs of the consumer for correct information and programs about physical activity and health, university and college exercise science departments have developed new areas of study in exercise physiology and fitness.
- Organizations like the American College of Sports Medicine and the National Strength and Conditioning Association have developed certification programs to establish a standard of knowledge and skill to be achieved by those who lead health-related exercise programs.

STUDY QUESTIONS

1. Identify two of the most prolific scientists in your personal area of interest in exercise physiology and briefly describe what they have done. Use a research database at the library to find your references.
2. Pick a topic of interest in exercise physiology and describe how a molecular biologist might approach it compared to a scientist interested in doing studies with humans.
3. Societal factors can have a major impact on career goals. Briefly describe the factors currently influencing one of the following professions: physical educator, physician, physical therapist, athletic trainer, and fitness professional. These might include academic programs, certification and licensure, demographics of the population, and changes in health care in the country.
4. Identify the primary professional organization with which you will associate. Find out if the organization has a membership category for students, and what you would receive if you chose to join.

SUGGESTED READINGS

Bassett, D. R., Jr. 2002. Scientific contributions of A. V. Hill: Exercise physiology pioneer. *Journal of Applied Physiology* 93: 1567–82.

Berryman, J. W. 1995. *Out of Many, One: A History of the American College of Sports Medicine.* Champaign, IL: Human Kinetics.

Gandevia, S. C. et al. 1995. *Fatigue: Neural and Muscular Mechanisms.* New York: Plenum Press.

Hill, A. V. 1966. *Trails and Trials in Physiology.* Baltimore: Williams & Wilkins.

Park, R. S. 1989. *Measurement of Physical Fitness: A Historical Perspective.* Washington, D.C.: ODPHP National Health Information Center.

Schmit-Nielsen, B. 1995. *August & Marie Krogh—Lives in Science.* New York: Oxford University Press.

Tipton, C. M. 2003. *Exercise Physiology—People and Ideas.* New York: Oxford University Press.

REFERENCES

1. American Alliance for Health, Physical Education, Recreation and Dance. 1980. *Lifetime Health Related Physical Fitness: Test Manual.* Reston, VA.
2. American College of Sports Medicine. 2006. *ACSM's Guidelines for Exercise Testing and Prescription,* 7th ed. Baltimore: Lippincott, Williams & Wilkins.
3. American Heart Association. 1992. Statement on exercise. *Circulation* 86:340–44.
4. Bassett, D. R. Jr., and E. T. Howley. 1997. Maximal oxygen uptake: "Classical" versus "contemporary" viewpoints. *Medicine and Science in Sports and Exercise* 29: 591–603.
5. Booth, F. W., M. V. Chakravarthy, S. E. Gordon, and E. E. Spangenburg, 2002. Waging war on physical inactivity: Using modern molecular ammunition against an ancient enemy. *Journal of Applied Physiology* 93:3–30.
6. Buskirk, E. R. 1987. Personal communication based on "Our extended family: Graduates from the Noll Lab for Human Performance Research." Noll Laboratory, Pennsylvania State University, University Park, PA 16802.
7. Buskirk, E. R. 1992. From Harvard to Minnesota: Keys to our history. In *Exercise and Sport Sciences Reviews,* vol. 20, 1–26, ed. J. O. Holloszy. Baltimore: Williams & Wilkins.
8. Buskirk, E. R., and C. M. Tipton. 1977. Exercise physiology. In *The History of Exercise and Sport Science,* 367–438, ed. J. D. Massengale and R. A. Swanson. Champaign, IL: Human Kinetics.
9. Chapman, C. B., and J. H. Mitchell. 1965. The physiology of exercise. *Scientific American* 212:88–96.
10. Clarke, H. H., and D. H. Clarke. 1978. *Developmental and Adapted Physical Education.* Englewood Cliffs, NJ: Prentice-Hall.
11. Cooper, K. H. 1968. *Aerobics.* New York: Bantam Books.
12. Dill, D. B. 1938. *Life, Heat, and Altitude.* Cambridge, MA: Harvard University Press.
13. Fenn, W. O., and H. Rahn, eds. 1964. *Handbook of Physiology: Respiration,* vol. 1. American Physiological Society, Washington, D.C.
14. Franks, B. Don. 1969. *Exercise and Fitness 1969.* Chicago, IL: The Athletic Institute.
15. Hackensmith, C. W. 1966. *History of Physical Education.* New York: Harper & Row.
16. Horvath, S. M., and E. C. Horvath. 1973. *The Harvard Fatigue Laboratory: Its History and Contributions.* Englewood Cliffs, NJ: Prentice-Hall.
17. Hunsicker, P. A. 1950. A survey of laboratory facilities in college physical education departments. *Research Quarterly* 21:420–23.
18. Huxley, T. H. 1948. *Selection from Essays.* Appleton-Century-Crofts, New York.
19. Ianuzzo, D., and R. S. Hutton. 1987. A prospectus for graduate students in muscle physiology and biochemistry. *Sports Medicine Bulletin* 22:17–18. Indianapolis: The American College of Sports Medicine.
20. Jackson, M.A. 1977. Bruno Balke welcomes—and creates—avalanches. *Physician and Sportsmedicine* 7: 93–98.
21. Kennedy, J. F. 1960. The soft American. *Sports Illustrated* 13:14–17.
22. Kroll, W. P. 1971. *Perspectives in Physical Education.* New York: Academic Press.
23. Lagrange, F. 1890. *Physiology of Bodily Exercise.* New York: D. Appleton and Company.
24. McKenzie, R. T. 1923. *Exercise in Education and Medicine.* Philadelphia: W. B. Saunders.
25 Montoye, H. J., and R. Washburn. 1980. Genealogy of scholarship among academy members. *The Academy Papers,* vol. 13, 94–101. Washington, D.C.: AAHPERD.
26. Montoye, H. J., and R. Washburn. 1980. Research quarterly contributors: An academic genealogy. *Research Quarterly for Exercise and Sport* 51:261–66.

27. Pate, R. R. et al. 1995. Physical activity and public health. *Journal of the American Medical Association* 273:402–07.

28. Powell, K. E., and R. S. Paffenbarger. 1985. Workshop on epidemiologic and public health aspects of physical activity and exercise: A summary. *Public Health Reports* 100:118–26.

29. Proceedings of the International Symposium on Physical Activity and Cardiovascular Health. 1967. *Canadian Medical Association Journal* 96:695–915.

30. Rowell, L. B. 1986. *Human Circulation: Regulation During Physical Stress.* New York: Oxford University Press.

31. Sargent, D. A. 1906. *Physical Education.* Boston: Ginn and Co.

32. Stainsby, W. N. 1987. Part two: "For what is a man profited?" *Sports Medicine Bulletin* 22:15. Indianapolis: The American College of Sports Medicine.

33. Thomas, C. K. et al. 1995. The scientific contributions of Brenda Bigland-Ritchie. *Advances in Experimental Medicine and Biology* 384:11–25.

34. Tipton, C. M. 1998. Contemporary exercise physiology: Fifty years after the closure of Harvard Fatigue Laboratory. In *Exercise and Sport Sciences Reviews*, vol. 26, 315–39, ed. J. O. Holloszy. Baltimore: Williams & Wilkins.

35. U. S. Department of Health and Human Services. 1996. *Physical Activity and Health: A Report of the Surgeon General.* Atlanta: U. S. Department of Health and Human Services, Centers for Disease Control and Prevention, National Center for Chronic Disease Prevention and Health Promotion.

36. U.S. Department of Health and Human Services and U.S. Department of Agriculture. 2005. *Dietary Guidelines for Americans.* Washington, D.C.: Author.

37. Van Dalen, D. B., and B. L. Bennett. 1971. A *World History of Physical Education: Cultural, Philosophical, Comparative,* 2d ed. Englewood Cliffs, NJ: Prentice-Hall.

CHAPTER 2

Control of the Internal Environment

■ Objectives

By studying this chapter, you should be able to do the following:

1. Define the terms *homeostasis* and *steady state*.
2. Diagram and discuss a biological control system.
3. Give an example of a biological control system.
4. Explain the term *negative feedback*.
5. Define what is meant by the gain of a control system.

■ Outline

Homeostasis: Dynamic Constancy   15

Control Systems of the Body   16

Nature of the Control Systems   17
   Negative Feedback   18
   Gain of a Control System   18

Examples of Homeostatic Control   18
   Regulation of Arterial Blood Pressure   18
   Regulation of Blood Glucose   19

Stress Proteins Assist in the Regulation of Cellular Homeostasis   19

Exercise: A Test of Homeostatic Control   21

■ Key Terms

biological control system
effector
gain
heat shock proteins

homeostasis
integrating center
negative feedback
receptor

steady state
stress proteins

RESEARCH FOCUS 2.1

How to Understand Graphs: A Picture Is Worth 1,000 Words

Throughout this book, we will use line graphs to illustrate important concepts in exercise physiology. Although these same concepts can be explained in words, graphs are useful visual tools that can illustrate complicated relationships in a way that is easy to understand. Let's briefly review the basic concepts behind the construction of a line graph.

A line graph is used to illustrate relationships between two variables; that is, how one thing is affected by another. You may recall from one of your math courses that a *variable* is the generic term for any characteristic that changes. For example, in exercise physiology, heart rate is a variable that changes as a function of exercise intensity. Figure 2.1 is a line graph illustrating the relationship between heart rate and exercise intensity. In this illustration, exercise intensity (independent variable) is placed on the x-axis (horizontal) and heart rate (dependent vari-

FIGURE 2.1
The relationship between heart rate and exercise intensity (expressed as a percent of $\dot{V}O_2$ max).

able) is located on the y-axis (vertical). Heart rate is considered the dependent variable because it changes as a function of exercise intensity. Since exercise intensity is independent of heart rate, it is the independent vari-

able. Note in figure 2.1 that heart rate increases as a linear (straight-line) function of the exercise intensity. This type of line graph makes it easy to see what happens to heart rate when exercise intensity is changed.

If you had a body temperature of 104° F (40° C) while sitting at rest, you would know that something is wrong. As children we learned that normal body temperature is 98.6° F (37° C) and that values above or below normal signify a problem. How does the body manage to maintain core temperature within a narrow range? Further, how is it that during exercise, when the body is producing great amounts of heat, we generally do not experience overheating problems?

Over 100 years ago, the French physiologist Claude Bernard observed that the "milieu interior" (internal environment) of the body remained remarkably constant despite a changing external environment. The fact that the body manages to maintain a relatively constant internal environment in spite of various stressors such as exercise, heat, cold, or fasting is not an accident but the result of many complex control systems. Control mechanisms that are responsible for maintaining a stable internal environment constitute a major chapter in exercise physiology, and it is helpful to examine their function in light of simple control theory. Therefore, the purpose of this chapter is to introduce the concept of "control systems" and to discuss

how the body maintains a rather constant internal environment during periods of stress. However, before you begin to read this chapter, take time to review Research Focus 2.1. This box provides an overview of how to interpret graphs and gain useful information from these important tools of science.

HOMEOSTASIS: DYNAMIC CONSTANCY

The term **homeostasis** was coined by Walter Cannon in 1932 and is defined as the maintenance of a constant or unchanging internal environment. A similar term, **steady state,** is often used by exercise physiologists to denote a steady physiological environment. Although the terms *steady state* and *homeostasis* are often used interchangeably, homeostasis generally refers to a relatively constant internal environment during unstressed conditions resulting from many compensating regulatory responses (1, 13, 19). In contrast, a steady state does not necessarily mean that the internal environment is completely normal, but simply

FIGURE 2.2 Changes in body core temperature during sixty minutes of submaximal exercise in a thermoneutral environment. Note that body temperature reaches a plateau (steady state) by approximately forty minutes of exercise.

FIGURE 2.3 Changes in arterial blood pressure across time during resting conditions. Notice that although the arterial pressure oscillates across time, the mean pressure remains unchanged.

that it is unchanging. In other words, a balance has been achieved between the demands placed on the body and the body's response to those demands. An example that is useful in distinguishing between these two terms is the case of body temperature during exercise. Figure 2.2 illustrates the changes in body core temperature during sixty minutes of constant-load submaximal exercise in a thermoneutral environment (i.e., low humidity and low temperature). Note that core temperature reaches a new and steady level within forty minutes after commencement of exercise. This plateau of core temperature represents a steady state, since temperature is constant; however, this constant temperature is above the normal resting body temperature and thus does not represent a true homeostatic condition. Therefore, the term *homeostasis* is generally reserved for describing normal resting conditions, and the term *steady state* is often applied to exercise wherein the physiological variable in question (i.e., body temperature) is unchanging but may not equal the "homeostatic" resting value.

Although the concept of homeostasis means that the internal environment is unchanging, this does not mean that the internal environment remains absolutely constant. In fact, most physiological variables vary around some "set" value, and thus homeostasis represents a rather dynamic constancy. An example of this dynamic constancy is the arterial blood pressure. Figure 2.3 shows the change in mean (average) arterial blood pressure during eight minutes of rest. Note the oscillatory change in arterial pressure, but the mean (average) arterial pressure remains around 93 mm Hg. The reason such an oscillation occurs in physiological variables is related to the "feedback" nature of biological control systems (9, 10, 18). This will be discussed later in the chapter in the Negative Feedback section.

IN SUMMARY

■ *Homeostasis* is defined as the maintenance of a constant or unchanging "normal" internal environment during unstressed conditions.

■ The term *steady state* is also defined as a constant internal environment, but this does not necessarily mean that the internal environment is at rest and normal. When the body is in a steady state, a balance has been achieved between the demands placed on the body and the body's response to those demands.

CONTROL SYSTEMS OF THE BODY

The body has literally hundreds of different control systems, and the overall goal of most is to regulate some physiological variable at or near a constant value (8, 13, 28). The most intricate of these control systems reside inside the cell itself. These cellular control systems regulate cell activities such as protein breakdown and synthesis, energy production, and maintenance of the appropriate amounts of stored nutrients (9, 25). Almost all organ systems of the body work to help maintain homeostasis (5, 10, 12, 18, 20, 24, 26). For example, the lungs (pulmonary system) and heart (circulatory system) work together to replenish oxygen and to remove carbon dioxide from the extracellular fluid. The fact that the cardiopulmonary system is usually able to maintain normal levels of oxygen and carbon dioxide even during periods of strenuous

Understanding How Biological Control Systems Operate During Exercise Is Important

An exciting area of research in exercise physiology centers around biological control systems. Indeed, many future investigations will be aimed at improving our understanding of how biological control systems regulate homeostasis during exercise. This type of research is termed "mechanistic" research because the goal of these studies is to determine the mechanism(s) of how a specific control system operates. For example, an important but unanswered question in physiology is, "How does the body regulate breathing during exercise to maintain constant blood levels of oxygen and carbon dioxide?" Given the importance of breathing to maintain homeostasis, it is not surprising that laboratories around the world continue to investigate how the body regulates breathing during exercise (see chapter 10). Mechanistic studies are critical to improving our understanding of both exercise physiology and how various diseases alter physiological function.

exercise is not an accident but the end result of a good control system.

Although much is known about how specific control systems of the body operate, the details of how many control systems work to maintain homeostasis remain a mystery. This is an active area of research in exercise physiology (see Research Focus 2.2).

NATURE OF THE CONTROL SYSTEMS

To develop a better understanding of how the body maintains a stable internal environment, let's begin with the analogy of a simple, nonbiological control system such as a thermostat-regulated heating and cooling system in a home. Suppose the thermostat is set at 20° C. Any change in room temperature away from the 20° C "set point" results in the appropriate response by either the furnace or the air conditioner to return the room temperature to 20° C. If the room temperature rises above the set point, the thermostat signals the air conditioner to start, which returns the room temperature to 20° C. In contrast, a decrease in temperature below the set point results in the thermostat signaling the heating system to begin operation (figure 2.4). In both cases the response by the heating or cooling systems was to correct the condition, low or high temperature, that initially turned it on.

A **biological control system** can be defined as a series of interconnected components that maintain a physical or chemical parameter of the body at a near constant value (13, 29). The general components of a biological control system are as follows: (1) a receptor, (2) an integrating center, and (3) an effector. Figure 2.5 represents the schematic of such a control system.

FIGURE 2.4 A thermostat-controlled heating/cooling system. An increase in temperature above the "set point" signals the air conditioner to turn on. In contrast, a decrease in room temperature below the set point results in turning on the furnace. This system illustrates a nonbiological control system.

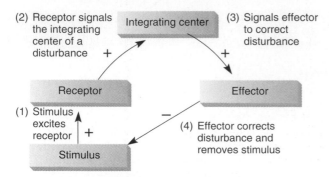

(1) Stimulus excites receptor

(2) Receptor signals the integrating center of a disturbance

(3) Signals effector to correct disturbance

(4) Effector corrects disturbance and removes stimulus

FIGURE 2.5 Schematic of the components that comprise a biological control system. The process begins with a change in the internal environment (stimulus), which excites a receptor to send information about the change to an integrating control center. The integrating center makes an assessment of the amount of response needed to correct the disturbance and sends the appropriate message to the effector. The effector is responsible for correcting the disturbance, and thus the stimulus is removed.

The signal to begin the operation of a control system is the stimulus (i.e., some detectable change in the environment), such as temperature, blood pressure, and so on. The stimulus excites a **receptor** (component capable of detecting change of the variable in question), which sends a message to the **integrating center,** which can be thought of as a control box. The integrating center assesses the strength of the stimulus and sends an appropriate output message to a component known as the **effector,** which is concerned with correcting the disturbance by responding in a manner that changes the internal environment back to normal. The return of the internal environment toward normal results in a decrease in the original stimulus that triggered the control system into action. This type of feedback is termed *negative feedback*.

Negative Feedback

Most control systems of the body operate via **negative feedback** (2, 9). An example of negative feedback can be seen in the respiratory system's regulation of the CO_2 concentration in extracellular fluid. In this case, an increase in extracellular CO_2 above normal levels triggers a receptor, which sends information to the respiratory control center (integrating center) to increase breathing. The effectors in this example are the respiratory muscles. This increase in breathing will reduce extracellular CO_2 concentrations back to normal, thus reestablishing homeostasis. The reason that this type of feedback is termed negative is that the response of the control system is negative (opposite) to the stimulus.

Gain of a Control System

The precision with which a control system maintains homeostasis is called the *gain* of the system. **Gain** can be thought of as the "capability" of the control system. This means that a control system with a large gain is more capable of correcting a disturbance in homeostasis than a control system with a low gain. As you might predict, the most important control systems of the body have large gains. For example, control systems that regulate body temperature, breathing (i.e., pulmonary system), and delivery of blood (i.e., cardiovascular system) all have large gains. The fact that these systems have large gains is not surprising, given that these control systems all deal with life-and-death issues.

IN SUMMARY

- A biological control system is composed of a receptor, an integrating center, and an effector.
- Most control systems act by way of negative feedback.
- The degree to which a control system maintains homeostasis is termed the *gain of the system*. A control system with a large gain is more capable of maintaining homeostasis than a system with a low gain.

EXAMPLES OF HOMEOSTATIC CONTROL

To better understand biological control systems, consider a few examples of homeostatic control.

Regulation of Arterial Blood Pressure

An excellent illustration of homeostatic control that uses negative feedback is the "baroreceptor system," which is responsible for the regulation of blood pressure. The baroreceptors are pressure-sensitive receptors located in the carotid arteries and in the arch of the aorta. When arterial blood pressure increases above normal levels, these baroreceptors are stimulated, and nerve impulses are transmitted to the cardiovascular control center in the medulla of the brain. In turn, the cardiovascular control center decreases the number of impulses transmitted to the heart, which lowers the amount of blood pumped by the heart and causes arterial pressure to return to normal (figure 2.6). In contrast, a reduction in arterial pressure reduces the number of impulses transmitted from the baroreceptors to the brain, which causes the cardiovascular control center to increase the number

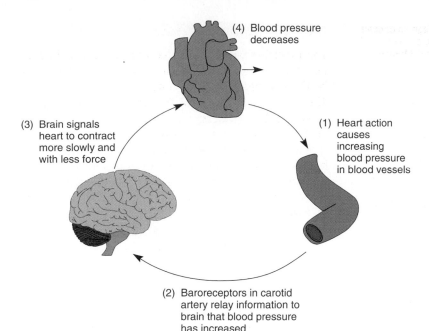

(4) Blood pressure decreases

(3) Brain signals heart to contract more slowly and with less force

(1) Heart action causes increasing blood pressure in blood vessels

(2) Baroreceptors in carotid artery relay information to brain that blood pressure has increased

FIGURE 2.6 Example of negative feedback mechanism to lower blood pressure. A similar mechanism helps to increase blood pressure if it decreases below normal.

of impulses transmitted to the heart to produce an increase in blood pressure (7).

Regulation of Blood Glucose

Homeostasis is also a function of the endocrine system (see chapter 5). The body contains eight major endocrine glands, which synthesize and secrete blood-borne chemical substances called hormones. Hormones are transported via the circulatory system throughout the body as an aid to regulate circulatory and metabolic functions (2, 11). An example of the endocrine system's role in the maintenance of homeostasis is the control of blood glucose levels. Indeed, in health, the blood glucose concentration is carefully regulated by the endocrine system. For example, the hormone insulin regulates cellular uptake and the metabolism of glucose and is therefore important in the regulation of the blood glucose concentration. After a large carbohydrate meal, the blood glucose level increases above normal (figure 2.7). The rise in blood glucose signals the pancreas to release insulin, which then lowers blood glucose by increasing cellular uptake. Failure of the blood glucose control system results in disease (diabetes) and is discussed in Clinical Applications 2.1.

Stress Proteins Assist in the Regulation of Cellular Homeostasis

A disturbance in cellular homeostasis occurs when a cell is faced with a "stress" that surpasses its ability to defend against this particular type of disturbance. A

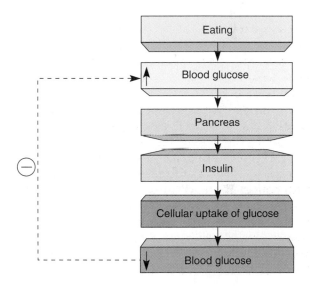

Eating

Blood glucose

Pancreas

Insulin

Cellular uptake of glucose

Blood glucose

FIGURE 2.7 Illustration of the regulation of blood glucose concentration. Changes in blood glucose concentration from the normal range regulate insulin secretion. Insulin, in turn, acts to regulate blood glucose levels (completing the negative feedback loop) and to maintain homeostasis. In this system the pancreas is both the sensor and the effector organ. It senses the change in blood glucose from normal and releases insulin appropriately.

classic illustration of how cells use control systems to combat stress (i.e., disturbances in homeostasis) is termed the "cellular stress response." The cellular stress response is a biological control system in cells that battles homeostatic disturbances by manufacturing proteins designed to defend against stress. A brief

Failure of a Biological Control System Results in Disease

Failure of any component of a biological control system results in a disturbance in homeostasis. A classic illustration of the failure of a biological control system is the disease diabetes. Although there are two forms of diabetes (type 1 and type 2), both types are characterized by abnormally high blood glucose levels (called hyperglycemia). In type 1 diabetes, the beta cells in the pancreas (beta cells produce insulin) become damaged. Hence, insulin is no longer produced and released into the blood to promote the transport of glucose into tissues. Therefore, damage to the pancreatic beta cells represents a failure of the "effector" component of this control system. If insulin cannot be released in response to an increase in blood glucose following a high-carbohydrate meal, glucose cannot be transported into body cells and the end result is hyperglycemia and diabetes.

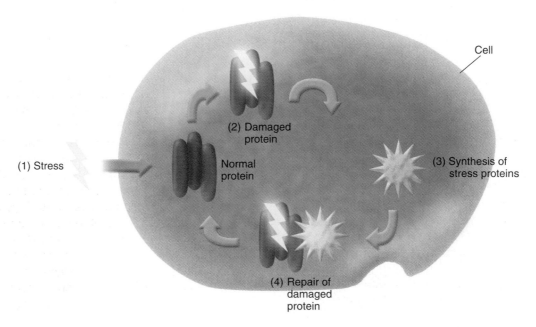

FIGURE 2.8 The cellular stress response. (1) Cellular stressors such as increased temperature, changes in pH, or, the production of free radicals produce (2) damage to functioning proteins. These damaged proteins signal the (3) synthesis of stress proteins. These stress proteins then (4) repair the damaged protein to restore homeostasis.

overview of the cellular stress response control system and how it protects cells against homeostatic disturbances follows.

At the cellular level, proteins are important in maintaining homeostasis. For example, proteins play critical roles in normal cell function by serving as intracellular transporters or as enzymes that catalyze chemical reactions. Damage to cellular proteins by stress (e.g., high temperature) can result in a disturbance in homeostasis. To combat this type of disruption in homeostasis, cells respond by rapidly manufacturing protective proteins called **stress proteins** (17). After synthesis, these stress proteins go to work to protect the cell by repairing damaged proteins and restoring homeostasis. Figure 2.8 provides an overview of how this control system regulates protein homeostasis in cells. The process starts with a stressor that results in protein damage. Stresses associated with exercise that are known to produce cellular protein damage include high temperatures, reduced cellular oxygen, low pH, and the production of free radicals. Damaged proteins become signals for the cell to produce stress proteins. After synthesis, these stress proteins work to repair damaged proteins and restore homeostasis. More details about stress proteins and their function in cells are provided in Research Focus 2.3.

RESEARCH FOCUS 2.3

Stress Proteins Help Maintain Cellular Homeostasis

Recent evidence demonstrates that when a cell is exposed to a stress that disturbs homeostasis, the cell responds by synthesizing "stress proteins." These stress proteins are designed to reduce cellular injury caused by the stress and restore homeostasis. The term *stress protein* refers to two families of proteins that are manufactured in cells in response to stress (e.g., high temperature). The larger and more thoroughly investigated of these families has been named **heat shock proteins.**

An Italian scientist discovered heat shock proteins after exposing flies to a hot environment. Several hours after this heat exposure, the flies responded by producing several new proteins. Hence, these molecules became known as heat shock proteins. However, heat is only one type of stress that disturbs cellular homeostasis and results in the synthesis of heat shock proteins. Indeed, many other stresses can promote the synthesis of heat shock proteins. Important

stresses that can damage proteins and promote the synthesis of heat shock proteins include low cellular energy levels, abnormal pH, alterations in cell calcium, and protein damage by free radicals (3, 15, 17). Since exercise can produce all of these stresses, it is not surprising that exercise scientists have become interested in the cellular response to stress and heat shock proteins. See reference 17 for a review of this topic.

EXERCISE: A TEST OF HOMEOSTATIC CONTROL

Muscular exercise can be considered a dramatic test of the body's homeostatic control systems, since exercise has the potential to disrupt many homeostatic variables. For example, during heavy exercise, skeletal muscle produces large amounts of lactic acid, which causes an increase in intracellular and extracellular acidity (6, 21–23, 27, 30, 31). This increase in acidity represents a serious challenge to the body's acid-base control system (4, 7) (see chapter 11). Additionally, heavy exercise results in large increases in muscle O_2 requirements, and large amounts of CO_2 are produced. These changes must be countered by increases in breathing (pulmonary ventilation) and blood flow to increase O_2 delivery to the exercising muscle and remove metabolically produced CO_2. Further, during heavy exercise the working muscles produce large amounts of heat that must be removed to prevent overheating. The body's control systems must respond rapidly to prevent drastic alterations in the internal environment.

In a strict sense, the body rarely maintains true homeostasis while performing intense exercise or during prolonged exercise in a hot or humid environment. Heavy exercise or prolonged work results in disturbances in the internal environment that are generally

too great for even the highest gain control systems to overcome, and thus a steady state is not possible. Severe disturbances in homeostasis result in fatigue and, ultimately, cessation of exercise (14, 16, 21, 22). Understanding how various body control systems minimize exercise-induced disturbances in homeostasis is extremely important to the exercise physiology student and is thus a major theme of this textbook. Specific details about individual control systems (e.g., circulatory, respiratory) that affect the internal environment during exercise are discussed in chapters 4 through 12. Further, improved exercise performance following exercise training is largely due to training adaptations that result in a better maintenance of homeostasis (22); this is discussed in chapter 13.

IN SUMMARY

- Exercise represents a challenge to the body's control systems to maintain homeostasis. In general, the body's many control systems are capable of maintaining a steady state during most types of submaximal exercise in a cool environment. However, intense exercise or prolonged work in a hostile environment (i.e., high temperature/humidity) may exceed the ability of a control system to maintain a steady state, and severe disturbances in homeostasis may occur.

STUDY QUESTIONS

1. Define the term *homeostasis*. How does it differ from the term *steady state*?

2. Cite an example of a biological homeostatic control system.

3. Draw a simple diagram that demonstrates the relationships between the components of a biological control system.
4. Briefly, explain the role of the receptor, the integrating center, and the effector organ in a biological control system.

5. Explain the term *negative feedback*. Give a biological example of negative feedback.
6. Discuss the concept of gain associated with a biological control system.

SUGGESTED READINGS

Brooks, G., T. Fahey, and K. Baldwin. 2005. *Exercise Physiology: Human Bioenergetics and Its Applications*, 4th ed. New York: McGraw-Hill Companies.

Fox, S. 2006. *Human Physiology*, 9th ed. New York: McGraw-Hill Companies.

Robergs, R., and S. Keteyian. 2003. *Fundamentals of Exercise Physiology: For Fitness, Performance, and Health*, 2nd ed. New York. McGraw-Hill Companies.

Widmaier, E., H. Raff, and K. Strang. 2006. *Vander's Human Physiology*, 10th ed. New York. McGraw-Hill Companies.

REFERENCES

1. Adolph, E. 1968. *Origins of Physiological Regulations*. New York: Academic Press.
2. Asterita, M. 1985. *Physiology of Stress*. New York: Human Sciences Press.
3. Benjamin, I., and E. Christians. 2002. Exercise, estrogen, and ischemic cardioprotection by heat shock protein 70. *Circulation Research* 90:833–35.
4. Brooks, G., T. Fahey, and K. Baldwin. 2005. *Exercise Physiology: Human Bioenergetics and Its Applications*, 4th ed. New York: McGraw-Hill.
5. Creager, J. 1992. *Human Anatomy and Physiology*. New York: McGraw-Hill Companies.
6. Edwards, R. H. T. 1983. Biochemical bases of fatigue in exercise performance: Catastrophe theory of muscular fatigue. In *Biochemistry of Exercise*, ed. H. Knuttgen, J. Vogel, and J. Poortmans. Champaign, IL: Human Kinetics.
7. Fox, S. 2006. *Human Physiology*. New York: McGraw-Hill Companies.
8. Frisancho, A. 1993. *Human Adaptation and Accommodation*. Ann Arbor: University of Michigan Press.
9. Garcia-Sainz, J. 1991. Cell responsiveness and protein kinase C: Receptors, G proteins, and membrane effectors. *News in Physiological Sciences* 6:169–73.
10. Guyton, A., and J. Hall. 2000. *Textbook of Medical Physiology*. Philadelphia: W. B. Saunders.
11. Hill, R., and G. Wyse. 1989. *Animal Physiology*. New York: Harper & Row.
12. Hole, J. 1992. *Human Anatomy and Physiology*. New York: McGraw-Hill Companies
13. Iyengar, S. 1984. *Computer Modeling of Complex Biological Systems*. Boca Raton, FL: CRC Press.
14. Jones, R. 1973. *Principles of Biological Regulation: An Introduction to Feedback Systems*. New York: Academic Press.
15. Kregel, K. 2002. Heat shock proteins: Modifying factors in physiological stress responses and acquired thermotolerance. *Journal of Applied Physiology* 92:2177–86.
16. Lindinger, M., and G. Heigenhauser. 1991. The roles of ion fluxes in skeletal muscle fatigue. *Canadian Journal of Physiology and Pharmacology* 69:246–53.
17. Locke, M. 1997. The cellular stress response to exercise: Role of stress proteins. *Exercise and Sport Sciences Reviews*, vol. 25, 105–36. Baltimore: Williams & Wilkins.
18. MacLaren, D. et al. 1989. A review of metabolic and physiological factors in fatigue. In *Exercise and Sport Sciences Reviews*, vol. 17, 29–66. Baltimore: Williams & Wilkins.
19. Marieb, E. 2002. *Human Anatomy and Physiology*. Menlo Park, CA: Benjamin-Cummings.
20. Mason, E. 1983. *Human Physiology*. Redwood City, CA: Benjamin-Cummings.
21. McCully, K. et al. 1991. Biochemical adaptations to training: Implications for resisting muscle fatigue. *Canadian Journal of Physiology and Pharmacology* 69:274–78.
22. Poortmans, J. 1983. The intracellular environment in peripheral fatigue. In *Biochemistry of Exercise*, ed. H. Knuttgen, J. Vogel, and J. Poortmans. Champaign, IL: Human Kinetics.
23. Sahlin, K. 1983. Effects of acidosis on energy metabolism and force generation in skeletal muscle. In *Biochemistry of Exercise*, ed. H. Knuttgen, J. Vogel, and J. Poortmans. Champaign, IL: Human Kinetics.
24. Schmidt-Nielson, K. 1997. *Animal Physiology: Adaptation and Environment*. New York: Cambridge University Press.
25. Sherwood, L. 1994. *Fundamentals of Human Physiology*. New York: West.
26. Siess, W. 1991. Multiple signal-transduction pathways synergize in platelet activation. *News in Physiological Sciences* 6:51–55.
27. Sjogaard, G. 1991. Role of potassium fluxes underlying muscle fatigue. *Canadian Journal of Physiology and Pharmacology* 69:238–45.
28. Spain, J. 1982. *Basic Microcomputer Models in Biology*. Redwood City, CA: Benjamin-Cummings.
29. Toates, F. 1975. *Control Theory in Biology and Experimental Psychology*. London: Hutchinson Education.
30. Vollestad, N., and O. Sejersted. 1988. Biochemical correlates of fatigue. *European Journal of Applied Physiology* 57:336–37.
31. Widmaier, E., H. Raff, and K. Strang. 2006. *Vander's Human Physiology*. New York. McGraw-Hill Companies.

CHAPTER 3

Bioenergetics

■ Objectives

By studying this chapter, you should be able to do the following:

1. Discuss the function of the cell membrane, nucleus, and mitochondria.
2. Define the following terms: (1) *endergonic reactions*, (2) *exergonic reactions*, (3) *coupled reactions*, and (4) *bioenergetics*.
3. Describe the role of enzymes as catalysts in cellular chemical reactions.
4. List and discuss the nutrients that are used as fuels during exercise.
5. Identify the high-energy phosphates.

6. Discuss the biochemical pathways involved in anaerobic ATP production.
7. Discuss the aerobic production of ATP.
8. Describe the general scheme used to regulate metabolic pathways involved in bioenergetics.
9. Discuss the interaction between aerobic and anaerobic ATP production during exercise.
10. Identify the enzymes that are considered rate limiting in glycolysis and the Krebs cycle.

■ Outline

Cell Structure   24

Biological Energy Transformation   25
   Cellular Chemical Reactions   25
   Oxidation-Reduction Reactions   27
   Enzymes   28

Fuels for Exercise   31

Carbohydrates   31
Fats   32
Proteins   32

High-Energy Phosphates   33

Bioenergetics   33
   Anaerobic ATP Production   33
   Aerobic ATP Production   38

Aerobic ATP Tally   46

Efficiency of Oxidative Phosphorylation   46

Control of Bioenergetics   46
   Control of ATP-PC System   47
   Control of Glycolysis   47
   Control of Krebs Cycle and Electron Transport Chain   48

Interaction Between Aerobic/ Anaerobic ATP Production   48

■ Key Terms

adenosine diphosphate (ADP)
adenosine triphosphate (ATP)
aerobic
anaerobic
ATPase
ATP-PC system
beta oxidation
bioenergetics
cell membrane
chemiosmotic hypothesis
coupled reactions
cytoplasm
electron transport chain

endergonic reactions
energy of activation
enzymes
exergonic reactions
FAD
glucose
glycogen
glycogenolysis
glycolysis
inorganic
inorganic phosphate (P_i)
isocitrate dehydrogenase
Krebs cycle

lactic acid
mitochondrion
molecular biology
NAD
nucleus
organic
oxidative phosphorylation
oxidation
phosphocreatine (PC)
phosphofructokinase (PFK)
reduction

Thousands of chemical reactions occur throughout the body during each minute of the day. Collectively, these reactions are called metabolism. Metabolism includes chemical pathways that result in the synthesis of molecules (anabolic reactions) as well as the breakdown of molecules (catabolic reactions).

Since energy is required by all cells, it is not surprising that cells possess chemical pathways that are capable of converting foodstuffs (i.e., fats, proteins, carbohydrates) into a biologically usable form of energy. This metabolic process is termed **bioenergetics.** In order for you to run, jump, or swim, skeletal muscle cells must be able to continuously extract energy from food nutrients. In fact, the inability to transform energy contained in foodstuffs into usable biological energy would limit performance in endurance activities. The explanation for this is simple. In order to continue to contract, muscle cells must have a continuous source of energy. When energy is not readily available, muscular contraction is not possible, and thus work must stop. Therefore, given the importance of cellular energy production during exercise, it is critical that the student of exercise physiology develop a thorough understanding of bioenergetics. It is the purpose of this chapter to introduce both general and specific concepts associated with bioenergetics.

CELL STRUCTURE

Cells were discovered in the seventeenth century by the English scientist Robert Hooke. Advancements in the microscope over the past 300 years have led to improvements in our understanding of cell structure and function. In order to understand bioenergetics, it is important to have some appreciation of cell structure and function. Four elements (an element is a basic chemical substance) compose over 95% of the human body. These include oxygen (65%), carbon (18%), hydrogen (10%), and nitrogen (3%) (21, 56). Additional elements found in rather small amounts in the body include sodium, iron, zinc, potassium, magnesium, chloride, and calcium. These various elements are linked together by chemical bonds to form molecules or compounds. Compounds that contain carbon are called **organic** compounds, while those that do not contain carbon are termed **inorganic.** For example, water (H_2O) lacks carbon and is thus inorganic. In contrast, proteins, fats, and carbohydrates contain carbon and are organic compounds.

As the basic functional unit of the body, the cell is a highly organized factory capable of synthesizing the large number of compounds necessary for normal cellular function. Figure 3.1 illustrates the structure of a typical cell. Note that not all cells are alike, nor do they all perform the same functions. The hypothetical cell pictured in figure 3.1 simply illustrates parts of cells that are contained in most cell types found in the body. In general, cell structure can be divided into three major parts:

1. **Cell membrane** The cell membrane (also called the plasma membrane) is a semipermeable barrier that separates the cell from the extracellular environment. The two most important functions of the cell membrane are to enclose the components of the cell and to regulate the passage of various types of substances in and out of the cell (21, 30).
2. **Nucleus** The nucleus is a large, round body within the cell that contains the cellular genetic components (genes). Genes are composed of double strands of deoxyribonucleic acids (DNA), which serve as the basis for the genetic code. In short, genes regulate protein synthesis, which determines cell composition and controls cellular activity. The field of **molecular biology** is concerned with understanding the composition and regulation of genes and is introduced in A Closer Look 3.1.
3. **Cytoplasm** (called sarcoplasm in muscle cells) This is the fluid portion of the cell between the nucleus and the cell membrane. Contained within the cytoplasm are various organelles (minute structures) that are concerned with specific cellular functions. One such organelle, the **mitochondrion,** is often called the powerhouse of the cell and is involved in the oxidative conversion of foodstuffs into usable cellular energy. Also contained in the cytoplasm are the enzymes that regulate the breakdown of glucose (i.e., glycolysis).

IN SUMMARY

- *Metabolism* is defined as the total of all cellular reactions that occur in the body; this includes both the synthesis of molecules and the breakdown of molecules.
- Cell structure includes the following three major parts: (1) cell membrane, (2) nucleus, and (3) cytoplasm (called sarcoplasm in muscle).
- The cell membrane provides a protective barrier between the interior of the cell and the extracellular fluid.
- Genes (located within the nucleus) regulate protein synthesis within the cell.
- The cytoplasm is the fluid portion of the cell and contains numerous organelles.

Secretory vesicle

Centriole

Nucleolus

Nucleus

Agranular endoplasmic reticulum

Golgi complex

Nuclear envelope

Mitochondrion

Lysosome

Chromatin

Plasma membrane

Microtubule

Granular endoplasmic reticulum

Cytoplasm (cytosol)

Ribosome

FIGURE 3.1 A typical cell and its major organelles.

BIOLOGICAL ENERGY TRANSFORMATION

All energy on earth comes from the sun. Plants use light energy from the sun to drive chemical reactions to form carbohydrates, fats, and proteins. Animals (including humans) then eat plants and other animals to obtain the energy required to maintain cellular activities.

Energy exists in several forms (e.g., electrical, mechanical, chemical, etc.) and all forms of energy are interchangeable (47, 49). For example, muscle fibers convert chemical energy obtained from carbohydrates, fats, or proteins into mechanical energy to perform movement. The bioenergetic process of converting chemical energy to mechanical energy requires a series of tightly controlled chemical reactions. Before discussing the specific reactions involved, we provide an overview of cellular chemical reactions.

Cellular Chemical Reactions

Energy transfer in the body occurs via the releasing of energy trapped within chemical bonds of various mol-

ecules. Chemical bonds that contain relatively large amounts of potential energy are often referred to as "high-energy bonds." As mentioned previously, bioenergetics is concerned with the transfer of energy from foodstuffs into a biologically usable form. This energy transfer in the cell occurs as a result of a series of chemical reactions. Many of these reactions require that energy be added to the reactants **(endergonic reactions)** before the reaction will "proceed." However, since energy is added to the reaction, the products contain more free energy than the original reactants.

Reactions that give off energy as a result of the chemical process are known as **exergonic reactions.** Figure 3.3 illustrates that the amount of total energy released via exergonic reactions is the same whether the energy is released in one single reaction (combustion) or many small, controlled steps that usually occur in cells (cellular oxidation).

Coupled Reactions Many of the chemical reactions that occur within the cell are called **coupled reactions.** Coupled reactions are reactions that are linked, with the liberation of free energy in one reaction being

Molecular Biology and Exercise Science

Molecular biology is one of the most rapidly growing scientific disciplines and is defined as the study of molecular structures and events underlying biological processes. Molecular biology is concerned with understanding the relationship between genes and the cellular characteristics that they determine.

Human cells contain approximately 20,000–25,000 genes, and each gene is responsible for the synthesis of a specific cellular protein. Cellular signals regulate protein synthesis by "turning on" or "turning off" specific genes. Therefore, understanding those factors that act as signals to promote or inhibit protein synthesis is of importance to exercise physiologists (7).

Figure 3.2 illustrates the process of protein synthesis in a cell. The process begins with a "signal" to "turn on" a gene. This signal starts the process of transcription. Transcription results in the formation of a message (called messenger RNA, or mRNA). This message, i.e., mRNA) leaves the nucleus and travels through the cytoplasm to a ribosome, which is the site of protein synthesis. Here, the mRNA is translated into a specific protein. Individual proteins differ in both structure and function; this is important because the types of proteins found in the cell determine cellular characteristics.

The technical revolution in the field of molecular biology offers another opportunity to make use of scientific information for the improvement of human performance. For example, exercise training results in modifications in the amounts and types of proteins synthesized in the exercised muscles (see chapter 13 for details). Indeed, it is well known that regular strength training results in an increase in muscle size due to an increase in contractile proteins. The techniques of molecular biology provide the exercise scientist with the "tools" to understand how exercise controls gene function. Ultimately, understanding how exercise promotes the synthesis of specific proteins in muscles will allow the exercise scientist to design the most effective training program to achieve the desired training effects.

FIGURE 3.2 Steps leading to protein synthesis: (1) DNA contains the information necessary to synthesize proteins; (2) transcription of DNA results in the formation of a message (called mRNA), which is a "blueprint" of the information needed to synthesize a protein; (3) mRNA leaves the nucleus and moves to the ribosome (site of protein synthesis); (4) amino acids (building blocks of proteins) are carried to the ribosome by transfer RNAs (tRNA); (5) the final step in protein synthesis is translation. In translation, the information contained within the mRNA is translated and amino acids are linked together in a chain, resulting in the formation of a specific protein.

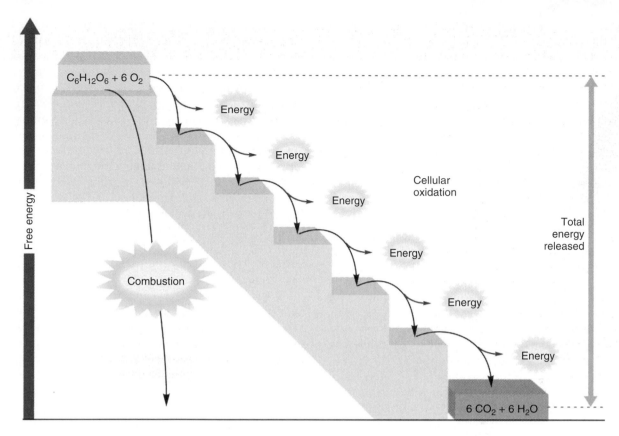

FIGURE 3.3 The breakdown of glucose into carbon dioxide and water via cellular oxidation results in a release of energy. Reactions that result in a release of free energy are termed exergonic.

used to "drive" a second reaction. Figure 3.4 illustrates this point. In this example, energy released by an exergonic reaction is used to drive an energy-requiring reaction (endergonic reaction) in the cell. This is like two meshed gears in which the turning of one (energy-releasing, exergonic gear) causes the movement of the second (endergonic gear). In other words, energy-liberating reactions are "coupled" to energy-requiring reactions. Oxidation-reduction reactions are an important type of coupled reaction and are discussed in the next section.

Oxidation-Reduction Reactions

The process of removing an electron from an atom or molecule is called **oxidation.** The addition of an electron to an atom or molecule is referred to as **reduction.** Oxidation and reduction are always coupled reactions because a molecule cannot be oxidized unless it donates electrons to another atom (or molecule). The atom or molecules that donates the electrons is known as the *reducing agent* whereas the one that accepts the electrons is called an *oxidizing agent.* Note that an atom (or molecule) can act as both an oxidizing agent and a reducing agent. For example, when molecules play both roles, they can gain elec-

Exergonic reactions   Endergonic reactions

FIGURE 3.4 Model showing the coupling of exergonic and endergonic reactions. Note that the energy given off by the exergonic reaction (drive shaft) powers the endergonic reactions (smaller gear)

trons in one reaction and then pass these electrons to another molecule to produce an oxidation-reduction reaction. Hence, coupled oxidation-reduction reactions are analogous to a bucket brigade, with electrons being passed along in the buckets.

Note that the term *oxidation* does not mean that oxygen participates in the reaction. This term is derived from the fact that oxygen tends to accept electrons and therefore acts as an oxidizing agent. This important property of oxygen is used by cells to produce a usable form of energy and will be discussed in detail in the section "Electron Transport Chain."

It is important to remember that oxidation-reduction reactions in cells often involve the transfer of hydrogen atoms rather than free electrons. This is true because a hydrogen atom contains one electron (and one proton in the nucleus). Therefore, an atom or molecule that loses a hydrogen atom also loses an electron and therefore is oxidized; the molecule that gains the hydrogen (and electron) is reduced. In many biological oxidation-reduction reactions, pairs of electrons are passed along between molecules as free electrons or as pairs of hydrogen atoms.

Two molecules play important roles in the transfer of hydrogens (and electrons): nicotinamide adenine dinucleotide and flavin adenine dinucleotide. Nicotinamide adenine dinucleotide is derived from the vitamin niacin (vitamin B$_3$) whereas flavin adenine dinucleotide comes from the vitamin riboflavin (B$_2$). The oxidized form of nicotinamide adenine dinucleotide is written as NAD whereas the reduced form is written as NADH. Similarly, the oxidized form of flavin adenine dinucleotide is written as FAD and the reduced form is abbreviated as FADH. An illustration of how NADH is formed from the reduction of NAD during a coupled oxidation-reduction reaction is shown in figure 3.5. Details of how NAD and FAD function as "carrier molecules" during bioenergetic reactions are discussed later in this chapter in the section "Electron Transport Chain".

Enzymes

The speed of cellular chemical reactions is regulated by catalysts called **enzymes.** Enzymes are proteins that play a major role in the regulation of metabolic pathways in the cell. Enzymes do not cause a reaction to occur, but simply regulate the rate or speed at which the reaction takes place. Further, the enzyme does not change the nature of the reaction nor its final result.

Chemical reactions occur when the reactants have sufficient energy to proceed. The energy required to initiate chemical reactions is called the **energy of activation** (11, 56). Enzymes work as catalysts by lowering the energy of activation. The end result is to increase the rate at which these reactions take place. Figure 3.6 illustrates this concept. Note that the energy of activation is greater in the noncatalyzed reaction on the left when compared to the enzyme-catalyzed reaction pictured on the right. By reducing the energy of activation, enzymes increase the speed of chemical reactions and therefore increase the rate of product formation.

The ability of enzymes to lower the energy of activation results from unique structural characteristics. In general, enzymes are large protein molecules with a three-dimensional shape. Each type of enzyme has characteristic ridges and grooves. The pockets that are formed from the ridges or grooves located on the enzyme are called active sites. These active sites are important, since it is the unique shape of the active site that causes a specific enzyme to adhere to a particular reactant molecule (called a substrate). The concept of how enzymes fit with a particular substrate molecule is analogous to the idea of a lock and key (figure 3.7). The shape of the enzyme's active site is specific for the shape of a particular substrate, which allows the two molecules (enzyme + substrate) to form a complex known as the enzyme-substrate complex. After the formation of the enzyme-substrate complex, the energy of activation needed for the reaction to occur is lowered, and the reaction is more easily brought to completion. This is followed by the dissociation of the enzyme and the product. The ability of an enzyme to work as a catalyst is not constant and can be modified by several factors and will be discussed shortly.

X–H$_2$ NAD

X   NADH + H$^+$ ------> NADH + H$^+$ Y

NAD   Y–H$_2$

NAD is oxidizing agent   **NADH is reducing agent**

FIGURE 3.5 This figure illustrates an oxidation-reduction reaction involving NAD and NADH. Note in the left portion of this figure that NAD is reduced to NADH + H$^+$ by accepting two hydrogens from a hydrogen donor (i.e., X-H$_2$). In the right side of this figure, notice that NADH + H$^+$ can then donate these hydrogens to another molecule (i.e., Y) to regenerate NAD. In this (coupled) oxidation-reduction reaction, NAD is the oxidizing agent and NADH is the reducing agent.

Noncatalyzed reaction   Catalyzed reaction

FIGURE 3.6 Enzymes catalyze reactions by lowering the energy of activation. That is, the energy required to start the reaction is reduced. Note the difference in the energy of activation in the catalyzed reaction versus the noncatalyzed reaction.

CLINICAL APPLICATIONS 3.1

Diagnostic Value of Measuring Enzyme Activity in the Blood

When tissues become diseased, dead cells often break open and release their enzymes into the blood. Since many of these intracellular enzymes are not normally found in blood, the presence of a specific enzyme in blood provides important diagnostic information regarding the source of the medical problem. In practice, the diagnostic test proceeds as follows. A doctor obtains a blood sample from the patient and forwards the sample to a clinical laboratory for analysis. The laboratory then determines the activity of a specific enzyme in a test tube by addition of the blood sample and appropriate substrates for the enzyme. The results of this test can often assist in making a diagnosis. For example, the finding that the blood sample contains high levels of the enzyme lactate dehydrogenase would suggest that the patient experienced a myocardial infarction (i.e., heart attack). Similarly, elevated blood levels of the enzyme creatine kinase would also indicate cardiac injury and would provide additional evidence that the patient suffered a heart attack. See table 3.1 for additional examples of the diagnostic usage for specific enzymes found in blood.

TABLE 3.1	Examples of the Diagnostic Value of Enzymes Found in Blood
Enzyme	**Diseases Associated with High Blood Levels of Enzyme**
Lactate dehydrogenase (cardiac-specific isoform)	Myocardial infarction
Creatine kinase	Myocardial infarction, muscular dystrophy
Alkaline phosphatase	Carcinoma of bone, Paget's disease, obstructive jaundice
Amylase	Pancreatitis, perforated peptic ulcer
Aldolase	Muscular dystrophy

(a) **Enzyme** and **substrates**   (b) **Enzyme-substrate complex**   (c) **Reaction products** and enzyme (unchanged)

FIGURE 3.7   The lock-and-key model of enzyme action. (*a*) Substrates A and B fit into active sites in the enzyme, forming an enzyme-substrate complex. (*b*) This complex then dissociates (*c*), releasing the products of the reaction and the free enzyme.

Note that cellular enzymes can often play a key role in diagnosing specific illnesses. For example, when tissues become damaged as a result of diseases, dead cells within these tissues can release enzymes into the blood. Many of these enzymes are not normally found in blood and therefore provide a clinical "clue" to diagnose the source of the illness. Details about the use of blood enzyme levels in the diagnosis of diseases are contained in Clinical Applications 3.1.

TABLE 3.2 Selected Examples of Specific Enzymes Representing Each of the Six Major Classes of Enzymes

Enzyme Class	Example of Enzyme Within this Class	Reaction Catalyzed
Oxidoreductases	Lactate dehydrogenase	Lactate + NAD $\leftrightarrow$ Pyruvate + NADH + H
Transferases	Hexokinase	Glucose + ATP $\rightarrow$ Glucose 6-phosphate + ADP
Hydrolases	Lipase	Triglyceride + 3 H_2O $\rightarrow$ Glycerol + 3 Fatty acids
Lyases	Carbonic anhydrase	Carbon dioxide + H_2O $\rightarrow$ Carbonic acid
Isomerases	Phosphoglycerate mutase	3-Phosphoglycerate $\rightarrow$ 2-Phosphoglycerate
Ligases	Pyruvate carboxylase	Pyruvate + HCO_3 + ATP $\rightarrow$ Oxaloacetate + ADP

Classification of Enzymes In the early days of biochemistry, enzymes were named by the scientist who discovered the enzyme. Often these names did not provide a clue to the function of the enzyme. Therefore, to reduce confusion, the International Union of Biochemistry developed a systematic naming system that classifies and names the enzyme according to the type of chemical reaction it catalyzes. In this scheme, enzymes are provided a systematic name and a numerical identification. In addition, a shorter version of the systematic name, called the recommended name, was provided for everyday use. Many of these recommended names for enzymes end with the suffix "ase" and reflect the both job category of the enzyme and the reaction it catalyzes. The "recommended" names for enzymes are used throughout this text. Using the International Union of Biochemistry classification, there are six classes of enzymes (44):

1. **Oxidoreductases** All of the enzymes in this class catalyze oxidation-reduction reactions. Subclasses in this group of enzymes include dehydrogenases, oxidases, oxygenases, reductases, peroxidases, and hydroxylases.
2. **Transferases** Transferases are enzymes that catalyze the transfer of elements from one molecule to another. Subclasses of this group include kinases, transcarboxylases, and transaminases.
3. **Hydrolases** These enzymes catalyze reactions in which the cleavage of bonds is accomplished by adding water. Subclasses of hydrolases include esterases, phosphatases, and pepidases.
4. **Lyases** Lyases catalyze reactions in which groups of elements (e.g., H_2O, CO_2, and NH_3) are removed to form a double bond or are added to an existing double bond. Synthases, deaminases, and decarboxylases are examples of lyases.
5. **Isomerases** This is a heterogeneous class of enzymes that catalyze reactions that result in the rearrangement of the structure of molecules.

Subclasses of this group of enzymes include mutases, isomerases, and epimerases.
6. **Ligases** Ligases catalyze bond formation between two substrate molecules. ATP provides energy for these reactions. The names of many ligases include synthetase or carboxylase.

Specific examples of each enzyme class as they relate to bioenergetics are contained in table 3.2

Factors that Alter Enzyme Activity The activity of an enzyme, as measured by the rate at which its substrates are converted into products, is influenced by several factors. Two of the more important factors include temperature and pH (pH is a measure of acidity) of the solution.

Individual enzymes have an optimum temperature at which they are most active. In general, a small rise in body temperature above normal (i.e., 37° C) increases the activity of most enzymes. This is useful during exercise, since muscular work results in an increase in body temperature. The resulting elevation in enzyme activity would enhance bioenergetics (ATP production) by speeding up the rate of reactions involved in the production of biologically useful energy. This point is illustrated in figure 3.8. Notice that enzyme activity is less than maximum at normal body temperature (37° C). Also, note that an exercise-induced increase in body temperature (e.g., 40° C) results in a temperature-induced increase in enzyme activity.

The pH of body fluids also has a large effect on enzyme activity. The relationship between pH and enzyme activity is similar to the temperature/enzyme activity relationship; that is, individual enzymes have a pH optimum. If the pH is altered from the optimum, the enzyme activity is reduced (figure 3.9). This has important implications during exercise. For example, during intense exercise, skeletal muscles can produce large amounts of lactic acid. Lactic acid is a relatively strong acid and quickly dissociates to release hydro-

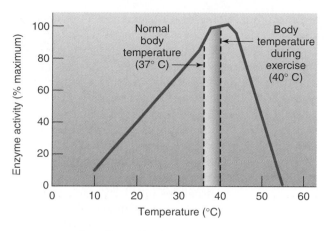

FIGURE 3.8 The effect of body temperature on enzyme activity. Notice that an optimal range of temperatures exists for enzyme activity. An increase or decrease in temperature away from the optimal temperature range results in diminished enzyme activity.

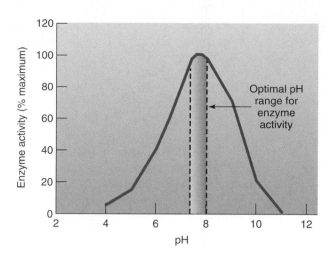

FIGURE 3.9 The effect of pH on enzyme activity. Note that every enzyme has a narrow range of optimal pH. An increase or decrease of pH away from this optimum range results in a decrease in enzyme activity.

gen ions and form lactate (see Closer Look 3.2). Accumulation of large quantities of hydrogen ions results in a decrease in the pH of body fluids below the optimum pH of important bioenergetic enzymes. The end result is a decreased ability to provide the energy (i.e., ATP) required for muscular contraction. In fact, extreme acidity is an important limiting factor in various types of intense exercise. This will be discussed again in chapter 19.

IN SUMMARY

- All energy on earth comes from the sun. Plants use this solar energy to perform chemical reactions to form carbohydrates, fats, and proteins. Animals consume plants and other animals to maintain the energy required to maintain cellular activities.
- Enzymes that serve as catalysts for these reactions regulate the speed of chemical reactions.
- Enzymes are classified into six categories based upon the type of reaction that the enzyme performs.
- Two important factors that regulate enzyme activity are temperature and pH. Individual enzymes have an optimum temperature and pH at which they are most active.

FUELS FOR EXERCISE

The body uses carbohydrate, fat, and protein nutrients consumed daily to provide the necessary energy to maintain cellular activities both at rest and during exercise. During exercise, the primary nutrients used for energy are fats and carbohydrates, with protein contributing a small amount of the total energy used (11, 18, 22, 23, 36, 50).

Carbohydrates

Carbohydrates are composed of atoms of carbon, hydrogen, and oxygen. Stored carbohydrates provide the body with a rapidly available form of energy, with 1 gram of carbohydrate yielding approximately 4 kcal of energy (46). As mentioned earlier, plants synthesize carbohydrates from the interaction of CO_2, water, and solar energy in a process called photosynthesis. Carbohydrates exist in three forms (42, 56): (1) monosaccharides, (2) disaccharides, and (3) polysaccharides. Monosaccharides are simple sugars such as glucose and fructose. **Glucose** is familiar to most of us and is often referred to as "blood sugar." It can be found in foods or can be formed in the digestive tract as a result of cleavage of more complex carbohydrates. Fructose is contained in fruits or honey and is considered to be the sweetest of the simple carbohydrates (42, 46).

Disaccharides are formed by combining two monosaccharides. For example, table sugar is called sucrose and is composed of glucose and fructose. Maltose, also a disaccharide, is composed of two glucose molecules. Sucrose is considered to be the most common dietary disaccharide in the United States and constitutes approximately 25% of the total caloric intake of most Americans (42). It occurs naturally in many carbohydrates such as cane sugar, beets, honey, and maple syrup.

Polysaccharides are complex carbohydrates that contain three or more monosaccharides. Polysaccharides may be rather small molecules (i.e., three monosaccharides) or relatively large molecules containing hundreds of monosaccharides. In general, polysaccharides are classified as either plant or animal polysaccharides. The two most common forms of plant polysaccharides are cellulose and starch. Humans lack the digestive enzymes necessary to digest cellulose, and thus cellulose forms fiber in the diet and is discarded as waste in the fecal material. On the other hand, starch, found in corn, grains, beans, potatoes, and peas, is easily digested by humans and is an important source of carbohydrate in the American diet (42). After ingestion, starch is broken down to form monosaccharides and may be used as energy immediately by cells or stored in another form within cells for future energy needs.

Glycogen is the term used for the polysaccharide stored in animal tissue. It is synthesized within cells by linking glucose molecules together using the action of the enzyme, glycogen synthase. Glycogen molecules are generally large and may consist of hundreds to thousands of glucose molecules. Cells store glycogen as a means of supplying carbohydrates as an energy source. For example, during exercise, individual muscle cells break down glycogen into glucose (this process is called **glycogenolysis**) and use the glucose as a source of energy for contraction. On the other hand, glycogenolysis also occurs in the liver, with the free glucose being released into the bloodstream and transported to tissues throughout the body.

Important to exercise metabolism is that glycogen is stored in both muscle fibers and the liver. However, total glycogen stores in the body are relatively small and can be depleted within a few hours as a result of prolonged exercise. Therefore, glycogen synthesis is an ongoing process within cells. Diets low in carbohydrates tend to hamper glycogen synthesis, while high-carbohydrate diets enhance glycogen synthesis (see chapter 23).

Fats

Although fats contain the same chemical elements as carbohydrates, the ratio of carbon to oxygen in fats is much greater than that found in carbohydrates. Stored body fat is an ideal fuel for prolonged exercise, since fat molecules contain large quantities of energy per unit of weight. One gram of fat contains about 9 kcal of energy, which is over twice the energy content of either carbohydrates or protein (46, 59, 61). Fats are insoluble in water and can be found in both plants and animals. In general, fats can be classified into four general groups: (1) fatty acids, (2) triglycerides, (3) phospholipids, and (4) steroids. Fatty acids consist of long chains of carbon atoms linked to a carboxyl group at one end (a carboxyl group contains a carbon, oxygen, and hydrogen group). Importantly, fatty acids

are the primary type of fat used by muscle cells for energy.

Fatty acids are stored in the body as triglycerides. Triglycerides are composed of three molecules of fatty acids and one molecule of glycerol (not a fat but a type of alcohol). Although the largest storage site for triglycerides is fat cells, these molecules are also stored in many cell types, including skeletal muscle. In times of need, they can be broken down into their component parts with fatty acids being used as energy substrates by muscle and other tissues. The process of breaking down triglycerides into fatty acids and glycerol is termed lipolysis and is regulated by a family of enzymes called lipases. The glycerol released by lipolysis is not a direct energy source for muscle, but can be used by the liver to synthesize glucose. Therefore, the entire triglyceride molecule is a useful source of energy for the body.

Phospholipids are not used as an energy source by skeletal muscle during exercise (48, 67). Phospholipids are lipids combined with phosphoric acid and are synthesized in virtually every cell in the body. The biological roles of phospholipids vary from providing the structural integrity of cell membranes to providing an insulating sheath around nerve fibers (59, 61).

The final classification of fats is the steroids. Again, these fats are not used as energy sources during exercise, but will be mentioned briefly to provide a clearer understanding of the nature of biological fats. The most common steroid is cholesterol (42, 46). Cholesterol is a component of all cell membranes. It can be synthesized in every cell in the body and, of course, can be consumed in foods. In addition to its role in membrane structure, cholesterol is needed for the synthesis of the sex hormones estrogen, progesterone, and testosterone (20, 26). Although cholesterol has many "useful" biological functions, high blood cholesterol levels have been implicated in the development of coronary artery disease (67) (see chapter 18).

Proteins

Proteins are composed of many tiny subunits called amino acids. At least twenty different types of amino acids are needed by the body to form various tissues, enzymes, blood proteins, and so on. Nine amino acids, called essential amino acids, cannot be synthesized by the body and therefore must be consumed in foods. Proteins are formed by linking amino acids by chemical bonds called peptide bonds. As a potential fuel source, proteins contain approximately 4 kcal per gram (46). In order for proteins to be used as substrates for the formation of high-energy compounds, they must be broken down into their constituent amino acids. Proteins may contribute energy for exercise in two ways. First, the amino acid alanine can be converted in the liver to glucose, which can then be used to synthesize glycogen. Liver glycogen can be degraded into glucose and transported to working skeletal muscle via the circulation. Second, many amino acids (e.g., isoleucine, alanine, leucine, valine) can be converted into metabolic intermediates (i.e., compounds that may directly participate in bioenergetics) in muscle cells and directly contribute as fuel in the bioenergetic pathways (38, 42, 44, 59).

IN SUMMARY

- The body uses carbohydrate, fat, and protein nutrients consumed daily to provide the necessary energy to maintain cellular activities both at rest and during exercise. During exercise, the primary nutrients used for energy are fats and carbohydrates, with protein contributing a relatively small amount of the total energy used.
- Glucose is stored in animal cells as a polysaccharide called glycogen.
- Fatty acids are the primary form of fat used as an energy source in cells. Fatty acids are stored as triglycerides in muscle and fat cells.

HIGH-ENERGY PHOSPHATES

The immediate source of energy for muscular contraction is the high-energy phosphate compound **adenosine triphosphate (ATP)** (62). Although ATP is not the only energy-carrying molecule in the cell, it is the most important one, and without sufficient amounts of ATP most cells die quickly.

The structure of ATP consists of three main parts: (1) an adenine portion, (2) a ribose portion, and (3) three linked phosphates (figure 3.10). The formation of ATP occurs by combining **adenosine diphosphate (ADP)** and **inorganic phosphate (P_i)** and requires a rather large amount of energy. Some of this energy is stored in the chemical bond joining ADP and P_i. Accordingly, this bond is called a high-energy bond. When the enzyme **ATPase** breaks this bond, energy is released, and this energy can be used to do work (e.g., muscular contraction):

$$ATP \xrightarrow{\text{ATPase}} ADP + P_i + Energy$$

ATP is often called the universal energy donor. It couples the energy released from the breakdown of foodstuffs into a usable form of energy required by all cells. For example, figure 3.11 presents a model depicting ATP as the universal energy donor in the cell. The cell uses exergonic reactions (breakdown of foodstuffs) to form ATP via endergonic reactions. This newly formed ATP can then be used to drive the

FIGURE 3.10 The structural formation of adenosine triphosphate (ATP).

energy-requiring processes in the cell. Therefore, energy-liberating reactions are linked to energy-requiring reactions like two meshed gears.

BIOENERGETICS

Muscle cells store limited amounts of ATP. Therefore, because muscular exercise requires a constant supply of ATP to provide the energy needed for contraction, metabolic pathways must exist in the cell with the capability to produce ATP rapidly. Indeed, muscle cells can produce ATP by any one or a combination of three metabolic pathways: (1) formation of ATP by **phosphocreatine (PC)** breakdown, (2) formation of ATP via the degradation of glucose or glycogen (called glycolysis), and (3) oxidative formation of ATP. Formation of ATP via the PC pathway and glycolysis does not involve the use of O_2; these pathways are called **anaerobic** (without O_2) pathways. Oxidative formation of ATP by the use of O_2 is termed **aerobic** metabolism. A detailed discussion of the operation of the three metabolic pathways involved in the formation of ATP during exercise follows.

Anaerobic ATP Production

The simplest and, consequently, the most rapid method of producing ATP involves the donation of a

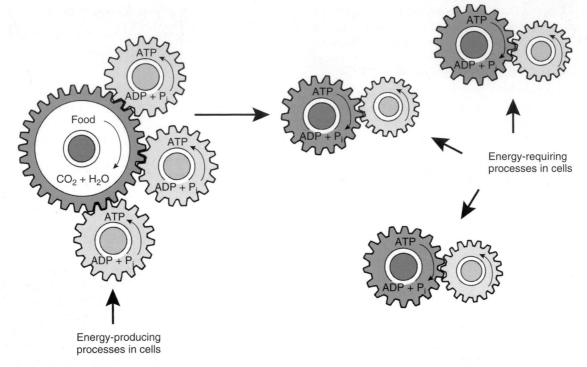

FIGURE 3.11 Model of ATP serving as the universal energy donor that drives the energy needs of the cell. On the left, the energy released from the breakdown of foodstuffs is used to form ATP. On the right, the energy released from the breakdown of ATP is used to "drive" the energy needs of the cell.

phosphate group and its bond energy from PC to ADP to form ATP (6, 13, 16, 27, 68):

$$PC + ADP \xrightarrow[\text{Creatine kinase}]{} ATP + C$$

The reaction is catalyzed by the enzyme creatine kinase. As rapidly as ATP is broken down to ADP + P_i at the onset of exercise, ATP is reformed via the PC reaction. However, muscle cells store only small amounts of PC, and thus the total amount of ATP that can be formed via this reaction is limited. The combination of stored ATP and PC is called the **ATP-PC system** or the "phosphagen system." It provides energy for muscular contraction at the onset of exercise and during short-term, high-intensity exercise (i.e., lasting less than five seconds). PC reformation requires ATP and occurs only during recovery from exercise (12, 17).

The importance of the ATP-PC system in athletics can be appreciated by considering short-term, intense exercise such as sprinting 50 meters, high jumping, performing a rapid weight-lifting move, or a football player racing 10 yards downfield. All of these activities require only a few seconds to complete and thus need a rapid supply of ATP. The ATP-PC system provides a simple one-enzyme reaction to produce ATP for these types of activities. The fact that depletion of PC is likely to limit short-term, high-intensity exercise has led to the suggestion that ingesting large amounts of creatine can improve exercise performance (see The Winning Edge 3.1).

A second metabolic pathway capable of producing ATP rapidly without the involvement of O_2 is termed **glycolysis.** Glycolysis involves the breakdown of glucose or glycogen to form two molecules of pyruvic acid or lactic acid (figure 3.13). Simply stated, glycolysis is an anaerobic pathway used to transfer bond energy from glucose to rejoin P_i to ADP. This process involves a series of enzymatically catalyzed, coupled reactions. Glycolysis occurs in the sarcoplasm of the muscle cell and produces a net gain of two molecules of ATP and two molecules of pyruvic or lactic acid per glucose molecule (see A Closer Look 3.2).

Let's consider glycolysis in more detail. First, the reactions between glucose and pyruvate can be considered as two distinct phases: (1) an energy investment phase, and (2) an energy generation phase (figure 3.13). The first five reactions make up the "energy investment phase" where stored ATP must be used to form sugar phosphates. Although the end result of glycolysis is energy producing (exergonic), glycolysis must be "primed" by the addition of ATP at two points at the beginning of the pathway (figures 3.14 and 3.15). The purpose of the ATP priming is to add phosphate groups (called phosphorylation) to glucose and to fructose 6-phosphate. Note that if glycolysis begins with glycogen as the substrate, the addition of only one ATP is required. That is, glycogen does not require phosphorylation by ATP, but is phosphorylated by inorganic phosphate instead

Exercise Physiology Applied to Sports

Does Creatine Supplementation Improve Exercise Performance?

The depletion of phosphocreatine (PC) may limit exercise performance during short-term, high-intensity exercise (e.g., 100- to 200-meter dash) because the depletion of PC results in a reduction in the rate of ATP production by the ATP-PC system. Studies have shown that ingestion of large amounts of creatine monohydrate (20 grams/day) over a five-day period results in increased stores of muscle PC (5, 24, 33, 40, 69). This creatine supplementation has been shown to improve performance in laboratory settings during short duration (<30 seconds), high-intensity stationary cycling exercise (24, 33, 40, 69). However, results on the influence of creatine supplementation on performance during short-duration running and swimming are not consistent (5, 24, 33, 40, 69). This may be due to the fact that creatine supplementation results in a weight gain due to water retention. Therefore, this increase in body weight may impair performance in weight-bearing activities such as running.

Studies suggest that creatine supplementation in conjunction with resistance exercise training results in an enhanced physiologic adaptation to weight training (5, 53, 69). Specifically, these studies indicate that creatine supplementation combined with resistance training promotes an increase in both dynamic muscular strength and fat-free mass. Nonetheless, whether creatine supplementation improves isokinetic or isometric muscular strength remains controversial (5).

Does oral creatine supplementation result in adverse physiological side effects and pose health risks? Unfortunately, a definitive answer to this question is not available. Although anecdotal reports indicate that creatine supplementation can be associated with negative side effects such as nausea, neurological dysfunction, minor gastrointestinal distress, and muscle cramping, these reports are not scientifically documented (5, 24, 34, 69). At present, due to limited data, a firm conclusion about the long-term health risks of creatine supplementa-

tion cannot be reached. However, current evidence suggests that creatine supplementation for up to eight weeks does not appear to produce major health risks, but the safety of more prolonged creatine supplementation has not been established.

An important issue related to the use of creatine and other dietary supplements is the possibility of contamination within the product; that is, the supplement product may contain other chemical compounds in addition to creatine (39). Indeed, this is an important safety issue in the "over-the-counter supplement" industry as a large study has reported a high level of variability in the purity of over-the-counter products (39). For additional information on the safety of nutritional supplements, please see Maughan et al. (2004) in the Suggested Readings. For more information on creatine and exercise performance, see Bemben and Lamont (2005) in the Suggested Readings.

Lactic Acid or Lactate?

Exercise physiologists often use the terms "lactic acid" and "lactate" interchangeably. This is often confusing to students who ask, "Are lactic acid and lactate the same molecule?" The answer is that lactic acid and lactate are related but are technically different molecules. Here's the explanation. During high-intensity exercise, skeletal muscle can produce large amounts of lactic acid (see chapters 3

and 4). Once produced in the body, lactic acid rapidly ionizes by releasing a hydrogen ion; the remaining ionized molecule is called lactate (figure 3.12). You may recall from another science course that when acids dissociate and release hydrogen ions the remaining molecule is called the conjugate base of the acid. It follows that lactate is the conjugate base of lactic acid.

To summarize, exercising skeletal muscles can produce lactic acid; however, lactic acid is unstable and is rapidly converted to its conjugate base, lactate. Therefore, in simple terms, lactic acid is the parent molecule and lactate is the offspring. Remembering the relationship between lactic acid and lactate will reduce confusion when you read about these molecules in future chapters within this text.

$$H-\overset{\overset{\displaystyle H}{|}}{\underset{\underset{\displaystyle H}{|}}{C}}-\overset{\overset{\displaystyle OH}{|}}{\underset{\underset{\displaystyle H}{|}}{C}}-\overset{\displaystyle O}{\underset{\displaystyle OH}{C}} \;\rightleftharpoons\; H-\overset{\overset{\displaystyle H}{|}}{\underset{\underset{\displaystyle H}{|}}{C}}-\overset{\overset{\displaystyle OH}{|}}{\underset{\underset{\displaystyle H}{|}}{C}}-\overset{\displaystyle O}{\underset{\displaystyle O^-}{C}} \;+\; H^+$$

Lactic acid   Lactate

FIGURE 3.12 The ionization of lactic acid forms the conjugate base called lactate. At normal body pH, lactic acid will rapidly dissociate to form lactate. Therefore, although skeletal muscle produces lactic acid, lactic acid rarely exists in the body because this acid is converted to its conjugate base, lactate.

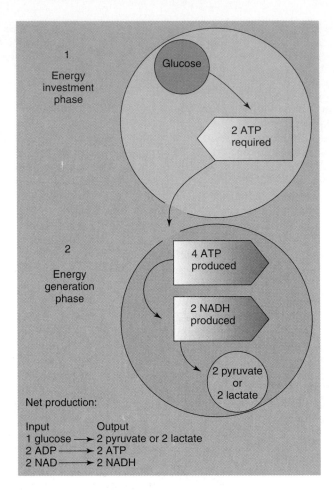

FIGURE 3.13 Illustration of the two phases of glycolysis and the products of glycolysis. From *Biochemistry* by Mathews and vanHolde. Copyright © 1990 by The Benjamin/Cummings Publishing Company. Reprinted by permission.

FIGURE 3.14 Illustration of the interaction between blood glucose and muscle glycogen for the provision of glucose for glycolysis. Regardless of the source of glucose for glycolysis, glucose must be phosphorylated to form glucose 6-phosphate as the first step in glycolysis. Note, however, that phosphorylation of glucose obtained from the blood requires 1 ATP, whereas the phosphorylation of glucose obtained from glycogen is achieved by using inorganic phosphate (P$_i$) located in the cell.

(figure 3.14). The last five reactions of glycolysis represent the "energy generation phase" of glycolysis. Figure 3.15 points out that two molecules of ATP are produced at each of two separate reactions near the end of the glycolytic pathway; thus, the net gain of glycolysis is two ATP if glucose is the substrate and three ATP if glycogen is the substrate.

Hydrogens are frequently removed from nutrient substrates in bioenergetic pathways and are transported by "carrier molecules." Two biologically important carrier molecules are **nicotinamide adenine dinucleotide (NAD)** and **flavin adenine dinucleotide (FAD).** Both NAD and FAD transport hydrogens and their associated electrons to be used for later generation of ATP in the mitochondrion via aerobic processes. In order for the chemical reactions in glycolysis to proceed, two hydrogens must be removed from glyceraldehyde 3-phosphate, which then combines with inorganic phosphate (P$_i$) to form 1,3-diphosphoglycerate. The hydrogen acceptor in this reaction is NAD (figure 3.15). Here, NAD accepts one

of the hydrogens, while the remaining hydrogen is free in solution. Upon accepting the hydrogen, NAD is converted to its reduced form, NADH. Adequate amounts of NAD must be available to accept the hydrogen atoms that must be removed from glyceraldehyde 3-phosphate if glycolysis is to continue (1, 12, 32). How is NAD reformed from NADH? There are two ways that the cell restores NAD from NADH. First, if sufficient oxygen (O$_2$) is available, the hydrogens from NADH can be "shuttled" into the mitochondria of the cell and can contribute to the aerobic production of ATP (see A Closer Look 3.3). Second, if O$_2$ is not available to accept the hydrogens in the mitochondria, pyruvic acid can accept the hydrogens to form **lactic acid** (figure 3.16). The enzyme that catalyzes this reaction is lactate dehydrogenase (LDH), with the end result being the formation of lactic acid and the reformation of NAD. Therefore, the reason for lactic acid formation is the "recycling" of NAD (i.e., NADH converted to NAD) so that glycolysis can continue.

Again, glycolysis is the breakdown of glucose into pyruvic acid or lactic acid with the net production of two or three ATP, depending on whether the pathway began with glucose or glycogen, respectively. Figure 3.15 summarizes glycolysis in a simple flowchart. Glucose is a six-carbon molecule and pyruvic acid and lactic acid are three-carbon molecules. This explains the production of two molecules of pyruvic acid or lactic acid from one molecule of glucose. Since O$_2$ is not directly involved in glycolysis, the pathway is considered anaerobic. However, in the presence of O$_2$ in the mitochondria, pyruvate can participate in the aerobic production of ATP. Thus, in addition to being an anaerobic pathway

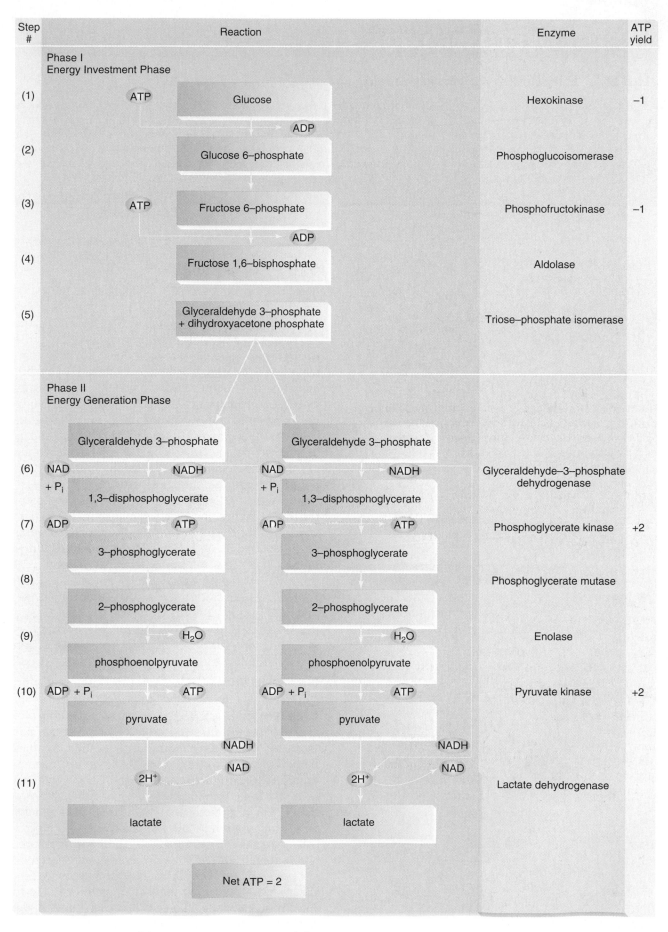

FIGURE 3.15 Summary of the anaerobic metabolism of glucose. Note that the end result of the anaerobic breakdown of one molecule of glucose is the production of two molecules of ATP and lactate.

A CLOSER LOOK 3.3

NADH Is "Shuttled" into Mitochondria

NADH generated during glycolysis must be converted back to NAD if glycolysis is to continue. As discussed in the text, the conversion of NADH to NAD can occur by pyruvic acid accepting the hydrogens (forming lactic acid) or "shuttling" the hydrogens from NADH across the mitochondrial membrane. The "shuttling" of hydrogens across the mitochondrial membrane requires a specific transport system. Figure 4.9 (see chapter 4) illustrates this process. This transport system is located within the mitochondrial membrane and transfers NADH-released hydrogens from the cytosol into the mitochondria where they can enter the electron transport chain.

FIGURE 3.16 The addition of two hydrogen atoms to pyruvic acid forms lactic acid and NAD, which can be used again in glycolysis. The reaction is catalyzed by the enzyme lactate dehydrogenase (LDH).

capable of producing ATP without O_2, glycolysis can be considered the first step in the aerobic degradation of carbohydrates. This will be discussed in detail in the next section, Aerobic ATP Production.

IN SUMMARY

- The immediate source of energy for muscular contraction is the high-energy phosphate ATP. ATP is degraded via the enzyme ATPase as follows:

$$\text{ATP} \xrightarrow{\text{ATPase}} \text{ADP} + \text{P}_i + \text{Energy}$$

- Formation of ATP without the use of O_2 is termed anaerobic metabolism. In contrast, the production of ATP using O_2 as the final electron acceptor is referred to as aerobic metabolism.
- Exercising skeletal muscles produce lactic acid. However, once produced in the body, lactic acid is rapidly converted to its conjugate base, lactate.
- Muscle cells can produce ATP by any one or a combination of three metabolic pathways: (1) ATP-PC system, (2) glycolysis, and (3) oxidative phosphorylation.
- The ATP-PC system and glycolysis are two anaerobic metabolic pathways that are capable of producing ATP without O_2.

Aerobic ATP Production

Aerobic production of ATP occurs inside the mitochondria and involves the interaction of two cooperating metabolic pathways: (1) the Krebs cycle and (2) the electron transport chain. The primary function of the **Krebs cycle** (also called the citric acid cycle) is to complete the oxidation (hydrogen removal) of carbohydrates, fats, or proteins using NAD and FAD as hydrogen (energy) carriers. The importance of hydrogen removal is that hydrogens (by virtue of the electrons that they possess) contain the potential energy in the food molecules. This energy can be used in the electron transport chain to combine ADP + P_i to reform ATP. Oxygen does not participate in the reactions of the Krebs cycle but is the final hydrogen acceptor at the end of the electron transport chain (i.e., water is formed, $H_2 + O \rightarrow H_2O$). The process of aerobic production of ATP is termed **oxidative phosphorylation.** It is convenient to think of aerobic ATP production as a three-stage process (figure 3.17). Stage 1 is the generation of a key two-carbon molecule, acetyl-CoA. Stage 2 is the oxidation of acetyl-CoA in the Krebs cycle. Stage 3 is the process of oxidative phosphorylation (i.e., ATP formation) in the electron transport chain (i.e., respiratory chain). A detailed look at the Krebs cycle and electron transport chain follows.

Krebs Cycle The Krebs cycle is named after the biochemist Hans Krebs, whose pioneering research has increased our understanding of this rather complex pathway. Entry into the Krebs cycle requires preparation of a two-carbon molecule, acetyl-CoA. Acetyl-CoA can be formed from the breakdown of either carbohydrates, fats, or proteins (figure 3.17). For the moment, let's focus on the formation of acetyl-CoA from pyruvate (pyruvate can be formed from both carbohydrates and proteins). Figure 3.18 depicts the cyclic nature of the reactions involved in the Krebs cycle. Note that pyruvate (three-carbon molecule) is broken down to form acetyl-CoA (two-carbon molecule) and the remaining carbon is given off as CO_2. Next, acetyl-CoA

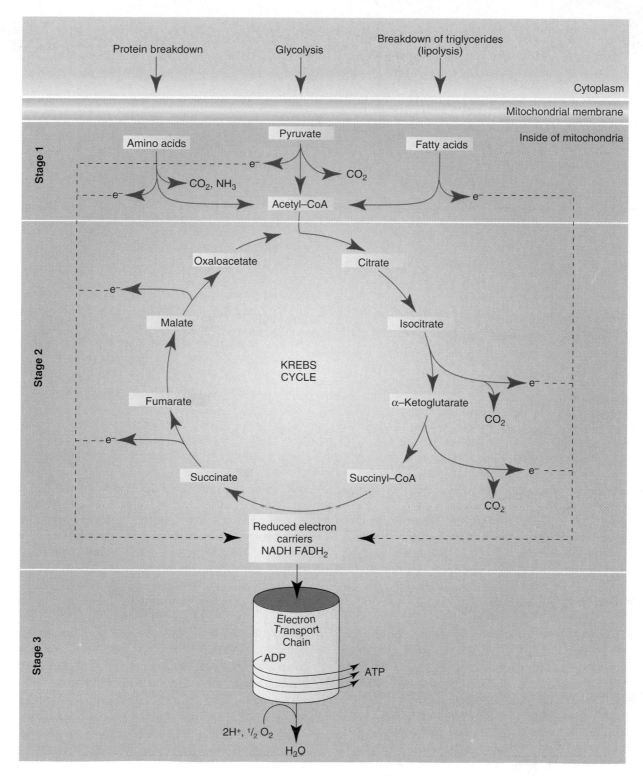

FIGURE 3.17 The three stages of oxidative phosphorylation. From Mathews and vanHolde, *Biochemistry*, Diane Bowen, Ed. Copyright© 1990 Benjamin/Cummings Publishing Company, Menlo Park, CA. Reprinted by permission.

combines with oxaloacetate (four-carbon molecule) to form citrate (six carbons). What follows is a series of reactions to regenerate oxaloacetate and two molecules of CO_2, and the pathway begins all over again.

For every molecule of glucose entering glycolysis, two molecules of pyruvate are formed, and in the presence of O_2, they are converted to two molecules of acetyl-CoA. This means that each molecule of glucose results in two turns of the Krebs cycle. With this in mind, let's examine the Krebs cycle in more detail. The primary function of the Krebs cycle is to remove hydrogens and the energy associated with those

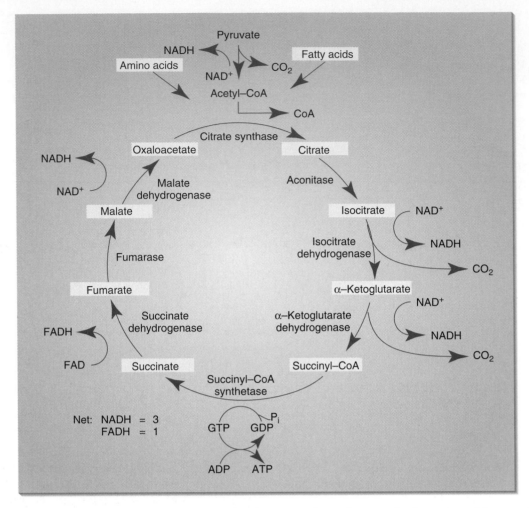

FIGURE 3.18 Compounds, enzymes, and reactions involved in the Krebs cycle. Note the formation of three molecules of NADH and one molecule of FADH per turn of the cycle.

hydrogens from various substrates involved in the cycle. Figure 3.18 illustrates that during each turn of the Krebs cycle, three molecules of NADH and one molecule of FADH are formed. For every pair of electrons passed through the electron transport chain from NADH to oxygen, enough energy is available to form 2.5 molecules of ATP (59, 65). For every FADH molecule that is formed, enough energy is available to produce 1.5 molecules of ATP. Thus, in terms of ATP production, FADH is not as energy rich as NADH.

In addition to the production of NADH and FADH, the Krebs cycle results in direct formation of an energy-rich compound, guanosine triphosphate (GTP) (59) (figure 3.18). GTP is a high-energy compound that can transfer its terminal phosphate group to ADP to form ATP. The direct formation of GTP in the Krebs cycle is called substrate-level phosphorylation, and it accounts for only a small amount of the total energy conversion in the Krebs cycle, since most of the Krebs cycle energy yield (i.e., NADH and FADH) is taken to the electron transport chain to form ATP.

Up to this point we have focused on the role that carbohydrates play in producing acetyl-CoA to enter the Krebs cycle. How do fats and proteins undergo aerobic metabolism? The answer can be found in figure 3.19. Note that fats (triglycerides) are broken down to form fatty acids and glycerol. These fatty acids can then undergo a series of reactions to form acetyl-CoA (called beta oxidation; see A Closer Look 3.4 for details) and thus enter the Krebs cycle (59, 61). Although glycerol can be converted into an intermediate of glycolysis in the liver, this does not occur to a great extent in human skeletal muscle. Therefore, glycerol is not an important direct muscle fuel source during exercise (22, 28).

As mentioned previously, protein is not considered a major fuel source during exercise, as it contributes only 2% to 15% of the fuel during exercise (18, 22, 36). Proteins can enter bioenergetic pathways in a variety of places. However, the first step is the breakdown of the protein into its amino acid subunits. What happens next depends on which amino acid is involved. For

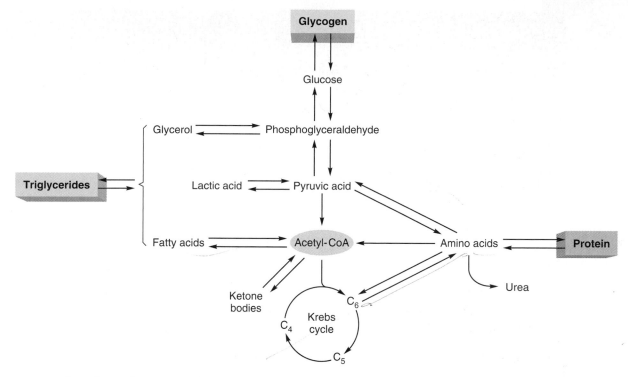

FIGURE 3.19 The relationships among the metabolism of proteins, carbohydrates, and fats. The overall interaction between the metabolic breakdown of these three foodstuffs is often referred to as the metabolic pool.

example, some amino acids can be converted to glucose or pyruvic acid, some to acetyl-CoA, and still others to Krebs-cycle intermediates. The role of proteins in bioenergetics is summarized in figure 3.19.

In summary, the Krebs cycle completes the oxidation of carbohydrates, fats, or proteins, produces CO_2, and supplies electrons to be passed through the electron transport chain to provide the energy for the aerobic production of ATP. Enzymes catalyzing Krebs-cycle reactions are located inside the mitochondria.

Electron Transport Chain The aerobic production of ATP (called oxidative phosphorylation) occurs in the mitochondria. The pathway responsible for this process is called the **electron transport chain** (also called the respiratory chain or cytochrome chain). Aerobic production of ATP is possible due to a mechanism that uses the potential energy available in reduced hydrogen carriers such as NADH and FADH to rephosphorylate ADP to ATP. The reduced hydrogen carriers do not directly react with oxygen. Instead, electrons removed from the hydrogen atoms are passed down a series of electron carriers known as cytochromes. During this passage of electrons down the cytochrome chain, enough energy is released to rephosphorylate ADP to form ATP at three different sites (57) (figure 3.20). Interestingly, as electrons pass down the electron transport chain, highly reactive

molecules called free radicals are formed. Large quantities of free radicals may be harmful to the muscle and contribute to muscle fatigue (4) (see Research Focus 3.1).

The hydrogen carriers that bring the electrons to the electron transport chain come from a variety of sources. Recall that two NADH are formed per glucose molecule that is degraded via glycolysis (figure 3.15). These NADH are outside the mitochondria, and their hydrogens must be transported across the mitochondrial membrane by special "shuttle" mechanisms. However, the bulk of the electrons that enter the electron transport chain come from those NADH and FADH molecules formed as a result of Krebs-cycle oxidation.

Figure 3.20 outlines the pathway for electrons entering the electron transport chain. Pairs of electrons from NADH or FADH are passed down a series of compounds that undergo oxidation and reduction, with enough energy being released to synthesize ATP at three places along the way. Notice that FADH enters the cytochrome pathway at a point just below the entry level for NADH (figure 3.20). This is important, because the level of FADH entry bypasses one of the sites of ATP formation, and thus each molecule of FADH that enters the electron transport chain has enough energy to form only 1.5 ATP. In contrast, NADH entry into the electron transport chain results in the

Free Radicals Are Formed During Aerobic Metabolism

Although the passage of electrons down the electron transport chain performs an essential role in the process of aerobic ATP production, this pathway also forms a product that may negatively influence muscle during exercise. Research has shown that the activation of the electron transport chain results in the formation of free radicals (52, 66). Free radicals are molecules that have an unpaired electron in their outer orbital which makes them highly reactive. That is, free radicals bind quickly to other molecules, and this combination results in damage to the molecule combining with the radical. For example, free radical formation in muscle during exercise might contribute to muscle fatigue and a reduction in the activity of several Krebs-cycle enzymes (2, 4, 35, 52, 55).

What determines how many free radicals are formed during exercise? The number of free radicals produced during exercise is directly linked to the rate of aerobic metabolism. Therefore, radicals are formed at high rates during high-intensity or prolonged exercise. More will be said about free radicals and fatigue in chapter 19, and the potential roles of antioxidants in improving exercise performance will be addressed in chapter 25. For additional information, see Powers et al. (2004) in the Suggested Readings.

FIGURE 3.20 ATP is formed during oxidative phosphorylation by the flow of hydrogen ions across the inner mitochondrial membrane. A maximum of two or three molecules of ATP are produced per pair of electrons donated, depending on the point at which a particular coenzyme enters the electron transport chain.

formation of 2.5 ATP (details will be mentioned later). At the end of the electron transport chain, oxygen accepts the electrons that are passed along and combines with hydrogen to form water. If O_2 is not available to accept those electrons, oxidative phosphorylation is not possible, and ATP formation in the cell must occur via anaerobic metabolism.

Again, note in figure 3.20 that ATP is formed at several points along the electron transport chain. How does this ATP formation occur? The mechanism to explain the aerobic formation of ATP is known as the **chemiosmotic hypothesis.** As electrons are transferred along the cytochrome chain, the energy released is used to "pump" hydrogens (protons; H^+) released from NADH and FADH from the inside of the mitochondria across the inner mitochondrial membrane (figure 3.22). This results in an accumulation of H^+ within the space between the inner and outer mitochondrial membranes. The accumulation of H^+ is a source of potential energy that can be captured and used to recombine P_i with ADP to form ATP (29). For example, this collection of H^+ is similar to the potential energy of water at the top of a dam; when the water accumulates and runs over the top of the dam, falling

A CLOSER LOOK 3.4

Beta Oxidation Is the Process of Converting Fatty Acids to Acetyl-CoA

Fats are stored in the body in the form of triglycerides within fat cells or in the muscle fiber itself. Release of fat from these storage depots occurs by the breakdown of triglycerides, which results in the liberation of fatty acids (see chapter 4). However, in order for fatty acids to be used as a fuel during aerobic metabolism, they must first be converted to acetyl-CoA. **Beta oxidation** is the process of oxidizing fatty acids to form acetyl-CoA. This occurs in the mitochondria and involves a series of enzymatically catalyzed steps, starting with an "activated fatty acid" and ending with the production of acetyl-CoA. A simple illustration of this process is presented in figure 3.21. This process begins with the "activation" of the fatty acid; the activated fatty acid is then transported into the mitochondria, where the process of beta oxidation begins. In short, beta oxidation is a sequence of four reactions that "chops" fatty acids into two carbon fragments forming acetyl-CoA. Once formed, acetyl-CoA then becomes a fuel source for the Krebs cycle and leads to the production of ATP via the electron transport chain.

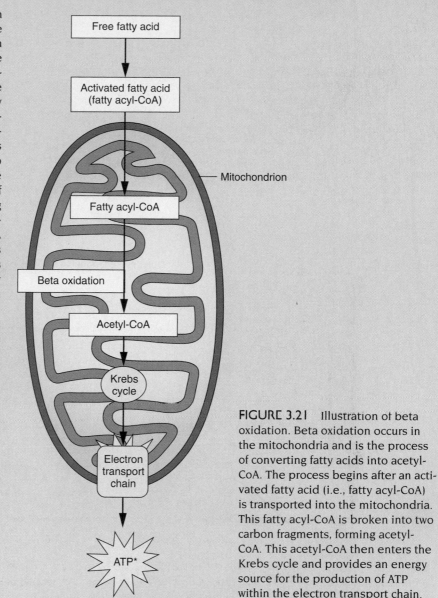

FIGURE 3.21 Illustration of beta oxidation. Beta oxidation occurs in the mitochondria and is the process of converting fatty acids into acetyl-CoA. The process begins after an activated fatty acid (i.e., fatty acyl-CoA) is transported into the mitochondria. This fatty acyl-CoA is broken into two carbon fragments, forming acetyl-CoA. This acetyl-CoA then enters the Krebs cycle and provides an energy source for the production of ATP within the electron transport chain.

water becomes kinetic energy, which can be used to do work (29).

Now for the details of how this potential energy is used to produce ATP. There are three pumps that move H^+ (i.e., protons) from mitochondrial matrix to the intermembrane space (figure 3.22). The first pump (using NADH) moves four H^+ into the intermembrane space for every two electrons that move along the electron transport chain. The second pump also transports four H^+ into the intermembrane space while the third pump moves only two H^+ into the intermembrane space. As a result, there is a higher concentration of H^+ within the intermembrane space compared to that in the matrix; this gradient creates a strong drive for these H^+ to diffuse back into the matrix. However, since the inner mitochondrial is not permeable to H^+, these ions can only cross the membrane through specialized H^+ channels (called *respiratory assemblies*). This idea is illustrated in figure 3.22. Notice that as H^+ cross the inner mitochondrial membrane through these channels, ATP is formed from the addition of phosphate to ADP (called *phosphorylation*). This occurs because the movement of H^+ across the inner mitochondrial membrane activates

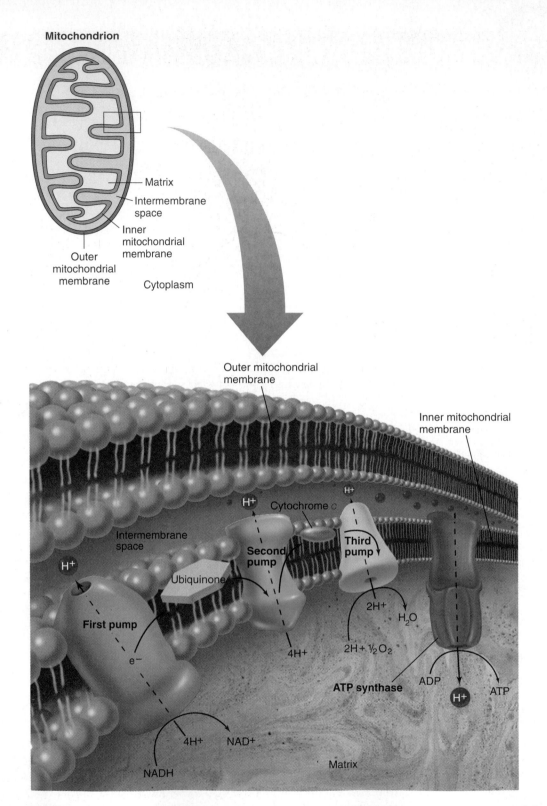

FIGURE 3.22 A schematic representation of the chemiosmotic theory. (*a*) A mitochondrion. (*b*) The matrix and the compartment between the inner and outer mitochondrial membranes showing how the electron transport system functions as H⁺ pumps. This results in a steep H⁺ gradient between the intermembrane space and the cytoplasm of the cell. The diffusion of H⁺ through ATP synthase results in the production of ATP.

A CLOSER LOOK 3.5

A New Look at the ATP Balance Sheet

Historically, it was believed that aerobic metabolism of one molecule of glucose resulted in the production of thirty-eight ATP. However, more recent studies indicate that this number overestimates the total ATP production and that only thirty-two molecules of ATP actually reach the cytoplasm (3, 20, 29). The explanation for this conclusion is that new evidence indicates that the energy provided by NADH and FADH is required not only for ATP production but also to transport ATP across the mitochondrial membrane. This added

energy cost of ATP metabolism reduces the estimates of the total ATP yield from glucose. Specific details of this process follow.

For many years it was believed that for every three H^+ produced, one molecule of ATP was produced and could be used for cellular energy. While it is true that approximately three H^+ must pass through the H^+ channels (i.e., respiratory assemblies) to produce one ATP, it is now known that another H^+ is required to move the ATP molecule across the mitochondrial membrane

into the cytoplasm. The ATP and H^+ are transported into the cytoplasm in exchange for ADP and P_i, which are transported into the mitochondria in order to reform ATP. Therefore, while the theoretical yield of ATP from glucose is thirty-eight molecules, the actual ATP yield, allowing for the energy cost of transport is only thirty-two molecules of ATP per glucose. For details of how these numbers are obtained, see the Aerobic ATP Tally section.

---

the enzyme ATP synthase, which is responsible for catalyzing the reaction:

$$ADP + P_i \rightarrow ATP$$

So, why is oxygen essential for the aerobic production of ATP? Remember that the purpose of the electron transport chain is to move electrons down a series of cytochromes to provide energy to drive ATP production in the mitochondria. The process, illustrated in figure 3.20, requires that each element in the electron transport chain undergo a series of oxidation-reduction reactions. If the last cytochrome (i.e., cytochrome a_3) remains in a reduced state, it would be unable to accept more electrons and the electron transport chain would stop. However, when oxygen is present, the last cytochrome in the chain can be oxidized by oxygen. That is, oxygen, derived from the air we breathe, allows electron transport to continue by functioning as the final electron acceptor of the electron transport chain. This oxidizes cytochrome a_3 and allows electron transport and oxidative phosphorylation to continue. At the last step in the electron transport chain, oxygen accepts two electrons that were passed along the electron transport chain from either NADH or FADH. This reduced oxygen molecule now binds with two protons (H^+) to form water (figures 3.20 and 3.22).

As mentioned earlier, NADH and FADH differ in the amount of ATP that can be formed from each of these molecules. Each NADH formed in the mitochondria donates two electrons to the electron transport system at the first proton pump (figure 3.22). These electrons are then passed to the second and third proton pumps until these electrons are finally passed along to oxygen. The first and second electron pumps transport four protons each, whereas the third electron pump transports two protons, for a total of ten. Because four protons are

required to produce and transport one ATP from the mitochondria to the cytoplasm, the total ATP production from one NADH molecule is 2.5 ATP (10 protons/4 protons per ATP = 2.5 ATP). Note that ATP molecules do not exist in halves and that the decimal fraction of ATP simply indicates an average number of ATP molecules that are produced per NADH.

Compared to NADH, each FADH molecule produces less ATP because the electrons from FADH are donated later in the electron transport chain than those by NADH (figure 3.21). Therefore, the electrons from FADH activate only the second and third proton pumps. Because the first proton pump is bypassed, the electrons from FADH result in the pumping of six protons (four by the second pump and two by the third pump). Since four protons are required to produce and transport one ATP from the mitochondria to the cytoplasm, the total ATP production from one FAD molecule is 1.5 ATP (10 protons/4 protons per ATP = 1.5 ATP). See A Closer Look 3.5 for more details on the quantity of ATP produced in cells.

IN SUMMARY

- Oxidative phosphorylation or aerobic ATP production occurs in the mitochondria as a result of a complex interaction between the Krebs cycle and the electron transport chain. The primary role of the Krebs cycle is to complete the oxidation of substrates and form NADH and FADH to enter the electron transport chain. The end result of the electron transport chain is the formation of ATP and water. Water is formed by oxygen-accepting electrons; hence, the reason we breathe oxygen is to use it as the final acceptor of electrons in aerobic metabolism.

TABLE 3.3	Aerobic ATP Tally from the Breakdown of One Molecule of Glucose		
Metabolic Process	High-Energy Products	ATP from Oxidative Phosphorylation	ATP Subtotal
Glycolysis	2 ATP	—	2 (total if anaerobic)
	2 NADH*	5	7 (if aerobic)
Pyruvic acid to acetyl-CoA	2 NADH	5	12
Krebs cycle	2 GTP	—	14
	6 NADH	15	29
	2 FADH**	3	32
			Grand total: 32 ATP

*2.5 ATP per NADH

**1.5 ATP per FADH

AEROBIC ATP TALLY

It is now possible to compute the overall ATP production as a result of the aerobic breakdown of glucose or glycogen. Let's begin by counting the total energy yield of glycolysis. Recall that the net ATP production of glycolysis was two ATP per glucose molecule. Further, when O_2 is present in the mitochondria, two NADH produced by glycolysis can then be shuttled into the mitochondria with the energy used to synthesize an additional five ATP (table 3.3). Thus, glycolysis can produce two ATP directly via substrate-level phosphorylation and an additional five ATP by the energy contained in the two molecules of NADH.

How many ATP are produced as a result of the oxidation-reduction activities of the Krebs cycle? Table 3.3 shows that two NADH are formed when pyruvic acid is converted to acetyl-CoA, which results in the formation of 5 ATP. Note that two GTP (similar to ATP) are produced via substrate-level phosphorylation. A total of six NADH and two FADH are produced in the Krebs cycle from one glucose molecule. Hence, the six NADH formed via the Krebs cycle results in the production of a total of 15 ATP (6 NADH × 2.5 ATP per NADH = 15 ATP), with three ATP being produced from the two FADH. Therefore, the total ATP yield for the aerobic degradation of glucose is thirty-two ATP. The aerobic ATP yield for glycogen breakdown is thirty-three ATP, since the net glycolytic production of ATP by glycogen is one ATP more than that of glucose.

EFFICIENCY OF OXIDATIVE PHOSPHORYLATION

How efficient is oxidative phosphorylation as a system of converting energy from foodstuffs into biologically usable energy? This can be calculated by computing the ratio of the energy contained in the ATP molecules produced via aerobic respiration divided by the total potential energy contained in the glucose molecule. For example, a mole (a mole is 1 gram molecular weight) of ATP, when broken down, has an energy yield of 7.3 kcal. The potential energy released from the oxidation of a mole of glucose is 686 kcal. Thus, an efficiency figure for aerobic respiration can be computed as follows (31):

$$\text{Efficiency of respiration} = \frac{32 \text{ moles ATP/mole glucose} \times 7.3 \text{ kcal/mole ATP}}{686 \text{ kcal/mole glucose}} \times 100 = 34\%$$

Therefore, the efficiency of aerobic respiration is approximately 34%, with the remaining 66% of the free energy of glucose oxidation being released as heat.

IN SUMMARY

- The aerobic metabolism of one molecule of glucose results in the production of 32 ATP molecules, whereas the aerobic ATP yield for glycogen breakdown is 33 ATP.
- The overall efficiency of aerobic respiration is approximately 34%, with the remaining 66% of the energy being released as heat.

CONTROL OF BIOENERGETICS

The biochemical pathways that result in the production of ATP are regulated by very precise control systems. Each of these pathways contains a number of reactions that are catalyzed by specific enzymes. In general, if ample substrate is available, an increase in the number of enzymes present results in an increased rate of chemical reactions. Therefore, the regulation of one or more enzymes in a biochemical pathway would provide a means of controlling the rate of that particular pathway. Indeed, metabolism is regulated by the control of enzymatic activity. Most metabolic pathways have one enzyme that is considered "rate limiting." This rate-limiting enzyme determines the speed of the particular metabolic pathway involved.

How does a rate-limiting enzyme control the speed of reactions? First, as a rule, rate-limiting enzymes are found early in a metabolic pathway. This position is important, since products of the pathway might accumulate if the rate-limiting enzyme were located near the end of a pathway. Second, the activity of rate-limiting enzymes is regulated by modulators. Modulators are substances that increase or decrease enzyme activity. Enzymes that are regulated by modulators are called allosteric enzymes. In the control of energy metabolism, ATP is the classic example of an inhibitor, while ADP and P_i are examples of substances that stimulate enzymatic activity (8). The fact that large amounts of cellular ATP would inhibit the metabolic production of ATP is logical, since large amounts of ATP would indicate that ATP usage in the cell is low. An example of this type of negative feedback is illustrated in figure 3.23. In contrast, an increase in cell levels of ADP and P_i (low ATP) would indicate that ATP utilization is high. Therefore, it makes sense that ADP and P_i stimulate the production of ATP to meet the increased energy need.

Control of ATP-PC System

Phosphocreatine breakdown is regulated by creatine kinase activity. Creatine kinase is activated when sarcoplasmic concentrations of ADP increase and is inhibited by high levels of ATP. At the onset of exercise, ATP is split into ADP + P_i to provide energy for muscular contraction. This immediate increase in ADP concentrations stimulates creatine kinase to trigger the breakdown of PC to resynthesize ATP. If exercise is continued, glycolysis and finally aerobic metabolism begin to produce adequate ATP to meet the muscles' energy needs. The increase in ATP concentration, coupled with a reduction in ADP concentration, inhibits creatine kinase activity (table 3.4). Regulation of the ATP-PC system is an example of a "negative feedback" control system, which was introduced in chapter 2.

Control of Glycolysis

Although several factors control glycolysis, the most important rate-limiting enzyme in glycolysis is **phosphofructokinase (PFK)** (51). Note that PFK is located near the beginning of glycolysis (figure 3.15). Table 3.4 lists known regulators of PFK. When exercise begins, ADP + P_i levels rise and enhance PFK activity, which serves to increase the rate of glycolysis. In contrast, at rest, when cellular ATP levels are high, PFK activity is inhibited and glycolytic activity is slowed. Further, high cellular levels of hydrogen ions, or citrate (produced via Krebs cycle) also inhibit PFK activity (58). Similar to the control of the ATP-PC system, regulation of PFK activity operates via negative feedback.

Another important regulatory enzyme in carbohydrate metabolism is phosphorylase, which is responsible for degrading glycogen to glucose. Although this enzyme is not technically considered a glycolytic enzyme, the reaction catalyzed by phosphorylase plays an important role in providing the glycolytic pathway with the necessary glucose at the origin of

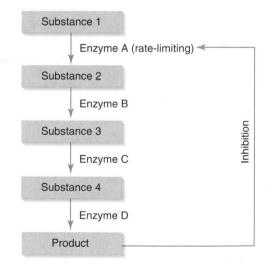

FIGURE 3.23 An example of a "rate-limiting" enzyme in a simple metabolic pathway. Here, a buildup of the product serves to inhibit the rate-limiting enzyme, which in turn slows down the reactions involved in the pathway.

Pathway	Rate-Limiting Enzyme	Stimulators	Inhibitors
ATP-PC system	Creatine kinase	ADP	ATP
Glycolysis	Phosphofructokinase	AMP, ADP, P_i, pH↑	ATP, CP, citrate, pH↓
Krebs cycle	Isocitrate dehydrogenase	ADP, Ca^{++}, NAD	ATP, NADH
Electron transport chain	Cytochrome oxidase	ADP, P_i	ATP

TABLE 3.4 Factors Known to Affect the Activity of Rate-Limiting Enzymes of Metabolic Pathways Involved in Bioenergetics

the pathway. With each muscle contraction, calcium (Ca^{++}) is released from the sarcoplasmic reticulum in muscle. This rise in sarcoplasmic Ca^{++} concentration indirectly activates phosphorylase, which immediately begins to break down glycogen to glucose for entry into glycolysis. Additionally, phosphorylase activity may be stimulated by high levels of the hormone epinephrine. Epinephrine is released at a faster rate during heavy exercise and results in the formation of the compound cyclic AMP (see chapter 5). It is cyclic AMP, not epinephrine, that directly activates phosphorylase. Thus, the influence of epinephrine on phosphorylase is indirect.

Control of Krebs Cycle and Electron Transport Chain

The Krebs cycle, like glycolysis, is subject to enzymatic regulation. Although several Krebs cycle enzymes are regulated, the rate-limiting enzyme is **isocitrate dehydrogenase.** Isocitrate dehydrogenase, like PFK, is inhibited by ATP and stimulated by increasing levels of ADP + P_i (59, 61). Further, growing evidence suggests that increased levels of calcium (Ca^{++}) in the mitochondria also stimulates isocitrate dehydrogenase activity (43). This is a logical signal to turn on energy metabolism in muscle cells, since an increase in free calcium in muscle is the signal to begin muscular contraction (see chapter 8).

The electron transport chain is also regulated by the amount of ATP and ADP + P_i present (6, 59). When exercise begins, ATP levels decline, ADP + P_i levels increase, and cytochrome oxidase is stimulated to begin aerobic production of ATP. When exercise stops, cellular levels of ATP increase and ADP + P_i concentrations decline, and thus the electron transport activity is reduced when normal levels of ATP, ADP, and P_i are reached.

IN SUMMARY

- Metabolism is regulated by enzymatic activity. An enzyme that regulates a metabolic pathway is termed the "rate-limiting" enzyme.
- The rate-limiting enzyme for glycolysis is phosphofructokinase, while the rate-limiting enzymes for the Krebs cycle and electron transport chain are isocitrate dehydrogenase and cytochrome oxidase, respectively.
- In general, cellular levels of ATP and ADP + P_i regulate the rate of metabolic pathways involved in the production of ATP. High levels of ATP inhibit further ATP production, while low levels of ATP and high levels of ADP + P_i stimulate ATP production. Evidence also exists that calcium may stimulate aerobic energy metabolism.

INTERACTION BETWEEN AEROBIC/ANAEROBIC ATP PRODUCTION

It is important to emphasize the interaction of anaerobic and aerobic metabolic pathways in the production of ATP during exercise. Although it is common to hear someone speak of aerobic versus anaerobic exercise, in reality the energy to perform most types of exercise comes from a combination of anaerobic and aerobic sources (11, 27, 42, 48). This point is illustrated in The Winning Edge 3.2. Notice that the contribution of anaerobic ATP production is greater in short-term, high-intensity activities, while aerobic metabolism predominates in longer activities. For example, approximately 90% of the energy to perform a 100-meter dash would come from anaerobic sources, with most of the energy coming via the ATP-PC system. Similarly, energy to run 400 meters (i.e., 55 seconds) would be largely anaerobic (70–75%). However, ATP and PC stores are limited, and thus glycolysis must supply much of the ATP during this type of an event (60).

On the other end of the energy spectrum, events like the marathon (i.e., 26.2-mile race) rely on aerobic production of ATP for the bulk of the needed energy. Where does the energy come from in events of moderate length (i.e., two to thirty minutes)? The Winning Edge 3.2 provides an estimation of the percentage anaerobic/aerobic yield in events over a wide range of durations. Although these estimates are based on laboratory measurements of running or exercising on a cycle ergometer, they can be related to other athletic events that require intense effort by comparing the length of time spent in the activity (see The Winning Edge 3.2).

In review, the shorter the duration of all-out activity, the greater the contribution of anaerobic energy production; conversely, the longer the duration, the greater the contribution of aerobic energy production. A more detailed discussion of the metabolic responses to various types of exercise is presented in chapter 4.

IN SUMMARY

- Energy to perform exercise comes from an interaction of anaerobic and aerobic pathways.
- In general, the shorter the activity (high intensity), the greater the contribution of anaerobic energy production. In contrast, long-term activities (low to moderate intensity) utilize ATP produced from aerobic sources.

THE WINNING EDGE 3.2

Exercise Physiology Applied to Sports

Contributions of Anaerobic/Aerobic Energy Production During Various Sporting Events

Because sports differ widely in both the intensity and the duration of physical effort, it is not surprising that the source of energy production differs widely between sporting events. Figure 3.24 provides an illustration of the anaerobic versus aerobic energy production during selected sports. Knowledge of the interaction between the anaerobic and aerobic energy production in exercise is useful to coaches and trainers in planning conditioning programs for athletes. See chapter 21 for more details.

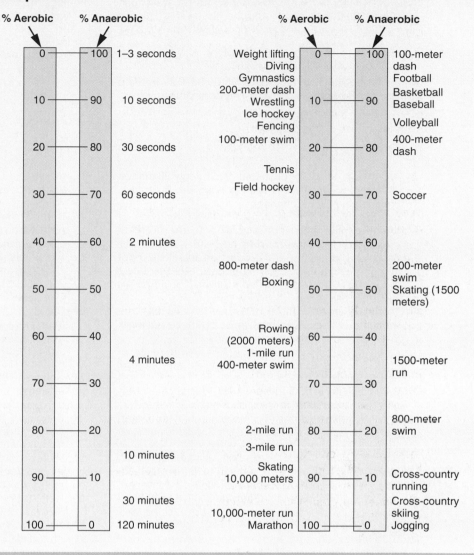

FIGURE 3.24 Contribution of anaerobic and aerobically produced ATP for use during sports.

STUDY QUESTIONS

1. List and briefly discuss the function of the three major components of cell structure.
2. Briefly explain the concept of coupled reactions.
3. Define the following terms: (1) bioenergetics, (2) endergonic reactions, and (3) exergonic reactions.
4. Discuss the role of enzymes as catalysts. What is meant by the expression "energy of activation"?
5. Briefly, identify the common forms of carbohydrates, proteins, and fats. What role does each play as an energy source during exercise?
6. Define the terms glycogen, glycogenolysis, and glycolysis.
7. What are high-energy phosphates? Explain the statement that "ATP is the universal energy donor."
8. Define the terms aerobic and anaerobic.
9. Briefly discuss the function of glycolysis in bioenergetics. What role does NAD play in glycolysis?
10. Discuss the operation of the Krebs cycle and the electron transport chain in the aerobic production of ATP. What is the function of NAD and FAD in these pathways?
11. What is the efficiency of the aerobic degradation of glucose?
12. How is bioenergetics controlled? What are rate-limiting enzymes and how do they operate?
13. What enzyme regulates glycolysis? The Krebs cycle?
14. Briefly, discuss the interaction of anaerobic versus aerobic ATP production during exercise.
15. Discuss the chemiosmotic theory of ATP production.
16. List and define the six classes of enzymes identified by the International Union of Biochemistry.
17. Briefly, discuss the impact of changes in both temperature and pH on enzyme activity.
18. Discuss the relationship between lactic acid and lactate.

SUGGESTED READINGS

Bemben, M., and H. Lamont. 2005. Creatine supplementation and exercise performance. *Sports Medicine* 35:107–25.

Brooks, G., T. Fahey, and K. Baldwin. 2005. *Exercise Physiology: Human Bioenergetics and Its Applications*, 4th ed. New York: McGraw-Hill Companies.

Fox, S. 2006. *Human Physiology*, 9th ed. New York: McGraw-Hill Companies.

Maughan, R., D. King, and T. Lea. 2004. Dietary supplements. *Journal of Sports Sciences* 22:95–113.

McKee, T., and J. McKee. 2003. *Biochemistry: The Molecular Basis of Life*, 3d ed. New York: McGraw-Hill Companies.

Powers, S., J. Quindry, K. DeRuisseau, and K. Hamilton. 2004. Exercise and dietary antioxidants. *Journal of Sports Sciences* 22:81–94.

Robergs, R., and S. Keteyian. 2003. *Fundamentals of Exercise Physiology: For Fitness, Performance, and Health*, 2d ed. New York: McGraw-Hill Companies.

Widmaier, E., H. Raff, and K. Strang. 2006. *Vander's Human Physiology*, 10th ed. New York: McGraw-Hill Companies.

REFERENCES

1. Armstrong, R. 1979. Biochemistry: Energy liberation and use. In *Sports Medicine and Physiology*, ed. R. Strauss. Philadelphia: W. B. Saunders.

2. Balaban, R., and F. Heineman. 1989. Interaction of oxidative phosphorylation and work in the heart, In vivo. *News in Physiological Sciences* 4:215–18.

3. Bangsbo, J. et al. 2001. ATP production and efficiency of human skeletal muscle during intense exercise: Effect of previous exercise. *American Journal of Physiology* 280:E956–64.

4. Barclay, J., and M. Hansel. 1991. Free radicals may contribute to oxidative skeletal muscle fatigue. *Canadian Journal of Physiology and Pharmacology* 69:279–84.

5. Bemben, M., and H. Lamont. 2005. Creatine supplementation and exercise performance: Recent findings. *Sports Medicine* 35:107–25.

6. Bessman, S., and C. Carpender. 1985. The creatine phosphate shuttle. *Annual Review of Biochemistry* 54:831–62.

7. Booth, F. 1989. Application of molecular biology in exercise physiology. In *Exercise and Sport Sciences Reviews*, vol. 17, 1–28. Baltimore: Williams & Wilkins.

8. Brazy, P., and L. Mandel. 1986. Does availability of inorganic phosphate regulate cellular oxidative metabolism? *News in Physiological Sciences* 1:100–2.

9. Brooks, G., T. Fahey, and K. Baldwin. 2005. *Exercise Physiology: Human Bioenergetics and Its Applications*, 4th ed. New York: McGraw-Hill Companies.

10. Brudnak, M. Creatine: Are the benefits worth the risk? 2004. *Toxicology Letters* 150:123–30.

11. Brooks, G., T. Fahey, and T. White. 2000. *Exercise Physiology: Human Bioenergetics and Its Applications*. Mountain View, CA: Mayfield.

12. Cerretelli, P., D. Rennie, and D. Pendergast. 1980. Kinetics of metabolic transients during exercise. *International Journal of Sports Medicine* 55:171–80.

13. Conley, K. 1994. Cellular energetics during exercise. *Advances in Veterinary Science and Comparative Medicine* 38a:1–39.

14. Cooper, C., N. Vollaard, T. Choueiri, and M. Wilson. 2002. Exercise, free radicals, and oxidative stress. *Biochemical Society Transactions* 30:280–85.

15. Davies, K., A. Quintanilha, G. Brooks, and L. Packer. 1982. Free radical and tissue damage produced by exercise. *Biochemistry and Biophysics Research Communications* 107:1198–1205.

16. De Zwaan, A., and G. Thillard. 1985. Low and high power output modes of anaerobic metabolism: Invertebrate and vertebrate categories. In *Circulation, Respiration, and Metabolism*, ed. R. Giles, 166–92. Berlin: Springer-Verlag.

17. di Prampero, P., U. Boutellier, and P. Pietsch. 1983. Oxygen deficit and stores at the onset of muscular exercise in humans. *Journal of Applied Physiology* 55:146–53.

18. Dolny, D., and P. Lemon. 1988. Effect of ambient temperature on protein breakdown during prolonged exercise. *Journal of Applied Physiology* 64:550–55.

19. Fox, S. 2006. *Human Physiology*, 9th ed. New York: McGraw-Hill Companies.

20. Fox, S. 2002. *Human Physiology*. New York: McGraw-Hill Companies.

21. Giese, A. 1979. *Cell Physiology*. Philadelphia: W. B. Saunders.

22. Gollnick, P. 1985. Metabolism of substrates: Energy substrate metabolism during exercise and as modified by training. *Federation Proceedings* 44:353–56.

23. Gollnick, P. et al. 1985. Differences in metabolic potential of skeletal muscle fibers and their significance for metabolic control. *Journal of Experimental Biology* 115:191–95.

24. Greenhaff, P. 1995. Creatine and its application as an ergogenic aid. *International Journal of Sports Nutrition* 5: (supplement), s100–s110.

25. Haller, C., K. Meier, and K. Olson. 2005. Siezures reported in association with use of dietary supplements. *Clinical Toxicology* 43:23–30.

26. Hole, J. 1995. *Human Anatomy and Physiology*. New York: McGraw-Hill Companies.

27. Holloszy, J. 1982. Muscle metabolism during exercise. *Archives of Physical and Rehabilitation Medicine* 63:231–34.

28. Holloszy, J., and E. Coyle. 1984. Adaptations of skeletal muscle to endurance exercise and their metabolic consequences. *Journal of Applied Physiology* 56:831–38.

29. Houston, M. 2001. *Biochemistry Primer for Exercise Science*. Champaign, IL: Human Kinetics.

30. Jain, M. 1972. *The Biomolecular Lipid Membrane: A System*. New York: Reinhold.

31. Jequier, E., and J. Flatt. 1986. Recent advances in human bioenergetics. *News in Physiological Sciences* 1:112–14.

32. Johnson, L. 1987. *Biology*. New York: McGraw-Hill Companies.

33. Juhn, M., and M. Tarnopolsky. 1998. Oral creatine supplementation and athletic performance: A critical review. *Clinical Journal of Sports Medicine* 8:286–97.

34. Juhn, M., and M. Tarnopolsky. 1998. Potential side effects of oral creatine supplementation: A critical review. *Clinical Journal of Sports Medicine* 8:298–304.

35. Lawler, J., S. Powers, T. Visser, H. Van Dijk, M. Kordus, and L. Ji. 1993. Acute exercise and skeletal muscle antioxidant and metabolic enzymes. Effects of fiber type and age. *American Journal of Physiology* 265:R1344–R1350.

36. Lemon, P., and J. Mullin. 1980. Effect of initial muscle glycogen levels on protein catabolism during exercise. *Journal of Applied Physiology* 48:624–29.

37. Mathews, C., K. van Holde, and K. Ahern. 1999. *Biochemistry*. San Francisco: Benjamin Cummings.

38. Mathews, C., and K. E. vanHolde. 1996. *Biochemistry*. Menlo Park, CA: Benjamin-Cummings.

39. Maughan, R., D. King, and T. Lea. 2004. Dietary supplements. *Journal of Sports Sciences* 22:95–113.

40. Maughan, R. 1995. Creatine supplementation and exercise performance. *International Journal of Sports Nutrition* 5:94–101.

41. McArdle, W., F. Katch, and V. Katch. 2004. *Exercise Physiology: Energy, Nutrition, and Human Performance*. Baltimore: Lippincott Williams & Wilkins.

42. McArdle, W., F. Katch, and V. Katch. 2001. *Exercise Physiology: Energy, Nutrition, and Human Performance*. Baltimore: Lippincott Williams & Wilkins.

43. McCormack, J., and R. Denton. 1994. Signal transduction by intramitochondrial calcium in mammalian energy metabolism. *News in Physiological Sciences* 9:71–76.

44. McGilvery, R. 1983. *Biochemistry: A Functional Approach*. Philadelphia: W. B. Saunders.

45. McKee, T., and J. McKee. 2003. *Biochemistry: The Molecular Basis of Life*, 3d ed. New York: McGraw-Hill Companies.

46. McMurray, W. 1977. *Essentials of Human Metabolism*. New York: Harper & Row.

47. Miller, F. 1987. *College Physics*. New York: Harcourt Brace Jovanovich.

48. Mole, P. 1983. Exercise metabolism. In *Exercise Medicine: Physiological Principles and Clinical Application*. New York: Academic Press.

49. Nave, C., and B. Nave. 1985. *Physics for the Health Sciences*. Philadelphia: W. B. Saunders.

50. Newsholme, E. 1979. The control of fuel utilization by muscle during exercise and starvation. *Diabetes* 28 (Suppl.):1–7.

51. Newsholme E., and A. Leech. 1988. *Biochemistry for the Medical Sciences*. New York: J. Wiley & Sons.

52. Powers, S., J. Quindry, K. DeRuisseau, and K. Hamilton. 2004. Exercise and dietary antioxidants. *Journal of Sports Sciences* 22:81–94.

53. Rawson, E., and J. Volek. 2003. Effects of creatine supplementation and resistance training on muscle strength and weightlifting performance. *Journal of Strength and Conditioning Research* 17:822–31.

54. Reid, M. 2001. Redox modulation of skeletal muscle contraction: What we know and what we don't. *Journal of Applied Physiology* 90:724–31.

55. Reid, M., K. Haack, K. Franchek, P. Valberg, L. Kobzik, and M. West. 1992. Reactive oxygen in skeletal muscle. I. Intracellular oxidant kinetics and fatigue in vitro. *Journal of Applied Physiology* 73:1797–1804.

56. Sears, C., and C. Stanitski. 1983. *Chemistry for the Health-Related Sciences*. Englewood Cliffs, NJ: Prentice-Hall.

57. Senior, A. 1988. ATP synthesis by oxidative phosphorylation. *Physiological Reviews* 68:177–216.

58. Spriet L. 1991. Phosphofructokinase activity and acidosis during short-term tetanic contractions. *Canadian Journal of Physiology and Pharmacology* 69:298–304.

59. Stanley W., and R. Connett. 1991. Regulation of muscle carbohydrate metabolism during exercise. *FASEB Journal* 5:2155–59.

60. Stryer, L. 2002. *Biochemistry*. New York: W. H. Freeman.

61. Suttie, J. 1977. *Introduction to Biochemistry*. New York: Holt, Rinehart & Winston.

62. Tullson, P., and R. Terjung. 1991. Adenine nucleotide metabolism in contracting skeletal muscle. *Exercise and Sport Science Reviews*, vol. 19, 507–37. Baltimore: Lippincott Williams & Wilkins.

63. Turrens, J. 2003. Mitochondrial formation of reactive oxygen species. *Journal of Physiology* 552.2:335–44.

64. Vincent, H., S. Powers, H. Demirel, J. Coombes, and H. Naito. 1999. Exercise training protects against contraction-induced lipid peroxidation in the diaphragm. *European Journal of Applied Physiology* 79:268–73.

65. Weibel, E. 1984. *The Pathway for Oxygen*. Cambridge: Harvard University Press.

66. West, J., ed. 2001. *Best and Taylor's Physiological Basis of Medical Practice*. Baltimore: Lippincott Williams & Wilkins.

67. West, J. 1985. *Best's and Taylor's Physiological Basis of Medical Practice*. Baltimore: Lippincott Williams & Wilkins.

68. Whipp, B., and M. Mahler. 1980. Dynamics of pulmonary gas exchange during exercise. In *Pulmonary Gas Exchange*, vol. 2, ed. J. West. New York: Academic Press.

69. Williams, M., and J. Branch. 1998. Creatine supplementation and exercise performance: An update. *Journal of the American College of Nutrition* 17:216–34.

CHAPTER 4

Exercise Metabolism

■ Objectives

By studying this chapter, you should be able to do the following:

1. Discuss the relationship between exercise intensity/duration and the bioenergetic pathways that are most responsible for the production of ATP during various types of exercise.

2. Define the term *oxygen deficit*.

3. Define the term *lactate threshold*.

4. Discuss several possible explanations for the sudden rise in blood-lactate concentration during incremental exercise.

5. List the factors that regulate fuel selection during different types of exercise.

6. Explain why fat metabolism is dependent on carbohydrate metabolism.

7. Define the term *oxygen debt*.

8. Give the physiological explanation for the observation that the O_2 debt is greater following intense exercise when compared to the O_2 debt following light exercise.

■ Outline

Energy Requirements Rest   53

Rest-to-Exercise Transitions   53

Recovery from Exercise: Metabolic Responses   54

Metabolic Responses to Exercise: Influence of Duration and Intensity   57

Short-Term, Intense Exercise   57
Prolonged Exercise   58
Incremental Exercise   58

Estimation of Fuel Utilization During Exercise   61

Factors Governing Fuel Selection   62

Exercise Intensity and Fuel Selection   62

Exercise Duration and Fuel Selection   63

Interaction of Fat/Carbohydrate Metabolism   64

Body Fuel Sources   65

■ Key Terms

anaerobic threshold
Cori cycle
EPOC
free fatty acid (FFA)
gluconeogenesis

graded exercise test
incremental exercise test
lactate threshold
lipase
lipolysis

maximal oxygen uptake ($\dot{V}O_2$ max)
oxygen debt
oxygen deficit
respiratory exchange ratio (R)

Exercise poses a serious challenge to the bioenergetic pathways in the working muscle. For example, during heavy exercise the body's total energy expenditure may increase fifteen to twenty-five times above expenditure at rest. Most of this increase in energy production is used to provide ATP for contracting skeletal muscles, which may increase their energy utilization 200 times over utilization at rest (1). Therefore, it is apparent that skeletal muscles have a great capacity to produce and use large quantities of ATP during exercise. This chapter will describe: (1) the metabolic responses at the beginning of exercise and during recovery from exercise; (2) the metabolic responses to high-intensity, incremental, and prolonged exercise; (3) the selection of fuels used to produce ATP; and (4) how exercise metabolism is regulated.

We begin with an overview of the energy requirements of the body at rest followed by a discussion of which bioenergetic pathways are activated at the onset of exercise.

ENERGY REQUIREMENTS AT REST

Recall that homeostasis is defined as a steady and unchanging internal environment (see chapter 2). During resting conditions, the healthy human body is in homeostasis and therefore the body's energy requirement is also constant. At rest, almost 100% of the energy (i.e., ATP) required to sustain bodily functions is produced by aerobic metabolism. It follows that resting blood lactate levels are also steady and low (e.g., <1.0 millimoles per liter).

Since the measurement of oxygen (O_2) consumption (oxygen consumed by the body) is an index of aerobic ATP production, measurement of O_2 consumption during rest provides an estimate of the body's "baseline" energy requirement. At rest, the total energy requirement of an individual is relatively low. For example, a 70-kilogram young adult would consume approximately 0.25 liters of oxygen each minute; this translates to a relative O_2 consumption of 3.5 ml of O_2 per kilogram (body weight) per minute. As mentioned earlier, muscular exercise can greatly increase the body's need for energy. Lets begin our discussion of exercise metabolism by considering which bioenergetic pathways are active during the transition from rest to exercise.

REST-TO-EXERCISE TRANSITIONS

Suppose you step onto a treadmill belt that is moving at 3 mph. Within one step, your muscles must increase their rate of ATP production from that required for

standing to that required for running at 3 mph. If they do not, you will fall off the back of the treadmill. What metabolic changes must occur in skeletal muscle at the beginning of exercise to provide the necessary energy to continue movement? Similar to measurement of O_2 consumption during rest, measurement of O_2 consumption during exercise can provide information about aerobic metabolism during exercise. For example, in the transition from rest to light or moderate exercise, O_2 consumption increases rapidly and reaches a steady state within one to four minutes (12, 23, 81) (figure 4.1). The fact that O_2 consumption does not increase instantaneously to a steady-state value suggests that anaerobic energy sources contribute to the overall production of ATP at the beginning of exercise. Indeed, there is much evidence to suggest that at the onset of exercise the ATP-PC system is the first active bioenergetic pathway, followed by glycolysis and, finally, aerobic energy production (4, 15, 37, 65, 88). However, after a steady state is reached, the body's ATP requirement is met via aerobic metabolism. The major point to be emphasized concerning the bioenergetics of rest-to-work transitions is that several energy systems are involved. In other words, the energy needed for exercise is not provided by simply turning on a single bioenergetic pathway, but rather by a mixture of several metabolic systems operating with considerable overlap.

The term **oxygen deficit** applies to the lag in oxygen uptake at the beginning of exercise. Specifically, the oxygen deficit is defined as the difference between oxygen uptake in the first few minutes of exercise and an equal time period after steady state has been obtained (77, 86). This is represented as the shaded area in the left-hand portion of figure 4.1. Note in figure 4.2 that the time to reach steady state is shorter in trained subjects than in untrained subjects (59, 81). This difference in the time course of oxygen uptake at the onset of exercise between trained and untrained subjects results in the trained subjects having a lower oxygen deficit when compared to the untrained. What is the explanation for this difference? It seems likely

FIGURE 4.1 The time course of oxygen uptake ($\dot{V}O_2$) in the transition from rest to submaximal exercise.

FIGURE 4.2 Differences in the time course of oxygen uptake ($\dot{V}O_2$) during the transition from rest to submaximal exercise between trained and untrained subjects. Note that the time to reach steady state is slower in untrained subjects. See text for details.

that the trained subjects have a better-developed aerobic bioenergetic capacity, resulting from either cardiovascular or muscular adaptations induced by endurance training (32, 59, 81, 86). (See Ask the Expert 4.1 for more information on this topic.) Practically speaking, this means that aerobic ATP production is active earlier at the beginning of exercise and results in less production of lactic acid in the trained individual when compared to the untrained individual. Chapter 13 provides a detailed analysis of this adaptation to training.

<hr>

IN SUMMARY

- In the transition from rest to light or moderate exercise, oxygen uptake increases rapidly, generally reaching a steady state within one to four minutes.
- The term *oxygen deficit* applies to the lag in oxygen uptake at the beginning of exercise.
- The failure of oxygen uptake to increase instantly at the beginning of exercise suggests that anaerobic pathways contribute to the overall production of ATP early in exercise. After a steady state is reached, the body's ATP requirement is met via aerobic metabolism.

RECOVERY FROM EXERCISE: METABOLIC RESPONSES

Metabolism remains elevated for several minutes immediately following exercise. The magnitude and duration of this elevated metabolism are influenced by

FIGURE 4.3 Oxygen deficit and debt during light/moderate exercise (*a*) and during heavy exercise (*b*).

the intensity of the exercise (6, 49, 86). This point is illustrated in figure 4.3. Note that oxygen uptake is greater and remains elevated for a longer time period following high-intensity exercise when compared to exercise of light-to-moderate intensity (49, 50). The reason(s) for this observation will be discussed shortly.

Historically, the term **oxygen debt** has been applied to mean the excess oxygen uptake above rest following exercise. The prominent British physiologist A. V. Hill (60) first used the term O_2 *debt* and reasoned that the excess oxygen consumed (above rest) following exercise was repayment for the O_2 deficit incurred at the onset of exercise. Evidence collected in the 1920s and 1930s by Hill and other researchers in Europe and the United States suggested that the oxygen debt could be divided into two portions: the rapid portion immediately following exercise (i.e., approximately two to three minutes post-exercise) and the slow portion, which persisted for greater than thirty minutes after exercise. The rapid portion is represented by the steep decline in oxygen uptake following exercise, and the slow portion is represented by the slow decline in O_2 across time following exercise (figure 4.3). The rationale for the two divisions of the O_2 debt was based on the belief that the rapid portion of the O_2 debt represented the oxygen that was required to resynthesize stored ATP and PC and replace tissue stores of O_2 (~20% of the O_2 debt), while the slow por-

ASK THE EXPERT 4.1

Oxygen Uptake Kinetics at the Onset of Constant Work-Rate Exercise: Questions and Answers with Dr. Bruce Gladden

Bruce Gladden, Ph.D., a professor in the Department of Exercise and Sport Sciences at Auburn University, is an internationally known expert in muscle metabolism during exercise. Dr. Gladden's research has addressed important questions relative to those factors that regulate oxygen consumption in skeletal muscle during exercise. Examples of Dr. Gladden's work can be found in prestigious international physiology journals. In this feature, Dr. Gladden answers questions about the time course of oxygen consumption at the onset of submaximal exercise.

QUESTION 1: What is so important about the response of oxygen consumption at the onset of submaximal, constant work-rate exercise?

DR. GLADDEN: First, it is critical to realize that oxygen consumption is a direct indicator of the energy supplied by oxidative phosphorylation (i.e., the oxidative or aerobic energy system). The fact that there is a "lag" or delay before oxygen consumption rises to a steady-state level tells us that aerobic metabolism (i.e., oxidative phosphorylation in the mitochondria) is not instantaneously activated at the onset of exercise. The importance of this response is that it can provide information about the control or regulation of oxidative

phosphorylation. Further, this delayed response tells us that the anaerobic energy systems must also be activated to supply the needed energy at the beginning of exercise.

QUESTION 2: Why is oxidative phosphorylation gradually activated at the onset of exercise rather than instantaneously activated?

DR. GLADDEN: Historically, two alternative hypotheses have been offered. First, it has been suggested that there is an inadequate oxygen supply to the contracting muscles at exercise onset. What this means is that in at least some mitochondria, at least some of the time, there may not be molecules of oxygen available to accept electrons at the end of the electron transport chains. Clearly, if this is correct, the oxidative phosphorylation rate, and therefore the whole body oxygen consumption, would be restricted. The second hypothesis holds that there is a delay because the stimuli for oxidative phosphorylation require some time to reach their final levels and to have their full effects for a given exercise intensity. Table 3.4 notes that the electron transport chain is stimulated by ADP and P_i. At the onset of exercise, the concentrations of ADP and P_i are barely above resting levels. The concentrations of ADP

and P_i will continue to rise as PC is broken down, gradually providing additional stimulation to "turn on" oxidative phosphorylation until this aerobic pathway is providing essentially 100% of the energy requirement of the exercise. The key point is that these regulators of oxidative phosphorylation rate do not instantaneously rise from resting concentrations to the steady-state concentration levels. This has sometimes been referred to as the "inertia of metabolism."

QUESTION 3: Which of these hypotheses is correct?

DR. GLADDEN: These two hypotheses are not mutually exclusive. My research with Dr. Bruno Grassi (University of Milano), Dr. Mike Hogan (University of California, San Diego), and others suggests that the most significant limitation lies within the second hypothesis—some "slowness" in the full expression of the metabolic signals. Nevertheless, oxygen supply limitation can also play a role, a role that likely becomes more important at higher exercise intensities. Oxygen should not be considered separately; it should be included as one of the regulators or controllers of oxidative phosphorylation.

---

tion of the debt was due to the oxidative conversion of lactic acid to glucose in the liver (~80% of the O$_2$ debt).

Contradicting previous beliefs, recent evidence has shown that only about 20% of the oxygen debt is used to convert the lactic acid produced during exercise to glucose (the process of glucose synthesis from noncarbohydrate sources is called **gluconeogenesis**) (14, 16). Therefore, the notion that the "slow" portion of the O$_2$ debt is due entirely to oxidative conversion of lactic acid to glucose does not appear to be accurate. Several investigators have argued that the term *oxygen debt* be eliminated from the literature, because the elevated oxygen consumption following exercise does not appear to be entirely due to the "borrowing" of oxy-

gen from the body's oxygen stores (14, 16, 20, 41). In recent years, several replacement terms have been suggested. One such term is **EPOC,** which stands for "excess post-exercise oxygen consumption" (20, 41).

If the EPOC is not exclusively used to convert lactic acid to glucose, why does oxygen consumption remain elevated post-exercise? Several possibilities exist. First, at least part of the O$_2$ consumed immediately following exercise is used to restore PC in muscle and O$_2$ stores in blood and tissues (12, 41). Restoration of both PC and oxygen stores in muscle is completed within two to three minutes of recovery (56). This is consistent with the classic view of the rapid portion of the oxygen debt. Further, heart rate

Removal of Lactic Acid Following Exercise

What happens to the lactic acid that is formed during exercise? Classical theory proposed that the majority of the post-exercise lactic acid was converted into glucose in the liver and resulted in an elevated post-exercise oxygen uptake (i.e., O_2 debt). However, recent evidence suggests that this is not the case and that lactic acid is mainly oxidized after exercise (14,16). That is, lactic acid is converted to pyruvic acid and used as a substrate by the heart and skeletal muscle. It is estimated that approximately 70% of the lactic acid produced during exercise is oxidized, while 20% is converted to glucose and the remaining 10% is converted to amino acids.

Figure 4.4 demonstrates the time course of lactic acid removal from the blood following strenuous exercise. Note that lactic acid removal is more rapid if continuous light exercise is performed as compared to a resting recovery. The explanation for these findings is linked to the fact that light exercise enhances oxidation of lactic acid by the working muscle (31, 44, 58). It is estimated that the optimum intensity of recovery exercise to promote

FIGURE 4.4 Blood lactate removal following strenuous exercise. Note that lactic acid can be removed more rapidly from the blood during recovery if the subject engages in continuous light exercise.

blood lactic acid removal is around 30% to 40% of $\dot{V}O_2$ max (31). Higher exercise intensities would likely result in an increased muscle production of lactic acid and therefore hinder removal.

Due to the increase in muscle oxidative capacity observed with endurance training, some authors have speculated that trained subjects might have a greater capacity to remove lactic acid during recovery from intense exercise (7, 9). Unfortunately, human studies examining the effects of training on the rate of blood lactate decline (following heavy exercise) have yielded conflicting results. However, two well-designed investigations have reported no differences in blood lactic acid disappearance between trained and untrained subjects during resting recovery from a maximal exercise bout (7, 38).

and breathing remain elevated above resting levels for several minutes following exercise; therefore, both of these activities require additional O_2 above resting levels. Other factors that may result in the EPOC are an elevated body temperature and specific circulating hormones. Increases in body temperature result in an increased metabolic rate (called the Q_{10} effect) (17, 54, 84). Further, it has been argued that high levels of epinephrine or norepinephrine result in increased oxygen consumption after exercise (42). However, both of these hormones are rapidly removed from the blood following exercise and therefore may not exist long enough to have a significant impact on the EPOC.

Earlier it was mentioned that the EPOC was greater following high-intensity exercise when compared to the EPOC following light-to-moderate work. This difference in EPOC is due to differences in the amount of body heat gained, the total PC depleted,

and the blood levels of epinephrine and norepinephrine (49). First, assuming similar ambient conditions (i.e., room temperature/relative humidity) and equal exercise time, high-intensity exercise will result in greater body heat gain than that gained by light exercise. Secondly, depletion of PC is dependent on exercise intensity. Since high-intensity exercise would utilize more PC, additional oxygen would be required during recovery for resynthesis. Finally, intense exercise results in greater blood concentrations of lactic acid, epinephrine, and norepinephrine when compared to light work. All of these factors may contribute to the EPOC being greater following intense exercise than following light exercise. Figure 4.5 contains a summary of factors thought to contribute to the "excess post-exercise oxygen consumption." Further, see A Closer Look 4.1 for more details on removal of lactic acid following exercise.

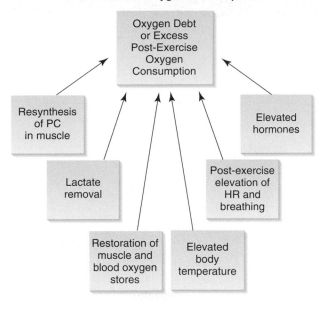

Factors Contributing to Excess Post-Exercise Oxygen Consumption

Oxygen Debt or Excess Post-Exercise Oxygen Consumption

Resynthesis of PC in muscle

Lactate removal

Restoration of muscle and blood oxygen stores

Elevated body temperature

Post-exercise elevation of HR and breathing

Elevated hormones

FIGURE 4.5 A summary of factors that might contribute to excess post-exercise oxygen consumption (EPOC). See text for details.

IN SUMMARY

- The oxygen debt (also called excess post-exercise oxygen consumption [EPOC]) is the O_2 consumption above rest following exercise.
- Several factors contribute to the EPOC. First, some of the O_2 consumed early in the recovery period is used to resynthesize stored PC in the muscle and replace O_2 stores in both muscle and blood. Other factors that contribute to the "slow" portion of the EPOC include an elevated body temperature, O_2 required to convert lactic acid to glucose (gluconeogenesis), and elevated blood levels of epinephrine and norepinephrine.

METABOLIC RESPONSES TO EXERCISE: INFLUENCE OF DURATION AND INTENSITY

The point was made in chapter 3 that short-term, high-intensity exercise lasting less than ten seconds utilizes primarily anaerobic metabolic pathways to produce ATP. In contrast, an event like the marathon makes primary use of aerobic ATP production to provide the needed ATP for work. However, events lasting longer than ten to twenty seconds and less than ten minutes generally produce the needed ATP for mus-

cular contraction via a combination of both anaerobic and aerobic pathways. In fact, most sports use a combination of anaerobic and aerobic pathways to produce the ATP needed for muscular contraction. The next three sections consider which bioenergetic pathways are involved in energy production in specific types of exercise.

Short-Term, Intense Exercise

The energy to perform short-term exercise of high intensity comes primarily from anaerobic metabolic pathways. Whether the ATP production is dominated by the ATP-PC system or glycolysis depends primarily on the length of the activity (1, 4, 65, 69). For example, the energy to run a 50-meter dash or to complete a single play in a football game comes principally from the ATP-PC system. In contrast, the energy to complete the 400-meter dash (i.e., fifty-five seconds) comes from a combination of the ATP-PC system, glycolysis, and aerobic metabolism, with glycolysis producing most of the ATP. In general, the ATP-PC system can supply almost all the needed ATP for work for events lasting one to five seconds; intense exercise lasting longer than five to six seconds begins to utilize the ATP-producing capability of glycolysis. It should be emphasized that the transition from the ATP-PC system to an increased dependence upon glycolysis during exercise is not an abrupt change but rather a gradual shift from one pathway to another.

Events lasting longer than forty-five seconds use a combination of all three energy systems (i.e., ATP-PC, glycolysis, and aerobic systems). This point was emphasized in figure 3.24 in chapter 3. In general, intense exercise lasting approximately sixty seconds utilizes 70%/30% (anaerobic/aerobic) energy production, while events lasting two minutes utilize anaerobic and aerobic bioenergetic pathways almost equally to supply the needed ATP (see figure 3.24).

IN SUMMARY

- During high-intensity, short-term exercise (i.e., two to twenty seconds), the muscle's ATP production is dominated by the ATP-PC system.
- Intense exercise lasting more than twenty seconds relies more on anaerobic glycolysis to produce much of the needed ATP.
- Finally, high-intensity events lasting longer than forty-five seconds use a combination of the ATP-PC system, glycolysis, and the aerobic system to produce the needed ATP for muscular contraction.

Prolonged Exercise

The energy to perform long-term exercise (i.e., more than ten minutes) comes primarily from aerobic metabolism. A steady-state oxygen uptake can generally be maintained during submaximal exercise of moderate duration. However, two exceptions to this rule exist. First, prolonged exercise in a hot/humid environment results in a "drift" upward of oxygen uptake; therefore, a steady state is not maintained in this type of exercise (84). Second, continuous exercise at a high relative work rate (i.e., >75% $\dot{V}O_2$ max) results in a slow rise in oxygen uptake across time (54) (figure 4.6). In each of these two types of exercise, the drift upward in $\dot{V}O_2$ is due principally to the effects of increasing body temperature and, to a lesser degree, to rising blood levels of the hormones epinephrine and norepinephrine (17, 41, 42, 54, 68). Both of these variables tend to increase the metabolic rate, resulting in increased oxygen uptake across time.

(a) Hot/humid environment

(b) High-intensity exercise

IN SUMMARY

- The energy to perform prolonged exercise (i.e., more than ten minutes) comes primarily from aerobic metabolism.
- A steady-state oxygen uptake can generally be maintained during prolonged, low-intensity exercise. However, exercise in a hot/humid environment or exercise at a high relative work rate results in an upward "drift" in oxygen consumption over time; therefore, a steady state is not obtained in these types of exercise.

FIGURE 4.6 Comparison of oxygen uptake ($\dot{V}O_2$) across time during prolonged exercise in a hot and humid environment (a) and during prolonged exercise at a high relative work rate (>75% $\dot{V}O_2$ max) (b). Note that in both conditions there is a steady "drift" upward in $\dot{V}O_2$. See text for description.

FIGURE 4.7 Changes in oxygen uptake ($\dot{V}O_2$) during an incremental exercise test. The observed plateau in $\dot{V}O_2$ represents $\dot{V}O_2$ max.

Incremental Exercise

The maximal capacity to transport and utilize oxygen during exercise (**maximal oxygen uptake**, or $\dot{V}O_2$ max) is considered by many exercise scientists to be the most valid measurement of cardiovascular fitness. Indeed, **incremental exercise tests** (also called **graded exercise tests**) are often employed by physicians to examine patients for possible heart disease and by exercise scientists to determine a subject's cardiovascular fitness. These tests are usually conducted on a treadmill or a cycle ergometer. However, an arm crank ergometer can be employed for testing paraplegics or athletes whose sport involves arm work (e.g., swimmers, rowers, etc.). The test generally begins with the subject performing a brief warm-up, followed by an increase in the work rate every one to three minutes until the subject cannot maintain the desired power output. This increase in work rate can be achieved on the treadmill by increasing either the speed of the treadmill or the incline. On the cycle or arm ergometer, the increase in power output is obtained by increasing the resistance against the flywheel.

Figure 4.7 illustrates the change in oxygen uptake during a typical incremental exercise test on a cycle ergometer. Oxygen uptake increases as a linear function of the work rate until $\dot{V}O_2$ max is reached. When $\dot{V}O_2$ max is reached, an increase in power output does not result in an increase in oxygen uptake; thus, $\dot{V}O_2$ max represents a "physiological ceiling" for the ability of the oxygen transport system to deliver O_2 to contracting muscles. The physiological factors that influence $\dot{V}O_2$ max include the following: (1) the maximum

FIGURE 4.8 Changes in blood lactic acid concentrations during incremental exercise. The sudden rise in lactate is known as the lactate threshold.

FIGURE 4.9 Failure of the mitochondrial "hydrogen shuttle" system to keep pace with the rate of glycolytic production of NADH + H$^+$ results in the conversion of pyruvic acid to lactic acid.

ability of the cardiorespiratory system to deliver oxygen to the contracting muscle; and (2) the muscle's ability to take up the oxygen and produce ATP aerobically. Both genetics and exercise training are known to influence V̇O$_2$ max; this will be discussed in chapter 13.

Lactate Threshold It is generally believed that most of the ATP production used to provide energy for muscular contraction during the early stages of an incremental exercise test comes from aerobic sources (74, 83, 92). However, as the exercise intensity increases, blood levels of lactic acid begin to rise in an exponential fashion (figure 4.8). This appears in untrained subjects around 50% to 60% of V̇O$_2$ max, while it occurs at higher work rates in trained subjects (i.e., 65%–80% V̇O$_2$ max) (47). Although there is disagreement on the point, many investigators believe that this sudden rise in lactic acid during incremental exercise represents a point of increasing reliance on anaerobic metabolism (i.e., glycolysis) (29, 99–103). A common term used to describe the point of a systematic rise in blood lactic acid during exercise is the **anaerobic threshold** (13, 30, 36, 61, 67, 82, 101, 102, 107). However, arguments over terminology exist, and this lactic acid inflection point has also been called the **lactate threshold** (31, 96).

Another commonly used term that is related to the lactate inflection point is the "onset of blood lactate accumulation" (abbreviated as OBLA). This term (OBLA) differs from the lactate threshold in one important way. Rather than defining the blood lactate inflection point, the OBLA is defined as the exercise intensity (or oxygen consumption) at which blood lactate levels reach 4 millimoles per liter (19, 57, 96). To avoid confusion, we will refer to the sudden rise in blood lactate levels during incremental exercise as the lactate threshold.

The basic argument against the term "anaerobic threshold" centers around the question of whether the rise in blood lactic acid during incremental exercise is due to a lack of oxygen (hypoxia) in the working muscle or occurs for other reasons. Historically, rising blood lactic acid levels have been considered an indication of increased anaerobic metabolism within the contracting muscle due to low levels of O$_2$ in the individual muscle cells (101, 102). However, whether the end product of glycolysis is pyruvic or lactic acid depends on a variety of factors. First, if the rate of glycolysis is rapid, then NADH production may exceed the transport capacity of the shuttle mechanisms that move hydrogens from the sarcoplasm into the mitochondria (93, 95, 106). Indeed, blood levels of epinephrine and norepinephrine begin to rise at 50% to 65% of V̇O$_2$ max during incremental exercise and have been shown to stimulate the glycolytic rate; this increase in glycolysis increases the rate of NADH production (95). Failure of the shuttle system to keep up with the rate of NADH production by glycolysis would result in pyruvic acid accepting some "unshuttled" hydrogens, and the formation of lactic acid could occur independent of whether the muscle cell had sufficient oxygen for aerobic ATP production (figure 4.9).

A second explanation for the formation of lactic acid in exercising muscle is related to the enzyme that catalyzes the conversion of pyruvate to lactic acid. The enzyme responsible for this reaction is lactate dehydrogenase (LDH), and it exists in several forms (different forms of the same enzyme are called isozymes). Recall that the reaction is as follows:

$$\underset{\text{Pyruvate}}{\overset{\displaystyle CH_3}{\underset{\displaystyle COO^-}{|\,C=O\,|}}} + NADH + H^+ \longleftrightarrow \underset{\text{Lactate}}{\overset{\displaystyle CH_3}{\underset{\displaystyle COO^-}{|\,H-C-OH\,|}}} + NAD$$

THE WINNING EDGE 4.1

Exercise Physiology Applied to Sports

Does Lactic Acid Cause Muscle Soreness?

A belief among some athletes and coaches is that lactic acid production during exercise is a primary cause of delayed-onset muscle soreness (i.e., soreness occurring twenty-four to forty-eight hours after exercise). Nonetheless, physiological evidence indicates that lactic acid is not a primary cause of this type of muscle soreness. Several lines of "physiological reasoning" can be used to support this position. First, although lactic acid production occurs in active skeletal muscle during high-intensity exercise, lactic acid removal from the muscle and blood is rapid following an exercise session. In fact, blood levels of lactic acid return to resting levels within sixty minutes after exercise (see A Closer Look 4.1). Therefore, it seems unlikely that lactic acid production during a single exercise bout would result in muscle soreness one or two days later.

A second argument against lactic acid causing delayed-onset muscle soreness is that if lactic acid production caused muscle soreness, power athletes would experience soreness after each workout. Clearly, this is not the case. Indeed, well-conditioned power athletes (e.g., track sprinters) rarely experience muscle soreness after a routine training session.

If lactic acid is not the cause of delayed-onset muscle soreness, what is the cause? Growing evidence indicates that this type of muscle soreness originates from microscopic injury to muscle fibers. This kind of injury results in a slow cascade of biochemical events leading to inflammation and edema within the injured muscles. Because these events are slow to develop, the resulting pain generally doesn't appear until twenty-four to forty-eight hours after exercise. Details of the events leading to delayed-onset muscle soreness are discussed in chapter 21.

This reaction is reversible in that lactic acid can be converted back to pyruvic acid under the appropriate conditions. Human skeletal muscle can be classified into three different fiber types (see chapter 8). One of these is a "slow" fiber (sometimes called slow-twitch), whereas the remaining two are called "fast" fibers (sometimes called fast-twitch). As the names imply, fast fibers are recruited during intense, rapid exercise, while slow fibers are used primarily during low-intensity activity. The LDH isozyme found in fast fibers has a greater affinity for attaching to pyruvic acid, promoting the formation of lactic acid (62, 92). In contrast, slow fibers contain an LDH form that promotes the conversion of lactic acid to pyruvic acid. Therefore, lactic acid formation might occur in fast fibers during exercise simply because of the type of LDH present. Thus, lactic acid production would again be independent of oxygen availability in the muscle cell. Early in an incremental exercise test it is likely that slow fibers are the first called into action. However, as the exercise intensity increases, the amount of muscular force developed must be increased. This increased muscular force is supplied by recruiting more and more fast fibers. Therefore, the involvement of more fast fibers may result in increased lactic acid production and thus may be responsible for the lactate threshold.

A final explanation for the lactate threshold may be related to the rate of removal of lactic acid from the blood during incremental exercise. When a researcher removes a blood sample from an exercising subject, the concentration of lactic acid in that sample is the difference between the amount of lactic acid entry into the blood and the rate of lactic acid removal from the blood. At any given time during exercise, some muscles are producing lactic acid and releasing it into the blood, and some tissues (e.g., liver, skeletal muscles, heart, etc.) are removing lactic acid. Therefore, the concentration of lactic acid in the blood at any given time can be expressed mathematically in the following way:

$$\text{Blood lactic acid concentration} = \text{Lactic acid entry into the blood} - \text{Blood lactic acid removal}$$

Thus, a rise in the blood lactic acid concentration can occur due to either an increase in lactic acid production or a decrease in lactic acid removal. Recent evidence suggests that the rise in blood lactic acid levels in animals during incremental exercise may be the result of both an increase in lactic acid production and a decrease in the rate of lactic acid removal (15, 35). See chapter 13 for a discussion of how endurance training affects lactic acid production. Also, see The Winning Edge 4.1.

To summarize, controversy exists over both the terminology and the mechanism to explain the sudden rise in blood lactic acid concentrations during incremental exercise. It is possible that any one or a combination of the explanations (including lack of O_2) might explain the lactate threshold. Figure 4.10 contains a summary of possible mechanisms to explain the lactate threshold. The search for definitive evidence to explain the mechanism(s) altering the blood

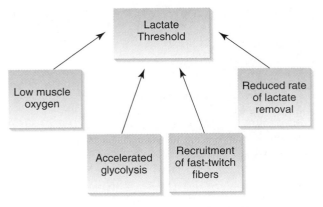

Potential causes of lactate threshold

FIGURE 4.10 Possible mechanisms to explain the lactate threshold during incremental exercise. See text for details.

lactate concentration during incremental exercise will continue for years to come.

Practical Use of the Lactate Threshold Regardless of the physiological mechanism to explain the lactate threshold, the point of exponential rise in lactic acid during graded exercise has important implications for predicting sports performance and perhaps in planning training programs for endurance athletes. For example, several studies have demonstrated that the lactate threshold used in combination with other physiological measurements (e.g., $\dot{V}O_2$ max), is a useful predictor of success in distance running (39, 75). Further, the lactate threshold might serve as a guideline for coaches and athletes in planning the level of exercise intensity needed to optimize training results. This will be discussed in more detail in chapters 16 and 21.

IN SUMMARY

- Oxygen uptake increases in a linear fashion during incremental exercise until $\dot{V}O_2$ max is reached.
- The point at which blood lactic acid rises systematically during graded exercise is termed the lactate threshold or anaerobic threshold.
- Controversy exists over the mechanism to explain the sudden rise in blood lactic acid concentrations during incremental exercise. It is possible that any one or a combination of the following factors might provide an explanation for the lactate threshold: (1) low muscle oxygen, (2) accelerated glycolysis, (3) recruitment of fast fibers, and (4) a reduced rate of lactate removal.
- The lactate threshold has practical uses such as in performance prediction and as a marker of training intensity.

ESTIMATION OF FUEL UTILIZATION DURING EXERCISE

A noninvasive technique that is commonly used to estimate the percent contribution of carbohydrate or fat to energy metabolism during exercise is the ratio of carbon dioxide output $\dot{V}CO_2$) to the volume of oxygen consumed $\dot{V}O_2$) (40, 105). This ratio $\dot{V}CO_2/\dot{V}O_2$) is called the **respiratory exchange ratio (R).** During steady-state conditions, the $\dot{V}CO_2/\dot{V}O_2$ ratio is often termed the respiratory quotient (RO). For simplicity, we will refer to the $\dot{V}CO_2/\dot{V}O_2$ ratio as the respiratory exchange ratio (R). How can the R be used to estimate whether fat or carbohydrate is being used as a fuel? The answer is related to the fact that fat and carbohydrate differ in the amount of O_2 used and CO_2 produced during oxidation. When using R as a predictor of fuel utilization during exercise, the role that protein contributes to ATP production during exercise is ignored. This is reasonable, since protein generally plays a small role as a substrate during physical activity. Therefore, the R during exercise is often termed a "nonprotein R."

Let's consider the R for fat first. When fat is oxidized, O_2 combines with carbon to form CO_2 and joins with hydrogen to form water. The chemical relationship is as follows:

Fat (palmitic acid) $C_{16}H_{32}O_2$
Oxidation: $C_{16}H_{32}O_2 + 23\ O_2 \rightarrow 16\ CO_2 + 16\ H_2O$
Therefore, the $R = \dot{V}CO_2 \div \dot{V}O_2 = 16\ CO_2 \div 23\ O_2$
$= 0.70$

In order for R to be used as an estimate of substrate utilization during exercise, the subject must have reached a steady state. This is important because only during steady-state exercise are the $\dot{V}CO_2$ and $\dot{V}O_2$ reflective of O_2 and CO_2 exchange in the tissues. For example, if a person is hyperventilating (i.e., breathing too much for a particular metabolic rate), excessive CO_2 loss could bias the ratio of $\dot{V}CO_2$ to $\dot{V}O_2$ and invalidate the use of R to estimate which fuel is being consumed.

Carbohydrate oxidation also results in a predictable ratio of the volume of oxygen consumed to the amount of CO_2 produced. The oxidation of carbohydrate results in an R of 1.0:

Glucose $= C_6H_{12}O_6$
Oxidation: $C_6H_{12}O_6 + 6\ O_2 \rightarrow 6\ CO_2 + 6\ H_2O$
$R = \dot{V}CO_2 \div \dot{V}O_2 = 6\ CO_2 \div 6\ O_2 = 1$

Fat oxidation requires more O_2 than does carbohydrate oxidation. This is due to the fact that carbohydrate contains more O_2 than does fat (96).

It is unlikely that either fat or carbohydrate would be the only substrate used during most types of

TABLE 4.1	Percentage of Fat and Carbohydrate Metabolized as Determined by a Nonprotein Respiratory Exchange Ratio (R)	
R	% Fat	% Carbohydrate
0.70	100	0
0.75	83	17
0.80	67	33
0.85	50	50
0.90	33	67
0.95	17	83
1.00	0	100

FIGURE 4.11 Illustration of the "crossover" concept. Note that as the exercise intensity increases, there is a progressive increase in the contribution of carbohydrate (CHO) as a fuel source.

submaximal exercise. Therefore, the exercise R would likely be somewhere between 1.0 and 0.70. Table 4.1 lists a range of R values and the percentage of fat or carbohydrate metabolism they represent. Note that a nonprotein R of 0.85 represents a condition wherein fat and carbohydrate contribute equally as energy substrates. Further, notice that the higher the R, the greater the role of carbohydrate as an energy source, and the lower the R, the greater the contribution of fat.

IN SUMMARY

- The respiratory exchange ratio (R) is the ratio of carbon dioxide produced to the oxygen consumed ($\dot{V}CO_2/\dot{V}O_2$).
- In order for R to be used as an estimate of substrate utilization during exercise, the subject must have reached a steady state. This is important because only during steady-state exercise are the CO_2 and O_2 reflective of metabolic exchange of gases in tissues.

FACTORS GOVERNING FUEL SELECTION

Proteins contribute less than 2% of the substrate used during exercise of less than one hour's duration. However, the role of proteins as a fuel source may increase slightly during prolonged exercise (i.e., three to five hours' duration). During this type of exercise, the total contribution of protein to the fuel supply may reach 5% to 10% during the final minutes of work (11, 20, 64, 71, 72, 87, 104). Therefore, proteins play only a minor role as a substrate during exercise, with fat and carbohydrate serving as the major sources of energy during activity in the healthy individual consuming a balanced diet. Whether fat or carbohydrate is the primary substrate during work is determined by several fac-

tors, including diet and the intensity and duration of exercise. For example, high-fat and low-carbohydrate diets promote a high rate of fat metabolism. In regard to exercise intensity, low-intensity exercise relies primarily on fat as fuel, whereas carbohydrate is the primary energy source during high-intensity exercise. Fuel selection is also influenced by the duration of exercise. During low-intensity, prolonged exercise, there is a progressive increase in the amount of fat oxidized by the working muscles. In the next two sections we discuss the influence of exercise intensity and duration on fuel selection in detail.

Exercise Intensity and Fuel Selection

Again, fats are a primary fuel source for muscle during low-intensity exercise (i.e., <30% $\dot{V}O_2$ max), whereas carbohydrate is the dominant substrate during high-intensity exercise (i.e., >70% $\dot{V}O_2$ max) (21, 26, 79, 91). The influence of exercise intensity on muscle fuel selection is illustrated in figure 4.11. Note that as the exercise intensity increases, there is a progressive increase in carbohydrate metabolism and a decrease in fat metabolism. Also, notice that as the exercise intensity increases, there is an exercise intensity at which the energy derived from carbohydrate exceeds that of fat; this work rate has been labeled the "crossover" point (21). That is, as the exercise intensity increases above the crossover point, there is a progressive shift from fat to carbohydrate metabolism.

What causes this shift from fat to carbohydrate metabolism as the exercise intensity increases? Two primary factors are involved: (1) recruitment of fast fibers and (2) increasing blood levels of epinephrine. As the exercise intensity increases, more and more fast muscle fibers are recruited (45). These fibers have

Regulation of Glycogen Breakdown During Exercise

Much of the carbohydrate broken down via glycolysis during moderate- to high-intensity exercise comes from intramuscular glycogen stores. Glycogen storage in muscle is dependent on the availability of glucose and the activity of the enzyme glycogen synthetase. Elevated blood levels of insulin and glucose along with high glycogen synthetase activity promote glycogen storage in muscle.

The breakdown of glycogen (glycogenolysis) into individual glucose molecules is dependent on the enzyme phosphorylase (94). In nonworking muscle, phosphorylase is generally found in an inactive form and thus must be "activated" before glycogen breakdown can occur. This activation of phosphorylase is regulated by two mechanisms (figure 4.12). First, the mechanism that best

explains the activation of phosphorylase at the beginning of exercise and during low-intensity exercise is linked to the protein molecule "calmodulin." Calmodulin is found in many tissues including muscle and is activated at the onset of exercise by the release of calcium from the sarcoplasmic reticulum (see chapter 8). Active calmodulin then activates phosphorylase, which promotes glycogenolysis (see chapter 5 for details of calmodulin activity).

The second system that can activate phosphorylase during exercise is controlled by the hormone epinephrine. Epinephrine binds to a receptor on the cell membrane, which results in the formation of "cyclic AMP," which then activates phosphorylase (chapter 5 contains additional information on cyclic AMP). This mechanism is opera-

tive during high-intensity or prolonged exercise, but is too slow to explain the immediate glycogenolysis at the onset of muscular contraction.

In summary, the breakdown of muscle glycogen into glucose during exercise is regulated by the activity of the enzyme phosphorylase. Activation of phosphorylase at the beginning of exercise is regulated by the calcium/calmodulin system whereas the epinephrine/cyclic AMP system plays an important role during prolonged or high-intensity exercise. Also, note that a small number of people are born without the enzyme phosphorylase. This genetic disorder impairs the victim's ability to use glycogen as an energy source during exercise and is discussed in Clinical Applications 4.1.

---

an abundance of glycolytic enzymes but few mitochondrial and lipolytic enzymes (enzymes responsible for fat breakdown). In short, this means that fast fibers are better equipped to metabolize carbohydrates than fats. Therefore, the increased recruitment of fast fibers results in greater carbohydrate metabolism and less fat metabolism (21).

A second factor that regulates carbohydrate metabolism during exercise is epinephrine. As exercise intensity increases, there is a progressive rise in blood levels of epinephrine (see chapter 5). High levels of epinephrine increase muscle glycogen breakdown, carbohydrate metabolism (i.e., glycolysis increases), and lactate production (21) (see A Closer Look 4.2). This increased production of lactate inhibits fat metabolism by reducing the availability of fat as a substrate (98). The lack of fat as a substrate for working muscles under these conditions dictates that carbohydrate will be the primary fuel (see A Closer Look 4.3).

Exercise Duration and Fuel Selection

During prolonged, low-intensity exercise (i.e., greater than thirty minutes), there is a gradual shift from carbohydrate metabolism toward an increasing reliance

FIGURE 4.12 The breakdown of muscle glycogen during exercise is regulated by two separate mechanisms: (1) epinephrine-cyclic AMP (cAMP) pathway, and (2) calcium-calmodulin pathway. Both pathways activate the enzyme phosphorylase, which degrades glycogen into glucose for entry into glycolysis. See text in A Closer Look 4.2 for details.

McArdle's Syndrome: A Genetic Error in Muscle Glycogen Metabolism

McArdle's syndrome is a genetic disease in which the patient is born without the enzyme phosphorylase. This metabolic disorder prevents the individual from breaking down muscle glycogen as a fuel source during exercise. This inability to use glycogen during exercise also prevents the muscle from producing lactate, as indicated by the observation that blood lactate levels do not increase in McArdle's patients during high-intensity exercise.

An unfortunate side effect of this genetic disorder is that McArdle's patients often complain of exercise intolerance and muscle pain during exertion. This clinical observation provides a practical illustration of the importance of muscle glycogen as an energy source during exercise. Further, the study of McArdle's patients during exercise has provided new insight into several important issues related to skeletal muscle metabolism and respiratory control during exercise.

FIGURE 4.14 Shift from carbohydrate metabolism toward fat metabolism during prolonged exercise.

on fat as a substrate (5, 46, 63, 70, 79, 85). Figure 4.14 demonstrates this point.

What factors control the rate of fat metabolism during prolonged exercise? Fat metabolism is regulated by those variables that control the rate of fat breakdown (a process called **lipolysis**). Triglycerides are broken down into **free fatty acids (FFAs)** and glycerol by enzymes called **lipases.** These lipases are generally inactive until stimulated by the hormones epinephrine, norepinephrine, and glucagon (63). For example, during low-intensity, prolonged exercise, blood levels of epinephrine rise, which increases lipase activity and thus promotes lipolysis. This increase in lipolysis results in an increase in blood and muscle levels of FFA and promotes fat metabolism. In general, lipolysis is a slow process, and an increase in fat metabolism occurs only after several minutes of exercise. This point is illustrated in figure 4.14 by the slow increase in fat metabolism across time during prolonged submaximal exercise.

The mobilization of FFA into the blood is inhibited by the hormone insulin and high blood levels of lactic acid. Insulin inhibits lipolysis by direct inhibition of lipase activity. Normally, blood insulin levels decline during prolonged exercise (see chapter 5). However, if a high-carbohydrate meal or drink is consumed thirty to sixty minutes prior to exercise, blood glucose levels rise and more insulin is released from the pancreas. This elevation in blood insulin results in diminished lipolysis and a reduction in fat metabolism.

Interaction of Fat/Carbohydrate Metabolism

During short-term exercise it is unlikely that muscle stores of glycogen or blood glucose levels would be depleted. However, during prolonged exercise (e.g., greater than two hours) muscle and liver stores of glycogen can reach very low levels (20, 25, 45, 52, 90). This is important because depletion of muscle and blood carbohydrate stores results in muscular fatigue (52). Why do low muscle glycogen levels produce fatigue? Recent evidence suggests the following answer. Depletion of available carbohydrate reduces the rate of glycolysis, and therefore the concentration of pyruvic acid in the muscle is also reduced (52). This lowers the rate of aerobic production of ATP by reducing the number of Krebs-cycle compounds (intermediates). In human muscle with adequate glycogen stores, submaximal exercise (i.e., 70% $\dot{V}O_2$ max) results in a ninefold increase (above resting values) in the number of Krebs-cycle intermediates (90). This elevated pool of Krebs-cycle intermediates is required for the Krebs cycle to "speed up" in an effort to meet the high ATP demands during exercise. Pyruvic acid (produced via glycolysis) is important in providing this increase in Krebs-cycle intermediates. For example, pyruvic acid is a precursor of several Krebs-cycle intermediates (e.g., oxaloacetate, malate). When the

A CLOSER LOOK 4.3

Exercise and Fat Metabolism: Is Low-Intensity Exercise Best for Burning Fat?

What intensity of exercise is optimal for burning fat? It is often assumed that the intensity of exercise must be kept very low to burn fat as a fuel. It is true that at low exercise intensities a high percentage of the total energy expenditure during exercise is derived from fat. It follows that as the exercise intensity increases, the percentage of fat used as fuel decreases (figure 4.11). However, a key point to consider is that the total rate of fat oxidation during exercise is typically greatest at higher exercise intensities that are below the lactate threshold. An appreciation of this point can be gained from figures 4.11 and 4.13. For example, during exercise at 20% of $\dot{V}O_2$ max, it is estimated that about 60% of the total energy expended would come from fat (figure 4.11). By comparison, during exercise at 50% of $\dot{V}O_2$ max, about 40% of the total energy expended would be obtained from fat (figure 4.11). Nonetheless, because the total rate of energy expenditure is 2.5 times greater at 50% $\dot{V}O_2$ max compared to 20% $\dot{V}O_2$ max, the absolute amount of fat metabolized is 33% higher during exercise at 50% $\dot{V}O_2$ max (figure 4.13).

Therefore, expressing energy derived from fat as a percentage without consideration of the total energy expenditure is often misleading.

FIGURE 4.13 Illustration of the rate of fat metabolism during exercise at varying intensities in an untrained subject.* Note that when comparing exercise at 20, 50, 80, and 100% of $\dot{V}O_2$ max, the greatest absolute amount of fat was metabolized at 50% of $\dot{V}O$ max. Therefore, when designing an exercise program to reduce body fat stores, it is important to consider both the total rate of energy expenditure and the percentage of energy that is derived from fat metabolism. It is important to appreciate that this illustration is not intended to represent the "ideal" exercise intensity for all subjects to optimize fat metabolism. It is simply intended to make the point that there is an optimal exercise intensity to use fat as a fuel source and that this intensity depends upon both the percentage of energy derived from fat and the total rate of energy expenditure.

*The data presented in this example are based upon measurements obtained from an untrained male subject (body weight = 89 kilograms; $\dot{V}O_2$ max = 4.0 liters/min; lactate threshold = 60% of $\dot{V}O_2$ max).

rate of glycolysis is reduced due to the unavailability of substrate, pyruvic acid levels in the sarcoplasm decline, and the levels of Krebs-cycle intermediates decrease as well. This decline in Krebs-cycle intermediates slows the rate of Krebs-cycle activity, with the end result being a reduction in the rate of aerobic ATP production. This reduced rate of muscle ATP production limits muscular performance and may result in fatigue.

It is important to appreciate that a reduction in Krebs-cycle intermediates (due to glycogen depletion) results in a diminished rate of ATP production from fat metabolism, since fat can only be metabolized via Krebs-cycle oxidation. Hence, when carbohydrate stores are depleted in the body, the rate at which fat is metabolized is also reduced (90). Therefore, "fats burn in the flame of carbohydrates" (95). The role that depletion of body carbohydrate stores may play in limiting performance during prolonged exercise is introduced in The Winning Edge 4.2 and is further dis-

cussed in both chapters 19 and 23.

Body Fuel Sources

In this section we outline the storage sites in the body for carbohydrates, fats, and proteins. Further, we will define the role that each of these fuel storage sites plays in providing energy during exercise. Finally, we will discuss the use of lactate as a fuel source during work.

Sources of Carbohydrate During Exercise Carbohydrate is stored as glycogen in both the muscle and the liver (see table 4.2). Muscle glycogen stores provide a direct source of carbohydrate for muscle energy metabolism, whereas liver glycogen stores serve as a means of replacing blood glucose. For example, when blood glucose levels decline during prolonged exercise, liver glycogenolysis is stimulated and glucose is released into the blood. This glucose

THE WINNING EDGE 4.2

Exercise Physiology Applied to Sports

Carbohydrate Feeding via Sports Drinks Improves Endurance Performance

The depletion of muscle and blood carbohydrate stores can contribute to muscular fatigue during prolonged exercise. Therefore, can the ingestion of carbohydrates during prolonged exercise improve endurance performance? The clear answer to this question is yes! Studies investigating the effects of carbohydrate feeding through "sports drinks" have convincingly shown that

carbohydrate feedings during submaximal (i.e., <70% $\dot{V}O_2$ max), long-duration (e.g., >90 minutes) exercise can improve endurance performance (27, 76). How much carbohydrate is required to improve performance? In general, carbohydrate feedings of 30 to 60 grams per hour are required to enhance performance.

Can carbohydrate feedings also improve exercise performance during shorter-duration exercise (i.e., thirty to sixty minutes)? A definitive answer to

this question is not currently available. However, research from the University of Texas indicates that carbohydrate ingestion improved exercise performance by 6.5% during sixty minutes of exercise at 80% $\dot{V}O_2$ max (10). Based on these promising results, additional studies investigating the effects of carbohydrate feedings on performance during high-intensity exercise are warranted.

TABLE 4.2	Principal Storage Sites of Carbohydrate and Fat in the Body of a Healthy, Nonobese (20% Body Fat), 70-kg Male Subject

Note that dietary intake of carbohydrate influences the amount of glycogen stored in both the liver and muscle. Mass units for storage are grams (g) and kilograms (kg). Energy units are kilocalories (kcal) and kilojoules (kJ). Data are from references 30, 31, and 62.

	CARBOHYDRATE (CHO)		
Storage Site	**Mixed Diet**	**High-CHO Diet**	**Low-CHO Diet**
Liver glycogen	60 g (240 kcal or 1,005 kJ)	90 g (360 kcal or 1,507 kJ)	<30 g (120 kcal or 502 kJ)
Glucose in blood and extracellular fluid	10 g (40 kcal or 167 kJ)	10 g (40 kcal or 167 kJ)	10 g (40 kcal or 167 kJ)
Muscle glycogen	350 g (1,400 kcal or 5,860 kJ)	600 g (2,400 kcal or 10,046 kJ)	300 g (1,200 kcal or 5,023 kJ)

FAT			
Storage Site	**Mixed Diet**		
Adipocytes	14 kg (107,800 kcal or 451,251 kJ)		
Muscle	0.5 kg (3,850 kcal or 16,116 kJ)		

can then be transported to the contracting muscle and used as fuel.

Carbohydrate used as a substrate during exercise comes from both glycogen stores in muscle and from blood glucose (24, 28, 45, 66, 94). The relative contribution of muscle glycogen and blood glucose to

energy metabolism during exercise varies as a function of the exercise intensity and duration. Blood glucose plays the greater role during low-intensity exercise, whereas muscle glycogen is the primary source of carbohydrate during high-intensity exercise (see figure 4.15). As mentioned earlier, the increased

FIGURE 4.16 Percentage of energy derived from the four major sources of fuel during submaximal exercise (i.e., 65%–75% $\dot{V}O_2$ max). Data are from trained endurance athletes.

FIGURE 4.15 Influence of exercise intensity on muscle fuel source. Data are from highly trained endurance athletes.

glycogen usage during high-intensity exercise can be explained by the increased rate of glycogenolysis that occurs due to recruitment of fast-twitch fibers and elevated blood epinephrine levels.

During the first hour of submaximal prolonged exercise, much of the carbohydrate metabolized by muscle comes from muscle glycogen. However, as muscle glycogen levels decline across time, blood glucose becomes an increasingly important source of fuel (see figure 4.16).

Sources of Fat During Exercise When an individual consumes more energy (i.e., food) than he or she expends, this additional energy is stored in the form of fat. A gain of 3,500 kcal of energy results in the storage of 1 pound of fat. Most fat is stored in the form of triglycerides in adipocytes (fat cells), but some is stored in muscle cells as well (see table 4.2). As mentioned earlier, the major factor that determines the role of fat as a substrate during exercise is its availability to the muscle cell. In order to be metabolized, triglycerides must be degraded to FFA (three molecules) and glycerol (one molecule). When triglycerides are split, FFA can be converted into acetyl-CoA and enter the Krebs cycle.

Which fat stores are used as a fuel source varies as a function of the exercise intensity and duration. For example, plasma FFAs (i.e., FFA from adipocytes) are the primary source of fat during low-intensity exercise. At higher work rates, metabolism of muscle triglycerides increases (see figure 4.15). At exercise intensities between 65% and 85% $\dot{V}O_2$ max, the contribution of fat as a muscle fuel source is approximately equal between plasma FFA and muscle triglycerides (26, 55, 89).

The contribution of plasma FFA and muscle triglycerides to exercise metabolism during prolonged exercise is summarized in figure 4.16. Note that at the beginning of exercise, the contribution of plasma FFA and muscle triglycerides is equal. However, as the duration of exercise increases, there is a progressive rise in the role of plasma FFA as a fuel source.

Sources of Protein During Exercise To be used as a fuel source, proteins must first be degraded into amino acids. Amino acids can be supplied to muscle from the blood or from the amino acid pool in the fiber itself. Again, the role that protein plays as a substrate during exercise is small and is principally dependent on the availability of branch-chained amino acids and the amino acid alanine (8, 51). Skeletal muscle can directly metabolize branched-chain amino acids (e.g., valine, leucine, isoleucine) to produce ATP (48, 64). Further, in the liver, alanine can be converted to glucose and returned via the blood to skeletal muscle to be utilized as a substrate.

Any factor that increases the amino acid pool (amount of available amino acids) in the liver or in skeletal muscle can theoretically enhance protein metabolism (64, 73). One such factor is prolonged exercise (i.e., more than two hours). Numerous investigators have demonstrated that enzymes capable of degrading muscle proteins (proteases) are activated during long-term exercise (2, 33, 34, 80). The mechanism responsible for activation of these proteases during prolonged exercise appears to be exercise-induced increases in calcium levels within muscle fibers during exercise (2, 78). Indeed, several families of proteases

The Cori Cycle: Lactate as a Fuel Source

During exercise some of the lactic acid that is produced by skeletal muscles is transported to the liver via the blood (53, 97). Upon entry into the liver, lactate can be converted to glucose via gluconeogensis. This "new" glucose can be released into the blood and transported back to skeletal muscles to be used as an energy source during exercise. The cycle of lactate-to-glucose between the muscle and liver is called the **Cori cycle** and is illustrated in figure 4.17.

FIGURE 4.17 The Cori cycle. The sequence of steps is indicated by the numbers 1–9 beginning with exercise.

are activated by increases in cellular levels of calcium (2, 78). Regardless of the mechanism responsible for protease activation during exercise, the practical aspect of this finding is that during the course of prolonged exercise, proteases become activated and amino acids are liberated from their parent proteins. This rise in the amino acid pool results in an increase in the use of amino acids as fuel during exercise (79).

Lactate as a Fuel Source During Exercise For many years, lactate was considered to be a waste product of glycolysis with limited metabolic use. However, new evidence has shown that lactate is not necessarily a waste product but can play a beneficial role during exercise by serving as both a substrate for the liver to synthesize glucose (see A Closer Look 4.4) and as a direct fuel source for skeletal muscle and the heart (15, 16, 55). That is, in slow skeletal muscle fibers and the heart, lactate removed from the blood can be converted to pyruvate, which can then be transformed to acetyl-CoA. This acetyl-CoA can then enter the Krebs cycle and contribute to oxidative metabolism. The concept that lactate can be produced in one tissue and then transported to another to be used as an energy source has been termed the "lactate shuttle" (13–16, 18). See Ask the Expert 4.2 for more details on the lactate shuttle.

IN SUMMARY

- The regulation of fuel selection during exercise is under complex control and is dependent upon several factors, including diet and the intensity and duration of exercise.
- In general, carbohydrates are used as the major fuel source during high-intensity exercise.
- During prolonged exercise, there is a gradual shift from carbohydrate metabolism toward fat metabolism.
- Proteins contribute less than 2% of the fuel used during exercise of less than one hour's duration. During prolonged exercise (i.e., three to five hours' duration), the total contribution of protein to the fuel supply may reach 5% to 10% during the final minutes of prolonged work.

ASK THE EXPERT 4.2

Lactate Production in Skeletal Muscle and the Lactate Shuttle: Questions and Answers with Dr. George Brooks

George Brooks, Ph.D., *a professor in the Department of Integrative Biology at the University of California-Berkeley, is an internationally known expert in carbohydrate metabolism during exercise. Dr. Brooks first coined the term "lactate shuttle" in 1985, and his laboratory has performed much of the original research that defines the role that lactate plays as a fuel source during exercise. Here, Dr. Brooks answers questions related to the production and fate of lactic acid produced in skeletal muscle during exercise.*

QUESTION 1: The mechanism(s) to explain lactate production in skeletal muscle during submaximal exercise has been a topic of discussion for over two decades. In your view, what role, if any, does oxygen availability in the muscle play in lactate production during submaximal, incremental exercise?

DR. BROOKS: It would be a mistake to say that oxygen plays no role, because oxygen lack can cause glycolytic flux to increase. However, we know that glycolysis takes place all the time, even at rest, and especially after eating carbohydrate energy sources. So, I look at the situation differently.

Traditionally, we think of nonoxidative (glycolytic) metabolism and aerobic (oxidative phosphorylation) metabolism as two independent processes. However, via the lactate shuttle concept, I have come to think of lactate as the link between glycolysis and aerobic metabolism. Remembering that gluconeogenesis and aerobic metabolism are oxygen dependent, oxygen is key to lactate removal.

QUESTION 2: During submaximal exercise, which body tissues receive the most benefit from circulating lactate?

DR. BROOKS: This is a very good question, but hard to answer. Most lactate disposal is by oxidation, so cell sites such as working muscle and heart receive great benefit. In fact, in our studies with exercising humans, lactate became an important fuel for the heart. However, the heart can probably account for 10% of lactate disposal during exercise, so the role of lactate as a fuel for working muscle is probably more important. Then, in terms of quantitation, after working muscle, I would say that the liver and kidneys are most important. Conversion to glucose accounts for 20% to 25% of lactate removal, and gluconeogenesis accounts for 20% to 25% of glucose production in people with good liver glycogen stores. Therefore, in priority order, the body tissues that receive the most benefit from circulating lactate during exercise are: (1) working muscle, (2) liver and kidney, and (3) heart.

STUDY QUESTIONS

1. Identify the predominant energy systems used to produce ATP during the following types of exercise:
   a. short-term, intense exercise (i.e., less than ten seconds' duration)
   b. 400-meter dash
   c. 20-kilometer race (i.e., 12.4 miles)
2. Graph the change in oxygen uptake during the transition from rest to steady-state, submaximal exercise. Label the oxygen deficit. Where does the ATP come from during the transition period from rest to steady state?
3. Graph the change in oxygen uptake and blood lactate concentration during incremental exercise. Label the point on the graph that might be considered the lactate threshold or lactate inflection point.
4. Discuss several possible reasons why blood lactate begins to rise rapidly during incremental exercise.
5. Briefly, explain how the respiratory exchange ratio is used to estimate which substrate is being utilized during exercise. What is meant by the term *nonprotein* R?
6. List two factors that play a role in the regulation of carbohydrate metabolism during exercise.
7. List those variables that regulate fat metabolism during exercise.
8. Define the following terms: (a) *triglyceride*, (b) *lipolysis*, and (c) *lipases*.
9. Graph the change in oxygen uptake during recovery from exercise. Label the oxygen debt.
10. How does modern theory of EPOC differ from the classical oxygen debt theory proposed by A. V. Hill?
11. Discuss the influence of exercise intensity on muscle fuel selection.
12. How does the duration of exercise influence muscle fuel selection?

SUGGESTED READINGS

Brooks, G., T. Fahey, and K. Baldwin. 2005. *Exercise Physiology: Human Bioenergetics and Its Applications*, 4th ed. New York: McGraw-Hill Companies.

Fox, S. 2006. *Human Physiology*, 9th ed. New York: McGraw-Hill Companies.

Gladden, L. B. 2004. Lactate metabolism: A new paradigm for the third millennium. *Journal of Physiology* 558:5–30.

McKee, T., and J. McKee. 2003. *Biochemistry: The Molecular Basis of Life*, 3rd ed. New York: McGraw-Hill Companies.

Mooren, F., and K. Volker, eds. 2005. *Molecular and Cellular Exercise Physiology*. Champaign, IL: Human Kinetics.

Svedahl, K., and B. MacIntosh. 2003. Anaerobic threshold: the concept and methods of measurement. *Canadian Journal of Applied Physiology* 28:299–323.

Widmaier, E., H. Raff, and K. Strang. 2006. *Vander's Human Physiology*, 10th ed. New York: McGraw-Hill Companies.

REFERENCES

1. Armstrong, R. 1979. Biochemistry: Energy liberation and use. In *Sports Medicine and Physiology*, ed. R. Strauss. Philadelphia: W. B. Saunders.

2. Arthur, G. et al. 1999. Exercise promotes a subcellular resdistribution of calcium-stimulated protease activity in striated muscle. *Canadian Journal of Physiology and Pharmacology* 77:42–47.

3. Åstrand, P., ed. *Texbook of Work Physiology*. 2003. Champaign, IL: Human Kinetics Publishers.

4. Åstrand, P., and K. Rodahl. 1986. *Textbook of Work Physiology*. New York: McGraw-Hill Companies.

5. Ball-Burnett, M., H. Green, and M. Houston. 1991. Energy metabolism in human slow and fast twitch fibers during prolonged cycle exercise. *Journal of Physiology* (London) 437:257–67.

6. Barnard, R., and M. Foss. 1969. Oxygen debt: Effect of beta adrenergic blockade on the lactacid and alactacid components. *Journal of Applied Physiology* 27:813–16.

7. Bassett, D. et al. 1991. Rate of decline in blood lactate after cycling exercise in endurance-trained and untrained subjects. *Journal of Applied Physiology* 70:1816–20.

8. Bates, P. et al. 1980. Exercise and protein turnover in the rat. *Journal of Physiology* (London) 303:41P.

9. Belcastro, A., and A. Bonen. 1975. Lactic acid removal rates during controlled and uncontrolled recovery exercise. *Journal of Applied Physiology* 39:932–36.

10. Below, P., R. Mora-Rodriguez, J. Gonzalez-Alonso, and E. Coyle. 1995. Fluid and carbohydrate ingestion independently improve performance during 1 hour of intense exercise. *Medicine and Science in Sports and Exercise*. 27:200–10.

11. Berg, A., and J. Keul. 1980. Serum alanine during long-lasting exercise. *International Journal of Sports Medicine* 1:199–202.

12. Boutellier, U. et al. 1984. Aftereffects of chronic hypoxia on O_2 kinetics and on O_2 deficit and debt. *European Journal of Applied Physiology* 53:87–91.

13. Brooks, G. 1985. Anaerobic threshold: Review of the concept and directions for future research. *Medicine and Science in Sports and Exercise* 17:22–23.

14. ———. 1985. Lactate: Glycolytic end product and oxidative substrate during sustained exercise in mammals—the lactate shuttle. In *Circulation, Respiration, and Metabolism*, ed. R. Giles. Berlin: Springer-Verlag.

15. ———. 1986. Lactate production under fully aerobic conditions: The lactate shuttle during rest and exercise. *Federation Proceedings* 45:2924–29.

16. ———. 1986. The lactate shuttle during exercise and recovery. *Medicine and Science in Sports and Exercise* 18:360–68.

17. Brooks, G. et al. 1971. Temperature, skeletal muscle, mitochondrial functions, and oxygen debt. *American Journal of Physiology* 220:1053–59.

18. Brooks, G., H. Dubouchaud, M. Brown, J. Sicurello, and C. Butz. 1999. Role of mitochondrial lactate dehydrogenase shuttle and lactate oxidation in the intracellular lactate shuttle. *Proceedings of the National Academy of Sciences* USA, 1129–34.

19. Brooks, G., T. Fahey, and K. Baldwin. 2005. *Exercise Physiology: Human Bioenergetics and Its Applications*, 4th ed. New York: McGraw-Hill Companies.

20. Brooks, G., T. Fahey, and T. White. 2000. *Exercise Physiology: Human Bioenergetics and Its Applications*. New York: McGraw-Hill Companies.

21. Brooks, G., and J. Mercier. 1994. Balance of carbohydrate and lipid utilization during exercise: The "crossover" concept. *Journal of Applied Physiology* 76:2253–61.

22. Buckley, J. P. Bourdon, and S. Woolford. 2003. *Journal of Science Medicine in Sport* 6:408–21.

23. Cerretelli, P. et al. 1977. Oxygen uptake transients at the onset and offset of arm and leg work. *Respiration Physiology* 30:81–97.

24. Coggin, A. 1991. Plasma glucose metabolism during exercise in humans. *Sports Medicine* 11:102–24.

25. Coyle, E. 1986. Muscle glycogen utilization during prolonged strenuous exercise when fed carbohydrate. *Journal of Applied Physiology* 61:165–72.

26. ———. 1995. Substrate utilization during exercise in active people. *American Journal of Clinical Nutrition* 61:(Suppl.) 968s–979s.

27. Coyle, E., and S. Montain. 1992. Carbohydrate and fluid ingestion during exercise: Are there tradeoffs? *Medicine and Science in Sports and Exercise* 24:671–78.

28. Coyle, E. F. et al. 1991. Carbohydrate metabolism during intense exercise when hyperglycemic. *Journal of Applied Physiology* 70:834–40.

29. Davis, J. 1985. Anaerobic threshold: Review of the concept and directions for future research. *Medicine and Science in Sports and Exercise* 17:6–18.

30. Davis, J. et al. 1976. Anaerobic threshold and maximal aerobic power for three modes of exercise. *Journal of Applied Physiology* 41:544–50.

31. Dodd, S. et al. 1984. Blood lactate disappearance at various intensities of recovery exercise. *Journal of Applied Physiology* 57:1462–65.

32. Dodd, S. et al. 1988. Effects of beta-blockade on ventilation and gas exchange during the rest-to-work transition. *Aviation, Space, and Environmental Medicine* 59:255–58.

33. Dohm, G. et al. 1978. Changes in tissue protein levels as a result of endurance exercise. *Life Sciences* 23:845–50.

34. Dohm, G. et al. 1981. Influence of exercise on free amino acid concentrations in rat tissues. *Journal of Applied Physiology* 50:41–44.

35. Donovan, C., and G. Brooks. 1983. Endurance training affects lactate clearance, not lactate production. *American Journal of Physiology* 244:E83–E92.

36. England, P. et al. 1985. The effect of acute thermal dehydration on blood lactate accumulation during incremental exercise. *Journal of Sports Sciences* 2:105–11.

37. Essen, B., and L. Kaijser. 1978. Regulation of glycolysis in intermittent exercise in man. *Journal of Physiology* 281:499–511.

38. Evans, B., and K. Cureton. 1983. Effect of physical conditioning on blood lactate disappearance after supramaximal exercise. *British Journal of Sports Medicine* 17:40–45.

39. Farrell, P. et al. 1979. Plasma lactate accumulation and distance running performance. *Medicine and Science in Sports* 11:338–44.

40. Fox, S. 2006. *Human Physiology*, 9th ed. New York: McGraw-Hill Companies.

41. Gaesser, G., and G. Brooks. 1984. Metabolic bases of excess post-exercise oxygen consumption: A review. *Medicine and Science in Sports and Exercise* 16:29–43.

42. Gladden, B., W. Stainsby, and B. MacIntosh. 1982. Norepinephrine increases canine muscle O_2 during recovery. *Medicine and Science in Sports and Exercise* 14:471–76.

43. Gladden, L. B. 2004. Lactate metabolism: A new paradigm for the third millennium. *Journal of Physiology* 558:5–30.

44. Gladden, L. B. 1991. Net lactate uptake during progressive steady-level contractions in canine muscle. *Journal of Applied Physiology* 71:514–20.

45. Gollnick, P. 1985. Metabolism of substrates: Energy substrate metabolism during exercise and as modified by training. *Federation Proceedings* 44:353–56.

46. Gollnick, P., and B. Saltin. 1988. Fuel for muscular exercise: Role of fat. In *Exercise, Nutrition, and Energy Metabolism*, ed. E. Horton and R. Terjung, 72–88. New York: Macmillan.

47. Gollnick, P., W. Bayly, and D. Hodgson. 1986. Exercise intensity, training, diet, and lactate concentration in muscle and blood. *Medicine and Science in Sports and Exercise* 18:334–40.

48. Goodman, M. 1988. Amino acid and protein metabolism. In *Exercise, Nutrition, and Energy Metabolism*, ed. E. Horton and R. Terjung, 89–99. New York: Macmillan.

49. Gore, C., and R. Withers. 1990. Effect of exercise intensity and duration on post-exercise metabolism. *Journal of Applied Physiology* 68:2362–68.

50. ———. 1990. The effect of exercise intensity and duration on the oxygen deficit and excess post-exercise oxygen consumption. *European Journal of Applied Physiology* 60:169–74.

51. Graham, T. et al. 1995. Skeletal muscle amino acid metabolism and ammonia production during exercise. In *Exercise Metabolism*, 131–75. Champaign, IL: Human Kinetics.

52. Green, H. 1991. How important is endogenous muscle glycogen to fatigue during prolonged exercise? *Canadian Journal of Physiology and Pharmacology* 69:290–97.

53. Green, H. et al. 2002. Increases in muscle MCT are associated with reductions in muscle lactate after a single exercise session in humans. *American Journal of Physiology* 282:E154–60.

54. Hagberg, J., J. Mullin, and F. Nagle. 1978. Oxygen consumption during constant load exercise. *Journal of Applied Physiology* 45:381–84.

55. Hargreaves, M. 1995. Skeletal muscle carbohydrate metabolism during exercise. In *Exercise Metabolism*, 41–72. Champaign, IL: Human Kinetics.

56. Harris, R. et al. 1976. The time course of phosphocreatine resynthesis during recovery of the quadriceps muscle in man. *Pflugers Archives* 367:137–42.

57. Heck, H., and A. Mader. 1985. Justification of the 4-mmol/l lactate threshold. *International Journal of Sports Medicine* 6:117–30.

58. Hermanson, L., and I. Stensvold. 1972. Production and removal of lactate during exercise in man. *Acta Physiologica Scandinavica* 86:191–201.

59. Hickson, R., H. Bomze, and J. Holloszy. 1978. Faster adjustment of O_2 uptake to the energy requirement of exercise in the trained state. *Journal of Applied Physiology* 44:877–81.

60. Hill, A. 1914. The oxidative removal of lactic acid. *Journal of Physiology* (London) 48:x–xi.

61. Hollman, W. 1985. Historical remarks on the development of the aerobic-anaerobic threshold up to 1966. *International Journal of Sports Medicine* 6:109–16.

62. Holloszy, J. 1982. Muscle metabolism during exercise. *Archives of Physical and Rehabilitation Medicine* 63:231–34.

63. ———. 1990. Utilization of fatty acids during exercise. In *Biochemistry of Exercise* VII, ed. A. W. Taylor et al., 319–28. Champaign, IL: Human Kinetics.

64. Hood, D., and R. Terjung. 1990. Amino acid metabolism during exercise and following endurance training. *Sports Medicine* 9:23–35.

65. Hultman, E. 1973. Energy metabolism in human muscle. *Journal of Physiology* (London) 231:56.

66. Hultman, E., and H. Sjoholm. 1983. Substrate availability. In *Biochemistry of Exercise*, ed. H. Knuttgen, J. Vogel, and J. R. Poortmans. Champaign, IL: Human Kinetics.

67. Jones, N., and R. Ehrsam. 1982. The anaerobic threshold. *Exercise and Sports Science Review* 10:49–83.

68. Kalis, J. et al. 1988. Effects of beta blockade on the drift in O_2 consumption during prolonged exercise. *Journal of Applied Physiology* 64:753–58.

69. Knuttgen, H., and B. Saltin. 1972. Muscle metabolites and oxygen uptake in short-term submaximal exercise in man. *Journal of Applied Physiology* 32:690–94.

70. Ladu, M., H. Kapsas, and W. Palmer. 1991. Regulation of lipoprotein lipase in muscle and adipose tissue during exercise. *Journal of Applied Physiology* 71:404–9.

71. Lemon, P., and F. Mullin. 1980. Effect of initial glycogen levels on protein metabolism during exercise. *Journal of Applied Physiology* 48:624–29.

72. Lemon, P., and R. Nagle. 1980. Effects of exercise on protein and amino acid metabolism. *Medicine and Science in Sports and Exercise* 13:141–49.

73. MacLean, D. et al. 1991. Plasma and muscle amino acid and ammonia responses during prolonged exercise. *Journal of Applied Physiology* 70:2095–2103.

74. Mader, A., and H. Heck. 1986. A theory of the metabolic origin of the anaerobic threshold. *International Journal of Sports Medicine* 7:45–65.

75. Marti, B., T. Abelin, and H. Howald. 1987. A modified fixed blood lactate threshold for estimating running speed for joggers in 16-Km races. *Scandavian Journal of Sports Sciences* 9:41–45.

76. Maughan, R. 1991. Carbohydrate-electrolyte solutions during prolonged exercise. Perspectives in exercise science and sports medicine. In *Ergogenics: Enhancements of Performance in Exercise and Sport*, vol. 4, ed. D. Lamb and M. Williams, 35–76. New York: McGraw-Hill Companies.

77. Medbo, J. et al. 1988. Anaerobic capacity determined maximal accumulated O_2 deficit. *Journal of Applied Physiology* 64:50–60.

78. Menconi, M. et al. 2004. Treatment of cultured myotubes with the calcium ionophore A23187 increases proteasome activity via a CaMk II-caspase-calpain-dependent mechanism. *Surgery* 136:135–42.

79. Mooren, F., and K. Volker, eds. 2005. *Molecular and Cellular Exercise Physiology*. Champaign, IL: Human Kinetics.

80. Ordway, G. et al. 2000. Chronic contractile activity upregulates the proteasome system in rabbit skeletal muscle. *Journal of Applied Physiology* 88:1134–41.

81. Powers, S., S. Dodd, and R. Beadle. 1985. Oxygen uptake kinetics in trained athletes differing in O_2 max. *European Journal of Applied Physiology* 39:407–15.

82. Powers, S., S. Dodd, and R. Garner. 1984. Precision of ventilatory and gas exchange alterations as a predictor

of the anaerobic threshold. *European Journal of Applied Physiology* 52:173–77.

83. Powers, S. et al. 1983. Effects of caffeine ingestion on metabolism and performance during graded exercise. *European Journal of Applied Physiology* 560:301–7.

84. Powers, S., E. Howley, and R. Cox. 1982. Ventilatory and metabolic reactions to heat stress during prolonged exercise. *Journal of Sports Medicine and Physical Fitness* 22:32–36.

85. Powers, S., W. Riley, and E. Howley. 1980. A comparison of fat metabolism in trained men and women during prolonged aerobic work. *Research Quarterly for Exercise and Sport* 52:427–31.

86. Powers, S. et al. 1987. Oxygen deficit-debt relationships in ponies during submaximal treadmill exercise. *Respiratory Physiology* 70:251–63.

87. Refsum, H., L. Gjessing, and S. Stromme. 1978. Changes in plasma amino acid distribution and urine amino acid excretion during prolonged heavy exercise. *Scandinavian Journal of Clinical and Laboratory Investigation* 39:407–13.

88. Riley, W., S. Powers, and H. Welch. 1981. The effect of two levels of muscular work on urinary creatinine excretion. *Research Quarterly for Exercise and Sport* 52:339–47.

89. Romijin, J. et al. 1993. Regulation of endogenous fat and carbohydrate metabolism in relation to exercise intensity. *American Journal of Physiology* 265:E380–E391.

90. Sahlin, K., A. Katz, and S. Broberg. 1990. Tricarboxylic acid cycle intermediates in human muscle during prolonged exercise. *American Journal of Physiology* 259:C834–C841.

91. Saltin, B., and P. Gollnick. 1988. Fuel for muscular exercise: Role of carbohydrate. In *Exercise, Nutrition, and Energy Metabolism*, ed. E. Horton and R. Terjung, 45–71. New York: Macmillan.

92. Skinner, J., and T. McLellan. 1980. The transition from aerobic to anaerobic exercise. *Research Quarterly* 51:234–48.

93. Stainsby, W. 1986. Biochemical and physiological bases for lactate production. *Medicine and Science in Sports and Exercise* 18:341–43.

94. Stanley, W., and R. Connett. 1991. Regulation of muscle carbohydrate metabolism during exercise. FASEB *Journal* 5:2155–59.

95. Stryer, L. 1995. *Biochemistry*. New York: W. H. Freeman.

96. Svedahl, K., and B. MacIntosh. 2003. Anaerobic threshold: The concept and methods of measurement. *Canadian Journal of Applied Physiology* 28: 299–323.

97. Tonouchi, M. et al. 2002. Muscle contraction increases lactate transport while reducing sarcolemmal MCT4, but not MCT1. *American Journal of Physiology* 282: E1062–69.

98. Turcotte, L. et al. 1995. Lipid metabolism during exercise. In *Exercise Metabolism*, 99–130. Champaign, IL: Human Kinetics.

99. Wasserman, K. 1986. Anaerobiosis, lactate, and gas exchange during exercise: The issues. *Federation Proceedings* 45:2904–9.

100. Wasserman, K., W. Beaver, and B. Whipp. 1986. Mechanisms and pattern of blood lactate increase during exercise in man. *Medicine and Science in Sports and Exercise* 18:344–52.

101. Wasserman, K., and M. McIlroy. 1964. Detecting the threshold of anaerobic metabolism. *American Journal of Cardiology* 14:844–52.

102. Wasserman, K. et al. 1973. Anaerobic threshold and respiratory gas exchange during exercise. *Journal of Applied Physiology* 35:236–43.

103. Wasserman, K., B. Whipp, and J. Davis. 1981. Respiratory physiology of exercise: Metabolism, gas exchange, and ventilatory control. In *International Review of Physiology, Respiratory Physiology III*, ed. J. Widdicombe. Baltimore: University Park Press.

104. White, T., and G. Brooks. 1981. (C^{14}) Glucose, alanine, and leucine oxidation in rats at rest and two intensities of running. *Journal of Physiology* 240:R147–R152.

105. Widmaier, E., H. Raff, and K. Strang. 2006. *Vander's Human Physiology*, 10th ed. New York: McGraw-Hill Companies.

106. Wilson, D. et al. 1977. Effect of oxygen tension on cellular energetics. *American Journal of Physiology* 233:C135–C140.

107. Yoshida, T. 1986. Effect of dietary modifications on the anaerobic threshold. *Sports Medicine* 3:4–9.

CHAPTER 5

Hormonal Responses to Exercise

■ Objectives

By studying this chapter, you should be able to do the following:

1. Describe the concept of hormone-receptor interaction.
2. Identify the four factors influencing the concentration of a hormone in the blood.
3. Describe the mechanism by which steroid hormones act on cells.
4. Describe the "second messenger" hypothesis of hormone action.
5. Describe the role of the hypothalamus-releasing factors in the control of hormone secretion from the anterior pituitary gland.
6. Describe the relationship of the hypothalamus to the secretion of hormones from the posterior pituitary gland.
7. Identify the site of release, stimulus for release, and the predominant action of the following hormones: epinephrine, norepinephrine, glucagon, insulin, cortisol, aldosterone, thyroxine, growth hormone, estrogen, and testosterone.
8. Discuss the use of testosterone (an anabolic steroid) and growth hormone on muscle growth and their potential side effects.
9. Contrast the role of plasma catecholamines with intracellular factors in the mobilization of muscle glycogen during exercise.
10. Graphically describe the changes in the following hormones during graded and prolonged exercise and discuss how those changes influence the four mechanisms used to maintain the blood glucose concentration: insulin, glucagon, cortisol, growth hormone, epinephrine, and norepinephrine.
11. Describe the effect of changing hormone and substrate levels in the blood on the mobilization of free fatty acids from adipose tissue.

■ Outline

Neuroendocrinology   74
   Blood Hormone
      Concentration   75
   Hormone-Receptor
      Interaction   76

Hormones: Regulation
and Action   78
   Hypothalamus and the
      Pituitary Gland   79

Thyroid Gland   81
Parathyroid Gland   82
Adrenal Gland   82
Pancreas   85
Testes and Ovaries   86

Hormonal Control of
Substrate Mobilization
During Exercise   92

Muscle-Glycogen
   Utilization   92
Blood Glucose Homeostasis
   During Exercise   93
Hormone-Substrate
   Interaction   100

acromegaly
adenylate cyclase
adrenal cortex
adrenocorticotrophic hormone (ACTH)
aldosterone
alpha receptors
anabolic steroid
androgenic steroid
androgens
angiotensin I and II
anterior pituitary
antidiuretic hormone (ADH)
beta receptors
calcitonin
calmodulin
catecholamines
cortisol
cyclic AMP
diabetes mellitus
diacylglycerol

endocrine gland
endorphin
epinephrine (E)
estrogens
follicle-stimulating hormone (FSH)
G protein
glucagon
glucocorticoids
growth hormone (GH)
hormone
hypothalamic somatostatin
hypothalamus
inositol triphosphate
insulin
insulin-like growth factors (IGFs)
luteinizing hormone (LH)
mineralocorticoids
neuroendocrinology
norepinephrine (NE)
pancreas

phosphodiesterase
phospholipase C
pituitary gland
posterior pituitary gland
prolactin
protein kinase C
releasing hormone
renin
second messenger
sex steroids
somatomedins
somatostatin
steroids
testosterone
thyroid gland
thyroid-stimulating hormone (TSH)
thyroxine (T_4)
triiodothyronine (T_3)

As presented in chapter 4, the fuels for muscular exercise include muscle glycogen and fat, plasma glucose and free fatty acids, and to a lesser extent, amino acids. These fuels must be provided at an optimal rate for activities as diverse as the 400-meter run and the 26-mile, 385-yard marathon, or performance will suffer. What controls the mixture of fuel used by the muscles? What stimulates the adipose tissue to release more FFA? How is the liver made aware of the need to replace the glucose that is being removed from the blood by exercising muscles? If glucose is not replaced, a hypoglycemic (low blood glucose) condition will occur. Hypoglycemia is a topic of crucial importance in discussing exercise as a challenge to homeostasis. Blood glucose is the primary fuel for the central nervous system (CNS), and without optimal CNS function during exercise, the chance of fatigue and the risk of serious injury increase. While blood glucose was used as an example, it should be noted that sodium, calcium, potassium, and water concentrations, as well as blood pressure and pH, are also maintained within narrow limits during exercise. It should be no surprise then that there are a variety of automatic control systems maintaining these variables within these limits. Chapter 2 presented an overview of automatic control systems that maintain homeostasis. This chapter will expand on that by providing information on **neuroendocrinology,** a branch of physiology dedicated to the systematic study of control systems. The first part of the chapter will present a brief introduction to each hormone, indicate the factors controlling its secretion, and discuss its role in homeostasis. Following that, we will discuss how hormones control the delivery of carbohydrates and fats during exercise.

NEUROENDOCRINOLOGY

The two major homeostatic systems involved in the control and regulation of various functions (cardiovascular, renal, metabolic, etc.) are the nervous and endocrine systems. Both are structured to sense information, organize an appropriate response, and then deliver the message to the proper organ or tissue. Often the two systems work together to maintain homeostasis, and the term *neuroendocrine response* is reflective of that interdependence. The two systems differ in the way the message is delivered: The endocrine system releases hormones into the blood to circulate to tissues, while nerves use neurotransmitters to relay messages from one nerve to the other, or from a nerve to a tissue.

Endocrine glands release **hormones** (chemical messengers) directly into the blood, which carries the hormone to a tissue to exert an effect. It is the binding of the hormone to a specific protein receptor that allows the hormone to exert its effect. In that way the hormone can circulate to all tissues while affecting only a few—those with the specific receptor.

Hormones can be divided into several classes based on chemical makeup: amino acid derivatives, peptides/protein, and **steroids.** The chemical structure influences the way in which the hormone is transported in the blood and the manner in which it exerts its effect on the tissue. For example, while steroid hormones' lipid-like structure requires that they be transported bound to plasma protein (to "dissolve" in the plasma), that same lipid-like structure allows them to diffuse through cell membranes to exert their effects. This will be discussed in detail in a later section, Stimulation of DNA in the Nucleus. Hormones exist in very small quantities in the blood and are measured in microgram (10^{-6} g), nanogram (10^{-9} g), and picogram (10^{-12} g) amounts. It wasn't until the 1950s that analytical techniques were improved to the point of allowing one to measure these low plasma concentrations (92).

Blood Hormone Concentration

The effect a hormone exerts on a tissue is directly related to the concentration of the hormone in the plasma and the number of active receptors to which it can bind. The hormone concentration in the plasma is dependent upon the following factors:

- the rate of secretion of the hormone from the endocrine gland,
- the rate of metabolism or excretion of the hormone,
- the quantity of transport protein (for some hormones), and
- changes in the plasma volume.

Control of Hormone Secretion   The rate at which a hormone is secreted from an endocrine gland is dependent on the magnitude of the input and whether it is stimulatory or inhibitory in nature. The input in every case is a chemical one, be it an ion (e.g., Ca^{++}) or a substrate (e.g., glucose) in the plasma, a neurotransmitter such as acetylcholine or norepinephrine, or another hormone. Most endocrine glands are under the direct influence of more than one type of input, which may either reinforce or interfere with each other's effect. An example of this interaction is found in the control of insulin release from the pancreas. Figure 5.1 shows that the pancreas, which produces insulin, responds to changes in plasma glucose and amino acids, norepinephrine released from sympathetic neurons as well as circulating epinephrine, parasympathetic neurons, which release acetylcholine, and a variety of hormones. Elevations of plasma glucose and amino acids increase insulin secretion (+), while an increase in sympathetic nervous system activity (epinephrine and norepinephrine) decreases (−) insulin secretion. It is this magnitude of inhibitory versus excitatory input that determines whether there will be an increase or a decrease in the secretion of insulin.

Metabolism and Excretion of Hormones   The concentration of a hormone in the plasma is also influenced by the rate at which it is metabolized (inac-

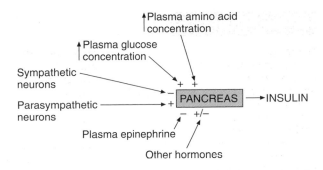

FIGURE 5.1   The secretion of a hormone can be modified by a number of factors, some exerting a positive influence and others, a negative influence. From A. J. Vander et al., *Human Physiology: The Mechanisms of Body Function*, 4th ed. Copyright © 1985 McGraw-Hill, Inc., New York. Reprinted by permission.

tivated) and/or excreted. Inactivation can take place at or near the receptor, or in the liver, the major site for hormone metabolism. In addition, the kidneys can metabolize a variety of hormones, or excrete them in their free (active) form. In fact, the rate of excretion of a hormone in the urine has been used as an indicator of its rate of secretion during exercise (10, 35, 68, 69). Since blood flow to the kidneys and liver decreases during exercise, the rate at which hormones are inactivated or excreted decreases. This results in an elevation of the plasma level of the hormone over and above that due to higher rates of secretion.

Transport Protein   The concentration of some hormones is influenced by the quantity of transport protein in the plasma. Steroid hormones and thyroxine are transported bound to plasma proteins. In order for a hormone to exert its effect on a cell it must be "free" to interact with the receptor, and not "bound" to the transport protein. The amount of free hormone is dependent on the quantity of transport protein and the capacity and affinity of the protein to bind the hormone molecules. Capacity refers to the maximal quantity of hormone that can be bound to the transport protein, and affinity refers to the tendency of the transport protein to bind to the hormone. An increase in the quantity, capacity, or affinity of transport protein would reduce the amount of free hormone and its effect on tissue (46, 80). For example, high levels of estrogen during pregnancy increase the quantity of thyroxine's transport protein, causing a reduction in free thyroxine. The thyroid gland produces more thyroxine to counteract this effect.

Plasma Volume   Changes in plasma volume will change the hormone concentration independent of changes in the rate of secretion or inactivation of the hormone. During exercise, plasma volume decreases due to the movement of water out of the cardiovascular system. This causes an increase in the concentration of hormones in the plasma, which can be "corrected" based on changes in plasma volume (80).

IN SUMMARY

- Endocrine glands release hormones directly into the blood to alter the activity of tissues possessing receptors to which the hormone can bind.
- The free plasma hormone concentration determines the magnitude of the effect at the tissue level.
- The free hormone concentration can be changed by altering the rate of secretion or inactivation of the hormone, the quantity of transport protein, and the plasma volume.

Hormone-Receptor Interaction

Hormones are carried by the circulation to all tissues, but they affect only certain tissues. Tissues responsive to specific hormones have specific protein receptors capable of binding those hormones. These protein receptors should not be viewed as static fixtures associated with cells, but like any cellular structures, they are subject to change. The number of receptors varies from 500 to 100,000 per cell, depending on the receptor. Receptor number may decrease when exposed to a chronically elevated level of a hormone (*down-regulation*), resulting in a diminished response for the same hormone concentration. The opposite case, chronic exposure to a low concentration of a hormone, may lead to an increase in receptor number (*up-regulation*), with the tissue becoming very responsive to the available hormone. Since there is a finite number of receptors on or in a cell, a situation can arise in which the concentration of a hormone is so high that all receptors are bound to the hormone; this is called *saturation*. Any additional increase in the plasma hormone concentration will have no additional effect (38). Further, since the receptors are specific to a hormone, any chemical similar in "shape" will compete for the limited receptor sites. A major way in which endocrine function is studied is to use chemicals (drugs) to block receptors and observe the consequences. For example, patients with heart disease may receive a drug that blocks the receptors to which epinephrine (adrenaline) binds; this prevents the heart rate from getting too high during exercise. After the hormone binds to a receptor, cellular activity is altered by a variety of mechanisms.

Mechanisms of Hormone Action Mechanisms by which hormones modify cellular activity include:

- alteration of membrane transport mechanisms,
- stimulation of DNA in the nucleus to initiate the synthesis of a specific protein, and
- activation of special proteins in the cells by "second messengers."

Membrane Transport After binding to a receptor on a membrane, the major effect of some hormones is to activate carrier molecules in or near the membrane to increase the movement of substrates or ions from outside to inside the cell. For example, insulin binds to receptors on the surface of the cell and mobilizes glucose transporters located in the membrane of the cell. The transporters link up with glucose on the outside of the cell membrane where the concentration of glucose is high, and the glucose transporter diffuses to the inside of the membrane to release glucose for use in the cell (76). If an individual does not have adequate insulin, as exists in uncontrolled diabetes, glucose accumulates in the plasma because the glucose transporters in the membrane are not activated.

Stimulation of DNA in the Nucleus Due to their lipid-like nature, steroid hormones diffuse easily through cell membranes, where they become bound to a protein receptor in the cytoplasm of the cell. Figure 5.2 shows that the steroid-receptor complex enters the nucleus and binds to a specific protein linked to DNA, which contains the instruction codes for protein synthesis. This initiates the steps leading to the synthesis of a specific messenger RNA (mRNA) that carries the codes from the nucleus to the cytoplasm where the specific protein is synthesized. While thyroid hormones are not steroid hormones, they act in a similar manner. These processes—the activation of DNA and the synthesis of specific protein—take time to turn on (making the hormones involved "slow-acting" hormones), but their effects are longer lasting than those generated by "second messengers" (54).

Second Messengers Many hormones, because of their size or highly charged structure, cannot easily cross cell membranes. These hormones exert their effects by binding to a receptor on the membrane surface and activating a **G protein** located in the membrane of the cell. The G protein is the link between the hormone-receptor interaction on the surface of the membrane and the subsequent events inside the cell. The G protein may open an ion channel to allow Ca^{++} to enter the cell, or it may activate an enzyme in the membrane. If the G protein activates **adenylate cyclase**, then **cyclic AMP** (cyclic 3',5'-adenosine monophosphate) is formed from ATP (see figure 5.3).

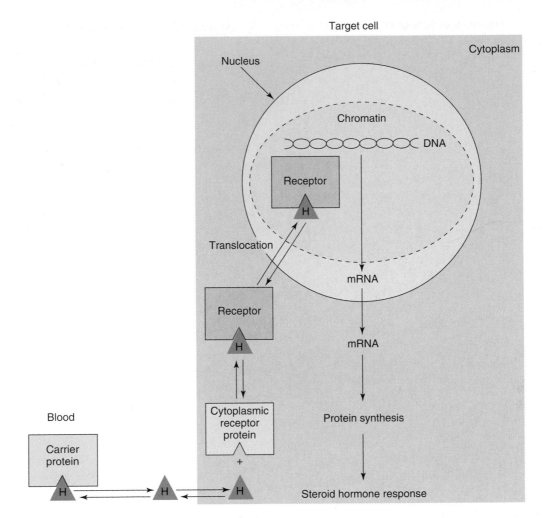

FIGURE 5.2 The mechanism by which steroid hormones act on target cells. The steroid hormone, represented by the triangle with the letter H, binds to a cytoplasmic receptor to be transported to the nucleus, where it stimulates DNA to bring about a change in cellular activity.

FIGURE 5.3 The cyclic AMP "second messenger" mechanism by which hormones act on target cells.

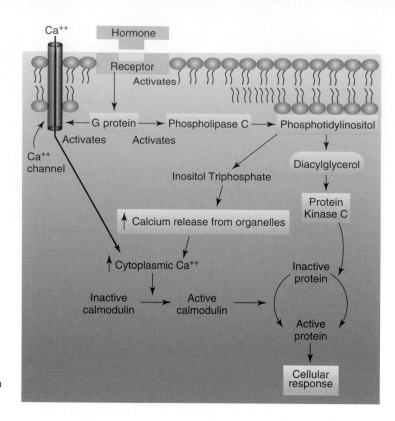

FIGURE 5.4 Calcium and phospholipase C second messenger mechanisms by which hormones act on target cells.

In turn, the cyclic AMP concentration increases in the cell and activates proteins, which directly alter cellular activity. For example, this mechanism is used to convert glycogen to glucose in the muscle, and triglycerides to free fatty acids and glycerol in adipose tissue. The cyclic AMP is inactivated by **phosphodiesterase,** an enzyme that converts cyclic AMP to 5'AMP. Factors that interfere with phosphodiesterase activity, such as caffeine, would increase the effect of the hormone by allowing cyclic AMP to exert its effect for a longer period of time. For example, caffeine may exert this effect on adipose tissue, causing free fatty acids to be mobilized at a faster rate (see chapter 25).

If the G protein activates a Ca^{++} ion channel, then Ca^{++} enters the cell and binds to and activates a protein called **calmodulin.** The activated calmodulin influences cellular activity in much the same way as cyclic AMP does (see figure 5.4). Lastly, a G protein may activate a membrane-bound enzyme **phospholipase C.** When this occurs, a phospholipid in the membrane, phosphatidylinositol, is hydrolyzed into two intracellular molecules, **inositol triphosphate,** which causes Ca^{++} release from intracellular stores, and **diacylglycerol.** The diacylglycerol activates **protein kinase C** that, in turn, activates proteins in the cell (see figure 5.4). Cyclic AMP, Ca^{++}, inositol triphosphate, and diacylglycerol are viewed as **second messengers** in the events following the hormone's

binding to a receptor on the cell membrane. These second messengers should not be viewed as being independent of one another, because changes in one can affect the action of the others (143).

IN SUMMARY

- The hormone-receptor interaction triggers events at the cell, and changing the concentration of the hormone, the number of receptors on the cell, or the affinity of the receptor for the hormone will all influence the magnitude of the effect.
- Hormones bring about their effects by altering membrane transport, stimulating DNA to increase protein synthesis, and activating second messengers (cyclic AMP, Ca^{++}, inositol triphosphate, and diacylglycerol).

HORMONES: REGULATION AND ACTION

This section will present the major endocrine glands, their hormones and how they are regulated, the effects the hormones have on tissues, and how some of the hormones respond to exercise. This information is essential in order to discuss the role of the neuroendocrine system in the mobilization of fuel for exercise.

Hypothalamus and the Pituitary Gland

The **pituitary gland** is located at the base of the brain, attached to the **hypothalamus.** The gland has two lobes, the anterior lobe (adenohypophysis), which is a true endocrine gland, and the posterior lobe (neurohypophysis), which is neural tissue extending from the hypothalamus. Both lobes are under the direct control of the hypothalamus. In the case of the **anterior pituitary,** hormone release is controlled by chemicals (**releasing hormones** or factors) that originate in neurons located in the hypothalamus. These releasing hormones stimulate or inhibit the release of specific hormones from the anterior pituitary. The posterior pituitary gland receives its hormones from special neurons originating in the hypothalamus. The hormones move down the axon to blood vessels in the posterior hypothalamus where they are discharged into the general circulation (81).

Anterior Pituitary Gland The anterior pituitary hormones include **adrenocorticotrophic hormone (ACTH), follicle-stimulating hormone (FSH), luteinizing hormone (LH), malanocyte-stimulating hormone (MSH), thyroid-stimulating hormone (TSH), growth hormone (GH),** and **prolactin.** Figure 5.5 shows each hormone and its target tissue. While prolactin directly stimulates the breast to produce milk, the majority of the hormones secreted from the anterior pituitary control the release of other hormones. TSH controls the rate of thyroid hormone formation and secretion from the thyroid gland; ACTH stimulates the production and secretion of cortisol in the adrenal cortex; LH stimulates the production of testosterone in the testes and estrogen in the ovary; and GH stimulates the release of **somatomedins,** or as they are commonly called today, **insulin-like growth factors (IGFs),** from the liver and other tissues. In fact, it is the IGF-1 produced in muscle that is associated with muscle hypertrophy (58, 88). However, as we will see, growth hormone exerts important effects on protein, fat, and carbohydrate metabolism (81).

Growth Hormone Growth hormone (GH) is secreted from the anterior pituitary gland and exerts profound effects on the growth of all tissues through the action of IGFs. Growth hormone secretion is controlled by releasing hormones secreted from the hypothalamus. Growth hormone-releasing hormone (GHRH) stimulates GH release from the anterior pituitary, while another factor, **hypothalamic somatostatin,** inhibits it. The GH and IGF levels in blood exert a negative feedback effect on the continued secretion of GH. As shown in figure 5.6, additional input to the hypothalamus that can influence the secretion of GH includes exercise, stress (broadly defined), a low plasma-glucose concentration, and sleep (142).

GH and IGFs stimulate tissue uptake of amino acids, the synthesis of new protein, and long bone growth. In addition, GH spares plasma glucose by:

- opposing the action of insulin to reduce the use of plasma glucose,
- increasing the synthesis of new glucose in the liver (gluconeogenesis), and
- increasing the mobilization of fatty acids from adipose tissue.

Given these characteristics, it should be no surprise that GH increases with exercise to help maintain the plasma glucose concentration (this will be covered in detail in a later section, Permissive and Slow Acting Hormones). Growth hormone, because of its role in protein synthesis, is being used by some athletes to enhance muscle mass and by the elderly to slow down the aging process. However, there are problems with this approach (see A Closer Look 5.1).

IN SUMMARY

- The hypothalamus controls the activity of both the anterior pituitary and posterior pituitary glands.
- GH is released from the anterior pituitary gland and is essential for normal growth.
- GH increases during exercise to mobilize fatty acids from adipose tissue and to aid in the maintenance of blood glucose.

Posterior Pituitary Gland The **posterior pituitary gland** releases two hormones, oxytocin and **antidiuretic hormone (ADH),** which is also called *vasopressin.* Oxytocin is a powerful stimulator of smooth muscle, especially at the time of childbirth, and is also involved in the milk "let down" response needed for the release of milk from the breast.

Antidiuretic Hormone Antidiuretic hormone (ADH) does what its name implies: It reduces water loss from the body. ADH favors the reabsorption of water from the kidney tubules back into the capillaries to maintain body fluid. There are two major stimuli that result in an increased secretion of ADH:

- high plasma osmolality (a low water concentration) that can be caused by excessive sweating without water replacement, and
- a low plasma volume, which can be due either to the loss of blood or to inadequate fluid replacement.

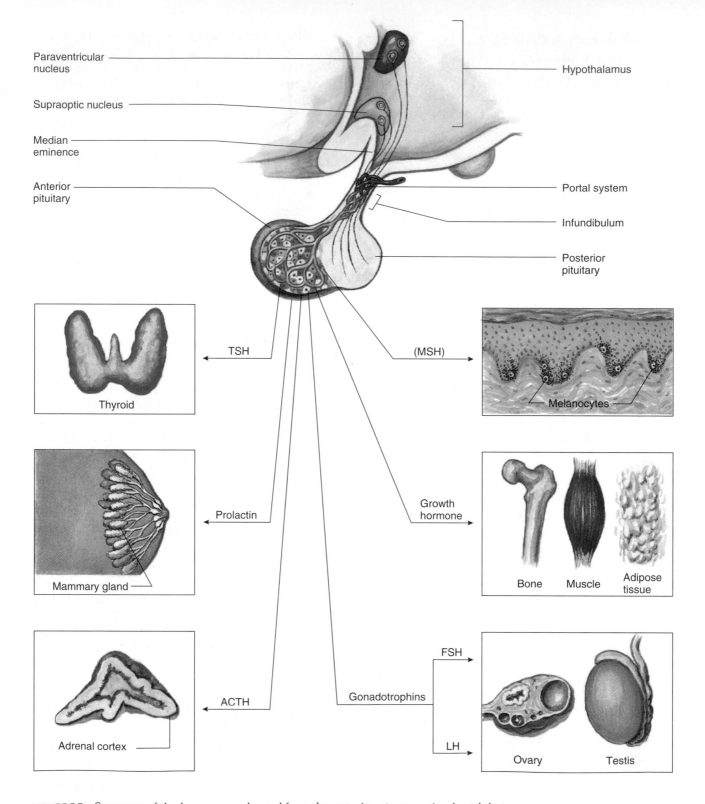

Paraventricular nucleus

Supraoptic nucleus

Median eminence

Anterior pituitary

Hypothalamus

Portal system

Infundibulum

Posterior pituitary

TSH

Thyroid

(MSH)

Melanocytes

Prolactin

Mammary gland

Growth hormone

Bone   Muscle   Adipose tissue

ACTH

Adrenal cortex

Gonadotrophins

FSH

LH

Ovary   Testis

FIGURE 5.5 Summary of the hormones released from the anterior pituitary gland, and their target tissues.

There are osmoreceptors in the hypothalamus that sense the water concentration in the interstitial fluid. When the plasma has a high concentration of particles (low water concentration), the osmoreceptors shrink, and a neural reflex to the hypothalamus stimulates ADH release, which causes a reduction in water loss at the kidney. If the osmolality of the plasma is normal, but the volume of plasma is low, stretch receptors in the left atrium initiate a reflex leading to ADH release to attempt to maintain body fluid. During exercise, plasma volume decreases and osmolality increases, and for exercise intensities in excess of 60% of $\dot{V}O_2$

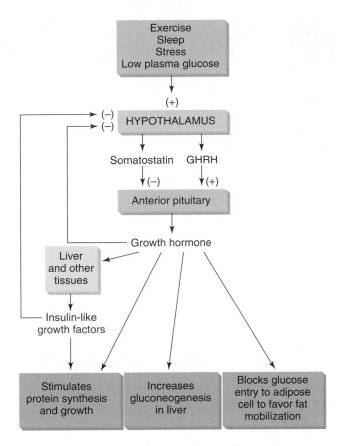

FIGURE 5.6 Summary of the positive and negative input to the hypothalamus, influencing growth hormone secretion. From A. J. Vander et al., *Human Physiology: The Mechanisms of Body Function*, 4th ed. Copyright© 1985 McGraw-Hill, Inc., New York. Reprinted by permission.

max, ADH secretion is increased as shown in figure 5.7 (21). This favors the conservation of water to maintain plasma volume (145).

Thyroid Gland

The **thyroid gland** is stimulated by TSH to synthesize two iodine-containing hormones: **triiodothyronine (T_3)** and **thyroxine (T_4)**. T_3 contains three iodine atoms and T_4 contains four. TSH is also the primary stimulus for the release of T_3 and T_4 into the circulation, where they are bound to plasma proteins. Remember, it is the "free" hormone concentration (that which is not bound to plasma proteins) that is important in bringing about an effect on tissue. T_4 is released from the thyroid gland in much larger amounts compared to T_3. However, after release, most of the T_4 is converted to T_3, the more potent of the thyroid hormones.

Thyroid Hormones Thyroid hormones are central in establishing the overall metabolic rate (i.e., a hypothyroid [low T_3] individual would be characterized as being lethargic and hypokinetic). It is this effect

FIGURE 5.7 Percent change in the plasma antidiuretic hormone (ADH) concentration with increasing exercise intensity.

of the hormone that has been linked to weight-control problems, but only a small percentage of obese individuals are hypothyroid. T_3 and T_4 act as permissive hormones in that they permit other hormones to exert their full effect. There is a relatively long latent period between the time T_3 and T_4 are elevated and the time when their effects are observed. The latent period is six to twelve hours for T_3 and two to three days for T_4. However, once initiated, their effects are long lasting (54). The control of T_3 and T_4 secretion is another example of the negative feedback mechanism introduced in chapter 2. As the plasma concentrations of T_3 and T_4 increase, they inhibit the release of TSH-releasing hormone from the hypothalamus as well as TSH itself. This self-regulating system ensures the necessary level of T_3 and T_4 for the maintenance of a normal metabolic rate. During exercise the "free" hormone concentration increases due to changes in the binding characteristic of the transport protein, and the hormones are taken up at a faster rate by tissues. In order to counter the higher rate of removal of T_3 and T_4, TSH secretion increases and causes an increased secretion of these hormones from the thyroid gland (138). Evidence suggests that resistance training has little effect on the pituitary (TSH)-thyroid (T_3, T_4) function (2).

- Thyroid hormones T_3 and T_4 are important for maintaining the metabolic rate and allowing other hormones to bring about their full effect.

Calcitonin The thyroid gland also secretes **calcitonin,** which is involved in a minor way in the regulation of plasma calcium (Ca^{++}), a crucial ion for normal muscle and nerve function. The secretion of this hormone is controlled by another negative feedback

A CLOSER LOOK 5.1

Growth Hormone and Performance

An excess of growth hormone (GH) during childhood is tied to gigantism, while an inadequate secretion causes dwarfism. The latter condition requires the administration of GH (along with other growth-promoting hormones) during the growing years if the child is to regain his or her normal position on the growth chart. GH was originally obtained by extracting it from the pituitary glands of cadavers—an expensive and time-consuming proposition. Due to the success of genetic engineering, recombinant human GH (rhGH) is now available in large quantities.

If an excess of GH occurs during adulthood, a condition called acromegaly occurs. The additional GH during adulthood does not affect growth in height, since the epiphyseal growth plates at the ends of the long bones have closed. Unfortunately, the excess GH causes permanent deformities, as seen in a thickening of the bones in the face, hands, and feet. Until recently, the usual cause of acromegaly was a tumor in the anterior pituitary gland that resulted in excess secretion of GH. This is no longer the case. In an unfortunate drive to take advantage of the muscle-growth-stimulating effects of GH, athletes are injecting the now readily available human GH, along with other hormones (see A Closer Look 5.3). Evidence exists showing that GH increases protein synthesis in muscle; however, it is connective tissue protein (collagen) that is increased more than contractile protein. Consistent with these observations is the fact that strength gains do not parallel gains in muscle size (98). Similar observations have been made in studies involving GH-deficient adults who were injected with GH during a resistance-training program (133, 154). As with all hormones that have multiple effects, the user can't have one effect without the other. Chronic use of GH may lead to diabetes, hyperlipidemia, arthritis, cardiomegaly, carpal tunnel compression, muscle disease, and shortened life span (47, 98, 151, 154, 158). Concern over the use of GH is so great that some people are recommending that it be reclassified as a "controlled substance" to reduce its availability (23, 136). Fortunately, the European Union and the International Olympic Committee have funded a research project, GH-2000, to develop new tests to distinguish natural GH from rhGH (127). However, Rennie (114) makes an interesting counterpoint to this action: Since there is no evidence that GH is a muscle-building hormone, does all the attention promote its abuse? This would be a good paper for the class to read to debate the merits of this view.

---

mechanism. As the plasma Ca^{++} concentration increases, calcitonin release is increased. Calcitonin blocks the release of Ca^{++} from bone and stimulates Ca^{++} excretion at the kidneys to lower the plasma Ca^{++} concentration. As the Ca^{++} concentration is decreased, the rate of calcitonin secretion is reduced.

Parathyroid Gland

Parathyroid hormone is the primary hormone involved in plasma Ca^{++} regulation. The parathyroid gland releases parathyroid hormone in response to a low plasma Ca^{++} concentration. The hormone stimulates bone to release Ca^{++} into the plasma and simultaneously increases the renal absorption of Ca^{++}; both raise the plasma Ca^{++} level. Parathyroid hormone also stimulates the kidney to convert a form of vitamin D (vitamin D$_3$) into a hormone that increases the absorption of Ca^{++} from the gastrointestinal tract. Exercise increases the concentration of parathyroid hormone in the plasma (94, 95).

Adrenal Gland

The adrenal gland is really two different glands, the adrenal medulla, which secretes the **catecholamines, epinephrine (E),** and **norepinephrine (NE),** and the **adrenal cortex,** which secretes steroid hormones.

Adrenal Medulla   The adrenal medulla is part of the sympathetic nervous system. Eighty percent of the gland's hormonal secretion is epinephrine, which affects receptors in the cardiovascular and respiratory systems, gastrointestinal (GI) tract, liver, other endocrine glands, muscle, and adipose tissue. E and NE are involved in the maintenance of blood pressure and the plasma glucose concentration. Their role in the cardiovascular system is discussed in chapter 9, and their involvement in the mobilization of substrate for exercise is discussed later in this chapter in *Fast-Acting Hormones*. E and NE also respond to strong emotional stimuli, and they form the basis for Cannon's "fight or flight" hypothesis of how the body responds to challenges from the environment (15). Cannon's view was that the activation of the sympathetic nervous system prepared you either to confront a danger or to flee from it. Statements by sportscasters such as "The adrenalin must really be pumping now" are a rough translation of this hypothesis.

E and NE bind to adrenergic (from adrenaline, the European name for epinephrine) receptors on target tissues. The receptors are divided into two major classes: **alpha** (α) and **beta** (β), with subgroups (α_1 and α_2; β_1 and β_2). E and NE bring about their effects via the second messenger mechanisms mentioned earlier. The response generated in the target tissue, both size and direction (inhibitory or excitatory), is dependent

TABLE 5.1 Physiological Responses to Epinephrine and Norepinephrine: Role of Adrenergic Receptor Type

Receptor Type	Effect of E/NE	Membrane-Bound Enzyme	Intracellular Mediator	Effects on Various Tissues
β_1	E = NE	Adenylate cyclase	↑cyclic AMP	↑Heart rate ↑Glycogenolysis ↑Lipolysis
β_2	E >>> NE	Adenylate cyclase	↑ cyclic AMP	↑Bronchodilation ↑Vasodilation
α_1	E ≥ NE	Phospholipase C	↑Ca^{++}	↑Phosphodiesterase ↑Vasoconstriction
α_2	E ≥ NE	Adenylate cyclase	↓ cyclic AMP	Opposes action of β_1 and β_2 receptors

Adapted from J. Tepperman and H. M. Tepperman. 1987. *Metabolic and Endocrine Physiology*, 5th ed. Chicago: Year Book Medical Publishers.

on the receptor type and whether E or NE is involved. This is an example of how important the receptors are in determining the cell's response to a hormone. Table 5.1 summarizes the effects of E and NE relative to the type of adrenergic receptor involved (128). The different receptors cause changes in the cell's activity by increasing or decreasing the cyclic AMP or Ca^{++} concentrations. From this table it can be seen that if a cell experienced a loss of β_1 receptors and a gain in α_2 receptors, the same epinephrine concentration would bring about very different effects in the cell.

IN SUMMARY

- The adrenal medulla secretes the catecholamines epinephrine (E) and norepinephrine (NE). E is the adrenal medulla's primary secretion (80%), while NE is primarily secreted from the adrenergic neurons of the sympathetic nervous system.
- Epinephrine and norepinephrine bind to α- and β-adrenergic receptors and bring about changes in cellular activity (e.g., increased heart rate, mobilization of fatty acids from adipose tissue) via second messengers.

Adrenal Cortex The adrenal cortex secretes a variety of steroid hormones having rather distinct physiological functions. The hormones can be grouped into three different categories:

- **mineralocorticoids** (aldosterone), involved in the maintenance of the Na^+ and K^+ concentrations in plasma,
- **glucocorticoids** (cortisol), involved in plasma glucose regulation, and
- **sex steroids (androgens** and **estrogens),** which support prepubescent growth, with

androgens being associated with postpubescent sex drive in women.

The chemical precursor common to all of these steroid hormones is cholesterol, and while the final active hormones possess minor structural differences, their physiological functions differ greatly.

Aldosterone Aldosterone (mineralocorticoid) is an important regulator of Na^+ reabsorption and K^+ secretion at the kidney. Aldosterone is directly involved in Na^+/H_2O balance and, consequently, plasma volume and blood pressure (see chapter 9). There are two levels of control over aldosterone secretion. The release of aldosterone from the adrenal cortex is controlled directly by the plasma K^+ concentration. An increase in K^+ concentration increases aldosterone secretion, which stimulates the kidney's active transport mechanism to secrete K^+ ions. This control system uses the negative feedback loop we have already seen. Aldosterone secretion is also controlled by another more complicated mechanism. A decrease in plasma volume, a fall in blood pressure at the kidney, or an increase in sympathetic nerve activity to the kidney stimulates special cells in the kidney to secrete an enzyme called **renin.** Renin enters the plasma and converts renin substrate (angiotensinogen) to **angiotensin I,** which is, in turn, converted to **angiotensin II** by angiotensin-converting enzyme (ACE) in the lungs. Angiotensin II is a powerful vasoconstrictor, and individuals with hypertension may be prescribed an ACE inhibitor to lower blood pressure. Angiotensin II stimulates aldosterone release, which increases Na^+ reabsorption. The stimuli for aldosterone and ADH secretion are also the signals that stimulate thirst, a necessary ingredient to restore body fluid volume. During light exercise there is little or no change in plasma renin activity or aldosterone (99). However, when a heat load is imposed during light exercise,

FIGURE 5.8 Parallel increases in renin activity, angiotensin II, and aldosterone with increasing intensities of exercise. Data are expressed as the percent change from resting values.

both renin and aldosterone secretion are increased (40). When exercise intensity approaches 50% $\dot{V}O_2$ max (figure 5.8), renin, angiotensin, and aldosterone increase in parallel, showing the linkage within this homeostatic system (99, 138). Further, liver production of renin substrate increases to maintain the plasma concentration (103).

Cortisol The primary glucocorticoid secreted by the adrenal cortex is **cortisol.** Cortisol contributes to the maintenance of plasma glucose during long-term fasting and exercise by a variety of mechanisms:

- promoting the breakdown of tissue protein (by inhibiting protein synthesis) to form amino acids, which are then used by the liver to form new glucose (gluconeogenesis),
- stimulating the mobilization of free fatty acids from adipose tissue,
- stimulating liver enzymes involved in the metabolic pathway leading to glucose synthesis, and
- blocking the entry of glucose into tissues, forcing those tissues to use more fatty acids as fuel (54, 142).

A summary of cortisol's actions and its regulation is presented in figure 5.9. Cortisol secretion is controlled in the same manner as thyroxine. The hypothalamus secretes corticotrophic-releasing hormone (CRH), which causes the anterior pituitary gland to secrete more ACTH into the general circulation. ACTH binds to receptors on the adrenal cortex and increases cortisol secretion. As the cortisol level increases, CRH and ACTH are inhibited in another negative feedback system. However, the hypothalamus, like any brain

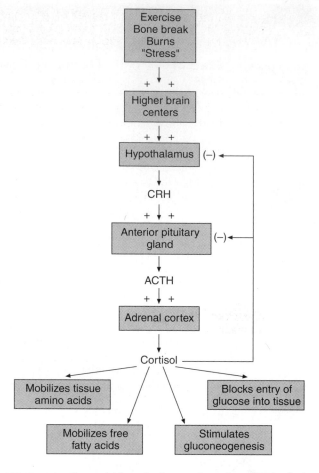

FIGURE 5.9 Control of cortisol secretion, showing the balance of positive and negative input to the hypothalamus, and cortisol's influence on metabolism.

center, receives neural input from other areas of the brain. This input can influence the secretion of hypothalamic-releasing hormones beyond the level seen in a negative feedback system. Over fifty years ago, Hans Selye observed that a wide variety of stressful events such as burns, bone breaks, and heavy exercise led to predictable increases in ACTH and cortisol; he called this response the *General Adaptation Syndrome* (GAS). A key point in this response was the release of ACTH and cortisol to aid in the adaptation. His GAS had three stages: (a) the *alarm reaction*, involving cortisol secretion, (b) the *stage of resistance*, where repairs are made, and (c) the *stage of exhaustion*, in which repairs are not adequate, and sickness or death results (125). The usefulness of the GAS is seen in times of "stress" caused by tissue damage. Cortisol stimulates the breakdown of tissue protein to form amino acids, which can then be used at the site of the tissue damage for repair. While it is clear that muscle tissue is a primary source of amino acids, the functional overload of muscle with resistance or endurance training can prevent the muscle atrophy the glucocorticoids

Endorphins and Exercise

The reader may be familiar with the expression "runner's high" as a description of the good feeling some individuals experience during long-distance runs. This experience has been linked to **endorphins**, endogenous, morphine-like substances that interact with opiate receptors in the brain areas involved in the transmission of information about pain. β-endorphin is formed in the anterior pituitary from β-lipotrophin, which is itself generated during the formation of adrenocorticotrophic hormone (ACTH) (142). Given the close relationship between these substances and ACTH, which is the cornerstone of Selye's General Adaptation Syndrome, investigators became interested in how plasma levels of β-lipotrophin and β-endorphin would respond to exercise stress. Studies conducted in the early

1980s found that exercise caused parallel changes in plasma ACTH and β-endorphin (39). A summary of the early work in this area supported this observation, showing an elevation in β-lipotrophin/β-endorphin with exercise in men (36) and women (101). As chemical techniques improved to separate β-endorphin from β-lipotrophin, other studies were conducted. One study found no changes in β-endorphin in subjects who exercised at 60% $\dot{V}O_2$ max for one hour (91). This has been confirmed in both trained and untrained subjects who showed elevated plasma β-endorphin levels only when the exercise intensity exceeded 70% $\dot{V}O_2$ max. Further, the higher the intensity, the shorter the duration needed to cause the elevation (48, 49). While there is support for the change in β-endorphin

to be linked to lactate levels above 4 mM (onset of blood lactate accumulation), trained subjects had the same β-endorphin response as untrained subjects, even though lactate levels were lower in the trained subjects (49, 123). The results support the proposition that β-endorphins may be related to changes in mood and pain threshold during endurance exercise. However, the plasma levels may not adequately reflect the influence of these substances on neuroendocrine function in the brain (139). Consistent with this cautious interpretation, Morgan (107) emphasizes the need to explore alternative hypotheses in studying the effect of exercise on mood changes. The reader is referred to a paper that does just that (139).

---

can cause (4, 62, 63). Could the GAS be linked to the "runner's high" experienced during long-term exercise? See A Closer Look 5.2 for details.

IN SUMMARY

- The adrenal cortex secretes aldosterone (mineralocorticoid), cortisol (glucocorticoid), and estrogens and androgens (sex steroids).
- Aldosterone regulates Na^+ and K^+ balance. Aldosterone secretion increases with strenuous exercise, driven by the renin-angiotensin system.
- Cortisol responds to a variety of stressors, including exercise, to ensure that fuel (glucose and free fatty acids) is available, and to make amino acids available for tissue repair.

Pancreas

The **pancreas** is both an exocrine and an endocrine gland. The exocrine secretions include digestive enzymes and bicarbonate, which are secreted into ducts leading to the small intestine. The hormones, released from groups of cells in the endocrine portion of the pancreas called the islets of Langerhans, include **insulin, glucagon,** and **somatostatin.**

Insulin   Insulin is secreted from beta (β) cells of the islets of Langerhans. Insulin is the most important hormone during the absorptive state, when nutrients are entering the blood from the small intestine. Insulin stimulates tissues to take up nutrient molecules such as glucose and amino acids and store them as glycogen, proteins, and fats. Insulin's best-known role is in the facilitated diffusion of glucose across cell membranes. A lack of insulin causes an accumulation of glucose in the plasma, since the tissues cannot take it up. The plasma glucose concentration can become so high that reabsorption mechanisms in the kidney are overwhelmed and glucose is lost to the urine, taking large volumes of water with it. This condition is called **diabetes mellitus.**

As mentioned earlier in this chapter, insulin secretion is influenced by a wide variety of factors: plasma glucose concentration, plasma amino acid concentration, sympathetic and parasympathetic nerve stimulation, and various hormones. The rate of secretion of insulin is dependent on the level of excitatory and inhibitory input to the beta cells of the pancreas (see figure 5.1). The blood glucose concentration is a major source of input that is part of a simple negative feedback loop; as the plasma glucose concentration increases (following a meal), the beta cells directly monitor this increase and secrete additional insulin to enhance tissue uptake of glucose. This increased uptake lowers the plasma glucose concentration, and insulin secretion is reduced (54, 92).

Glucagon   Glucagon, secreted from the alpha (α) cells in the islets of Langerhans, exerts an effect opposite that of insulin. Glucagon secretion increases in response to a low plasma glucose concentration, which is monitored by the alpha cells. Glucagon stimulates both the mobilization of glucose from liver stores (glycogenolysis) and free fatty acids from adipose tissue (to spare blood glucose as a fuel). Lastly, along with cortisol, glucagon stimulates gluconeogenesis in the liver. Glucagon secretion is also influenced by factors other than the glucose concentration, notably the sympathetic nervous system (137). A complete description of the role of insulin and glucagon in the maintenance of blood glucose during exercise is presented later in this chapter in Fast-Acting Hormones.

IN SUMMARY

- Insulin is secreted by the β cells of the islets of Langerhans in the pancreas and promotes the storage of glucose, amino acids, and fats.
- Glucagon is secreted by the α cells of the islets of Langerhans in the pancreas and promotes the mobilization of glucose and fatty acids.

Somatostatin   Pancreatic somatostatin is secreted by the delta cells of the islets of Langerhans. Pancreatic somatostatin secretion is increased during the absorptive state, and it modifies the activity of the GI tract to control the rate of entry of nutrient molecules into the circulation. It may also be involved in the regulation of insulin secretion (137).

Testes and Ovaries

Testosterone and estrogen are the primary sex steroids secreted by the testis and ovary, respectively These hormones are not only important in establishing and maintaining reproductive function, they determine the secondary sex characteristics associated with masculinity and femininity.

Testosterone   Testosterone is secreted by the interstitial cells of the testes and is controlled by interstitial cell stimulating hormone (ICSH—also known as LH), which is produced in the anterior pituitary. LH is, in turn, controlled by a releasing hormone secreted by the hypothalamus. Sperm production from the seminiferous tubules of the testes requires follicle-stimulating hormone (FSH) from the anterior pituitary and testosterone. Figure 5.10 shows testosterone secre-

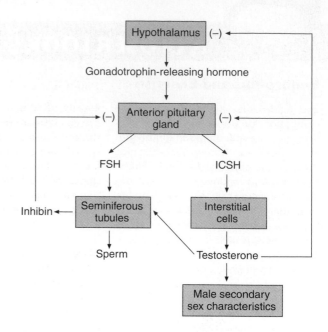

FIGURE 5.10   Control of testosterone secretion and sperm production by hypothalamus and anterior pituitary.

tion to be controlled by a negative feedback loop involving the anterior pituitary gland and the hypothalamus. Sperm production is controlled, in part, by another negative feedback loop involving the hormone inhibin (92, 142).

Testosterone is both an **anabolic** (tissue building) and **androgenic** (promoter of masculine characteristics) **steroid** because it stimulates protein synthesis and is responsible for the characteristic changes in boys at adolescence that lead to the high muscle-mass to fat-mass ratio. The plasma testosterone concentration is increased 10% to 37% during prolonged submaximal work (144), during exercise taken to maximum levels (25), and during endurance or strength training workouts (78). Some feel that these small changes are due to a reduction in plasma volume, or to a decrease in the rate of inactivation and removal of testosterone (138). However, others have concluded on the basis of a parallel increase in the LH concentration that the increase in plasma testosterone is due to an increased rate of production (25). While the testosterone response to exercise is small, and the concentration returns to resting values two hours after exercise (78), there is evidence that the resting plasma concentration is lower in both endurance-trained and resistance-trained males (6, 56). In one study, high-mileage (108 km · wk^{-1}) runners had lower levels of testosterone, sperm count, and sperm motility compared to moderate-mileage (54 km · wk^{-1}) runners (30). However, values were still in the normal range. Most readers probably recognize testosterone or one of its synthetic analogs as one of the most abused drugs in the drive to increase muscle

Anabolic Steroids and Performance

Testosterone, as both an anabolic and an androgenic steroid, causes size changes as well as male secondary sexual characteristics, respectively. Due to these combined effects, scientists developed steroids to maximize the anabolic effects and minimize the androgenic effects. However, these effects can never be completely separated. These synthetic steroids were developed to promote tissue growth in patients who had experienced atrophy as a result of prolonged bed rest. Before long the thought occurred that these anabolic steroids might be helpful in developing muscle mass and strength in athletes.

Numerous studies were conducted to determine whether or not these steroids would bring about the desired changes, but a consensus was not achieved (5, 150, 151). The variation in results in published studies was related to the different tests used to measure body composition and strength, the study participants (novice or experienced), the length of the study, and training methods (155). In most of these studies the scientists used the recommended therapeutic dosage, as required by committees approving research with human subjects. Unfortunately, the "results" of many personal studies conducted in various gyms and weight-training facilities throughout the world disagreed with these scientific results. Why the disagreement in results between the controlled scientific studies and these latter "studies"? In the weight room it was not uncommon for a person looking for greater "strength through chemistry" to take 10 to 100 times the recom-

mended dosage! In effect, it was difficult to compare the results of the controlled scientific studies with those done in the gym. When such a comparison was done using supraphysiologic doses of testosterone, the investigators reported greater increases in fat-free mass, muscle mass, and strength for the groups receiving testosterone compared to the groups receiving a placebo (9). In addition, such changes follow a dose-response relationship (8).

By the mid-1980s, the steroid problem had reached a level that prompted both professional and college sport teams to institute testing of athletes to control drug use. Olympic and Pan-American athletes were also tested to disqualify those who used the steroid. The problem escalated when athletes started to take pure testosterone rather than the anabolic steroid. Part of the reason for the switch was to reduce the chance of detection when drug testing was conducted, and part was related to the availability of testosterone. The loss of the gold medal by Canadian sprinter Ben Johnson in the 1988 Olympic Games indicates that testing has caught up with some of those who break the rules.

Like the GH example presented in A Closer Look 5.1, the use of testosterone or synthetic anabolic steroids can bring about undesirable effects. Females taking anabolic steroids experience an increase in male secondary sex characteristics, (including deepening of voice and beard growth), clitoral enlargement, and a disruption in menstrual function (156). Adverse reactions to chronic anabolic steroid use in males include (a) a decrease in

testicular function, including a reduction in sperm production, (b) gynaecomastia—breast development, (c) liver dysfunction, and (d) mood or behavioral changes (3, 7, 90, 156). Given that the use of anabolic steroids has a detrimental effect on ventricular wall mass (29, 140), blood lipids (3, 89, 106, 156), and glucose tolerance (3, 156), the risk of heart disease is also increased. These changes can be invoked by short-term use, but they revert to normal values upon discontinuance of the drug (3, 156). Although special attention has been directed at the habitual long-term user, there are questions about the validity of extrapolating from short-term studies to long-term consequences (155).

Finally, the use of androstenedione, a precursor of testosterone, has been promoted as a natural alternative to anabolic steroid use. Interestingly, the only sex steroid hormone to increase was estrogen. Plasma testosterone did not increase, and strength and muscle adaptations to resistance training were not different compared to a control (83). The abuse of anabolic steroids (and other drugs) by professional athletes gained unwanted high-level visibility when Major League Baseball (MLB) players and owners had to appear before the U.S. Congress in early 2005. Later that year, Congress proposed legislation to require professional sports to follow the same drug restrictions as Olympic athletes. See Hartgens and Kuipers' recent review of anabolic steroids in the Suggested Readings. Lastly, visit the World Anti-Doping Agency's Web site for a list of prohibited substances (www.wada-ama.org/en/).

mass and performance. Such use is not without its problems (see A Closer Look 5.3).

Estrogen Estrogen is a group of hormones that exerts similar physiological effects. These hormones include estradiole, estrone, and estriol. Estrogen stimulates breast development, female fat deposition, and other secondary sex characteristics (see figure 5.11). During the early part of the menstrual cycle

called the *follicular phase*, LH stimulates the production of androgens in the follicle, which are subsequently converted to estrogens under the influence of FSH. Following ovulation, the *luteal phase* of the menstrual cycle begins, and both estrogens and progesterone are produced by the corpus luteum, a secretory structure occupying the space where the ovum was located (142). How does exercise affect these hormones, and vice versa? In one study (79), the plasma levels of LH,

FIGURE 5.11 Role of estrogen in the development of female secondary sex characteristics and maturation of the ovum.

FIGURE 5.12 Percent change (from resting values) in the plasma FSH, LH, progesterone, and estradiol concentrations during graded exercise in the follicle and luteal phases of the menstrual cycle.

FSH, estradiol, and progesterone were measured at rest and at three different work rates during both the follicular and luteal phases of the menstrual cycle. The patterns of response of these hormones during graded exercise were very similar in the two phases of the menstrual cycle (79). Figure 5.12 shows only small changes in progesterone and estradiol with increasing intensities of work. Given that LH and FSH changed little or not at all during the luteal phase, the small increases in progesterone and estradiol were believed to be due to changes in plasma volume and to a decreased rate of removal rather than an increased rate of secretion (12, 138).

The effect of the phase of the menstrual cycle on exercise metabolism is not clear cut. Some studies have shown that the pattern of substrate use (11) and the respiratory exchange ratio (31) are the same for the two phases of the menstrual cycle. Further, amenorrheic subjects (31) or those taking oral contraceptives (11) responded similarly to eumenorrheic control subjects. In contrast, there is evidence that estradiol decreases glycogen use and increases lipid use to result in an increase in performance (13, 82). Other studies support this observation. Investigators report lower rates of carbohydrate oxidation for exercise at 35% and 60% $\dot{V}O_2$ max (but not at 75% $\dot{V}O_2$ max) during the midluteal phase of the menstrual cycle, compared to the midfollicular phase (57). Consistent with the role that estrogen might play in this process, women who were matched for maximal aerobic power and training with men had a lower rate of glycogen use during a moderate-intensity, prolonged treadmill run

test (134). This finding was supported in a study showing that women (42) respond differently than men (41) to training-induced changes in exercise metabolism. There is clearly a need for additional research to explain discrepancies across studies and to propose a mechanism of action (119, 135). In contrast to this discrepancy, there is general agreement that there are no menstrual cycle phase effects on $\dot{V}O_2$ max, and the lactate, plasma volume, heart rate, and ventilation responses to exercise (152). Further, there does not appear to be an increased risk of heat illness during the luteal phase of the menstrual cycle, even though body temperature is higher (100).

Although the changes in estrogen and progesterone during an acute exercise bout are small, concern is being raised about the effect of chronic heavy exercise on the menstrual cycle of distance runners, gymnasts, and ballet dancers. For example, it has been shown that 29% of endurance athletes have pri-

ASK THE EXPERT 5.1

Reproductive Disorders in Female Athletes
Questions and Answers with Dr. Anne B. Loucks

Dr. Loucks *is Professor of Biological Sciences at Ohio University. She is a productive researcher in the area of reproductive disorders in female athletes, the author of numerous research articles and reviews on this topic, and is recognized internationally as an expert in the field. Dr. Loucks was involved in the development and revision of the American College of Sports Medicine's position stand on the Female Athlete Triad. Based on her reputation as an excellent teacher as well as a recognized researcher, Dr. Loucks was selected to deliver one of the prestigious President's Lectures at the 2002 annual meeting of the American College of Sports Medicine.*

QUESTION #1: Over the past 30 years a great deal of attention has focused on low body fatness as the primary cause of reproductive disorders in female athletes. How has that view changed?

ANSWER: Amongst reproductive endocrinologists that view has been replaced by the opinion that the primary cause of reproductive disorders in female athletes is inadequate daily energy availability, defined as dietary energy intake minus exercise energy expenditure. This implies that a reduction in dietary energy intake is not necessary to induce reproductive disorders, if exercise energy expenditure is high enough. It also implies that reproductive disorders can be prevented by dietary supplementation without any moderation of an exercise regimen.

QUESTION #2: What was the crucial experiment that provided that insight?

ANSWER: There was not one experiment. Rather there was an overwhelming accumulation of scientific criticisms of the reasoning underlying the body fatness hypothesis itself. Many observational studies have found no consistent difference in body composition between regularly menstruating and amenorrheic athletes. In addition, observations in field biology indicate that reproductive function in mammals is dependent on energy availability. Further, animal experiments show that reproductive disorders can be reversed by manipulating energy availability, without any change in body fatness. Finally, several clinical studies were able to disrupt or prevent the disruption of the reproductive system in regularly menstruating women by manipulating energy availability.

QUESTION #3: What do you see as the most important issues remaining to be solved?

ANSWER: The brain depends specifically on blood glucose for energy, and working muscle competes very aggressively against the brain for that glucose. There is some evidence to suggest that the factor controlling reproductive function in women is actually carbohydrate availability rather than energy availability in general. That should be clarified. There is evidence that some women may be much more sensitive to reductions in energy (or carbohydrate) availability than others. It would be helpful to be able to identify those at greater risk so that precautions can be taken to sustain their energy (or carbohydrate) availability. And, of course, effective intervention strategies need to be developed to prevent and to reverse reproductive disorders in athletes.

---

mary (delay of menarche until age sixteen) or secondary (absence of menstruation in women who have had normal menstrual cycles) amenorrhea (147). Special attention is now being directed at the issue of secondary amenorrhea (27). Athletic amenorrhea is associated with chronically low estradiol levels, which can have a deleterious effect on bone mineral content. Osteoporosis, usually associated with the elderly (see chapter 17), is common in athletes with amenorrhea (65). Interested readers are referred to Loucks's review of the possible causes of exercise-induced menstrual cycle irregularities (96). What is most interesting is that exercise itself may not suppress reproductive function, but rather the impact of the energy cost of the exercise on energy availability. For some first-hand insights into this issue, see Ask the Expert 5.1.

Table 5.2 contains a summary of the information on each of the endocrine glands, their secretion(s),

actions, controlling factors, the stimuli that elicit a response, and the effect of exercise on the hormonal response. This would be a good place to stop and review before proceeding to the discussion of the hormonal control of muscle glycogen mobilization and the maintenance of the plasma glucose concentration during exercise.

IN SUMMARY

- Testosterone and estrogen establish and maintain reproductive function and determine secondary sex characteristics.
- Chronic exercise (training) can decrease testosterone levels in males and estrogen levels in females. The latter adaptation has potentially negative consequences related to osteoporosis.

TABLE 5.2 Summary of Endocrine Glands, Their Hormones, Their Action, Factors Controlling Their Secretion, Stimuli That Elicit a Response, and the Effect of Exercise

Endocrine Gland	Hormone	Action	Controlling Factors	Stimuli	Exercise Effect
Anterior pituitary	Growth hormone (GH)	Increases growth, FFA mobilization, and gluconeogenesis; decreases glucose uptake	Hypothalamic GH-releasing hormone; hypothalamic somatostatin	Exercise; "stress"; low blood glucose	↑
	Thyroid-stimulating hormone (TSH)	Increases T_3 and T_4 production and secretion	Hypothalamic TSH-releasing hormone	Low plasma T_3 and T_4	↑
	Adrenocorticotrophic hormone (ACTH)	Increases cortisol synthesis and secretion	Hypothalamic ACTH-releasing hormone	"Stress"; bone breaks; heavy exercise; burns etc.	?
	Gonadotrophins: follicle-stimulating hormone (FSH); luteinizing hormone (LH)	Female: estrogen and progesterone production and ovum development Male: testosterone production and sperm development	Hypothalamic gonadotrophic-releasing hormone Females: plasma estrogen and progesterone Males: plasma testosterone	Cyclic or intermittent firing of neurons in the hypothalamus	Small or no change
	Prolactin	Increases breast milk production	Prolactin-inhibiting hormone (dopamine)	Sucking of nipple	?
	Endorphins	Blocks pain by acting on opiate receptors in brain	ACTH-releasing hormone ???	"Stress"	↑ for exercise ≥ 70% $\dot{V}O_2$ max
Posterior pituitary	Antidiuretic hormone (ADH) (vasopressin)	Decreases water loss at kidney; increases peripheral resistance	Hypothalamic neurons	Plasma volume; plasma osmolality	↑
	Oxytocin	Decreases uterine contractions; milk "let down"	Hypothalamic neurons	Uterine receptors; sucking of nipple	?
Thyroid	Triiodothyronine (T_3); thyroxine (T_4)	Increases metabolic rate, mobilization of fuels, growth	TSH; plasma T_3 and T_4	Low T_3 and T_4	↑ "Free" T_3 and T_4
	Calcitonin	Decreases plasma calcium	Plasma calcium	Elevated plasma calcium	?
Parathyroid	Parathyroid hormone	Increases plasma calcium	Plasma calcium	Low plasma calcium	↑

TABLE 5.2 (Continued)

Endocrine Gland	Hormone	Action	Controlling Factors	Stimuli	Exercise Effect
Adrenal cortex	Cortisol	Increases gluconeogenesis, FFA mobilization and protein synthesis; decreases glucose utilization	ACTH	See ACTH, above	↑ Heavy exercise; ↓ light exercise
	Aldosterone	Increases potassium secretion and sodium reabsorption at kidney	Plasma potassium concentration and renin-angiotensin system	Low blood pressure and plasma volume; elevated plasma potassium and sympathetic activity to kidney	↑
Adrenal medulla	Epinephrine (80%); norepinephrine (20%)	Increases glycogenolysis, FFA mobilization, heart rate, stroke volume, and peripheral resistance	Output of baroreceptors; glucose receptor in hypothalamus; brain and spinal centers	Low blood pressure, and blood glucose; too much "stress"; emotion	↑
Pancreas	Insulin	Increases glucose, amino acid, and FFA uptake into tissues	Plasma glucose and amino acid concentrations; autonomic nervous system	Elevated plasma glucose and amino acid concentrations; decreased epinephrine and norepinephrine	↓
	Glucagon	Increases glucose and FFA mobilization; gluconeogenesis	Plasma glucose and amino acid concentrations; autonomic nervous system	Low plasma glucose and amino acid concentrations; elevated epinephrine and norepinephrine	↑
Testes	Testosterone	Protein synthesis; secondary sex characteristics; sex drive; sperm production	FSH and LH (ICSH)	Increased FSH and LH	Small ↑
Ovaries	Estrogen	Fat deposition; secondary sex characteristics; ovum development	FSH and LH	Increased FSH and LH	Small ↑

HORMONAL CONTROL OF SUBSTRATE MOBILIZATION DURING EXERCISE

The type of substrate and the rate at which it is utilized during exercise depend to a large extent on the intensity and duration of the exercise. During strenuous exercise there is an obligatory demand for carbohydrate oxidation that must be met; fatty acid oxidation cannot substitute. In contrast, there is an increase in fat oxidation during prolonged, moderate exercise as carbohydrate fuels are depleted (66). While diet and the training state of the person are important (see chapters 13, 21, and 23), the factors of intensity and duration of exercise ordinarily have prominence. Because of this, our discussion of the hormonal control of substrate mobilization during exercise will be divided into two parts. The first part will deal with the control of muscle glycogen utilization, and the second part with the control of glucose mobilization from the liver and free fatty acids (FFA) from adipose tissue.

Muscle-Glycogen Utilization

At the onset of most types of exercise, and for the entire duration of very strenuous exercise, muscle glycogen is the primary carbohydrate fuel for muscular work (122). The intensity of exercise, which is inversely related to exercise duration, determines the rate at which muscle glycogen is used as a fuel. Figure 5.13 shows a series of lines describing the rates of glycogen breakdown for various exercise intensities expressed as a percent of $\dot{V}O_2$ max (122). The heavier the exercise, the faster glycogen is broken down. This process of glycogen breakdown (glycogenolysis) is initiated by second messengers, which activate protein kinases in the muscle cell (described in figure 5.3). Plasma epinephrine, a powerful stimulator of cyclic AMP formation when bound to β-adrenergic receptors on a cell, was believed to be primarily responsible for glycogenolysis. Figure 5.14 also shows a family of lines, the slopes of which describe how fast plasma E changes with increasing intensities of exercise (85). Clearly, the data presented in figures 5.13 and 5.14 are consistent with the view that there is a linkage between changes in plasma E during exercise and the increased rate of glycogen degradation. However, there is more to this story.

In order to test the hypothesis that glycogenolysis in muscle is controlled by circulating E during exercise, investigators had subjects take propranolol, a drug that blocks both β_1- and β_2-adrenergic receptors on the cell membrane. This procedure should block glycogenolysis since cyclic AMP formation would be affected. In the control experiment, subjects worked

FIGURE 5.13 Glycogen depletion in the quadriceps muscle during bicycle exercise of increasing exercise intensities.

FIGURE 5.14 Changes in the plasma epinephrine concentration during exercises of different intensities and durations.

for two minutes at an intensity of exercise that caused the muscle glycogen to be depleted to half its initial value, and the muscle lactate concentration to be elevated tenfold. Surprisingly, as shown in figure 5.15, when the subjects took the propranolol and repeated the test on another day, there was no difference in glycogen depletion or lactate formation (59). Other experiments have also shown that β-adrenergic blocking drugs have little effect on slowing the rate of glycogen breakdown during exercise (141). How can this be?

As mentioned in chapter 3, enzymatic reactions in a cell are under the control of both intracellular and extracellular factors. In the aforementioned example with propranolol, plasma E may not have been able to activate adenylate cyclase to form the cyclic AMP needed to activate the protein kinases to initiate glycogen breakdown. However, when a muscle cell is

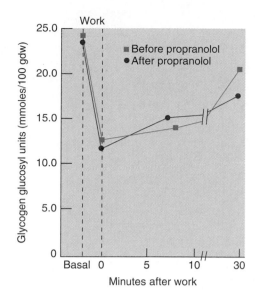

FIGURE 5.15 Changes in muscle glycogen due to two minutes of work at 1,200 kpm/min, before and after propranolol administration. Blocking the beta-adrenergic receptors had no effect on glycogen breakdown.

FIGURE 5.16 The breakdown of muscle glycogen, glycogenolysis, can be initiated by either the Ca++-calmodulin mechanism or the cyclic AMP mechanism. When a drug blocks the β-receptor, glycogenolysis can still occur.

stimulated to contract, Ca++, which is stored in the sarcoplasmic reticulum, floods the cell. Some Ca++ ions are used to initiate contractile events (see chapter 8), but other Ca++ ions bind to calmodulin, which, in turn, activates the protein kinases needed for glycogenolysis (see figure 5.4). In this case, the increased intracellular Ca++ (rather than cAMP) is the initial event stimulating muscle glycogen breakdown. Figure 5.16 summarizes these events. Experiments in which the increased secretion of catecholamines was blocked during exercise confirmed the propranolol experiments, showing that an intact sympathoadrenal system was not necessary to initiate glycogenolysis in skeletal muscle (17).

Observations of glycogen depletion patterns support this view. Individuals who do heavy exercise with one leg will cause elevations in plasma E, which circulates to all muscle cells. The muscle glycogen, however, is depleted only from the exercised leg (71), suggesting that intracellular factors (e.g., Ca++) are more responsible for these events. Further, in experiments in which individuals engaged in intermittent, intense exercise interspersed with a rest period (interval work), the glycogen was depleted faster from fast-twitch fibers (33, 34, 50). The plasma E concentration should be the same outside both fast- and slow-twitch muscle fibers, but the glycogen was depleted at a faster rate from the fibers used in the activity. This is reasonable, since a "resting" muscle fiber should not be using glycogen (or any other fuel) at a high rate. The rate of glycogenolysis would be expected to parallel the rate at which ATP is used by the muscle, and this has been shown to be the case, independent of E

(113). This discussion does not mean that E cannot or does not cause glycogenolysis (18, 153). There is ample evidence to show that a surge of E will, in fact, cause this to occur (77, 128, 129, 130).

IN SUMMARY

■ Glycogen breakdown to glucose in muscle is under the dual control of epinephrine-cyclic AMP and Ca++-calmodulin. The latter's role is enhanced during exercise due to the increase in Ca++ from the sarcoplasmic reticulum. In this way the delivery of fuel (glucose) parallels the activation of contraction.

Blood Glucose Homeostasis During Exercise

As mentioned in the introduction, a focal point of hormonal control systems is the maintenance of the plasma glucose concentration during times of inadequate carbohydrate intake (fasting/starvation) and accelerated glucose removal from the circulation (exercise). In both cases, body energy stores are used to meet the challenge, and the hormonal response to these two different situations, exercise and starvation, is quite similar.

The plasma glucose concentration is maintained through four different processes that:

■ mobilize glucose from liver glycogen stores,

■ mobilize plasma FFA from adipose tissue to spare plasma glucose,

■ synthesize new glucose in the liver (gluconeogenesis) from amino acids, lactic acid, and glycerol, and

■ block glucose entry into cells to force the substitution of FFA as a fuel.

The overall aim of these four processes is to provide fuel for work while maintaining the plasma glucose concentration. This is a major task when you consider that the liver may have only 80 grams of glucose before exercise begins, and the rate of blood glucose oxidation approaches 1 g/min in heavy exercise or in prolonged ($\geq$3 hours) moderate exercise (20, 24).

While the hormones will be presented separately, keep in mind that each of the four processes is controlled by more than one hormone, and all four processes are involved in the adaptation to exercise. Some hormones act in a "permissive" way, or are "slow acting," while others are "fast-acting" controllers of substrate mobilization. For this reason, this discussion of the hormonal control of plasma glucose will be divided into two sections, one dealing with permissive and slow-acting hormones, and the other dealing with fast-acting hormones.

Permissive and Slow-Acting Hormones Thyroxine, cortisol, and growth hormone are involved in the regulation of carbohydrate, fat, and protein metabolism. These hormones are discussed in this section because they either facilitate the actions of other hormones or respond to stimuli in a slow manner. Remember that to act in a permissive manner the hormone concentration doesn't have to change. However, as you will see, there are certain stressful situations in which permissive hormones can achieve such elevated plasma concentrations that they act directly to influence carbohydrate and fat metabolism rather than to simply facilitate the actions of other hormones.

Thyroid Hormones. The discussion of substrate mobilization during exercise must include the thyroid hormones T_3 and T_4, whose free concentrations do not change dramatically from resting to the exercising state. As mentioned earlier, T_3 and T_4 are important in establishing the overall metabolic rate and in allowing other hormones to exert their full effect (permissive hormone). They accomplish this latter function by influencing either the number of receptors on the surface of a cell (for other hormones to interact with), or the affinity of the receptor for the hormone. For example, without T_3, epinephrine has little effect on the mobilization of free fatty acids from adipose tissue. During exercise there is an increase in "free" T_3 due to changes in the binding characteristics of the transport protein (138). T_3 and T_4 are removed from the plasma by tissues during exercise at a greater rate than at rest. In turn, TSH secretion from the anterior pituitary is increased to stimulate the secretion of T_3 and T_4 from the thyroid gland to maintain the plasma level (45). Low levels of T_3 and T_4 (hypothyroid state) would interfere with the ability of other hormones to mobilize fuel for exercise (109, 138).

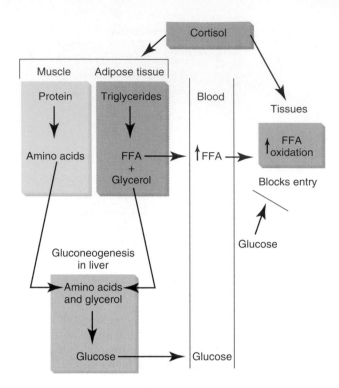

FIGURE 5.17 Role of cortisol in the maintenance of plasma glucose.

Cortisol The primary glucocorticoid in humans is cortisol. As figure 5.17 shows, cortisol stimulates FFA mobilization from adipose tissue, mobilizes tissue protein to yield amino acids for glucose synthesis in the liver (gluconeogenesis), and decreases the rate of glucose utilization by cells (54). There are problems, however, when attempting to describe the cortisol response to exercise. Given the General Adaptation Syndrome (GAS) of Selye, events other than exercise can influence the cortisol response. Imagine how a naive subject might view a treadmill test on first exposure. The wires, noise, nose clip, mouthpiece, and blood sampling could all influence the level of arousal of the subject and result in a cortisol response that is not related to a need to mobilize additional substrate. Results supporting such a proposition were reported in the following study (112). Twelve subjects walked on a treadmill at five times their resting metabolic rate (5 METs) for thirty minutes, and blood samples were taken for cortisol analysis. Ten of the twelve subjects showed a decrease in cortisol due to the exercise, while the other two, who were anxious, had an increase. Clearly, the perception of the subject can influence the cortisol response to mild exercise.

As exercise intensity increases, one might expect the cortisol secretion to increase. This is true, but only within certain limits. For example, Bonen (10) showed that the urinary excretion of cortisol was not changed by exercise at 76% $\dot{V}O_2$ max for ten minutes, but was

FIGURE 5.18 Percent change (from resting values) in the plasma cortisol concentration with increasing exercise intensity.

FIGURE 5.19 Role of plasma growth hormone in the maintenance of plasma glucose.

increased about twofold when the duration was extended to thirty minutes. Davies and Few (26) extended our understanding of the cortisol response to exercise when they studied subjects who completed several one-hour exercise bouts. Each test was set at a constant intensity between 40% and 80% $\dot{V}O_2$ max. Exercise at 40% $\dot{V}O_2$ max resulted in a decrease in plasma cortisol over time, while the response was considerably elevated for exercise at 80% $\dot{V}O_2$ max. Figure 5.18 shows the plasma cortisol concentration measured at sixty minutes into each of the exercise tests plotted against % $\dot{V}O_2$ max. When the exercise intensity exceeded 60% $\dot{V}O_2$ max, the cortisol concentration increased; below that, the cortisol concentration decreased. What caused these changes? Using radioactive cortisol as a tracer, the researchers found that during light exercise cortisol was removed faster than the adrenal cortex secreted it, and during intense exercise the increase in plasma cortisol was due to a higher rate of secretion that could more than match the rate of removal, which had doubled.

What is interesting is that for low-intensity, long-duration exercise where the effects of cortisol would go a long way in maintaining the plasma glucose concentration, the concentration of cortisol does not change very much. Even if it did, the effects on metabolism would not be immediately noticeable. The direct effect of cortisol is mediated through the stimulation of DNA and the resulting mRNA formation, which leads to protein synthesis, a slow process. In essence, cortisol, like thyroxine, exerts a permissive effect on substrate mobilization during acute exercise, allowing other fast-acting hormones such as epinephrine and glucagon to deal with glucose and FFA mobilization. Support for this was provided in a study in which a drug was used to lower plasma cortisol before

and during submaximal exercise; the overall metabolic response was not affected compared to a normal cortisol condition (28). Given that athletic competitions (triathlon, ultra marathon, most team sports) can result in tissue damage, the reason for changes in the plasma cortisol concentration might not be for the mobilization of fuel for exercising muscles. In these situations cortisol's role in dealing with tissue repair might come to the forefront.

Growth Hormone Growth hormone plays a major role in the synthesis of tissue protein, acting either directly or through the enhanced secretion of IGFs from the liver. However, GH can also influence fat and carbohydrate metabolism. Figure 5.19 shows that growth hormone supports the action of cortisol; it decreases glucose uptake by tissue, increases FFA mobilization, and enhances gluconeogenesis in the liver. The net effect is to preserve the plasma glucose concentration.

Describing the plasma GH response to exercise is as difficult as describing cortisol's response to exercise, since GH can also be altered by a wide variety of physical, chemical, and psychological stresses (22, 52, 132). Given that, the earlier comments about cortisol should be kept in mind. Figure 5.20a shows plasma GH to increase with increasing intensities of exercise, achieving, at maximal work, values twenty-five times those at rest (132). Figure 5.20b shows the plasma GH concentration to increase over time during sixty minutes of exercise at 60% $\dot{V}O_2$ max (14). What is interesting, compared to other hormonal responses, is that the trained runners had a higher response compared to a group of nonrunners (see *Fast-Acting Hormones*). By sixty minutes, values for both groups were about five to six times those measured at rest. It must be added that the increased GH response at the same workload, shown by trained individuals, has not been universally observed. Some report lower responses following training (131). In conclusion, GH, a hormone primarily concerned with protein synthesis, can achieve plasma

FIGURE 5.20 (*a*) Percent change (from resting values) in the plasma growth hormone concentration with increasing exercise intensity. (*b*) Percent change (from resting values) in the plasma growth hormone concentration during exercise at 60% V̇O₂ max for runners and nonrunners (controls).

concentrations during exercise that can exert a direct but "slow-acting" effect on carbohydrate and fat metabolism.

IN SUMMARY

- The hormones thyroxine, cortisol, and growth hormone act in a permissive manner to support the actions of other hormones during exercise.
- Growth hormone and cortisol also provide a "slow-acting" effect on carbohydrate and fat metabolism during exercise.

Fast-Acting Hormones In contrast to the aforementioned "permissive" and slow-acting hormones, there are very fast-responding hormones whose actions

FIGURE 5.21 Role of catecholamines in substrate mobilization.

quickly return the plasma glucose to normal. Again, while each will be presented separately, they behave collectively and in a predictable way during exercise to maintain the plasma glucose concentration (19).

Epinephrine and Norepinephrine Epinephrine and norepinephrine have already been discussed relative to muscle glycogen mobilization. However, as figure 5.21 shows, they are also involved in the mobilization of glucose from the liver, FFA from adipose tissue, and may interfere with the uptake of glucose by tissues (118). Although plasma NE can increase ten- to twentyfold during exercise and can achieve a plasma concentration that can exert a physiological effect (126), the primary means by which NE acts is when released from sympathetic neurons onto the surface of the tissue under consideration. The plasma level of NE is usually taken as an index of overall sympathetic nerve activity, but there is evidence that muscle sympathetic nerve activity during exercise may be a better indicator than that of plasma NE (124). Epinephrine, released from the adrenal medulla, is viewed as the primary catecholamine in the mobilization of glucose from the liver.

Figure 5.22 shows plasma E and NE to increase linearly with duration of exercise (70, 110). These changes are related to cardiovascular adjustments to exercise, as well as to the mobilization of fuel. These responses favor the mobilization of glucose and FFA to maintain the plasma glucose concentration. While it is sometimes difficult to separate the effect of E from NE, E seems to be more responsive to changes in the plasma glucose concentration. A low plasma glucose concentration stimulates a receptor in the hypothalamus to increase E secretion while having only a modest effect on plasma NE. In contrast, when the blood pressure is challenged, as during an increased heat load, the primary catecholamine involved is norepinephrine (110). Epinephrine binds to β-adrenergic receptors on the liver and stimulates the breakdown of liver glycogen to form glucose for release into the plasma. For example, when arm exer-

FIGURE 5.22 Percent change (from resting values) in the plasma epinephrine and norepinephrine concentrations during exercise at ~60% $\dot{V}O_2$ max.

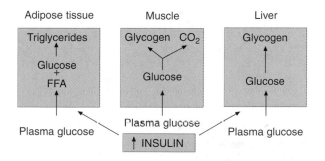

FIGURE 5.23 Changes in plasma epinephrine and norepinephrine responses to a fixed workload over seven weeks of endurance training.

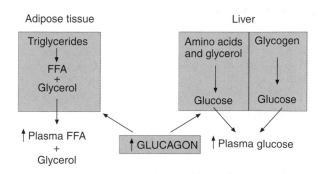

FIGURE 5.24 Effect of insulin and glucagon on glucose and fatty acid uptake and mobilization.

cise is added to existing leg exercise, the adrenal medulla secretes a large amount of E. This causes the liver to release more glucose than muscles are using, and the blood glucose concentration actually increases (87). What happens if we block the effects of E and NE? If β-adrenergic receptors are blocked with propranolol (a β-adrenergic receptor blocking drug), the plasma glucose concentration is more difficult to maintain during exercise, especially if the subject has fasted (141). In addition, since the propranolol blocks β-adrenergic receptors on adipose tissue cells, less FFAs are released and the muscles have to rely more on the limited carbohydrate supply for fuel (44).

Figure 5.23 shows that endurance training causes a very rapid decrease in the plasma E and NE responses to a fixed exercise bout. Within three weeks, the concentration of both catecholamines is greatly reduced (148). Paralleling this rapid decrease in E and NE with endurance exercise training is a reduction in glucose mobilization (102). In spite of this, the plasma glucose concentration is maintained because there is also a reduction in glucose uptake by muscle at the same fixed workload following endurance training (116, 149). Interestingly, during a very stressful event a trained individual has a greater capacity to secrete E than an untrained individual (86). In addition, when exercise is performed at the same relative workload (% $\dot{V}O_2$ max) after training (in contrast to the same fixed workload as in figure 5.23), the plasma NE concentration is higher (53). This suggests that physical training, which stimulates the sympathetic nervous system on a regular basis, increases its capacity to respond to extreme challenges (84).

Insulin and Glucagon These two hormones will be discussed together, since they respond to the same stimuli but exert opposite actions relative to the mobilization of liver glucose and adipose tissue FFA. In fact, it is the ratio of glucagon to insulin that provides control over the mobilization of these fuels (19, 143). Figure 5.24 shows insulin to be the primary hormone involved in the uptake and storage of

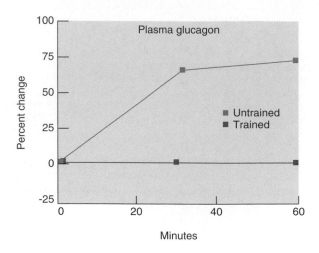

FIGURE 5.25 (*a*) Percent change (from resting values) in the plasma insulin concentration with increasing intensities of exercise. (*b*) Percent change (from resting values) in the plasma insulin concentration during prolonged exercise at 60% V̇O₂ max showing the effect of endurance training on that response.

FIGURE 5.26 Percent change (from resting values) in the plasma glucagon concentration during prolonged exercise at 60% V̇O₂ max showing the effect of endurance training on that response.

glucose and FFA, and glucagon to cause the mobilization of those fuels from storage, as well as increase gluconeogenesis.

Given that insulin is directly involved in the uptake of glucose into tissue, and that glucose uptake by muscle can increase seven- to twentyfold during exercise (37), what should happen to the insulin concentration during exercise? Figure 5.25a shows that the insulin concentration decreases during exercise of increasing intensity (43, 60, 111); this, of course, is an appropriate response. If exercise were associated with an increase in insulin, the plasma glucose would be taken up into all tissues (including adipose tissue) at a faster rate, leading to an immediate hypoglycemia. The lower insulin concentration during exercise favors the mobilization of glucose from the liver and FFA from adipose tissue, both of which are necessary to maintain the plasma glucose concentration. Figure 5.25b shows that the plasma insulin concentration decreases during moderate-intensity, long-term exercise (55).

With plasma insulin decreasing with long-term exercise, it should be no surprise that the plasma glucagon concentration increases (55). This increase in plasma glucagon (shown in figure 5.26) favors the mobilization of FFA from adipose tissue and glucose from the liver, as well as an increase in gluconeogenesis. Overall, the reciprocal responses of insulin and glucagon favor the maintenance of the plasma glucose concentration at a time when the muscle is using plasma glucose at a high rate. Figure 5.26 also shows that following an endurance training program the glucagon response to a fixed exercise task is diminished to the point that there is no increase during exercise. In effect, endurance training allows the plasma glucose concentration to be maintained with little or no change in insulin and glucagon. This is related in part to an increase in glucagon sensitivity in the liver (32), a decrease in glucose uptake by muscle (116), and an increase in the muscle's use of fat as a fuel.

These findings raise several questions. If the plasma glucose concentration is relatively constant during exercise, and the plasma glucose concentration is a primary stimulus for insulin and glucagon secretion, what causes the insulin secretion to decrease and glucagon secretion to increase? The answer lies in the multiple levels of control over hormonal secretion mentioned earlier in the chapter (see figure 5.1). There is no question that changes in the plasma glucose concentration provide an important level of control over the secretion of glucagon and insulin (44). However, when the plasma glucose concentration is relatively constant, the sympathetic nervous system can modify the secretion of insulin and glucagon. Figure 5.27 shows that E and NE stimulate α-adrenergic receptors on the beta cells of the pancreas to decrease insulin secretion during

PANCREAS

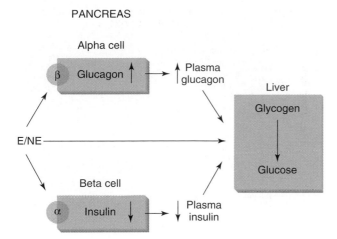

FIGURE 5.27 Effect of epinephrine and norepinephrine on insulin and glucagon secretion from the pancreas during exercise.

FIGURE 5.28 Effect of increased sympathetic nervous system activity on free fatty acid and glucose mobilization during submaximal exercise.

exercise when the plasma glucose concentration is normal. Figure 5.27 also shows that E and NE stimulate β-adrenergic receptors on the alpha cells of the pancreas to increase glucagon secretion when the plasma glucose concentration is normal. These effects have been confirmed through the use of adrenergic receptor blocking drugs. When phentolamine, an α-adrenergic receptor blocker, is given, insulin secretion increases with exercise. When propranolol, a β-adrenergic receptor blocker, is given, the glucagon concentration remains the same or decreases with exercise (97). Figure 5.28 summarizes the effect the sympathetic nervous system has on the mobilization of fuel for muscular work. Endurance training decreases the sympathetic nervous system response to a fixed exercise bout, resulting in less stimulation of adrenergic receptors on the pancreas, and less change in insulin and glucagon.

The observation that plasma insulin decreases with prolonged, submaximal exercise raises another question. How can exercising muscle take up glucose seven to twenty times faster than at rest if the insulin concentration is decreasing? Part of the answer lies in the large (ten- to twentyfold) increase in blood flow to muscle during exercise. Glucose delivery is the product of muscle blood flow and the blood glucose concentration. Therefore, during exercise, more glucose and insulin are delivered to muscle than at rest, and because the muscle is using glucose at a higher rate, a gradient for its facilitated diffusion is created (74, 116, 149). Another part of the answer relates to exercise-induced changes in the number of glucose transporters in the membrane. It has been known for some time that acute (a single bout) and chronic (training program) exercise increase a muscle's sensi-

tivity to insulin such that less insulin is needed to have the same effect on glucose uptake into tissue (61, 75). The effects of insulin and exercise on glucose transport are additive, suggesting that two separate pools of glucose transporters are activated or translocated in the membrane (51, 73, 75, 146). Interestingly, hypoxia brings about the same effect as exercise, but it is not an additive effect, suggesting that hypoxia and exercise recruit the same transporters (16). What is there about exercise that could cause these changes in glucose transporters?

Part of the answer lies in the high intramuscular Ca^{++} concentration that exists during exercise. The Ca^{++} appears to recruit inactive glucose transporters such that more glucose is transported for the same concentration of insulin (16, 67, 74). This improved glucose transport remains following exercise and facilitates the filling of muscle glycogen stores (see chapter 23). Repeated exercise bouts (training) reduce whole-body insulin resistance, making exercise an important part of therapy for the diabetic (74, 105, 157). Consistent with this, bed rest (104) and limb immobilization (115) increase insulin resistance. However, it is clear that glucose transporters in contracting muscle are regulated by more than changes in the calcium concentration. Factors such as protein kinase C, nitric oxide, AMP-activated protein kinase, and others play a role (117, 120, 121).

In summary, figures 5.29a and 5.29b show the changes in epinephrine, norepinephrine, growth hormone, cortisol, glucagon, and insulin to exercise of varying intensity and duration. The decrease in insulin and the increase in all the other hormones favor the

FIGURE 5.29 (*a*) Summary of the hormonal responses to exercise of increasing intensity. (*b*) Summary of the hormonal responses to moderate exercise of long duration.

mobilization of glucose from the liver, FFA from adipose tissue, and gluconeogenesis in the liver, while inhibiting the uptake of glucose. These combined actions maintain homeostasis relative to the plasma glucose concentration so that the central nervous system and the muscles can have the fuel they need.

IN SUMMARY

- Plasma glucose is maintained during exercise by increasing liver glucose mobilization, using more plasma FFA, increasing gluconeogenesis, and decreasing glucose uptake by tissues. The decrease in plasma insulin and the increase in plasma E, NE, GH, glucagon, and cortisol during exercise control these mechanisms to maintain the glucose concentration.
- Glucose is taken up seven to twenty times faster during exercise than at rest—even with the decrease in plasma insulin. The increases in intracellular Ca^{++} and other factors are associated with an increase in the number of glucose transporters that increase the membrane transport of glucose.
- Training causes a reduction in E, NE, glucagon and insulin responses to exercise.

Hormone-Substrate Interaction

In the examples mentioned previously, insulin and glucagon responded as they did during exercise with a normal plasma glucose concentration due to the influence of the sympathetic nervous system. It must be mentioned that if there were a sudden change in the plasma glucose concentration during exercise, these

hormones would respond to that change. For example, if the ingestion of glucose before exercise caused an elevation of plasma glucose, the plasma concentration of insulin would increase. This hormonal change would reduce FFA mobilization and force the muscle to use additional muscle glycogen (1).

During intense exercise, plasma glucagon, GH, cortisol, E, and NE are elevated and insulin is decreased. These hormonal changes favor the mobilization of FFA from adipose tissue that would spare carbohydrate and help maintain the plasma glucose concentration. If this is the case, why does plasma FFA use decrease with increasing intensities of exercise (119)? Part of the answer seems to be that there is an upper limit in the adipose cell's ability to deliver FFA to the circulation during exercise. For example, in trained subjects, the rate of release of FFA from adipose tissue was the highest at 25% $\dot{V}O_2$ max, and decreased at 65% and 85% $\dot{V}O_2$ max (119). Given the fact that the adipose cell is under stronger hormonal stimulation at the higher work rates, the FFA actually appears to be "trapped" in the adipose cell (65, 119). This may be due to a variety of factors, one of which is lactate. Figure 5.30a shows that as the blood lactate concentration increases, the plasma FFA concentration decreases (72). The elevated lactate has been linked to an increase in alpha glycerol phosphate, the activated form of glycerol needed to make triglycerides. In effect, as fast as the FFA becomes available from the breakdown of triglycerides, the alpha glycerol phosphate recycles the FFA to generate a new triglyceride molecule (see figure 5.30b). The result is that the FFAs are not released from the adipose cell (108). Other explanations of the reduced availability of adipose tissue FFA during heavy exercise include a reduced blood supply to adipose tissue resulting in less FFA to transport to muscle (119), and an inade-

FIGURE 5.30 (*a*) Changes in plasma free fatty acids due to increases in lactic acid. (*b*) Effect of lactic acid on the mobilization of free fatty acids from the adipose cell.

quate amount of albumin, the plasma protein needed to transport the FFA in the plasma (65). The result is that FFAs are not released from the adipose cell, the plasma FFA level falls, and the muscle must use more carbohydrate as a fuel. One of the effects of endurance training is to decrease the lactate concentration at any fixed work rate. Such an adaptation would reduce the inhibition of this mobilization of FFA from adipose tissue and allow the trained person to use more fat as a fuel, thus sparing the limited carbohydrate stores and improving performance.

IN SUMMARY

■ The plasma FFA concentration decreases during heavy exercise even though the adipose cell is stimulated by a variety of hormones to increase triglyceride breakdown to FFA and glycerol. This may be due to (a) the high levels of lactate during heavy exercise that promote the resynthesis of triglycerides, (b) an inadequate blood flow to adipose tissue, or (c) insufficient albumin needed to transport the FFA in the plasma.

STUDY QUESTIONS

1. Draw and label a diagram of a negative feedback mechanism for hormonal control using cortisol as an example.
2. List the factors that can influence the blood concentration of a hormone.
3. Discuss the use of testosterone and growth hormone as aids to increase muscle size and strength, and discuss the potential long-term consequences of such use.
4. List each endocrine gland, the hormone(s) secreted from that gland, and its (their) action(s).
5. Describe the two mechanisms by which muscle glycogen is broken down to glucose (glycogenolysis) for use in glycolysis. Which one is activated at the same time as muscle contraction?
6. Identify the four mechanisms involved in maintaining the blood glucose concentration.
7. Draw a summary graph of the changes in the following hormones with exercise of increasing intensity or duration: epinephrine, norepinephrine, cortisol, growth hormone, insulin, and glucagon.
8. What is the effect of training on the responses of epinephrine, norepinephrine, and glucagon to the same exercise task?
9. Briefly explain how glucose can be taken into the muscle at a high rate during exercise when plasma insulin is reduced. Include the role of glucose transporters.
10. Explain how free fatty acid mobilization from the adipose cell decreases during maximal work in spite of the cell being stimulated by all the hormones to break down triglycerides.
11. Discuss the effect of glucose ingestion on the mobilization of free fatty acids during exercise.

SUGGESTED READING

Hartgens, F., and H. Kuipers. 2004. Effects of androgenic-anabolic steroids in athletes. *Sports Medicine* 34(8):513–54.

REFERENCES

1. Ahlborg, G., and P. Felig. 1976. Influence of glucose ingestion on fuel-hormone response during prolonged exercise. *Journal of Applied Physiology* 41:683–88.
2. Alen, M., A. Pakarinen, and K. Hakkinen. 1993. Effects of prolonged training on serum thyrotropin and thyroid hormones in elite strength athletes. *Journal of Sports Science* 11:493–97.
3. Alen, M., and P. Rahkila. 1988. Anabolic-androgenic steroid effects on endocrinology and lipid metabolism in athletes. *Sports Medicine* 6:327–32.
4. Almon, R. R., and D. C. Dubois. 1990. Fiber-type discrimination in disuse and glucocorticoid-induced atrophy. *Medicine and Science in Sports and Exercise* 22(3):304–11.
5. American College of Sports Medicine. 1984. The use of anabolic-androgenic steroids in sports. In *Position Stands and Opinion Statements*. Indianapolis: The American College of Sports Medicine.
6. Arce, J. C., M. M. De Souza, L. S. Pescatello, and A. A. Luciano. 1993. Subclinical alterations in hormone and semen profile in athletes. *Fertility-Sterility* 59:398–404.
7. Bahrke, M. S., C. E. Yesalis III, and J. E. Wright. 1990. Psychological and behavioural effects of endogenous testosterone levels and anabolic-androgenic steroids among males: A review. *Sports Medicine* 10(5):303–37.
8. Bhasin, S., L. Woodhouse, T. Storer, and W. Androgen. 2003. Effects on body composition. *Science Direct* S63–S71.
9. Bhasin, S., T. W. Storer, N. Berman, C. Callegari, B. Clevenger, J. Phillips, T. J. Bunnell, R. Tricker, A. Shirazi, and R. Casaburi. 1996. The effects of supraphysiologic doses of testosterone on muscle size and strength in normal men. *New England Journal of Medicine* 335(1):1–7.
10. Bonen, A. 1976. Effects of exercise on excretion rates of urinary free cortisol. *Journal of Applied Physiology* 40:155–58.
11. Bonen, A., F. W. Haynes, and T. E. Graham. 1991. Substrate and hormonal responses to exercise in women using oral contraceptives. *Journal of Applied Physiology* 70(5):1917–27.
12. Bunt, J. C. 1986. Hormonal alterations due to exercise. *Sports Medicine* 3:331–45.
13. ———. 1990. Metabolic actions of estradiol: Significance for acute and chronic exercise responses. *Medicine and Science in Sports and Exercise* 22(3):286–90.
14. Bunt, J. C. et al. 1986. Sex and training differences in human growth hormone levels during prolonged exercise. *Journal of Applied Physiology* 61:1796–1801.
15. Cannon, W. B. 1953. *Bodily Changes in Pain, Hunger, Fear and Rage*. 2d ed. Boston: Charles T. Branford Company.
16. Cartee, G. D., A. G. Douen, T. Ramlal, A. Klip, and J. O. Holloszy. 1991. Stimulation of glucose transport in skeletal muscle by hypoxia. *Journal of Applied Physiology* 70(4):1593–1600.
17. Cartier, L., and P. D. Gollnick. 1985. Sympathoadrenal system and activation of glycogenolysis during muscular exercise. *Journal of Applied Physiology* 58:1122–27.
18. Christensen, N. J., and H. Galbo. 1983. Sympathetic nervous activity during exercise. *Annual Review of Physiology* 45:139–53.
19. Coggan, A. R. 1991. Plasma glucose metabolism during exercise in humans. *Sports Medicine* 11:102–24.
20. Coggan, A. R., and E. F. Coyle. 1991. Carbohydrate ingestion during prolonged exercise: Effects on metabolism and performance. In *Exercise and Sport Sciences Reviews*, vol. 19, ed. J. Holloszy, 1–40. Baltimore: Lippincott Williams & Wilkins.
21. Convertino, V. A., L. C. Keil, and J. E. Greenleaf. 1983. Plasma volume, renin and vasopressin responses to graded exercise after training. *Journal of Applied Physiology: Respiratory, Environmental and Exercise Physiology* 54:508–14.
22. Copinschi, G. et al. 1967. Effect of various blood-sampling procedures on serum levels of immuno-reactive human growth hormone. *Metabolism: Clinical and Experimental* 16:402–9.
23. Cowart, V. S. 1988. Human growth hormone: The latest ergogenic aid. *Physician and Sportsmedicine* 16(3):175–85.
24. Coyle, E. F. 1995. Substrate utilization during exercise in active people. *American Journal of Clinical Nutrition* 61(suppl.):968S–979S.
25. Cumming, D. C. et al. 1986. Reproductive hormone increases in response to acute exercise in men. *Medicine and Science in Sports and Exercise* 18:369–73.
26. Davies, C. T. M., and J. D. Few. 1973. Effects of exercise on adrenocorticol function. *Journal of Applied Physiology* 35:887–91.
27. De Cree, C. 1998. Sex steroid metabolism and menstrual irregularities in the exercising female. A review. *Sports Medicine* 25:369–406.
28. Del Corral, Pedro, E. T. Howley, M. Hartsell, M. Ashraf, and M. S. Younger. 1998. Metabolic effects of low cortisol during exercise in humans. *Journal of Applied Physiology* 84:939–47.
29. De Piccoli, B., F. Giada, A. Benettin, F. Sartori, and E. Piccolo. 1991. Anabolic steroid use in body builders: An echocardiographic study of left ventricle morphology and function. *Journal of Sports Medicine* 12(4):408–12.
30. De Souza, M. J., J. C. Arce, L. S. Pescatello, H. S. Scherzer, and A. A. Luciano. 1994. Gonadal hormones and semen quality in male runners. *International Journal of Sports Medicine* 15:383–91.
31. De Souza, M. J., M. S. Maguire, K. R. Rubin, and C. M. Maresh. 1990. Effects of menstrual phase and amenorrhea on exercise performance in runners. *Medicine and Science in Sports and Exercise* 22(5):575–80.
32. Drouin, R., C. Lavoie, J. Bourque, F. Ducros, D. Poisson, and J. L. Chiasson. 1998. Increased hepatic glucose production response to glucagon in trained subjects. *American Journal of Physiology* 274 (1 Pt 1):E23–28.
33. Edgerton, V. R. et al. 1975. Glycogen depletion in specific types of human skeletal muscle fibers in intermittent and continuous exercise. In *Metabolic Adaptation to Prolonged Physical Exercise*, ed. H. Howald and J. R. Poortmans, 402–15. Verlag Basel, Switzerland: Birkhauser.
34. Essen, B. 1978. Glycogen depletion of different fibre types in human skeletal muscle during intermittent and continuous exercise. *Acta Physiologica Scandinavica* 103:446–55.
35. Euler, U. S. von. 1969. Sympatho-adrenal activity and physical exercise. In *Biochemistry of Exercise, Medicine and Sport 3*, ed. J. R. Poortmans, 170–81. New York: Karger, Basal.
36. Farrell, P. A. 1985. Exercise and endorphins—male responses. *Medicine and Science in Sports and Exercise* 17:89–93.
37. Felig, P., and J. Wahren. 1975. Fuel homeostasis in exercise. *The New England Journal of Medicine* 293:1078–84.
38. Fox, S. I. 2002. *Human Physiology*. New York: McGraw-Hill Companies.
39. Fraioli, F. et al. 1980. Physical exercise stimulates marked concomitant release of β-endorphin and adrenocorticotrophic hormone (ACTH) in peripheral blood in man. *Experientia* 36:987–89.
40. Francesconi, R. P., M. Sawka, and K. B. Pandolf. 1983. Hypohydration and heat acclimatization: Plasma renin and aldosterone during exercise. *Journal of Applied Physiology: Respiratory, Environmental and Exercise Physiology* 55:1790–94.

41. Friedlander, A. L., G. A. Casazza, M. A. Horning, M. J. Huie, and G. A. Brooks. 1997. Training-induced alterations of glucose flux in men. *Journal of Applied Physiology* 82:1360–69.

42. Friedlander, A. L., G. A. Casazza, M. A. Horning, M. J. Huie, M. F. Piacentini, J. K. Trimmer, and G. A. Brooks. 1998. Training-induced alterations of carbohydrate metabolism in women: Women respond differently from men. *Journal of Applied Physiology* 85:1176–86.

43. Galbo, H., J. J. Holst, and N. J. Christensen. 1975. Glucagon and plasma catecholamine responses to graded and prolonged exercise in man. *Journal of Applied Physiology* 38:70–76.

44. Galbo, H. et al. 1976. Glucagon and plasma catecholamines during beta-receptor blockade in exercising man. *Journal of Applied Physiology* 40:855–63.

45. Galbo, H. et al. 1977. Thyroid and testicular hormone responses to graded and prolonged exercise in man. *European Journal of Applied Physiology* 36:101–6.

46. Ganong, W. F. 1979. *Review of Medical Physiology.* Los Altos, CA: Lange Medical Publications.

47. Godfrey, R. J., Z. Madgwich., and G. P. Whyte. 2003. The exercise-induced growth hormone response in athletes. *Sport Medicine* 32(8):599–613.

48. Goldfarb, A. H., B. D. Hatfield, D. Armstrong, and J. Potts. 1990. Plasma beta-endorphin concentration: Response to intensity and duration of exercise. *Medicine and Science in Sports and Exercise* 22(2):241–44.

49. Goldfarb, A. H., B. D. Hatfield, J. Potts, and D. Armstrong. 1991. Beta-endorphin time course response to intensity of exercise: Effect of training status. *Journal of Sports Medicine* 12(3):264–68.

50. Gollnick, P. D. et al. 1975. Glycogen depletion patterns in human skeletal muscle fibers after varying types and intensities of exercise. In *Metabolic Adaptation to Prolonged Physical Exercise*, ed. H. Howald and J. R. Poortmans, 416–21. Verlag Basel, Switzerland: Birkhauser.

51. Goodyear, L. J., and B. B. Kahn. 1998. Exercise, glucose transport, and insulin sensitivity. *Annual Review of Medicine* 49:235–61.

52. Greenwood, F. C., and J. Landon. 1966. Growth hormone secretion in response to stress in man. *Nature* 210:540–41.

53. Greiwe, J. S., R. C. Hickner, S. D. Shah, P. E. Cryer, and J. O. Holloszy. 1999. Norepinephrine response to exercise at the same relative intensity before and after endurance exercise training. *Journal of Applied Physiology* 86:531–35.

54. Guyton, A. C. 1986. *Textbook of Medical Physiology*, 7th ed. Philadelphia: W. B. Saunders.

55. Gyntelberg, F. et al. 1977. Effect of training on the response of plasma glucagon to exercise. *Journal of Applied Physiology: Respiratory, Environmental and Exercise Physiology* 43:302–5.

56. Hackney, A. C. 1989. Endurance training and testosterone levels. *Sports Medicine* 8(2):117–27.

57. Hackney, A. C., M. A. McCracken-Compton, and B. Ainsworth. 1994. Substrate responses to submaximal exercise in the midfollicular and midluteal phases of the menstrual cycle. *International Journal of Sport Nutrition* 4:299–308.

58. Hameed, M., S. D. R. Harridge, and G. Goldspink. 2002. Sarcopenia and hypertrophy: A role for insulin-like growth factor-I in aged muscle? *Exercise and Sport Sciences Reviews* 15–19.

59. Harris, R. C., J. Bergström, and E. Hultman. 1971. The effect of propranolol on glycogen metabolism during exercise. In *Muscle Metabolism During Exercise*, ed. B. Pernow and B. Saltin, 301–5. New York: Plenum Press.

60. Hartley, L. H. et al. 1972. Multiple hormonal responses to graded exercise in relation to physical training. *Journal of Applied Physiology* 33:602–6.

61. Heath, G. W. et al. 1983. Effect of exercise and lack of exercise on glucose tolerance and insulin sensitivity. *Journal of Applied Physiology: Respiratory, Environmental and Exercise Physiology* 55:512–17.

62. Hickson, R. C., S. M. Czerwinski, M. T. Falduto, and A. P. Young. 1990. Glucocorticoid antagonism by exercise and androgenic-anabolic steroids. *Medicine and Science in Sports and Exercise* 22(3):331–40.

63. Hickson, R. C., and J. R. Marone. 1993. Exercise and inhibition of glucocorticoid-induced muscle atrophy. In *Exercise and Sport Sciences Reviews*, vol. 21, ed. J. O. Holloszy, 135–68, Baltimore: Lippincott Williams & Wilkins.

64. Highet, R. 1989. Athletic amenorrhea: An update on aetiology, complications, and management. *Sports Medicine* 7:82–108.

65. Hodgetts, V., S. W. Coppack, K. N. Frayn, and T. D. R. Hockaday. 1991. Factors controlling fat mobilization from human subcutaneous adipose tissue during exercise. *The American Physiological Society*, 445.

66. Holloszy, J. O., W. M. Kohrt, and P. A. Hansen. 1998. The regulation of carbohydrate and fat metabolism during and after exercise. *Frontiers of Bioscience* 3:D1011–27.

67. Holloszy, J. O., and H. T. Narahara. 1967. Enhanced permeability of sugar associated with muscle contraction: Studies of the role of Ca^{++}. *Journal of General Physiology* 50:551–62.

68. Howley, E. T. 1976. The effect of different intensities of exercise on the excretion of epinephrine and norepinephrine. *Medicine and Science in Sports* 8:219–22.

69. ———. 1980. The excretion of catecholamines as an index of exercise stress. In *Exercise in Health and Disease*, ed. F. J. Nagle and H. J. Montoye, 171–83. Springfield, IL: Charles C Thomas.

70. Howley, E. T. et al. 1983. Effect of hyperoxia on metabolic and catecholamine responses to prolonged exercise. *Journal of Applied Physiology: Respiratory, Environmental and Exercise Physiology* 54:54–63.

71. Hultman, E. 1967. Physiological role of muscle glycogen in man with special reference to exercise. In *Circulation Research XX and XXI*, ed. C. B. Chapman, 1–99 and 1–114. New York: The American Heart Association.

72. Issekutz, B., and H. Miller. 1962. Plasma free fatty acids during exercise and the effect of lactic acid. *Proceedings of the Society of Experimental Biology and Medicine* 110:237–39.

73. Ivy, J. L. 1997. Role of exercise training in the prevention and treatment of insulin resistance and non-insulin-dependent diabetes mellitus. *Sports Medicine* 24:321–36.

74. Ivy, J. 1987. The insulin-like effects of muscle contraction. In *Exercise and Sport Sciences Reviews*, ed. K. B. Pandolf, vol. 15, 29–51. New York: Macmillan.

75. Ivy, J. L. et al. 1983. Exercise training and glucose uptake by skeletal muscle in rats. *Journal of Applied Physiology: Respiratory, Environmental and Exercise Physiology* 55:1393–96.

76. James, D. E. 1995. The mammalian facilitative glucose transporter family. *International Union Physiology of Science/American Physiology Society* 10:67–71.

77. Jasson, E., P. Hjemdahl, and L. Kaijser. 1986. Epinephrine-induced changes in carbohydrate metabolism during exercise in male subjects. *Journal of Applied Physiology* 60:1466–70.

78. Jensen, J., H. Oftebro, B. Breigan, A. Johnsson, K. Ahlin, H. D. Meen, S. B. Stromme, and H. A. Dahl. 1991. Comparison of changes in testosterone concentrations after strength and endurance exercise in well trained men. *European Journal of Applied Physiology and Occupational Physiology* 63:467–71.

79. Jurkowski, J. E. et al. 1978. Ovarian hormonal responses to exercise. *Journal of Applied Physiology: Respiratory, Environmental and Exercise Physiology* 44:109–14.

80. Kargotich, S., C. Goodman, D. Keast, R. W. Fry, P. Garcia-Webb, P. M. Crawford, and A. R. Morton. 1997. Influence of exercise-induced plasma volume changes on the interpretation of biochemical data following high-intensity exercise. *Clinical Journal of Sports Medicine* 7:185–91.

81. Keizer H. A., and A. D. Rogol. 1990. Physical exercise and menstrual cycle alterations: What are the mechanisms? *Sports Medicine* 10(4):218–35.

82. Kendrick, Z. V., and G. S. Ellis. 1991. Effect of estradiol on tissue glycogen metabolism and lipid availability in exercised male rats. *Journal of Applied Physiology* 71(5):1694–99.

83. King, D. S., R. L. Sharp, M. D. Vukovich, G. A. Brown, T. A. Reifenrath, N. L. Uhl, and K. A. Parsons. 1999. Effect of oral androstenedione on serum testosterone and adaptations to resistance training in young men: A randomized controlled trial. *Journal of the American Medical Association* 281:2020–28.

84. Kjaer, M. 1998. Adrenal medulla and exercise training. *European Journal of Applied Physiology* 77:195–99.

85. Kjaer, M. 1989. Epinephrine and some other hormonal responses to exercise in man: With special reference to physical training. *International Journal of Sports Medicine* 10:2–15.

86. Kjaer, M., and H. Galbo. 1988. Effects of physical training on the capacity to secrete epinephrine. *Journal of Applied Physiology* 64:11–16.

87. Kjaer, M., B. Kiens, M. Hargreaves, and E. A. Richter. 1991. Influence of active muscle mass on glucose homeostasis during exercise in humans. *Journal of Applied Physiology* 71(2):552–57.

88. Kostek, M. C., M. J. Delmonico, J. B. Reucgekm, S. M. Roth, S. M. Douglass, R. E. Ferrell, and B. F. Hurley. 2005. Muscle strength response to strength training is influenced by insulin-like growth factor 1 genotype in older adults. *Journal of Applied Physiology* 98:2147–54.

89. Kuipers, H., J. A. G. Wijnen, F. Hartgens, and S. M. M. Willems. 1991. Influence of anabolic steroids on body composition, blood pressure, lipid profile and liver functions in body builders. *International Journal of Sports Medicine* 12(4):413–18.

90. Kutscher, E. C., B. C. Lund, and P. J. Perry. 2002. Anabolic steroids: A review for the clinician. *Sports Medicine* 32:285–96.

91. Langenfeld, M. E., L. S. Hart, and P. C. Kao. 1987. Plasma β-endorphin responses to one-hour bicycling and running at 60% max. *Medicine and Science in Sports and Exercise* 19:83–86.

92. Laycock, J. F., and P. H. Wise. 1983. *Essential Endocrinology.* New York: Oxford University Press.

93. Lebrun, C. M. 1994. The effect of the phase of the menstrual cycle and the birth control pill on athletic performance. *Clinical Sports Medicine* 13:419–41.

94. Ljunghall, S. et al. 1986. Prolonged low-intensity exercise raises the serum parathyroid hormone levels. *Clinical Endocrinology* 25:535–42.

95. Ljunghall, S. et al. 1988. Increase in serum parathyroid hormone levels after prolonged exercise. *Medicine and Science in Sports and Exercise* 20:122–25.

96. Loucks, A. B. 2001. Physical health of the female athlete: Observations, effects, and causes of reproductive disorders. *Canadian Journal of Applied Physiology* 26 (Suppl.): S176–85.

97. Luyckx, A. S., and P. J. Lefebvre. 1974. Mechanisms involved in the exercise-induced increase in glucagon secretion in rats. *Diabetes* 23:81–93.

98. Macintyre, J. G. 1987. Growth hormone and athletes. *Sports Medicine* 4:129–42.

99. Maher, J. T. et al. 1975. Aldosterone dynamics during graded exercise at sea level and high altitude. *Journal of Applied Physiology* 39:18–22.

100. Marsh, S. A., and D. G. Jenkins. 2002. Physiological responses to the menstrual cycle: Implications for the development of heat illness in female athletes. *Sports Medicine* 32(10):601–14.

101. McArthur, J. W. 1985. Endorphins and exercise in females: Possible connection with reproductive dysfunction. *Medicine and Science in Sports and Exercise* 17:82–88.

102. Mendenhall, L. A., S. C. Swanson, D. L. Habash, and A. R. Coggan. 1994. Ten days of exercise training reduces glucose production and utilization during moderate-intensity exercise. *American Journal of Physiology* 266(1 Pt 1):E136–E143.

103. Metsrinne, K. 1988. Effect of exercise on plasma renin substrate. *International Journal of Sports Medicine* 9:267–69.

104. Mikines, K. J., E. A. Richter, F. Dela, and H. Galbo. 1991. Seven days of bed rest decrease insulin action on glucose uptake in leg and whole body. *Journal of Applied Physiology* 70(3):1245–54.

105. Mikines, K. J., B. Sonne, B. Tronier, and H. Galbo. 1989. Effects of acute exercise and detraining on insulin action in trained men. *Journal of Applied Physiology* 66(2):704–11.

106. Moffatt, R. J., M. B. Wallace, and S. P. Sady. 1990. Effects of anabolic steroids on lipoprotein profiles of female weight lifters. *Physician and Sportsmedicine* 18(9):106–15.

107. Morgan, W. P. 1985. Affective beneficence of vigorous physical activity. *Medicine and Science in Sports and Exercise* 17:94–100.

108. Paul, P. 1970. FFA metabolism of normal dogs during steady-state exercise at different work loads. *Journal of Applied Physiology* 28:127–32.

109. ———. 1971. Uptake and oxidation of substrates in the intact animal during exercise. In *Muscle Metabolism During Exercise*, ed. B. Pernow and B. Saltin, 225–48. New York: Plenum Press.

110. Powers, S. K., E. T. Howley, and R. H. Cox. 1982. A differential catecholamine response during prolonged exercise and passive heating. *Medicine and Science in Sports and Exercise* 14:435–39.

111. Pruett, E. D. R. 1970. Glucose and insulin during prolonged work stress in men living on different diets. *Journal of Applied Physiology* 28:199–208.

112. Raymond, L. W., J. Sode, and J. R. Tucci. 1972. Adrenocorticotrophic response to non-exhaustive muscular exercise. *Acta Endocrinologica* 70:73–80.

113. Ren, J. M., and E. Hultman. 1990. Regulation of phosphorylase a activity in human skeletal muscle. *Journal of Applied Physiology* 69(3):919–23.

114. Rennie, M. J. 2003. Claims for the anabolic effects of growth hormone: A case of the emperor's new clothes? *British Journal of Sports Medicine* 37:100–05.

115. Richter, E. A., B. Kiens, M. Mizuno, and S. Strange. 1989. Insulin action in human thighs after one-legged immobilization. *Journal of Applied Physiology* 67(1):19–23.

116. Richter, E. A., S. Kristiansen, J. Wojtaszewski, J. R. Daugaard, S. Asp, P. Hespel, and B. Kiens. 1998. Training effects of muscle glucose transport during exercise. *Advances in Experimental and Medical Biology* 441:107–16.

117. Richter, E. A., W. Derave, and J.F.P. Wojtaszewski. 2001. Glucose, exercise and insulin: Emerging concepts. *Journal of Physiology* 535:313–22.

118. Rizza, R. et al. 1979. Differential effects of epinephrine on glucose production and disposal in man. *American Journal of Physiology* 237:E356–E362.

119. Romijn, J. A., E. F. Coyle, L. S. Sidossis, A. Gastaldelli, J. F. Horowitz, E. Endert, and R. R. Wolfe. 1993. Regulation of endogenous fat and carbohydrate metabolism in relation to exercise intensity and duration. *The American Physiological Society* E380–E391.

120. Ryder, J. W., A. V. Chibalin, and J. R. Zierath. 2001. Intracellular mechanisms underlying increases in glucose uptake in response to insulin or exercise in skeletal muscle. *Acta Physiologica Scandinavica* 171:249–57.

121. Sakamoto, K. and L. Goodyear. 2002. Exercise effects on muscle insulin signaling and action. Invited review: intracellular signaling in contracting skeletal muscle. *Journal of Applied Physiology* 93:369–83.

122. Saltin, B., and J. Karlsson. 1971. Muscle glycogen utilization during work of different intensities. In *Muscle Metabolism During Exercise*, ed. B. Pernow and B. Saltin, 289–99. New York: Plenum Press.

123. Schwarz, L., and W. Kindermann. 1992. Changes in β-endorphin levels in response to aerobic and anaerobic exercise. *Sports Medicine* 13(1):25–36.

124. Seals, D. R., R. G. Victor, and A. L. Mark. 1988. Plasma norepinephrine and muscle sympathetic discharge during rhythmic exercise in humans. *Journal of Applied Physiology* 65(2):940–44.

125. Selye, H. 1976. *The Stress of Life*. New York: McGraw-Hill.

126. Silverberg, A. B. et al. 1978. Norepinephrine: Hormone and neurotransmitter in man. *American Journal of Physiology* 234:E252–E256.

127. Sonksen, P. H. 2001. Insulin, growth hormone and sport. *Journal of Endocrinology* 170:13–25.

128. Spriet, L. L., J. M. Ren, and E. Hultman. 1988. Epinephrine infusion enhances muscle glycogenolysis during prolonged electrical stimulation. *Journal of Applied Physiology* 64:1439–44.

129. Stainsby, W. N., C. Sumners, and G. M. Andrew. 1984. Plasma catecholamines and their effect on blood lactate and muscle lactate output. *Journal of Applied Physiology* 57:321–25.

130. Stainsby, W. N., C. Sumners, and P. D. Eitzman. 1985. Effects of catecholamines on lactic acid output during progressive working contractions. *Journal of Applied Physiology* 59:1809–14.

131. Stokes, K. 2003. Growth hormone responses to submaximal and sprint exercise. *Growth Hormone and IGF Research.* 13:225–238.

132. Sutton, J., and L. Lazarus. 1976. Growth hormone in exercise: Comparison of physiological and pharmacological stimuli. *Journal of Applied Physiology* 41:523–27.

133. Taafe, D. R., L. Pruitt, J. Reim, R. L. Hintz, G. Butterfield, A. R. Hoffman, and R. Marcus. 1994. Effect of recombinant human growth hormone on the muscle strength response to resistance exercise in elderly men. *Journal of Clinical Endocrinology Metabolism* 79:1361–66.

134. Tarnopolsky, L. J., J. D. MacDougall, S. A. Atkinson, M. A. Tarnopolsky, and J. R. Sutton. 1990. Gender differences in substrate for endurance exercise. *Journal of Applied Physiology* 68(1):302–8.

135. Tate, C. A., and R. W. Holtz. 1998. Gender and fat metabolism during exercise: A review. *Canadian Journal of Applied Physiology* 23:570–82.

136. Taylor, W. M. 1988. Synthetic human growth hormone: A call for federal control. *Physician and Sportsmedicine* 16(3): 189–92.

137. Tepperman, J., and H. M. Tepperman. 1987. *Metabolic and Endocrine Physiology*, 5th ed. Chicago: Year Book Medical Publishers.

138. Terjung, R. 1979. Endocrine response to exercise. In *Exercise and Sport Sciences Reviews*, vol. 7, ed. R. S. Hutton and D. I. Miller, 153–79. New York: Macmillan.

139. Thorn, P., J. S. Floras, P. Hoffmann, and D. R. Seals. 1990. Endorphins and exercise: Physiological mechanisms and clinical implications. *Medicine and Science in Sports and Exercise* 22(4):417–28.

140. Urhausen, A., R. Holpes, and W. Kindermann. 1989. One- and two-dimensional echocardiography in bodybuilders using anabolic steroids. *European Journal of Applied Physiology* 58:633–40.

141. Van Baak, M. A. 1988. β-adrenoceptor blockade and exercise: An update *Sports Medicine* 4:209–25.

142. Vander, A. J., J. H. Sherman, and D. S. Luciano. 1985. *Human Physiology: The Mechanisms of Body Function*, 4th ed. New York: McGraw-Hill Companies.

143. Voet, D., and J. G. Voet. 1995. *Biochemistry*. New York: John Wiley & Sons.

144. Vogel, R. B. et al. 1985. Increase of free and total testosterone during submaximal exercise in normal males. *Medicine and Science in Sports and Exercise* 17:119–23.

145. Wade, C. E. 1984. Response, regulation, and actions of vasopressin during exercise: A review. *Medicine and Science in Sports and Exercise* 16:506–11.

146. Wallberg-Henriksson, H., S. H. Constable, D. A. Young, and J. O. Holloszy. 1988. Glucose transport into rat skeletal muscle: Interaction between exercise and insulin. *Journal of Applied Physiology* 65(2):909–13.

147. Weicker, H. et al. 1984. Changes in sexual hormones with female top athletes. *International Journal of Sports Medicine* 5:200–02.

148. Winder, W. W. et al. 1978. Time course of sympathoadrenal adaptation to endurance exercise training in man. *Journal of Applied Physiology: Respiratory, Environmental and Exercise Physiology* 45:370–74.

149. Wojtaszewski, J. F., and E. A. Richter. 1998. Glucose utilization during exercise: Influence of endurance training. *Acta Physiologica Scandinavica* 162:351–58.

150. Wright, J. E. 1980. Anabolic steroids and athletics. In *Exercise and Sport Sciences Reviews*, vol. 8, ed. R. S. Hutton and D. I. Miller, 149–202. New York: Macmillan.

151. ———. 1982. *Anabolic Steroids and Sports*, vol. 2. New York: Sports Science Consultants.

152. Xanne A. K., De Jonge, Janse. 2003. Effects of the menstrual cycle on exercise performance. *Sports Medicine* 33(11):833–51.

153. Yakovlev, N. N., and A. A. Viru. 1985. Adrenergic regulation of adaptation to muscular activity. *International Journal of Sports Medicine* 6:255–65.

154. Yarasheski, K. E. 1994. Growth hormone effects on metabolism, body composition, muscle mass, and strength. *Exercise Sports Science Review* 22:285–312.

155. Yesalis, C. E., and M. S. Bahrke. 1995. Anabolic-androgenic steroids: Current issues. *Sports Medicine* 19:341–57.

156. Yesalis, C. E., J. E. Wright, and M. S. Bahrke. 1989. Epidemiological and policy issues in the measurement of the long term health effects of anabolic-androgenic steroids. *Sports Medicine* 8(3):129–38.

157. Young, J. C., J. Enslin, and B. Kuca. 1989. Exercise intensity and glucose tolerance in trained and nontrained subjects. *Journal of Applied Physiology* 67(1):39–43.

158. Zachwieja, J. J., and K. E. Yarasheski. 1999. Does growth hormone therapy in conjunction with resistance exercise increase muscle force production and muscle mass in men and women aged 60 years or older? *Physical Therapy* 79:76–82.

CHAPTER 6

Measurement of Work, Power, and Energy Expenditure

■ Objectives

By studying this chapter, you should be able to do the following:

1. Define the terms *work*, *power*, *energy*, and *net efficiency*.

2. Give a brief explanation of the procedure used to calculate work performed during: (a) cycle ergometer exercise and (b) treadmill exercise.

3. Describe the concept behind the measurement of energy expenditure using: (a) direct calorimetry and (b) indirect calorimetry.

4. Discuss the procedure used to estimate energy expenditure during horizontal treadmill walking and running.

5. Define the following terms: (a) kilogram-meter, (b) relative $\dot{V}O_2$, (c) MET, and (d) open-circuit spirometry.

6. Describe the procedure used to calculate net efficiency during steady-state exercise.

■ Outline

Units of Measure   107
   Metric System   107
   SI Units   107

Work and Power Defined   107
   Work   107
   Power   108

Measurement of Work and Power   109

Bench Step   109
Cycle Ergometer   110
Treadmill   110

Measurement of Energy Expenditure   111
   Direct Calorimetry   111
   Indirect Calorimetry   112

Estimation of Energy Expenditure   112

Calculation of Exercise Efficiency   115
   Factors That Influence Exercise Efficiency   115

Running Economy   117

■ Key Terms

cycle ergometer
direct calorimetry
ergometer
ergometry
indirect calorimetry

kilocalorie (kcal)
MET
net efficiency
open-circuit spirometry
percent grade

power
relative $\dot{V}O_2$
SI units
work

Measurement of energy expenditure and power output has many applications in exercise science. For example, adequate knowledge of the energy requirements of physical activities (e.g., running) is important to a coach in planning a training and dietary program for athletes. This same information can be used by an exercise specialist to prescribe exercise for adults entering a fitness program. Therefore, an understanding of human energy expenditure, how it is measured, and its practical significance is critical for the physical therapist, coach, physical educator, exercise specialist, or exercise physiologist. It is the purpose of this chapter to discuss those concepts necessary for understanding the measurement of human work output and the associated energy expenditure.

UNITS OF MEASURE

Metric System

In the United States, the English system of measurement remains in common use. In contrast, the metric system, which is used in many other countries, is the standard system of measurement for scientists, and is used by many scientific journals. In the metric system, the basic units of length, volume, and mass are the meter, the liter, and the gram, respectively. The main advantage of the metric system is that subdivisions or multiples of its basic units are expressed in factors of 10 using prefixes attached to the basic unit. Students not familiar with the metric system should refer to table 6.1 for a list of the basic prefixes used in metric measurements.

SI Units

An ongoing problem in exercise science is the failure of scientists to standardize units of measurement employed in presenting research data. In an effort to eliminate this problem, a uniform system of reporting scientific measurement has been developed through international cooperation. This system, known as System International units, or **SI units,** has been endorsed by numerous exercise and sports medicine

journals for the publication of research data (25, 26). The SI system ensures standardization in the reporting of scientific data and makes comparison of published values easy. Table 6.2 contains SI units of importance in the measurement of exercise performance.

IN SUMMARY

- The metric system is the system of measurement used by scientists to express mass, length, and volume.
- In an effort to standardize terms for the measurement of energy, force, work, and power, scientists have developed a common system of terminology called System International (SI units).

WORK AND POWER DEFINED

Work

Work is defined by the physicist as the product of force times distance:

$$\text{Work} = \text{Force} \times \text{distance}$$

If you lift a 5-kilogram (kg) weight (1 kg = 2.2 lbs) upward over the vertical distance of 2 meters (m), the work performed would be:

$$\text{Work} = 5 \text{ kp} \times 2 \text{ m}$$
$$= 10 \text{ kpm}$$

Here, the force exerted by the 5-kg weight is 5 kiloponds (kp), and the distance traveled is 2 meters, with the resulting amount of work performed being expressed in kilopond-meters (kpm). The explanation for the shift from kg to kp in the example just given is that kg is a measure of mass, not force. That is, 1 kp is

TABLE 6.1	Common Metric Prefixes

mega: one million (1,000,000)
kilo: one thousand (1,000)
centi: one-hundredth (0.01)
milli: one-thousandth (0.001)
micro: one-millionth (0.000001)
nano: one-billionth (0.000000001)
pico: one-trillionth (0.000000000001)

TABLE 6.2	SI Units of Importance in the Measurement of Human Exercise Performance

Units for Quantifying Human Exercise	SI Unit
Mass	kilogram (kg)
Distance	meter (m)
Time	second (s)
Force	Newton (N)
Work	joule (J)
Energy	joule (J)
Power	watt (W)
Velocity	meters per second $(m \cdot s^{-1})$
Torque	newton-meter $(N \cdot m)$

TABLE 6.3 Common Units Used to Express the Amount of Work Performed or Energy Expended

Term	Abbreviation	Conversion Table
Kilogram-meter	kgm	1 kgm = 9.81 joules
		1 kgm = 7.23 ft-lbs
		1 kgm = 9.81 × 10 ergs
		1 kgm = 2.34 × 10^{-3} kcal
Kilopond-meter	kpm	1 kpm = 1 kgm
Kilocalorie	kcal	1 kcal = 4,186 joules
		1 kcal = 426.8 kpm
		1 kcal = 3,087 ft-lbs
Joule[*]	J	1 J = 2.38 × 10^{-4} kcal
		1 J = 0.737 ft-lbs
		1 J = 0.101 kgm
Foot-pounds	ft-lbs	1 ft-lb = 0.1383 kgm

[*]The joule is the basic unit adopted by the System International (called SI unit) for expression of energy expenditure or work.

TABLE 6.4 Common Terms and Units Used to Express Power

Term	Abbreviation	Conversion Table
Watt[*]	W	1 W = 0.001 kilowatt
		1 W = 1 J $\cdot$ s^{-1}
		1 W = 6.12 kpm $\cdot$ min^{-1}
Horsepower	hp	1 hp = 745.1 W
		1 hp = 745.7 J $\cdot$ s^{-1}
		1 hp = 10.69 kcal $\cdot$ min^{-1}
Kilopond-meter $\cdot$ min^{-1}	kpm $\cdot$ min^{-1}	1 kpm $\cdot$ min^{-1} = 0.163 W

[*]The watt is the basic unit adopted by the System International (called SI units) for expression of power.

the force acting upon the mass of 1 kg at the normal acceleration of gravity.

Although SI units are the preferred units for quantifying exercise performance, note that there are a number of traditional units that can be used to express both work and energy expenditure. Table 6.3 contains a list of terms that are in common use today. The SI unit for work is joules; 1 kpm of work is equal to 9.81 joules. Therefore, in the previous example, 10 kpm is equal to 98.1 joules (see table 6.3 for other unit conversions).

It is often difficult to compute how much work is performed during sporting events. For instance, a shot-putter performs work, since the shot has mass and is moved vertically; however, the exact amount of vertical displacement of the shot is difficult to measure without sophisticated photographic equipment, and thus the computation of work performed is not a simple problem. In contrast, a weight lifter performing a clean and jerk is lifting a known amount of weight over a fixed vertical distance, making the calculation of work quite easy.

Power

Power is the term used to describe how much work is accomplished per unit of time. The SI unit for power is the watt (W) and is defined as 6.12 kpm $\cdot$ min^{-1}. Power can be calculated as:

$$Power = Work \div time$$

The concept of power is important, since it describes the rate at which work is being performed (work rate). It is the work rate or power output that describes the intensity of exercise. Given enough time, any healthy adult could perform a total work output of 2,000 kpm (19.6 kilojoules). However, only a few highly trained athletes could perform this amount of work in sixty seconds (s). Calculation of power output using this example can be done as follows:

$$Power = 2,000\ kpm \div 60\ s$$
$$= 33.33\ kpm \cdot s^{-1}$$

Expressed in SI units, this power output is 326.8 W (e.g., 1 W = 0.102 kpm $\cdot$ s^{-21}). Table 6.4 contains a list of traditional ways that power can be expressed other than in SI units.

MEASUREMENT OF WORK AND POWER

Bench Step

The term **ergometry** refers to the measurement of work output. The word **ergometer** refers to the appa-ratus or device used to measure a specific type of work. Many types of ergometers are in use today in exercise physiology laboratories (figure 6.1). A brief introduction to commonly used ergometers follows.

One of the earliest ergometers used to measure work capacity in humans was the bench step. This ergometer is still in use today and simply involves the subject stepping up and down on a bench at a specified rate. Calculation of the work performed during bench stepping is very easy. Suppose a 70-kg man steps up and down on a 50-centimeter (0.5 meter)

(a) (b) (c)

(d) (e)

FIGURE 6.1 Illustrations of five different ergometers used in the measurement of human work output and power. (*a*) A bench step. (*b*) Friction-braked cycle ergometer. (*c*) Electrically braked cycle ergometer. This type of cycle ergometer is capable of maintaining a constant power output even when the cranking speed is varied. Maintaining a constant work output is possible because this ergometer has an electronic resistance mechanism that can vary the resistance on the flywheel with a change in pedaling speed. (*d*) Motor-driven treadmill. Both the treadmill elevation and the horizontal speed of walking/running can be adjusted by electronic controls. (*e*) Arm crank ergometer. Arm crank ergometry can be used to measure work output with the arms and is based on the same principle as cycle ergometry.

bench for ten minutes at a rate of thirty steps per minute. The amount of work performed during this ten-minute task can be computed as follows:

Force = 70 kp (i.e., body weight = 70 kg)
Distance = 0.5 m·step^{-1} × 30 steps·min^{-1}
  × 10 min = 150 m
Therefore, total work performed = 70 kp × 150 m
  = 10,500 kpm or
  ~103 kilojoules
  (see table 6.3 for
  conversions)

The power output can be calculated as:

Power = 10,500 kpm ÷ 10 min
  = 1,050 kpm·min^{-1} or 171.6 W

Cycle Ergometer

One of the most popular ergometers is the **cycle ergometer** (20). This type of ergometer is a stationary exercise bicycle that permits accurate measurement of the amount of work performed. A common type of cycle ergometer is the Monark friction-braked cycle, which incorporates a belt wrapped around the wheel (called a flywheel) (figure 6.1b). The belt can be loosened or tightened to provide a change in resistance. Distance traveled can be determined by computing the distance covered per revolution of the pedals (6 meters per revolution on a standard Monark cycle) times the number of pedal revolutions. Consider the following example for the computation of work and power using the cycle ergometer. Calculate work given:

Duration of exercise = 10 min
Resistance against flywheel = 1.5 kp
Distance traveled per pedal revolution = 6 m
Pedalling speed = 60 rev·min^{-1}
Therefore, the total revolutions in 10 min = 10 min × 60 rev·min^{-1}
Hence, total work = 1.5 kp × (6 m·rev^{-1} × 600 rev)
  = 5,400 kpm or 52.97 kilojoules

The power output in this example is computed by dividing the total work performed by time:

Power = 5,400 kpm ÷ 10 min
  = 540 kpm·min^{-1} or 88.2 W

Treadmill

Calculation of the work performed while a subject runs or walks on a treadmill is not generally possible when the treadmill is horizontal. Although running horizontally on a treadmill requires energy, the vertical displacement of the body's center of gravity is not easily measured. Therefore, the measurement of work performed during horizontal walking or running is complicated. However, quantifiable work is being performed

TABLE 6.5	Determination of Percent Grade from Angles of Incline	
Degrees	**Sine**	**Percent Grade**
1	0.0175	1.75
2	0.0349	3.49
3	0.0523	5.23
4	0.0698	6.98
5	0.0872	8.72
6	0.1045	10.45
7	0.1219	12.19
8	0.1392	13.92
9	0.1564	15.64
10	0.1736	17.36

when walking or running up a slope, and calculating the amount of work done is a simple task. The incline of the treadmill is expressed in units called "percent grade." **Percent grade** is defined as the amount of vertical rise per 100 units of belt travel. For instance, a subject walking on a treadmill at a 10% grade travels 10 meters vertically for every 100 meters of the belt travel. Percent grade is calculated by multiplying the sine of the treadmill angle by 100. Examples of this calculation are presented in table 6.5. In practice, the treadmill angle (expressed in degrees) can be determined by simple trigometric computations, or by using a measurement device called an inclinometer (10).

To calculate the work output during treadmill exercise, you must know both the subject's body weight and the distance traveled vertically. Vertical travel can be computed by multiplying the distance the belt traveled by the percent grade. This can be written as:

Vertical displacement = % grade × distance

where percent grade is expressed as a fraction and the total distance traveled is calculated by multiplying the treadmill speed (m · min^{-1}) by the total minutes of exercise (figure 6.2). Consider the following sample calculation of work output during treadmill exercise. Calculate work given:

Subject's body weight = 70 kg (i.e., force = 70 kp)
Treadmill speed = 200 m · min^{-1}
Treadmill angle = 7.5% grade (7.5% ÷ 100 = 0.075
  as fractional grade)
Exercise time = 10 min
Total vertical distance traveled = 200 m · min^{-1}
  × 0.075 × 10 min
  = 150 m
Therefore, total work performed = 70 kp × 150 m
  = 10,500 kpm or
  ~103 kilojoules

Axle-to-axle distance
(hypotenuse)

Vertical
rise

θ

Fixed rear-axle treadmill
Grade = Sine θ = Rise ÷ Hypotenuse

FIGURE 6.2 Determination of the "percent grade" on an inclined treadmill. Theta (θ) represents the angle of inclination. Percent grade is computed as the sine of angle $\theta \times 100$.

MEASUREMENT OF ENERGY EXPENDITURE

Measurement of an individual's energy expenditure at rest or during a particular activity has many practical applications. One direct application applies to exercise-assisted weight-loss programs. Clearly, knowledge of the energy cost of walking, running, or swimming at various speeds is useful to individuals who use these modes of exercise as an aid in weight loss. Further, an industrial engineer might measure the energy cost of various tasks around a job site and use this information in making the appropriate job assignments to workers (18, 38). In this regard, the engineer might recommend that the supervisor assign those jobs that demand large energy requirements to workers who are physically fit and possess high work capacities. In general, there are two techniques employed in the measurement of human energy expenditure: (1) direct calorimetry and (2) indirect calorimetry.

Direct Calorimetry

When the body uses energy to do work, heat is liberated. This production of heat by cells occurs via both cellular respiration (bioenergetics) and cell work.

Temperature measurement

Airflow into chamber

Airflow out of chamber (measurement of evaporative heat loss)

Circulating "jacket" of water

Direct calorimetry

FIGURE 6.3 Diagram of a simple calorimeter used to measure metabolic rate by measuring the production of body heat. This method of determining metabolic rate is called direct calorimetry.

The general process can be drawn schematically as (6, 39, 40):

$$\text{Foodstuff} + O_2 \rightarrow \text{ATP} + \text{heat}$$
$$\downarrow \text{cell work}$$
$$\text{Heat}$$

The process of cellular respiration was discussed in detail in chapter 3. Note that the rate of heat production in an animal is directly proportional to the metabolic rate. Therefore, measuring heat production (calorimetry) by an animal gives a direct measurement of metabolic rate.

The SI unit to measure heat energy is the joule. However, a common unit employed to measure heat energy is the calorie (see table 6.3). A calorie is defined as the amount of heat required to raise the temperature of one gram of water by one degree Celsius. Since the calorie is very small, the term **kilocalorie (kcal)** is generally used to express energy expenditure and the energy value of foods. One kcal is equal to 1,000 calories. In converting kcals to SI units, 1 kcal is equal to 4,186 joules or 4.186 Kilojoules(kJ) (see table 6.3 for conversions). The process of measuring an animal's metabolic rate via the measurement of heat production is called **direct calorimetry,** and has been used by scientists since the eighteenth century. This technique involves placing the animal in a tight chamber (called a calorimeter), which is insulated from the environment (usually by a jacket of water surrounding the chamber), and allowance is made for the free exchange of O_2 and CO_2 from the chamber (figure 6.3). The animal's body heat raises the temperature of the water circulating around the chamber. Therefore, by measuring the volume of water flowing through the chamber per minute and the temperature change of the water per unit of time, the amount of heat production can be computed. In addition, heat is lost from the animal by evaporation of water from the skin and respiratory passages. This heat loss can be measured and added back to the total heat picked up by the water to yield an estimate of the rate of energy utilization by the animal (6, 10).

Indirect Calorimetry

Although direct calorimetry is considered to be a precise technique for the measurement of metabolic rate, construction of a chamber that is large enough for humans is expensive. Also, the use of direct calorimetry to measure metabolic rate during exercise is complicated since the ergometer used may produce heat. Fortunately, another procedure can be used to measure metabolic rate. This technique is termed **indirect calorimetry** because it does not involve the direct measurement of heat production. The principle of indirect calorimetry can be explained by the following relationship:

$$\text{Foodstuffs} + O_2 \longrightarrow \text{Heat} + CO_2 + H_2O$$
$$\text{(Indirect calorimetry)} \qquad \text{(Direct calorimetry)}$$

Since a direct relationship exists between O_2 consumed and the amount of heat produced in the body, measuring O_2 consumption provides an estimate of metabolic rate (4, 6, 16). In order to convert the amount of O_2 consumed into heat equivalents, it is necessary to know the type of nutrient (i.e., carbohydrate, fat, or protein) that was metabolized. The energy liberated when fat is the only foodstuff metabolized is 4.7 kcal (or 19.7 kJ) $\cdot$ 1 O_2^{-1}, while the energy released when only carbohydrates are used is 5.05 kcal (or 21.13 kJ) $\cdot$ 1 O_2^{-1}. Although it is not exact, the caloric expenditure of exercise is often estimated to be approximately 5 kcal (or 21 kJ) per liter of O_2 consumed (23). Therefore, a person exercising at an oxygen consumption of 2.0 $\ell \cdot \text{min}^{-1}$ would expend approximately 10 kcal (or 42 kJ) of energy per minute.

The most common technique used to measure oxygen consumption today is termed **open-circuit spirometry.** Modern-day, open-circuit spirometry employs computer technology and is shown diagrammatically in figure 6.4 (34). The laboratory equipment used to measure oxygen consumption is illustrated in the accompanying photo. The volume of air inspired is measured with a device that is capable of measuring gas volumes. The expired gas from the subject is channeled to a small mixing chamber to be analyzed for O_2 and CO_2 content by electronic gas analyzers. Information concerning the volume of air inspired and the fraction of O_2 and CO_2 in the expired gas is sent to a digital computer by way of a device called an analog-to-digital converter (converts a voltage signal to a dig-

FIGURE 6.4 Modern open-circuit spirometry utilizing electronic gas analyzers and computer technology. Computerized open-circuit spirometer for measurement of oxygen consumption and carbon dioxide production.

ital signal). The computer is programmed to perform the necessary calculations of $\dot{V}O_2$ (volume of O_2 consumed per min) and the volume of carbon dioxide produced ($\dot{V}CO_2$). In short, $\dot{V}O_2$ is calculated in the following way:

$$\dot{V}O_2 = [\text{volume of } O_2 \text{ inspired}] - [\text{volume of } O_2 \text{ expired}]$$

See appendix A for details of $\dot{V}O_2$ and $\dot{V}CO_2$ calculations.

IN SUMMARY

- Measurement of energy expenditure at rest or during exercise is possible using either direct or indirect calorimetry.
- Direct calorimetry uses the measurement of heat production as an indication of metabolic rate.
- Indirect calorimetry estimates metabolic rate via the measurement of oxygen consumption.

ESTIMATION OF ENERGY EXPENDITURE

Researchers studying the oxygen cost (O_2 cost = $\dot{V}O_2$ at steady state) of exercise have demonstrated that it is possible to estimate the energy expended during physical activity with reasonable precision (9, 11, 12, 20, 33). Walking, running, and cycling are activities

A CLOSER LOOK 6.1

Estimation of the O_2 Requirement of Treadmill Walking

The O_2 requirement of horizontal treadmill walking can be estimated with reasonable accuracy for speeds between 50 and 100 m · min^{-1} using the following formula (1):

$$\dot{V}O_2 \text{ (ml · kg}^{-1}\text{· min}^{-1}) = 0.1 \text{ ml · kg}^{-1}\text{· min}^{-1}/(\text{m · min}^{-1}) \times \text{speed (m · min}^{-1}) + 3.5 \text{ ml · kg}^{-1}\text{· min}^{-1} \text{ (resting } \dot{V}O_2)$$

This equation tells us that the O_2 requirement of walking increases as a linear function of walking speed. The slope of the line is 0.1 and the Y intercept is 3.5 ml · kg^{-1} · min^{-1} (resting $\dot{V}O_2$). The O_2 cost of grade walking is:

$$\dot{V}O_2 \text{ (ml · kg}^{-1}\text{· min}^{-1}) = 1.8 \text{ ml · kg}^{-1}\text{· min}^{-1} \times \text{speed (m · min}^{-1}) \times \% \text{ grade (expressed as a fraction)}$$

The total O_2 requirement of graded treadmill walking is the sum of the horizontal O_2 cost and the vertical O_2 cost. For example, the O_2 cost of walking at 80 m · min^{-1} at 5% grade would be:

$$\text{Horizontal } O_2 \text{ cost} = 0.1 \text{ ml · kg}^{-1}\text{· min}^{-1} \times 80 \text{ m min}^{-1} + 3.5 \text{ ml · kg}^{-1}\text{· min}^{-1}$$
$$= 11.5 \text{ ml · kg}^{-1}\text{· min}^{-1}$$
$$\text{Vertical } O_2 \text{ cost} = 1.8 \text{ ml · kg}^{-1}\text{· min}^{-1} \times (0.05 \times 80) = 7.2 \text{ ml · kg}^{-1}\text{· min}^{-1}$$

Hence, the total O_2 requirement of walking would amount to:

$$11.5 \text{ ml · kg}^{-1}\text{· min}^{-1} + 7.2 \text{ ml · kg}^{-1}\text{· min}^{-1} = 18.7 \text{ ml · kg}^{-1}\text{· min}^{-1}$$

This O_2 requirement can be expressed in METs by dividing the measured (or estimated) $\dot{V}O_2$ (ml · kg^{-1} · min^{-1}) by 3.5 ml · kg^{-1} · min^{-1} per MET:

$$18.7 \text{ ml · kg}^{-1}\text{· min}^{-1} \div 3.5 \text{ ml · kg}^{-1}\text{· min}^{-1} \text{ per MET} = 5.3 \text{ METs}$$

Formulas are taken from reference 1.

FIGURE 6.5 The relationship between speed and $\dot{V}O_2$ cost is linear for both walking and running. Note that x equals the walking/running speed in meters · min^{-1}.

that have been studied in detail. The O_2 requirements of walking and running graphed as a function of speed are presented in figure 6.5. Note that the relationships between the relative O_2 requirement (ml · kg^{-1} · min^{-1}) and walking/running speed are straight lines (2, 20). A similar relationship exists for cycling (see figure 6.6).

The fact that this relationship is linear over a wide range of speeds is convenient and makes the calculation of the O_2 cost (or energy cost) very easy (see A Closer Look 6.1, 6.2, and 6.3 for examples). Estimation of the energy expenditure of other types of activities is more complex (figure 6.7). For example, estimation of energy expenditure during tennis is dependent on whether the match is singles or doubles, and is also influenced by the participants' skill level. Nonetheless, a gross estimate of the energy expended during a tennis match is possible. Appendix B contains a list of activities and their estimated energy costs.

The need to express the energy cost of exercise in simple units has led to the development of the term *metabolic equivalent* (MET) (often called "MET"). The concept of a MET is simple. One **MET** is equal to resting $\dot{V}O_2$, which is approximately 3.5 ml · kg^{-1} · min^{-1} (2, 4). Thus, the energy cost of exercise can be described in multiples of resting $\dot{V}O_2$ (i.e., METs), which will simplify the quantification of exercise energy requirement. For example, a physical activity requiring a 10-MET energy expenditure (i.e., ten times resting metabolic rate) represents a $\dot{V}O_2$ of 35 ml · kg^{-1} · min^{-1} (10 METs × 3.5 ml · kg^{-1} · min^{-1} per MET = 35 ml · kg^{-1} · min^{-1}). The absolute oxygen requirement of an activity requiring 10 METs can be calculated by multiplying the individual's body weight times the $\dot{V}O_2$ (ml · kg^{-1} · min^{-1}).

A CLOSER LOOK 6.2

Estimation of the O₂ Requirement of Treadmill Running

The O_2 requirements of horizontal treadmill running for speeds greater than 134 m · min^{-1} can be estimated in a manner similar to the procedure used to estimate the O_2 requirement for treadmill walking. It is also possible to estimate the O_2 requirement for running up a grade. This calculation is done in two parts:

1. First, the O_2 cost of the horizontal component is calculated using the following formula:

$$\dot{V}O_2 \text{ (ml · kg}^{-1} \text{· min}^{-1}) = 0.2 \text{ ml · kg}^{-1} \text{· min}^{-1}/\text{m · min}^{-1} \times \text{speed (m · min}^{-1}) + 3.5 \text{ ml · kg}^{-1} \text{· min}^{-1} \text{ (resting } \dot{V}O_2)$$

2. Second, the O_2 requirement of the vertical component is computed using the relationship that running 1 m/min vertically requires 0.9 ml · kg^{-1} · min^{-1}. The vertical velocity is computed by multiplying running speed by the fractional grade. Therefore, the formula to estimate the O_2 cost of vertical treadmill work while running is as follows:

$$\dot{V}O_2 \text{ (ml · kg}^{-1} \text{· min}^{-1}) = 0.9 \text{ ml · kg}^{-1} \text{ per m · min}^{-1} \times \text{vertical velocity (m · min}^{-1})$$

Formulas are taken from reference 1.

A CLOSER LOOK 6.3

Estimation of the O₂ Requirement of Cycling

Similar to the energy cost of walking and running, the oxygen requirement of cycling is also linear (straight line) over a wide range of work rates (figure 6.6). Because of this linear relationship, the O_2 requirement of cycling can be easily estimated for power outputs between 50 and 200 watts (i.e., 300 and 1,200 kg · m · min^{-1}). The total O_2 cost of cycling on a cycle ergometer is comprised of three components. These include the resting O_2 consumption, the O_2 demand associated with unloaded cycling (i.e., energy cost of moving the legs), and an O_2 require-ment that is directly proportional to the external load on the cycle. An explanation of how the O_2 cost of these components is computed follows.

First, the resting O_2 consumption is estimated at 3.5 ml · kg^{-1} · min^{-1}. Second, at a cranking speed of 50–60 rpm, the oxygen cost of unloaded cycling is also approximately 3.5 ml · kg^{-1} · min^{-1}. Finally, the relative O_2 cost of cycling against an external load is approximately 1.8 ml · min^{-1} × work rate × body mass^{-1}. Putting these three components together, the collective formula to compute the O_2 of cycling is:

$$\dot{V}O_2 \text{ (ml · kg}^{-1} \text{· min}^{-1}) = 1.8 \text{ (work rate)} \times M^{-1} + 7$$

Where:

work rate on the cycle ergometer is expressed in kilopond-meter · min^{-1}

M is body mass in kilograms

7 is the sum of resting O_2 consumption (3.5) and the O_2 cost of unloaded cycling (3.5)

Formulas are from reference 2.

FIGURE 6.6 The relationship between work rate and $\dot{V}O_2$ cost is linear for cycling over a wide range of workloads. This figure illustrates the relative oxygen cost (i.e., $\dot{V}O_2$ per kilogram of body mass) of cycling for 70-kilogram individual.

FIGURE 6.7 Measurement of oxygen consumption during exercise can be performed with the use of a computerized metabolic cart.

Therefore, the oxygen requirement for a 60-kg individual performing a 10-MET activity would be:

$$\dot{V}O_2 \ (ml \cdot min^{-1} = 35 \ ml \cdot kg^{-1} \cdot min^{-1} \times 60 \ kg$$
$$= 2,100 \ ml \cdot min^{-1}$$

IN SUMMARY

- The energy cost of horizontal treadmill walking or running can be estimated with reasonable accuracy, since the O_2 requirements of both walking and running increase as a linear function of speed.
- The need to express the energy cost of exercise in simple terms has led to the development of the term MET. One MET is equal to the resting $\dot{V}O_2$ (3.5 ml $\cdot$ kg^{-1} $\cdot$ min^{-1}).

CALCULATION OF EXERCISE EFFICIENCY

Exercise physiologists have long searched for ways to mathematically describe the efficiency of human movement. Although disagreement exists as to the most valid technique of calculating efficiency, the efficiency of exercise is often described by the term **net efficiency** (7, 8, 12, 32, 33, 41, 42). Net efficiency is defined as the mathematical ratio of work output divided by the energy expended above rest:

$$\% \ net \ efficiency = \frac{Work \ output}{Energy \ expended \ above \ rest} \times 100$$

No machine is 100% efficient, since some energy is lost due to friction of the moving parts. Likewise, the human machine is not 100% efficient because energy is lost as heat. It is estimated that the gasoline automobile engine operates with an efficiency of approximately 20% to 25%. Similarly, net efficiency for humans exercising on a cycle ergometer ranges from 15% to 27%, depending on work rate (14, 17, 33, 37, 42).

To compute net efficiency during cycle ergometer or treadmill exercise requires measurement of work output and an appraisal of the subject's energy expenditure during the exercise and at rest. It should be emphasized that $\dot{V}O_2$ measurements must be made during steady-state conditions. The work rate on the cycle ergometer or treadmill is calculated as discussed earlier and is generally expressed in kpm $\cdot$ min^{-1}. The energy expenditure during these types of exercise is usually estimated by first measuring $\dot{V}O_2$ (liter $\cdot$ min^{-1}) using open-circuit spirometry, and then converting it to either kcal or kJ (i.e., 5 kcal or 21 kJ = 1 liter O_2). In order to do the computation using the net-efficiency formula, both numerator and denominator must be expressed in similar terms. Since the numerator (work output) is expressed in kJ and energy expenditure is also expressed in kJ, no conversion of units is required. Consider the following sample calculation of net efficiency during submaximal, steady-state cycle ergometer exercise using kJ as both work and energy units. Given:

Resistance against the cycle flywheel = 2 kp
Cranking speed = 50 rpm
Steady-state resting $\dot{V}O_2 = 0.25\ell \cdot min^{-1}$
Steady-state exercise $\dot{V}O_2 = 1.5\ell \cdot min^{-1}$
Distance traveled per revolution = 6 m
Therefore:
Work rate = [(2 kp) × (50 rpm × 6 m/rev)]
= 600 kpm $\cdot$ min^{-1} or 5.89 kJ
Energy expenditure = [$\dot{V}O_2(\ell \cdot min^{-1}) \times 21kJ \cdot \ell^{-1}$]
= 26.25 kJ
note: $\dot{V}O_2 = (1.5\ell \cdot min^{-1} - 0.25\ell \cdot min^{-1})$

Hence, net efficiency $= \dfrac{5.89 \ kJ \cdot min^{-1}}{26.25 kJ \cdot min^{-1}} \times 100\%$

$$= 22.4\%$$

Factors That Influence Exercise Efficiency

The efficiency of exercise is influenced by several factors: (1) the exercise work rate, (2) the speed of movement, and (3) the fiber composition of the muscles performing the exercise. A brief discussion of each of these factors follows.

Work Rate and Exercise Efficiency Figure 6.8 depicts the changes in net efficiency during cycle ergometry exercise as a function of work rate. Note

FIGURE 6.8 Changes in net efficiency during arm crank ergometry as a function of work rate.

FIGURE 6.9 Relationship between energy expenditure and work rate. Note that energy expenditure increases as a curvilinear function of work rate.

that efficiency decreases as the work rate increases (14, 33). This is because the relationship between energy expenditure and work rate is curvilinear rather than linear (see figure 6.9) (17, 33). That is, as the work rate increases, total body energy expenditure increases out of proportion to the work rate; this results in a lowered efficiency.

Movement Speed and Efficiency Research has shown that there is an "optimum" speed of movement for any given work rate. Recent evidence suggests that the optimum speed of movement increases as the power output increases (9). In other words, at higher power outputs, a greater speed of movement is required to obtain optimum efficiency. At low-to-moderate work

FIGURE 6.10 Effects of decreasing or increasing speed of movement on exercise efficiency. Note an optimum speed of movement for maximum efficiency at any given work rate.

rates, a pedaling speed of 40 to 60 rpm is generally considered optimum during arm or cycle ergometry (13, 15, 17, 30, 33, 36). Note that any change in the speed of movement away from the optimum results in a decrease in efficiency (figure 6.10). This decline in efficiency at low speeds of movement is probably due to inertia (33). That is, there may be an increased energy cost of performing work when movements are slow and the limbs involved must repeatedly stop and start. The decline in efficiency associated with high-speed movement (low work rates) may be because increasing speeds might augment muscular friction and thus increase internal work (7, 33).

Fiber Type and Efficiency People differ greatly in their net efficiency during cycle ergometer exercise. Why? Recent evidence suggests that subjects with a high percentage of slow muscle fibers display a higher exercise efficiency compared to subjects with a high percentage of fast muscle fibers (see chapter 8 for a discussion of muscle fiber types) (21, 24, 28, 35). The physiological explanation for this observation is that slow muscle fibers are more efficient than fast fibers. That is, slow fibers require less ATP per unit of work performed compared to fast fibers.

The significance of a high exercise efficiency is that superior efficiency can improve exercise performance. Indeed, studies have shown that endurance performance is improved by a high exercise efficiency (21). This can be explained by the fact that, compared to subjects with a relatively low efficiency, subjects with high efficiency can generate a greater power output at any rate of energy expenditure. In other words, a high exercise efficiency improves endurance performance by increasing the power output produced for a given amount of ATP used.

- Net efficiency is defined as the mathematical ratio of work performed divided by the energy expenditure above rest, and is expressed as a percentage:

$$\% \text{ Net efficiency} = \frac{\text{Work output}}{\text{Energy expended above rest}} \times 100$$

- The efficiency of exercise decreases as the exercise work rate increases. This occurs because the relationship between work rate and energy expenditure is curvilinear.
- To achieve maximal efficiency at any work rate, there is an optimal speed of movement.
- Exercise efficiency is greater in subjects who possess a high percentage of slow muscle fibers compared to subjects with a high percentage of fast fibers. This is due to the fact that slow muscle fibers are more efficient than fast fibers

RUNNING ECONOMY

As discussed previously, the computation of work is not generally possible during horizontal treadmill running, and thus a calculation of exercise efficiency cannot be performed. However, the measurement of the steady-state $\dot{V}O_2$ requirement (O_2 cost) of running at various speeds offers a means of comparing running economy (not efficiency) between two runners or groups of runners (19, 20, 29). Figure 6.11 compares the O_2 cost of running between a group of highly trained male and female distance runners at slow running speeds (i.e., slower than race pace). A runner who exhibits poor running economy would require a higher $\dot{V}O_2$ (ml · kg^{-1} · min^{-1}) at any given running speed than an economical runner. Notice that the O_2 cost of running labeled on the ordinate (y-axis) is expressed as $\dot{V}O_2$ in ml · kg^{-1} · min^{-1}. Expressing $\dot{V}O_2$ as a function of the body weight is referred to as **relative $\dot{V}O_2$**, and it is appropriate when describing the O_2 cost of weight-bearing activities such as running, climbing steps, walking, or ice skating.

Do gender differences exist in running economy? This issue has been studied by numerous investiga-

FIGURE 6.11 Comparison of the oxygen cost of horizontal treadmill running between highly trained men and women distance runners.

tors, with mixed findings. Figure 6.11 illustrates the results of one of these studies (20). This study compared the oxygen cost of running between highly trained men and women distance runners. The runners were matched for maximal aerobic power and the number of years of training experience. The similar slopes of the two lines suggests that running economy is comparable for highly trained men and women distance runners at slow running speeds (20). However, recent evidence suggests that at fast "race pace" speeds, male runners may be more economical than females (12). The reason for this apparent gender variation in running economy is unclear and requires further study (31).

- Although it is not easy to compute efficiency during horizontal running, the measurement of the O_2 cost of running (ml · kg^{-1} · min^{-1}) at any given speed offers a measure of running economy.
- Running economy does not differ between highly trained men and women distance runners at slow running speeds. However, at fast "race pace" speeds, male runners may be more economical than females. The reasons for these differences are unclear.

STUDY QUESTIONS

1. Define the following terms:
   a. work
   b. power
   c. percent grade

   d. relative $\dot{V}O_2$
   e. net efficiency
   f. metric system
   g. SI units

2. Calculate the total amount of work performed in five minutes of exercise on the cycle ergometer, given the following:

Resistance on the flywheel = 2.5 kp
Cranking speed = 60 rpm
Distance traveled per revolution = 6 meters

3. Compute total work and power output per minute for ten minutes of treadmill exercise, given the following:

Treadmill grade = 15%
Horizontal speed = 200 m · min⁻¹
Subject's weight = 70 kg

4. Briefly, describe the procedure used to estimate energy expenditure using (a) direct calorimetry and (b) indirect calorimetry.

5. Compute the estimated energy expenditure during horizontal treadmill walking for the following examples:
   a. Treadmill speed = 50 m · min⁻¹
      Subject's weight = 62 kg
   b. Treadmill speed = 100 m · min⁻¹
      Subject's weight = 75 kg
   c. Treadmill speed = 80 m · min⁻¹
      Subject's weight = 60 kg

6. Calculate the estimated O_2 cost of horizontal treadmill running for a 70-kg subject at 150, 200, and 235 m · min⁻¹.

7. Calculate net efficiency, given the following:

Exercise $\dot{V}O_2$ = 3.0ℓ · min⁻¹
Resting exercise $\dot{V}O_2$ = 0.3ℓ · min⁻¹
Work rate = 1200 kpm · min⁻¹ (196 W)

8. Calculate the power output during one minute of cycle ergometer exercise, given the following:

Resistance on the flywheel = 5.0 kp
Cranking speed = 50 rpm
Distance traveled per revolution = 6 meters

9. Calculate the total work performed during ten minutes of cycle ergometer exercise, given the following:

Resistance on the flywheel = 2.0 kp
Cranking speed = 70 rpm
Distance traveled per revolution = 6 meters

10. Calculate net efficiency, given the following:

Resting $\dot{V}O_2$ = 0.3ℓ · min⁻¹
Exercise $\dot{V}O_2$ = 2.1ℓ · min⁻¹
Work rate = 900 kpm · min⁻¹

11. Compute the power output for three minutes of treadmill exercise, given the following:

Treadmill grade = 10%
Horizontal speed = 100 m · min⁻¹
Subject's weight = 60 kg

12. Calculate the power output (expressed in watts) for a subject who performed ten minutes of cycle ergometer exercise at:

Resistance on the flywheel = 2.0 kp
Cranking speed = 60 rpm
Distance traveled per revolution = 6 meters

13. Compute the oxygen cost of cycling at work rates of 300, 450, 500, and 750 kilopond-meters · min⁻¹ for a 60-kilogram person.

SUGGESTED READINGS

American College of Sports Medicine. 2005. *Guidelines for Exercise Testing and Prescription*. Baltimore: Lippincott, Williams & Wilkins.

American College of Sports Medicine Metabolic Calculations Tutorial (CD-ROM). L. Kaminisky. 2000.

Brooks, G., T. Fahey, and K. Baldwin. 2005. *Exercise Physiology: Human Bioenergetics and Its Applications*, ed 4. New York: McGraw-Hill Companies.

Gore, C., (ed). 2000. *Physiological tests for Elite Athletes*. Champaign, IL: Human Kinetics Publishers.

Morrow, J. et al. 2005. *Measurement and Evaluation of Human Performance*. Champaign, IL: Human Kinetics Publishers.

Powers, S., S. Dodd, and V. Noland. 2006. *Total Fitness and Wellness*. San Francisco: Benjamin Cummings.

REFERENCES

1. American College of Sports Medicine. 2005. *Guidelines for Exercise Testing and Prescription*. Baltimore: Lippincott, Williams & Wilkins.

2. American College of Sports Medicine. 2000. *ACSM's Guidelines for Exercise Testing and Prescription*. Baltimore: Lippincott, Williams & Wilkins.

3. Astrand, P., ed. 2003. *Textbook of Work Physiology*. 2003. Champaign, IL: Human Kinetics Publishers.

4. Åstrand, P., and K. Rodahl. 1986. *Textbook of Work Physiology*. New York: McGraw-Hill Companies.

5. Brooks, G., T. Fahey, and K. Baldwin. 2005. *Exercise Physiology: Human Bioenergetics and Its Applications*, 4th ed. New York. McGraw-Hill Companies.

6. Brooks, G. et al. 2000. *Exercise Physiology: Human Bioenergetics and Its Applications*. New York: McGraw-Hill Companies.

7. Cavanagh, P., and R. Kram. 1985. Mechanical and muscular factors affecting the efficiency of human movement. *Medicine and Science in Sports and Exercise* 17:326–31.

8. ———. 1985. The efficiency of human movement—a statement of the problem. *Medicine and Science in Sports and Exercise* 17:304–8.

9. Coast, J., and H. G. Welch. 1985. Linear increase in optimal pedal rate with increased power output in cycle ergometry. *European Journal of Applied Physiology* 53:339–42.

10. Consolazio, C., R. Johnson, and L. Pecora. 1963. *Physiological Measurements of Metabolic Function in Man*. New York: McGraw-Hill Companies.

11. Daniels, J. 1985. A physiologist's view of running economy. *Medicine and Science in Sports and Exercise* 17:332–38.

12. Daniels, J., and N. Daniels. 1992. Running economy of elite male and elite female distance runners. *Medicine and Science in Sports and Exercise* 24:483–89.

13. Deschenes, M. R. et al. 2000. Muscle recruitment patterns regulate physiological responses during exercise of the same intensity. *American Journal of Physiology* 279: R2229–36.

14. Donovan, C., and G. Brooks. 1977. Muscular efficiency during steady-rate exercise: Effects of speed and work rate. *Journal of Applied Physiology* 43:431–39.

15. Ferguson, R. A. et al. 2001. Muscle oxygen uptake and energy turnover during dynamic exercise at different contraction frequencies in humans. *Journal of Physiology* 536:261–71.

16. Fox, E., M. Foss, and S. Keteyian. 1998. *Fox's Physiological Basis for Exercise and Sport*. New York: McGraw-Hill Companies.

17. Gaesser, G., and G. Brooks. 1975. Muscular efficiency during steady-rate exercise: Effects of speed and work rate. *Journal of Applied Physiology* 38:1132–39.

18. Grandjean, E. 1982. *Fitting the Task to the Man: An Ergonomic Approach*. New York: International Publications Service.

19. Hagan, R. et al. 1980. Oxygen uptake and energy expenditure during horizontal treadmill running. *Journal of Applied Physiology* 49:571–75.

20. Hopkins, P., and S. Powers. 1982. Oxygen uptake during submaximal running in highly trained men and women. *American Corrective Therapy Journal* 36:130–32.

21. Horowitz, J. et al. 1994. High efficiency of type I muscle fibers improves performance. *International Journal of Sports Medicine*. 15:152–57.

22. Howley, E., and B. Franks. 2003. *Health Fitness Instructor's Handbook*. Champaign, IL: Human Kinetics.

23. Howley, E., and B. D. Franks. 1997. *Health/Fitness Instructor's Handbook*. Champaign, IL: Human Kinetics.

24. Hunter, G. R. et al. 2001. Muscle metabolic economy is inversely related to exercise intensity and type II myofiber distribution. *Muscle and Nerve* 24:654–61.

25. Knuttgen, H. 1978. Force, power, and exercise. *Medicine and Science in Sports and Exercise* 10:227–28.

26. Knuttgen, H., and P. Komi. 1992. Basic definitions for exercise. In *Strength and Power in Sport*, ed. P. Komi. Oxford: Blackwell Scientific Publications.

27. Lakomy, H. 1986. Measurement of work and power output using friction loaded cycle ergometers. *Ergonomics* 29:509–17.

28. Luciá, A. et al. 2002. Determinants of O_2 kinetics at high power outputs during a ramp exercise protocol. *Medicine and Science in Sports and Exercise* 34: 326–31.

29. Margaria, R. et al. 1963. Energy cost of running. *Journal of Applied Physiology* 18:367–70.

30. Michielli, D., and M. Stricevic. 1977. Various pedalling frequencies at equivalent power outputs. *New York State Medical Journal* 77:744–46.

31. Morgan, D., and M. Craib. 1992. Physiological aspects of running economy. *Medicine and Science in Sports and Exercise* 24:456–61.

32. Moseley, L., and A. E. Juekendrup. 2001. The reliability of cycling efficiency. *Medicine and Science in Sports and Exercise* 33:621–27.

33. Powers, S., R. Beadle, and M. Mangum. 1984. Exercise efficiency during arm ergometry: Effects of speed and work rate. *Journal of Applied Physiology* 56:495–99.

34. Powers, S. et al. 1987. Measurement of oxygen uptake in the non-steady state. *Aviation, Space, and Environmental Medicine* 58:323–27.

35. Scheurermann, B. W., J. H. McConnell, and T. J. Barstow. 2002. EMG and oxygen uptake responses during slow and fast ramp exercise in humans. *Experimental Physiology* 87:91–100.

36. Seabury, J., W. Adams, and M. Ramey. 1977. Influence of pedalling rate and power output on energy expenditure during bicycle ergometry. *Ergonomics* 20:491–98.

37. Shephard, R. 1982. *Physiology and Biochemistry of Exercise*. New York: Praeger.

38. Singleton, W. 1982. *The Body at Work*. London: Cambridge University Press.

39. Spence, A., and E. Mason. 1992. *Human Anatomy and Physiology*. Menlo Park, CA: Benjamin-Cummings.

40. Stegeman, J. 1981. *Exercise Physiology: Physiological Bases of Work and Sport*. Chicago: Year Book Publishers.

41. Stuart, M. et al. 1980. Efficiency of trained subjects differing in maximal oxygen uptake and type of training. *Journal of Applied Physiology* 50:444–49.

42. Whipp, B., and K. Wasserman. 1969. Efficiency of muscular work. *Journal of Applied Physiology* 26:644–48.

CHAPTER 7

The Nervous System: Structure and Control of Movement

■ Objectives

By studying this chapter, you should be able to do the following:

1. Discuss the general organization of the nervous system.
2. Describe the structure and function of a nerve.
3. Draw and label the pathways involved in a withdrawal reflex.
4. Define depolarization, action potential, and repolarization.
5. Discuss the role of position receptors in the control of movement.
6. Describe the role of the vestibular apparatus in maintaining equilibrium.
7. Discuss the brain centers involved in voluntary control of movement.
8. Describe the structure and function of the autonomic nervous system.

■ Outline

General Nervous System Functions   121

Organization of the Nervous System   121
　Structure of the Neuron   122
　Electrical Activity in Neurons   122

Sensory Information and Reflexes   129
　Proprioceptors   129

Muscle Chemoreceptors   130
　Reflexes   130

Somatic Motor Function   131

Vestibular Apparatus and Equilibrium   132

Motor Control Functions of the Brain   132
　Brain Stem   133
　Cerebrum   133
　Cerebellum   134

Motor Functions of the Spinal Cord   134

Control of Motor Functions   135

Autonomic Nervous System   136

Exercise Enhances Brain Health   137

■ Key Terms

action potential
afferent fibers
autonomic nervous system
axon
brain stem
cell body
central nervous system (CNS)
cerebellum
cerebrum
conductivity

dendrites
efferent fibers
EPSP
IPSP
irritability
kinesthesia
motor cortex
motor unit
neuron
parasympathetic nervous system

peripheral nervous system (PNS)
proprioceptors
reciprocal inhibition
resting membrane potential
Schwann cell
spatial summation
sympathetic nervous system
synapses
temporal summation
vestibular apparatus

The nervous system provides the body with a rapid means of internal communication that allows us to move about, talk, and coordinate the activity of billions of cells. Thus, neural activity is critically important in the body's ability to maintain homeostasis. The purpose of this chapter is to present an overview of the nervous system, with emphasis on neural control of voluntary movement. We will begin with a brief discussion of the functions of the nervous system.

GENERAL NERVOUS SYSTEM FUNCTIONS

The nervous system is the body's means of perceiving and responding to events in the internal and external environments. Receptors capable of sensing touch, pain, temperature changes, and chemical stimuli send information to the **central nervous system (CNS)** concerning changes in our environment. The CNS may respond to these stimuli in several ways. The response may be involuntary movement (e.g., rapid removal of a hand from a hot surface), or alteration in the rate of release of some hormone from the endocrine system (see chapter 5). In addition to integrating body activities and controlling voluntary movement, the nervous system is responsible for storing experiences (memory) and establishing patterns of response based on previous experiences (learning). A summary of the functions of the nervous system follows (11, 35, 36):

1. Control of the internal environment (nervous system works with endocrine system)
2. Voluntary control of movement
3. Programming of spinal cord reflexes
4. Assimilation of experiences necessary for memory and learning

ORGANIZATION OF THE NERVOUS SYSTEM

Anatomically, the nervous system can be divided into two main parts: the CNS and the **peripheral nervous system (PNS).** The CNS is that portion of the nervous system contained in the skull (brain) and the spinal cord; the PNS consists of nerve cells **(neurons)** outside the CNS (see figure 7.1).

The PNS can be further subdivided into two sections: (1) the sensory portion and (2) the motor portion. The sensory division is responsible for transmission of neuron impulses from sense organs (receptors) to the CNS. These sensory nerve fibers, which conduct information toward the CNS, are called **afferent fibers.** The motor portion of the PNS can be

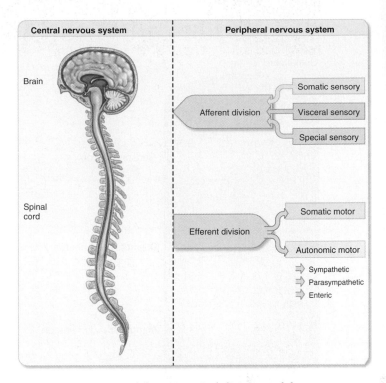

FIGURE 7.1 Overview of the anatomical divisions of the nervous system.

further subdivided into the somatic motor division (which innervates skeletal muscle) and autonomic motor division (which innervates involuntary effector organs like smooth muscle in the gut, cardiac muscle, and glands). Motor nerve fibers, which conduct impulses away from the CNS, are referred to as **efferent fibers.** The relationships between the CNS and the PNS are visualized in figure 7.2.

IN SUMMARY

- The nervous system is the body's means of perceiving and responding to events in the internal and external environments. Receptors capable of sensing touch, pain, temperature, and chemical stimuli send information to the CNS concerning changes in our environment. The CNS responds by either voluntary movement or a change in the rate of release of some hormone from the endocrine system, depending on which response is appropriate.
- The nervous system is divided into two major divisions: (1) the central nervous system and (2) the peripheral nervous system. The central nervous system includes the brain and the spinal cord, whereas the peripheral nervous system includes the nerves outside the central nervous system.

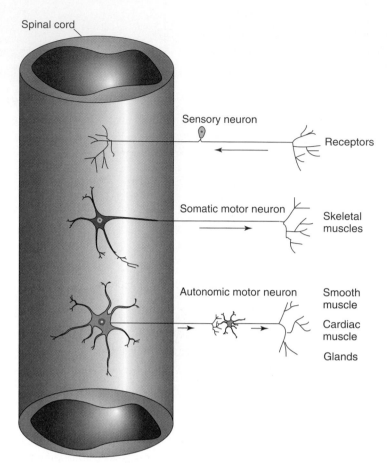

CNS   PNS

Spinal cord

Sensory neuron

Receptors

Somatic motor neuron

Skeletal muscles

Autonomic motor neuron

Smooth muscle

Cardiac muscle

Glands

FIGURE 7.2 The relationship between the motor and sensory fibers of the peripheral nervous system (PNS) and the central nervous system (CNS).

Structure of the Neuron

The functional unit of the nervous system is the neuron. Anatomically, neurons can be divided into three regions: (1) **cell body,** (2) **dendrites,** and (3) **axon** (see figure 7.3). The center of operation for the neuron is the cell body, or soma, which contains the nucleus. Narrow, cytoplasmic attachments extend from the cell body and are called dendrites. Dendrites serve as a receptive area that can conduct electrical impulses toward the cell body. The axon (also called the nerve fiber) carries the electrical message away from the cell body toward another neuron or effector organ. Axons vary in length from a few millimeters to a meter (11, 17). Each neuron has only one axon; however, the axon can divide into several collateral branches that terminate at other neurons, muscle cells, or glands (figure 7.3). Contact points between an axon of one neuron and the dendrite of another neuron are called **synapses** (see figure 7.4).

In large nerve fibers like those innervating skeletal muscle, the axons are covered with an insulating layer of cells called **Schwann cells.** The membranes of Schwann cells contain a large amount of a lipid-protein substance called myelin, which forms a dis-

continuous sheath that covers the outside of the axon. The gaps or spaces between the myelin segments along the axon are called nodes of Ranvier and play an important role in neural transmission. In general, the larger the diameter of the axon, the greater the speed of neural transmission (11, 17). Thus, those axons with large myelin sheaths conduct impulses more rapidly than small, nonmyelinated fibers. Damage or destruction of myelin along myelinated nerve fibers results in nervous system dysfunction. Indeed, damage to myelin is the basis for the neurological disease multiple sclerosis (see Clinical Applications 7.1 for more information about multiple sclerosis).

Electrical Activity in Neurons

Neurons are considered "excitable tissue" because of their specialized properties of irritability and conductivity. **Irritability** is the ability of the dendrites and neuron cell body to respond to a stimulus and convert it to a neural impulse. **Conductivity** refers to the transmission of the impulse along the axon. A nerve impulse can be thought of as an electrical signal

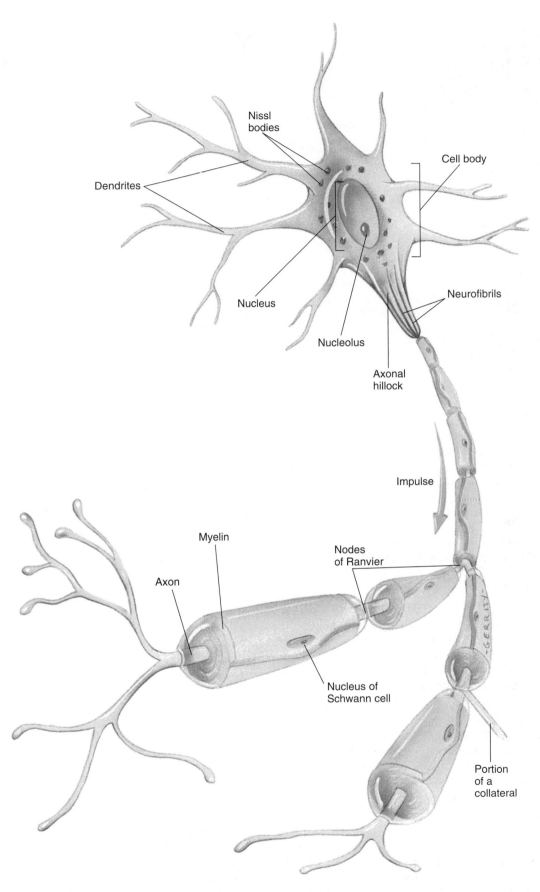

FIGURE 7.3 The parts of a neuron.

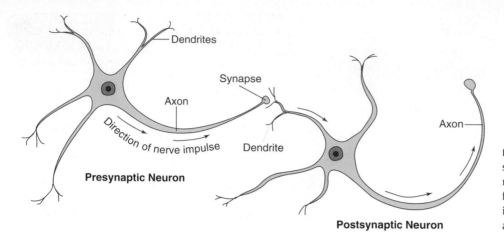

FIGURE 7.4 An illustration of synaptic transmission. For a nerve impulse to continue from one neuron to another, it must cross the synaptic cleft at a synapse.

Dendrites

Synapse

Axon

Direction of nerve impulse

Dendrite

Presynaptic Neuron

Axon

Postsynaptic Neuron

CLINICAL APPLICATIONS 7.1

Multiple Sclerosis and Nervous System Function

Multiple sclerosis (MS) is a neurological disease that progressively destroys the myelin sheaths of axons in multiple areas of the central nervous system (10, 14). Although the exact cause of MS is not known, the MS-mediated destruction of myelin has an inherited (i.e., genetic) component and is due to an immune system attack on myelin. Destruction of the myelin sheath prohibits the normal conduction of nerve impulses, resulting in a progressive loss of nervous system function. The pathology of MS is characterized by general fatigue, muscle weakness, poor motor control, loss of balance, and mental depression (43). Therefore, patients with MS often have difficulties in performing activities of daily living and suffer from a low quality of life.

Although there is no known cure for MS, growing evidence indicates that regular exercise, including both endurance and resistance exercise, can improve the functional capacity of patients suffering from this neurological disorder (43, 44). For example, recent studies reveal that MS patients engaging in a regular exercise program exhibit increased muscular strength and endurance resulting in an improved quality of life (44). Importantly, regular exercise may also reduce the mental depression associated with MS (43).

---

carried the length of the axon. This electrical signal is initiated via some stimulus that causes a change in the normal electrical charge of the neuron.

Resting Membrane Potential At rest, all cells (including neurons) are negatively charged on the inside of the cell with respect to the charge on the exterior of the cell. This negative charge is the result of an unequal distribution of charged ions (ions are elements with a positive or negative charge) across the cell membrane. Thus, a neuron is said to be polarized, and this electrical charge difference is called the **resting membrane potential.** The magnitude of the resting membrane potential varies from −5 to −100 mv depending upon the cell type; in neurons, the resting membrane potential is generally in the range of −40 mv to −75 mv (38) (figure 7.5).

Let's discuss the resting membrane potential in more detail. Cellular proteins, phosphate groups, and other nucleotides are negatively charged (anions) and are fixed inside the cell because they cannot penetrate the cell membrane. Since these negatively charged molecules are unable to leave the cell, they attract positively charged ions (cations) from the extracellular fluid. This results in an accumulation of a net positive charge on the outside surface of the membrane and a net negative charge on the inside surface of the membrane (11, 18).

The magnitude of the resting membrane potential is primarily determined by two factors: (1) the permeability of the plasma membrane to different ion species and (2) the difference in ion concentrations between the intracellular and extracellular fluids (45). Although numerous intracellular and extracellular ions exist, sodium, potassium, and chloride ions are present in the greatest concentrations and therefore play the most important role in generating the resting membrane potential (37, 45). The concentrations of

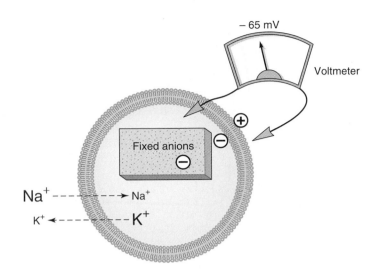

FIGURE 7.5 Illustration of the resting membrane potential in cells. Compared to the outside of the cell, more negatively charged (fixed) ions exist inside the cell; this results in a negative resting membrane potential. Also, notice that both sodium and potassium can diffuse across the plasma member with potassium diffusing from the inside of the cell to the extracellular fluid, whereas sodium diffuses into the cell from the extracellular fluid.

FIGURE 7.6 Concentrations of ions across a typical cell membrane. Although the body contains many different ions, sodium, potassium, and chloride ions exist in the largest concentrations and therefore play the most important roles in determining the resting membrane potential in cells.

sodium, potassium, chloride, and calcium are illustrated in figure 7.6. Notice that the concentration of sodium is much greater on the outside of the cell, whereas the concentration of potassium is much greater on the inside of the cell. For comparative purposes, the intracellular and extracellular concentration of calcium is also illustrated.

The permeability of the neuron membrane to potassium, sodium, and other ions is regulated by proteins within the membrane that function as channels that can be opened or closed by "gates" within the channel. This concept is illustrated in figure 7.7. Notice that ions can move freely across the cell membrane when the channel is open, whereas closure of the channel gate prevents ion movement. Since the concentration of potassium (+ charge) is high inside the cell and the concentration of sodium (+ charge) is high outside the cell, a change in the membrane's permeability to either potassium or sodium would result in a movement of these charged ions down their concentration gradients. That is, sodium would enter the cell and potassium would leave the cell. At rest, almost all of the sodium channels are closed, whereas a few potassium channels are open. This means that there are more potassium ions leaving the cell than sodium ions "leaking" into the cell. This results in a net loss of positive charges from the inside of the membrane, thus making the resting membrane potential negative. In short, the negative membrane

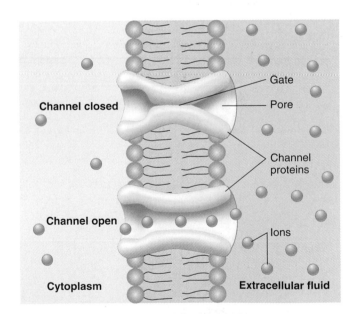

FIGURE 7.7 Illustration of channels that regulate ion passage across the plasma membrane. Ion channels are composed of proteins that span the entire membrane from the inside to the outer surface. Ion passage through the channels is regulated by the opening or closing of "gates" that serve as doors in the middle of the channel. For example, when channels are open (i.e., gate is open) ions are free to pass through the channel (lower portion of figure). In contrast, when the channel gate is closed, ions' movement through the channel is halted (upper portion of figure).

potential in a resting neuron is due primarily to the diffusion of potassium out of the cell, caused by: (1) the higher permeability of the membrane for potassium than sodium and (2) the concentration gradient for potassium from inside to outside the cell.

As mentioned previously, a small number of ions are always moving across the cell membrane. If potassium ions continued to diffuse out of the cell and the sodium ions continued to diffuse into the cell, the concentration gradients for these ions would decrease. This would result in a loss of the negative membrane potential. What prevents this from happening? The cell membrane has a sodium/potassium pump that uses energy from ATP to maintain the intracellular/extracellular concentrations by pumping sodium out of the cell and potassium into the cell. Interestingly, this pump not only maintains the concentration gradients that are needed to maintain the resting membrane potential, but it also helps to generate the potential since it exchanges three sodium ions for every two potassium ions (43) (figure 7.8).

Action Potential A neural message is generated when a stimulus of sufficient strength reaches the neuron membrane and opens sodium gates, which

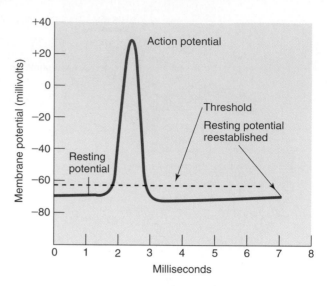

FIGURE 7.9 An action potential is produced by an increase in sodium conductance into the neuron. As sodium enters the neuron, the change becomes more and more positive, and an action potential is generated.

allows sodium ions to diffuse into the neuron, making the inside more and more positive (depolarizing the cell). When depolarization reaches a critical value called "threshold," the sodium gates open wide and an **action potential,** or nerve impulse, is formed (see figures 7.9 and 7.10a). Once an action potential has been generated, a sequence of ionic exchanges occurs along the axon to propagate the nerve impulse. This ionic exchange along the neuron occurs in a sequential fashion at the nodes of Ranvier (figure 7.3).

Repolarization occurs immediately following depolarization, resulting in a return of the resting membrane potential with the nerve ready to be stimulated again (figure 7.9). How does repolarization occur? Depolarization, with a slight time delay, causes a brief increase in membrane permeability to potassium. As a result, potassium leaves the cell rapidly, making the inside of the membrane more negative (see figure 7.10b). Secondly, after the depolarization stimulus is removed, the sodium gates within the cell membrane close, and sodium entry into the cell is slowed (therefore, few positive charges are entering the cell). The combined result of these activities quickly restores the resting membrane potential to the original negative charge.

All-or-None Law The development of a nerve impulse is considered to be an "all-or-none" response and is referred to as the "all-or-none" law of action potentials. This means that if a nerve impulse is initiated, the impulse will travel the entire length of the

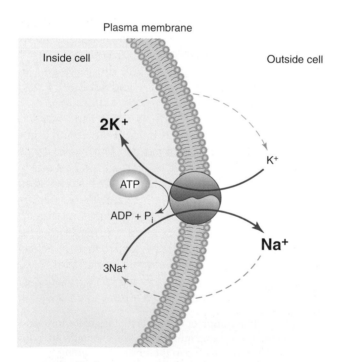

FIGURE 7.8 Exchange of sodium and potassium across the plasma membrane by the sodium/potassium pump. The sodium/potassium pump requires energy (ATP) and is therefore an active transport pump that moves 3 molecules of sodium out of the cell and returns 2 molecules of potassium into the cell. The dashed arrows indicate the direction of passive transport (diffusion) and the solid arrows indicate the direction of active transport.

FIGURE 7.10 (a) When a polarized nerve fiber is stimulated, sodium channels open, some sodium ions diffuse inward, and the membrane is depolarized. (b) When the potassium channels open, potassium ions diffuse outward, and the membrane is repolarized.

axon without a decrease in voltage. In other words, the neural impulse is just as strong after traveling the length of the axon as it was at the initial point of stimulation.

A mechanical analogy of the all-or-none law is the firing of a gun (43). That is, the speed of the bullet leaving the gun does not depend upon how hard you pulled the trigger. Indeed, firing a gun is all or none; you cannot fire a gun halfway.

Neurotransmitters and Synaptic Transmission

As mentioned previously, neurons communicate with other neurons at junctions called synapses. A synapse is a small gap (20–30 nanometers) between the synaptic endfoot of the presynaptic neuron and a dendrite of a postsynaptic neuron (see figure 7.11). Communication between neurons occurs via a process called synaptic transmission, and it happens when sufficient amounts of a specific neurotransmitter (a neurotransmitter is a chemical messenger that neurons use to communicate with each other) are released from synaptic vesicles contained in the presynaptic neuron. The nerve impulse results in the synaptic vesicles releasing stored neurotransmitter into the synaptic cleft. Neurotransmitters that cause the depolarization of membranes are termed *excitatory transmitters*. After release into the synaptic cleft, these neurotransmitters bind to "receptors" on the target membrane, which produces a series of graded depolarizations in the dendrites and cell body (1, 2, 18, 22, 28, 34). These graded depolarizations are known as excitatory postsynaptic potentials **(EPSPs).** If sufficient amounts of the neurotransmitter are released, the postsynaptic neuron is depolarized to threshold and an action potential is generated.

There are two ways in which EPSPs can bring the postsynaptic neuron to threshold: (1) temporal summation and (2) spatial summation. The summing of several EPSPs from a single presynaptic neuron over a short time period is termed **temporal summation** ("temporal" refers to time). The number of EPSPs required to bring the postsynaptic neuron to threshold varies, but it is estimated that the addition of up to fifty EPSPs might be required to produce an action potential within some neurons (37). Nonetheless, one means by which an action potential can be generated is through rapid, repetitive excitation from a single excitatory presynaptic neuron.

A second means of achieving an action potential at the postsynaptic membrane is to sum EPSPs from several different presynaptic inputs (i.e., different points in space) and is known as **spatial summation.** In spatial summation, concurrent EPSPs come into a postsynaptic neuron from numerous different excitatory inputs. As with temporal summation, up to fifty EPSPs arriving simultaneously on the postsynaptic membrane may be required to produce an action potential (37).

Sending neuron

Nerve impulse

Axon

Endfeet

Neural impulse

Dendrite

Receiving neuron

Neural impulse

Endfoot
(or terminal bouton)

Synaptic vesicle

Synaptic cleft

Neurotransmitter
molecule

Presynaptic membrane

Postsynaptic membrane

FIGURE 7.11   The basic structure of a chemical synapse. In this idealized drawing, the basic elements of the synapse can be seen: the terminal of the presynaptic axon containing synaptic vesicles, the synaptic cleft, and the postsynaptic membrane. From A. J. Vander et al. *Human Physiology: The Mechanisms of Body Function*, 8th edition. Copyright 2001 McGraw-Hill, Inc., New York. Reprinted by permission.

A common neurotransmitter, which also happens to be the transmitter at the nerve/muscle junction, is acetylcholine. Upon release into the synaptic cleft, acetylcholine binds to receptors on the postsynaptic membrane and opens "channels," which allow sodium to enter the nerve or muscle cell. When enough sodium enters the postsynaptic membrane of a neuron or muscle, depolarization results. In order to prevent chronic depolarization of the postsynaptic neuron, the neurotransmitter must be broken down into less-active molecules via enzymes found in the synaptic cleft. In the case of acetylcholine, the degrading enzyme is called acetylcholinesterase. This enzyme breaks down acetylcholine into acetyl and choline and thus removes the stimulus for depolarization (11). Following breakdown of the neurotransmitter, the postsynaptic membrane repolarizes and is prepared to receive additional neurotransmitters and generate a new action potential. Note that not all neurotransmitters are excitatory. In fact, some neurotransmitters have just the opposite effect of excitatory transmitters (28). These inhibitory transmitters cause a hyperpolarization (increased negativity) of the postsynaptic membrane. This hyperpolarization of the membrane is called an inhibitory postsynaptic potential, or **IPSP.** The end result of an IPSP is that the neuron develops a more negative resting membrane potential, is pushed further from threshold, and thus resists depolarization. In general, whether a neuron reaches threshold or not is dependent on the ratio of the number of EPSPs to the number of IPSPs. For example, a neuron that is simultaneously bombarded by an equal number of EPSPs and IPSPs will not reach threshold and generate an action potential. On the other hand, if the EPSPs outnumber the IPSPs, the neuron is moved toward threshold and an action potential may be generated.

Acetylcholine is an interesting example of a neurotransmitter that can be both inhibitory and excitatory. While acetylcholine produces depolarization of skeletal muscle, it causes a hyperpolarization of the heart, slowing the heart rate. This occurs because the combination of acetylcholine with receptors in the heart causes the opening of membrane channels that allow potassium to diffuse out of the cell. Therefore, an outward diffusion of potassium produces a hyperpolarization of heart tissue, and the membrane potential is moved further away from the threshold valve.

IN SUMMARY

- Nerve cells are called neurons and are divided anatomically into three parts: (1) the cell body, (2) dendrites, and (3) the axon. Axons are generally covered by Schwann cells, with gaps between these cells called nodes of Ranvier.
- Neurons are specialized cells that respond to physical or chemical changes in their environment. At rest, neurons are negatively charged in the interior with respect to the electrical charge outside the cell. This difference in electrical charge is called the resting membrane potential.
- A neuron "fires" when a stimulus changes the permeability of the membrane, allowing sodium to enter at a high rate, which depolarizes the cell. When the depolarization reaches threshold, an action potential or nerve impulse is initiated. Repolarization occurs immediately following depolarization due to an increase in membrane permeability to potassium and a decreased permeability to sodium.
- Neurons communicate with other neurons at junctions called synapses. Synaptic trans-

mission occurs when sufficient amounts of a specific neurotransmitter are released from the presynaptic neuron. Upon release, the neurotransmitter binds to a receptor on the postsynaptic membrane.
- Neurotransmitters can be excitatory or inhibitory. An excitatory transmitter increases neuronal permeability to sodium and results in excitatory postsynaptic potentials (EPSPs). Inhibitory neurotransmitters cause the neuron to become more negative (hyperpolarized). This hyperpolarization of the membrane is called an inhibitory postsynaptic potential (IPSP).

SENSORY INFORMATION AND REFLEXES

The CNS receives a constant bombardment of messages from receptors throughout the body about changes in both the internal and external environment. These receptors are "sense organs" that "change" forms of energy in the "real world" into the energy of nerve impulses, which are conducted to the CNS by sensory neurons. A complete discussion of sense organs is beyond the scope of this chapter, so we will limit our discussion to those receptors responsible for position sense and muscle chemoreceptors (i.e., receptors that are sensitive to changes in the chemical environment of muscles). Receptors that provide the CNS with information about body position are called **proprioceptors,** or kinesthetic receptors, and include muscle spindles, Golgi tendon organs, and joint receptors. Muscle spindles and Golgi tendon organs are discussed in chapter 8, so our discussion will center around joint receptors, chemoreceptors, and neural reflexes.

Proprioceptors

The term **kinesthesia** means conscious recognition of the position of body parts with respect to one another as well as recognition of limb-movement rates (24, 26, 31). These functions are accomplished by extensive sensory devices in and around joints. There are three principal types of proprioceptors: (1) free nerve endings, (2) Golgi-type receptors, and (3) pacinian corpuscles. The most abundant of these are free nerve endings, which are sensitive to touch and pressure. These receptors are stimulated strongly at the beginning of movement; they adapt (i.e., become less sensitive to stimuli) slightly at first, but then transmit a steady signal until the movement is complete (5, 12). A second type of position receptor, Golgi-type receptors (not to be confused with Golgi tendon organs found in muscle tendons), are found in ligaments around joints. These receptors are not as abundant as free nerve endings, but they work in a similar manner (11, 35). Pacinian corpuscles are found in the tissues around joints and adapt rapidly following the initiation of movement. This rapid adaptation presumably helps detect the rate of joint rotation (11, 35). To summarize, the joint receptors work together to provide the body with a conscious means of recognition of the orientation of body parts as well as feedback about the rates of limb movement.

Muscle Chemoreceptors

Numerous studies have demonstrated the existence of muscle chemoreceptors (19, 20, 21, 27). These receptors are a type of free nerve ending and are sensitive to changes in the chemical environment surrounding muscle and send information to the CNS via slow conducting fibers classified as group III (myelinated) and group IV (unmyelinated) fibers. Scientific debate continues about the complete list of factors that stimulate muscle chemoreceptors. However, changes in the concentration of hydrogen ions, carbon dioxide, and/or potassium around muscle are known to be potent stimulators of these receptors. The physiological role of muscle chemoreceptors is to provide the CNS with information about the metabolic rate of muscular activity. This information may be important in the regulation of the cardiovascular and pulmonary responses to exercise (3, 21, 27) and will be discussed in chapters 9 and 10.

Reflexes

A reflex arc is the nerve pathway from the receptor to the CNS and from the CNS along a motor pathway back to the effector organ. Reflex contraction of skeletal muscles can occur in response to sensory input and is not dependent on the activation of higher brain centers. One purpose of a reflex is to provide a rapid means of removing a limb from a source of pain. Consider the case of a person touching a sharp object. The obvious reaction to this painful stimulus is to quickly remove the hand from the source of pain. This rapid removal is accomplished via reflex action. Again, the pathways for this neural reflex are as follows (17): (1) first, a sensory nerve (pain receptor) sends a nerve impulse to the spinal column; (2) second, interneurons within the spinal cord are excited and in turn stimulate motor neurons; (3) finally, the excited interneurons cause depolarization of specific motor neurons, which control the flexor muscles necessary to withdraw the limb from the point of injury. The antagonistic muscle group (e.g., extensors) is simultaneously inhibited via IPSPs. This simultaneous excitatory and inhibitory activity is known as **reciprocal inhibition** (see figure 7.12).

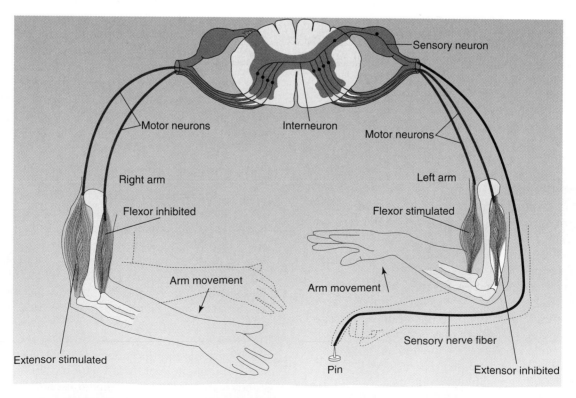

FIGURE 7.12 When the flexor muscle on one side of the body is stimulated to contract via a withdrawal reflex, the extensor on the opposite side also contracts.

Another interesting feature of the withdrawal reflex is that the opposite limb is extended to support the body during the removal of the injured limb. This event is called the crossed-extensor reflex and is illustrated by the left portion of figure 7.12. Notice that the extensors are contracting as the flexors are inhibited.

IN SUMMARY

■ Proprioceptors are position receptors located in joint capsules, ligaments, and muscles. The three most abundant joint and ligament receptors are free nerve endings, Golgi-type receptors, and pacinian corpuscles. These receptors provide the body with a conscious means of recognizing the orientation of body parts as well as feedback about the rates of limb movement.

■ Muscle chemoreceptors are sensitive to changes in the chemical environment surrounding muscle and send information back to the CNS about the metabolic rate of muscular activity.

■ Reflexes provide the body with a rapid, unconscious means of reacting to some stimuli.

SOMATIC MOTOR FUNCTION

The term *somatic* refers to the outer (i.e., nonvisceral) regions of the body. The somatic motor portion of the peripheral nervous system is responsible for carrying neural messages from the spinal cord to skeletal muscle fibers. These neural messages are the signals for muscular contraction to occur. Muscular contraction will be discussed in detail in chapter 8.

The organization of the somatic motor nervous system is illustrated in figure 7.13. The somatic neuron that innervates skeletal muscle fibers is called a motor neuron (also called an alpha motor neuron). Note (figure 7.13) that the cell body of motor neurons is located within the spinal cord. The axon of the motor neuron leaves the spinal cord as a spinal nerve and extends to the muscle that it is responsible for innervating. Once the axon reaches the muscle, the axon splits into collateral branches; each collateral branch innervates a single muscle fiber. Each motor neuron and all the muscle fibers that it innervates is known as a **motor unit.**

When a single motor neuron is activated, all of the muscle fibers that it innervates are stimulated to contract. However, note that the number of muscle fibers that a motor neuron innervates is not constant and varies from muscle to muscle. The number of muscle

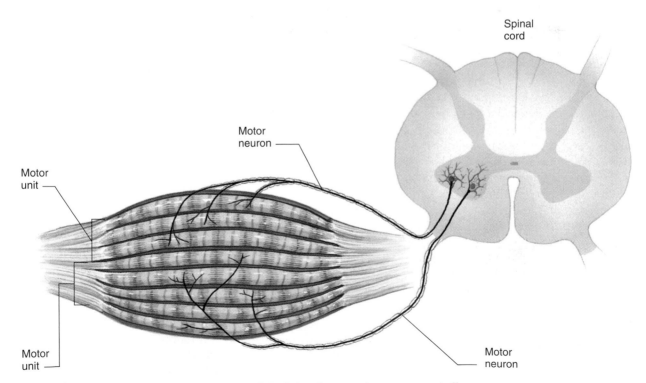

FIGURE 7.13 Illustration of a motor unit. A motor unit is defined as a motor neuron and all the muscle fibers it innervates.

fibers innervated by a single motor neuron is called the innervation ratio (i.e., number of muscle fibers/ motor neuron). In muscle groups that require fine motor control, the innervation ratio is low. For example, the innervation ratio of the extraocular muscles (i.e., muscles that regulate eye movement) is 23/1. In contrast, innervation ratios of large muscles that are not involved in fine motor control (e.g., leg muscles) may range from 1,000/1 to 2,000/1.

IN SUMMARY

- The somatic motor portion of the peripheral nervous system is responsible for carrying neural messages from the spinal cord to skeletal muscle fibers.
- A motor neuron and all the muscle fibers that it innervates are known as a motor unit.
- The number of muscle fibers innervated by a single motor neuron is called the innervation ratio (i.e., number of muscle fibers/motor neuron).

VESTIBULAR APPARATUS AND EQUILIBRIUM

The **vestibular apparatus,** an organ located in the inner ear, is responsible for maintaining general equilibrium. Although a detailed discussion of the anatomy of the vestibular apparatus will not be presented here, a brief discussion of the function of the vestibular apparatus is appropriate. The receptors contained within the vestibular apparatus are sensitive to any change in head position or movement direction (18, 32). Movement of the head excites these receptors, and nerve impulses are sent to the CNS regarding this change in position. Specifically, these receptors provide information about linear acceleration and angular acceleration. This mechanism allows us to have a sense of acceleration or deceleration when running or traveling by car. Further, a sense of angular acceleration helps us maintain balance when the head is turning or spinning (e.g., performing gymnastics or diving).

The neural pathways involved in the control of equilibrium are outlined in figure 7.14. Any head movement results in the stimulation of receptors in the vestibular apparatus, which transmits neural information to the cerebellum and the vestibular nuclei located in the brain stem. Further, the vestibular nuclei relay a message to the oculomotor center (controls eye movement) and to neurons in the spinal cord that control movements of the head and limbs.

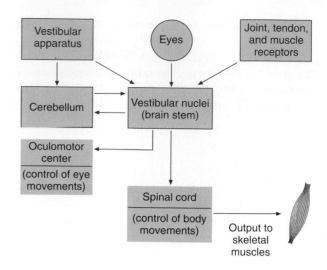

FIGURE 7.14 The role of the vestibular apparatus in the maintenance of equilibrium and balance.

Thus, the vestibular apparatus controls head and eye movement during physical activity, which serves to maintain balance and visually track the events of movement. In summary, the vestibular apparatus is sensitive to the position of the head in space and to sudden changes in the direction of body movement. Its primary function is to maintain equilibrium and preserve a constant plane of head position. Failure of the vestibular apparatus to function properly would prevent the accurate performance of any athletic task that requires head movement. Since most sporting events require at least some head movement, the importance of the vestibular apparatus is obvious.

IN SUMMARY

- The vestibular apparatus is responsible for maintaining general equilibrium and is located in the inner ear. Specifically, these receptors provide information about linear and angular acceleration.

MOTOR CONTROL FUNCTIONS OF THE BRAIN

The brain can be conveniently subdivided into three parts: the brain stem, cerebrum, and cerebellum. Figure 7.15 demonstrates the anatomical relationship of these components. Each of these structures makes important contributions to the regulation of movement. The next several paragraphs will outline the brain's role in regulating the performance of sports skills.

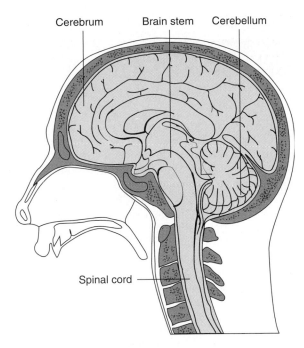

Cerebrum   Brain stem   Cerebellum

Spinal cord

FIGURE 7.15 The anatomical relationship among the cerebrum, the cerebellum, and the brain stem.

Brain Stem

The **brain stem** is located inside the base of the skull just above the spinal cord. It consists of a complicated series of nerve tracts and nuclei (clusters of neurons), and is responsible for many metabolic functions, cardiorespiratory control, and some highly complex reflexes. The major structures of the brain stem are the medulla, pons, and midbrain. In addition, there is a series of complex neurons scattered throughout the brain stem that is collectively called the *reticular formation*. The reticular formation receives and integrates information from all regions of the CNS and works with higher brain centers in controlling muscular activity (7, 43).

In general, the neuronal circuits in the brain stem are thought to be responsible for the control of eye movement and muscle tone, equilibrium, support of the body against gravity, and many special reflexes. One of the most important roles of the brain stem in control of locomotion is that of maintaining postural tone. That is, centers in the brain stem provide the nervous activity necessary to maintain normal upright posture and therefore support the body against gravity. It is clear that the maintenance of upright posture requires that the brain stem receive information from several sensory modalities (e.g., vestibular receptors, pressure receptors of the skin, vision). Damage to any portion of the brain stem results in impaired movement control (9, 18) (see A Closer Look 7.1).

Cerebrum

The **cerebrum** is the large dome of the brain that is divided into right and left cerebral hemispheres. The outermost layer of the cerebrum is called the *cerebral cortex* and is composed of tightly arranged neurons. Although the cortex is only about one-fourth of an inch thick, it contains over eight million neurons. The cortex performs three very important motor behavior

A CLOSER LOOK 7.1

Parkinson's Disease and Motor Function

Much of our present information concerning the regulation of motor control has come from those disorders involving various areas of the brain. When an area of the CNS malfunctions, the resulting impairment of motor control gives neuroscientists a better understanding of the function of the affected area. The basal ganglia are a series of clusters of neurons located in both cerebral hemispheres. One of the important functions of the basal ganglia (also called BASAL nuclei) is to aid in the regulation of movement. Parkinson's disease is a disorder of the basal ganglia that results in a decrease in the synthesis of a neurotransmitter called dopamine. Dopamine's function in the basal ganglia appears to be one of inhibiting the amount of muscular activity as an aid in the control of various muscular activities. Patients with Parkinson's disease have a reduction in the amount of discharge from the basal ganglia, which results in involuntary movement or tremors. Further, although Parkinson's patients can frequently carry out rapid movements normally, these individuals often have great difficulty in performing slow movements. This observation supports the concept that the basal ganglia are important in the conduct of slow voluntary movement. Parkinson's disease is often treated by administering drugs that stimulate the production of dopamine.

The cause of Parkinson's disease isn't known. It has been attributed to exposure to certain chemicals and to severe and frequent injury to the brain, such as occurred in heavyweight boxing champion Muhammad Ali (38).

Head Injuries in Sports

Although head injuries can occur in many different types of sports, sports with the greatest risk of head injury include football, gymnastics, ice hockey, wrestling, and boxing. Other sporting activities with a significant risk for head injury include horse racing, motorcycle and automobile racing, martial arts, soccer, and rugby.

A forceful blow to the head during sports (e.g., a football collision) can result in a brain injury that can be classified as minor or major, depending upon the amount of damage to brain tissue. One of the most serious head injuries associated with sports is an intracranial hemorrhage (i.e., bleeding in the brain) (4). In fact, intracranial hemorrhage is the leading cause of death in athletes today (reviewed in 4). This type of injury can occur when an athlete sustains a hard blow to the head (e.g., baseball player struck in the head by a pitch) that results in damage to blood vessels in the brain. Several different categories of intracranial hemorrhages can occur, and the risk of serious injury or death varies across the different types (30).

Another common type of head injury in sports is the concussion. At present, there is not universal agreement on the definition of a concussion (4). However, a concussion is generally considered to be a "clinical syndrome characterized by impairment of neural functions" (e.g., loss of consciousness, disturbed vision, or loss of equilibrium). Concussions generally occur due to a blow to the head (e.g., punch to the head in boxing). For additional information on head injuries in sports, see Bailes and Hudson (2001) and Cross and Serenelli (2003) in the Suggested Readings.

functions (11, 35): (1) the organization of complex movement, (2) the storage of learned experiences, and (3) the reception of sensory information. We will limit our discussion to the role of the cortex in the organization of movement. The portion of the cerebral cortex that is most concerned with voluntary movement is the **motor cortex.** Although the motor cortex plays a significant role in motor control, it appears that input to the motor cortex from subcortical structures (i.e., cerebellum, etc.) is absolutely essential for coordinated movement to occur (15, 35). Thus, the motor cortex can be described as the final relay point upon which subcortical inputs are focused. After the motor cortex sums these inputs, the final movement plan is formulated and the motor commands are sent to the spinal cord. This "movement plan" can be modified by both subcortical and spinal centers, which supervise the fine details of the movement.

Cerebellum

The **cerebellum** lies behind the pons and medulla and has a convoluted appearance (figure 7.15). Although complete knowledge about cerebellar function is not currently available, much is known about the role of this structure in movement control. It is clear that the cerebellum plays an important role in coordinating and monitoring complex movement. This work is accomplished via connections leading from the cerebellum to the motor cortex, the brain stem, and the spinal cord. Evidence exists to suggest that the primary role of the cerebellum is to aid in the control of movement in response to feedback from

proprioceptors (35). Further, the cerebellum may initiate fast, ballistic movements via its connection with the motor cortex (15). Damage to the cerebellum results in poor movement control and muscular tremor that is most severe during rapid movement. Head injuries due to sport-related injuries can lead to damage and dysfunction in both the cerebrum and/or cerebellum. For an overview of sport-related head injuries, see Clinical Applications 7.2.

IN SUMMARY

- The brain can be subdivided into three parts: (1) the brain stem, (2) the cerebrum, and (3) the cerebellum.
- The motor cortex controls motor activity with the aid of input from subcortical areas.

MOTOR FUNCTIONS OF THE SPINAL CORD

One motor function of the spinal cord has already been discussed (withdrawal reflex). The precise role of spinal reflexes in the control of movement is still being debated. However, there is increasing evidence that normal motor function is influenced by spinal reflexes. In fact, some authors claim that reflexes play a major role in the control of voluntary movements. These investigators believe that the events that underlie volitional movement are built on a variety of spinal reflexes (15, 41). Support for this idea comes from the demonstration that spinal reflex neurons are directly affected by descending neural traffic from the brain stem and cortical centers.

The spinal cord makes a major contribution to the control of movement by the preparation of spinal centers to perform the desired movement. The spinal mechanism by which a voluntary movement is translated into appropriate muscle action is termed *spinal tuning*. Spinal tuning appears to operate in the following way: Higher brain centers of the motor system are concerned with only the general parameters of movement. The specific details of the movement are refined at the spinal cord level via interaction of spinal cord neurons and higher brain centers. In other words, although the general pattern of the anticipated movement is controlled by higher motor centers, additional refinement of this movement may occur by a complex interaction of spinal cord neurons and higher centers (8, 35, 41). Thus, it appears that spinal centers play an important role in volitional movement.

IN SUMMARY

- Evidence exists that the spinal cord plays an important role in voluntary movement with groups of neurons controlling certain aspects of motor activity.
- The spinal mechanism by which a voluntary movement is translated into appropriate muscle action is termed *spinal tuning*.

CONTROL OF MOTOR FUNCTIONS

Watching a highly skilled athlete perform a sports skill is exciting, but it really does not help us to appreciate the complex integration of the many parts of the nervous system required to perform this act. A pitcher throwing a baseball seems to the observer to be accomplishing a simple act, but in reality this movement consists of a complex interaction of higher brain centers with spinal reflexes performed together with precise timing. How the nervous system produces a coordinated movement has been one of the major unresolved mysteries facing neurophysiologists for many decades. Although progress has been made toward answering the basic question of "How do humans control voluntary movement?" much is still unknown about this process. Our purpose here will be to provide the reader with a simplistic overview of the brain and the control of movement.

Traditionally, it was believed that the motor cortex controlled voluntary movement with little input

from subcortical areas (33, 39). Recent evidence suggests that this is not the case (15, 35). Although the motor cortex is the final executor of movement programs, it appears that the motor cortex does not give the initial signal to move, but rather is at the end of the chain of neurophysiological events involved in volitional movement (15). The first step in performing a voluntary movement occurs in subcortical and cortical motivational areas, which play a key role in consciousness. This conscious "prime drive" sends signals to the so-called association areas of the cortex (not motor cortex), which forms a "rough draft" of the planned movement from a stock of stored subroutines (8). Information concerning the nature of the plan of movement is then sent to both the cerebellum and the basal ganglia (clusters of neurons located in the cerebral hemispheres) (see figure 7.16). These structures cooperate to convert the "rough draft" into precise temporal and spatial excitation programs (15). The cerebellum is possibly more important for making fast movements, while the basal ganglia are more responsible for slow or deliberate movements. From the cerebellum and basal ganglia the precise program is sent through the thalamus to the motor cortex, which forwards the message down to spinal neurons for "spinal tuning" and finally to skeletal muscle (13). Feedback to the CNS from muscle receptors and proprioceptors allows for modification of motor programs if necessary. The ability to change movement

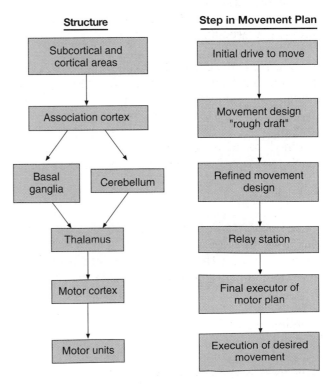

FIGURE 7.16 Block diagram of the structures and processes leading to voluntary movement.

patterns allows the individual to correct "errors" in the original movement plan.

To summarize, the control of voluntary movement is complex and requires the cooperation of many areas of the brain as well as several subcortical areas. Recent evidence suggests that the motor cortex does not by itself formulate the signals required to initiate voluntary movement. Instead, the motor cortex receives input from a variety of cortical and subcortical structures. Feedback to the CNS from muscle and joint receptors allows for adjustments to improve the movement pattern. Much is still unknown about the details of the control of complex movement, and this topic provides an exciting frontier for future research.

IN SUMMARY

- Control of voluntary movement is complex and requires the cooperation of many areas of the brain as well as several subcortical areas.
- The first step in performing a voluntary movement occurs in subcortical and cortical motivational areas, which send signals to the association cortex, which forms a "rough draft" of the planned movement.
- The movement plan is then sent to both the cerebellum and the basal ganglia. These structures cooperate to convert the "rough draft" into precise temporal and spatial excitation programs.
- The cerebellum is important for making fast movements, while the basal ganglia are more responsible for slow or deliberate movements.
- From the cerebellum and basal ganglia the precise program is sent through the thalamus to the motor cortex, which forwards the message down to spinal neurons for "spinal tuning" and finally to skeletal muscle.
- Feedback to the CNS from muscle receptors and proprioceptors allows for the modification of motor programs if necessary.

AUTONOMIC NERVOUS SYSTEM

The **autonomic nervous system** plays an important role in maintaining the constancy of the body's internal environment. In contrast to somatic motor nerves, autonomic motor nerves innervate effector organs (e.g., smooth muscle, cardiac muscle), which are not usually under voluntary control. Autonomic motor nerves innervate cardiac muscle, glands, and smooth muscle found in airways, the gut, and blood vessels. In general, the autonomic nervous system operates below the conscious level, although some individuals apparently can learn to control some portions of this system. Although involuntary, it appears that the function of the autonomic nervous system is closely linked to emotion. For example, all of us have experienced an increase in heart rate following extreme excitement or fear. Further, the secretions of digestive glands and sweat glands are affected by periods of excitement. It should not be surprising that participation in intense exercise results in an increase in autonomic activity.

The autonomic nervous system can be separated both functionally and anatomically into two divisions: (1) **sympathetic** division and (2) **parasympathetic** division (see figure 7.17). Most organs receive dual innervation, by both the parasympathetic and sympathetic branches of the autonomic nervous system (43). In general, the sympathetic portion of the autonomic nervous system tends to activate an organ (e.g., increases heart rate), while parasympathetic impulses tend to inhibit it (e.g., slows heart rate). Therefore, the activity of a particular organ can be regulated according to the ratio of sympathetic/parasympathetic impulses to the tissue. In this way, the autonomic nervous system may regulate the activities of involuntary muscles and glands in accordance with the needs of the body (see chapter 5).

The sympathetic division of the autonomic nervous system has its cell bodies of the preganglionic neurons (a ganglion is a group of cell bodies outside of the CNS) in the thoracic and lumbar regions of the spinal cord. These fibers leave the spinal cord and enter the sympathetic ganglia (figure 7.17). The neurotransmitter between the preganglionic neurons and postganglionic neurons is acetylcholine. Postganglionic sympathetic fibers leave these sympathetic ganglia and innervate a wide variety of tissues. The neurotransmitter released at the effector organ is primarily norepinephrine. Recall from chapter 5 that norepinephrine exerts its action on the effector organ by binding to either an alpha or a beta receptor on the membrane of the target organ (6). Following sympathetic stimulation, norepinephrine is removed in a variety of ways. First, much of the norepinephrine is taken back up into the postganglionic fiber, while the remaining portion will be broken down into nonactive by-products (6, 16, 40, 42).

The parasympathetic division of the autonomic nervous system has its cell bodies located within the brain stem and the sacral portion of the spinal cord. Parasympathetic fibers leave the brain stem and the spinal cord and converge on ganglia in a wide variety of anatomical areas. Acetylcholine is the neurotransmitter in both preganglionic and postganglionic fibers. After parasympathetic nerve stimulation, acetylcholine is released and rapidly degraded by the enzyme acetyl-cholinesterase.

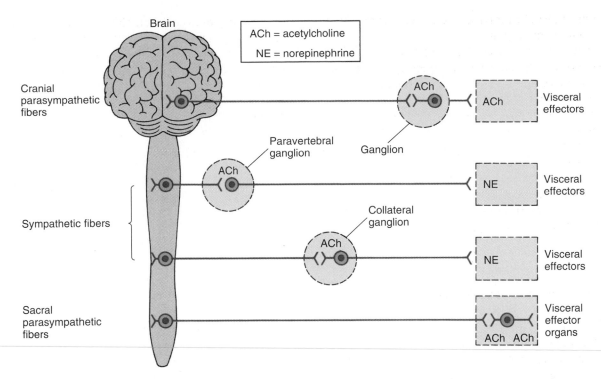

FIGURE 7.17 A simple schematic demonstrating the neurotransmitters of the autonomic nervous system. ACh = acetylcholine; NE = norepinephrine.

EXERCISE ENHANCES BRAIN HEALTH

While it is well known that regular exercise can benefit overall health, research now indicates that exercise can also improve brain (cognitive) function, particularly in later life. Maintaining brain health throughout life is an important goal and both mental stimulation (e.g., reading) and exercise are interventions that can contribute to good brain health. Therefore, daily exercise is a simple and inexpensive way to help maintain the health of the central nervous system.

How strong is the scientific evidence to support the concept that exercise improves brain function? In short, the research evidence is very convincing. Indeed, over the past decade, many studies on humans have demonstrated the benefits of exercise on brain health and function, particularly in aging populations (25). For example, a recent five-year study in humans has concluded that exercise improves brain function and reduces the risk of cognitive impairment associated with aging (23). Further, it is clear that regular exercise can protect the brain against disease (e.g., Alzheimer's disease) and certain types of brain injury (e.g., stroke) (25).

How does exercise enhance brain health? It appears that exercise maintains neuronal health by improving blood flow to the brain and by increasing brain levels of growth factors that promote optimal function of neurons. Many of the positive effects of exercise on the brain are realized in the hippocampus, a brain region that is important for learning and memory. Because voluntary exercise provides benefits to this important area of the brain, many gerontologists (doctors that specialize in treating older people) now recommend daily exercise for their patients. For more details on exercise and brain function, see McAuley et al. (2004) in the Suggested Readings.

> **IN SUMMARY**
>
> - The autonomic nervous system is responsible for maintaining the constancy of the body's internal environment.
> - Anatomically and functionally, the autonomic nervous system can be divided into two divisions: (1) the sympathetic division and (2) the parasympathetic division.
> - In general, the sympathetic portion (releasing norepinephrine) tends to excite an organ, while the parasympathetic portion (releasing acetylcholine) tends to inhibit the same organ.
> - Research indicates that exercise can improve brain (cognitive) function, particularly in older individuals.

STUDY QUESTIONS

1. Identify the location and functions of the central nervous system.
2. Draw a simple chart illustrating the organization of the nervous system.
3. Define *synapses*.
4. Define *membrane potential* and *action potential*.
5. Discuss an IPSP and an EPSP. How do they differ?
6. What are proprioceptors? Give some examples.
7. Describe the location and function of the vestibular apparatus.
8. What is meant by the term *spinal tuning*?
9. List the possible motor functions played by the brain stem, the motor cortex, and the cerebellum.
10. Describe the divisions and functions of the autonomic nervous system.
11. Define the terms *motor unit* and *innervation ratio*.
12. Briefly describe the positive benefits of exercise on brain function.
13. How does regular exercise maintain neuronal health?

SUGGESTED READINGS

Bailes J., and V. Hudson. 2001. Classification of sports-related head trauma: A spectrum of mild to severe injury. *Journal of Athletic Training* 36:236–43.

Brooks, G., T. Fahey, and K. Baldwin. 2005. *Exercise Physiology: Human Bioenergetics and Its Application*, 4th ed. New York: McGraw-Hill Companies.

Cross, K., and C. Serenelli. 2003. Training and equipment to prevent head and neck injuries. *Clinics in Sports Medicine* 22:639–67.

Fox, S. 2006. *Human Physiology*, 9th ed. New York: McGraw-Hill Companies.

McAuley, E., A. Kramer, and S. Colombe. 2004. Cardiovascular fitness and neurocognitive function in older adults: A brief review. *Brain, Behavior and Immunity* 18:214–20.

Paxinos, G., and J. Mai. 2003. *The Human Nervous System*. New York. Academic Press.

White, L., and R. Dressendorfer. 2004. Exercise and multiple sclerosis. *Sports Medicine* 34:1077–1100.

Widmaier, E., H. Raff, and K. Strang. 2006. *Vander's Human Physiology*, 10th ed. New York: McGraw-Hill Companies.

REFERENCES

1. Barchas, J. D. et al. 1978. Behavioral neurochemistry: Neuroregulators and behavioral states. *Science* 200:964.
2. Barde, Y. A., D. Edgar, and H. Thoen. 1983. New neurotropic factors. *Annual Review of Physiology* 45:601.
3. Busse, M., N. Maassen, and H. Konrad. 1991. Relation between plasma K^+ and ventilation during incremental exercise after glycogen depletion and repletion in man. *Journal of Physiology* (London) 443:469–76.
4. Cantu, R. 1991. Minor head injuries in sports. *Adolescent Medicine*. 2:141–54.
5. Clark, F., and P. Burgess. 1975. Slowly adapting receptors in the cat knee joint: Can they signal joint angle? *Journal of Neurophysiology* 38:1448–63.
6. Collins, S., M. Caron, and R. Lefkowitz. 1991. Regulation of adrenergic receptor responsiveness through modulation of receptor gene expression. *Annual Review of Physiology* 53:497–508.
6a. Cotman, C., and N. Berchtold. 2002. Exercise: A behavioral intervention to enhance brain health and plasticity. *Trends in Neuroscience* 25:295–301.
7. Delong, M., and P. Strick. 1974. Relation of the basal ganglia, cerebellum, and motor cortex units to ramp and ballistic limb movements. *Brain Research* 71:327–35.
8. Dietz, V. 1992. Human neuronal control of automatic functional movements interaction between central programs and afferent input. *Physiological Reviews* 72:33–69.
9. Eccles, J. C. 1977. *The Understanding of the Brain*. New York: McGraw-Hill Companies.
10. Fox, S. 2006. *Human Physiology*, 9th ed. New York: McGraw-Hill.
11. Fox, S. I. 2002. *Human Physiology*. New York: McGraw-Hill Companies.
12. Goodwin, G., D. McCloskey, and P. Mathews. 1972. The contribution of muscle afferents to kinesthesia shown by vibration-induced illusions of movement and by the effects of paralyzing joint afferents. *Brain* 95:705–48.
13. Grillner, S. 1981. Control of locomotion in bipeds, tetrapods, and fish. In *Handbook of Physiology*. The Nervous System. Motor Control. Section 1, vol. II, part 2, 1179–1236. Washington, D.C.: American Physiological Society.
14. Hafler, D. et al. 2005. Multiple sclerosis. *Immunology Review* 204:208–31.
15. Henatsch, H., and H. Langer. 1985. Basic neurophysiology of motor skills in sport: A review. *International Journal of Sports Medicine* 6:2–14.
16. Hoffman, B., and R. Lefkowitz. 1980. Alpha and beta receptor subtypes. *New England Journal of Medicine* 302:1390.
17. Hole, J. 1995. *Human Anatomy and Physiology*. 7th ed. New York: McGraw-Hill Companies.
18. Kandel, E., J. Schwartz, and T. Jessell, eds. 2000. *Principles of Neural Science*. Stamford: Appleton & Lange.
19. Kaufman, M., K. Rybicki, T. Waldrop, and G. Ordway. 1984. Effect of ischemia on responses of group III and IV afferents to contraction. *Journal of Applied Physiology* 57:644–50.
20. Kaufman, M., K. Rybicki, T. Waldrop, G. Ordway, and J. Mitchell. 1984. Effects of static and rhythmic twitch contractions on the discharge of group III and IV muscle afferents. *Cardiovascular Research* 18:663–68.
21. Kniffki, K., S. Mense, and R. Schmidt. 1981. Muscle receptors with fine afferent fibers which may evoke circulatory reflexes. *Circulation Research* 48 (Suppl.):25–31.
22. Krieger, D. T., and J. B. Martin. 1981. Brain peptides. *New England Journal of Medicine* 304:876.
23. Laurin, D. et al. 2001. Physical activity and risk of cognitive impairment and dementia in elderly persons. *Archives Neurology* 58:498–504.

24. Mathews, P. 1977. Muscle afferents and kinesthesia. *British Medical Bulletin* 33:137–42.

25. McAuley, E., A. Kramer, and S. Colombe. 2004. Cardiovascular fitness and neurocognitive function in older adults: A brief review. *Brain, Behavior and Immunity.* 18:214–20.

26. ———. 1982. Where does Sherrington's muscle sense originate? *Annual Review of Neuroscience* 5:189–218.

27. McCloskey, D., and J. Mitchell. 1972. Reflex cardiovascular and respiratory responses originating in exercising muscle. *Journal of Physiology* (London) 224:173–86.

28. Nicoll, R., R. Malenka, and J. Kauer. 1990. Functional comparison of neurotransmitter receptor subtypes in mammalian central nervous system. *Physiological Reviews* 70:513–65.

29. Nowak, T., and G. Handford. 2003. *Pathophysiology: Concepts and Applications for Health Care Professionals.* New York: McGraw-Hill.

30. Nowak, T., and A. Handford. 1999. *Essentials of Pathophysiology.* New York: McGraw-Hill Companies.

31. O'Donovan, M. 1985. Developmental regulation of motor function. *Medicine and Science in Sports and Exercise* 17:35–43.

32. Pozzo, T., A. Berthoz, L. Lefort, and E. Vittle. 1991. Head stabilization during various locomotor tasks in humans. II. Patients with bilateral peripheral vestibular deficits. *Brain Research* 85:208–17.

33. Prochazka, A. 1989. Sensorimotor gain control: A basic strategy of motor systems. *Progressive Neurobiology* 33: 281–307.

34. Redman, S. 1986. Monosynaptic transmission in the spinal cord. *News in Physiological Sciences* 1:171–74.

35. Sage, G. H. 1984. *Motor Learning and Control: A Neuropsychological Approach.* New York: McGraw-Hill Companies.

36. Seeley, R., T. Stephen, and P. Tate. 2003. *Anatomy and Physiology.* New York: McGraw-Hill Companies.

37. Sherwood, L. 1993. *Fundamentals of Physiology.* St. Paul, MN.: West.

38. Shier, D., J. Butler, and R. Lewis. 2003. *Hole's Human Anatomy and Physiology.* New York: McGraw-Hill Companies.

39. Smith, J. C., J. Feldman, and B. Schmidt. 1988. Neural mechanisms generating locomotion studied in mammalian brain stem–spinal cord in vitro. *FASEB Journal* 2:2283–88.

40. Snyder, S. H. 1980. Brain peptides as neurotransmitters. *Science* 209:976.

41. Soechting, J., and M. Flanders. 1991. Arm movements in three-dimensional space: Computation, theory, and observation. In *Exercise and Sport Science Reviews*, vol. 19, ed. J. Holloszy, 389–418. Baltimore: Lippincott Williams & Wilkins.

42. Stjarne, L. 1986. New paradigm: Sympathetic neurotransmission by lateral interaction between secretory units? *News in Physiological Sciences* 1:103–6.

43. White, L., and R. Dressendorfer. 2004. Exercise and multiple sclerosis. *Sports Medicine* 34:1077–1100.

44. White, L. et al. 2004. Resistance training improves strength and functional capacity in persons with multiple sclerosis. *Multiple Sclerosis* 10:668–72.

45. Widmaier, E., H. Raff, and K. Strang. 2006. *Vander's Human Physiology,* 10th ed. New York: McGraw-Hill Companies.

CHAPTER 8

Skeletal Muscle: Structure and Function

■ Objectives

By studying this chapter, you should be able to do the following:

1. Draw and label the microstructure of skeletal muscle.
2. Outline the steps leading to muscle shortening.
3. Define the terms *concentric* and *isometric*.
4. Discuss the following terms: (1) *twitch*, (2) *summation*, and (3) *tetanus*.
5. Discuss the major biochemical and mechanical properties of human skeletal muscle fiber types.
6. Discuss the relationship between skeletal muscle fiber types and performance.

7. List and discuss those factors that regulate the amount of force exerted during muscular contraction.
8. Graph the relationship between movement velocity and the amount of force exerted during muscular contraction.
9. Discuss the structure and function of a muscle spindle.
10. Describe the function of a Golgi tendon organ.

■ Outline

Structure of Skeletal Muscle   141

Neuromuscular Junction   143

Muscular Contraction   144
   Overview of the Sliding
      Filament Model   144
   Energy for Contraction   145
   Regulation of Excitation-
      Contraction Coupling   145

Fiber Types   149
   Biochemical and Contractile
      Characteristics of Skeletal
      Muscle   149

Characteristics of Individual
      Fiber Types   152
   Fiber Types and
      Performance   154

Alterations in Skeletal Muscle
Due to Exercise, Inactivity
and Aging   155
   Exercise-Induced Changes in
      Skeletal Muscles   155
   Muscle Atrophy Due to
      Inactivity   155
   Age-Related Changes in
      Skeletal Muscle   157

Muscle Actions   158

Speed of Muscle Action
and Relaxation   159

Force Regulation
in Muscle   160

Force-Velocity/Power-Velocity
Relationships   161

Receptors in Muscle   163
   Muscle Spindle   163
   Golgi Tendon Organs   164

actin
concentric action
dynamic
eccentric action
endomysium
end-plate potential (EPP)
epimysium
extensors
fasciculi
fast-twitch fibers
flexors
Golgi tendon organs (GTOs)
intermediate fibers

isometric action
lateral sac
motor neurons
motor unit
muscle action
muscle spindle
myofibrils
myosin
neuromuscular junction
perimysium
sarcolemma
sarcomeres
sarcoplasmic reticulum

satellite cells
sliding filament model
slow-twitch fibers
summation
terminal cisternae
tetanus
transverse tubules
tropomyosin
troponin
twitch
type I fibers
type IIa fibers
type IIx fibers

The human body contains over 400 skeletal muscles, which constitute 40% to 50% of the total body weight (40, 53, 54). Skeletal muscle performs three important functions: (1) force generation for locomotion and breathing, (2) force generation for postural support, and (3) heat production during periods of cold stress. The most obvious function of skeletal muscle is to enable an individual to move freely and breathe. Skeletal muscles are attached to bones by tough connective tissue called tendons. One end of the muscle is attached to a bone that does not move (origin), while the opposite end is fixed to a bone (insertion) that is moved during muscular contraction. A variety of different movements are possible, depending on the type of joint and muscles involved. Muscles that decrease joint angles are called **flexors,** while muscles that increase joint angles are called **extensors.**

Given the role of skeletal muscles in determining sports performance, a thorough understanding of muscle structure and function is important to the exercise scientist, physical educator, physical therapist, and coach. It is the purpose of this chapter to discuss the structure and function of skeletal muscle.

STRUCTURE OF SKELETAL MUSCLE

Skeletal muscle is composed of several kinds of tissue. These include muscle cells (called fibers) themselves, nerve tissue, blood, and various types of connective tissue. Figure 8.1, displays the relationship between muscle and the various connective tissues. Individual muscles are separated from each other and held in position by connective tissue called *fascia*. There are three separate layers of connective tissue found in skeletal muscle. The outermost layer that surrounds the entire muscle is called the **epimysium.**

As we move inward from the epimysium, connective tissue called the **perimysium** surrounds individual bundles of muscle fibers (note: for muscle, the terms *cell* and *fiber* are often used interchangeably). These individual bundles of muscle fibers are called a **fascicle.** Each muscle fiber within the fasciculus is surrounded by connective tissue called the **endomysium.** Just below the endomysium and surrounding each muscle fiber is another layer of protective tissue called the external lamina (also called the basement membrane).

Despite their unique shape, muscle fibers have many of the same organelles that are present in other cells. That is, they contain mitochondria, lysosomes, and so on. However, unlike most other cells in the body, muscle cells are multinucleated (i.e., have many nuclei). One of the most distinctive features of the microscopic appearance of skeletal muscles is their striated appearance (see figure 8.2). These stripes are produced by alternating light and dark bands that appear across the length of the fiber.

Each individual muscle fiber is a thin, elongated cylinder that generally extends the length of the muscle. The cell membrane surrounding the muscle fiber cell is called the **sarcolemma.** Located above the sarcolemma and below the external lamina are a group of muscle precursor cells called satellite cells. **Satellite cells** are undifferentiated cells that play a key role in muscle growth and repair (106). If muscle fibers are destroyed (i.e., due to injury or disease), they cannot be replaced by cell division. Nonetheless, it is possible that new fibers can be formed from activated satellite cells that are capable of undergoing differentiation and developing into mature muscle fibers (106). Moreover, satellite cells contribute to muscle growth during strength training by dividing and contributing nuclei to existing muscle fibers. Increasing the number of nuclei within muscle fibers enhances the fibers' ability to synthesize proteins and, therefore, assists in muscle growth (106).

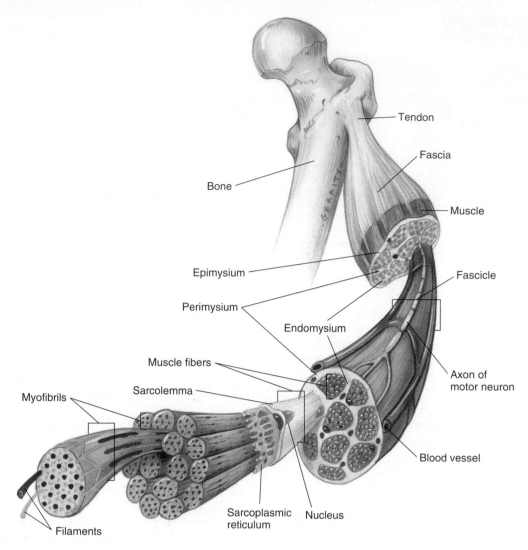

FIGURE 8.1 Connective tissue surrounding skeletal muscle.

Beneath the sarcolemma lies the sarcoplasm (also called cytoplasm), which contains the cellular proteins, organelles, and myofibrils. **Myofibrils** are numerous threadlike structures that contain the contractile proteins (figure 8.2). In general, myofibrils are composed of two major types of protein filaments: (1) thick filaments composed of the protein **myosin** and (2) thin filaments composed primarily of the protein **actin.** The arrangement of these two protein filaments give skeletal muscle its striated appearance (figure 8.2). Located on the actin molecule itself are two additional proteins, troponin and tropomyosin. These proteins make up only a small portion of the muscle, but they play an important role in the regulation of the contractile process.

Myofibrils can be further subdivided into individual segments called **sarcomeres.** Sarcomeres are divided from each other by a thin sheet of structural proteins called a Z *line.* Myosin filaments are located primarily within the dark portion of the sarcomere, which is called the A *band,* while actin filaments occur principally in the light regions of the sarcomere called I *bands* (figure 8.2). In the center of the sarcomere there is a portion of the myosin filament with no overlap of the actin. This is the H *zone.*

Within the sarcoplasm of muscle is a network of membranous channels that surrounds each myofibril and runs parallel with it. These channels are called the **sarcoplasmic reticulum** and are storage sites for calcium, which plays an important role in muscular contraction (see figure 8.3). Another set of membranous channels called the **transverse tubules** extends inward from the sarcolemma and passes completely through the fiber. These transverse tubules pass between two enlarged portions of the sarcoplasmic reticulum called the **terminal cisternae.** All of

Myofibril

Skeletal muscle fiber

Z line — Z line

|←—— Sarcomere ——→|

Filaments of actin

(a)

H zone — M line — Z line

(b)

|I band|←—— A band ——→|I band|←—— A band ——→|

Myosin (thick) filaments

Actin (thin) filaments

(c)

FIGURE 8.2 The microstructure of muscle. Note that a skeletal muscle fiber contains numerous myofibrils, each consisting of units called sarcomeres.

these parts serve a function in muscular contraction and will be discussed in further detail later in this chapter.

NEUROMUSCULAR JUNCTION

Each skeletal muscle cell is connected to a nerve fiber branch coming from a nerve cell. These nerve cells are called **motor neurons,** and they extend outward from the spinal cord. The motor neuron and all the muscle fibers it innervates are called a **motor unit.** Stimulation from motor neurons initiates the contraction process. The site where the motor neuron and muscle cell meet is called the **neuromuscular junction.** At this junction the sarcolemma forms a pocket that is called the *motor end plate* (see figure 8.4,).

The end of the motor neuron does not physically make contact with the muscle fiber, but is separated by a short gap called the *neuromuscular cleft*. When a nerve impulse reaches the end of the motor nerve, the neurotransmitter acetylcholine is released and diffuses across the synaptic cleft to bind with receptor

sites on the motor end plate. This causes an increase in the permeability of the sarcolemma to sodium, resulting in a depolarization called the **end-plate potential (EPP).** The EPP is always large enough to exceed threshold and is the signal to begin the contractile process.

IN SUMMARY

■ The human body contains over 400 voluntary skeletal muscles, which constitute 40% to 50% of the total body weight. Skeletal muscle performs three major functions: (1) force production for locomotion and breathing, (2) force production for postural support, and (3) heat production during cold stress.

■ Individual muscle fibers are composed of hundreds of threadlike protein filaments called myofibrils. Myofibrils contain two major types of contractile protein: (1) actin (part of the thin filaments) and (2) myosin (major component of the thick filaments).

Sarcolemma

Triad of the reticulum:

Terminal cisternae

Transverse tubule

Sarcoplasmic reticulum

Mitochondria

Waldrop

Myofibrils

A band

I band

Z line

Nucleus

FIGURE 8.3 Within the sarcoplasm of muscle is a network of channels called the sarcoplasmic reticulum and the transverse tubules.

continued

- Motor neurons extend outward from the spinal cord and innervate individual muscle fibers. The site where the motor neuron and muscle cell meet is called the neuromuscular junction. Acetylcholine is the neurotransmitter that stimulates the muscle fiber to depolarize, which is the signal to start the contractile process.

MUSCULAR CONTRACTION

Muscular contraction is a complex process involving a number of cellular proteins and energy production systems. The final result is a sliding of actin over myosin, which causes the muscle to shorten and therefore develop tension. Although complete details of muscular contraction at the molecular level continue to be debated, the basic process of muscular contraction is well defined. The process of muscular contraction is best explained by the **sliding filament model** of contraction (31, 32, 82, 101).

Overview of the Sliding Filament Model

The general process of muscular contraction is illustrated in figure 8.5. Muscle fibers contract by a shortening of their myofibrils due to actin sliding over myosin. This results in a reduction in the distance from Z line to Z line. Understanding the details of how

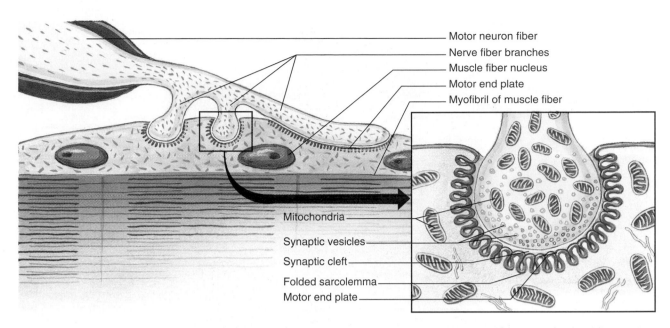

Motor neuron fiber
Nerve fiber branches
Muscle fiber nucleus
Motor end plate
Myofibril of muscle fiber

Mitochondria
Synaptic vesicles
Synaptic cleft
Folded sarcolemma
Motor end plate

FIGURE 8.4 The connecting point between a motor neuron and a single muscle fiber is called the neuromuscular junction. The neurotransmitter acetylcholine is stored in synaptic vesicles at the end of the nerve fiber.

muscular contraction occurs requires an appreciation of the microscopic structure of the myofibril. Note that the "heads" of the myosin cross-bridges are oriented toward the actin molecule (see figure 8.6). The actin and myosin filaments slide across each other during muscular contraction due to the action of the numerous cross-bridges extending out as "arms" from myosin and attaching to actin in a "strong binding state." It was previously believed that the myosin cross-bridges were not attached to actin when skeletal muscle is not contracting. However, recent evidence shows that myosin cross-bridges are always attached to actin, but the strength of the attachment varies from a "weak" bond to a "strong" bond. These two states of myosin-actin bonding are referred to as the weak binding state and the strong binding state. Force development and muscular contraction occur only when the cross-bridges are in the strong binding state. The development of this strong binding state results in an orientation of cross-bridges so that when they attach to actin on each side of the sarcomere, they can pull the actin from each side toward the center. This "pulling" of actin over the myosin molecule results in muscle shortening and the generation of force.

The term *excitation-contraction coupling* refers to the sequence of events in which a nerve impulse (action potential) reaches the muscle membrane and leads to muscle shortening by cross-bridge activity. This process will be discussed step-by-step next. Let's begin with a discussion of the energy source for contraction.

Energy for Contraction

The energy for muscular contraction comes from the breakdown of ATP by the enzyme myosin ATPase (26, 43, 49, 55). This enzyme is located on the "head" of the myosin cross-bridge. Recall that the bioenergetic pathways responsible for the synthesis of ATP were discussed earlier in chapter 3; they are summarized in figure 8.7. The breakdown of ATP to ADP + P_i and the release of energy serves to energize the myosin cross-bridges, which in turn pull the actin molecules over myosin and thus shorten the muscle (32, 63, 82, 83, 101).

Note that a single contraction cycle or "power stroke" of all the cross-bridges in a muscle would shorten the muscle by only 1 percent of its resting length (83). Since some muscles can shorten up to 60% of their resting length, it is clear that the contraction cycle must be repeated over and over again (83).

Regulation of Excitation-Contraction Coupling

Relaxed muscles are easily stretched, which demonstrates that at rest, actin and myosin are not firmly attached and therefore exist in the weak binding state. What regulates the interaction of actin and myosin and thus regulates muscle contraction? The first step in the process of muscular contraction begins with a nerve impulse arriving at the neuromuscular junction. The action potential from the motor neuron causes the release of acetylcholine into the synaptic cleft of

Relaxed muscle

1. Actin and myosin myofilaments in a relaxed muscle (*right*) and a contracted muscle (*#4 below*) are the same length. Myofilaments do not change length during muscle contraction.

Myosin myofilament   Actin myofilament   Sarcomere

Contracting muscle

2. During contraction, actin myofilaments at each end of the sarcomere slide past the myosin myofilaments toward each other. As a result, the Z disks are brought closer together, and the sarcomere shortens.

Actin myofilaments move toward each other

Sarcomere shortens as Z disks move toward each other

Contracting muscle

3. As the actin myofilaments slide over the myosin myofilaments, the H zones (*yellow*) and the I bands (*blue*) narrow. The A bands, which are equal to the length of the myosin myofilaments, do not narrow, because the length of the myosin myofilaments does not change.

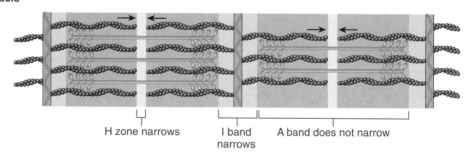

H zone narrows   I band narrows   A band does not narrow

Fully contracted muscle

4. In a fully contracted muscle, the ends of the actin myofilaments overlap and the H zone disappears.

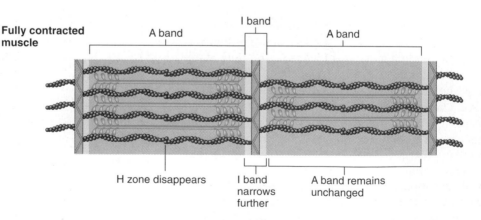

H zone disappears   I band narrows further   A band remains unchanged

FIGURE 8.5 The sliding filament theory of contraction. As contraction occurs, the Z lines are brought closer together. The A bands remain the same length, but the I and H bands get progressively narrower as shortening continues.

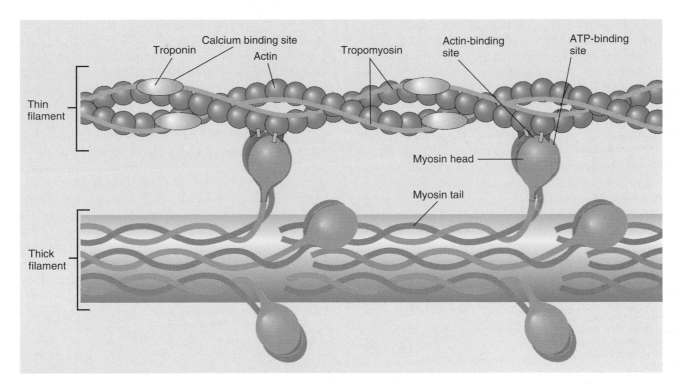

FIGURE 8.6 Proposed relationships among troponin, tropomyosin, myosin cross-bridges, and calcium. Note that when Ca^{++} binds to troponin, tropomyosin is removed from the active sites on actin, and cross-bridge attachment can occur.

FIGURE 8.7 The three sources of ATP production in muscle during contraction: (1) phosphocreatine, (2) glycolysis, and (3) oxidative phosphorylation. From A. J. Vander et al., *Human Physiology: The Mechanisms of Body Function*, 8th ed. Copyright © 2001 McGraw-Hill, Inc., New York. Reprinted by permission.

the neuromuscular junction; acetylcholine binds to receptors on the motor end plate, producing an end-plate potential that leads to depolarization of the muscle cell (83). This depolarization (i.e., excitation) is conducted down the transverse tubules deep into the muscle fiber. When the action potential reaches the sarcoplasmic reticulum, calcium is released and diffuses into the muscle to bind to a protein called *troponin*. This is the "trigger" step in the control of muscular contraction, since the regulation of contraction

is a function of two regulatory proteins, **troponin** and **tropomyosin,** which are located on the actin molecule. Troponin and tropomyosin regulate muscular contraction by controlling the interaction of actin and myosin.

To understand how troponin and tropomyosin control muscular contraction, one needs to appreciate the anatomical relationship between actin, troponin, and tropomyosin (see figure 8.6). Notice that the actin filament is formed from many protein subunits arranged in a double row and twisted. Tropomyosin is a thin molecule that lies in a groove between the double rows of actin. Attached directly to the tropomyosin is the protein troponin. This arrangement allows troponin and tropomyosin to work together to regulate the attachment of the actin and myosin cross-bridges. In a relaxed muscle, tropomyosin blocks the active sites on the actin molecule where the myosin cross-bridges must attach to form a strong binding state to produce a contraction. The trigger for contraction to occur is linked to the release of stored calcium (Ca^{++}) from a region of the sarcoplasmic reticulum termed the **lateral sac,** or sometimes called the *terminal cisternae* (65, 97). In a resting (relaxed) muscle the concentration of Ca^{++} in the sarcoplasm is very low. However, when a nerve impulse arrives at the neuromuscular junction, it travels down the transverse tubules to the sarcoplasmic reticulum and causes the release of Ca^{++}. Much of this Ca^{++} binds to troponin (see figure 8.6), which causes a position change in tropomyosin such that the active

sites on the actin are uncovered. This permits the strong binding of a "cocked or energized" myosin cross-bridge on the actin molecule. The strong cross-bridge binding initiates the release of energy stored within the myosin molecule; this produces an angular movement of each cross-bridge, resulting in muscle shortening. Attachment of "fresh" ATP to the myosin cross-bridges breaks the strong binding state of the myosin cross-bridge bound to actin and results in a weak binding state. The enzyme, ATPase, again hydrolyzes (i.e., breaks down) the ATP attached to the myosin cross-bridge and provides the energy necessary for cocking (i.e., energizing) the myosin cross-bridge for reattachment to another active site on an actin molecule. This contraction cycle can be repeated as long as free Ca^{++} is available to bind to troponin and ATP can be hydrolyzed to provide the energy. Failure of the muscle to maintain adequate Ca^{++} levels or to hydrolyze ATP results in a disturbance of muscle homeostasis, and fatigue occurs (see A Closer Look 8.1).

A CLOSER LOOK 8.1

Muscle Fatigue

Short-term, high-intensity exercise or prolonged, submaximal exercise can result in a decline in muscle force production. This decrease in muscle force production is known as fatigue. Specifically, muscular fatigue is defined as a reduction in maximal force production of the muscle and is characterized by a reduced ability to perform work (figure 8.8)

What are the factors that contribute to muscle fatigue? At present, a complete answer to this question is unavailable. Indeed, exercise physiologists do not universally agree upon the exact mechanism(s) responsible for muscle fatigue (23, 39, 66, 102, 104). However, it is clear that the causes of muscle fatigue are complex and may vary depending upon the type of exercise performed. For example, muscle fatigue resulting from high-intensity exercise lasting approximately 60 seconds (e.g., sprinting 400 meters) may be due to several factors including an accumulation of lactate, hydrogen ions, ADP, inorganic phosphate, and free radicals within the active muscle fibers

FIGURE 8.8
Muscular fatigue is characterized by a reduced ability to generate force.

(23, 39, 102, 104). Collectively, the accumulation of these metabolites results in a disruption of muscle homeostasis and impairs muscle force production in several different ways (39, 102, 104).

Muscular fatigue that occurs in the later stages of an endurance event lasting 2 to 4 hours (i.e., marathon running) may also involve an accumulation of free radicals in the muscle, but other factors such as disturbances in muscle/extracellular electrolyte homeostasis and depletion of muscle glycogen may also contribute to this type of muscle fatigue (39, 102, 104). Further, evidence suggests that the central nervous system may also contribute to this category of muscle fatigue. The role of the central nervous system in muscle fatigue has become known as "central fatigue." Central fatigue occurs when the subconscious brain reduces motor drive (i.e., neural activation) to the contracting muscles during exercise (66). This reduced motor drive results in a decreased number of muscle fibers activated and, therefore, a decline in muscle force production. Muscle fatigue and the limiting factors to exercise performance are discussed in more detail in chapter 19.

The signal to stop contraction is the absence of the nerve impulse at the neuromuscular junction. When this occurs, an energy-requiring Ca^{++} *pump* located within the sarcoplasmic reticulum begins to move Ca^{++} back into the sarcoplasmic reticulum. This removal of Ca^{++} from troponin causes tropomyosin to move back to cover the binding sites on the actin molecule, and cross-bridge interaction ceases. Figure 8.9 illustrates the basic steps involved in muscle contraction and relaxation.

A Closer Look 8.2 contains a step-by-step summary of the events that occur during excitation and muscular contraction. For a detailed discussion of molecular events involved in skeletal muscle contraction, see references 11, 32, 35, 82, 83, and 101. Time spent learning the microstructure of muscle and the events that lead to contraction will pay dividends later, as this material is important to a thorough understanding of exercise physiology.

IN SUMMARY

- The process of muscular contraction can be best explained by the sliding filament model, which proposes that muscle shortening occurs due to movement of the actin filament over the myosin filament.
- The steps leading to muscular contraction are (see figure 8.10 for a detailed, step-by-step illustration):
  a. The nerve impulse travels down the transverse tubules and reaches the sarcoplasmic reticulum, and Ca^{++} is released.
  b. Ca^{++} binds to the protein troponin.
  c. Ca^{++} binding to troponin causes a position change in tropomyosin away from the "active sites" on the actin molecule and permits a strong binding state between actin and myosin.
  d. Muscular contraction occurs by multiple cycles of cross-bridge activity. Shortening will continue as long as energy is available and Ca^{++} is free to bind to troponin.
- When neural activity ceases at the neuromuscular junction, Ca^{++} is removed from the sarcoplasm and actively pumped into the sarcoplasmic reticulum by the Ca^{++} pump. This results in tropomyosin moving to cover the active site on actin, and the muscle relaxes.

FIBER TYPES

Human skeletal muscle can be divided into several different classes based on the histochemical or biochemical characteristics of the individual fibers. (How

fibers are "typed" is discussed in A Closer Look 8.3, page 152.) Although some confusion exists concerning the nomenclature of fiber types, historically, muscle fibers have been classified into two general categories: (1) fast (also called fast-twitch) fibers or (2) slow (also called slow-twitch) fibers (20, 21, 33, 34, 62). Though some muscle groups are known to be composed of predominantly fast or slow fibers, most muscle groups in the body contain an equal mixture of both slow and fast fiber types. The percentage of the respective fiber types contained in skeletal muscles can be influenced by genetics, blood levels of hormones, and the exercise habits of the individual. From a practical standpoint, the fiber composition of skeletal muscles plays an important role in performance in both power and endurance events (13, 92).

Biochemical and Contractile Characteristics of Skeletal Muscle

Before discussing the specific characteristics of muscle fiber types, we should briefly discuss the key biochemical and contractile properties of skeletal muscle.

Biochemical Properties of Muscle In general, the two key biochemical characteristics of muscle that are important to muscle function are (1) the oxidative capacity and (2) the type of ATPase isoform. The oxidative capacity of a muscle fiber is determined by the number of mitochondria, the number of capillaries surrounding the fiber, and the amount of myoglobin within the fiber. A large number of mitochondria provides a greater capacity to produce ATP aerobically. A high number of capillaries surrounding a muscle fiber insures that the fiber will receive adequate oxygen during periods of contractile activity. Finally, myoglobin is similar to hemoglobin in the blood in that it binds O_2, and it also acts as a "shuttle" mechanism for O_2 between the cell membrane and the mitochondria. Therefore, a high myoglobin concentration improves the delivery of oxygen from the capillary to the mitochondria where it will be used. Collectively, the significance of these biochemical characteristics is that a muscle fiber with a high concentration of myoglobin along with a high number of mitochondria and capillaries will have a high aerobic capacity and therefore will be fatigue resistant.

The second important biochemical characteristic of muscle fiber is the ATPase activity. Many isoforms of ATPase exist, and the various isoforms differ in their activities (i.e., speed that they degrade ATP). Muscle fibers that contain ATPase isoforms with high ATPase activity will degrade ATP rapidly; this results in a high

Step-by-Step Summary of Excitation-Contraction Coupling

Excitation

The process of excitation is illustrated in steps 1 and 2 in figure 8.9 and involves two processes:

1. The generation of an action potential in a motor neuron causes the release of acetylcholine into the synaptic cleft of the neuromuscular junction.
2. Acetylcholine binds with receptors on the motor end-plate, producing an end-plate potential, which leads to a depolarization that is conducted down the transverse tubules deep into the muscle fiber. This depolarization results in calcium being released from the sarcoplasmic reticulum.

Contraction

The steps involved in muscular contraction are illustrated in figure 8.10 and are listed in sequential order here (82, 101):

1. In the resting state, the myosin cross-bridges remain connected to actin in a weak binding state (no force generation; step 1, figure 8.10).
2. When the depolarization (i.e., neural stimulation) reaches the sarcoplasmic reticulum, Ca^{++} is released into the sarcoplasm. The Ca^{++} then binds to troponin, which causes a shift in the position of tropomyosin to uncover the "active sites" on the actin. The "energized" or "cocked" myosin cross-bridge then forms a

strong bond (i.e., strong binding state) at the active site on actin (step 2, figure 8.10).
3. Inorganic phosphate is now released from the myosin cross-bridge and the energized cross-bridge pulls the actin molecule (step 3, figure 8.10).
4. Cross-bridge movement is completed by the release of ADP from the myosin cross-bridge. Note, at this point within the contraction cycle, the myosin cross-bridge remains in the strong binding state with actin (step 4, figure 8.10).
5. Attachment of ATP to the myosin cross-bridge allows the myosin cross-bridge to break the strong binding state and form a weak bind-

FIGURE 8.9 Illustration of the steps involved in muscle excitation, contraction, and relaxation. From A. J. Vander et al., *Human Physiology: The Mechanisms of Body Function*, 8th ed. Copyright © 2001 McGraw-Hill, Inc., New York. Reprinted by permission.

ing state. In this weak binding state, ATP is broken down to ADP + P_i + energy, and the released energy is used to "energize" the myosin cross-bridge (step 5, figure 8.10).

This contraction cycle can be repeated as long as Ca^{++} and ATP are present (i.e., step 5 moves to step 2 and the cycle continues). The contraction cycle is broken when

action potentials stop and the sarcoplasmic reticulum actively removes Ca^{++} from the sarcoplasm (i.e., step 5 moves to step 1).

FIGURE 8.10 Steps leading to muscular contraction. See text for details.

speed of muscle shortening. Conversely, muscle fibers with low ATPase activities shorten at slow speeds.

Contractile Properties of Skeletal Muscle In comparing the contractile properties of muscle fiber types, three performance characteristics are important: (1) maximal force production, (2) speed of contraction, and (3) muscle fiber efficiency. Let's discuss each of these characteristics briefly.

First, maximal force production of a muscle fiber is compared by expressing how much force the fiber produces per unit of fiber cross-sectional area (spe-

cific tension). In other words, specific tension is the force production divided by the size of the fiber (e.g., specific force = force/fiber cross-sectional area).

The contraction speed of muscle fibers is compared by measuring the maximal shortening velocity (called Vmax) of individual fibers. Vmax represents the highest speed at which a fiber can shorten. Since muscle fibers shorten by cross-bridge movement (called cross-bridge cycling), Vmax is determined by the rate of cross-bridge cycling. Again, a key biochemical factor that regulates fiber Vmax is the myosin ATPase activity. Fibers with high myosin

A CLOSER LOOK 8.3

How Are Skeletal Muscle Fibers Typed?

The relative percentage of fast or slow fibers contained in a particular muscle can be estimated by removing a small piece of muscle (via a procedure called a *biopsy*) and performing histochemical or biochemical analysis of the individual muscle cells. An early method used a histochemical procedure that divides muscle fibers into three categories based on the specific "isoform" of myosin ATPase enzyme found in the fiber. This technique applies a chemical stain that darkens muscle cells that contain high concentrations of the type of ATPase found in slow muscles. Using this technique, slow (type I) fibers become dark, while type IIa fibers remain light in color. The shade of type IIx fibers tends to fall somewhere between the type I and IIa fibers. Hence, this technique provides a means of determining these three fiber types at the same time. Figure 8.11 is an example of a muscle cross section after histochemical staining, showing type I, IIa, and IIx fibers.

Another means of determining the percentage of the various muscle fiber types is by identifying the specific type of myosin found in the muscle using a technique called *gel electrophoresis*. At present, three different types of myosins (called myosin isoforms) have been reported in adult human skeletal muscle (e.g., type I, type IIa, type IIx). The functional differences between these myosin isoforms explain why fast fibers shorten more rapidly than slow fibers (11, 58). For example, the myosin isoform found in fast fibers has a high ATPase activity; this promotes a rapid breakdown of ATP and provides the needed energy for a high speed of muscle shortening (i.e., high Vmax). In contrast, the myosin isoform found in slow fibers has a low ATPase activity and therefore shortens at a slower rate compared to fast fibers. For details of the different types of myosins found in skeletal muscle see references 65 and 71.

One of the inherent problems with fiber typing in humans is that a muscle biopsy is usually performed on only one muscle group. Therefore, a single sample from one muscle may not be representative of the entire body. A further complication is that fiber types tend to be layered within muscle, and thus a small sample of muscle taken from a single area of the muscle may not be truly representative of the total fiber population of the muscle biopsied (5, 94). Therefore, it is difficult to make a definitive statement concerning the whole body percentage of a particular fiber type based on the staining of a single muscle biopsy.

FIGURE 8.11 Histochemical staining of a cross-sectional area of muscle. The darkest cells are type I fibers and the lightest-colored cells are type IIa fibers. The cells with the brown appearance are type IIx fibers.

ATPase activities (e.g., fast fibers) possess a high Vmax, whereas fibers with low myosin ATPase activities possess a low Vmax (e.g., slow fibers).

The efficiency of a muscle fiber is a measure of the muscle fiber's economy. That is, an efficient fiber would require less energy to perform a certain amount of work compared to a less-efficient fiber. In practice, this measurement is made by dividing the amount of energy used (i.e., ATP used) by the amount of force produced.

Characteristics of Individual Fiber Types

It is generally agreed that three individual human skeletal muscle fibers exist (two subtypes of fast fibers—identified as type IIx and IIa; and a slow fiber—identified as type I). Note that the fastest muscle fiber in humans has historically been called a type IIb fiber. However, new evidence suggests that the fastest fiber in humans should be renamed and called

RESEARCH FOCUS 8.1

The Fastest Fiber in Human Skeletal Muscle Is a Type IIx Fiber and Not a Type IIB Fiber

The fastest skeletal muscle fiber in many animals is the type IIb fiber. For several years it was believed that fastest fiber in human skeletal muscle was also a "type IIb" fiber. However, recent research has revealed that human skeletal muscle probably does not contain type IIb fibers and that the fastest muscle fiber in humans is the type IIx fiber. The story behind this change in scientific thinking follows.

In the late 1980s, German and Italian scientists discovered a new fast muscle fiber in rodent skeletal muscle (9, 88). This fiber was named a "type IIx fiber" and the existence of this fiber has since been confirmed by many laboratories (25, 28, 47, 69, 89, 96, 103). Since the discovery of the type IIx fiber in rodents, it has been determined that the type of myosin contained in the fastest muscle fiber in humans is

similar in structure to that contained in the rodent type IIx fiber (87, 89). Hence, scientists now believe that the fastest skeletal muscle fiber type in humans is the type IIx fiber and not the type IIb fiber as originally thought. Therefore, throughout this textbook we will refer to type IIx fibers as the fastest skeletal muscle fiber type in humans.

---

a type IIx fiber. The rationale for this name change is discussed in Research Focus 8.1. While it seems possible that human skeletal muscles may contain more than three fiber types, we will discuss only the three fiber types that have been carefully studied. Let's begin our discussion of muscle fiber types by examining the biochemical and contractile properties of both slow and fast fibers.

Slow Fibers   One type of slow fiber has been identified in humans—type I. **Type I fibers** (also called slow-oxidative or **slow-twitch fibers**) contain large numbers of oxidative enzymes (i.e., high mitochondrial volume) and are surrounded by more capillaries than any of the fibers. In addition, type I fibers contain higher concentrations of myoglobin than fast fibers. The high concentration of myoglobin, the large number of capillaries, and the high mitochondrial enzyme activities provide type I fibers with a large capacity for aerobic metabolism and a high resistance to fatigue.

In terms of contractile properties, type I fibers possess a slower Vmax compared to fast fibers (see figure 8.12). Further, it appears that type I fibers produce a lower specific tension compared to fast fibers (see A Closer Look 8.4). Finally, type I fibers are more efficient than fast fibers.

Fast Fibers   Two subtypes of fast fibers exist in humans: (1) type IIx, and (2) type IIa. **Type IIx fibers** (sometimes called **fast-twitch fibers** or fast-glycolytic fibers) have a relatively small number of mitochondria, a limited capacity for aerobic metabolism, and are less resistant to fatigue than slow fibers (44, 70). However, these fibers are rich in glycolytic enzymes, which provide them with a large anaerobic capacity (67).

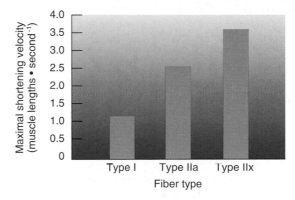

FIGURE 8.12   Comparison of maximal shortening velocities between fiber types. Data are from reference 17.

The specific tension of type IIx fibers is similar to type IIa fibers but is greater than type I fibers. Further, the myosin ATPase activity in type IIx fibers is higher than other fiber types, resulting in the highest Vmax of all fiber types. The speed of contraction differences between slow and fast fibers is illustrated in figure 8.12.

Type IIx fibers are less efficient than all other fiber types. This low efficiency is due to the high ATPase activity, which results in a greater energy expenditure per unit of work performed.

A second type of fast fiber is the **type IIa fiber** (also called **intermediate fibers** or fast-oxidative glycolytic fibers). These fibers contain biochemical and fatigue characteristics that are between type IIx and type I fibers. Therefore, conceptually, type IIa fibers can be viewed as a mixture of both type I and type IIx fiber characteristics. However, note that type IIa fibers are extremely adaptable. That is, with endurance

A CLOSER LOOK 8.4

Do Fast Fibers Exert More Force Than Slow Fibers?

The question, "Do fast muscle fibers exert more force than slow fibers?" has been a topic of research for many years. Although controversial, recent research using single rat muscle fibers demonstrates that the maximal specific force production (force per cross-sectional area) of fast muscle fibers (types IIx and IIa) is 10% to 20% greater than the force produced by slow (type I) fibers (17).

What is the physiological explanation for the observation that fast fibers exert more force than slow fibers? The amount of force generated by a muscle fiber is directly related to the number of myosin cross-bridges in the strong binding state (i.e., force generating state) at any given time. That is, the more cross-bridges generating force, the greater the force production. Therefore, it appears that fast fibers exert more force than slow fibers because they contain more myosin cross-bridges per cross-sectional area of fiber than slow fibers.

TABLE 8.1	Characteristics of Human Skeletal Muscle Fiber Types		
	FAST FIBERS		**SLOW FIBERS**
Characteristic	**Type IIx**	**Type IIa**	**Type I**
Number of mitochondria	Low	High/moderate	High
Resistance to fatigue	Low	High/moderate	High
Predominant energy system	Anaerobic	Combination	Aerobic
ATPase activity	Highest	High	Low
Vmax (speed of shortening)	Highest	Intermediate	Low
Efficiency	Low	Moderate	High
Specific tension	High	High	Moderate

training, they can increase their oxidative capacity to levels equal with type I. For more details on muscle fiber characteristics, see references 8, 14, 46, and 71.

IN SUMMARY

- Human skeletal muscle fiber types can be divided into three general classes of fibers based on their biochemical and contractile properties. Two categories of fast fibers exist, type IIx and type IIa. One type of slow fiber exists, type I fibers.
- The biochemical and contractile properties characteristic of all muscle fiber types are summarized in table 8.1.
- Although classifying skeletal muscle fibers into three general groups is a convenient system to study the properties of muscle fibers, it is important to appreciate that human skeletal muscle fibers exhibit a wide range of contractile and biochemical properties. That is, the biochemical and contractile properties of type IIx, type IIa, and type I fibers represent a continuum instead of three neat packages.

Fiber Types and Performance

Descriptive studies have demonstrated several interesting facts concerning the percentages of fast and slow muscle fibers found in humans. First, there are no apparent sex or age differences in fiber distribution (67). Secondly, the average sedentary man or woman possesses approximately 47% to 53% slow fibers. Thirdly, it is commonly believed that successful power athletes (e.g., sprinters, fullbacks, etc.) possess a large percentage of fast fibers, whereas endurance athletes generally have a high percentage of slow fibers (27, 34, 99). Table 8.2 presents some examples of the percentage of slow and fast fibers found in successful athletes.

It is clear from table 8.2 that considerable variation in the percentage of various fiber types exists even among successful athletes competing in the same event or sport. In other words, two equally successful 10,000-meter runners might differ in the percentage of slow fibers that each possesses. For example, runner A might be found to possess 70% slow fibers, while runner B might contain 85% slow fibers. This observation demonstrates that an individ-

TABLE 8.2	Typical Muscle Fiber Composition in Elite Athletes	
Sport	% Slow Fibers (Type I)	% Fast Fibers (Types IIx and IIa)
Distance runners	70–80	20–30
Track sprinters	25–30	70–75
Nonathletes	47–53	47–53

Data from references 17 and 77.

ual's muscle fiber composition is not the only variable that determines success in athletic events. In fact, it is generally believed that success in athletic performance is due to a complex interaction of psychological, biochemical, neurological, cardiopulmonary, and biomechanical factors (18, 19, 60, 105).

IN SUMMARY

- Successful power athletes (e.g., sprinters) generally possess a large percentage of fast muscle fibers and therefore, a low percentage of slow, type I fibers.
- In contrast to power athletes, endurance athletes (e.g., marathoners) typically possess a high percentage of slow muscle fibers and a low percentage of fast fibers.

ALTERATIONS IN SKELETAL MUSCLE DUE TO EXERCISE, INACTIVITY, AND AGING

Skeletal muscle is a highly plastic tissue. That is, the size and biochemical makeup of a skeletal muscle fiber can be modified by several factors. For example, muscle composition and function can be altered in response to increased physical activity, inactivity, and due to the aging process. In this section, we provide a brief summary of the major changes that occur in skeletal muscle in response to exercise training, muscular inactivity, and during aging. We begin with a discussion of the effects of exercise training on skeletal muscle.

Exercise-Induced Changes In Skeletal Muscles

Specific details of muscle adaptation to different types of exercise training will be discussed later in chapter 13. Our purpose here is to provide a brief overview of exercise-induced changes in skeletal muscle to establish the foundation for a more detailed understanding of this important topic later in the text. The muscle's response to increased physical activity is specific to the type of exercise training. For example, it is well known that the primary adaptation to strength training (weight lifting) is to increase both muscle size and force production (3, 41, 54, 64, 86, 98). This increase in muscle size is primarily due to muscle fiber enlargement (hypertrophy), although some researchers argue that strength training may also promote a small increase in muscle fiber number (hyperplasia) (59, 93, 100). In contrast to strength training, endurance exercise (e.g., long-distance running) does not increase muscle size or strength but results in an increase in muscle oxidative capacity (e.g., mitochondrial number increases) (103).

A frequently asked question is, can exercise training alter skeletal muscle fiber types? In the past, researchers remained divided on the answer. For example, several older studies concluded that endurance exercise training did not promote the conversion of fast fibers to slow fibers (7, 8, 36, 42 50, 57). Nonetheless, recent investigations using more advanced techniques to study muscle fiber adaptation have shown that regular and rigorous exercise training results in alterations in skeletal muscle fiber types. Interestingly, both endurance training and resistance exercise training result in a fast-to-slow shift in muscle fiber type (2, 68, 80, 90, 96). Also, note that resistance-training-induced changes in muscle fiber type are often small and typically result in a reduction of the percentage of type IIx fibers and an increase in the percentage of type IIa fibers (2). (See figure 8.13). This transformation of type IIx to type IIa is considered a fast-to-slow shift because the movement is from the fastest fiber type (i.e., type IIx) toward a slower, and more oxidative fiber type (i.e., type IIa).

Does endurance exercise training result in an increase in the percentage of slow, type I fibers? At one time it was believed that endurance training does not increase the number of type I fibers (80, 96). However, more recent research reveals that long-duration endurance exercise training is capable of promoting a type IIx to type I fiber shift in skeletal muscle (26, 69, 90). Interestingly, it appears that exercise-training-induced fast-to-slow changes in muscle fiber types occurs in distinct stages. That is, during the training-induced shift of type IIx fibers to type I fibers, type IIx fibers are first changed to a type IIa fiber (69). If training persists, this newly formed type IIa fiber can then be converted into a type I fiber, resulting in a complete type IIx to type I fiber transformation (69).

Muscle Atrophy Due to Inactivity

It is well known that muscle disuse results in atrophy. This type of muscle atrophy can result from periods of prolonged bed rest, immobilization of a limb (i.e.,

ASK THE EXPERT 8.1

Effects of Space Flight on Human Skeletal Muscle
Questions and Answers with Dr. Kenneth Baldwin

Kenneth Baldwin, Ph.D. *is a professor in the Department of Physiology and Biophysics at the University of California–Irvine. Dr. Baldwin is an internationally respected scientist and is a leader in both the American Physiological Society and the American College of Sports Medicine. To date, Dr. Baldwin has published over 150 research articles in a variety of muscle-related topics. Much of Dr. Baldwin's research has focused on the effects of inactivity on skeletal muscle. Specifically, Dr. Baldwin's research team has performed many of the "landmark" studies that describe the impact of space flight on skeletal muscle structure and function. In this box feature, Dr. Baldwin answers questions related to the effects of prolonged space flight on skeletal muscle structure and function.*

QUESTION #1: During space travel, astronauts are exposed to low levels of gravity; this low-gravity environment results in an "unloading" of their skeletal muscles. What effect does prolonged space travel have on skeletal muscle size and function?

ANSWER: During exposure to the environment of space flight, the load placed on antigravity muscles in the lower extremities (i.e., leg muscles) is greatly reduced. As a result, these muscles undergo atrophy, resulting in a reduction in muscle fiber size. This loss in fiber cross-sectional area results in reduced strength and endurance. So, the end result is that the astronaut cannot generate sufficient muscular power to sustain physical activity for long periods of time.

QUESTION #2: How does eight weeks of space travel alter locomotor muscle fiber type in astronauts?

ANSWER: Prolonged space flight results in several changes to skeletal muscle fibers. One reason for the loss in muscle endurance in astronauts following space flight is associated with a decrease in the size of type I (i.e., slow-twitch fibers). Also, many of these type I fibers are converted to fast, type II fibers (i.e., fast-twitch fibers). One key feature of all fast-twitch fibers is that they have low endurance because of their low capacity for aerobic metabolism, which is a key feature in establishing endurance in all muscle cells. The reason for the fiber-type switching during space flight is very complicated, but it has to do with

down-regulating genes that control slow-twitch properties and up-regulating those genes that confer a fast-twitch property.

QUESTION #3: What countermeasures can be applied during space travel to reduce the effects of low gravity on skeletal muscle atrophy?

ANSWER: In order to prevent atrophy, loss of strength, and fiber-type transformation in astronauts exposed to prolonged space flight, one must impose regular resistance exercise (i.e., similar to resistance training on earth) on the target muscles. That is, skeletal muscles must be loaded several times each day with sufficient force to prevent or slow down the unloading condition that appears to be responsible for the atrophy/fiber-typing changes. Thus, the astronauts must be conditioned with resistance-training devices specifically designed for space flight environments.

For more details on the effects of space flight on skeletal muscle performance, please see "Ask the Expert 19.1" (chapter 19) for questions and answers with Dr. Robert Fitts.

---

casting due to broken bone), or the reduced loading of a muscle that occurs during space flight. From a practical perspective, disuse muscle atrophy results in a loss of muscular strength that is proportional to the degree of the atrophy.

Why do muscles atrophy during periods of disuse? Research has shown that during the first two days of muscle disuse, most of the initial atrophy occurs due to a reduction in muscle protein synthesis (16). After this initial period of atrophy, subsequent atrophy occurs primarily due to increased muscle protein breakdown (16, 91). Therefore, muscle atrophy resulting from prolonged muscle disuse occurs due to both a reduction in protein synthesis and an increase in the rate of muscle protein breakdown (16, 29, 81, 91).

Although muscle atrophy results in a loss of muscle mass and strength, this loss is not permanent and can be reversed by returning the muscle to normal use (i.e., reloading the muscle). A rapid and effective means of restoring normal muscle size and function after a period of disuse atrophy is to begin a program of resistance exercise training (i.e., weight lifting). Resistance exercise provides the muscle with an overload stimulus and promotes an increase in protein synthesis that results in both muscle hypertrophy and an increase in muscular strength.

For more details on the effects of inactivity on skeletal muscle size and function, see Ask the Expert 8.1 for a discussion of the impact of space flight on skeletal muscle.

A CLOSER LOOK 8.5

Muscle Atrophy Due to Disuse

It is well known that muscle disuse results in atrophy. This type of muscle atrophy can result from periods of prolonged bed rest, immobilization of a limb, or the reduced loading of a muscle that occurs during space flight. From a practical perspective, disuse atrophy results in a loss of muscular strength that is proportional to the degree of the atrophy.

Why do muscles atrophy during periods of disuse? Research has shown that during the first several days of muscle disuse, most of this initial atrophy occurs due to a reduction in muscle protein synthesis (16). After this beginning period of atrophy, subsequent atrophy occurs primarily due to increased muscle protein breakdown. Therefore, muscle atrophy resulting from prolonged muscle disuse occurs due to both a reduction in protein synthesis and an increase in the rate of muscle protein breakdown (16).

Although muscle atrophy results in a loss of muscle mass and strength, this loss is not permanent and can be reversed by returning the muscle to normal use (i.e., reloading the muscle). A rapid and effective means of restoring normal muscle size and function after a period of disuse atrophy is to begin a program of resistance exercise training. Resistance training provides the muscle with an overload stimulus and promotes an increase in protein synthesis that results in both muscle hypertrophy and an increase in muscular strength.

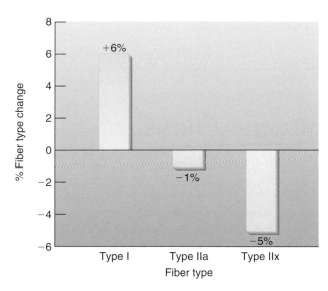

FIGURE 8.13 Effects of 16 weeks of endurance exercise training (i.e., 3–4 days/week at 50–60% V̇O₂ max) on human skeletal muscle fiber types. Note that exercise training promoted a significant fast-to-slow shift in muscle fiber type resulting in a net reduction in the percent of fast type IIx fibers and an increase in the percent of slow, type I fibers. Data are from Short et al. (90).

Age-Related Changes in Skeletal Muscle

Aging is associated with a loss of muscle mass (called sarcopenia). The age-related decline in muscle mass appears to have two phases. The first is a "slow" phase of muscle loss, in which 10% of muscle mass is lost from age 25 to 50 years. Thereafter, there is a rapid loss in muscle mass. In fact, from age 50 to 80 years, an additional 40% of muscle mass is lost. Thus, by age 80, one-half of the total muscle mass is lost (15). Also, aging results in a loss of fast fibers (particularly type IIx) and an increase in slow fibers (96). See references 15 and 25 for a review.

The loss of muscle size and strength observed in inactive older adults is not isolated to aging populations. A classic example of disuse muscle atrophy in young individuals is the reduction in muscle size observed in a broken limb during the period of immobilization imposed by the plaster "cast" (4). This simple example further illustrates that skeletal muscle is a highly "plastic" tissue that responds to both use and disuse (1, 45, 73, 74, 79). See A Closer Look 8.5 for details.

Does aging impair skeletal muscle's ability to adapt to physical training? The answer to this question is no. Although a loss of muscle mass occurs in aging humans, this decline in muscle size is due not only to the aging process but is often due to atrophy associated with limited physical activity in older individuals. Although regular exercise cannot completely eliminate the age-related loss of muscle, regular exercise can improve muscular endurance and strength in the elderly in a manner similar to that observed in young people (12, 15, 48, 75, 76, 77, 90, 96).

Scientists continue to search for safe and practical ways to increase skeletal muscle mass in elderly people. A new and exciting technique that can restore muscular strength in the elderly involves gene

Gene Therapy Can Restore the Age-Related Loss of Muscle Mass

One of the consequences of aging is the loss of skeletal muscle strength and mass. As discussed in the text, humans can lose up to one-half of their muscle mass and strength between the ages of 25 and 80 years. Unfortunately, this large loss of muscular strength reduces the quality of life for older people. Therefore, the prevention of this age-related loss in muscle mass is important. It is well known that resistance exercise training (i.e., weight training) can improve muscular strength in older people. Nonetheless, due to orthopedic or other health problems, many older people cannot engage in rigorous resistance training programs. Therefore, other methods of restoring muscular strength must be used by people who are not capable of performing heavy exercise. A promising approach to restoring the age-related loss of muscle

mass in the elderly is gene therapy. Recall that a gene is a segment of DNA with a unique order of nucleotide bases that encodes for a specific protein. Gene therapy is the technique of introducing a functioning gene into a human cell to correct a genetic error or to repair an acquired dysfunction of an existing gene. Effective gene therapy requires the transfer of foreign genes into a target cell and expression of this gene in the cell. A brief explanation of how gene therapy can be used to restore muscle mass during aging follows.

Insulin-like growth factor I (IGF-I) is a protein that is important in promoting the growth of skeletal muscle. Recent studies have shown that systemic administration of IGF-I results in muscle hypertrophy in animals. The hypertrophy occurs due to an increase in muscle protein synthesis and a reduction in

protein breakdown. Although the mechanisms responsible for the loss of muscle mass with aging continue to be investigated, it is believed that the decreased production of IGF-I associated with aging is a contributory factor (10). Therefore, increasing the production of IGF-I in older individuals could be an effective strategy to stop the age-related loss of skeletal muscle mass. In this regard, insertion of IGF-I genes (i.e., gene therapy) into skeletal muscle fibers of old animals has been shown to be an effective treatment for blocking the age-related loss of muscular strength (10). Therefore, the transfer of IGF-I genes into skeletal muscles could be a useful therapy for preventing the loss of skeletal muscle strength due to aging.

---

replacement therapy. This procedure is discussed in Clinical Applications 8.1.

IN SUMMARY

- Both endurance and resistance exercise training have been shown to promote a fast-to-slow shift in skeletal muscle fiber types. However, this exercise-induced shift in fiber type is typically small and does not result in a complete transformation of all fast fibers (type II) into slow fibers (type I).
- Prolonged periods of muscle disuse (bed rest, limb immobilization, etc.) result in muscle atrophy. This inactivity-induced atrophy results in a loss of muscle protein due to a reduction in protein synthesis and an increase in the rate of muscle protein breakdown.
- Aging is associated with a loss of muscle mass. This age-related loss of muscle mass is slow from age 25 to 50 years but increases rapidly after 50 years of age.
- Regular exercise training can improve skeletal muscle strength and endurance in the elderly but cannot completely eliminate the age-related loss of muscle mass.

MUSCLE ACTIONS

The process of skeletal muscle force generation has historically been referred to as a "muscle contraction." However, to describe both lengthening and shortening actions of a muscle as a contraction can be confusing. Therefore, the term **muscle action** has been proposed to describe the process of muscle force development. This term is now commonly used to describe different types of muscular contractions.

Several different types of muscle actions exist. For example, it is possible for skeletal muscle to generate force without a large amount of muscle shortening. This might occur when an individual pulls against a wire attached to the wall of a building (see figure 8.14b). What happens here is that muscle tension increases, but the wire does not move, and therefore neither does the body part that applies the force. This kind of muscle force development is called an **isometric action** and is referred to as a static exercise. Isometric actions are common in the postural muscles of the body, which act to maintain a static body position during periods of standing or sitting.

In contrast to isometric muscle actions, most types of exercise or sports activities require muscle actions that result in the movement of body parts.

(a)

(b)

FIGURE 8.14 (a) Isometric actions occur when a muscle exerts force but does not shorten. (b) Isotonic actions occur when a muscle contracts and shortens.

TABLE 8.3	Summary of the Classifications of Exercise and Muscle Action Types	
Type of Exercise	Muscle Action	Muscle Length Change
Dynamic	Concentric	Decreases
	Eccentric	Increases
Static	Isometric	No change

Exercise that involves movement of body parts is called **dynamic** exercise (formally called isotonic exercise). Two types of muscle actions can occur during dynamic exercise: (1) concentric and (2) eccentric. A muscle action that results in muscular shortening with movement of a body part is called a **concentric action** (figure 8.14a). An **eccentric action** occurs when a muscle is activated and force is produced but the muscle lengthens. Table 8.3 summarizes the classifications of exercise and muscle action types.

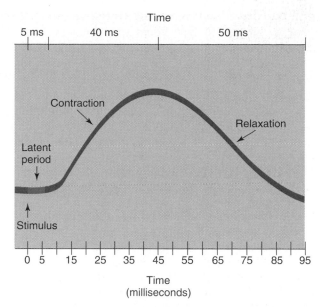

FIGURE 8.15 A recording of a simple twitch. Note the three time periods (latent period, contraction, and relaxation) following the stimulus.

SPEED OF MUSCLE ACTION AND RELAXATION

If a muscle is given a single stimulus, such as a brief electrical shock applied to the nerve innervating it, the muscle responds with a simple **twitch**. The movement of the muscle can be recorded on a special recording device, and the time periods for contraction and relaxation can be studied. Figure 8.15 demonstrates the time course of a simple twitch in an isolated frog muscle. Notice that the twitch can be divided into three phases. First, immediately after the stimulus, there is a brief latent period (lasting a few milliseconds) prior to the beginning of muscle shortening. The second phase of the twitch is the contraction phase, which lasts approximately 40 milliseconds. Finally, the muscle returns to its original length during the relaxation period, which lasts about 50 milliseconds and thus is the longest of the three phases.

The timing of the phases in a simple twitch varies among muscle fiber types. The variability in speed of contraction arises from differences in the responses of the individual fiber types that make up muscles. Individual muscle fibers behave much like individual neurons in that they exhibit all-or-none responses to stimulation. To contract, an individual muscle fiber must receive an appropriate amount of stimulation. However, fast fibers contract in a shorter time period when stimulated than do slow fibers. The explanation for this observation is as follows: The speed of shortening is greater in fast fibers than in slow fibers because the sarcoplasmic reticulum in fast fibers releases Ca^{++} at a faster rate, and fast fibers possess a higher ATPase activity compared to the slow fiber types (34, 37, 86). The higher ATPase activity results in a more rapid splitting of ATP and a quicker release of the energy required for contraction.

FORCE REGULATION IN MUSCLE

As stated earlier, the amount of force generated in a single muscle fiber is related to the number of myosin cross-bridges making contact with actin. However, the amount of force exerted during muscular contraction in a group of muscles is complex and dependent on three primary factors: (1) number and types of motor units recruited, (2) the initial length of the muscle, and (3) the nature of the neural stimulation of the motor units (6, 21, 24, 37). A discussion of each of these factors follows.

First, variations in the strength of contraction within an entire muscle depend on both the type and the number of muscle fibers that are stimulated to contract (i.e., recruited). If only a few motor units are recruited, the force is small. If more motor units are stimulated the force increases. Figure 8.16 illustrates this point. Note that as the stimulus is increased, the force of contraction is increased due to the recruitment of additional motor units. Also, recall that fast fibers exert a greater specific force than do slow fibers. Therefore, the types of motor units recruited also influence force production.

A second factor that determines the force exerted by a muscle is the initial length of the muscle at the time of contraction. There exists an "ideal" length of the muscle fiber. The explanation for the existence of an ideal length is related to the overlap between actin and myosin. For instance, when the resting length is longer than optimal, the overlap between actin and myosin is limited and few cross-bridges can attach. This concept is illustrated in figure 8.17. Note that when the muscle is stretched to the point where there is no overlap of actin and myosin, cross-bridges cannot attach and thus tension cannot be developed. At the other extreme, when the muscle is shortened to about 60% of its resting length, the Z lines are very close to the thick myosin filaments, and thus only limited additional shortening can occur.

A final factor that can affect the amount of force a muscle exerts upon contraction is the nature of the neural stimulation. Simple muscle twitches studied under experimental conditions reveal some interesting, fundamental properties about how muscles function. However, normal body movements involve sustained contractions that are not simple twitches. The sustained contractions involved in normal body movements can be closely replicated in the laboratory if a series of stimulations are applied to the muscle. The recording pictured in figure 8.18, represents what occurs when successive stimuli are applied to the muscle. The first few contractions represent simple twitches. Note that as the frequency of stimulations is increased, the muscle does not have time to relax between stimuli and the force appears to be additive. This response is called **summation** (addition of successive twitches). If the frequency of stimuli is increased further, individual contractions are blended together in a single, sustained contraction called **tetanus.** A tetanic contraction will continue until the stimuli are stopped or the muscle fatigues.

Muscular contractions that occur during normal body movements are tetanic contractions. These sustained contractions result from a series of rapidly repeated neural impulses conducted by the motor neurons that innervate those motor units involved in the movement. It is important to appreciate that in the body, neural impulses to various motor units do not arrive at the same time as they do in the laboratory-induced tetanic contraction. Instead, various motor units are stimulated to contract at different times. Thus, some motor units are contracting while some are relaxing. This type of tetanic contraction results in a smooth contraction and aids in sustaining a coordinated muscle contraction.

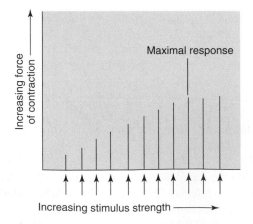

FIGURE 8.16 The relationship between increasing stimulus strength and the force of contraction. Weak stimuli do not activate many motor units and do not produce great force. In contrast, increasing the stimulus strength recruits more and more motor units and thus produces more force.

FIGURE 8.17 Length-tension relationships in skeletal muscle. Note that an optimal length of muscle exists, which will produce maximal force when stimulated. Lengths that are above or below this optimal length result in a reduced amount of force when stimulated.

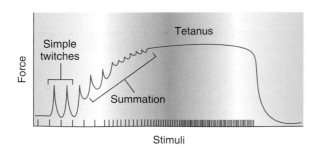

FIGURE 8.18 Recording showing the change from simple twitches to summation, and finally tetanus. Peaks to the left represent simple twitches, while increasing the frequency of the stimulus results in summation of the twitches, and finally tetanus.

FORCE-VELOCITY/POWER-VELOCITY RELATIONSHIPS

In most physical activities, muscular force is applied through a range of movement. For instance, an athlete performing the shot put applies force against the shot over a specified range of movement prior to release. How far the shot travels is a function of both the speed of the shot upon release and the angle of release. Since success in many athletic events is dependent on speed, it is important to appreciate some of the basic concepts underlying the relationship between muscular force and the speed of movement. The relationship

FIGURE 8.19 Muscle force-velocity relationships. Note that at any given speed of movement, muscle groups with a high percentage of fast fibers exert more *force* than those with muscle groups that contain primarily slow fibers.

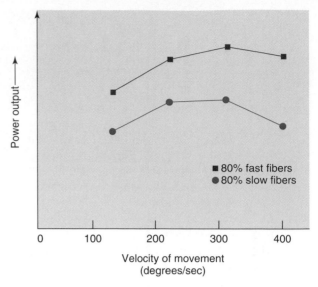

FIGURE 8.20 Muscle power-velocity relationships. In general, the power produced by a muscle group increases as a function of velocity of movement. At any given speed of movement, muscles that contain a large percentage of fast fibers produce more *power* than those muscles that contain primarily slow fibers.

between speed of movement and muscular force is shown in figure 8.19. Two important points emerge from an examination of figure 8.19:

1. At any absolute force exerted by the muscle, the velocity or speed of movement is greater in muscles that contain a high percentage of fast fibers when compared to muscles that possess predominantly slow fibers.
2. The maximum velocity of muscle shortening is greatest at the lowest force (i.e., resistance against the muscle). In short, the greatest speed of movement is generated at the lowest workloads (13, 56). This principle holds true for both slow and fast fibers.

The data contained in figure 8.19 also demonstrate that fast fibers are capable of producing greater muscular force at a faster speed than slow fibers. The biochemical mechanism to explain this observation is related to the fact that fast fibers possess higher ATPase activity than do slow fibers (34, 37). Therefore, ATP is broken down more rapidly in fast fibers when compared to slow fibers. Further, calcium release from the sarcoplasmic reticulum is faster following neural stimulation in fast fibers than in slow fibers (37, 84).

The relationship between force and movement speed has practical importance for the physical therapist, athlete, or physical educator. The message is simply that athletes who possess a high percentage of fast fibers would seem to have an advantage in power-type athletic events. This may explain why successful sprinters and weight lifters typically possess a relatively high percentage of fast fibers.

As might be expected, the fiber-type distribution in muscle influences the power-velocity curve (see figure 8.20). The peak power that can be generated by muscle is greater in muscle that contains a high percentage of fast fibers than in muscle that is largely composed of slow fibers. As with the force-velocity curve, two important points should be retained from the examination of the power-velocity curve:

1. At any given velocity of movement, the peak power generated is greater in muscle that contains a high percentage of fast fibers than in muscle with a high percentage of slow fibers. This difference is due to the aforementioned biochemical differences between fast and slow fibers. Again, athletes who possess a high percentage of fast fibers can generate more power than athletes with predominantly slow fibers.
2. The peak power generated by any muscle increases with increasing velocities of movement up to a movement speed of 200 to 300 degrees/ second. The reason for the plateau of power output with increasing movement speed is that muscular force decreases with increasing speed of movement (see figure 8.19). Therefore, with any given muscle group there is an optimum speed of movement that will elicit the greatest power output.

- The amount of force generated during muscular contraction is dependent on the following factors: (1) types and number of motor units recruited, (2) the initial muscle length, and (3) the nature of the motor units' neural stimulation.
- The addition of muscle twitches is termed *summation*. When the frequency of neural stimulation to a motor unit is increased, individual contractions are fused together in a sustained contraction called *tetanus*.
- The peak force generated by muscle decreases as the speed of movement increases. However, in general, the amount of power generated by a muscle group increases as a function of movement velocity.

RECEPTORS IN MUSCLE

Skeletal muscle contains several types of sensory receptors. These include chemoreceptors, muscle spindles, and Golgi tendon organs (61). Chemoreceptors are specialized free nerve endings that send information to the central nervous system in response to changes in muscle pH, concentrations of extracellular potassium, and changes in O_2 and CO_2 tensions. Chemoreceptors may play a role in cardiopulmonary regulation during exercise and will be discussed in more detail in chapters 9 and 10.

In order for the nervous system to properly control skeletal muscle movements, it must receive continuous sensory feedback from the contracting muscle. This sensory feedback includes (1) information concerning the tension developed by a muscle and (2) an account of the muscle length. **Golgi tendon organs (GTOs)** provide the central nervous system with feedback concerning the tension developed by the muscle, while the **muscle spindle** provides sensory information concerning the relative muscle length (52, 61). A discussion of each sensory organ follows.

Muscle Spindle

As previously stated, the muscle spindle functions as a length detector. Muscle spindles are found in large numbers in most human locomotor muscles (52). Muscles that require the finest degree of control, such as the muscles of the hands, have the highest density of spindles. In contrast, muscles that are responsible for gross movements (e.g., quadriceps) contain relatively few spindles.

The muscle spindle is composed of several thin muscle cells (called *intrafusal fibers*) that are surrounded by a connective tissue sheath. Like normal skeletal muscle fibers (called *extrafusal fibers*), muscle spindles insert into connective tissue within the muscle. Therefore, muscle spindles run parallel with muscle fibers (see figure 8.21).

Muscle spindles contain two types of sensory nerve endings. The primary endings respond to dynamic changes in muscle length. The second type of sensory ending is called the secondary ending, and it does not respond to rapid changes in muscle length, but provides the central nervous system with continuous information concerning static muscle length.

In addition to the sensory neurons, muscle spindles are innervated by gamma motor neurons, which stimulate the intrafusal fibers to contract simultaneously along with extrafusal fibers. Gamma motor neuron stimulation causes the central region of the intrafusal fibers to shorten, which serves to tighten the spindle. The need for contraction of the intrafusal fibers can be explained as follows: When skeletal muscles are shortened by motor neuron stimulation, muscle spindles are passively shortened along with the skeletal muscle fibers. If the intrafusal fibers did not compensate accordingly, this shortening would result in "slack" in the spindle and make them less sensitive. Therefore, their function as length detectors would be compromised.

Muscle spindles are responsible for the observation that rapid stretching of skeletal muscles results in a reflex contraction. This is called the *stretch reflex* and is present in all muscles, but is most dramatic in the extensor muscles of the limbs. The so-called knee-jerk reflex is often evaluated by the physician by tapping the patellar tendon with a rubber mallet. The blow by the mallet stretches the entire muscle and thus "excites" the primary nerve endings located in muscle spindles. The neural impulse from the muscle spindle synapses at the spinal cord level with a motor neuron, which then stimulates the extrafusal fibers of the extensor muscle, resulting in an isotonic contraction.

The function of the muscle spindle is to assist in the regulation of movement and to maintain posture. This is accomplished by the muscle spindle's ability to detect and cause the central nervous system (CNS) to respond to changes in the length of skeletal muscle fibers. The following practical example shows how the muscle spindle assists in the control of movement. Suppose a student is holding a single book in front of him or her with the arm extended. This type of load poses a tonic stretch on the muscle spindle, which sends information to the CNS concerning the final length of the extrafusal muscle fibers. If a second book is suddenly placed upon the first book, the muscles

1. Muscle spindles detect stretch of the muscle.

2. Sensory neurons conduct action potentials to the spinal cord.

3. Sensory neurons synapse with alpha motor neurons.

4. Stimulation of the alpha motor neurons causes the muscle to contract and resist being stretched.

FIGURE 8.21 The structure of muscle spindles and their location in skeletal muscle.

would be suddenly stretched (arm would drop) and a burst of impulses from the muscle spindle would alert the CNS about the change in muscle length (and thus load). The ensuing reflex would recruit additional motor units to raise the arm back to the original position. Generally, this type of reflex action results in an overcompensation. That is, more motor units are recruited than are needed to bring the arm back to the original position. However, immediately following the overcompensation movement, an additional adjustment rapidly occurs and the arm is quickly returned to the original position.

Golgi Tendon Organs

The Golgi tendon organs (GTOs) continuously monitor the tension produced by muscle contraction. Golgi tendon organs are located within the tendon and thus are in series with the extrafusal fibers (figure 8.22). In essence, GTOs serve as "safety devices" that help prevent excessive force during muscle contraction. When activated, GTOs send information to the spinal cord via sensory neurons, which in turn excite inhibitory neurons (i.e., send IPSPs). This inhibitory disynaptic reflex (i.e., two synapses are involved) helps prevent

excessive muscle contractions and provides a finer control over skeletal movements. This process is pictured in figure 8.22.

It seems likely that GTOs play an important role in the performance of strength activities. For instance, the amount of force that can be produced by a muscle group may be dependent on the ability of the individual to voluntarily oppose the inhibition of the GTO. It seems possible that the inhibitory influences of the GTO could be gradually reduced in response to strength training (105). This would allow an individual to produce a greater amount of muscle force and, in many cases, improve sport performance.

IN SUMMARY

- The muscle spindle functions as a length detector in muscle.
- Golgi tendon organs continuously monitor the tension developed during muscular contraction. In essence, Golgi tendon organs serve as safety devices that help prevent excessive force during muscle contractions.

1. Golgi tendon organs detect tension applied to a tendon.

2. Sensory neurons conduct action potentials to the spinal cord.

3. Sensory neurons synapse with inhibitory interneurons that synapse with alpha motor neurons.

4. Inhibition of the alpha motor neurons causes muscle relaxation, relieving the tension applied to the tendon.

Muscle contraction increases tension applied to tendons. In response, action potentials are conducted to the spinal cord.

Sensory neuron

Tendon

Muscle

Golgi tendon organ

To brain

Sensory neuron

Inhibitory interneuron

Alpha motor neuron

Golgi tendon organ

Golgi tendon reflex

FIGURE 8.22   The Golgi tendon organ. The Golgi tendon organ is located in series with muscle and serves as a "tension monitor" that acts as a protective device for muscle. See text for details.

STUDY QUESTIONS

1. List the principal functions of skeletal muscles.
2. List the principal proteins contained in skeletal muscle.
3. Outline the contractile process. Use a step-by-step format illustrating the entire process, beginning with the nerve impulse reaching the neuromuscular junction.
4. Outline the mechanical and biochemical properties of human skeletal muscle fiber types.
5. Discuss those factors thought to be responsible for regulating force during muscular contractions.
6. Define the term *summation*.
7. Graph a simple muscle twitch and a contraction that results in tetanus.
8. Discuss the relationship between force and speed of movement during a muscular contraction.
9. Describe the general anatomical design of a muscle spindle and discuss its physiological function.
10. Discuss the function of Golgi tendon organs in monitoring muscle tension.

SUGGESTED READINGS

Brooks, G., T. Fahey, and K. Baldwin. 2005. *Exercise Physiology: Human Bioenergetics and Its Applications*, 4th ed. New York: McGraw-Hill Companies.

Cairns, S., A. Knicker, M. Thompson, and G. Sjogaard. 2005. Evaluation of models used to study neuromuscular fatigue. *Exercise and Sport Science Reviews* 33:9–16.

Fox, S. 2006. *Human Physiology*. New York: McGraw-Hill Companies.

Leiber, R. 2002. *Skeletal Muscle Structure, Function, and Plasticity: The Physiological Basis of Rehabilitation*. New York: Lippincott, Williams & Wilkins.

MacIntosh, B., P. Gardiner, and A. McComas. 2005. *Skeletal Muscle–Form and Function*. Champaign, IL: Human Kinetics Publishers.

Powers, S., A. Kavazis, and K. DeRuisseau. 2005. Mecha-

nisms of disuse muscle atrophy: Role of oxidative stress. *American Journal of Physiology* 288:R337–44.

Short, K. et al. 2005. Changes in myosin heavy chain mRNA and protein expression in human skeletal muscle with age and endurance training. *Journal of Applied Physiology* 99:95–102.

Westerblad, H., and D. Allen. 2003. Cellular mechanisms of skeletal muscle fatigue. *Advances in Experimental Medicine and Biology* 538:563–70.

Widmaier, E., H. Raff, and K. Strang. 2006. *Vander's Human Physiology*, 10th ed. New York: McGraw-Hill Companies.

Wozniak, A. et al. 2005. Signaling satellite-cell activation in skeletal muscle: Markers, models, stretch, and potential alternative pathways. *Muscle Nerve* 31:283–300.

REFERENCES

1. Abernethy, P., R. Thayer, and A. Taylor. 1990. Acute and chronic responses of skeletal muscle to endurance and sprint exercise: A review. *Sports Medicine* 10:365–89.
2. Adams, G. et al. 1993. Skeletal muscle myosin heavy chain composition and resistance training. *Journal of Applied Physiology*. 74:911–15.
3. Alway, S. et al. 1990. Muscle cross-sectional area and torque in resistance trained subjects. *European Journal of Applied Physiology* 60:86–90.
4. Appell, H. 1990. Muscular atrophy following immobilisation: A review. *Sports Medicine* 10:42–58.
5. Armstrong, R. et al. 1983. Differential inter- and intramuscular responses to exercise: Considerations in use of the biopsy technique. In *Biochemistry of Exercise*, eds. H. Knuttgen, J. Vogel, and J. Poortmans, 775–80. Champaign, IL: Human Kinetics.
6. Armstrong, R., and H. Laughlin. 1985. Muscle function during locomotion in mammals. In *Circulation, Respiration, and Metabolism*, ed. R. Giles, 56–63. New York: Springer-Verlag.
7. Bagby, G., W. Sembrowich, and P. Gollnick. 1972. Myosin ATPase and fiber type composition from trained and untrained rat skeletal muscle. *Journal of Applied Physiology* 223:1415–17.
8. Baldwin, K. et al. 1972. Respiratory capacity of white, red, and intermediate muscle: Adaptive response to exercise. *Journal of Applied Physiology* 222:373–78.
9. Bar, A., and D. Pette. 1988. Three fast myosin heavy chains in adult rat skeletal muscle. *FEBS Letters*. 235:153–54.
10. Barton-Davis, E. et al. 1998. Viral mediated expression of insulin-like growth factor I blocks the age-related loss of skeletal muscle function. *Proceedings of the National Academy of Sciences* 95:15603–7.
11. Billeter, R., and H. Hoppeler. 1992. Muscular basis of strength. In *Strength and Power in Sport*, ed. P. Komi, 39–63. Oxford: Blackwell Scientific Publishing.
12. Black, R. 1991. Muscle strength as an indicator of the habitual level of physical activity. *Medicine and Science in Sports and Exercise* 23:1375–81.
13. Bobbert, M., G. Ettema, and P. Huijing. 1990. The force-length relationship of a muscle-tendon complex: Experimental results and model calculations. *European Journal of Applied Physiology* 61:323–29.
14. Booth, F., and D. Thomason. 1991. Molecular and cellular adaptation of muscle in response to exercise: Perspectives of various models. *Physiological Reviews* 71:541–85.
15. Booth, F., and S. Weeden. 1993. Structural aspects of aging human skeletal muscle. In *Musculoskeletal Soft-tissue Aging: Impact on Mobility*, ed. J. Buckwalter, V. Goldberg, and S. Woo. Rosemont, IL: American Academy of Orthopaedic Surgeons.
16. Booth, F. W., and D. S. Criswell. 1997. Molecular events underlying skeletal muscle atrophy and the development of effective countermeasures. *International Journal of Sports Medicine* 18 (Suppl. 4): S265–69.
17. Bottinelli, R., M. Canepari, C. Reggiani, and G. Stienen. 1994. Myofibrillar ATPase activity during isometric contractions and isomyosin composition in rat single skinned muscle fibers. *Journal of Physiology* (London). 481:663–75.
18. Brooks, G., T. Fahey, T. White, and K. Baldwin. 2000. *Exercise Physiology: Human Bioenergetics and Its Applications*. New York: McGraw-Hill Companies.
19. ———. 1987. *Fundamentals of Human Performance*. New York: Macmillan.
20. Buchthal, F., and H. Schmalbruch. 1970. Contraction times and fiber types in intact human muscle. *Acta Physiologica Scandanavica* 79:435–40.
21. Burke, R. 1986. The control of muscle force: Motor unit recruitment and firing pattern. In *Human Muscle Power*, ed. N. Jones, N. McCartney, and A. McComas, 97–105. Champaign, IL: Human Kinetics.
22. Caiozzo, V. et al. 1993. Single fiber analyses of Type IIa myosin heavy chain distribution in hyper- and hypothyroid soleus. *American Journal of Physiology*. 265:C842–49.
23. Cairns, S., A. Knicker, M. Thompson, and G. Sjogaard. 2005. Evaluation of models used to study neuromuscular fatigue. *Exercise and Sport Science Reviews* 33:9–16.
24. Carlson, F., and D. Wilkie. 1974. *Muscle Physiology*. Englewood Cliffs, NJ: Prentice-Hall.
25. Carmeli, E., R. Coleman, and A. Z. Reznick. 2002. The biochemistry of aging muscle. *Experimental Gerontology* 37:477–89.
26. Conley, K. 1994. Cellular energetics during exercise. *Advances in Veterinary Science and Comparative Medicine*. 38A:1–39.
27. Costill, D., W. Fink, and M. Pollock. 1976. Muscle fiber composition and enzyme activities of elite distance runners. *Medicine and Science in Sports* 8:96.
28. Demirel, H., S. Powers, H. Naito, M. Hughes, and J. Coombes. 1999. Exercise-induced alterations in skeletal muscle myosin heavy chain phenotype: dose-response relationship. *Journal of Applied Physiology* 86:1002–8.
29. DeRuisseau, K., Kavazis, M. Deering, D. Falk, D. Van Gammeren, T. Yimlamai, G. Ordway, and S. Powers. 2005. Mechanical ventilation induces alterations of the ubiquitin-proteasome pathway in the diaphragm. *Journal of Applied Physiology* 98:1314–21.
30. Devor, S., and T. White. 1995. Myosin heavy chain phenotype in regenerating skeletal muscle is affected by thyroid hormone. *Medicine and Science in Sports and Exercise* 27:674–81.
31. Ebashi, S. 1976. Excitation-contraction coupling. *Annual Review of Physiology* 38:293–309.
32. ———. 1991. Excitation-contraction coupling. *Annual Review of Physiology* 53:1–16.
33. Edgerton, V. et al. 1983. Muscle fiber activation and recruitment. In *Biochemistry of Exercise*, ed. H. Knuttgen, J. Vogel, and J. Poortmans, 31–49. Champaign, IL: Human Kinetics.
34. Edgerton, V. et al. 1986. Morphological basis of skeletal muscle power output. In *Human Muscle Power*, ed. N. Jones, N. McCartney, and A. McComas, 43–58. Champaign, IL: Human Kinetics.
35. Edman, K. 1992. Contractile performance of skeletal muscle fibers. In *Strength and Power in Sport*, ed. P. Komi, 96–114. Oxford: Blackwell Scientific Publishing.
36. Edstrom, L., and L. Grimby. 1986. Effect of exercise on the motor unit. *Muscle and Nerve* 9:104–26.
37. Faulker, J., D. Claflin, and K. McCully. 1986. Power output of fast and slow fibers from human skeletal muscles. In *Human Muscle Power*, ed. N. Jones, N. McCartney, and A. McComas, 81–90. Champaign, IL: Human Kinetics.
38. Fauteck, S., and S. Kandarian. 1995. Sensitive detection of myosin heavy chain composition in skeletal muscle under different loading conditions. *American Journal of Physiology* 37:C419–C424.

39. Fitts, R. 1994. Cellular mechanisms of muscle fatigue. *Physiological Reviews* 74:49–94.

40. Fox, S. 2002. *Human Physiology*. New York: McGraw-Hill Companies.

41. Goldspink, G. 1992. Cellular and molecular aspects of adaptation in skeletal muscle. In *Strength and Power in Sport*, ed. P. Komi, 211–29. London: Blackwell Scientific Publishing.

42. Gollnick, P. 1985. Metabolism of substrates: Energy substrate metabolism during exercise and as modified by training. *Federation Proceedings* 44:353–56.

43. Gollnick, P., and B. Saltin. 1983. Hypothesis: Significance of skeletal muscle oxidative capacity with endurance training. *Clinical Physiology* 2:1–12.

44. Green, H. 1986. Muscle power: Fiber type recruitment, metabolism, and fatigue. In *Human Muscle Power*, ed. N. Jones, N. McCartney, and A. McComas, 65–79. Champaign, IL: Human Kinetics.

45. Grinton, S. et al. 1992. Exercise training-induced increases in expiratory muscle oxidative capacity. *Medicine and Science in Sports and Exercise* 24:551–55.

46. Gunning, P., and E. Hardeman. 1991. Multiple mechanisms regulate muscle fiber diversity. FASEB *Journal* 5:3064–70.

47. Hameed, M., S. Harridge, and G. Goldspink. 2002. Sarcopenia and hypertrophy: A role for insulin-like growth factor-I in aged muscle? *Exercise and Sport Science Reviews* 30:15–19.

48. Hammeren, J. et al. 1992. Exercise training-induced alterations in skeletal muscle oxidative and antioxidant enzyme activity in senescent rats. *International Journal of Sports Medicine* 13:412–16.

49. Holloszy, J. 1982. Muscle metabolism during exercise. *Archives of Physical and Rehabilitation Medicine* 63:231–34.

50. Hoppeler, H. 1986. Exercise-induced ultrastructure changes in skeletal muscle. *International Journal of Sports Medicine* 7:187–204.

51. Hughes, S. et al. 1993. Three slow myosin heavy chains sequentially expressed In developing mammalian skeletal muscle. *Developmental Biology* 158:183–99.

52. Hunt, C. 1991. Mammalian muscle spindle: Peripheral mechanisms. *Physiological Reviews* 70:643–63.

53. Johnson, L. 1987. *Biology*. New York: McGraw-Hill Companies.

54. Johnson, T., and K. Klueber. 1991. Skeletal muscle following tonic overload: Functional and structural analysis. *Medicine and Science in Sports and Exercise* 23:49–55.

55. Kodama, T. 1985. Thermodynamic analysis of muscle ATPase mechanisms. *Physiological Reviews* 65:468–540.

56. Kojima, T. 1991. Force-velocity relationship of human elbow flexors in voluntary isotonic contraction under heavy loads. *International Journal of Sports Medicine* 12: 208–13.

57. Larsson, L. 1982. Physical training effects on muscle morphology in sedentary males at different ages. *Medicine and Science in Sports and Exercise* 14:203.

58. Lowey, S. 1986. Cardiac and skeletal muscle myosin polymorphism. *Medicine and Science in Sports and Exercise* 18:284–91.

59. MacDougall, J. 1992. Hypertrophy or hyperplasia. In *Strength and Power in Sport*, ed. P. Komi, 230–38. London: Blackwell Scientific Publishing.

60. McArdle, W., F. Katch, and V. Katch. 2001. *Exercise Physiology: Energy, Nutrition, and Human Performance*. Baltimore: Lippincott Williams & Wilkins.

61. McCloskey, D. et al. 1987. Sensing position and movements of the fingers. *News in Physiological Sciences* 2:226–30.

62. MacIntosh, B., P. Gardiner, and A. McComas. 2005. *Skeletal Muscle—Form and Function*. Champaign, IL: Human Kinetics Publishers.

63. Metzger, J. 1992. Mechanism of chemomechanical coupling in skeletal muscle during work. In *Energy Metabolism in Exercise and Sport*, ed. D. Lamb and C. Gisolfi, 1–43. New York: McGraw-Hill Companies.

64. Milesky, A. et al. 1991. Changes in muscle fiber size and composition in response to heavy-resistance exercise. *Medicine and Science in Sports and Exercise* 23:1042–49.

65. Moss, R., G. Diffee, and M. Greaser. 1995. Contractile properties of skeletal muscle fibers in relation to myofibrillar protein isoforms. *Review of Physiology, Biochemistry, and Pharmacology* 126:1–63.

66. Noakes, T., and A. St Clair Gibson. 2004. Logical limitations to the catastrophe models of fatigue during exercise in humans. *British Journal of Sports Medicine* 38:648–59.

67. Pette, D. 1980. *Plasticity of Muscle*. New York: Walter de Gruyter.

68. ———. 1984. Activity-induced fast-to-slow transitions in mammalian muscle. *Medicine and Science in Sports and Exercise* 16:517–28.

69. ———. 2001. Historical perspectives: Plasticity of mammalian skeletal muscle. *Journal of Applied Physiology* 90:1119–24.

70. Pette, D., and C. Spamer. 1986. Metabolic properties of muscle fibers. *Federation Proceedings* 45:2910–14.

71. Pette, D., and R. Staron. 1990. Cellular and molecular diversities of mammalian skeletal muscle fibers. *Review of Physiology, Biochemistry, and Pharmacology* 116:1–76.

72. Pette, D., and G. Vrbova. 1992. Adaptation of mammalian muscle fibers to chronic electrical stimulation. *Review of Physiology, Biochemistry, and Pharmacology* 120: 115–202.

73. Powers, S. et al. 1990. Endurance-training-induced cellular adaptations in respiratory muscles. *Journal of Applied Physiology* 69:648–50.

74. Powers, S. et al. 1990. Regional metabolic differences in the rat diaphragm. *Journal of Applied Physiology* 68: 2114–18.

75. Powers, S. et al. 1991. Age-related changes in enzyme activity in the rat diaphragm. *Respiration Physiology* 83: 1–10.

76. Powers, S. et al. 1992. Aging and exercise-induced cellular alterations in the rat diaphragm. *American Journal of Physiology* 32:R1093–R1098.

77. Powers, S. et al. 1992. Aging and respiratory muscle metabolic plasticity: Effects of endurance training. *Journal of Applied Physiology* 72:1068–73.

78. Powers, S. et al. 1992. Diaphragmatic fiber type specific adaptation to endurance training. *Respiration Physiology* 89:195–207.

79. Powers, S. et al. 1992. High intensity exercise training-induced metabolic alterations in respiratory muscles. *Respiration Physiology* 89:169–77.

80. Powers, S. et al. 1995. Role of beta-adrenergic mechanisms in exercise training-induced metabolic changes in respiratory and locomotor muscle. *International Journal of Sports Medicine* 16:13–18.

81. Powers, S., A. Kavazis, and K. DeRuisseau. 2005. Mechanisms of disuse muscle atrophy: Role of oxidative stress. *American Journal of Physiology* 288:R337–R344.

82. Rayment, I. et al. 1993. Structure of the actin myosin complex and its implications for muscle contraction. *Science* 261:58–65.

83. Ruegg, J. 1992. *Calcium in Muscle Activation*. Berlin: Springer-Verlag.

84. Ruegg, J. C. 1987. Excitation-contraction coupling in fast- and slow-twitch muscle fibers. *International Journal of Sports Medicine* 8:360–64.

85. Saltin, B. et al. 1977. Fiber types and metabolic potentials of skeletal muscles in sedentary man and endurance runners. *Annals of New York Academy of Sciences* 301:3–29.

86. Saltin, B., and P. Gollnick. 1983. Skeletal muscle adaptability: Significance for metabolism and performance. In *Handbook of Physiology*, ed. L. Peachy, R. Adrian, and S. Geiger. Section 10: Skeletal Muscle, chapter 19, 555–631. Bethesda, MD: American Physiological Society.

87. Sant'Ana Pereira, J., S. Ennion, A. Moorman, G. Goldspink, and A. Sargeant. 1994. The predominant fast myHC's in human skeletal muscle corresponds to the rat IIa and IIx and not IIb. *Annual Meeting of Society For Neuroscience*. Abstract. A26.

88. Schiaffino, S., L. Gorza, L. Saggin, S. Ausoni, M. Vianello, K. Gundersen, and T. Lomo. 1989. Three myosin heavy chain isoforms in type 2 skeletal muscle fibers. *Journal of Muscle Research and Cell Motility* 10:197–205.

89. Schiaffino, S., and C. Reggiani. 1994. Myosin isoforms in mammalian skeletal muscle. *Journal of Applied Physiology* 77:493–501.

90. Short, K. et al. 2005. Changes in myosin heavy chain mRNA and protein expression in human skeletal muscle with age and endurance training. *Journal of Applied Physiology* 99:95–102.

91. Shanely, R., D. Van Gammeren, K. DeRuisseau, A. Zergeroglu, M. McKenzie, K. Yarasheski, and S. Powers. 2004. Mechanical ventilation depresses protein synthesis in the rat diaphragm. *American Journal of Respiratory and Critical Care Medicine* 170:994–99.

92. Simoneau, J. et al. 1986. Inheritance of human skeletal muscle and anaerobic capacity adaptation to high-intensity intermittent training. *International Journal of Sports Medicine* 7:167–71.

93. Sjostrom, M. et al. 1991. Evidence of fiber hyperplasia in human skeletal muscles from healthy young men? *European Journal of Applied Physiology* 62:301–4.

94. Snow, D., and R. Harris. 1985. Thoroughbreds and greyhounds: Biochemical adaptations in creatures of nature and man. In *Circulation, Respiration, and Metabolism*, ed. R. Giles, 227–39. New York: Springer-Verlag.

95. Staron, R. et al. 1989. Muscle hypertrophy and fast fiber conversions in heavy resistance-trained women. *European Journal of Applied Physiology* 60:71–79.

96. Sullivan, V. et al. 1995. Myosin heavy chain composition in young and old rat skeletal muscle: Effects of endurance exercise. *Journal of Applied Physiology* 78:2115–20.

97. Tate, C., M. Hyek, and G. Taffet. 1991. The role of calcium in the energetics of contracting skeletal muscle. *Sports Medicine* 12:208–17.

98. Tesch, P. 1992. Short and long-term histochemical and biochemical adaptations in muscle. In *Strength and Power in Sport*, ed. P. Komi, 239–48. Oxford: Blackwell Scientific Publishing.

99. Tesch, P., A. Thorsson, and P. Kaiser. 1984. Muscle capillary supply and fiber type characteristics in weight and power lifters. *Journal of Applied Physiology* 56:35–38.

100. Umnova, M., and T. Seene. 1991. The effect of increased functional load on the activation of satellite cells in the skeletal muscles of adult rats. *International Journal of Sports Medicine* 12:501–4.

101. Vale, R. 1994. Getting a grip on myosin. *Cell* 78:733–37.

102. Vandenboom, R. 2004. The myofibrillar complex and fatigue: A review. *Canadian Journal of Applied Physiology* 29:330–56.

103. Vincent, H., S. Powers, H. Demirel, J. Coombes, and H. Naito. 1999. Exercise training protects against contraction-induced lipid peroxidation in the diaphragm. *European Journal of Applied Physiology*. 79:268–73.

104. Westerblad, H., and D. Allen. 2003. Cellular mechanisms of skeletal muscle fatigue. *Advances in Experimental Medicine and Biology* 538:563–70.

105. Wilmore, J., and D. Costill. 1993. *Training for Sport and Activity: The Physiological Basis of the Conditioning Process.* Champaign, IL: Human Kinetics.

106. Wozniak, A. et al. 2005. Signaling satellite-cell activation in skeletal muscle: Markers, models, stretch, and potential alternative pathways. *Muscle Nerve* 31:283–300.

CHAPTER 9

Circulatory Responses to Exercise

■ Objectives

By studying this chapter, you should be able to do the following:

1. Give an overview of the design and function of the circulatory system.

2. Describe the cardiac cycle and the associated electrical activity recorded via the electrocardiogram.

3. Discuss the pattern of redistribution of blood flow during exercise.

4. Outline the circulatory responses to various types of exercise.

5. Identify the factors that regulate local blood flow during exercise.

6. List and discuss those factors responsible for regulation of stroke volume during exercise.

7. Discuss the regulation of cardiac output during exercise.

■ Outline

Organization of the Circulatory System 170
  Structure of the Heart 170
  Pulmonary and Systemic Circuits 171

Heart: Myocardium and Cardiac Cycle 171
  Myocardium 171
  Cardiac Cycle 174
  Arterial Blood Pressure 176
  Factors That Influence Arterial Blood Pressure 177
  Electrical Activity of the Heart 178

Cardiac Output 181
  Regulation of Heart Rate 182

Regulation of Stroke Volume 183

Hemodynamics 186
  Physical Characteristics of Blood 186
  Relationships Among Pressure, Resistance, and Flow 186
  Sources of Vascular Resistance 187

Changes in Oxygen Delivery to Muscle During Exercise 188
  Changes in Cardiac Output During Exercise 188
  Changes in Arterial-Mixed Venous O_2 Content During Exercise 189

Redistribution of Blood Flow During Exercise 189
Regulation of Local Blood Flow During Exercise 190

Circulatory Responses to Exercise 192
  Emotional Influence 192
  Transition from Rest to Exercise 192
  Recovery from Exercise 192
  Incremental Exercise 192
  Arm versus Leg Exercise 193
  Intermittent Exercise 194
  Prolonged Exercise 194

Regulation of Cardiovascular Adjustments to Exercise 195

arteries
arterioles
atrioventricular node (AV node)
autoregulation
capillaries
cardiac accelerator nerves
cardiac output
cardiovascular control center

central command
diastole
diastolic blood pressure
double product
electrocardiogram (ECG)
intercalated discs
mixed venous blood
myocardium

pulmonary circuit
sinoatrial node (SA node)
stroke volume
systole
systolic blood pressure
vagus nerve
veins
venules

One of the major challenges to homeostasis posed by exercise is the increased muscular demand for oxygen; during heavy exercise the demand may be fifteen to twenty-five times greater than at rest. The primary purpose of the cardiorespiratory system is to deliver adequate amounts of oxygen and remove wastes from body tissues. In addition, the circulatory system transports nutrients and aids in temperature regulation. It is important to note that the respiratory system and the circulatory system function together as a "coupled unit"; the respiratory system adds oxygen and removes carbon dioxide from the blood, while the circulatory system is responsible for the delivery of oxygenated blood and nutrients to tissues in accordance with their needs. Stated another way, the "cardiopulmonary system" works to maintain oxygen and carbon dioxide homeostasis in body tissues.

In order to meet the increased oxygen demands of muscle during exercise, two major adjustments of blood flow must be made: (1) an increased **cardiac output** (i.e., increased amount of blood pumped per minute by the heart) and (2) a redistribution of blood flow from inactive organs to the active skeletal muscles. However, while the needs of the muscles are being met, other tissues, such as the brain, cannot be denied blood flow. This is accomplished by maintaining blood pressure, the driving force of the blood. A thorough understanding of the cardiovascular responses to exercise is important for the student of exercise physiology. Therefore, it is the purpose of this chapter to describe the design and function of the circulatory system and how it responds during exercise.

ORGANIZATION OF THE CIRCULATORY SYSTEM

The human circulatory system is a closed loop that circulates blood to all body tissues. Circulation of blood requires the action of a muscular pump, the heart, that creates the "pressure head" needed to move blood through the system. Blood travels away from the heart in **arteries** and returns to the heart by way of **veins.** The system is considered "closed" because arteries and veins are continuous with each other through smaller vessels. Arteries branch extensively to form a "tree" of smaller vessels. As the vessels become microscopic they form **arterioles,** which eventually develop into "beds" of much smaller vessels called **capillaries.** Capillaries are the smallest and most numerous of blood vessels; all exchanges of oxygen, carbon dioxide, and nutrients between tissues and the circulatory system occur across capillary beds. Blood passes from capillary beds to small venous vessels called **venules.** As venules move back toward the heart they increase in size and become veins. Major veins empty directly into the heart. The mixture of venous blood from both the upper and lower body that accumulates in the right side of the heart is termed **mixed venous blood.** Mixed venous blood therefore represents an average of venous blood from the entire body.

Structure of the Heart

The heart is divided into four chambers and is often considered to be two pumps in one. The right atrium and right ventricle form the right pump, while the left atrium and left ventricle combine to make the left pump (see figure 9.1). The right side of the heart is separated from the left side by a muscular wall called the interventricular septum. This septum prevents the mixing of blood from the two sides of the heart.

Blood movement within the heart is from the atria to the ventricles, and from the ventricles blood is pumped into the arteries. To prevent backward movement of blood, the heart contains four, one-way valves. The right and left atrioventricular valves connect the atria with the right and left ventricles, respectively (figure 9.1). These valves are also known as the tricuspid valve (right atrioventricular valve) and the bicuspid valve (left atrioventricular valve). Backflow from the arteries into the ventricles is prevented by the pulmonary semilunar valve (right ventricle) and the aortic semilunar valve (left ventricle).

Superior vena cava

Pulmonary valve

Right pulmonary artery

Right pulmonary veins

Right atrium

Tricuspid valve

Right ventricle

Inferior vena cava

Aorta

Left pulmonary artery

Pulmonary trunk

Left pulmonary veins

Left atrium

Bicuspid valve

Chordae tendineae

Papillary muscle

Left ventricle

Interventricular septum

FIGURE 9.1 Anterior view of the heart.

Pulmonary and Systemic Circuits

As mentioned previously, the heart can be considered as two pumps in one. The right side of the heart pumps blood that is partially depleted of its oxygen content and contains an elevated carbon dioxide content as a result of gas exchange in the various tissues of the body. This blood is delivered from the right heart into the lungs through the **pulmonary circuit.** At the lungs, oxygen is loaded into the blood and carbon dioxide is released. This "oxygenated" blood then travels to the left side of the heart and is pumped to the various tissues of the body via the systemic circuit (figure 9.2).

IN SUMMARY

- The purposes of the cardiovascular system are the following: (1) the transport of O_2 to tissues and removal of wastes, (2) the transport of nutrients to tissues, and (3) the regulation of body temperature.
- The heart is two pumps in one. The right side of the heart pumps blood through the pulmonary circulation, while the left side of the heart delivers blood to the systemic circulation.

HEART: MYOCARDIUM AND CARDIAC CYCLE

To better appreciate how the circulatory system adjusts to the stress of exercise, it is important to understand elementary details of heart muscle structure as well as the electrical and mechanical activities of the heart.

Myocardium

The wall of the heart is composed of three layers: (1) an outer layer called the epicardium, (2) a muscular middle layer, the myocardium, and (3) an inner layer known as the endocardium (see figure 9.3). It is the **myocardium,** or heart muscle, that is responsible for contracting and forcing blood out of the heart. The myocardium receives its blood supply via the right and left coronary arteries. These vessels branch off the aorta and encircle the heart. The coronary veins run alongside the arteries and drain all coronary blood into a larger vein called the coronary sinus, which deposits blood into the right atrium.

Maintaining a constant blood supply to the heart via the coronary arteries is critical because, even at

Lungs
Pulmonary capillaries

Pulmonary circulation

Pulmonary trunk and arteries

Pulmonary veins

Vena cavae

Aorta

Right atrium

Left atrium

Right ventricle

Left ventricle

Systemic circulation

Systemic veins

Systemic arteries

Systemic arterioles, capillaries, and venules in all organs and tissues except the lungs

FIGURE 9.2 Illustration of the systemic and pulmonary circulations. As depicted from the color change from blue to red, blood becomes fully oxygenated as it flows through the lungs and then loses some oxygen (color changes from red to blue) as it flows through the other organs and tissues.

rest, the heart has a high demand for oxygen and nutrients. When coronary blood flow is disrupted (i.e., blockage of a coronary blood vessel) for more than several minutes, permanent damage to the heart occurs. This type of injury results in the death of cardiac muscle cells and is commonly called a heart attack or myocardial infarction (see chapter 17). The number of heart cells that die from this insult determines the severity of a heart attack. That is, a "mild" heart attack may damage only a small portion of the heart, whereas a "major" heart attack may destroy a large number of heart cells (fibers). A major heart attack greatly diminishes the heart's pumping capacity; therefore, minimizing the amount of injury to the heart during a heart attack is important. In this regard, new evidence indicates that exercise training can provide cardiac protection against damage during a heart attack (see Clinical Applications 9.1).

Heart muscle differs from skeletal muscle in several ways. First, cardiac muscle fibers are shorter than skeletal muscle fibers and are connected in a tight series. Further, cardiac fibers are typically branched, whereas skeletal muscle fibers are elongated and do not branch. Also, cardiac muscle contraction is involuntary, whereas skeletal muscle contractions are under voluntary control.

Another difference between cardiac fibers and skeletal muscle fibers is that, unlike skeletal muscle fibers, heart muscle fibers are all interconnected via **intercalated discs.** These intercellular connections permit the transmission of electrical impulses from one fiber to another. Intercalated discs are nothing more than leaky membranes that allow ions to cross from one fiber to another. Therefore, when one heart fiber is depolarized to contract, all connecting heart fibers also become excited and contract as a unit. This arrangement is called a *functional syncytium*. Heart muscle cells in the atria are separated from ventricular muscle cells by a layer of connective tissue that does not permit the transmission of electrical impulses. Hence, the atria contract separately from the ventricles.

One more difference between heart and skeletal muscle fibers is that human heart fibers cannot be divided into different fiber types. The ventricular myocardium is considered to be a homogenous muscle containing one primary fiber type that has similarities to the type I, slow fiber found in skeletal muscle. In this regard, heart muscle fibers are highly aerobic and contain large numbers of mitochondria. Note, however, that cardiac muscle fibers contain many more mitochondria than type I, slow skeletal muscle fibers. This fact highlights the importance of continuous aerobic metabolism in the heart.

Although heart muscle and skeletal muscle differ in many ways, they are also similar in several ways. For example, both heart and skeletal muscle fibers are striated and contain the same contractile proteins: actin and myosin. Further, both heart and skeletal muscle fibers require calcium to activate the myofilaments (5, 6) and both fibers contract via the sliding filament model of contraction (see chapter 8). In addition, like skeletal muscle, heart muscle can alter its force of contraction as a function of the degree of overlap actin-myosin filaments due to changes in fiber length. Table 9.1 contains a point-by-point comparison of the structural/functional similarities and differences between cardiac and skeletal muscle fibers.

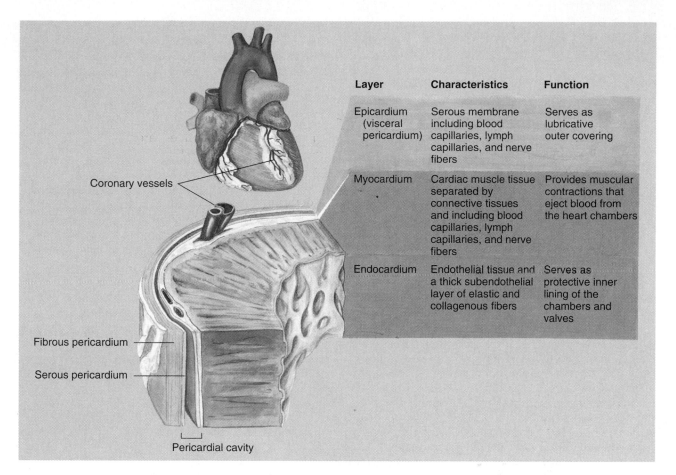

Layer	Characteristics	Function
Epicardium (visceral pericardium)	Serous membrane including blood capillaries, lymph capillaries, and nerve fibers	Serves as lubricative outer covering
Myocardium	Cardiac muscle tissue separated by connective tissues and including blood capillaries, lymph capillaries, and nerve fibers	Provides muscular contractions that eject blood from the heart chambers
Endocardium	Endothelial tissue and a thick subendothelial layer of elastic and collagenous fibers	Serves as protective inner lining of the chambers and valves

Coronary vessels

Fibrous pericardium

Serous pericardium

Pericardial cavity

FIGURE 9.3 The heart wall is composed of three distinct layers: (1) epicardium, (2) myocardium, and (3) endocardium.

TABLE 9.1	A Comparison of the Structural and Functional Differences/Similarities Between Heart Muscle and Skeletal Muscle

Structual Comparison	Heart Muscle	Skeletal Muscle
Contractile proteins: actin and myosin	Present	Present
Shape of muscle fibers	Shorter than skeletal muscle fibers and branching	Elongated—no branching
Nuclei	Single	Multiple
Z discs	Present	Present
Striated	Yes	Yes
Cellular junctions	Yes—intercalated discs	No junctional complexes
Connective tissue	Endomysium	Epimysium, perimysium, and endomysium

Functional Comparision		
Energy production	Aerobic (primarily)	Aerobic and anaerobic
Calcium source (for contraction)	Sarcoplasmic reticulum and extracellular calcium	Sarcoplasmic reticulum
Neural control	Involuntary	Voluntary
Regeneration potential	None—no satellite cells present	Some possibilities via satellite cells

Exercise Training Protects the Heart

It is widely believed that regular exercise training is cardioprotective. Indeed, many epidemiological studies have provided evidence that regular exercise can reduce the incidence of heart attacks and that the survival rate of heart attack victims is greater in active people than in sedentary ones. Recent experiments using animal models have provided direct evidence that regular endurance exercise training reduces the amount of myocardial damage that occurs during a heart attack (11, 31, 23, 45, 59). The protective effect of exercise is illustrated in figure 9.4. Notice that exercise training can reduce the magnitude of cardiac injury during a heart attack by approximately 60%. This is significant, because the number of cardiac cells that are destroyed during a heart attack determines the patient's chances of a full, functional recovery.

How does exercise training alter the heart and provide cardioprotec-

FIGURE 9.4 Regular endurance exercise protects the heart against cell death during a heart attack. Note that during a myocardial infarction (i.e., heart attack), exercise-trained individuals suffer significantly less cardiac injury compared to untrained individuals. Data are from reference 87.

tion during a heart attack? A definitive answer to this question is not available. Nonetheless, new evidence suggests that the exercise-training-induced improvement in the heart's ability to resist permanent injury during a heart attack is linked to improvements in the heart's antioxidant capacity (i.e., the ability to remove free radicals) and an elevation in heat shock proteins in the myocardium (12, 42, 47, 59, 60). These heat shock proteins are also called stress proteins and were introduced in chapter 2. See Ask the Expert 9.1 (page 175) for practical information about these stress proteins and exercise-induced cardioprotection.

Cardiac Cycle

The cardiac cycle refers to the repeating pattern of contraction and relaxation of the heart. The contraction phase is called **systole** and the relaxation period is called **diastole.** Generally, when these terms are used alone, they refer to contraction and relaxation of the ventricles. However, note that the atria also contract and relax; therefore, there is an atrial systole and diastole. Atrial contraction occurs during ventricular diastole and atrial relaxation occurs during ventricular systole. The heart thus has a two-step pumping action. The right and left atria contract together, which empties atrial blood into the ventricles. Approximately 0.1 seconds after the atrial contraction, the ventricles contract and deliver blood into both the systemic and pulmonary circuits.

At rest, contraction of the ventricles during systole ejects about two-thirds of the blood in the ventricles, leaving about one-third in the ventricles. The ventricles then fill with blood during the next diastole. A healthy, twenty-one-year-old female might have an average resting heart rate of 75 beats per minute. This

means that the total cardiac cycle lasts 0.8 seconds, with 0.5 seconds spent in diastole and the remaining 0.3 seconds dedicated to systole (35) (see figure 9.5). If the heart rate increases from 75 beats per minute to 180 beats per minute (e.g., heavy exercise), there is a reduction in the time spent in both systole and diastole (22, 28). This point is illustrated in figure 9.5. Note that a rising heart rate results in a greater time reduction in diastole, while systole is less affected.

Pressure Changes During the Cardiac Cycle

During the cardiac cycle, the pressure within the heart chambers rises and falls. When the atria are relaxed, blood flows into them from the venous circulation. As these chambers fill, the pressure inside gradually increases. Approximately 70% of the blood entering the atria during diastole flows directly into the ventricles through the atrioventricular valves before the atria contract. Upon atrial contraction, atrial pressure rises and forces most of the remaining 30% of the atrial blood into the ventricles.

Pressure in the ventricles is low while they are filling, but when the atria contract, the ventricular

ASK THE EXPERT 9.1

Exercise Training and Cardiac Protection
Questions and Answers with Dr. Joe Starnes

Joe Starnes, Ph. D., professor in the Department of Kinesiology and Health at the University of Texas–Austin, is an internationally known researcher in the field of cardiovascular physiology. Much of Dr. Starnes's research has focused on the effects of exercise on protection of the heart during a heart attack. Specifically, Dr. Starnes's research team has performed many of the "landmark" studies that explore the effects of endurance exercise on cardiac protection. In this box feature, Dr. Starnes answers questions related to exercise-induced cardiac protection.

QUESTION 1: Historically, it has been believed that weeks or months of regular exercise is required for training adaptation to occur in the heart. However, your recent research challenges this concept. Based on your research findings, how rapidly does the heart adapt after beginning an exercise-training program?

ANSWER: A single bout of appropriate exercise will stimulate the heart to increase the synthesis of protective proteins. Most of these proteins fall into a category called *stress proteins.* Within twenty-four hours after the exercise bout, the proteins can increase enough to protect the heart against a variety of physical stresses.

QUESTION 2: Recent research in your laboratory has explored the dose-response relationship between exercise intensity and cardiac protection. Is high-intensity exercise training superior to low- or moderate-intensity exercise in providing cardiac protection?

ANSWER: It appears that a certain threshold of intensity has to be reached before realizing intrinsic cardioprotection. We have found that exercising at a moderate intensity for sixty minutes provides a considerable improvement in cardioprotection. Increasing the intensity above this provides only modest additional improvements in intrinsic cardioprotection. Low-intensity exercise appears to result in little, if any, intrinsic cardioprotection. However,

exercise at lower intensities or for shorter durations may still provide significant indirect protection to the heart by improving the cholesterol profile in the blood and by lowering blood pressure.

QUESTION 3: It is clear that regular exercise training protects the heart against injury during a heart attack. However, your research indicates that exercise-induced cardioprotection is lost following the stoppage of regular training. How quickly after the cessation of exercise training does the heart lose the cardioprotective benefits of exercise?

ANSWER: As with most exercise-related adaptations, the reversibility principle applies to exercise-induced cardioprotection. When the exercise training stops, the stimulus to increase the synthesis of the protective proteins also stops. In less than a week, the level of the protective proteins will return to pre-exercise levels and the exercise-enhanced cardioprotection is lost.

FIGURE 9.5 Increases in heart rate during exercise are achieved primarily through a decrease in the time spent in diastole; however, at high heart rates, the length of time spent in systole also decreases.

pressure increases slightly. Then as the ventricles contract, the pressure rises sharply, which closes the atrioventricular valves and prevents backflow into the atria. As soon as ventricular pressure exceeds the pressure of the pulmonary artery and the aorta, the pulmonary and aortic valves open and blood is forced into both pulmonary and systemic circulations.

Figure 9.6, page 000, illustrates the changes in ventricular pressure as a function of time during the resting cardiac cycle. Note the occurrence of two heart sounds that are produced by the closing of the atrioventricular valves (first heart sound) and the closing of the aortic and pulmonary valves (second heart sound).

FIGURE 9.6 Relationship among pressure, volume, and heart sounds during the cardiac cycle. Notice the change in ventricular pressure and volume during the transition from systole to diastole.

Arterial Blood Pressure

Blood exerts pressure throughout the vascular system, but is greatest within the arteries where it is generally measured and used as an indication of health. Blood pressure is the force exerted by blood against the arterial walls and is determined by how much blood is pumped and the resistance to blood flow.

Arterial blood pressure can be estimated by the use of a sphygmomanometer (see A Closer Look 9.1, page 177). The normal blood pressure of an adult male is 120/80, while that of adult females tends to be lower (110/70). The larger number in the expression of blood pressure is the systolic pressure expressed in millimeters of mercury (mm Hg). The lower number in the blood pressure ratio is the diastolic pressure, again expressed in mm Hg. **Systolic blood pressure** is the pressure generated as blood is ejected from the heart during ventricular systole. During ventricular relaxation (diastole), the arterial blood pressure decreases and represents **diastolic blood pressure.** The difference between systolic and diastolic blood pressure is called the *pulse pressure.*

The average pressure during a cardiac cycle is called *mean arterial pressure.* Mean arterial blood pressure is important because it determines the rate of blood flow through the systemic circuit.

Determination of mean arterial pressure is not easy. It is not a simple average of systolic and diastolic

pressure, since diastole generally lasts longer than systole. However, mean arterial pressure can be estimated at rest in the following way:

Mean arterial pressure = DBP + .33 (pulse pressure)

Here, DBP is the diastolic blood pressure, and the pulse pressure is the difference between systolic and diastolic pressures. Let's consider a sample calculation of mean arterial pressure at rest.

For example, suppose an individual has a blood pressure of 120/80 mm Hg. The mean arterial pressure would be:

**Mean arterial pressure = 80 mm Hg
+ .33(120 − 80)
= 80 mm Hg + 13
= 93 mm Hg**

Note that this equation cannot be used to compute mean arterial blood pressure during exercise because it is based on the timing of the cardiac cycle at rest. That is, arterial blood pressure rises during systole and falls during diastole across the cardiac cycle. Therefore, in order to accurately estimate the average arterial blood pressure at any time, systolic and diastolic blood pressure must be measured and the amount of time spent in both systole and diastole must be known. Recall that the time spent in systole and diastole differs between rest and exercise. For example, the formula estimates that the time spent in systole occupies 33% of the total cardiac cycle at rest. However, during maximal exercise, systole may account for 66% of the total cardiac cycle time. Therefore, any formula designed to estimate mean arterial blood pressure must be adjusted to reflect the time spent in systole and diastole.

Approximately 20% of all adults in the United States have hypertension, which is defined as blood pressure in excess of the normal range for the person's age and sex (22). Blood pressures above 140/90 are considered to be indicators of hypertension (22, 28). Hypertension is generally classified into one of two categories: (1) primary, or essential hypertension, and (2) secondary hypertension. The cause of primary hypertension is unknown. This type of hypertension constitutes 90% of all reported cases of hypertension in the United States. Secondary hypertension is a result of some known disease process, and thus the hypertension is "secondary" to another disease.

Hypertension can result in a variety of health problems. For example, hypertension increases the workload on the left ventricle resulting in an adaptive increase in the muscle mass of the left heart (called left ventricular hypertrophy). In the early phases of hypertension-induced left ventricular hypertrophy, the increase in cardiac mass helps to maintain the

Measurement of Arterial Blood Pressure

Arterial blood pressure is not usually measured directly but is estimated using an instrument called a sphygmomanometer (see figure 9.7). This device consists of an inflatable arm cuff connected to a column of mercury. The cuff can be inflated by a bulb pump, with the pressure in the cuff measured by the rising column of mercury. For example, a pressure of 100 mm of mercury (mm Hg) would be enough force to raise the column of mercury upward a distance of 100 mm.

Blood pressure is measured in the following way: The rubber cuff is placed around the upper arm so it surrounds the brachial artery. Air is pumped into the cuff so that the pressure around the arm exceeds arterial pressure. Since the pressure applied around the arm is greater than arterial pressure, the brachial artery is squeezed shut and blood flow is stopped. If a stethoscope is placed over the brachial artery (just below the cuff), no sounds are heard, since there is no blood flow. However, if the air control valve is slowly opened to release air, the pressure in the cuff begins to decline, and soon the pressure around the arm reaches a point that is equal to or just slightly below arterial pressure. At this point blood begins to spurt through the artery and a sharp sound (known as *Korotkoff sounds*) can be heard through the stethoscope. The pressure (i.e., height of mercury column) at which the first tapping sound is heard represents systolic blood pressure.

FIGURE 9.7 A sphygmomanometer is used to measure arterial blood pressure.

As the cuff pressure continues to decline, a series of increasingly louder sounds can be heard. When the pressure in the cuff is equal to or slightly below diastolic blood pressure, the sounds heard through the stethoscope cease. Therefore, resting diastolic blood pressure represents the height of the mercury column when the sounds disappear.

heart's pumping ability. However, with time, this left ventricular hypertrophy changes the organization and function of cardiac muscle fibers resulting in diminished pumping capacity of the heart which can lead to heart failure. Further, the presence of hypertension is a major risk factor for developing arteriosclerosis and heart attacks. Finally, hypertension also increases the risk of kidney damage and the rupture of a cerebral blood vessel resulting in localized brain injury (i.e., a stroke).

Factors That Influence Arterial Blood Pressure

Mean arterial blood pressure is determined by two factors: (1) cardiac output and (2) total vascular resistance. Cardiac output is the amount of blood pumped from the heart, and total vascular resistance is the sum of resistance to blood flow provided by all systemic blood vessels. Mathematically, mean arterial blood is defined as the product of cardiac output and total vascular resistance as given in the following equation:

Mean arterial blood pressure = (cardiac output × total vascular resistance)

Therefore, an increase in either cardiac output or vascular resistance results in an increase in mean arterial blood pressure. In the body, mean arterial blood pressure depends on a variety of physiological factors, including cardiac output, blood volume, resistance to flow, and blood viscosity. These relationships are summarized in figure 9.8. An increase in any of these variables results in an increase in arterial blood pressure. Conversely, a decrease in any of these variables causes a decrease in blood pressure.

How is blood pressure regulated? Acute (short-term) regulation of blood pressure is achieved by the sympathetic nervous system, whereas long-term regulation of blood pressure is primarily a function of the kidneys (8). The kidneys regulate blood pressure by their control of blood volume.

Pressure receptors (called *baroreceptors*) in the carotid artery and the aorta are sensitive to changes in arterial blood pressure. An increase in arterial pressure triggers these receptors to send impulses to the cardiovascular control center, which responds by decreasing sympathetic activity. A reduction in sympathetic activity may lower cardiac output and/or reduce vascular resistance, which in turn lowers blood pressure. Conversely, a decrease in blood pressure results in a reduction of baroreceptor activity to the brain. This causes the cardiovascular control center to respond by increasing sympathetic outflow, which raises blood pressure back to normal. For a complete discussion of blood-pressure regulation, see Widmaier et al. (2006) and Fox (2006) in the Suggested Readings.

Electrical Activity of the Heart

Many myocardial cells have the unique potential for spontaneous electrical activity (i.e., each has an intrinsic rhythm). However, in the normal heart, spontaneous electrical activity is limited to a special region located in the right atrium. This region, called the **sinoatrial node (SA node),** serves as the pacemaker for the heart (see figure 9.9). Spontaneous electrical activity in the SA node occurs due to a decay of the resting membrane potential via inward diffusion of sodium during diastole. When the SA node reaches the depolarization threshold and "fires," the wave of depolarization spreads over the atria, resulting in atrial contraction. The wave of atrial depolarization

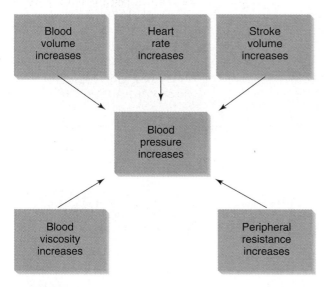

FIGURE 9.8 Some factors that influence arterial blood pressure.

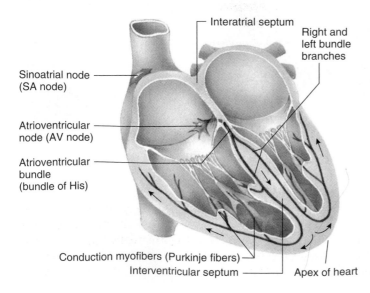

FIGURE 9.9 Conduction system of the heart.

Diagnostic Use of the ECG During Exercise

Cardiologists are physicians who specialize in diseases of the heart and vascular system. One of the diagnostic procedures commonly used to evaluate cardiac function is to make ECG measurements during an incremental exercise test (usually on a treadmill). This allows the physician to observe changes in blood pressure as well as changes in the patient's ECG during periods of stress.

The most common cause of heart disease is the collection of fatty plaque (called atherosclerosis) inside coronary vessels. This collection of plaque reduces blood flow to the myocardium. The adequacy of blood flow to the heart is relative—it depends on the metabolic demand placed on the heart. An obstruction to a coronary artery, for example, may allow sufficient blood flow at rest, but may be inadequate

Normal

Ischemia

FIGURE 9.10
Depression of the S-T segment of the electrocardiogram as a result of myocardial ischemia.

during exercise due to increased metabolic demand placed on the heart. Therefore, a graded exercise test may serve as a "stress test" to evaluate cardiac function.

An example of an abnormal exercise ECG is illustrated in figure 9.10. Myocardial ischemia (reduced blood flow) may be detected by changes in

the S-T segment of the ECG. Notice the depressed S-T segment in the picture on the right when compared to the normal ECG on the left. This S-T segment depression suggests to the physician that ischemic heart disease may be present and that additional diagnostic procedures may be warranted.

cannot directly cross into the ventricles but must be transported by way of specialized conductive tissue. This specialized conductive tissue radiates from a small mass of muscle tissue called the **atrioventricular node (AV node).** This node, located in the floor of the right atrium, connects the atria with the ventricles by a pair of conductive pathways called the right and left bundle branches (figure 9.9). Note that atrial-mediated depolarization of the SA node is delayed by approximately 0.10 seconds. This time delay is important because it allows atrial contraction to empty atrial blood into the ventricles prior to ventricular depolarization and contraction. Upon reaching the ventricles, these conductive pathways branch into smaller fibers called Purkinje fibers. The Purkinje fibers then spread the wave of depolarization throughout the ventricles.

A recording of the electrical changes that occur in the myocardium during the cardiac cycle is called an **electrocardiogram (ECG).** Analysis of ECG waveforms allows the physician to evaluate the heart's ability to conduct impulses and therefore determine if electrical problems exist. Further, analysis of the ECG during exercise is often used in the diagnosis of coronary artery disease (see A Closer Look 9.2). Figure 9.11 illustrates a normal ECG pattern. Notice that the ECG pattern contains several different deflections, or

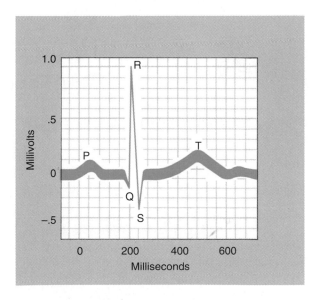

FIGURE 9.11 The normal electrocardiogram during rest.

waves, during each cardiac cycle. Each of these distinct waveforms is identified by different letters. The first deflection on the EKG is called the P wave and represents the depolarization of the atria. The second wave, the QRS complex, represents the depolarization

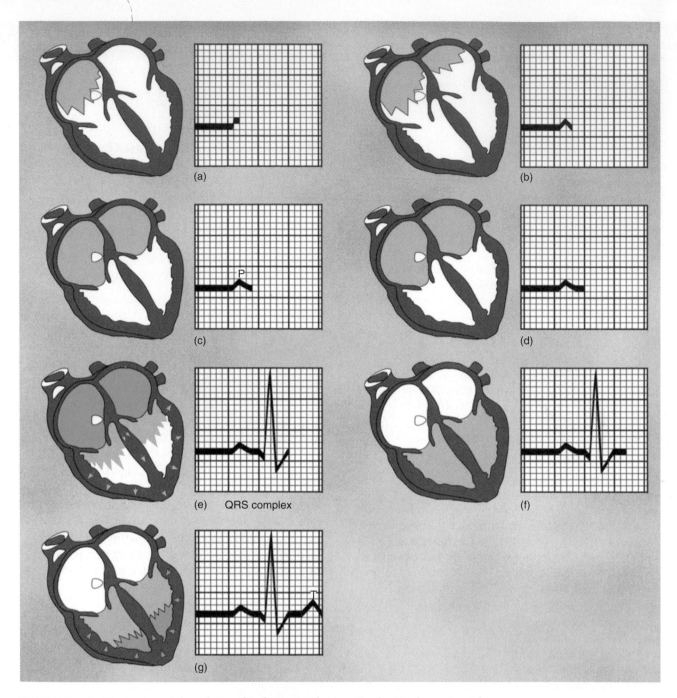

FIGURE 9.12 An illustration of the relationship between the heart's electrical events and the recording of the ECG. Panels *a–d* illustrate atrial depolarization and the formation of the P-wave. Panels *e–f* illustrate ventricular depolarization and formation of the QRS complex. Finally, panel *g* illustrates repolarization of the ventricles and formation of the T wave.

of the ventricles and occurs approximately 0.10 seconds following the P wave. The final deflection, the T wave, is the result of ventricular repolarization. Notice that atrial repolarization is usually not visible on the EKG because it occurs at the same time as the QRS complex (figure 9.12). In other words, atrial repolarization is "hidden" by the QRS complex.

Finally, figure 9.13 illustrates the relationship between changes in the intraventricular pressure and the ECG. Note that the QRS complex (i.e., depolarization of the ventricles) occurs at the beginning of systole, whereas the T wave (i.e., repolarization of the ventricles) occurs at the beginning of diastole. Also, notice that the rise in intraventricular pressure at the beginning of systole results in the first heart sound due to closure of the atrioventricular valves (AV valves) and that the fall in intraventricular pressure at the end of systole results in the second heart sound due to the closure of the aortic and pulmonary semi-lunar valves.

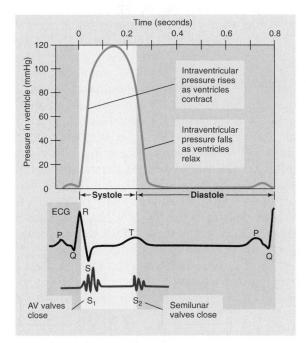

FIGURE 9.13 The relationship between changes in the intraventricular pressure and the ECG. Notice that the QRS complex (i.e., depolarization of the ventricles) occurs at the beginning of systole and the rise in ventricular pressure. Further, note that the T wave (repolarization of the ventricles) occurs at the same time that the ventricles relax at the beginning of diastole.

IN SUMMARY

- The contraction phase of the cardiac cycle is called *systole* and the relaxation period is called *diastole*.
- The pacemaker of the heart is the SA node.
- The average blood pressure during a cardiac cycle is called *mean arterial blood pressure*.
- Blood pressure can be increased by one or all of the following factors:
  a. increase in blood volume,
  b. increase in heart rate,
  c. increased blood viscosity,
  d. increase in stroke volume, and/or
  e. increased peripheral resistance.
- A recording of the electrical activity of the heart during the cardiac cycle is called the *electrocardiogram* (ECG).

CARDIAC OUTPUT

Cardiac output ($\dot{Q}$) is the product of the heart rate (HR) and the **stroke volume** (SV) (amount of blood pumped per heartbeat):

$$\dot{Q} = HR \times SV$$

Thus, cardiac output can be increased due to a rise in either heart rate or stroke volume. During exercise in the upright position (e.g., running, cycling, etc.), the increase in cardiac output is due to an increase in both heart rate and stroke volume. Table 9.2 presents typical values at rest and during maximal exercise for heart rate, stroke volume, and cardiac out-

TABLE 9.2	Typical Resting and Maximal Exercise Values for Stroke Volume (SV), Heart Rate (HR), and Cardiac Output ($\dot{Q}$) for College-Age Untrained Subjects and Trained Endurance Athletes (Body Weights for Males are 70 kg and for Females, 50 kg.)					
Subject	**HR (beat/min)**		**SV (ml/beat)**		**$\dot{Q}$ (l/min)**	
Rest						
Untrained male	72	×	70	=	5.00	
Untrained female	75	×	60	=	4.50	
Trained male	50	×	100	=	5.00	
Trained female	55	×	80	=	4.50	
Max Exercise						
Untrained male	200	×	110	=	22.0	
Untrained female	200	×	90	=	18.0	
Trained male	190	×	180	=	34.2	
Trained female	190	×	125	=	23.9	

Note that values are rounded off. Data from references 4, 22, and 68.

put in both untrained and highly trained endurance athletes. The gender differences in stroke volume and cardiac output are due mainly to differences in body sizes between men and women (4) (see table 9.2).

Regulation of Heart Rate

During exercise, the quantity of blood pumped by the heart must change in accordance with the elevated skeletal muscle oxygen demand. Since the SA node controls heart rate, changes in heart rate often involve factors that influence the SA node. The two most prominent factors that influence heart rate are the parasympathetic and sympathetic nervous systems (34, 64, 73, 80).

The parasympathetic fibers that supply the heart arise from neurons in the **cardiovascular control center** in the medulla oblongata and make up a portion of the **vagus nerve.** Upon reaching the heart, these fibers make contact with both the SA node and the AV node (see figure 9.14). When stimulated, these nerve endings release acetylcholine, which causes a decrease in the activity of both the SA and AV nodes due to hyperpolarization (i.e., moving the resting membrane potential further from threshold). The end result is a reduction of heart rate. Therefore, the parasympathetic nervous system acts as a braking system to slow down heart rate.

Even at rest, the vagus nerves carry impulses to the SA and AV nodes (22, 28, 54). This is often referred to as *parasympathetic tone.* As a consequence, changes in parasympathetic activity can cause heart rate to increase or decrease. For instance, a decrease in parasympathetic tone to the heart can elevate heart rate, while an increase in parasympathetic activity causes a slowing of heart rate.

Studies have shown that the initial increase in heart rate during exercise, up to approximately 100 beats per minute, is due to a withdrawal of parasympathetic tone (68). At higher work rates, stimulation of the SA and AV nodes by the sympathetic nervous system is responsible for increases in heart rate (68). Sympathetic fibers reach the heart by means of the **cardiac accelerator nerves,** which innervate both the SA node and the ventricles (figure 9.13). Endings of these fibers release norepinephrine upon stimulation, which act on beta receptors in the heart and cause an increase in both heart rate and the force of myocardial contraction. (See Clinical Applications 9.2.)

At rest, a normal balance between parasympathetic tone and sympathetic activity to the heart is maintained by the cardiovascular control center in the

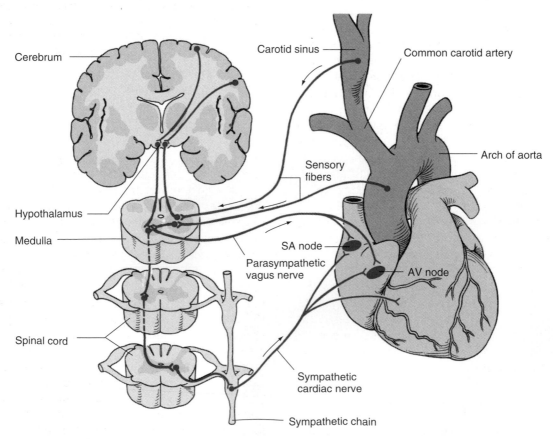

FIGURE 9.14 The activities of the SA and AV nodes can be altered by both the sympathetic and parasympathetic nervous systems.

CLINICAL APPLICATIONS 9.2

Beta-Blockade and Exercise Heart Rate

Beta-adrenergic blocking medications (beta-blockers) are commonly prescribed for patients with coronary artery disease and/or hypertension. Although there are many different classes of these drugs, all of these medications compete with epinephrine and norepinephrine for beta-adrenergic receptors in the heart. The end result is that beta-blockers reduce heart rate and the vigor of myocardial contraction, thus reducing the oxygen requirement of the heart.

In clinical exercise physiology, it is important to appreciate that all beta-blocking drugs will decrease resting heart rate as well as exercise heart rate. Indeed, individuals on beta-blocking medications will exhibit lower exercise heart rates during both submaximal and maximal exercise. This is an important fact that should be considered when prescribing exercise and interpreting the exercise test results of individuals using beta-blocking medications.

medulla oblongata. The cardiovascular control center receives impulses from various parts of the circulatory system relative to changes in important parameters (e.g., blood pressure, blood oxygen tension, etc.), and it relays motor impulses to the heart in response to a changing cardiovascular need. For example, an increase in resting blood pressure above normal stimulates pressure receptors in the carotid arteries and the arch of the aorta, which in turn send impulses to the cardiovascular control center (figure 9.13). In response, the cardiovascular control center increases parasympathetic activity to the heart to slow the heart rate and reduce cardiac output. This reduction in cardiac output causes blood pressure to decline back toward normal.

Another regulatory reflex involves pressure receptors located in the right atrium. In this case, an increase in right atrial pressure signals the cardiovascular control center that an increase in venous return has occurred; hence, in order to prevent a backup of blood in the systemic venous system, an increase in cardiac output must result. The cardiovascular control center responds by sending sympathetic accelerator nerve impulses to the heart, which increases heart rate and cardiac output. The end result is that the increase in cardiac output lowers right atrial pressure back to normal, and venous blood pressure is reduced.

Finally, a change in body temperature can influence heart rate. An increase in body temperature above normal results in an increase in heart rate, while a lowering of body temperature below normal causes a reduction in heart rate (7, 22, 28, 40, 68, 70, 72). This topic will be discussed in chapter 12.

Regulation of Stroke Volume

Stroke volume, at rest or during exercise, is regulated by three variables: (1) the end-diastolic volume (EDV), which is the volume of blood in the ventricles at the

FIGURE 9.15 An illustration of the relationship between ventricular end-diastolic volume and stroke volume. Notice the increase in stroke volume when venous return increases above the normal resting level.

end of diastole; (2) the average aortic blood pressure; and (3) the strength of ventricular contraction.

EDV is often referred to as "preload," and it influences stroke volume in the following way. Two physiologists, Frank and Starling, demonstrated that the strength of ventricular contraction increased with an enlargement of EDV (i.e., stretch of the ventricles). This relationship has become known as the Frank-Starling law of the heart. The increase in EDV results in a lengthening of cardiac fibers, which improves the force of contraction in a manner similar to that seen in skeletal muscle (discussed in chapter 8). The mechanism to explain the influence of fiber length on cardiac contractility is that an increase in the length of cardiac fibers increases the number of myosin cross-bridge interactions with actin resulting in increased force production. A rise in cardiac contractility results in an increase in the amount of blood pumped per beat and the relationship between EDV volume and stroke volume is illustrated in figure 9.15.

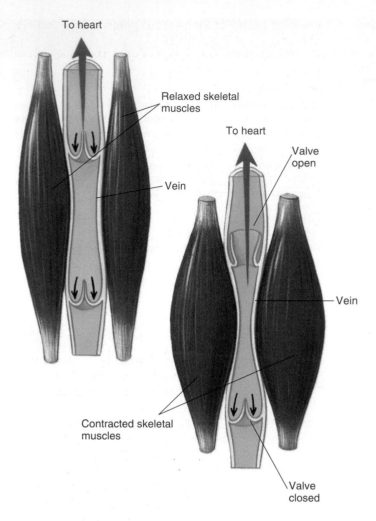

FIGURE 9.16 The action of the one-way venous valves. Contraction of skeletal muscles helps to pump blood toward the heart, but is prevented from pushing blood away from the heart by closure of the venous valves.

The principal variable that influences EDV is the rate of venous return to the heart. An increase in venous return results in a rise in EDV and therefore an increase in stroke volume. Increased venous return and the resulting increase in EDV play a key role in the increase in stroke volume observed during upright exercise (28).

What factors regulate venous return during exercise? There are three principal mechanisms for increasing venous return during exercise: (1) constriction of the veins (venoconstriction), (2) pumping action of contracting skeletal muscle (called the muscle pump), and (3) pumping action of the respiratory system (respiratory pump).

1. *Venoconstriction*. Venoconstriction increases venous return by reducing the volume capacity of the veins to store blood. The end result of a reduced volume capacity in veins is to move blood back toward the heart. Venoconstriction occurs via a reflex sympathetic constriction of smooth muscle in veins draining skeletal muscle, which is controlled by the cardiovascular control center (4, 28, 53, 68).

2. *Muscle pump*. The muscle pump is a result of the mechanical action of rhythmic skeletal muscle contractions. As muscles contract, they compress veins and push blood back toward the heart. Between contractions, blood refills the veins and the process is repeated. Blood is prevented from flowing away from the heart between contractions by one-way valves located in large veins (figure 9.16). During sustained muscular contractions (isometric exercise), the muscle pump cannot operate, and venous return is reduced.

3. *Respiratory pump*. The rhythmic patter of breathing also provides a mechanical pump by which venous return is promoted. The respiratory pump works in the following way. During inspiration, the pressure within the thorax (chest) decreases and abdominal pressure increases. This creates a flow of venous blood from the abdominal region into the thorax and therefore promotes venous return. Although quiet breathing (rest) aids in venous return, the role of the respiratory pump is enhanced during exercise due to the greater respiratory rate and depth. Indeed, recent evidence indicates that the respiratory pump is the

predominant factor that promotes venous return to the heart during upright exercise (50).

A second variable that affects stroke volume is the aortic pressure (mean arterial pressure). In order to eject blood, the pressure generated by the left ventricle must exceed the pressure in the aorta. Therefore, aortic pressure or mean arterial pressure (called *afterload*) represents a barrier to the ejection of blood from the ventricles. Stroke volume is thus inversely proportional to the afterload; that is, an increase in aortic pressure produces a decrease in stroke volume. However, it is noteworthy that afterload is minimized during exercise due to arteriole dilation. This arteriole dilation in the working muscles reduces afterload and makes it easier for the heart to pump a large volume of blood.

The final factor that influences stroke volume is the effect of circulating epinephrine-norepinephrine and direct sympathetic stimulation of the heart by cardiac accelerator nerves. Both of these mechanisms increase cardiac contractility by increasing the amount of calcium available to the myocardial cell (22, 28, 68). In particular, epinephrine and norepinephrine both increase in entry of extracellular calcium into the cardiac muscle fiber. The relationship between sympathetic stimulation of the heart and stroke volume is illustrated in figure 9.17. Notice that compared to control conditions (i.e., limited sympathetic stimulation), an increase in sympathetic stimulation of the heart increases stroke volume at any level of EDV.

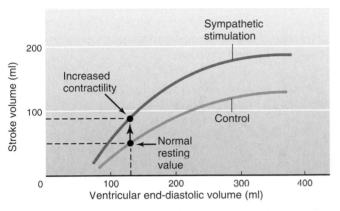

FIGURE 9.17 Effects of sympathetic stimulation of the heart on stroke volume. Note that sympathetic stimulation results in an increase in stroke at any given diastolic volume; that is, sympathetic stimulation increases ventricular contractility via an increased level of intracellular calcium resulting in a higher myosin cross-bridge interaction with actin.

- Cardiac output is the product of heart rate and stroke volume ($\dot{Q}$ = HR × SV). Figure 9.18 summarizes those variables that influence cardiac output during exercise.
- The pacemaker of the heart is the SA node. SA node activity is modified by the parasympathetic nervous system (slows HR) and the sympathetic nervous system (increases HR).
- Heart rate increases at the beginning of exercise due to a withdrawal of parasympathetic tone. At higher work rates, the increase in heart rate is achieved via an increased sympathetic outflow to the SA nodes.
- Stroke volume is regulated via: (1) end-diastolic volume, (2) aortic blood pressure, and (3) the strength of ventricular contraction.
- Venous return increases during exercise due to: (1) venoconstriction, (2) the muscle pump, and (3) the respiratory pump.

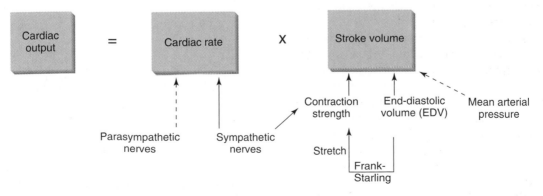

FIGURE 9.18 Factors that regulate cardiac output. Variables that stimulate cardiac output are shown by solid arrows, while factors that reduce cardiac output are shown by dotted arrows.

100

Plasma

White blood cells and platelets

Percent 42

Red blood cells

Hematocrit = 42%

0

FIGURE 9.19 Blood cells become packed at the bottom of the test tube when blood is centrifuged; this leaves the plasma at the top of the tube. The percentage of whole blood that is comprised of blood cells is termed the hematocrit.

HEMODYNAMICS

One of the most important features of the circulatory system to remember is that the system is a continuous "closed loop." Blood flow through the circulatory system results from pressure differences between the two ends of the system. In order to understand the physical regulation of blood flow to tissues, it is necessary to appreciate the interrelationships between pressure, flow, and resistance. The study of these factors and the physical principles of blood flow is called *hemodynamics*.

Physical Characteristics of Blood

Blood is composed of two principal components, plasma and cells. Plasma is the "watery" portion of blood that contains numerous ions, proteins, and hormones. The cells that make up blood are red blood cells (RBCs), platelets, and white blood cells. Red blood cells contain hemoglobin used for the transport of oxygen (see chapter 10). Platelets play an important role in blood clotting, and white blood cells are important in preventing infection.

The percentage of the blood that is composed of cells is called the *hematocrit*. That is, if 42% of the blood is cells and the remainder is plasma, the hematocrit is 42% (see figure 9.19). On a percentage basis, RBCs constitute the largest fraction of cells found in blood. Therefore, the hematocrit is principally influenced by increases or decreases in RBC numbers. The average hematocrit of a normal college-age male is 42%, while the hematocrit of a normal college-age female averages approximately 38%. These values vary among individuals and are dependent on a number of variables.

Blood is several times more viscous than water, and this viscosity increases the difficulty with which blood flows through the circulatory system. One of the major contributors to viscosity is the concentration of RBCs found in the blood. Therefore, during periods of anemia (decreased RBCs), the viscosity of blood is lowered. Conversely, an increase in hematocrit results in an elevation in blood viscosity. The potential influence of changing blood viscosity on performance will be discussed in chapter 25.

Relationships Among Pressure, Resistance, and Flow

As mentioned earlier, blood flow through the vascular system depends in part on the difference in pressure at the two ends of the system. If the pressures at the two ends of the vessel are equal, there will be no flow. In contrast, if the pressure is higher at one end of the vessel than the other, blood will flow from the region of higher pressure to the region of lower pressure. The rate of flow is proportional to the pressure difference $(P_1 - P_2)$ between the two ends of the tube. Figure 9.20 illustrates the "pressure head" driving blood flow in the systemic circulatory system under resting conditions. Here, the mean arterial pressure is 100 mm Hg (i.e., this is the pressure of blood in the aorta), while the pressure at the opposite end of the circuit (i.e., pressure in the right atrium) is 0 mm Hg. Therefore, the driving pressure across the circulatory system is 100 mm Hg (100 − 0 = 100).

It should be pointed out that the flow rate of blood through the vascular system is proportional to the pressure difference across the system, but is inversely proportional to the resistance. Inverse proportionality is expressed mathematically by the placement of this variable in the denominator of a fraction, since a fraction decreases when the denominator increases. Therefore, the relationship between blood flow, pressure, and resistance is given by the equation:

$$\text{Blood flow} = \frac{\Delta \text{ Pressure}}{\text{Resistance}}$$

where Δ pressure means the difference in pressure between the two ends of the circulatory system. Notice that blood flow can be increased by either an increase in blood pressure or a decrease in resistance. A five-fold increase in blood flow could be generated by increasing pressure by a factor of five; however, this large increase in blood pressure would be hazardous to health. Fortunately, increases in blood flow during exercise are achieved primarily by a decrease in resistance with a small rise in blood pressure.

FIGURE 9.20 The flow of blood through the systemic circuit is dependent on the pressure difference (ΔP) between the aorta and the right atrium. In this illustration, the mean pressure in the aorta is 100 mm Hg, while the pressure in the right atrium is 0 mm Hg. Therefore, the "driving" pressure across the circuit is 100 mm Hg (100 − 0 = 100).

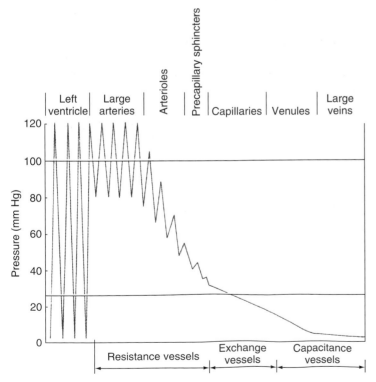

FIGURE 9.21 Pressure changes across the systemic circulation. Notice the large pressure drop across the arterioles.

What factors contribute to the resistance of blood flow? Resistance to flow is directly proportional to the length of the vessel and the viscosity of blood. However, the most important variable determining vascular resistance is the diameter of the blood vessel, since vascular resistance is inversely proportional to the fourth power of the radius of the vessel:

$$\text{Resistance} = \frac{\text{Length} \times \text{viscosity}}{\text{Radius}^4}$$

In other words, an increase in either vessel length or blood viscosity results in a proportional increase in resistance. However, reducing the radius of a blood vessel by one-half would increase resistance sixteen-fold (i.e., $2^4 = 16$)!

Sources of Vascular Resistance

Under ordinary circumstances, the viscosity of blood and the length of the blood vessels are not manipulated in normal physiology. Therefore, the primary factor regulating blood flow through organs must be the radius of the blood vessel. Since the effect of changes in radius on changes in flow rate are magnified by a power of four, blood can be diverted from one organ system to another by varying degrees of vasoconstriction and vasodilation. This principle is used during heavy exercise to divert blood toward contracting skeletal muscle and away from less-active tissue. This concept will be discussed in detail in the next section, Changes in Oxygen Delivery to Muscle During Exercise.

The greatest vascular resistance in blood flow occurs in arterioles. This point is illustrated in figure 9.21. Note the large drop in arterial pressure that occurs across the arterioles; approximately 70% to 80% of the decline in mean arterial pressure occurs across the arterioles.

IN SUMMARY

- Blood is composed of two principal components, plasma and cells.
- Blood flow through the vascular system is directly proportional to the pressure at the two ends of the system and inversely proportional to resistance:

$$\text{Blood flow} = \frac{\Delta \text{ Pressure}}{\text{Resistance}}$$

- The most important factor determining resistance to blood flow is the radius of the blood vessel. The relationship between vessel radius, vessel length, blood viscosity, and flow is:

$$\text{Resistance} = \frac{\text{Length} \times \text{viscosity}}{\text{Radius}^4}$$

- The greatest vascular resistance to blood flow is offered in the arterioles.

CHANGES IN OXYGEN DELIVERY TO MUSCLE DURING EXERCISE

During intense exercise, the metabolic need for oxygen in skeletal muscle increases many times over the resting value (4). In order to meet this rise in oxygen demand, blood flow to the contracting muscle must increase. As mentioned earlier, increased oxygen delivery to exercising skeletal muscle is accomplished via two mechanisms: (1) an increased cardiac output and (2) a redistribution of blood flow from inactive organs to the working skeletal muscle.

Changes in Cardiac Output During Exercise

Cardiac output increases during exercise in direct proportion to the metabolic rate required to perform the exercise task. This is pointed out in figure 9.22. Note that the relationship between cardiac output and percent maximal oxygen uptake is essentially linear. The increase in cardiac output during exercise in the upright position is achieved by an increase in both stroke volume and heart rate. However, note that in untrained or moderately trained subjects, stroke volume does not increase beyond a workload of 40% to 50% of $\dot{V}O_2$ max (figure 9.22). Therefore, at work rates greater than 40% to 50% $\dot{V}O_2$ max, the rise in cardiac output in these individuals is achieved by increases in heart rate alone (4, 19, 25, 66, 82) (see Research Focus 9.1). The examples presented in figure 9.21 for maximal heart rate, stroke volume, and cardiac output are typical values for a 70-kg, active (but not highly trained) college-age male. See table 9.2 for examples of maximal stroke volume and cardiac output for trained men and women.

Maximal cardiac output tends to decrease in a linear fashion in both men and women after thirty years of age (25, 29). This is primarily due to a decrease in maximal heart rate with age (25). For example, since cardiac output equals heart rate times stroke volume, any decrease in heart rate would result in a decrease in cardiac output. The decrease in maximal heart rate with age can be estimated by the following formula:

$$\text{Max HR} = 220 - \text{age (years)}$$

According to this formula, a twenty-year-old subject might have a maximal heart rate of 200 beats per minute (220 − 20 = 200), whereas a fifty-year-old would have a maximal heart rate of 170 beats per minute (220 − 50 = 170). However, this is only an estimate, and values can be actually 20 beats · min^{-1} higher or lower.

FIGURE 9.22 Pressure changes in blood pressure, stroke volume, cardiac output, heart rate, and the arterial–mixed venous oxygen difference as a function of relative work rates. See text for details.

Changes in Arterial-Mixed Venous O_2 Content During Exercise

Note in figure 9.21 the change in the arterial–mixed venous oxygen difference (a $-\ \bar{v} O_2$ diff) that occurs during exercise. The a $-\ \bar{v} O_2$ difference represents the

Stroke Volume Does Not Plateau in Endurance Athletes

It is widely accepted that during incremental exercise, stroke volume in active or untrained subjects reaches a plateau at a submaximal work rate (i.e., approximately 40% $\dot{V}O_2$ max). The physiological explanation for this plateau in stroke volume is that at high heart rates, the time available for ventricular filling is decreased. Therefore, diastole and end-diastolic volume decrease. However, new evidence suggests that during incremental work rates the stroke volume of endurance athletes (e.g., highly trained distance runners) does not plateau but continues to increase to $\dot{V}O_2$ max (26, 90). What is the explanation for this observation? It appears that compared to untrained subjects, endurance athletes have improved ventricular filling during heavy exercise due to increased venous return. This increase in end-diastolic volume results in an increased force of ventricular contraction (Frank-Starling law) and an increase in stroke volume.

amount of O_2 that is taken up from 100 ml of blood by the tissues during one trip around the systemic circuit. An increase in the $a - \bar{v} O_2$ difference during exercise is due to an increase in the amount of O_2 taken up and used for the oxidative production of ATP by skeletal muscle. The relationship between cardiac output ($\dot{Q}$), $a - \bar{v} O_2$ diff, and oxygen uptake is given by the Fick equation:

$$\dot{V}O_2 = \dot{Q} \times (a - \bar{v} \, O_2 \text{ diff})$$

Simply stated, the Fick equation says that $\dot{V}O_2$ is equal to the product of cardiac output and the $a - \bar{v} O_2$ diff. This means that an increase in either cardiac output or $a - \bar{v} O_2$ diff would elevate $\dot{V}O_2$.

Redistribution of Blood Flow During Exercise

In order to meet the increased oxygen demand of the skeletal muscles during exercise, it is necessary to increase muscle blood flow while at the same time reducing blood flow to less active organs such as the liver, kidneys, and GI tract. Figure 9.23 points out that the change in blood flow to muscle and the splanchnic (pertaining to the viscera) circulation is dictated by the exercise intensity (metabolic rate). That is, the increase in muscle blood flow during exercise and the decrease in splanchnic blood flow change as a linear function of % $\dot{V}O_2$ max (66, 68).

Figure 9.24 illustrates the change in blood flow to various organ systems between resting conditions and during maximal exercise. Several important points need to be stressed. First, at rest, approximately 15% to 20% of total cardiac output is directed toward skeletal muscle (4, 22, 68). However, during

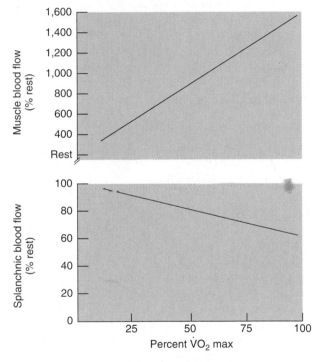

FIGURE 9.23 Changes in muscle and splanchnic blood flow as a function of exercise intensity. Notice the large increase in muscle blood flow as the work rate increases. Data from L. Rowell, *Human Circulation Regulating During Physical Stress.* 1986: Oxford University Press, New York, NY.

maximal exercise, 80% to 85% of total cardiac output goes to contracting skeletal muscle (45, 68, 77). This is necessary to meet the huge increase in muscle oxygen requirements during intense exercise. Second, notice that during heavy exercise, the percent of total cardiac

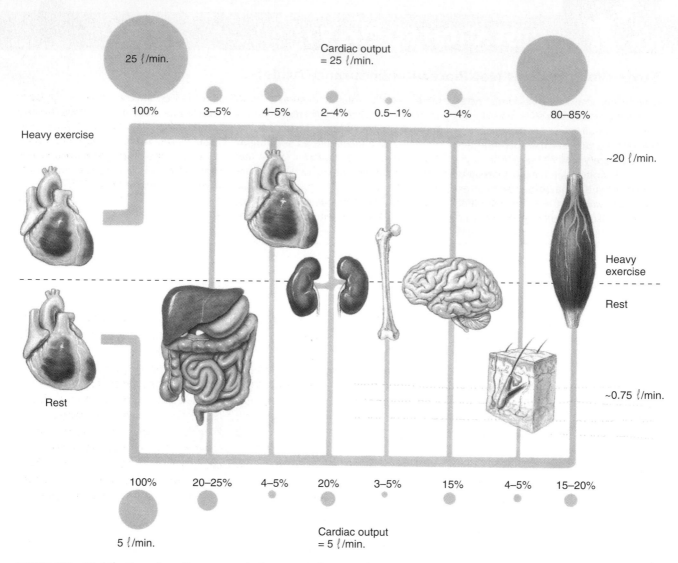

Cardiac output = 25 ℓ/min.

25 ℓ/min.

| 100% | 3–5% | 4–5% | 2–4% | 0.5–1% | 3–4% | 80–85% |

Heavy exercise

~20 ℓ/min.

Heavy exercise

Rest

~0.75 ℓ/min.

Rest

| 100% | 20–25% | 4–5% | 20% | 3–5% | 15% | 4–5% | 15–20% |

Cardiac output = 5 ℓ/min.

5 ℓ/min.

FIGURE 9.24 Distribution of cardiac output during rest and maximal exercise. At rest, the cardiac output is 5 ℓ/min. (bottom of figure); during maximum exercise, the cardiac output increased five-fold to 25 ℓ/min. Note the large increases in blood flow to the skeletal muscle and the reduction in flow to the liver/GI tract. From P. Åstrand K. Rodahl, *Textbook of Work Physiology*, 3d ed. Copyright© 1986 McGraw-Hill, Inc., New York. Reprinted by permission of the authors.

output that goes to the brain is reduced compared to that during rest. However, the absolute blood flow that reaches the brain is slightly increased above resting values; this is due to the elevated cardiac output during exercise (91). Further, although the percentage of total cardiac output that reaches the myocardium is the same during maximal exercise as it is at rest, the total coronary blood flow is increased due to the increase in cardiac output during heavy exercise. Finally, note the reduction in blood flow to the skin (79) and the abdominal organs that occurs during intense exercise when compared to resting conditions. This reduction in abdominal blood flow during heavy exercise is an important means of shifting blood flow away from "less-active" tissues and toward the working skeletal muscles.

Regulation of Local Blood Flow During Exercise

What regulates blood flow to various organs during exercise? Muscle as well as other body tissues have the unique ability to regulate their own blood flow in direct proportion to their metabolic needs. Blood flow to skeletal muscle during exercise is regulated in the following way. First, the arterioles in skeletal muscle have a high vascular resistance at rest. This is due to adrenergic sympathetic stimulation, which causes arteriole smooth muscle to contract (vasoconstriction) (75). This produces a relatively low blood flow to muscle at rest (4–5 ml per minute per 100 grams of muscle), but because muscles have a large mass, this accounts for 20% to 25% of total blood flow from the heart.

RESEARCH FOCUS 9.2

Nitric Oxide Is An Important Vasodilator

Research in the early 1990s led to the discovery of an important vasodilator called nitric oxide (see reference 56 for a review). Nitric oxide is produced in the endothelium of arterioles. After production, nitric oxide promotes smooth muscle relaxation in the arteriole, which results in vasodilation and therefore causes an increase in blood flow. Current evidence suggests that nitric oxide works in conjunction with other local factors in autoregulation of blood flow.

How important is nitric oxide in the autoregulation of muscle blood flow during exercise? At present, a definitive answer to this question is not available. Nonetheless, it seems likely that nitric oxide is one of several factors involved in regulation of muscle blood flow during exercise. Current speculation is that muscular contraction results in increased production of nitric oxide, which promotes vasodilation in those arterioles leading to the working muscle. Improving our understanding of the role of nitric oxide in the regulation of muscle blood flow is an exciting area for future research.

At the beginning of exercise, the initial skeletal muscle vasodilation that occurs is due to an intrinsic metabolic control (10, 83). This type of blood flow regulation is termed **autoregulation,** and it is thought to be the most important factor in regulating blood flow to muscle during exercise. The increased metabolic rate of skeletal muscle during exercise causes local changes such as decreases in oxygen tension, increases in CO_2 tension, nitric oxide, potassium and adenosine concentrations, and a decrease in pH (increase in acidity) (see Research Focus 9.2). These local changes work together to cause vasodilation of arterioles feeding the contracting skeletal muscle (10, 25, 56, 77). Vasodilation reduces the vascular resistance and therefore increases blood flow. As a result of these changes, blood delivery to contracting skeletal muscle during heavy exercise may rise fifteen to twenty times above that during rest (4, 7, 22, 74). Further, arteriole vasodilation is combined with "recruitment" of the capillaries in skeletal muscle. At rest, only 5% to 10% of the capillaries in skeletal muscle are open at any one time; however, during intense exercise, almost all of the capillaries in contracting muscle may be open (68).

The level of vasodilation that occurs in arterioles and small arteries leading to skeletal muscle is regulated by the metabolic need of the muscle. That is, the intensity of exercise and the number of motor units recruited determines the overall need for blood flow to the muscle. For example, during low-intensity exercise, a relatively small number of motor units will be recruited into action resulting in a relatively small demand for blood flow to these active muscle fibers. In contrast, high-intensity exercise would result in the recruitment of a large number of motor units and, therefore, result in increased production of local vasodilatory factors. Collectively, these changes would result in increased vasodilation of arterioles/small arteries and promote increased blood flow to the contracting muscle in order to match the metabolic demand.

While the vascular resistance in skeletal muscle decreases during exercise, vascular resistance to flow in the visceral organs and other inactivity tissue increases. This occurs due to an increased sympathetic output to these organs, which is regulated by the cardiovascular control center. As a result of the increase in visceral vasoconstriction during exercise (i.e., resistance increases), blood flow to the viscera can decrease to only 20% to 30% of resting values (68, 70).

IN SUMMARY

- Oxygen delivery to exercising skeletal muscle increases due to: (1) an increased cardiac output and (2) a redistribution of blood flow from inactive organs to the contracting skeletal muscles.
- Cardiac output increases as a linear function of oxygen uptake during exercise. During exercise in the upright position, stroke volume reaches a plateau at approximately 40% of $\dot{V}O_2$ max; therefore, at work rates above 40% $\dot{V}O_2$ max, the rise in cardiac output is due to increases in heart rate alone.
- During exercise, blood flow to contracting muscle is increased and blood flow to less active tissues is reduced.
- Regulation of muscle blood flow during exercise is primarily regulated by local factors (called *autoregulation*). Autoregulation refers to intrinsic control of blood flow by change in local metabolites (e.g., oxygen tension, pH, potassium, adenosine, and nitric oxide) around arterioles.

CIRCULATORY RESPONSES TO EXERCISE

The changes in heart rate and blood pressure that occur during exercise reflect the type and intensity of exercise performed, the duration of exercise, and the environmental conditions under which the work was performed. For example, heart rate and blood pressure, at any given oxygen uptake, are higher during arm work when compared to leg work. Further, exercise in a hot/humid condition results in higher heart rates when compared to the same exercise in a cool environment. The next several sections discuss the cardiovascular responses to exercise under varying conditions.

Emotional Influence

Submaximal exercise in an emotionally charged atmosphere results in higher heart rates and blood pressures when compared to the same work in a psychologically "neutral" environment (4, 33, 76). This emotional elevation in heart rate and blood pressure response to exercise is mediated by an increase in sympathetic nervous system activity. If the exercise is maximal (e.g., 400-meter dash), high emotion elevates the pre-exercise heart rate and blood pressure but does not generally alter the peak heart rate or blood pressure observed during the exercise itself.

Transition from Rest to Exercise

At the beginning of exercise there is a rapid increase in heart rate, stroke volume, and cardiac output. It has been demonstrated that heart rate and cardiac output begin to increase within the first second after muscular contraction begins (76) (see figure 9.25). If the work rate is constant and below the lactate threshold, a steady-state plateau in heart rate, stroke volume, and cardiac output is reached within two to three minutes. This response is similar to that observed in oxygen uptake at the beginning of exercise (see chapter 4).

Recovery from Exercise

Recovery from short-term, low-intensity exercise is generally rapid. This is illustrated in figure 9.25. Notice that heart rate, stroke volume, and cardiac output all decrease rapidly back toward resting levels following this type of exercise. Recovery speed varies from individual to individual, with well-conditioned subjects demonstrating better recuperative powers than untrained subjects. In regard to recovery heart rates, the slopes of heart-rate decay following exercise are generally the same for trained and untrained subjects. However, trained subjects recover faster follow-

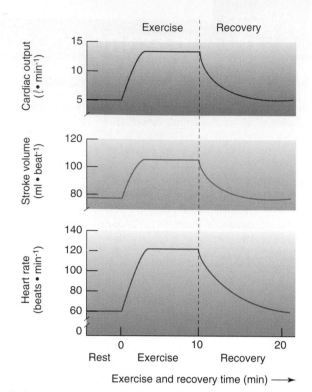

FIGURE 9.25 Changes in cardiac output, stroke volume, and heart rate during the transition from rest to submaximal constant intensity exercise and during recovery. See text for discussion. Data from L. Rowell, 1974, "Human Cardiovascular Adjustments to Exercise and Thermal Stress," American Physiological Society, Bethesda, MD: *Physiological Reviews*, 54:75–159; and L. Rowell, H*uman Circulation Regulating During Physical Stress*. 1986: Oxford University Press, New York, NY.

ing exercise since they don't achieve as high a heart rate as untrained subjects during a particular exercise.

Recovery from long-term exercise is much slower than the response depicted in figure 9.25. This is particularly true when the exercise is performed in hot/humid conditions, since an elevated body temperature delays the fall in heart rate during recovery from exercise (72).

Incremental Exercise

The cardiovascular responses to dynamic incremental exercise are illustrated in figure 9.22. Heart rate and cardiac output increase in direct proportion to oxygen uptake. Further, blood flow to muscle increases as a function of oxygen uptake (see figure 9.23). This ensures that as the need to synthesize ATP to supply the energy for muscular contraction increases, the supply of O_2 reaching the muscle rises. However, both cardiac output and heart rate reach a plateau at approximately 100% $\dot{V}O_2$ max (see figure 9.22). This point represents a maximal ceiling for oxygen transport to exercising skeletal muscles, and it is thought

| TABLE 9.3 | Changes in the Double Product (i.e., Heart Rate × Systolic Blood Pressure) During an Incremental Exercise Test in a Healthy 21-Year-Old Female Subject |

Note that the double product is a dimensionless term that reflects the relative changes in the workload placed on the heart during exercise and other forms of stress.

Condition	Heart Rate (beats · min⁻¹)	Systolic Blood Pressure (mm Hg)	Double Product
Rest	75	110	8,250
Exercise			
25% $\dot{V}O_2$ max	100	130	13,000
50% $\dot{V}O_2$ max	140	160	22,400
75% $\dot{V}O_2$ max	170	180	30,600
100% $\dot{V}O_2$ max	200	210	42,000

to occur simultaneously with the attainment of maximal oxygen uptake.

The increase in cardiac output during incremental exercise is achieved via a decrease in vascular resistance to flow and an increase in mean arterial blood pressure. The elevation in mean arterial blood pressure during exercise is due to an increase in systolic pressure, since diastolic pressure remains fairly constant during incremental work (see figure 9.22).

As mentioned earlier, the increase in heart rate and systolic blood pressure that occurs during exercise results in an increased workload on the heart. The increased metabolic demand placed on the heart during exercise can be estimated by examining the double product. The **double product** (also known as *rate-pressure product*) is computed by multiplying heart rate times systolic blood pressure:

Double product = heart rate × systolic blood pressure

Table 9.3 contains an illustration of changes in the double product during an incremental exercise test. The take-home message in table 9.3 is simply that increases in exercise intensity result in an elevation in both heart rate and systolic blood pressure; each of these factors increases the workload placed on the heart.

Careful examination of table 9.3 reveals that the double product during exercise at $\dot{V}O_2$ max is five times greater than the double product at rest. This implies that maximal exercise increases the workload on the heart by 500% over rest.

The practical application of the double product is that this measure can be used as a guideline to prescribe exercise for patients with coronary artery blockage. For example, suppose a patient develops chest pain (called angina pectoris) at a certain intensity of exercise due to myocardial ischemia at a double product of >30,000. Because chest pain appears at a double product of >30,000, the cardiologist or exercise

FIGURE 9.26 Comparison of mean arterial blood pressure and heart rate during submaximal rhythmic arm and leg exercise.

physiologist would recommend that this patient perform types of exercise that result in a double product of <30,000. This would reduce the risk of the patient developing chest pain due to a high metabolic demand on the heart.

Arm versus Leg Exercise

As mentioned earlier, at any given level of oxygen consumption, both heart rate and blood pressure are higher during arm work when compared to leg work (1, 2, 18, 41, 52, 65) (see figure 9.26). The explanation for the higher heart rate seems to be linked to a greater sympathetic outflow to the heart during arm work when compared to leg exercise (4). Additionally, isometric exercise also increases the heart rate above the expected value based on relative oxygen consumption (1, 2, 7, 37, 39, 41).

The relatively large increase in blood pressure for arm work is due to a vasoconstriction in the inactive muscle groups (4). For example, the larger the muscle group (e.g., legs) involved in performing the exercise, the more resistance vessels (arterioles) that are dilated. Therefore, this lower peripheral resistance is reflected in lower blood pressure (since cardiac output × resistance = pressure).

Intermittent Exercise

If exercise is discontinuous (e.g., interval training), the extent of the recovery of heart rate and blood pressure between bouts depends on the level of subject fitness, environmental conditions (temperature, humidity), and the duration and intensity of the exercise. With a relatively light effort in a cool environment, there is generally complete recovery between exercise bouts within several minutes. However, if the exercise is intense or the work is performed in a hot/humid environment, there is a cumulative increase in heart rate between efforts, and thus recovery is not complete (74). The practical consequence of performing repeated bouts of light exercise is that many repetitions can be performed. In contrast, the nature of high-intensity exercise dictates that a limited number of efforts can be tolerated.

Prolonged Exercise

Figure 9.27 illustrates the change in heart rate, stroke volume, and cardiac output that occurs during prolonged exercise at a constant work rate. Note that cardiac output is maintained at a constant level throughout the duration of the exercise. However, stroke volume declines while heart rate increases (7, 15, 32, 40, 58, 70, 72, 74). Figure 9.27 demonstrates that the ability to maintain a constant cardiac output in the face of declining stroke volume is due to the increase in heart rate being equal in magnitude to the decline in stroke volume.

The increase in heart rate and decrease in stroke volume observed during prolonged exercise is often referred to as *cardiovascular drift* and is due to the influence of rising body temperature on dehydration and a reduction in plasma volume (62, 68). A reduction in plasma volume acts to reduce venous return to the heart and therefore reduce stroke volume. If prolonged exercise is performed in a hot/humid environment, the increase in heart rate and decrease in stroke volume is exaggerated even more than depicted in figure 9.27 (57, 63). In fact, it is not surprising to find near-maximal heart rates during submaximal exercise

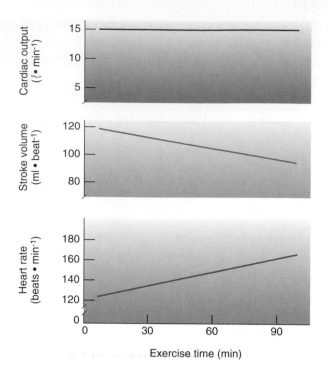

FIGURE 9.27 Changes in cardiac output, stroke volume, and heart rate during prolonged exercise at a constant intensity. Notice that cardiac output is maintained by an increase in heart rate to offset the fall in stroke volume that occurs during this type of work.

in the heat. For example, it has been demonstrated that during a 2.5-hour marathon race at a work rate of 70% to 75% $\dot{V}O_2$ max, maximal heart rates may be maintained during the last hour of the race (20).

Does prolonged exercise at high heart rates pose a risk for cardiac injury? The answer to this question is almost always "no" for healthy individuals. However, sudden cardiac deaths have occurred in individuals of all ages during exercise. See Clinical Applications 9.3 for more details on sudden death during exercise.

IN SUMMARY

- The changes in heart rate and blood pressure that occur during exercise are a function of the type and intensity of exercise performed, the duration of exercise, and the environmental conditions.
- The increased metabolic demand placed on the heart during exercise can be estimated by examining the double product.
- At the same level of oxygen consumption, heart rate and blood pressure are greater during arm exercise than during leg exercise.
- The increase in heart rate that occurs during prolonged exercise is called *cardiovascular drift*.

Sudden Cardiac Death During Exercise

Sudden death is defined as an unexpected, natural, and nonviolent death occurring within the first six hours following the beginning of symptoms. Note that not all sudden deaths are due to cardiac events. In fact, in the United States, only 30% of sudden deaths in people between 14 to 21 years of age are cardiac in origin (85). How many of these cases of sudden death occur during exercise? Each year, ten to thirteen cases of sudden cardiac death during exercise are reported in the United States. However, given that millions of people are actively engaged in sports and regular exercise in the United

States, the likelihood that a healthy person will die from sudden cardiac death is extremely small.

The causes of sudden cardiac death are diverse and vary as a function of age. For example, in children and adolescents, most sudden cardiac deaths occur due to lethal cardiac arrhythmias (abnormal heart rhythm). These arrhythmias can arise from genetic anomalies in coronary arteries, cardiomyopathy (wasting of cardiac muscle due to disease), and/or myocarditis (inflammation of the myocardium)(85). In adults, coronary heart disease and cardiomyopathy are the most common

causes of sudden cardiac death (85). Similar to sudden deaths in children, sudden cardiac deaths in adults are also generally associated with lethal cardiac arrhythmias.

Can a medical exam identify people at risk for sudden cardiac death during exercise? Yes. The combination of a medical history and a complete medical exam by a qualified physician can usually identify individuals with undetected heart disease or genetic defects that would place them at risk for sudden death during exercise.

REGULATION OF CARDIOVASCULAR ADJUSTMENTS TO EXERCISE

The cardiovascular adjustments at the beginning of exercise are rapid. Within one second after the commencement of muscular contraction there is a withdrawal of vagal outflow to the heart, which is followed by an increase in sympathetic stimulation of the heart (68). At the same time, there is a vasodilation of arterioles in active skeletal muscles and a reflex increase in the resistance of vessels in less active areas. The end, result is an increase in cardiac output to ensure that blood flow to muscle matches the metabolic needs (see figure 9.28). What is the signal to "turn on" the cardiovascular system at the onset of exercise? This question has puzzled physiologists for many years (27). At present, a complete answer is not available. However, recent advances in understanding cardiovascular control have led to the development of the *central command theory* (13, 16, 17, 52, 78, 86, 87).

The term **central command** refers to a motor signal developed within the brain. The central command theory of cardiovascular control argues that the initial cardiovascular changes at the beginning of dynamic exercise (e.g., cycle ergometer exercise) are due to centrally generated cardiovascular motor signals, which set the general pattern of the cardiovascular response. However, it is believed that cardiovascular activity can be and is modified by heart mechanoreceptors, muscle chemoreceptors, muscle mechano-

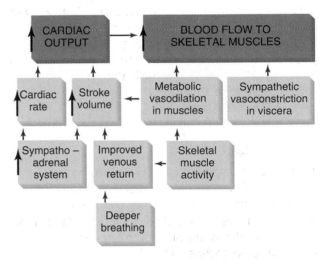

FIGURE 9.28 A summary of cardiovascular responses to exercise.

receptors, and pressure-sensitive receptors (baroreceptors) located within the carotid arteries and the aortic arch (30, 43, 48, 51, 69, 71, 80). Muscle chemoreceptors are sensitive to increases in muscle metabolites (e.g., potassium, lactic acid, etc.) and send messages to higher brain centers to "fine-tune" the cardiovascular responses to exercise (7, 24, 36–49, 55). This type of peripheral feedback to the cardiovascular control center (medulla oblongata) has been termed the *exercise pressor reflex* (14, 51).

Muscle mechanoreceptors (e.g., muscle spindles, Golgi tendon organs) are sensitive to the force and speed of muscular movement. These receptors, like

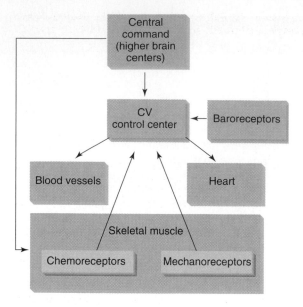

FIGURE 9.29 A summary of cardiovascular control during exercise. See text for discussion.

muscle chemoreceptors, send information to higher brain centers to aid in modification of the cardiovascular responses to a given exercise task (67, 68, 84, 88).

Finally, baroreceptors, which are sensitive to changes in arterial blood pressure, may also send afferent information back to the cardiovascular control center to add precision to the cardiovascular activity during exercise. These pressure receptors are important, since they regulate arterial blood pressure around an elevated systemic pressure during exercise (67, 68).

In review, the central command theory proposes that the initial signal to the cardiovascular system at the beginning of exercise comes from higher brain centers. However, fine-tuning of the cardiovascular response to a given exercise test is accomplished via a series of feedback loops from muscle chemoreceptors, muscle mechanoreceptors, and arterial baroreceptors (see figure 9.29). The fact that there appears to be some overlap among these three feedback systems during submaximal exercise suggests that redundancy in cardiovascular control exists (67, 68). This is not surprising considering the importance of matching blood flow to the metabolic needs of exercising skeletal muscle. Whether or not one or many of these feedback loops becomes more important during heavy exercise is not currently known and poses an interesting question for future research.

IN SUMMARY

- The central command theory of cardiovascular control during exercise proposes that the initial signal to "drive" the cardiovascular system at the beginning of exercise comes from higher brain centers.
- Although central command is the primary drive to increase heart rate during exercise, the cardiovascular response to exercise is fine-tuned by feedback from muscle chemoreceptors, muscle mechanoreceptors, and arterial baroreceptors to the cardiovascular control center.

STUDY QUESTIONS

1. What are the major purposes of the cardiovascular system?
2. Briefly, outline the design of the heart. Why is the heart often called "two pumps in one"?
3. Outline the cardiac cycle and the associated electrical activity recorded via the electrocardiogram.
4. Graph the heart rate, stroke volume, and cardiac output response to incremental exercise.
5. What factors regulate heart rate during exercise? Stroke volume?
6. How does exercise influence venous return?
7. What factors determine local blood flow during exercise?
8. Graph the changes that occur in heart rate, stroke volume, and cardiac output during prolonged exercise. What happens to these variables if the exercise is performed in a hot/humid environment?
9. Compare heart rate and blood pressure responses to arm and leg work at the same oxygen uptake. What factors might explain the observed differences?
10. Explain the central command theory of cardiovascular regulation during exercise.

SUGGESTED READINGS

Brooks, G., T. Fahey, and K. Baldwin. 2005. *Exercise Physiology: Human Bioenergetics and Its Application*, 4th ed. New York: McGraw-Hill Companies.

Coyle, E., and J. Gonzalez-Alonso. 2001. Cardiovascular drift during prolonged exercise: New perspectives. *Exercise and Sport Sciences Reviews* 29:88–92.

Delp, M., and D. O'Leary. 2004. Integrative control of the skeletal muscle microcirculation in the maintenance of arterial pressure during exercise. *Journal of Applied Physiology* 97:1112–18.

Fox, S. 2006. *Human Physiology*, 9th ed. New York: McGraw-Hill Companies.

Guyton, A., and J. Hall. 2005. *Textbook of Medical Physiology*. New York: Elsevier/Saunders.

Powers, S., J. Quindry, and K. Hamilton. 2004. Aging, exercise, and cardioprotection. *Annuals of New York Academy of Science* 1019:462–70.

Thomas, G., and S. Segal. 2004. Neural control of muscle blood flow during exercise. *Journal of Applied Physiology* 97:731–38.

Vella, C. A., and R. Robergs. 2005. A review of the stroke volume response to upright exercise in healthy subjects. *British Journal of Sports Medicine* 39(4):190–95.

Widmaier, E., H. Raff, and K. Strang. 2006. *Vander's Human Physiology*, 10th ed. New York: McGraw-Hill Companies.

REFERENCES

1. Asmussen, E. 1981. Similarities and dissimilarities between static and dynamic exercise. *Circulation Research* 48 (Suppl. 1):3–10.
2. Åstrand, P. et al. 1965. Intra-arterial blood pressure during exercise with different muscle groups. *Journal of Applied Physiology* 20:253–57.
3. Åstrand, P-O., K. Rodahl, H. Dahl, and S. Strome. 2003. *Textbook of Work Physiology*. Champaign, IL: Human Kinetics Publishers.
4. Åstrand, P., and K. Rodahl. 1986. *Textbook of Work Physiology*. New York: McGraw-Hill Companies.
5. Bers, D. 1991. Calcium regulation in cardiac muscle. *Medicine and Science in Sports and Exercise* 23:1157–62.
6. Brady, A. 1991. Mechanical properties of isolated cardiac myocytes. *Physiological Reviews* 71:413–28.
7. Brengelmann, G. 1983. Circulatory adjustments to exercise and heat stress. *Annual Review of Physiology* 45: 191–212.
8. Cowley, A. 1992. Long-term control of arterial blood pressure. *Physiological Reviews* 72:231–300.
9. Coyle, E., and J. Gonzalez-Alonso. 2001. Cardiovascular drift during prolonged exercise: New perspectives. *Exercise and Sport Sciences Reviews* 29:88–92.
10. Delp, M., and D. O'Leary. 2004. Integrative control of the skeletal muscle microcirculation in the maintenance of arterial pressure during exercise. *Journal of Applied Physiology* 97:1112–18.
11. Demirel, H., S. Powers, C. Caillaud, J. Coombes, L. Fletcher, I. Vrabas, H. Naito, J. Jessup, and L. Ji. 1998. Exercise training reduces myocardial lipid peroxidation following short-term ischemia-reperfusion. *Medicine and Science in Sports and Exercise*. 30:1211–16.
12. Demirel, H. et al. 2001. Short-term exercise improves myocardial tolerance to in vivo ischemia-reperfusion in the rat. *Journal of Applied Physiology* 91:2205–12.
13. Dormer, J., and H. L. Stone. 1982. Fastigial nucleus and its possible role in the cardiovascular response to exercise. In *Circulation, Neurobiology and Behavior*, ed. O. Smith, R. Galosy, and S. Weiss. New York: Elsevier.
14. Duncan, G., R. Johnson, and D. Lambie. 1981. Role of sensory nerves in the cardiovascular and respiratory changes with isometric forearm exercise in man. *Clinical Science* 60:145–55.
15. Ekelund, L., and A. Holmgren. 1964. Circulatory and respiratory adaptation during long-term, non-steady-state exercise, in the sitting position. *Acta Physiologica Scandanavica* 62:240–55.
16. Eldridge, F., D. Milhorn, and T. Waldrop. 1981. Exercise hyperpnea and locomotion: Parallel activation from the hypothalamus. *Science* 211:844–46.
17. Eldridge, F. et al. 1985. Stimulation by central command of locomotion, respiration, and circulation during exercise. *Respiratory Physiology* 59:313–37.
18. Eston, R., and D. Brodie. 1986. Responses to arm and leg ergometry. *British Journal of Sports Medicine* 20:4–6.
19. Fox, E., M. Foss, and S. Keteyian. 1998. *Fox's Physiological Basis for Exercise and Sport*. New York: McGraw-Hill Companies.
20. Fox, E., and D. Costill. 1972. Estimated cardiorespiratory responses during marathon running. *Archives of Environmental Health* 24:315–24.
21. Fox, S. 2006. *Human Physiology*, 9th ed. New York: McGraw-Hill Companies.
22. Fox, S. 2002. *Human Physiology*. New York: McGraw-Hill Companies.
23. French, J., J. Quindry, D. Falk, J. Staib, Y. Lee, K. Wang, and S. Powers. 2005. Ischemia-reperfusion induced calpain activation and SERCA2a degradation are attenuated by exercise training and calpain inhibition. *American Journal of Physiology* 90:H128–H136, 2006.
24. Freund, P., S. Hobbs, and L. Rowell. 1978. Cardiovascular responses to muscle ischemia in man—dependency on muscle mass. *Journal of Applied Physiology* 45:762–67.
25. Gerstenblith, G., D. Renlund, and E. Lakatta. 1987. Cardiovascular response to exercise in younger and older men. *Federation Proceedings* 46:1834–39.
26. Gledhill, N. et al. 1994. Endurance athletes' stroke volume does not plateau: Major advantage is diastolic function. *Medicine and Science in Sports and Exercise* 26: 1116–21.
27. Gorman, M., and H. Sparks. 1991. The unanswered question. *News in Physiological Sciences* 6:191–93.
28. Guyton, A., and J. E. Hall. 2002. *Textbook of Medical Physiology*. Philadelphia: W. B. Saunders.
29. Hagberg, J. 1987. Effect of training on the decline of O_2 max with aging. *Federation Proceedings* 46:1830–33.
30. Hainsworth, R. 1991. Reflexes from the heart. *Physiological Reviews* 71:617–58.
31. Hamilton, K., J. Quindry, J. French, J. Staib, J. Hughes, J. Mehta, and S. Powers. 2004. MnSOD antisense treatment and exercise-induced protection against arrhythmias. *Free Radicals in Biology and Medicine* 37:1360–68.
32. Hartley, L. 1977. Central circulatory function during prolonged exercise. *Annals of New York Academy of Sciences* 301:189–94.
33. Herd, J. 1991. Cardiovascular response to stress. *Physiological Reviews* 71:305–30.
34. Hirst, G., F. Edwards, N. Bramich, and M. Klemm. 1991. Neural control of cardiac pacemaker potentials. *News in Physiological Sciences* 6:185–90.
35. Hole, J. 1995. *Human Anatomy and Physiology*. New York: McGraw-Hill Companies.
36. Johansson, B. 1962. Circulatory responses to stimulation of somatic afferents. *Acta Physiologica Scandanavica* (Suppl. 198):1–91.
37. Kaufman, M. et al. 1983. Effects of static muscular contraction on impulse activity of groups III and IV afferents in cats. *Journal of Applied Physiology* 55:105–12.
38. Kaufman, M. et al. 1984. Effect of ischemia on responses of group III and IV afferents to contraction. *Journal of Applied Physiology* 57:644–50.
39. Kaufman, M. et al. 1984. Effects of static and rhythmic twitch contractions on the discharge of group III and IV muscle afferents. *Cardiovascular Research* 18:663–68.
40. Kenny, W. L. 1988. Control of heat-induced cutaneous vasodilation in relation to age. *European Journal of Applied Physiology* 57:120–25.
41. Kilbom, A., and T. Brunkin. 1976. Circulatory effects of isometric muscle contractions, performed separately and in combination with dynamic exercise. *European Journal of Applied Physiology* 36:7–27.

42. Kirchoff, S. R., S. Gupta, and A. A. Knowlton. 2002. Cytosolic heat shock protein 60, apoptosis, and myocardial injury. *Circulation* 105:2899–2904.

43. Kjaer, M., and N. Secher. 1992. Neural influence on cardiovascular and endocrine responses to static exercise in humans. *Sports Medicine* 13:303–9.

44. Kniffki, K., S. Mense, and R. Schmidt. 1981. Muscle receptors with fine afferent fibers which may evoke circulatory reflexes. *Circulation Research* 48 (Suppl. 1):25–31.

45. Laughlin, M. H., and R. Korthius 1987. Control of muscle blood flow during sustained physiological exercise. *Canadian Journal of Applied Sports Sciences* 12 (Suppl.): 775–835.

46. Lennon, S., J. Quindry, K. Hamilton, J. French, J. Hughes, J. Mehta, and S. Powers. 2004. Elevated MnSOD is not required for exercise-induced cardioprotection. *American Journal of Physiology* 287:H975–H980.

47. Lepore, D. et al. 2001. Role of priming stresses and Hsp70 in protection from ischemia-reperfusion injury in cardiac and skeletal muscle. *Cell Stress & Chaperones* 6:93–96.

48. Marshall, J. 1994. Peripheral chemoreceptors and cardiovascular regulation. *Physiological Reviews* 74:543–79.

49. McCloskey, D., and J. Mitchell. 1972. Reflex cardiovascular and respiratory responses originating in exercising muscle. *Journal of Physiology* (London) 224:173–86.

50. Miller, J., D. Pegelow, A. Jacques, and J. Dempsey. 2005. Skeletal muscle pump versus respiratory muscle pump: Modulation of venous return from the locomotor limb in humans. *Journal of Physiology* 563:925–43.

51. Mitchell, J. 1990. Neural control of the circulation during exercise. *Medicine and Science in Sports and Exercise* 22: 141–54.

52. Mitchell, J. et al. 1980. The role of muscle mass in the cardiovascular response to static contraction. *Journal of Physiology* (London) 309:45–54.

53. Monos, E., V. Berczi, and G. Nadasy. 1995. Local control of veins: Biomechanical, metabolic, and humoral aspects. *Physiological Reviews* 75:611–53.

54. Opie, L., B. Swynghedauw, H. Taegtmeyer, C. Ruegg, and E. Carmeliet. 1991. *The Heart: Physiology and Metabolism.* Philadelphia: Lippincott-Raven Publishers.

55. Paterson, D., and A. Morton. 1986. Maximal aerobic power, ventilatory and respiratory compensation thresholds during arm cranking and bicycle ergometry. *Australian Journal of Science and Medicine in Sport* 18:11–15.

56. Pearson, P., and P. Vanhoutte. 1993. Vasodilator and vasoconstrictor substances produced by the endothelium. *Review of Physiology, Biochemistry, and Pharmacology.* 122:2–37.

57. Powers, S., E. Howley, and R. Cox. 1982. A differential catecholamine response to prolonged exercise and passive heating. *Medicine and Science in Sports* 14:435–39.

58. ———. 1982. Ventilatory and metabolic responses to heat stress during prolonged exercise. *Journal of Sports Medicine and Physical Fitness* 22:32–36.

59. Powers, S., H. Demirel, H. Vincent, J. Coombes, H. Naito, K. Ward, R. Shanely, and J. Jessup. 1998. Exercise training improves myocardial tolerance to in vivo ischemia-reperfusion in the rat. *American Journal of Physiology.* 275:R1468–77.

60. Powers, S. K., M. Locke, and H. A. Demirel. 2001. Exercise, heat shock proteins, and myocardial protection from I-R injury. *Medicine and Science in Sports and Exercise* 33:386–92.

61. Powers, S., J. Quindry, and K. Hamilton. 2004. Aging, exercise, and cardioprotection. *Annuals of New York Academy of Science* 1019:462–70.

62. Raven, P., and G. Stevens. 1988. Cardiovascular function during prolonged exercise. In *Perspectives in Exercise Science and Sports Medicine: Prolonged Exercise,* ed. D. Lamb and R. Murray, 43–71. Indianapolis: Benchmark Press.

63. Ridge, B., and F. Pyke. 1986. Physiological responses to combinations of exercise and sauna. *Australian Journal of Science and Medicine in Sports* 18:25–28.

64. Rosen, M., E. Anyukhovsky, and S. Steinberg. 1991. Alpha-adrenergic modulation of cardiac rhythm. *News in Physiological Sciences* 6:135–38.

65. Rosiello, R., D. Mahler, and J. Ward. 1987. Cardiovascular responses to rowing. *Medicine and Science in Sports and Exercise* 19:239–45.

66. Rowell, L. 1974. Human cardiovascular adjustments to exercise and thermal stress. *Physiological Reviews* 54: 75–159.

67. ———. 1980. What signals govern the cardiovascular response to exercise? *Medicine and Science in Sports and Exercise* 12:307–15.

68. ———. 1986. *Human Circulation Regulation during Physical Stress.* New York: Oxford University Press.

69. ———. 1992. Reflex control of the circulation during exercise. *International Journal of Sports Medicine* 13 (Suppl. 1):S25–S27.

70. Rowell, L., L. Hermansen, and J. Blackmon. 1976. Human cardiovascular and respiratory responses to graded muscle ischemia. *Journal of Applied Physiology* 41: 693–701.

71. Rowell, L., and D. O'Leary. 1990. Reflex control of the circulation during exercise: Chemoreflexes and mechanoreflexes. *Journal of Applied Physiology* 69:407–18.

72. Rubin, S. 1987. Core temperature regulation of heart rate during exercise in humans. *Journal of Applied Physiology* 62:1997–2002.

73. Saul, J. 1990. Beat-to-beat variations of heart rate reflect modulation of cardiac autonomic outflow. *News in Physiological Sciences* 5:32–37.

74. Sawka, M., R. Knowlton, and J. Critz. 1979. Thermal and circulatory responses to repeated bouts of prolonged running. *Medicine and Science in Sports* 11:177–80.

75. Seals, D., and R. Victor. 1991. Regulation of muscle sympathetic nerve activity during exercise in humans. In *Exercise and Sport Science Reviews,* ed. J. Holloszy, 313–50. Baltimore: Lippincott Williams & Wilkins.

76. Shephard, R. 1981. *Physiology and Biochemistry of Exercise.* New York: Praeger.

77. Sjogaard, G., G. Sauard, and C. Juel. 1988. Muscle blood flow during isometric activity and its relation to muscle fatigue. *European Journal of Applied Physiology* 57:327–35.

78. Smith, O., R. Rushmer, and E. Lasher. 1960. Similarity of cardiovascular responses to exercise and to diencephalic stimulation. *American Journal of Physiology* 198: 1139–42.

79. Smolander, J., J. Saalo, and O. Korhonen. 1991. Effect of workload on cutaneous vascular response to exercise. *Journal of Applied Physiology* 71:1614–19.

80. Spyer, K. 1994. Central nervous mechanisms contributing to cardiovascular control. *Journal of Physiology* (London). 474:1–19.

81. Suga, H. 1990. Ventricular energetics. *Physiological Reviews* 70:247–77.

82. Sullivan, M., F. Cobb, and M. Higginbotham. 1991. Stroke volume increases by similar mechanisms during upright exercise in normal men and women. *American Journal of Cardiology* 67:1405–12.

83. Thomas, G., and S. Segal. 2004. Neural control of muscle blood flow during exercise. *Journal of Applied Physiology* 97:731–38.

84. Tibes, V. 1977. Reflex inputs to the cardiovascular and respiratory centers from dynamically working canine muscles. *Circulation Research* 41:332–41.

85. Virmani, R., A. Burke, and A. Farb. 2001. Sudden cardiac death. *Cardiovascular Pathology* 10:211–18.

86. Williamson, J. 1995. Instantaneous heart rate increase with dynamic exercise: Central command and muscle-heart reflex contributions. *Journal of Applied Physiology* 78:1273–79.

87. Williamson, J. W. et al. 2002. Brain activation by central command during actual and imagined handgrip under hypnosis. *Journal of Applied Physiology* 92:1317–24.

88. Wyss, C. et al. 1983. Cardiovascular responses to graded reductions in hindlimb perfusion in exercising dogs. *American Journal of Physiology* 245:H481–H486.

89. Yamashita, N. et al. 1999. Exercise provides direct biphasic cardioprotection via manganese superoxide dismutase activation. *Journal of Experimental Medicine* 189:1699–1706.

90. Zhou, B. et al. 2001. Stroke volume does not plateau during graded exercise in elite male distance runners. *Medicine and Science in Sports and Exercise* 33:1849–54.

91. Zobl, E. et al. 1965. Effect of exercise on the cerebral circulation and metabolism. *Journal of Applied Physiology* 20:1289–93.

CHAPTER 10

Respiration During Exercise

■ Objectives

By studying this chapter, you should be able to do the following:

1. Explain the principal physiological function of the pulmonary system.

2. Outline the major anatomical components of the respiratory system.

3. List the major muscles involved in inspiration and expiration at rest and during exercise.

4. Discuss the importance of matching blood flow to alveolar ventilation in the lung.

5. Explain how gases are transported across the blood-gas interface in the lung.

6. Discuss the major transportation modes of O_2 and CO_2 in the blood.

7. Discuss the effects of increasing temperature, decreasing pH, and increasing levels of 2–3 DPG on the oxygen-hemoglobin dissociation curve.

8. Describe the ventilatory response to constant load, steady-state exercise. What happens to ventilation if exercise is prolonged and performed in a high-temperature/humid environment?

9. Describe the ventilatory response to incremental exercise. What factors are thought to contribute to the alinear rise in ventilation at work rates above 50% to 70% of $\dot{V}O_2$ max?

10. Identify the location and function of chemoreceptors and mechanoreceptors that are thought to play a role in the regulation of breathing.

11. Discuss the neural-humoral theory of respiratory control during exercise.

■ Outline

Function of the Lung   201

Structure of the Respiratory System   201
    Conducting Zone   202
    Respiratory Zone   204

Mechanics of Breathing   204
    Inspiration   204
    Expiration   204
    Airway Resistance   206

Pulmonary Ventilation   207

Pulmonary Volumes and Capacities   208

Diffusion of Gases   210

Blood Flow to the Lung   211

Ventilation-Perfusion Relationships   212

O_2 and CO_2 Transport in Blood   213
    Hemoglobin and O_2 Transport   213
    Oxyhemoglobin Dissociation Curve   213
    O_2 Transport in Muscle   215
    CO_2 Transport in Blood   215

Ventilation and Acid-Base Balance   217

Ventilatory and Blood-Gas Responses to Exercise   217
    Rest-to-Work Transitions   217
    Prolonged Exercise in a Hot Environment   217
    Incremental Exercise   218

Control of Ventilation   219
    Ventilatory Regulation at Rest   219
    Ventilatory Control During Submaximal Exercise   222

Ventilatory Control During
   Heavy Exercise   222

Do the Lungs Adapt to Exercise
Training?   224

Does the Pulmonary System
Limit Maximal Exercise
Performance?   224

■ Key Terms

alveolar ventilation ($\dot{V}_A$)
alveoli
anatomical dead space
aortic bodies
Bohr effect
bulk flow
carotid bodies
cellular respiration
deoxyhemoglobin

diaphragm
diffusion
hemoglobin
myoglobin
oxyhemoglobin
partial pressure
pleura
pulmonary respiration
residual volume (RV)

respiration
spirometry
tidal volume
total lung capacity (TLC)
ventilation
ventilatory threshold (Tvent)
vital capacity (VC)

The word **respiration** can have two definitions in physiology. These definitions can be divided into two separate but related subdivisions: (1) **pulmonary respiration** and (2) **cellular respiration.** Pulmonary respiration refers to ventilation (breathing) and the exchange of gases (O_2 and CO_2) in the lungs. Cellular respiration relates to O_2 utilization and CO_2 production by the tissues (see chapter 3). This chapter is concerned with pulmonary respiration, and the term *respiration* is used in the text as a synonym for pulmonary respiration. Since the respiratory, or pulmonary, system plays a key role in maintaining blood-gas homeostasis (i.e., O_2 and CO_2 tensions) during exercise, an understanding of lung function during work is important for the student of exercise physiology. It is the purpose of this chapter to discuss the design and function of the respiratory system during exercise.

large surface area within the lungs and a very short diffusion distance between blood and gas in the lungs. The fact that the O_2 and CO_2 tension in the blood leaving the lung is almost in complete equilibrium with the O_2 and CO_2 tension found within the lung is testimony to the high efficiency of normal lung function.

The respiratory system also plays an important role in the regulation of the acid-base balance during heavy exercise. This important topic will be discussed later in this chapter and again in chapter 11.

IN SUMMARY

■ The primary function of the pulmonary system is to provide a means of gas exchange between the environment and the body. Further, the respiratory system plays an important role in the regulation of the acid-base balance during exercise.

FUNCTION OF THE LUNG

The primary purpose of the respiratory system is to provide a means of gas exchange between the external environment and the body. That is, the respiratory system provides the individual with a means of replacing O_2 and removing CO_2 from the blood. The exchange of O_2 and CO_2 between the lung and blood occurs as a result of ventilation and diffusion. The term **ventilation** refers to the mechanical process of moving air into and out of the lungs. **Diffusion** is the random movement of molecules from an area of high concentration to an area of lower concentration. Since O_2 tension in the lung is greater than in the blood, O_2 moves from the lungs into the blood. Similarly, the tension of CO_2 in the blood is greater than the tension of CO_2 in the lungs, and thus CO_2 moves from the blood into the lung and is expired. Diffusion in the respiratory system occurs rapidly because there is a

STRUCTURE OF THE RESPIRATORY SYSTEM

The human respiratory system consists of a group of passages that filter air and transport it into the lungs, where gas exchange occurs within microscopic air sacs called **alveoli.** The major components of the respiratory system are pictured in figure 10.1. The organs of the respiratory system include the nose, nasal cavity, pharynx, larynx, trachea, bronchial tree, and the lungs themselves. The anatomical position of the lungs relative to the major muscle of inspiration, the diaphragm, is pictured in figure 10.2. Note that both the right and left lungs are enclosed by a set of membranes called **pleura.** The visceral pleura adheres to the outer surface of the lung, whereas the parietal pleura lines the thoracic walls and the diaphragm.

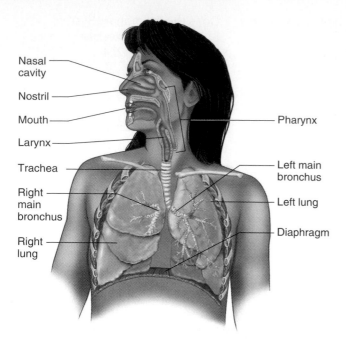

Nasal cavity
Nostril
Mouth
Larynx
Trachea
Right main bronchus
Right lung
Pharynx
Left main bronchus
Left lung
Diaphragm

FIGURE 10.1 Major organs of the respiratory system.

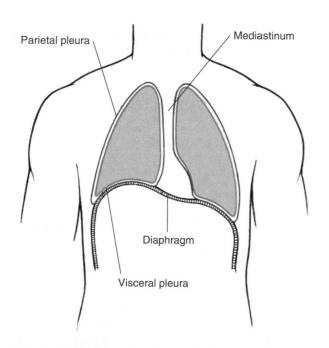

Parietal pleura
Mediastinum
Diaphragm
Visceral pleura

FIGURE 10.2 Position of the lungs, diaphragm, and pleura.

These two pleura are separated by a thin layer of fluid that acts as a lubricant, allowing a gliding action of one pleura on the other. The pressure in the pleural cavity (intrapleural pressure) is less than atmospheric and becomes even lower during inspiration, causing air to inflate the lungs. The fact that intrapleural pressure is less than atmospheric is important, since it prevents the collapse of the fragile air sacs within the lungs. More will be said about this later.

Conducting Zone

The air passages of the respiratory system are divided into two functional zones: (1) the conducting zone and (2) the respiratory zone (see figure 10.3). The conducting zone includes all those anatomical structures (e.g., trachea, bronchial tree, bronchioles) that air passes through to reach the respiratory zone. The region of the lung where gas exchange occurs is labeled the respiratory zone and includes the respiratory bronchioles and alveolar sacs. Respiratory bronchioles are included in this region, since they contain small clusters of alveoli.

Air enters the trachea from the pharynx (throat), which receives air from both the nasal and oral cavities. In general, humans breathe through the nose until ventilation is increased to approximately 20 to 30 liters per minute, at which time the mouth becomes the primary passageway for air (32). In order for gas to enter or leave the trachea, it must pass through a valvelike opening called the *epiglottis*, which is located between the vocal cords.

The trachea branches into two primary bronchi (right and left) that enter each lung. The bronchial tree then branches several more times before forming bronchioles (bronchioles are small branches of the segmental bronchi). The bronchioles then branch several times before they become the alveolar ducts leading to the alveolar sacs and respiratory zone of the lung (see figure 10.4).

The conducting zone of the respiratory system not only serves as a passageway for air, but also functions to humidify and filter the air as it moves toward the respiratory zone of the lung. Regardless of the temperature or humidity of the environment, the air that reaches the lung is warmed and is saturated with water vapor (63). This warming and humidification of air serves to protect body temperature and prevents the delicate lung tissue from desiccation (drying out).

The role of the conducting zone and the respiratory zone in filtration of the inspired gas is critical in preventing lung damage due to the collection of inhaled particles in the respiratory zone. These filtration and cleaning processes are achieved via two principal means. First, mucus, secreted by the cells of the conducting zone, traps small, inhaled particles. This mucus is moved toward the oral cavity via tiny fingerlike projections called *cilia*. These cilia move in a wavelike fashion, which propels the mucus at a rate of 1 to 2 centimeters/minute. When a particle becomes trapped in the mucus, it is moved toward the pharynx via ciliary action, where it can be either swallowed or expectorated.

A second means of protecting the lung from foreign particles is by the action of cells called *macrophages* that reside primarily in the alveoli (94). These macrophages literally engulf particles that

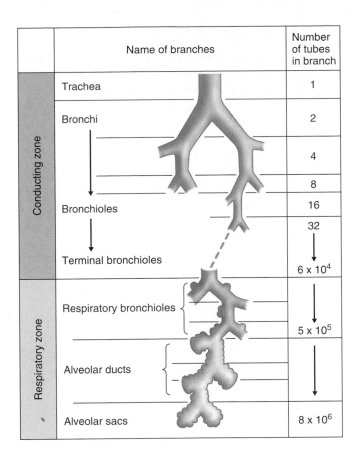

	Name of branches	Number of tubes in branch
Conducting zone	Trachea	1
	Bronchi	2
		4
		8
	Bronchioles	16
		32
	Terminal bronchioles	6×10^4
Respiratory zone	Respiratory bronchioles	5×10^5
	Alveolar ducts	
	Alveolar sacs	8×10^6

FIGURE 10.3 The conducting zones and respiratory zones of the pulmonary system.

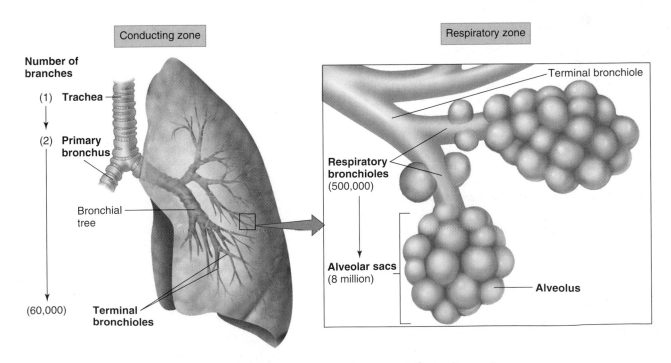

Conducting zone

Respiratory zone

Number of branches

(1) **Trachea**

(2) **Primary bronchus**

Bronchial tree

(60,000) **Terminal bronchioles**

Terminal bronchiole

Respiratory bronchioles (500,000)

Alveolar sacs (8 million)

Alveolus

FIGURE 10.4 The bronchial tree consists of the passageways that connect the trachea and the alveoli.

Type I alveolar cell

Fluid with surfactant

Type II alveolar cell

Alveolus

White blood cell

Macrophage

Red blood cell

Capillary

FIGURE 10.5 Relationship between type II alveolar cells and the alveolus.

reach the alveoli. The cleansing action of both the cilia and macrophages has been shown to be hindered by cigarette smoke and certain types of air pollution (63).

Respiratory Zone

Gas exchange in the lungs occurs across about 300 million tiny (0.25–0.50 mm diameter) alveoli. The enormous number of these structures provides the lung with a large surface area for diffusion. It is estimated that the total surface area available for diffusion in the human lung is 60 to 80 square meters, or about the size of a tennis court. The rate of diffusion is further assisted by the fact that each alveolus is only one cell layer thick, so that the total *blood-gas barrier* is only two cell layers thick (alveolar cell and capillary cell) (see figure 10.5).

Although the 300 million alveoli provide the ideal structure for gas exchange, the fragility of these tiny "bubbles" presents some problems for the lung. For example, because of the surface tension (pressure exerted due to the properties of water) of the liquid lining the alveoli, relatively large forces develop, which tend to collapse alveoli. Fortunately, some of the alveolar cells (called type II, see figure 10.5) synthesize and release a material called *surfactant*, which lowers the surface tension of the alveoli and thus prevents their collapse (57).

■ Anatomically, the pulmonary system consists of a group of passages that filter air and transport it into the lungs where gas exchange occurs within tiny air sacs called *alveoli*.

MECHANICS OF BREATHING

As previously mentioned, movement of air from the environment to the lungs is called pulmonary ventilation and occurs via a process known as **bulk flow.** Bulk flow refers to the movement of molecules along a passageway due to a pressure difference between the two ends of the passageway. Thus, inspiration occurs due to the pressure in the lungs (intrapulmonary) being reduced below atmospheric pressure. Conversely, expiration occurs when the pressure within the lungs exceeds atmospheric pressure. The means by which this pressure change within the lungs is achieved will be discussed within the next several paragraphs.

Inspiration

Any muscle capable of increasing the volume of the chest is considered to be an inspiratory muscle. The **diaphragm** is the most important muscle of inspiration and is the only skeletal muscle considered essential for life (28, 32, 63, 84, 85, 87). This thin, dome-shaped muscle inserts into the lower ribs and is innervated by the phrenic nerves. When the diaphragm contracts, it forces the abdominal contents downward and forward. Further, the ribs are lifted outward (see figure 10.6). The outcome of these two actions is to reduce intrapleural pressure, which in turn causes the lungs to expand. This expansion of the lungs results in a reduction in intrapulmonary pressure below atmospheric, which allows airflow into the lungs.

During normal, quiet breathing the diaphragm performs most of the work of inspiration. However, during exercise, accessory muscles of inspiration are called into play (66, 67, 93). These include the external intercostal muscles, pectoralis minor, the scalene muscles, and the sternocleidomastoids (see figure 10.7). Collectively, these muscles assist the diaphragm in increasing the volume of the thorax, which aids in inspiration (see A Closer Look 10.1).

Expiration

Expiration is passive during normal, quiet breathing. That is, no muscular effort is necessary for expiration to occur at rest. This is true because the lungs and chest walls are elastic and tend to return to equilibrium position after expanding during inspiration (98). During exercise and voluntary hyperventilation,

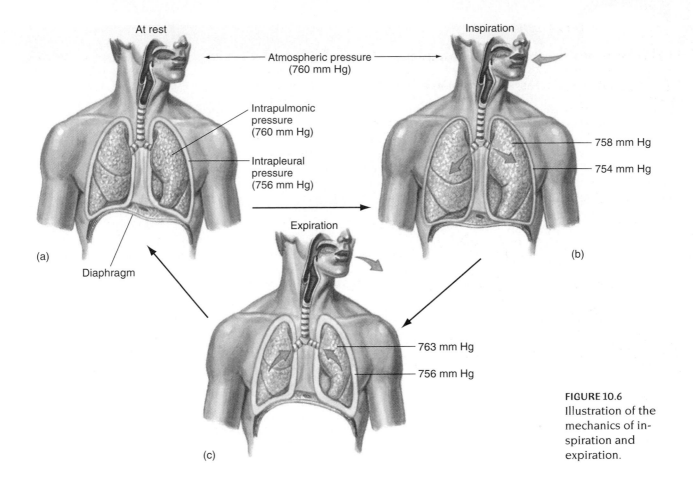

At rest

Atmospheric pressure
(760 mm Hg)

Intrapulmonic
pressure
(760 mm Hg)

Intrapleural
pressure
(756 mm Hg)

(a)

Diaphragm

Inspiration

758 mm Hg

754 mm Hg

(b)

Expiration

763 mm Hg

756 mm Hg

(c)

FIGURE 10.6
Illustration of the
mechanics of in-
spiration and
expiration.

Muscles of inspiration

Muscles of expiration

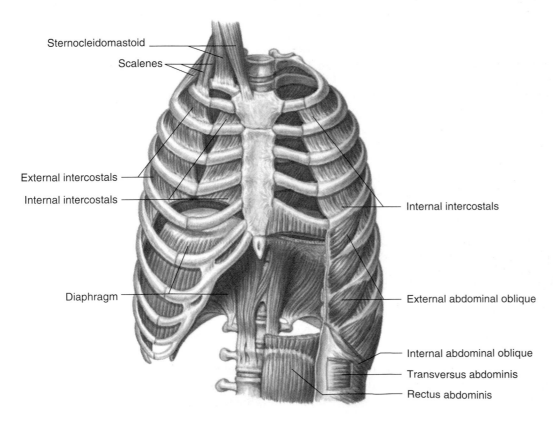

Sternocleidomastoid

Scalenes

External intercostals

Internal intercostals

Diaphragm

Internal intercostals

External abdominal oblique

Internal abdominal oblique

Transversus abdominis

Rectus abdominis

FIGURE 10.7 The
muscles of respira-
tion. The principal
muscles of inspira-
tion are shown on
the left side of the
trunk; the principal
muscles of expira-
tion are shown on
the right side.

A CLOSER LOOK 10.1

Respiratory Muscles and Exercise

Respiratory muscles are skeletal muscles that are functionally similar to locomotor muscles. Their primary task is to act upon the chest wall to move gas in and out of the lungs to maintain arterial blood gas and pH homeostasis. The importance of normal respiratory muscle function can be appreciated by considering that respiratory muscle failure due to disease or spinal cord injury would result in the inability to ventilate the lungs and maintain blood gas and pH levels within an acceptable range.

Muscular exercise results in an increase in pulmonary ventilation, and therefore an increased workload is placed on respiratory muscles. Historically, it has been believed that respiratory muscles do not fatigue during exercise. However, growing evidence indicates that both prolonged exercise (e.g., >120 minutes) and high-intensity exercise (90%–100% $\dot{V}O_2$ max) can promote respiratory muscle fatigue (60, 74, 75). The impact of respiratory muscle fatigue on exercise performance will be discussed later in this chapter.

Do respiratory muscles adapt to regular exercise training in a similar manner to locomotor skeletal muscles? The answer to this question is yes! Regular endurance exercise training increases respiratory muscle oxidative capacity and improves respiratory muscle endurance (74, 75, 92, 103, 104). Further, new evidence reveals that regular exercise training also increases the oxidative capacity of upper airway muscles (95a). This is important because these muscles play a key role in maintaining open airways to reduce the work of breathing during exercise. The effects of exercise training on skeletal muscles will be discussed in detail in chapter 13. For more information on respiratory muscle adaptation to exercise, see Powers and Shanely (2004) in the Suggested Readings.

CLINICAL APPLICATIONS 10.1

Exercise-Induced Asthma

Asthma is a disease that promotes a reversible narrowing of the airways (called a bronchospasm). This reduction in airway diameter results in an increased work of breathing, and individuals suffering from asthma generally report being short of breath (called dyspnea).

Although there are many potential causes of asthma (26), some asthmatic patients develop a bronchospasm during or immediately after exercise. This type of asthma is called "exercise-induced asthma." When an individual experiences an asthma attack during exercise, breathing becomes labored and a wheezing sound is often heard during expiration. If the asthmatic attack is severe, it becomes impossible for the individual to exercise at even low intensities because of the dyspnea associated with the increased work of breathing. Asthma is an excellent example of how even a small decrease in airway diameter can result in a large increase in breathing resistance. See Beck et al. (2002) and Anderson and Kippelen (2005) in the Suggested Readings and chapter 17 for more details.

---

expiration becomes active. The most important muscles involved in expiration are those found in the abdominal wall, which include the rectus abdominus and the internal oblique (66, 93, 114). When these muscles contract, the diaphragm is pushed upward and the ribs are pulled downward and inward. This results in an increase in intrapulmonary pressure and expiration occurs.

Airway Resistance

At any given rate of airflow into the lungs, the pressure difference that must be developed depends on the resistance of the airways. Airflow through the airways of the respiratory system can be mathematically defined by the following relationships:

$$\text{Airflow} = \frac{P_1 - P_2}{\text{Resistance}}$$

where $P_1 - P_2$ is the pressure difference at the two ends of the airway, and resistance is the resistance to flow offered by the airway. Airflow is increased any time there is an increase in the pressure gradient across the pulmonary system, or if there is a decrease in airway resistance. This same relationship for blood flow was discussed in chapter 9.

What factors contribute to airway resistance? By far the most important variable contributing to airway

Exercise and Chronic Obstructive Lung Disease

Chronic obstructive lung disease (COPD) is clinically identified by a decreased expiratory airflow resulting from increased airway resistance. Although COPD and asthma both result in blockage of the airways, these diseases differ in one key feature. Asthma is a reversible narrowing of the airways; that is, asthma can come and go. In contrast, COPD is a constant narrowing of the airways. Although COPD patients can experience some variation in airway blockage, these individuals always experience some level of airway obstruction.

Note that COPD is often the result of a combination of two-separate lung diseases: (1) chronic bronchitis and (2) emphysema. Each of these individual diseases results in increased airway obstruction. Chronic bronchitis is a lung disorder that results in a constant production of mucus within airways, resulting in airway blockage. Emphysema causes a decreased elastic support of the airways, resulting in airway collapse and increased airway resistance. Two of the greatest risk factors in developing COPD are tobacco smoking and a family history of emphysema (112).

Because COPD patients have a constant narrowing of the airways, this airway resistance places an increased workload on respiratory muscles to move gas in and out of the lung. Recognition of this increased work of breathing leads to the sensation of being short of breath (dyspnea). Because the magnitude of dyspnea is closely linked to the amount of work performed by respiratory muscles, dyspnea in COPD patients is greatly increased during exercise. In patients with severe COPD, dyspnea may become so debilitating that the patient has difficulty in performing routine activities of daily living (e.g., walking to the bathroom, showering, etc.). See West (2001) in the Suggested Readings for more details on COPD and exercise.

---

resistance is the diameter of the airway. Airways that are reduced in size due to disease (chronic obstructive lung disease, asthma, etc.) offer more resistance to flow than healthy, open airways. Recall from chapter 9 that if the radius of a blood vessel (or airway) is reduced by one-half, the resistance to flow is increased sixteen times! Therefore, one can easily understand the effect of obstructive lung diseases (e.g., exercise-induced asthma) on increasing the work of breathing, especially during exercise when pulmonary ventilation is ten to twenty times greater than at rest (see Clinical Applications 10.1 and 10.2).

IN SUMMARY

- The major muscle of inspiration is the diaphragm. Air enters the pulmonary system due to intrapulmonary pressure being reduced below atmospheric pressure (bulk flow). At rest, expiration is passive. However, during exercise, expiration becomes active, using muscles located in the abdominal wall (e.g., rectus abdominus and internal oblique).
- The primary factor that contributes to airflow resistance in the pulmonary system is the diameter of the airway.

PULMONARY VENTILATION

Before beginning a discussion of ventilation, it is helpful to define some commonly used pulmonary physiology symbols:

1. V is used to denote volume.
2. $\dot{V}$ means volume per unit of time (generally one minute).
3. The subscripts $_{T, D, A, I, E}$ are used to denote tidal, dead space, alveolar, inspired, and expired, respectively.

Pulmonary ventilation refers to the movement of gas into and out of the lungs. The amount of gas ventilated per minute is the product of the frequency of breathing (f) and the amount of gas moved per breath (**tidal volume**):

$$\dot{V} = V_T \times f$$

In a 70-kg man the $\dot{V}$ at rest is generally around 7.5 liters/minute, with a tidal volume of 0.5 liters and a frequency of 15. During maximal exercise, ventilation may reach 120 to 175 liters per minute, with a frequency of 40 to 50 and a tidal volume of approximately 3 to 3.5 liters.

It is important to understand that not all of the air that passes the lips reaches the alveolar gas compartment, where gas exchange occurs. Part of each breath remains in conducting airways (trachea, bronchi, etc.) and thus does not participate in gas exchange. This "unused" ventilation is called dead-space ventilation (V_D), and the space it occupies is known as **anatomical dead space**. The volume of inspired gas that reaches the respiratory zone is referred to as **alveolar ventilation ($\dot{V}_A$)**. Thus, total minute ventilation can be subdivided into dead space ventilation and alveolar ventilation:

$$\dot{V} = \dot{V}_A + \dot{V}_D$$

Note that pulmonary ventilation is not equally distributed throughout the lung. The basal (bottom) region of the lung receives more ventilation than the apex (top region), particularly during quiet breathing (63). This changes to some degree during exercise, with the apical (top) regions of the lung receiving an increased percentage of the total ventilation (54).

FIGURE 10.8 Photograph of a computerized spirometer used to measure lung volumes. Courtesy of Sensormedics Corp.

IN SUMMARY

- Pulmonary ventilation refers to the amount of gas moved into and out of the lungs.
- The amount of gas moved per minute is the product of tidal volume times breathing frequency.

PULMONARY VOLUMES AND CAPACITIES

Pulmonary volumes can be measured via a technique known as **spirometry.** Using this procedure, the subject breathes into a device that is capable of measuring inspired and expired gas volumes. Modern spirometers use computer technology to measure pulmonary volumes and the rate of expired airflow (see figure 10.8). Figure 10.9 is a spirogram showing the measurement of tidal volumes during quiet breathing and the various lung volumes and capacities that are defined in table 10.1. Several of these terms require special mention. First, **vital capacity (VC)** is defined as the maximum amount of gas that can be expired after a maximum inspiration. Secondly, the **residual volume (RV)** is the volume of gas remaining in the lungs after a maximum expiration. Finally, **total lung capacity (TLC)** is defined as the amount of gas in the lungs after a maximum inspira-

tion, and is the sum of the two lung volumes (VC + RV) just mentioned.

Clinically, spirometry is useful in diagnosing obstructive lung diseases such as chronic obstructive lung disease (COPD). For example, because of increased airway resistance, COPD patients will have a diminished vital capacity and a reduced rate of expired airflow during a maximal expiratory effort. Further, because of increased airway resistance and airway closure during expiration, COPD patients cannot expire as much gas as healthy individuals; this results in trapped gas in the lungs and an abnormally high residual volume.

A specific illustration of how spirometry can detect airway obstruction in patients is as follows. One of the easiest spirometric tests to detect airway blockage is the measurement of forced expiratory volume

FIGURE 10.9 A spirogram showing lung volumes and capacities at rest.

TABLE 10.1 Definitions of Terms Used to Describe Lung Volumes and Capacities

Term	Definitions
Lung Volumes	
Tidal volume	The volume of gas inspired or expired during an unforced respiratory cycle
Inspiratory reserve	The volume of gas that can be inspired at the end of a tidal inspiration
Expiratory reserve	The volume of gas that can be expired at the end of a tidal expiration
Residual volume	The volume of gas left in the lungs after a maximal expiration
Lung Capacities	
Total lung capacity	The total amount of gas in the lungs at the end of a maximal inspiration
Vital capacity	The maximum amount of gas that can be expired after a maximum inspiration
Inspiratory capacity	The maximum amount of gas that can be inspired at the end of a tidal expiration
Functional residual capacity	The amount of gas remaining in the lungs after a normal quiet tidal expiration

Lung volumes are the four, nonoverlapping components of the total lung capacity. Lung capacities are the sum of two or more lung volumes.

Forced Expiratory Volume and Vital Capacity

COPD
FEV1 = 1.0 liters
VC = 3.0 liters
FEV1/VC = 1.0/3.0 × 100 = 33%

Normal
FEV1 = 4.0 liters
VC = 5.0 liters
FEV1/VC = 4.0/5.0 × 100 = 80%

FIGURE 10.10 A spirogram illustrating the use of forced expired airflow to diagnose airway obstruction. Notice the marked difference in both the forced expired volume in 1 second (FEV1) and the vital capacity (VC) between the normal individual and the patient with chronic obstructive lung disease (COPD). See text for details.

and vital capacity (VC). The forced expiratory volume (called FEV1) is the volume of gas expired in 1 second by a forced (maximal effort) expiration from a full inspiration. Vital capacity is the total amount of gas that can be expired during a maximal expiration following a full inspiration. A simple way to make these measures is illustrated in figure 10.8. The patient is comfortably seated in front of the spirometer and breathes through a rubber mouthpiece connected to the spirometer. The patient breathes in maximally and then maximally exhales. The spirometer records the expired volume of gas against time during the expiratory effort.

Figure 10.10 compares the measurements of FEV1 and VC in both a normal, healthy individual and a patient with COPD. Notice, in the normal individual, the vital capacity is 5.0 liters and the FEV1 was 4.0 liters. Therefore, the FEV in this healthy individual is 80% of the VC (i.e., 4.0/5.0 × 100 = 80%). Indeed, the normal ratio of FEV1 to VC in healthy individual is 80% or higher.

Now, let's analyze the measurement of FEV1 and VC in the patient with COPD. Notice that the rate at which air was expired in the COPD patient is much slower than the healthy subject, so that only 1.0 liter of air is expired in the first second. Moreover, the vital capacity in the COPD patient is only 3.0 liters. Therefore, in this patient, the ratio of forced expired volume to vital capacity (1.0/3.0 × 100) is 33%. This value is much lower than the normal values for a normal individual (i.e., 80%) and is typical of a COPD patient with severe airway obstruction. For more information on the impact of COPD on exercise tolerance, see Clinical Applications 10.2.

IN SUMMARY

- Pulmonary volumes can be measured using spirometry.
- Vital capacity is the maximum amount of gas that can be expired after a maximal inspiration.
- Residual volume is the amount of gas left in the lungs after a maximal expiration.

DIFFUSION OF GASES

Prior to discussing diffusion of gases across the alveolar membrane into the blood, it is necessary to introduce the concept of **partial pressure.** According to Dalton's law, the total pressure of a gas mixture is equal to the sum of the pressures that each gas would exert independently. Thus, the pressure that each gas exerts independently can be calculated by multiplying the fractional composition of the gas by the absolute pressure (barometric pressure). Let's consider an example calculating the partial pressure of oxygen in air at sea level. The barometric pressure at sea level is 760 mm Hg (barometric pressure is the force exerted by the weight of the gas contained within the atmosphere). The composition of air is generally considered to be:

Gas	Percentage	Fraction
Oxygen	20.93	.2093
Nitrogen	79.04	.7904
Carbon dioxide	0.03	.0003
Total	100.0	

Therefore, the partial pressure of oxygen (PO_2) at sea level can be computed as:

$$PO_2 = 760 \times .2093$$
$$PO_2 = 159 \text{ mm Hg}$$

In a similar manner, the partial pressure of nitrogen can be calculated to be:

$$PN_2 = 760 \times .7904$$
$$PN_2 = 600.7 \text{ mm Hg}$$

Since O_2, CO_2, and N_2 make up almost 100% of the atmosphere, the total barometric pressure (P) can be computed as:

$$P \text{ (dry atmosphere)} = PO_2 + PN_2 + PCO_2$$

Diffusion of a gas across tissues is described by Fick's law of diffusion, which states that the rate of gas transfer (V gas) is proportional to the tissue area, the diffusion coefficient of the gas, and the difference in the partial pressure of the gas on the two sides of the tissue, and is inversely proportional to the thickness:

$$V \text{ gas} = \frac{A}{T} \times D \times (P_1 - P_2)$$

where A is the area, T is the thickness of the tissue, D is the diffusion coefficient of the gas, and $P_1 - P_2$ is the difference in the partial pressure between the two sides of the tissue. In simple terms, the rate of diffusion for any single gas is greater when the surface area for diffusion is large and the "driving pressure" between the two sides of the tissue is high. In contrast, an increase in tissue thickness impedes diffusion. The lung is well designed for the diffusion of gases across the alveolar membrane into and out of the blood.

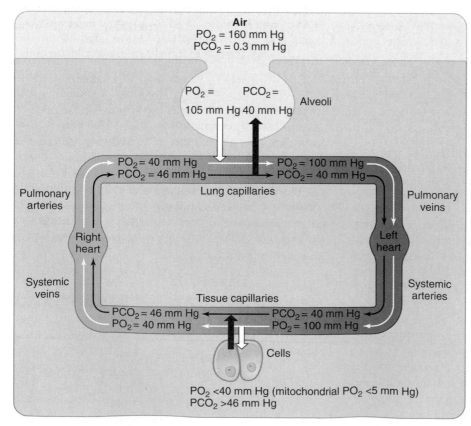

FIGURE 10.11 Partial pressures of oxygen (PO_2) and carbon dioxide (PCO_2) in blood as a result of gas exchange in lung and gas exchange between capillaries and tissues. Note that the alveolar PO_2 of 105 is a result of mixing atmospheric air (i.e., 159 mm Hg at sea level) with existing alveolar gas along with water vapor.

First, the total surface area available for diffusion is large. Secondly, the alveolar membrane is extremely thin. The fact that the lung is an ideal organ for gas exchange is important, since during maximal exercise the rate of O_2 uptake and CO_2 output may increase twenty to thirty times above resting condition.

The amount of O_2 or CO_2 dissolved in blood obeys Henry's law and is dependent on the temperature of blood, the partial pressure of the gas, and the solubility of the gas. Since the temperature of the blood does not change a great deal during exercise (i.e., 1–3°C), and the solubility of the gas remains constant, the major factor that determines the amount of dissolved gas is the partial pressure.

Figure 10.11 illustrates gas exchange via diffusion across the alveolar-capillary membranes and at the tissue level. Note that the PCO_2 and PO_2 of blood entering the lung are approximately 46 and 40 mm Hg, respectively. In contrast, the PCO_2 and PO_2 in alveolar gas are around 40 and 105 mm Hg, respectively. As a consequence of the difference in partial pressure across the blood-gas interface, CO_2 leaves the blood and diffuses into the alveolus, and O_2 diffuses from the alveolus into the blood. Blood leaving the lung has a PO_2 of approximately 100 mm Hg and a PCO_2 of 40 mm Hg.

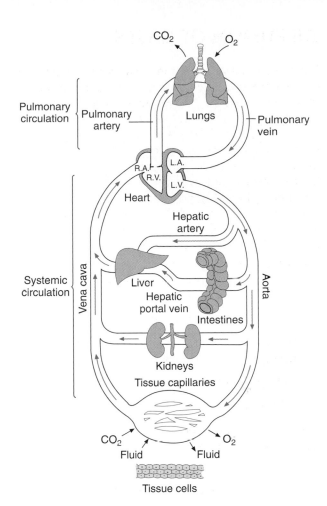

FIGURE 10.12 The pulmonary circulation is a low-pressure system that pumps mixed venous blood through the pulmonary capillaries for gas exchange. After the completion of gas exchange, this oxygenated blood is returned to the left heart chambers to be circulated throughout the body.

IN SUMMARY

- Gas moves across the blood-gas interface in the lung due to simple diffusion.
- The rate of diffusion is described by Fick's law which states: the volume of gas that moves across a tissue is proportional to the area for diffusion and the difference in partial pressure across the membrane, and is inversely proportional to membrane thickness.

BLOOD FLOW TO THE LUNG

The pulmonary circulation begins at the pulmonary artery, which receives venous blood from the right ventricle (recall that this is mixed venous blood). Mixed venous blood is then circulated through the pulmonary capillaries where gas exchange occurs, and this oxygenated blood is returned to the left atrium via the pulmonary vein to be circulated throughout the body (see figure 10.12).

In the adult, the right ventricle of the heart (like the left) has an output of approximately 5 liters/minute. Therefore, the rate of blood flow throughout the pulmonary circulation is equal to that of the systemic circulation. The pressures in the pulmonary circulation are relatively low when compared to those in the systemic circulation (see chapter 9). This low-

pressure system is due to low vascular resistance in the pulmonary circulation (63). An interesting feature of pulmonary circulation is that during periods of increased pulmonary blood flow during exercise, the resistance in the pulmonary vascular system falls due to the distension of vessels and the recruitment of previously unused capillaries. This decrease in pulmonary vascular resistance allows lung blood flow to increase during exercise with relatively small increases in pulmonary arterial pressure.

When we are standing, considerable inequality of blood flow exists within the human lung due to gravity. For example, in the upright position, blood flow decreases almost linearly from bottom to top, reaching very low values at the top (apex) of the lung (see figure 10.13). This distribution may be altered during exercise and with a change in posture. During light exercise, blood flow to the apex of the lung is increased (21). This is advantageous for improved gas exchange and will be discussed in the next section,

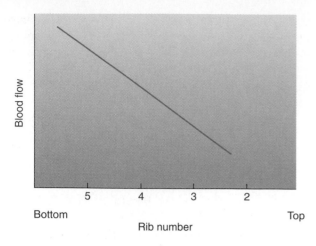

FIGURE 10.13 Regional blood flow within the lung. Note that there is a linear decrease in blood flow from the lower regions of the lung toward the upper regions.

FIGURE 10.14 The relationship between ventilation and blood flow (ventilation/perfusion ratios) at the top (apex) and the base of the lung. The ratios indicate that the base of the lung is overperfused relative to ventilation and that the apex is underperfused relative to ventilation. This uneven matching of blood flow to ventilation results in less than perfect gas exchange.

Ventilation-Perfusion Relationships. When an individual is supine, blood flow becomes uniform within the lung. In contrast, measurements of blood flow in humans who are suspended upside down show that blood flow to the apex of the lung greatly exceeds that found in the base.

IN SUMMARY

- The pulmonary circulation is a low-pressure system with a rate of blood flow equal to that in the systemic circuit.
- In a standing position, most of the blood flow to the lung is distributed to the base of the lung due to gravitational force.

VENTILATION-PERFUSION RELATIONSHIPS

Thus far we have discussed pulmonary ventilation, blood flow to the lungs, and diffusion of gases across the blood-gas barrier in the lung. It seems reasonable to assume that if all these processes were adequate, normal gas exchange would occur in the lung. However, normal gas exchange requires a matching of ventilation to blood flow (perfusion, Q). In other words, an alveolus can be well ventilated, but if blood flow to the alveolus does not adequately match ventilation, normal gas exchange does not occur. Indeed, mismatching of ventilation and perfusion is responsible for most of the problems of gas exchange that occur due to lung diseases.

The ideal ventilation-to-perfusion ratio (V/Q) is 1.0 or slightly greater. That is, there is a one-to-one matching of ventilation to blood flow, which results in optimum gas exchange. Unfortunately, the V/Q ratio is generally not equal to 1.0 throughout the lung, but varies depending on the section of the lung being considered (28, 40, 63, 111). This concept is illustrated in figure 10.14, where the V/Q ratio at the apex and the base of the lung is calculated for resting conditions.

Let's discuss the V/Q ratio in the apex of the lung first. Here, the ventilation (at rest) in the upper region of the lung is estimated to be 0.24 liters/minute, while the blood flow is considered to be 0.07 liters/minute. Thus, the V/Q ratio is 3.3 (i.e., 0.24/0.07 = 3.3). A large V/Q ratio represents a disproportionately high ventilation relative to blood flow, which results in poor gas exchange. In contrast, the ventilation at the base of the lung (figure 10.14) is 0.82 liters/minute, with a blood flow of 1.29 liters/minute (V/Q ratio = 0.82/1.29 = 0.63). A V/Q ratio less than 1.0 represents a greater blood flow than ventilation to the region in question. Although V/Q ratios less than 1.0 are not indicative of ideal conditions for gas exchange, in most cases V/Q ratios greater than 0.50 are adequate to meet the gas exchange demands at rest (111).

What effect does exercise have on the V/Q ratio? The complete answer to this question is not currently available. However, it appears that light exercise may improve the V/Q relationship, while heavy exercise may result in a small V/Q inequality, and thus a minor impairment in gas exchange (54). Whether the increase in V/Q inequality is due to low ventilation or low perfusion is not clear. The possible effects of this V/Q mismatch on blood gases will be discussed later in the chapter.

- Efficient gas exchange between the blood and the lung requires proper matching of blood flow to ventilation (called *ventilation-perfusion relationships*).
- The ideal ratio of ventilation to perfusion is 1.0 or slightly greater, since this ratio implies a perfect matching of blood flow to ventilation.

O_2 AND CO_2 TRANSPORT IN BLOOD

Although some O_2 and CO_2 are transported as dissolved gases in the blood, the major portion of O_2 and CO_2 transported via blood is done by O_2 combining with hemoglobin and CO_2 being transformed into bicarbonate (HCO_3). A complete discussion of how O_2 and CO_2 are transported in blood follows.

Hemoglobin and O_2 Transport

Approximately 99% of the O_2 transported in the blood is chemically bound to **hemoglobin,** which is a protein contained in the red blood cells (erythrocytes). Each molecule of hemoglobin can transport four O_2 molecules. The binding of O_2 to hemoglobin forms **oxyhemoglobin;** hemoglobin that is not bound to O_2 is referred to as **deoxyhemoglobin.**

The amount of O_2 that can be transported per unit volume of blood is dependent on the concentration of hemoglobin. Normal hemoglobin concentration for a healthy male and female is approximately 150 grams and 130 grams, respectively, per liter of blood. When completely saturated with O_2, each gram of hemoglobin can transport 1.34 ml of O_2 (63). Therefore, if hemoglobin is 100% saturated with O_2, the healthy male and female can transport approximately 200 ml and 174 ml of O_2, respectively, per liter of blood at sea level.

Oxyhemoglobin Dissociation Curve

The combination of O_2 with hemoglobin in the lung (alveolar capillaries) is sometimes referred to as *loading*, and the release of O_2 from hemoglobin at the tissues is called *unloading*. Loading and unloading is thus a reversible reaction:

Deoxyhemoglobin + O_2 ⟷ Oxyhemoglobin

The factors that determine the direction of this reaction are (1) the PO_2 of the blood and (2) the affinity or bond strength between hemoglobin and O_2. A high PO_2 drives the reaction to the right, while low PO_2 and a reduced affinity of hemoglobin for O_2 moves the reaction to the left. For example, a high PO_2 in the lungs results in an increase in arterial PO_2 and the formation of oxyhemoglobin (i.e., reaction moves right). In contrast, a low PO_2 in the tissue results in a decrease of PO_2 in the systemic capillaries, and thus unloads O_2 to be used by the tissues (reaction moves left).

The effect of PO_2 on the combination of O_2 with hemoglobin can be best illustrated by the oxyhemoglobin dissociation curve, which is presented in figure 10.15. This sigmoidal (S shaped) curve has several interesting features. First, the percent hemoglobin saturated with O_2 (% HbO_2) increases sharply up to an arterial PO_2 of 40 mm Hg. At PO_2 values above 40 mm Hg, the increase in % HbO_2 rises slowly to a plateau around 90 to 100 mm Hg, at which the % HbO_2 is approximately 97%. At rest, the body's O_2 requirements

FIGURE 10.15 The relationship between the partial pressure of O_2 in blood and the relative saturation of hemoglobin with O_2 is pictured here in the oxygen-hemoglobin dissociation curve. Notice the relatively steep portion of the curve up to PO_2 values of 40 mm Hg, after which there is a gradual rise to reach a plateau.

are relatively low, and only about 25% of the O_2 transported in the blood is unloaded to the tissues. In contrast, during intense exercise, the mixed venous PO_2 may reach a value of 18 to 20 mm Hg, and the tissues may extract up to 90% of the O_2 carried by hemoglobin.

The shape of the oxyhemoglobin dissociation curve is well designed to meet human O_2 transport needs. The relatively flat portion of the curve (above a PO_2 of approximately 90 mm Hg) allows arterial PO_2 to oscillate from 90 to 100 mm Hg without a large drop in % HbO_2. This is important, since there is a decline in arterial PO_2 with aging and upon ascent to altitude. At the other end of the curve (steep portion, 0–40 mm Hg), small changes in PO_2 result in a release of large amounts of O_2 from hemoglobin. This is critical during exercise when tissue O_2 consumption is high.

Effect of pH on O_2-Hb Dissociation Curve   In addition to the effect of blood PO_2 on O_2 binding to hemoglobin, a change in acidity, temperature, or red blood cell (RBC) levels of 2,3-diphosphoglyceric acid (2–3 DPG) can affect the loading/unloading reaction. First, let's consider the effect of changing blood acid-base status on hemoglobin's affinity for O_2. The strength of the bond between O_2 and hemoglobin is weakened by a decrease in blood pH (increased acidity), which results in increased unloading of O_2 to the tissues. This is represented by a "right" shift in the oxyhemoglobin curve and is called the **Bohr effect** (see figure 10.16). A right shift in the oxyhemoglobin

dissociation curve might be expected during heavy exercise due to the rise in blood lactic acid levels observed in this type of work. After being produced in the muscle cell, lactic acid gives up a proton (H^+), which results in the decrease in pH. The mechanism to explain the Bohr effect is the fact that protons bind to hemoglobin, which reduces its O_2 transport capacity. Therefore, when there is a higher-than-normal concentration of H^+ in the blood (a condition called *acidosis*), there is a reduction in hemoglobin affinity for O_2. This facilitates the unloading of O_2 to the tissues during exercise since the acidity level is higher in muscles.

Temperature Effect on O_2-Hb Dissociation Curve
Another factor that affects hemoglobin affinity for O_2 is temperature. At a constant pH, the affinity of hemoglobin for O_2 is inversely related to blood temperature. That is, a decrease in temperature results in a left shift in the oxyhemoglobin curve, while an increase in temperature causes a right shift of the curve. This means that an increase in blood temperature weakens the bond between O_2 and hemoglobin, which assists in the unloading of O_2 to muscle. Conversely, a decrease in blood temperature results in a stronger bond between O_2 and hemoglobin, which hinders O_2 release. The effect of increasing blood temperature on the oxyhemoglobin dissociation curve is presented in figure 10.17. During exercise, increased heat production in the contracting muscle would promote a right

FIGURE 10.16   The effect of changing blood pH on the shape of the oxygen-hemoglobin dissociation curve. A decrease in pH results in a rightward shift of the curve (Bohr effect), while an increase in pH results in a leftward shift of the curve.

FIGURE 10.17   The effect of changing blood temperature on the shape of the oxygen-hemoglobin dissociation curve. An increase in temperature results in a rightward shift in the curve, while a decrease in blood temperature results in a leftward shift in the curve.

FIGURE 10.18 Comparison of the dissociation curve for myoglobin and hemoglobin. The steep myoglobin dissociation demonstrates a higher affinity for O_2 than hemoglobin.

shift in the oxyhemoglobin dissociation curve and facilitate unloading of O_2 to the tissue.

2–3 DPG and the O_2-Hb Dissociation Curve   A final factor that potentially can affect the shape of the oxyhemoglobin dissociation curve is the concentration of 2–3 DPG in red blood cells (RBCs). Red blood cells are unique in that they do not contain a nucleus or mitochondria. Therefore, they must rely on anaerobic glycolysis to meet the cell's energy needs. A byproduct of RBC glycolysis is the compound 2–3 DPG, which can combine with hemoglobin and reduce hemoglobin's affinity for O_2 (i.e., right shift in oxyhemoglobin dissociation curve).

Red blood cell concentrations of 2–3 DPG are known to increase during exposure to altitude and in anemia (low blood hemoglobin) (63). However, reports in the literature about the acute effects of exercise on blood 2–3 DPG levels remain controversial. In an effort to resolve this issue, a group of Austrian researchers (65) performed a series of well-designed experiments that demonstrated that moderate exercise resulted in no change in blood levels of 2–3 DPG, and that severe exercise resulted in a small decrease in blood 2–3 DPG. Therefore, although an increase in blood 2–3 DPG can alter Hb-O_2 affinity, it appears that exercise at sea level does not increase 2–3 DPG in the red blood cell. Therefore, the right shift in the oxyhemoglobin curve during heavy exercise is not due to changes in 2–3 DPG but to the degree of acidosis and blood temperature elevation.

O_2 Transport in Muscle

Myoglobin is an oxygen-binding protein found in skeletal muscle fibers and cardiac muscle (not in blood) and acts as a "shuttle" to move O_2 from the muscle cell membrane to the mitochondria. Myoglobin is found in large quantities in slow-twitch fibers (i.e., high aerobic capacity), in smaller amounts in intermediate fibers, and in only limited amounts in fast-twitch fibers. Myoglobin is similar in structure to hemoglobin, but is about one-fourth the weight. The difference in structure between myoglobin and hemoglobin results in a difference in O_2 affinity between the two molecules. This point is illustrated in figure 10.18. Myoglobin has a greater affinity for O_2 than hemoglobin, and therefore the myoglobin-O_2 dissociation curve is much steeper than that of hemoglobin for PO_2 values below 20 mm Hg. The practical implication of the shape of the myoglobin-O_2 dissociation curve is that myoglobin discharges its O_2 at very low PO_2 values. This is important, since the PO_2 in the mitochondria of contracting skeletal muscle may be as low as 1 to 2 mm Hg.

Myoglobin O_2 stores may serve as an "O_2 reserve" during transition periods from rest to exercise. At the beginning of exercise, there is a time lag between the onset of muscular contraction and an increased O_2 delivery to the muscle. Therefore, O_2 bound to myoglobin prior to the initiation of exercise serves to buffer the O_2 needs of the muscle until the cardiopulmonary system can meet the new O_2 requirement. At the conclusion of exercise, myoglobin O_2 stores must be replenished, and this O_2 consumption above rest contributes to the O_2 debt (see chapter 4).

CO_2 Transport in Blood

Carbon dioxide is transported in the blood in three forms: (1) dissolved CO_2 (about 10% of blood CO_2 is transported this way), (2) CO_2 bound to hemoglobin (called carbaminohemoglobin; about 20% of blood CO_2 is transported via this form), and (3) bicarbonate

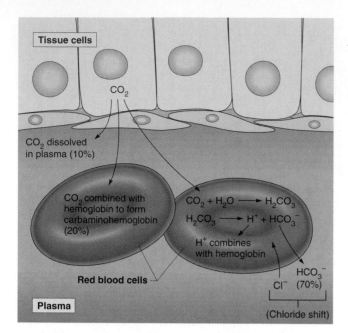

FIGURE 10.19 Carbon dioxide is released from the tissues and moves into the blood. Carbon dioxide is transported in three forms in the blood: (1) dissolved CO_2, (2) CO_2 combined with hemoglobin (carboxyhemoglobin), and (3) bicarbonate (HCO_3^-). Notice that as HCO_3^- moves out of the red blood cell, chloride (Cl^-) moves into the red blood cell (chloride shift) to maintain electrochemical balance in the cell.

FIGURE 10.20 Carbon dioxide is released from the blood into the pulmonary capillaries. At the time of CO_2 release in the lung, there is a "reverse chloride shift" and carbonic acid dissociates into CO_2 and H_2O.

(70% of CO_2 found in blood is transported as bicarbonate: HCO_3^-). The three forms of CO_2 transport in the blood are illustrated in figure 10.19.

Since most of the CO_2 that is transported in blood is transported as bicarbonate, this mechanism deserves special attention. Carbon dioxide can be converted to bicarbonate (within RBCs) in the following way:

$$
\begin{array}{ccccc}
 & \textbf{Carbonic} & & & \\
 & \textbf{anhydrase} & & & \\
\textbf{CO}_2 & \longleftrightarrow & \textbf{H}_2\textbf{CO}_3 & \longleftrightarrow & \textbf{H}^+ \\
\textbf{+} & & \textbf{Carbonic} & & \textbf{+} \\
\textbf{H}_2\textbf{O} & & \textbf{acid} & & \textbf{HCO}_3^-
\end{array}
$$

A high PCO_2 causes CO_2 to combine with water to form carbonic acid. This reaction is catalyzed by the enzyme carbonic anhydrase, which is found in RBCs. After formation, carbonic acid dissociates into a hydrogen ion and a bicarbonate ion. The hydrogen ion then binds to hemoglobin, and the bicarbonate ion diffuses out of the RBC into the plasma (figure 10.19). Since bicarbonate carries a negative charge (anion), the removal of a negatively charged molecule from a cell without replacement would result in an electrochemical imbalance across the cell membrane. This problem is avoided by the replacement of bicarbonate

by chloride (Cl^-), which diffuses from the plasma into the RBC. This exchange of anions occurs in the RBC as blood moves through the tissue capillaries, and is called the *chloride shift* (figure 10.19).

When blood reaches the pulmonary capillaries, the PCO_2 of the blood is greater than that of the alveolus, and thus CO_2 diffuses out of the blood across the blood-gas interface. At the lung, the binding of O_2 to Hb results in a release of the hydrogen ions bound to hemoglobin and promotes the formation of carbonic acid:

$$\textbf{H}^+ + \textbf{HCO}_3^- \longrightarrow \textbf{H}_2\textbf{CO}_3$$

Under conditions of low PCO_2 that exist at the alveolus, carbonic acid then dissociates into CO_2 and H_2O:

$$\textbf{H}_2\textbf{CO}_3 \longrightarrow \textbf{CO}_2 + \textbf{H}_2\textbf{O}$$

The release of CO_2 from the blood is summarized in figure 10.20.

IN SUMMARY

- Over 99% of the O_2 transported in blood is chemically bonded with hemoglobin. The effect of the partial pressure of O_2 on the combination of O_2 with hemoglobin is illustrated by the S-shaped O_2-hemoglobin dissociation curve.
- An increase in body temperature and a reduction in blood pH results in a right shift in

the O_2-hemoglobin dissociation curve and a reduced affinity of hemoglobin for O_2.

■ Carbon dioxide is transported in blood in three forms: (1) dissolved CO_2 (10% is transported in this way), (2) CO_2 bound to hemoglobin (called carbaminohemoglobin; about 20% of blood CO_2 is transported via this form), and (3) bicarbonate (70% of CO_2 found in blood is transported as bicarbonate [HCO_3^-]).

VENTILATION AND ACID-BASE BALANCE

Pulmonary ventilation can play an important role in removing H^+ from the blood by the HCO_3^- reaction discussed previously (99). For example, an increase in CO_2 in blood or body fluids results in an increase in hydrogen ion accumulation and thus a decrease in pH. In contrast, removal of CO_2 from blood or body fluids may decrease hydrogen ion concentration and thus increase pH. Recall that the CO_2-carbonic anhydrase reaction occurs as follows:

Lung

$$CO_2 + H_2O \longleftrightarrow H_2CO_3 \longleftrightarrow H^+ + HCO_3^-$$

Muscle

Therefore, an increase in pulmonary ventilation causes exhalation of additional CO_2 and results in a reduction of blood PCO_2 and a lowering of hydrogen ion concentration. On the other side, a reduction in pulmonary ventilation would result in a buildup of CO_2 and an increase in hydrogen ion concentration (pH would decrease). The role of the pulmonary system in acid-base balance will be discussed in detail in chapter 11.

IN SUMMARY

■ An increase in pulmonary ventilation causes exhalation of additional CO_2, which results in a reduction of blood PCO_2 and a lowering of hydrogen ion concentration (i.e., pH increases).

VENTILATORY AND BLOOD-GAS RESPONSES TO EXERCISE

Before discussing ventilatory control during exercise, we should examine the ventilatory response to several different types of exercise.

FIGURE 10.21 The changes in ventilation and partial pressures of O_2 and CO_2 in the transition from rest to steady-state submaximal exercise.

Rest-to-Work Transitions

The change in pulmonary ventilation observed in the transition from rest to constant-load submaximal exercise (i.e., below the lactate threshold) is pictured in figure 10.21. Note that expired ventilation ($\dot{V}_E$) increases abruptly at the beginning of exercise, followed by a slower rise toward a steady-state value (9, 22, 23, 38, 52, 80, 81, 115).

Figure 10.21 also points out that arterial tensions of PCO_2 and PO_2 are relatively unchanged during this type of exercise (33, 35, 109). However, note that arterial PO_2 decreases and arterial PCO_2 tends to increase slightly in the transition from rest to steady-state exercise (35). This observation suggests that the increase in alveolar ventilation at the beginning of exercise is not as rapid as the increase in metabolism.

Prolonged Exercise in a Hot Environment

Figure 10.22 illustrates the change in pulmonary ventilation during prolonged, constant-load, submaximal exercise (below the lactate threshold) in two different environmental conditions. The neutral environment represents exercise in a cool, low-relative-humidity environment (19°C, 45% relative humidity). The second condition represented in figure 10.22 is a hot/high-humidity environment, which hampers heat loss from the body. The major point to appreciate from figure 10.22 is that ventilation tends to "drift" upward during prolonged work. The mechanism to explain this increase in $\dot{V}_E$ during work in the heat is an

FIGURE 10.22 Changes in ventilation and blood gas tensions during prolonged, submaximal exercise in a hot/humid environment.

increase in blood temperature, which directly affects the respiratory control center (76).

Another interesting point to gain from figure 10.22 is that although ventilation is greater during exercise in a hot/humid environment when compared to work in a cool environment, there is little difference in arterial PCO_2 between the two types of exercise. This finding suggests that the increase in ventilation seen during work in the heat is due to an increase in breathing frequency and dead-space ventilation (28). This type of breathing in humans in hot weather is similar to the panting observed in dogs and cats during warm conditions (28).

Incremental Exercise

The ventilatory response for an elite male distance runner and an untrained college student during an incremental exercise test is illustrated in figure 10.23. In both subjects, ventilation increases as a linear function of oxygen uptake up to 50% to 75% of O_2 max, where ventilation begins to rise exponentially (108). This $\dot{V}_E$ "inflection point" has been called the **ventilatory threshold (Tvent)** (53, 73, 78).

An interesting point that emerges from figure 10.23 is the startling difference between the highly trained elite athlete and the untrained subject in arterial PO_2 during heavy exercise. The untrained subject is able to maintain arterial PO_2 within 10 to 12 mm Hg of the normal resting value, while the highly trained distance runner shows a decrease of 30 to 40 mm Hg at near-maximal work (28, 29, 32). This drop in arterial PO_2, often observed in the healthy, trained athlete, is similar to that observed in exercising patients who have severe lung disease. However, not all healthy,

elite endurance athletes develop low-arterial PO_2 values (low PO_2 is called *hypoxemia*) during heavy exercise. It appears that only about 40% to 50% of highly trained, male endurance athletes ($\dot{V}O_2$ max 4.5 ℓ/min or > 68 ml · kg · min^{-1}) show this marked hypoxemia (82, 88). In addition, the degree of hypoxemia observed in these athletes during heavy work varies considerably among individuals (29, 79, 88, 106). The reason for the subject differences is unclear.

By the late 1980s it became clear that 40% to 50% of elite, male endurance athletes were capable of developing exercise-induced hypoxemia. However, it was not known until the late 1990s that elite, female endurance athletes were also capable of developing exercise-induced hypoxemia (55, 56, 58). The incidence of exercise-induced hypoxemia in elite, female athletes appears to be similar to that of males in that 25% to 51% of all highly trained, female endurance athletes exhibit exercise-induced hypoxemia (55, 58).

Perhaps the most important question concerning exercise-induced hypoxemia in healthy athletes is, What factor(s) accounts for this failure of the pulmonary system? Unfortunately, a complete answer to this question is not available. Nonetheless, it appears that both ventilation-perfusion mismatch and diffusion limitations are likely contributors to exercise-induced hypoxemia in elite athletes (67, 88, 113). Diffusion limitations during intense exercise in elite athletes could occur due to a reduced amount of time that the red blood cells spend in the pulmonary capillary (28, 34). This short red blood cell transit time in the pulmonary capillaries is due to the high cardiac outputs achieved by these athletes during high-intensity exercise, and may be less than the time required for gas equilibrium to be achieved between the lung and blood (29, 91, 116).

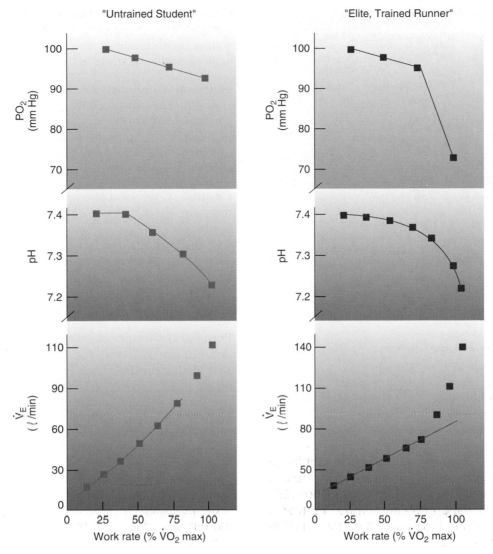

FIGURE 10.23 Changes in ventilation, blood-gas tensions, and pH during incremental exercise in a highly trained male distance runner and an untrained male college student.

CONTROL OF VENTILATION

Obviously, precise regulation of pulmonary gas exchange during rest and exercise is important in maintaining homeostasis by providing normal arterial O_2 content and maintenance of the acid-base balance within the body. Although the control of breathing has been actively studied by physiologists for many years, many unanswered questions remain. Let's begin our discussion of ventilatory control during exercise with a review of ventilatory regulation at rest.

Ventilatory Regulation at Rest

As mentioned earlier, inspiration and expiration are produced by the contraction and relaxation of the diaphragm during quiet breathing, and by accessory

muscles during exercise. Contraction and relaxation of these respiratory muscles are directly controlled by somatic motor neurons in the spinal cord. Motor neuron activity, in turn, is directly controlled by the respiratory control center in the medulla oblongata.

Respiratory Control Center The initial drive to inspire or expire comes from neurons located in the medulla oblongata (labeled as the "rhythmicity area" in figure 10.24). Discharges from some of these neurons produce inspiration, while discharges from other neurons produce expiration. These respiratory neurons act in a reciprocal way to produce a rhythmic pattern of breathing (12, 42, 95, 96). At rest, the cycle of inspiration and a passive expiration is built in, or intrinsic to, the neural activity of the medulla. However, neural activity in the medulla can be modified by

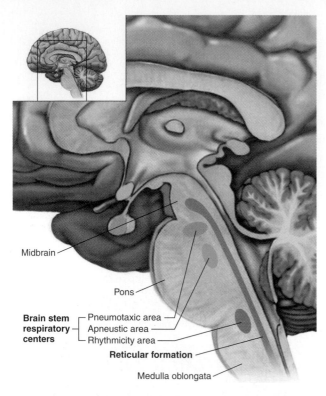

Midbrain

Pons

Brain stem respiratory centers
- Pneumotaxic area
- Apneustic area
- Rhythmicity area

Reticular formation

Medulla oblongata

FIGURE 10.24 Locations of the brain stem respiratory control centers.

neurons located outside the respiratory rhythmicity center.

Two additional areas located in the region of the brain stem, called the *pons*, contribute to respiratory control; these are the *apneustic area* and the *pneumotaxic area*. The apneustic area directly communicates with inspiratory neurons located in the rhythmicity area to stop inspiratory neuronal activity. Therefore, it is believed that the apneustic area functions as an "inspiratory cutoff switch" that terminates inspiration. Another group of respiratory neurons, the pneumotaxic area, fine-tunes the activity of the apneustic area (figure 10.24). The practical function of the apneustic/pneumotaxic areas is that they work in concert to regulate the depth of breathing (63).

Input to the Respiratory Control Center Several types of receptors are capable of modifying the actions of neurons contained in the respiratory control center. In general, input to the respiratory control center can be classified into two types: (1) neural and (2) humoral (blood-borne). Neural input refers to afferent or efferent input to the respiratory control center from neurons that are excited by means other than blood-borne stimuli. Humoral input to the respiratory control center refers to the influence of some blood-borne stimuli reaching a specialized chemoreceptor. This receptor reacts to the strength of the

stimuli and sends the appropriate message to the medulla. A brief overview of each of these receptors will be presented prior to a discussion of ventilatory control during exercise.

Humoral Chemoreceptors Chemoreceptors are specialized neurons that are capable of responding to changes in the internal environment. Traditionally, respiratory chemoreceptors are classified according to their location as being either *central chemoreceptors* or *peripheral chemoreceptors*.

Central Chemoreceptors The central chemoreceptors are located in the medulla (anatomically separate from the respiratory center) and are affected by changes in PCO_2 and H^+ of the cerebrospinal fluid (CSF). An increase in either PCO_2 or H^+ of the CSF results in the central chemoreceptors sending afferent input into the respiratory center to increase ventilation (33).

Peripheral Chemoreceptors The primary peripheral chemoreceptors are located in the aortic arch and at the bifurcation of the common carotid artery. The receptors located in the aorta are called **aortic bodies,** and those found in the carotid artery are **carotid bodies** (figure 10.25). These peripheral chemoreceptors respond to increases in arterial H^+ concentrations and PCO_2 (1, 5, 13, 117). Additionally, the carotid bodies are sensitive to increases in blood potassium levels and decreases in arterial PO_2 (19, 70). When comparing these two sets of peripheral chemoreceptors, it appears that the carotid bodies are more important (33, 63).

There is evidence that specialized (peripheral) chemoreceptors in the lungs of dogs and rabbits are sensitive to CO_2 and act to match ventilation with CO_2 return to the lungs (6, 11, 17, 49–51, 100, 102, 109, 110). In other words, an increase in CO_2 return to the lung stimulates lung receptors, which send a message to the respiratory control center to increase $\dot{V}_E$. This increase in $\dot{V}_E$ is hypothesized to be precisely matched to the amount of the CO_2 returned to the lung, and thus arterial PCO_2 remains constant. Do these lung CO_2 receptors exist in humans? At present, a definitive answer to this question is not available; exciting research in this area continues.

Effect of Blood PCO_2, PO_2, and Potassium on Ventilation How do the central and peripheral chemoreceptors respond to changes in chemical stimuli? The effects of increases in arterial PCO_2 on minute ventilation can be seen in figure 10.26. Note that $\dot{V}_E$ increases as a linear function of arterial PCO_2. In general, a 1 mm Hg rise in PCO_2 results in a 2 liter/minute increase in $\dot{V}_E$ (33). The increase in $\dot{V}_E$ that results from a rise in arterial PCO_2 is likely due to CO_2 stimulation

FIGURE 10.26 Changes in ventilation as a function of increasing arterial PCO_2. Notice that ventilation increases as a linear function of increasing PCO_2.

FIGURE 10.27 Changes in ventilation as a function of decreasing arterial PO_2. Note the existence of a "hypoxic threshold" for ventilation as arterial PO_2 declines.

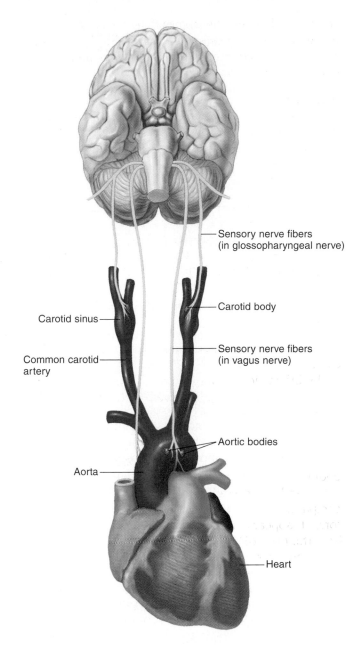

FIGURE 10.25 Illustration of the anatomical location of the peripheral chemoreceptors (i.e., aortic bodies and carotid bodies). The aortic chemoreceptors respond to arterial changes in arterial H^+ ion concentration (i.e., pH) and PCO_2. The carotid bodies also respond to arterial changes in arterial pH, PCO_2, and also changes in PO_2.

of both the carotid bodies and the central chemoreceptors (33, 71).

In healthy individuals breathing at sea level, changes in arterial PO_2 have little effect on the control of ventilation (63). However, exposure to an environment with a barometric pressure much lower than that at sea level (i.e., high altitude), can alter arterial PO_2 and stimulate the carotid bodies, which in turn signal

the respiratory center to increase ventilation. The relationship between arterial PO_2 and $\dot{V}_E$ is illustrated in figure 10.27. The point on the $PO_2/\dot{V}_E$ curve where $\dot{V}_E$ begins to rise rapidly is often referred to as the *hypoxic threshold* ("hypoxic" means low PO_2) (3). This hypoxic threshold usually occurs around an arterial PO_2 of 60 to 75 mm Hg. The chemoreceptors responsible for the increase in $\dot{V}_E$ following exposure to low PO_2 are the carotid bodies, since the aortic and central chemoreceptors in humans do not respond to changes in PO_2 (33, 63).

Recent evidence demonstrates that increases in blood levels of potassium stimulate the carotid bodies and promote an increase in ventilation (19, 70). Since blood potassium levels rise during exercise due to a net potassium efflux from the contracting muscle, some investigators have suggested that potassium may play a role in regulating ventilation during exercise (19, 70). More will be said about this later.

Neural Input to the Respiratory Control Center
Evidence obtained from animal experiments shows that neural input to the respiratory control center can

come from both efferent and afferent pathways. For example, it has been demonstrated in cats that impulses from the motor cortex (i.e., central command) can both control skeletal muscle and drive ventilation in proportion to the amount of work being performed (43, 44). In short, neural impulses originating in the motor cortex may pass through the medulla and "spill over," causing an increase in $\dot{V}_E$ that reflects the number of muscle motor units being recruited.

Afferent input to the respiratory control center during exercise may come from one of several peripheral receptors such as the muscle spindles, Golgi tendon organs, or joint pressure receptors (8, 62, 101). In addition, it is possible that special chemoreceptors located in muscle may respond to changes in potassium and H^+ concentrations and send afferent information to the respiratory control center. This type of input to the medulla is considered afferent neural information, since the stimuli is not humorally mediated. Finally, recent evidence suggests that the right ventricle of the heart contains mechanoreceptors that send afferent information back to the respiratory control center relative to increases in cardiac output (e.g., during exercise) (110). These mechanoreceptors might play important roles in providing afferent input to the respiratory control center at the onset of exercise.

Ventilatory Control During Submaximal Exercise

In the previous sections, we have discussed several possible sources of input to the respiratory control center. Unfortunately, at present, which of these factors is most responsible for ventilatory control during exercise remains controversial (8, 10, 18, 20, 27, 36, 41, 43, 47, 62, 72, 90, 109, 117). Nonetheless, it appears that ventilatory control during exercise has similarities to the control of the cardiovascular system. Indeed, there is growing evidence that the "primary" drive to increase ventilation during exercise is due to neural input from higher brain centers (central command) to the respiratory control center (31). However, the fact that arterial PCO_2 is tightly regulated during most types of submaximal exercise suggests that humoral chemoreceptors and afferent neural feedback from working muscles act to fine-tune breathing to match the metabolic rate and thus maintain a rather constant arterial PCO_2 (15, 16, 69, 109). Therefore, ventilation during exercise is regulated by several overlapping factors, which provides redundancy to the control system.

During prolonged exercise in a hot environment, ventilation can be influenced by factors other than those discussed previously. For example, the drift upward in $\dot{V}_E$ seen in figure 10.22 may be due to a direct influence of rising blood temperature on the respiratory control center, and rising blood cate-

*Act to fine-tune ventilation during exercise

FIGURE 10.28 A summary of respiratory control during submaximal exercise. See text for details.

cholamines (epinephrine and norepinephrine) stimulating the carotid bodies to increase $\dot{V}_E$ (76).

To summarize, the increase in ventilation during submaximal exercise is due to an interaction of both neural and humoral input to the respiratory control center. It seems likely that efferent neural mechanisms from higher brain centers (central command) provide the primary drive to breathe during exercise, with humoral chemoreceptors and neural feedback from working muscles providing a means of precisely matching ventilation with the amount of CO_2 produced via metabolism. This apparent redundancy in mechanisms is not surprising when one considers the important role that respiration plays in sustaining life and maintaining a steady state during exercise (48, 51). A summary of respiratory control during submaximal exercise appears in figure 10.28.

Ventilatory Control During Heavy Exercise

Controversy exists concerning the mechanism to explain the alinear rise in ventilation (ventilatory threshold) that occurs during an incremental exercise test. However, several factors may contribute to this rise. First, examination of figure 10.23 suggests that the alinear rise in $\dot{V}_E$ and the decrease in pH often occur simultaneously. Since rising H^+ levels in blood have been shown to stimulate the carotid bodies and increase $\dot{V}_E$, it has been proposed that the rise in blood lactate, which occurs during incremental exercise, is the stimulus causing the alinear rise in $\dot{V}_E$ (i.e., ventilatory threshold). Based on this belief, it is common for researchers to estimate the lactate threshold

A CLOSER LOOK 10.2

Training Reduces the Ventilatory Response to Exercise

Although exercise training does not alter the structure of the lung, endurance training does promote a decrease in ventilation during submaximal exercise at moderate-to-high-intensity work rates. For example, when comparisons are made at a fixed submaximal work rate, a training program can reduce exercise ventilation by 20% TO 30% below pretraining levels (24, 25)(see figure 10.29).

What is the mechanism to explain this training-induced reduction in exercise ventilation? A definitive answer is not known. However, it seems likely that this training effect is due to changes in the aerobic capacity of the locomotor skeletal muscles. These training-induced changes result in less production of lactic acid and probably less afferent feedback from the working muscles to stimulate breathing (24).

FIGURE 10.29 Illustration of the effects of endurance training on ventilation during exercise.

noninvasively by measurement of the ventilatory threshold (7, 20, 107, 108). However, several studies have shown that this technique is not perfect and that the ventilatory threshold and the lactate threshold do not always occur at the same work rate (45, 73).

What additional factors, other than rising blood lactate, might cause the alinear rise in $\dot{V}_E$ observed during incremental exercise? The close relationship between blood potassium levels and ventilation during heavy exercise has led several investigators to speculate that potassium is an important factor in controlling ventilation during heavy exercise (19, 64, 70). Certainly, other secondary factors, such as rising body temperature and blood catecholamines, might play a small contributory role to the increasing $\dot{V}_E$ during heavy exercise. Further, it is likely that neural input to the respiratory control center influences the ventilatory pattern during incremental exercise. For example, as exercise intensity increases, motor unit recruitment may occur in a nonlinear fashion and the associated efferent and afferent neural signals to the respiratory control center may promote the alinear rise in $\dot{V}_E$ seen at the ventilatory threshold (73).

To review, it is logical that the rise in blood lactate and reduction in blood pH observed at the lactate threshold can stimulate ventilation and thus may be a primary mechanism to explain the ventilatory thresh-

old. However, secondary factors such as an increase in blood potassium levels, rising body temperature, elevated blood catecholamines, and possible neural influences might also contribute to ventilatory control during heavy exercise (see A Closer Look 10.2).

IN SUMMARY

- The respiratory control center is contained in the medulla oblongata. At rest, the normal breathing pattern is determined by the intrinsic firing of inspiratory neurons. This can be modified by neurons outside the medulla oblongata. The apneustic center and the pneumotaxic center (both located in the pons) work together to regulate the depth of breathing by acting as a cutoff switch for inspiratory neurons.

- Input into the respiratory control center to increase ventilation can come from both neural and humoral sources. Neural input may come from higher brain centers, or it may arise from receptors in the exercising muscle. Humoral input may arise from central chemoreceptors, peripheral chemoreceptors, and/or lung CO_2 receptors. The central chemoreceptors are sensitive to increases in PCO_2 and decreases in pH.

continued

The peripheral chemoreceptors (carotid bodies are the most important) are sensitive to increases in PCO_2 and decreases in PO_2 or pH. Receptors in the lung that are sensitive to an increase in PCO_2 are hypothesized to exist.

■ The primary drive to increase ventilation during exercise probably comes from higher brain centers (central command). Also, humoral chemoreceptors and neural feedback from working muscles act to fine-tune ventilation.

■ Controversy exists concerning the mechanism to explain the alinear rise in ventilation (ventilatory threshold) that occurs during an incremental exercise test. However, it appears that the rise in blood H^+ concentration that occurs during this type of exercise provides the principal stimulus to increase ventilation via stimulation of the carotid bodies.

DO THE LUNGS ADAPT TO EXERCISE TRAINING?

It is well known that the muscular-skeletal system and the cardiovascular system are actively engaged during muscular exercise and that both organ systems undergo adaptive changes in response to regular endurance exercise. In contrast, it is generally believed that the lung in physically trained individuals is not significantly different from the lung in a sedentary individual (37, 59). More specifically, endurance exercise training (months to years) has no measurable effect on lung structure and resting pulmonary function that will improve pulmonary gas exchange during exercise (37, 59).

If both the cardiovascular system and skeletal muscles adapt to exercise training, why is the adaptability of pulmonary structures substantially less than these other links in the oxygen transport system? Unfortunately, a clear answer to this question is not available. Nonetheless, it is widely believed that the structural capacity of the normal lung is "overbuilt" and exceeds the demand for oxygen and carbon dioxide transport in young adults during exercise (37). Therefore, in most individuals, adaptation of the lung to exercise training is not required for the lung to adequately perform the job of maintaining blood-gas homeostasis during exercise. However, one exception to this rule is the highly trained and elite endurance athlete discussed earlier in this chapter. In these athletes, the inability of the lung to increase its gas exchange capabilities in response to exercise training results in a failure of the pulmonary system to match the high requirement for oxygen transfer across the blood-gas barrier during maximal exercise. This failure results in a reduction in the arterial oxygen content (i.e., hypoxemia). The impact of exercise-induced hypoxemia in elite athletes on exercise performance is discussed in the next section.

DOES THE PULMONARY SYSTEM LIMIT MAXIMAL EXERCISE PERFORMANCE?

Though some controversy exists (14), the pulmonary system is not generally considered to be the limiting factor during prolonged submaximal exercise (21, 28, 30, 39, 46). Although respiratory muscle failure can occur during certain disease states (e.g., obstructive lung disease), respiratory muscle fatigue is not thought to limit exercise in healthy humans exercising at low-to-moderate intensity at sea level (30, 39). Indeed, the major muscle of inspiration, the diaphragm, is a highly oxidative muscle that resists fatigue (84, 87, 89). The best evidence that the lungs and respiratory muscles are performing well during prolonged submaximal exercise (e.g., <75% $\dot{V}O_2$ max) is the observation that arterial oxygen content does not decrease during this type of work (86).

Historically, it has not been believed that the pulmonary system limits performance during high-intensity exercise at sea level (39, 46, 61). However, several recent studies question this idea. Indeed, new evidence suggests that the pulmonary system may limit exercise performance during high-intensity exercise (e.g., 95%–100% $\dot{V}O_2$ max) in trained and untrained healthy subjects. For example, unloading the respiratory muscles (e.g., breathing a low-density helium/oxygen gas) during heavy exercise (>90% $\dot{V}O_2$ max) improves exercise performance (60). This observation indicates that respiratory muscle fatigue may play a role in limiting human performance at extremely high work rates.

Indeed, new evidence now confirms that respiratory muscle fatigue does occur during high-intensity exercise (i.e., >10 minutes of exercise at 80% to 85% $\dot{V}O_2$ max) (4). For more details on respiratory muscle fatigue and exercise performance, see Ask the Expert 10.1.

The pulmonary system may also limit performance during high-intensity exercise in the elite endurance athlete who exhibits exercise-induced hypoxemia. Recall that in approximately 40% to 50% of elite endurance athletes, arterial PO_2 declines during heavy exercise to a level that negatively affects their ability to transport oxygen to the working muscles (83, 91, 116) (figure 10.23). In these athletes, the

ASK THE EXPERT 10.1

Respiratory Muscle Fatigue and Exercise Performance
Questions and Answers with Dr. Jerome Dempsey

Jerome Dempsey, Ph. D., a professor in the Department of Population Health Sciences at the University of Wisconsin–Madison, is an internationally known researcher in the field of pulmonary physiology and a leader in both the American Physiological Society and the American Thoracic Society. A significant portion of Dr. Dempsey's research has focused on respiratory muscle function during exercise and the regulation of pulmonary gas exchange during intense exercise. Without question, Dr. Dempsey's research team has performed many of the "classic" studies that explore the mechanisms responsible for exercise-induced hypoxemia in elite athletes and the effects of exercise on respiratory muscle function. Here, Dr. Dempsey answers questions related to the effects of respiratory muscle fatigue on both exercise performance and pulmonary gas exchange.

QUESTION 1: Recent work from your laboratory demonstrates that respiratory muscle fatigue can and does occur during exercise in humans. What types (i.e., intensity and duration) of exercise are most likely to promote respiratory muscle fatigue?

ANSWER: To date, the effects of all intensities and durations of exercise on respiratory muscle fatigue have not been investigated. Nonetheless, current evidence suggests that in healthy, trained and untrained subjects, the intensity of exercise must be very high (>80% $\dot{V}O_2$ max) and be sustained for ten minutes or longer to cause diaphragm fatigue. We believe that the fatigue process begins in the diaphragm after the first few minutes of heavy exercise and that >10 minutes of high-intensity (> 80% $\dot{V}O_2$ max) exercise can reduce maximal diaphragmatic force production by 15%–50%.

QUESTION 2: The role that respiratory muscle fatigue plays in human exercise performance has been debated for many years. In your view, does respiratory muscle fatigue limit human exercise tolerance in those exercise conditions in which respiratory muscle fatigue occurs?

ANSWER: Unfortunately, this is a complicated question and therefore the answer is not straightforward. We do know that mechanical unloading of the respiratory muscles (using a special mechanical ventilator) during high-intensity endurance exercise in healthy, fit subjects will prolong exercise time and decrease the subject's perception of breathing effort and limb muscle discomfort. So, what is it about respiratory muscle work during exercise that limits exercise performance? Since mechanical unloading of the respiratory muscles can prevent diaphragm fatigue, then perhaps diaphragm fatigue itself might cause exercise limitation. How might this occur? It is *not* a matter of diaphragm fatigue leading to arterial hypoxemia, because even without respiratory muscle unloading, there is sufficient alveolar hyperventilation and no hypoxemia. We believe the most important effect of high levels of respiratory muscle work leading to diaphragm fatigue is their effect on reducing blood flow (and, therefore, O_2 transport) to limb locomotor muscles. In support of this idea, we have recently shown that fatiguing respiratory muscles will elicit a reflex increase of sympathetically mediated vasoconstriction of limb muscle; this effect may account for the effects of changing respiratory muscle work during heavy exercise on limb blood flow.

QUESTION 3: Does respiratory muscle fatigue contribute to exercise-induced hypoxemia in elite endurance athletes?

ANSWER: Inadequate hyperventilation during exercise does contribute to many cases of exercise-induced arterial hypoxemia in elite athletes. However, the evidence does not indicate that diaphragm fatigue is a significant cause of this inadequate hyperventilation. In contrast, a significant portion of this reduced hyperventilation is due to airflow limitation by the airways in the face of very high ventilatory demand.

pulmonary system cannot keep pace with the need for respiratory gas exchange at workloads near $\dot{V}O_2$ max (28, 29, 34, 82, 83, 88). This failure in pulmonary gas exchange may limit exercise performance in these subjects (83). (see Research Focus 10.1.)

IN SUMMARY

- The pulmonary system does not limit exercise performance in healthy young subjects during prolonged submaximal exercise (e.g., work rates <90% $\dot{V}O_2$ max).
- In contrast to submaximal exercise, new evidence indicates that the repiratory system (i.e., respiratory muscle fatigue) may be a limiting factor in exercise performance at work rates >90% $\dot{V}O_2$ max. Further, incomplete pulmonary gas exchange may occur in some elite endurance athletes and limit exercise performance at high exercise intensities.

Exercise Physiology Applied to Sports

Do Nasal Strips Improve Athletic Performance?

The use of Breathe Right Nasal Strips™ (Band-Aid-like devices placed over the bridge of the nose) during athletic competition has become a common sight on athletic fields. These devices began to gain popularity in 1995 when professional football players started to use them during televised games. What are the physiological effects of these nasal strips, and can these devices improve athletic performance?

The purpose of these nasal strips is to hold the nostrils open and therefore reduce nasal airway resistance; this would theoretically increase airflow to the lungs. Initially, these devices were developed to help people with obstructive sleep apnea (i.e., stoppage of breathing).

While limited claims have been made by the manufacturer indicating that these devices improve athletic performance, some coaches and athletes believe that these devices improve athletic performance by improving airflow to the lungs and increasing oxygen delivery to the working muscles. However, to date, there is no convincing evidence that these devices increase pulmonary ventila-

tion during exercise and that performance is improved during either aerobic or anaerobic athletic events (66).

While it does not appear that these nasal strips provide a physiological benefit to the athlete, the potential psychological effect of using these strips is unknown. If using these nasal strips provides the athlete with the psychological advantage of believing that he or she can breathe easier, it seems likely that athletes will continue to use these devices in hopes of gaining an edge on their competitors.

STUDY QUESTIONS

1. What is the primary function of the pulmonary system? What secondary functions does it serve?
2. List and discuss the major anatomical components of the respiratory system.
3. What muscle groups are involved in ventilation during rest? During exercise?
4. What is the functional significance of the ventilation-perfusion ratio? How would a high V/Q ratio affect gas exchange in the lung?
5. Discuss those factors that influence the rate of diffusion across the blood-gas interface in the lung.
6. Graph the relationship between hemoglobin-O_2 saturation and the partial pressure of O_2 in the blood. What is the functional significance of the shape of the O_2-hemoglobin dissociation curve? What factors affect the shape of the curve?
7. Discuss the modes of transportation for CO_2 in the blood.
8. Graph the ventilatory response in the transition from rest to constant-load submaximal exercise. What happens to ventilation if the exercise is prolonged and performed in a hot/humid environment? Why?
9. Graph the ventilatory response to incremental exercise. Label the ventilatory threshold. What factor(s) might explain the ventilatory threshold?
10. List and identify the functions of the chemoreceptors that contribute to the control of breathing.
11. What neural afferents might also contribute to the regulation of ventilation during exercise?
12. Discuss the control of ventilation during exercise.

SUGGESTED READINGS

Anderson, S., and P. Kippelen. 2005. Exercise-induced bronchoconstriction: Pathogenesis. *Current Allergy and Asthma Reports* 5:116–22.

Beck K. et al. 2002. Exercise-induced asthma: Diagnosis, treatment, and regulatory issues. *Exercise and Sport Science Reviews* 30:1–3.

Brooks, G., T. Fahey, and K. Baldwin. 2005. *Exercise Physiology: Human Bioenergetics and Its Applications*, 4th ed. New York: McGraw-Hill Companies.

Fox, S. 2006. *Human Physiology*, 9th ed. New York: McGraw-Hill Companies.

Nielsen, H. 2003. Arterial desaturation during exercise in man: Implications for O_2 uptake and work capacity. *Scandinavian Journal of Medicine in Science and Sports* 13:339–58.

Powers, S., and R. Shanely. 2002. Exercise-induced changes in diaphragmatic bioenergetic and antioxidant capacity. *Exercise and Sport Science Reviews* 30:69–74.

West, J. 2001. *Pulmonary Physiology and Pathophysiology: An Integrated, Case-Based approach*. Hagerstown, MD: Lippincott, Williams & Wilkins.

Widmaier, E., H. Raff, and K. Strang. 2006. *Vander's Human Physiology*, 10th ed. New York: McGraw-Hill Companies.

REFERENCES

1. Allen, C., and N. Jones. 1984. Rate of change of alveolar carbon dioxide and the control of ventilation during exercise. *Journal of Physiology* (London) 355:1–9.
2. Anderson, S., and P. Kippelen. 2005. Exercise-induced bronchoconstriction: Pathogenesis. *Current Allergy and Asthma Reports* 5:116–22.
3. Asmussen, E. 1983. Control of ventilation in exercise. In *Exercise and Sport Science Reviews*, vol. 2., ed. R. Terjung. Philadelphia: Franklin Press.
4. Babcock, M. A. et al. 2002. Effects of respiratory muscle unloading on exercise-induced diaphragm fatigue. *Journal of Applied Physiology* 93:201–6.
5. Band, D. et al. 1980. Respiratory oscillations in arterial carbon dioxide tension as a signal in exercise. *Nature* 283:84–85.
6. Banzett, R., H. Coleridge, and J. Coleridge. 1978. Pulmonary CO_2 ventilatory reflex in dogs: Effective range of CO_2 and vagal cooling. *Respiration Physiology* 34:121–34.
7. Beaver, W., K. Wasserman, and B. Whipp. 1986. A new method for detecting anaerobic threshold by gas exchange. *Journal of Applied Physiology* 60:2020–27.
8. Fox, S. 2006. *Human Physiology*, 9th ed. New York: McGraw-Hill Companies.
9. Bennett, F., and W. Fordyce. 1985. Characteristics of the ventilatory exercise stimulus. *Respiration Physiology* 59:55–63.
10. Bennett, F., R. Tallman, and G. Grodins. 1984. Role of $\dot{V}CO_2$ in control of breathing in awake exercising dogs. *Journal of Applied Physiology* 56:1335–37.
11. Beon, J., W. Kuhlmann, and M. Fedde. 1980. Control of respiration in the chicken: Effects of venous CO_2 loading. *Respiration Physiology* 39:169–81.
12. Bianchi, A., M. Denavit-Saubie, and J. Champagnat. 1995. Central control of breathing in mammals: Neuronal circuitry, membrane properties, and neurotransmitters. *Physiological Reviews* 75:1–45.
13. Bisgard, G. et al. 1982. Role of the carotid body in hyperpnea of moderate exercise in goats. *Journal of Applied Physiology* 52:1216–22.
14. Boutellier, U., and P. Piwko. 1992. The respiratory system as an exercise limiting factor in normal sedentary subjects. *European Journal of Applied Physiology* 64:145–52.
15. Brice, A. et al. 1988. Is the hyperpnea of muscular contractions critically dependent upon spinal afferents? *Journal of Applied Physiology* 64:226–33.
16. Brice, A. et al. 1988. Ventilatory and PCO_2 responses to voluntary and electrically induced leg exercise. *Journal of Applied Physiology* 64:218–25.
17. Brown, H., K. Wasserman, and B. Whipp. 1976. Effect of beta-adrenergic blockade during exercise on ventilation and gas exchange. *Journal of Applied Physiology* 41:886–92.
18. Brown, D. et al. 1990. Ventilatory response of spinal cord-lesioned subjects to electrically induced exercise. *Journal of Applied Physiology* 68:2312–21.
19. Busse, M., N. Maassen, and H. Konrad. 1991. Relation between plasma K^+ and ventilation during incremental exercise after glycogen depletion and repletion in man. *Journal of Physiology* (London) 443:469–76.
20. Caozzo, V. et al. 1982. A comparison of gas exchange indices used to detect the anaerobic threshold. *Journal of Applied Physiology* 53:1184–89.
21. Capen, R. et al. 1990. Distribution of pulmonary capillary transit times in recruited networks. *Journal of Applied Physiology* 69:473–78.
22. Casaburi, R. et al. 1977. Ventilatory and gas exchange dynamics in response to sinusoidal work. *Journal of Applied Physiology* 42:300–11.
23. Casaburi, R. et al. 1978. Ventilatory control characteristics of the exercise hyperpnea discerned from dynamic forcing techniques. *Chest* 73:280–83.
24. Casaburi, R. et al. 1987. Mediation of reduced ventilatory response to exercise after endurance training. *Journal of Applied Physiology* 63:1533–38.
25. Clanton, T. et al. 1987. Effects of swim training on lung volumes and inspiratory muscle conditioning. *Journal of Applied Physiology* 62:39–46.
26. Coleridge, H., and J. Coleridge. 1995. Airway axon reflexes-where now? *News in Physiological Sciences* 10:91–96.
27. Dejours, P. 1964. Control of respiration in muscular exercise. In *Handbook of Physiology*, section 3, ed. W. Fenn. Washington: American Physiological Society.
28. Dempsey, J. 1986. Is the lung built for exercise? *Medicine and Science in Sports and Exercise* 18:143–55.
29. Dempsey, J. et al. 1982. Limitation to exercise capacity and endurance: Pulmonary system. *Canadian Journal of Applied Sports Sciences* 7:4–13.
30. Dempsey, J., E. Aaron, and B. Martin. 1988. Pulmonary function during prolonged exercise. In *Perspectives in Exercise and Sports Medicine: Prolonged Exercise*, ed. D. Lamb and R. Murray, 75–119. Indianapolis: Benchmark Press.
31. Dempsey, J., H. Forster, and D. Ainsworth. 1994. Regulation of hyperpnea, hyperventilation, and respiratory muscle recruitment during exercise. In *Regulation of Breathing*, ed. A. Pack and J. Dempsey, 1065–34. New York: Marcel Dekker.
32. Dempsey, J., and R. Fregosi. 1985. Adaptability of the pulmonary system to changing metabolic requirements. *American Journal of Cardiology* 55:59D–67D.
33. Dempsey, J., G. Mitchell, and C. Smith. 1984. Exercise and chemoreception. *American Review of Respiratory Disease* 129:31–34.
34. Dempsey, J., S. Powers, and N. Gledhill. 1990. Cardiovascular and pulmonary adaptation to physical activity. In *Exercise, Fitness, and Health: A Consensus of Current Knowledge*, ed. C. Bouchard et al., 205–16. Champaign, IL: Human Kinetics.
35. Dempsey, J., E. Vidruk, and G. Mitchell. 1985. Pulmonary control systems in exercise: Update. *Federation Proceedings* 44:2260–70.
36. Dempsey, J. et al. 1996. *Handbook of Physiology: Exercise*. Section 12: Integration of motor, circulatory, respiratory, and metabolic control. L. Rawl and J. Sheppard. New York: Oxford University Press.
37. Dempsey, J. et al. 2003. Pulmonary limitations to exercise in health. *Canadian Journal of Applied Physiology* 28 (Suppl):S2–S24.
38. Dodd, S. et al. 1988. Effects of acute beta-adrenergic blockade on ventilation and gas exchange during the rest-to-work transition. *Aviation, Space, and Environmental Medicine* 59:255–58.
39. Dodd, S. et al. 1989. Exercise performance following intense, short-term ventilatory work. *International Journal of Sports Medicine* 10:48–52.
40. Domino, K. et al. 1991. Pulmonary blood flow and ventilation-perfusion heterogeneity. *Journal of Applied Physiology* 71:252–58.
41. Duffin, J. 1994. Neural drives to breathing during exercise. *Canadian Journal of Applied Physiology* 19:289–304.

42. Duffin, J., K. Enzure, and J. Lipski. 1995. Breathing rhythm generation: Focus on the rostal ventrolateral medulla. *News in Physiological Sciences* 10:133–40.

43. Eldridge, F., D. Millhorn, and T. Waldrop. 1981. Exercise hyperpnea and locomotion: Parallel activation from the hypothalamus. *Science* 211:844–46.

44. Eldridge, F. et al. 1985. Stimulation by central command of locomotion, respiration, and circulation during exercise. *Respiration Physiology* 59:313–37.

45. England, P. et al. 1985. The effect of acute thermal dehydration on blood lactate accumulation during incremental exercise. *Journal of Sports Sciences* 2:105–11.

46. Fairburn, M. et al. 1991. Improved respiratory muscle endurance of highly trained cyclists and the effects on maximal exercise performance. *International Journal of Sports Medicine* 12:66–70.

47. Favier, R. et al. 1983. Ventilatory and circulatory transients during exercise: New arguments for a neurohumoral theory. *Journal of Applied Physiology* 54:647–53.

48. Forster, H., and L. Pan. 1991. Exercise hyperpnea: Characteristics and control. In *The Lung: Scientific Foundations*, vol. 2, ed. R. Crystal and J. West, 1553–64. New York: Raven Press.

49. Green, J., and N. Schmidt. 1984. Mechanism of hyperpnea induced by changes in pulmonary blood flow. *Journal of Applied Physiology* 56:1418–22.

50. Green, J., and M. Sheldon. 1983. Ventilatory changes associated with changes in pulmonary blood flow in dogs. *Journal of Applied Physiology* 54:997–1002.

51. Green, J. et al. 1986. Effect of pulmonary arterial PCO_2 on slowly adapting stretch receptors. *Journal of Applied Physiology* 60:2048–55.

52. Grucza, R., Y. Miyamoto, and Y. Nakazono. 1990. Kinetics of cardiorespiratory response to rhythmic-static exercise in men. *European Journal of Applied Physiology* 61:230–36.

53. Hagberg, J. et al. 1982. Exercise hyperventilation in patients with McArdle's disease. *Journal of Applied Physiology* 52:991–94.

54. Hammond, M. et al. 1986. Pulmonary gas exchange in humans during exercise at sea level. *Journal of Applied Physiology* 60:1590–98.

55. Harms, C. A. et al. 1998. Exercise-induced arterial hypoxemia in healthy young women. *Journal of Physiology* 507:619–28.

56. Harms, C. A. et al. 2000. Effect of exercise-induced arterial O_2 desaturation on $\dot{V}O_2$ max in women. *Medicine and Science in Sports and Exercise* 32:1101–8.

57. Hawgood, S., and K. Shiffer. 1991. Structures and properties of the surfactant-associated proteins. *Annual Review of Physiology* 53:375–94.

58. Hopkins, S. R. et al. 2000. Pulmonary gas exchange in women: Effects of exercise type and work increment. *Journal of Applied Physiology* 89:721–30.

59. Hopkins, S., and C. Harms. 2004. Gender and pulmonary gas exchange during exercise. *Exercise and Sport Science Reviews* 32:50–56.

60. Johnson, B., E. Aaron, M. Babcock, and J. Dempsey. 1996. Respiratory muscle fatigue during exercise: Implications for performance. *Medicine and Science in Sports and Exercise* 28:1129–37.

61. Johnson, B., and J. Dempsey. 1991. Demand vs. capacity in the aging pulmonary system. *Exercise and Sport Science Reviews* 19:171–210.

62. Kao, F. 1963. An experimental study of the pathways involved in exercise hyperpnea employing cross-circulation techniques. In *The Regulation of Human Respiration*, ed. D. Cunningham. Oxford: Blackwell.

63. Levitzky, M. 1999. *Pulmonary Physiology*. New York: McGraw-Hill Companies.

64. Lindinger, M., and G. Sjogaard. 1991. Potassium regulation during exercise. *Sports Medicine* 11:382–401.

65. Mairbaurl, H. et al. 1986. Regulation of red cell 2, 3-DPG and Hb-O_2-affinity during acute exercise. *European Journal of Applied Physiology* 55:174–80.

66. McParland, C., J. Mink, and C. Gallagher. 1991. Respiratory adaptations to dead space loading during maximal incremental exercise. *Journal of Applied Physiology* 70:55–62.

67. Nielsen, H. 2003. Arterial desaturation during exercise in man: Implications for O_2 uptake and work capacity. *Scandinavian Journal of Medicine in Science and Sports* 13:339–58.

68. O'kroy, J. A. et al. 2001. Effects of an external nasal dilator on the work of breathing during exercise. *Medicine and Science in Sports and Exercise* 33:454–58.

69. Pan, L. et al. 1995. Effect of multiple denervation on the exercise hyperpnea in awake ponies. *Journal of Applied Physiology* 79:302–11.

70. Paterson, D. 1992. Potassium and ventilation during exercise. *Journal of Applied Physiology* 72:811–20.

71. Paulev, P-E. et al. 1990. Modeling of alveolar carbon dioxide oscillations with or without exercise. *Japanese Journal of Physiology* 40:893–905.

72. Powers, S., and R. Beadle. 1985. Control of ventilation during submaximal exercise: A brief review. *Journal of Sports Sciences* 3:51–65.

73. ———. 1985. Onset of hyperventilation during incremental exercise: A brief review. *Research Quarterly for Exercise and Sport* 56:352–60.

74. Powers, S., J. Coombes, and H. Demirel. 1997. Exercise training–induced changes in respiratory muscles. *Sports Medicine* 24:120–31.

75. Powers, S., and D. Criswell. 1996. Adaptive strategies of respiratory muscles in response to endurance exercise. *Medicine and Science in Sports and Exercise* 28:1115–22.

76. Powers, S., E. Howley, and R. Cox. 1982. Ventilatory and metabolic reactions to heat stress during prolonged exercise. *Journal of Sports Medicine and Physical Fitness* 22:32–36.

77. Powers, S. et al. 1983. Effects of caffeine ingestion on metabolism and performance during graded exercise. *European Journal of Applied Physiology* 50:301–7.

78. Powers, S. et al. 1983. Ventilatory threshold, running economy, and distance running performance. *Research Quarterly for Exercise and Sport* 54:179–82.

79. Powers, S. et al. 1984. Hemoglobin desaturation during incremental arm and leg exercise. *British Journal of Sports Medicine* 18:212–16.

80. Powers, S. et al. 1985. Caffeine alters ventilatory and gas exchange kinetics during exercise. *Medicine and Science in Sports and Exercise* 18:101–6.

81. Powers, S. et al. 1987. Ventilatory and blood gas dynamics at onset and offset of exercise in the pony. *Journal of Applied Physiology* 62:141–48.

82. Powers, S. et al. 1988. Incidence of exercise-induced hypoxemia in the elite endurance athlete at sea level. *European Journal of Applied Physiology* 58:298–302.

83. Powers, S. et al. 1989. Effects of incomplete pulmonary gas exchange on O_2 max. *Journal of Applied Physiology* 66:2491–95.

84. Powers, S. et al. 1990. Endurance-training–induced cellular adaptations in respiratory muscles. *Journal of Applied Physiology* 68:2114–18.

85. Powers, S. et al. 1990. Regional metabolic differences in the rat diaphragm. *Journal of Applied Physiology* 69:648–50.

86. Powers, S. et al. 1991. Evidence for an alveolar-arterial PO_2 gradient threshold during incremental exercise. *International Journal of Sports Medicine* 12:313–18.

87. Powers, S. et al. 1992. Aging and respiratory muscle metabolic plasticity: Effects of endurance training. *Journal of Applied Physiology* 72:1068–73.

88. Powers, S. et al. 1992. Exercise-induced hypoxemia in athletes: Role of inadequate hyperventilation. *European Journal of Applied Physiology* 64:37–42.

89. Powers, S. et al. 1994. Regional training-induced alterations in diaphragmatic oxidative and antioxidant enzymes. *Respiration Physiology* 95:227–37.

90. Powers, S., M. Stuart, and G. Landry. 1988. Ventilatory and gas exchange dynamics in response to head-down tilt with and without venous occlusion. *Aviation, Space, and Environmental Medicine* 59:239–45.

91. Powers, S., and J. Williams. 1987. Exercise-induced hypoxemia in highly trained athletes. *Sports Medicine* 4:46–53.

92. Powers, S., and R. Shanely. 2002. Exercise-induced changes in diaphragmatic bioenergetic and antioxidant capacity. *Exercise and Sport Science Reviews* 30:69–74.

93. Ramonatxo, M. et al. 1991. Effect of resistive loads on pattern of respiratory muscle recruitment during exercise. *Journal of Applied Physiology* 71:1941–48.

94. Reynolds, H. 1991. Immunologic system in the respiratory tract. *Physiological Reviews* 71:1117–33.

95. Richter, D. 1982. Generation and maintenance of the respiratory rhythm. *Journal of Experimental Biology* 100:93–107.

96. Richter, D., D. Ballantyne, and J. Remmers. 1986. How is the respiratory rhythm generated? A model. *News in Physiological Sciences* 1:109–11.

97. Sheldon, M., and J. Green. 1982. Evidence for pulmonary CO_2 sensitivity on ventilation. *Journal of Applied Physiology* 52:1192–97.

98. Stamenovic, D. 1990. Micromechanical foundations of pulmonary elasticity. *Physiological Reviews* 70:1117–34.

99. Stringer, W., R. Casaburi, and K. Wasserman. 1992. Acid-base regulation during exercise in humans. *Journal of Applied Physiology* 72:954–61.

100. Suzuki, S., J. Suzuki, and T. Okubo. 1991. Expiratory muscle fatigue in normal subjects. *Journal of Applied Physiology* 70:2632–39.

101. Tibes, V. 1977. Reflex inputs to the cardiovascular and respiratory centers from dynamically working canine muscles. *Circulation Research* 41:332–41.

102. Trenchard, D., N. Russell, and H. Raybould. 1984. Nonmyelinated vagal lung receptors and reflex effects on respiration in rabbits. *Respiration Physiology* 55:63–79.

103. Vincent, H., S. Powers, H. Demirel, J. Coombes, and H. Naito. 1999. Exercise training protects against contraction-induced lipid peroxidation in the diaphragm. *European Journal of Applied Physiology* 79:268–73.

104. Vincent, H., S. Powers, D. Stewart, H. Demirel, R. A. Shanely, and Hisashi Naito. 2000. Short-term exercise training improves diaphragm antioxidant capacity and endurance. *European Journal of Applied Physiology* 81:67–74.

105. Vincent, H. K. et al. 2002. Adaptation of upper airway muscles to chronic endurance exercise. *American Journal of Respiratory and Critical Care Medicine* 166:287–93.

106. Warren, G. et al. 1991. Red blood cell pulmonary capillary transit time during exercise in athletes. *Medicine and Science in Sports and Exercise* 23:1353–61.

107. Wasserman, K. 1984. The anaerobic threshold measurement to evaluate exercise performance. *American Review of Respiratory Disease* 129:535–40.

108. Wasserman, K. et al. 1973. Anaerobic threshold and respiratory gas exchange during exercise. *Journal of Applied Physiology* 35:236–43.

109. Wasserman, K. et al. 1977. CO_2 flow to the lungs and ventilatory control. In *Muscular Exercise and the Lung*, ed. J. Dempsey and C. Reed. Madison: University of Wisconsin Press.

110. Weissman, M. et al. 1982. Cardiac output increase and gas exchange at the start of exercise. *Journal of Applied Physiology* 52:236–44.

111. West, J., and P. Wagner. 1991. Ventilation-perfusion relationships. In *The Lung: Scientific Foundations*, vol. 2, ed. R. Crystal and J. West, 1289–1305. New York: Raven Press.

112. West, J. B. 2001. *Pulmonary Physiology and Pathophysiology: An Integrated, Case-Based Approach*. Hagerstown, MD: Lippincott Williams & Wilkins.

113. Wetter, T. et al. 2002. Role of inflammatory mediators as a cause of exercise-induced arterial hypoxemia in young athletes. *Journal of Applied Physiology* 93:116–26.

114. Widmaier, E., H. Raff, and K. Strang. 2006. *Vander's Human Physiology*, 10th ed. New York: McGraw-Hill Companies.

115. Whipp, B., and S. Ward. 1990. Physiological determinants of pulmonary gas exchange kinetics during exercise. *Medicine and Science in Sports and Exercise* 22:62–71.

116. Williams, J., S. Powers, and M. Stuart. 1986. Arterial desaturation during heavy exercise in highly trained distance runners. *Medicine and Science in Sports and Exercise* 18:168–73.

117. Yamamoto, W., and M. Edwards. 1960. Homeostasis of carbon dioxide during intravenous infusion of carbon dioxide. *Journal of Applied Physiology* 15:807–18.

CHAPTER 11

Acid-Base Balance During Exercise

■ Objectives

By studying this chapter, you should be able to do the following:

1. Define the terms *acid*, *base*, and *p*H.

2. Discuss the importance of acid-base regulation to exercise performance.

3. List the principal intracellular and extracellular buffers.

4. Explain the role of respiration in the regulation of acid-base status during exercise.

5. Outline acid-base regulation during exercise.

6. Discuss the principal ways that hydrogen ions are produced during exercise.

■ Outline

Acids, Bases, and pH   231

Hydrogen Ion Production During Exercise   232

Importance of Acid-Base Regulation During Exercise   234

Acid-Base Buffer Systems   234
   Intracellular Buffers   234
   Extracellular Buffers   235

Respiratory Influence on Acid-Base Balance   236

Regulation of Acid-Base Balance via the Kidneys   236

Regulation of Acid-Base Balance During Exercise   237

■ Key Terms

acid
acidosis
alkalosis
base

buffer
hydrogen ions
ion
pH

respiratory compensation
strong acids
strong bases

Electrolytes that release **hydrogen ions** are called *acids* (an **ion** is any atom that is missing electrons or has gained electrons). Substances that readily combine with hydrogen ions are termed *bases*. In physiology, the concentration of hydrogen ions is expressed in pH units. The pH of body fluids must be regulated (i.e., normal arterial blood pH = 7.40 ± .02) in order to maintain homeostasis. Regulation of the pH of body fluids is extremely important since changes in hydrogen ion concentrations can alter the rates of enzyme-controlled metabolic reactions and modify numerous other normal body functions. Therefore, acid-base balance is primarily concerned with the regulation of hydrogen ion concentrations. Heavy exercise can present a serious challenge to hydrogen ion control systems due to lactic acid production, and hydrogen ions may limit performance in some types of intense activities (4, 5, 11, 15, 17, 20, 24, 29, 30, 33, 35). Given the potential detrimental influence of hydrogen ion accumulation on exercise performance, it is important that the student of exercise physiology have an understanding of acid-base regulation.

ACIDS, BASES, AND PH

In biological systems, one of the simplest but most important ions is the hydrogen ion. The concentration of the hydrogen ion influences the rates of chemical reaction, the shape and function of enzymes as well as other cellular proteins, and the integrity of the cell itself (7, 9, 13, 39, 43, 44).

An **acid** is defined as a molecule that can liberate hydrogen ions and thus can raise the hydrogen ion concentration of an aqueous solution above that of pure water. In contrast, a **base** is a molecule that is capable of combining with hydrogen ions and therefore lowers the hydrogen ion concentration of the solution.

Acids that tend to give up hydrogen ions (ionize) more completely are termed **strong acids.** For example, lactic acid produced during heavy exercise as a result of glycolysis is a relatively strong acid. At normal body pH, lactic acid tends to liberate almost all of its hydrogen ions and therefore elevates the hydrogen ion concentration of the body.

Bases that ionize completely are defined as **strong bases.** The bicarbonate ion HCO_3 is an example of a biologically important strong base. Bicarbonate ions are found in relatively large concentrations in blood and are capable of combining with hydrogen ions to form a weak acid called carbonic acid. The role of HCO_3 in the regulation of acid-base balance during exercise will be discussed later in the chapter.

As stated earlier, the concentration of hydrogen ions is expressed in pH units. The **pH** of a solution is defined as the negative logarithm of the hydrogen ion concentration (H^+). Recall that a logarithm is the

pH of Arterial Blood

Normal pH

Acidosis | Alkalosis

7.0   7.4   7.8

Survival range

FIGURE 11.1 The pH scale. If the pH of arterial blood drops below the normal value of 7.4, the resulting condition is termed acidosis. In contrast, if the pH increases above 7.4, blood alkalosis occurs.

exponent that indicates the power to which one number must be raised to obtain another number. For instance, the logarithm of 100 to the base 10 is 2. Thus, the definition of pH can be written mathematically as:

$$pH = -\log_{10} [H^+]$$

As an example, if the $[H^+]$ = 40 nM (0.000000040 M), then the pH would be 7.40.

A solution is considered neutral (in terms of acid-base status) if the concentration of H^+ and hydroxyl ions (OH^-) are equal. This is the case for pure water, in which the concentrations are both 0.00000010 M. Thus, the pH of pure water is:

$$pH \text{ (pure water)} = -\log_{10} [H^+]$$
$$= 7.0$$

Figure 11.1 shows the continuum of the pH scale. Note that as the hydrogen ion concentration increases, pH declines and the acidity of the blood increases, resulting in a condition termed **acidosis.** Conversely, as the hydrogen ion concentration decreases, pH increases and the solution becomes more basic (alkalotic). This condition is termed **alkalosis.** Conditions leading to acidosis or alkalosis are summarized in figure 11.2.

The normal arterial pH is 7.4 and in health, this value varies, less than 0.05 pH units. Interestingly, the body is more tolerant to acidosis than to alkalosis. The lowest pH that is consistent with survival is 6.8 (decrease of 0.6 pH units below normal) whereas the highest pH tolerated is 7.8 (an increase of 0.4 pH units) (37).

Failure to maintain acid-base homeostasis in the body can have lethal consequences. Indeed, even small changes in blood pH can have negative effects on the function of organ systems. For example, both increases and decreases in arterial pH can promote abnormal electrical activity in the heart, resulting in rhythm disturbances. In fact, large disturbances in arterial pH homeostasis have been associated with life-threatening rhythm disturbances in the heart (37). Numerous disease states can result in acid-base disturbances in the body and are introduced in Clinical Applications 11.1

Conditions and Diseases that Promote Metabolic Acidosis or Alkalosis

The normal arterial pH is 7.4 and in healthy individuals, this value is maintained within 0.05 pH units. As mentioned previously, failure to maintain acid-base homeostasis in the body can have serious consequences and can lead to dysfunction of essential organs. Indeed, even relatively small changes in arterial pH (i.e., 0.1–0.2 pH units) can have significant negative impact on organ function.

Metabolic acidosis occurs due to a gain in the amount of acid in the body. A number of conditions or disease states can promote metabolic acidosis. For example, long-term starvation (i.e., several days) can result in metabolic acidosis due to the production of ketoacids in the body as a by-product of fat metabolism. In extreme circumstances, the type of metabolic acidosis can result in death.

Diabetes is a common metabolic disease that promotes metabolic acidosis. Uncontrolled diabetes can result in a form of metabolic acidosis called diabetic ketoacidosis. Similar to starvation-induced acidosis, this form of acidosis is also due to the overproduction of ketoacids due to high levels of fat metabolism. Worldwide, numerous deaths occur each year from this form of acidosis (37).

Metabolic alkalosis results from a loss of acids from the body. Conditions leading to metabolic alkalosis include severe vomiting and diseases such as kidney disorders that result in a loss of acids (37). In both of these circumstances, the loss of acids results in an overabundance of bases in the body, leading to metabolic alkalosis.

FIGURE 11.2 Acidosis results from an accumulation of acids or a loss of bases. Alkalosis results from a loss of acids or an accumulation of bases.

IN SUMMARY

- Acids are defined as molecules that can liberate hydrogen ions, which increases the hydrogen ion concentration of an aqueous solution.
- Bases are molecules that are capable of combining with hydrogen ions.
- The concentration of hydrogen ions in a solution is quantified by pH units. The pH of a solution is defined as the negative logarithm of the hydrogen ion concentration:

$$pH = -\log_{10}[H^+]$$

HYDROGEN ION PRODUCTION DURING EXERCISE

Although small quantities of acids or bases are present in foods, the major threat to the pH of body fluids is acids formed in metabolic processes. These metabolic acids can be divided into three major groups (8, 20):

1. Volatile acids (e.g., carbon dioxide). Carbon dioxide, an end product in the oxidation of carbohydrates, fats, and proteins, can be regarded as an acid by virtue of its ability to react with water to form carbonic acid (H_2CO_3), which in turn dissociates to form H^+ and HCO_3^-:

$$CO_2 + H_2O \longleftrightarrow H_2CO_3 \longleftrightarrow H^+ + HCO_3$$

Because CO_2 is a gas and can be eliminated by the lungs, it is often referred to as a volatile acid. During the course of a day, the body produces large amounts of CO_2 due to normal metabolism. During exercise, metabolic production of CO_2 increases and therefore adds an additional "volatile acid" load on the body.

2. Fixed acids (e.g., sulfuric acid and phosphoric acid). Sulfuric acid is a product of the oxidation of certain amino acids, while phosphoric acid is formed in the metabolism of various phospholipids and nucleic acids. In contrast to CO_2, both sulfuric acid and phosphoric acid are nonvolatile and therefore are referred to as fixed acids. The production of fixed acids varies with the diet and

A CLOSER LOOK 11.1

Sport and Exercise-Induced Disturbances in Muscle Acid-Base Balance

What types of sports or exercise promote acid-base disturbances in skeletal muscle? In general, any sport or exercise activity requiring high-intensity muscular contractions that persist for 45 seconds or longer can produce significant amounts of hydrogen ions resulting in a decrease in muscle and blood pH. Table 11.1 provides a list of popular sports and the risk of developing muscle acid-base disturbances in each sport. Note that the risk of acid-base disturbances is classified as being high, moderate, or low. For sports classified in the low-to-moderate risk category (e.g., soccer), the risk of muscle acid-base distur-

bance is often connected to effort of the competitor. That is, an aggressive athlete that is constantly playing at 100% effort is more likely to develop an acid-base imbalance compared to the athlete that plays at "half speed" during the game. Also, note that track and field races like the 5,000 and 10,000 meter runs are listed as moderate and low-to-moderate risks for acid-base disturbances, respectively. In these types of track races, athletes may produce limited amounts of lactic acid during most of the race, but a sustained sprint to the finish during the last lap of these events could result in production of relatively large amounts

of lactic acid and, therefore, result in acid-base disturbances in the muscle and blood.

Since acid-base disturbances can contribute to muscle fatigue and limit exercise performance, it is not surprising that some exercise scientists have investigated the possibility that increasing the buffering capacity of the blood results in improved exercise performance. One approach to this problem is to ingest large quantities of a buffer prior to exercise. A detailed discussion of this topic can be found in The Winning Edge 11.1.

TABLE 11.1	Risk of Developing an Acid-Base Disturbance in Popular Sports
Sport	**Risk of Acid-Base Disturbance**
Baseball	Low
Basketball	Low-to-moderate
Boxing	Low-to-moderate
Cross-country skiing	Low
Football (American)	Low
100-meter sprint	Low
100-meter swim	High
400-meter run	High
800-meter run	High
1,500-meter run	Moderate-to-high
5,000-meter run	Moderate
10,000-meter run	Low-to-moderate
Marathon run	Low
Soccer	Low-to-moderate
Weight lifting (low repetitions)	Low
Volleyball	Low

normal resting conditions, both of these acids are further metabolized to CO_2 and therefore do not greatly influence the pH of body fluids. However, an exception to this rule occurs during heavy exercise (i.e., work above the lactate threshold). During periods of intense physical efforts, contracting skeletal muscles can produce large amounts of lactic acid, resulting in acidosis. In general, it appears that the production of lactic acid during heavy exercise presents the greatest challenge to maintaining pH homeostasis during exercise. Some metabolic processes that serve as sources of hydrogen ions are illustrated in figure 11.3.

While it is clear that high-intensity exercise of sufficient duration (i.e., >45 seconds) can produce large quantities of lactic acid, not all sports or exercise activities produce significant amounts of hydrogen ions. A detailed discussion of which sports or exercise activities pose the greatest risk of producing significant acid-base disturbances is contained in a Closer Look 11.1

is not greatly influenced by acute exercise. Hence, fixed acids are not a major contributor of hydrogen ions during heavy exercise.

3. Organic acids (e.g., lactic acid). Organic acids, such as lactic acid and acetoacetic acid, are formed in the metabolism of carbohydrates and fats, respectively (see chapters 3 and 4). Under

IN SUMMARY

- Metabolic acids can be subdivided into three major groups: (1) volatile acids (e.g., carbon dioxide), (2) fixed acids (e.g., sulfuric acid, phosphoric acid), and (3) organic acids (e.g., lactic acid).

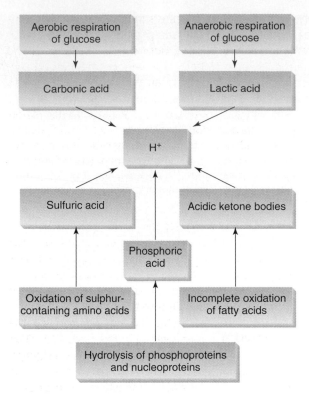

FIGURE 11.3 Sources of hydrogen ions due to metabolic processes.

IMPORTANCE OF ACID-BASE REGULATION DURING EXERCISE

As discussed earlier, heavy exercise results in the production of large amounts of lactic acid by the contracting skeletal muscle. Lactic acid, a strong acid, ionizes and releases hydrogen ions. These hydrogen ions can exert a powerful effect on other molecules due to their small size and positive charge. Hydrogen ions exert their influence by attaching to molecules and thus altering their original size and shape (5, 11, 14, 27, 36). This change in size and shape may alter the normal function of the molecule (enzyme) and therefore influence metabolism in an important way.

An increase in the intramuscular hydrogen ion concentration can impair exercise performance in at least two ways. First, an increase in the hydrogen ion concentration reduces the muscle cell's ability to produce ATP by inhibiting key enzymes involved in both anaerobic and aerobic production of ATP (5, 11, 16). Second, hydrogen ions compete with calcium ions for binding sites on troponin, thereby hindering the contractile process (5, 11, 42). This will be discussed again in chapter 19.

IN SUMMARY

- Failure to maintain acid-base homeostasis during exercise can impair performance by inhibiting metabolic pathways responsible for the production of ATP or by interfering with the contractile process in the working muscle.

ACID-BASE BUFFER SYSTEMS

From the preceding discussion, it is clear that a rapid accumulation of hydrogen ions during heavy exercise can negatively influence muscular performance. Therefore, it is important that the body have control systems capable of regulating acid-base status to prevent drastic decreases or increases in pH. How does the body regulate pH? One of the most important means of regulating hydrogen ion concentrations in body fluids is by the aid of buffers. A **buffer** resists pH change by removing hydrogen ions when the hydrogen ion concentration increases, and releasing hydrogen ions when the hydrogen ion concentration falls.

Buffers often consist of a weak acid and its associated base (called a conjugate base). The ability of individual buffers to resist pH change is dependent upon two factors. First, individual buffers differ in their intrinsic physiochemical ability to act as buffers. Simply stated, some buffers are better than others. A second factor influencing buffering capacity is the concentration of the buffer present. The greater the concentration of a particular buffer, the more effective the buffer can be in preventing pH change.

Intracellular Buffers

The first line of defense in protecting against pH change during exercise is in the cell itself. The most common intracellular buffers are proteins and phosphate groups (20). Many intracellular proteins contain ionizable groups that are weak acids capable of accepting hydrogen ions. Intracellular phosphocreatine (see chapter 3) has been shown to be a useful buffer at the onset of exercise (1). Further, weak phosphoric acids are found in relatively large concentrations in cells and also serve as an intracellular buffer system. In addition, bicarbonate in muscle has been demonstrated to be a useful buffer during exercise (14). A summary of the chemical action of intracellular buffer systems is presented in table 11.2.

Extracellular Buffers

The blood contains three principal buffer systems (14, 20): (1) proteins, (2) hemoglobin, and (3) bicarbonate.

Buffer System	Constituents	Actions
TABLE 11.2	**Chemical Acid-Base Buffer Systems**	
Bicarbonate system	Sodium bicarbonate ($NaHCO_3$)	Converts strong acid into weak acid
	Carbonic acid (H_2CO_3)	Converts strong base into weak base
Phosphate system	Sodium phosphate (Na_2HPO_4)	Converts strong acid into weak acid
Protein system	COO^- group of a molecule	Accepts hydrogens in the presence of excess acid
	NH_3 group of a molecule	Accepts hydrogens in the presence of excess acid

Blood proteins act as buffers in the extracellular compartment. Like intracellular proteins, these blood proteins contain ionizable groups that are weak acids and therefore act as buffers. However, because blood proteins are found in small quantities, their usefulness as buffers during heavy exercise is limited.

In contrast, hemoglobin is a particularly important protein buffer and is a major blood buffer during resting conditions. In fact, hemoglobin has approximately six times the buffering capacity of plasma proteins due to its high concentration (20). Also contributing to the effectiveness of hemoglobin as a buffer is the fact that deoxygenated hemoglobin is a better buffer than oxygenated hemoglobin. As a result, once hemoglobin becomes deoxygenated in the capillaries, it is better able to bind hydrogen ions formed when CO_2 enters the blood from the tissues. Thus, hemoglobin helps to minimize pH changes caused by loading of CO_2 into the blood.

The bicarbonate buffer system is probably the most important buffer system in the body (20). This fact has been exploited by some investigators who have demonstrated that an increase in blood bicarbonate concentration (ingestion of bicarbonate) results in an improvement in performance in some types of exercise (4, 17, 22) (see The Winning Edge 11.1).

THE WINNING EDGE 11.1

Exercise Physiology Applied to Sports

Ingestion of Sodium Buffers and Human Performance

Since exercise-induced disturbances in muscle acid-base balance has been linked to muscle fatigue and impaired sport performance, several studies have explored the possibility that ingestion of a sodium buffer can improve athletic performance. Although not all investigators have reported an improvement in human performance with the ingestion of sodium buffers (2), many studies have found that performance during high-intensity exercise is improved when athletes ingest a sodium buffer prior to exercise (3, 4, 22, 28, 30). Two buffers that have been studied extensively are sodium bicarbonate and sodium citrate. In general, results from several studies suggest that boosting the blood-buffering capacity by ingestion of these buffers increases time to exhaustion during high-intensity exercise (e.g., 80%–120% $\dot{V}O_2$ max). It seems likely that if ingestion of a buffer improves physical performance, it does so by increasing the extracellular buffering capacity, which in turn increases the transport of lactate and hydrogen ions out of the muscle fibers (32). This would reduce the interference of hydrogen ions on bioenergetic ATP production and/or the contractile process itself.

In deciding to use sodium bicarbonate or sodium citrate prior to a sporting event, an athlete should understand the risks associated with the procedure. Ingestion of sodium bicarbonate in the doses required to improve blood-buffering capacity can cause gastrointestinal problems including diarrhea and vomiting (4, 30). In contrast, the ingestion of sodium citrate has been reported to improve exercise performance without the same gastrointestinal side effects associated with sodium bicarbonate (19, 25). Regardless of the type of buffer ingested, extremely large does of any buffer could result in severe alkalosis and have serious health consequences. A final consideration in the use of any ergogenic aid is the legality of the drug. In regard to the use of acid-base buffers, numerous sport regulatory agencies have banned the use of sodium buffers during competition.

The bicarbonate buffer system involves the weak acid H_2CO_3, which undergoes the following dissociation reaction:

$$CO_2 + H_2O \longleftrightarrow H_2CO_3 \longleftrightarrow H^+ + HCO_3^-$$

The ability of carbonic acid (H_2CO_3) to act as a buffer is described mathematically by a relationship known as the Henderson-Hasselbalch equation:

$$pH = pKa + \log_{10}\left(\frac{HCO_3^-}{H_2CO_3}\right)$$

where pKa is the dissociation constant for H_2CO_3 and has a constant value of 6.1. In short, the Henderson-Hasselbalch equation states that the pH of a weak acid solution is determined by the ratio of the concentration of base (i.e., bicarbonate) in solution to the concentration of acid (i.e., carbonic acid). The normal pH of arterial blood is 7.4, and the ratio of bicarbonate to carbonic acid is 20 to 1. Let's consider an example using the Henderson-Hasselbalch equation to calculate arterial blood pH. Normally the concentration of blood bicarbonate is 24 m Eq/l and the concentration of carbonic acid is 1.2 m Eq/l. Therefore, the blood pH can be calculated as follows:

$$pH = pKa + \log_{10} 24/1.2$$
$$= 6.1 + \log_{10} 20$$
$$= 6.1 + 1.3$$
$$pH = 7.4$$

IN SUMMARY

■ The body maintains acid-base homeostasis by buffer-control systems. A buffer resists pH change by removing hydrogen ions when the pH declines and by releasing hydrogen ions when the pH increases.
■ The principal intracellular buffers are proteins, phosphate groups, and bicarbonate. Primary extracellular buffers are bicarbonate, hemoglobin, and blood proteins.

RESPIRATORY INFLUENCE ON ACID-BASE BALANCE

Recall that CO_2 is considered a volatile acid because it can be readily changed from CO_2 to carbonic acid. Also, recall that it is the partial pressure of CO_2 in the blood that determines the concentration of carbonic acid. For example, according to Henry's law, the concentration of a gas in solution is directly proportional to its partial pressure. That is, as the partial pressure

increases, the concentration of the gas in solution increases and vice versa.

Because CO_2 is a gas, it can be eliminated by the lungs. Therefore the respiratory system is an important regulator of blood carbonic acid and pH. To better understand the role of the lungs in acid-base balance, let's reexamine the carbonic acid dissociation equation:

$$CO_2 + H_2O \longleftrightarrow H_2CO_3 \longleftrightarrow H^+ + HCO_3^-$$

This relationship demonstrates that when the amount of CO_2 in the blood increases, the amount of H_2CO_3 increases, which lowers pH by elevating the acid concentration of the blood (i.e., the reaction moves to the right). In contrast, when the CO_2 content of the blood is lowered (i.e., CO_2 is "blown off" by the lungs), the pH of the blood increases because less acid is present (reaction moves to the left). Therefore, the respiratory system provides the body with a rapid means of regulating blood pH by controlling the amount of CO_2 present in the blood.

IN SUMMARY

■ Respiratory control of acid-base balance involves the regulation of blood PCO_2. An increase in blood PCO_2 lowers pH, whereas a decrease in blood PCO_2 increases pH.

REGULATION OF ACID-BASE BALANCE VIA THE KIDNEYS

Since the kidneys do not play an important part in acid-base regulation during short-term exercise, only a brief overview of the kidney's role in acid-base balance will be presented here. The principal means by which the kidneys regulate hydrogen ion concentration is by increasing or decreasing the bicarbonate concentration (6, 8, 18). When the hydrogen ion concentration increases in body fluids, the kidney responds by a reduction in the rate of bicarbonate excretion. This results in an increase in the blood bicarbonate concentration and therefore assists in buffering the increase in hydrogen ions. Conversely, when the pH of body fluids rises (hydrogen ion concentration decreases), the kidneys increase the rate of bicarbonate excretion. Therefore, by changing the amount of buffer present in body fluids, the kidneys aid in the regulation of the hydrogen ion concentration. The kidney mechanism involved in regulating the bicarbonate concentration is located in a portion of the kidney called the *tubule*, and acts through a series of complicated reactions and active transport across the tubular wall.

Why is the kidney not an important regulator of acid-base balance during exercise? The answer lies in the amount of time required for the kidney to respond to an acid-base disturbance. It takes several hours for the kidneys to react effectively in response to an increase in blood hydrogen ions (6–8). Therefore, the kidneys respond too slowly to be of major benefit in the regulation of hydrogen ion concentration during exercise.

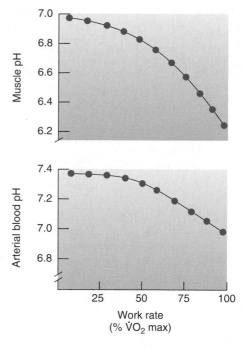

IN SUMMARY

- Although the kidneys play an important role in the long-term regulation of acid-base balance, the kidneys are not significant in the regulation of acid-base balance during exercise.

REGULATION OF ACID-BASE BALANCE DURING EXERCISE

During the final stages of an incremental exercise test or during near-maximal exercise of short duration, there is a decrease in both muscle and blood pH primarily due to the increase in the production of lactic acid by the muscle (10, 12, 23). This point is illustrated in figure 11.4, where the changes in blood and muscle pH during an incremental exercise test are graphed as a function of % $\dot{V}O_2$ max. Note that muscle and blood pH follow similar trends during this type of exercise, but that muscle pH is always 0.4 to 0.6 pH units lower than blood pH (21, 26). This is because muscle lactic acid concentration is higher than that of blood, and muscle buffering capacity is lower than that of blood.

The amount of lactic acid produced during exercise is dependent on: (1) the exercise intensity, (2) the amount of muscle mass involved, and (3) the duration of the work (10, 12). Exercise involving high-intensity leg work (e.g., running) may reduce arterial pH from 7.4 to a value of 7.0 within a few minutes (10, 15, 21, 31, 40). Further, repeated bouts of this type of exercise may cause blood pH to decline even further to a value of 6.8 (10). This blood pH value is the lowest ever recorded and would present a life-threatening situation if it were not corrected within a few minutes.

How does the body regulate acid-base balance during exercise? Since the primary source of hydrogen ions released during exercise is lactic acid produced within the working muscles, it is reasonable that the first line of defense against a rise in acid production would reside in the muscle itself. This is indeed the case. It is estimated that intracellular proteins con-

FIGURE 11.4 Changes in arterial blood pH and muscle pH during incremental exercise. Notice that arterial and muscle pH begin to fall together at work rates above 50% $\dot{V}O_2$ max.

tribute as much as 60% of the cell's buffering capacity, with an additional 20% to 30% of the total buffering capacity coming from muscle bicarbonate (20). The final 10% to 20% of muscle buffering capacity comes from intracellular phosphate groups.

Since the muscle's buffering capacity is limited, extracellular fluid (principally the blood) must possess a means of buffering hydrogen ions as well. The principal extracellular buffer and probably the most important buffer in the body is blood bicarbonate (20). Hemoglobin and blood proteins assist in this buffer process, but play only a minor role in blood buffering of lactic acid during exercise (20). Figure 11.5 illustrates the role of blood bicarbonate as a buffer during incremental exercise. Note that as blood lactic acid concentration increases, blood bicarbonate concentration decreases proportionally (41). Also note that at approximately 50% to 60% of $\dot{V}O_2$ max, blood pH begins to decline due to the rise in lactic acid production. This increase in blood hydrogen ion concentration stimulates the carotid bodies, which then signal the respiratory control center to increase alveolar ventilation (i.e., ventilatory threshold; see chapter 10). An increase in alveolar ventilation results in the reduction of blood PCO_2 and therefore acts to reduce the acid load produced by exercise. The overall process of respiratory assistance in buffering lactic

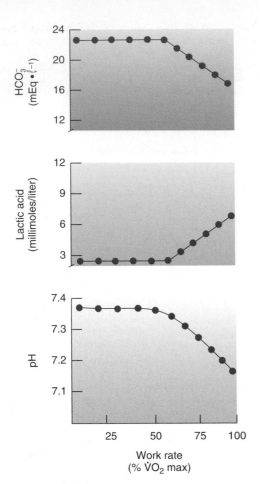

FIGURE 11.5 Changes in blood concentrations of lactic acid, bicarbonate, and pH as a function of work rate.

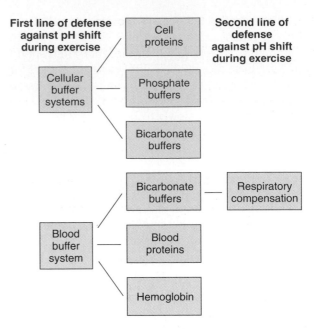

FIGURE 11.6 Lines of defense against pH change during intense exercise.

acid during exercise is referred to as **respiratory compensation** for metabolic acidosis.

- Figure 11.6 outlines the process of buffering exercise-induced acidosis.

- The first line of defense against exercise-produced hydrogen ions is the chemical buffer systems of the intracellular compartment and the blood. These buffer systems act rapidly to convert strong acids into weak acids.
- Intracellular buffering occurs with the aid of cellular proteins, bicarbonate, and phosphate groups.
- Blood buffering of hydrogen ions occurs through bicarbonate, hemoglobin, and blood proteins, with bicarbonate playing the most important role.
- The second line of defense against pH shift during exercise is respiratory compensation for metabolic acidosis.

STUDY QUESTIONS

1. Define the terms *acid, base, buffer, acidosis, alkalosis,* and *pH.*
2. Graph the pH scale. Label the pH values that represent normal arterial and intracellular pH.
3. List and briefly discuss the three major groups of acids formed by the body.
4. Why is the maintenance of acid-base homeostasis important to physical performance?
5. What are the principal intracellular and extracellular buffers?
6. Discuss respiratory compensation for metabolic acidosis. What would happen to blood pH if an individual began to hyperventilate at rest? Why?
7. Briefly, outline how the body resists pH change during exercise.

SUGGESTED READINGS

Bahrke, M. S., and C. Yesalis. 2002. *Performance-Enhancing Substances in Sport and Exercise.* Champaign, IL: Human Kinetics Publishers.

Brooks, G., T. Fahey, and K. Baldwin. 2005. *Exercise Physiology: Human Bioenergetics and Its Applications,* 4th ed. New York: McGraw-Hill Companies.

Fox, S. 2006. *Human Physiology*, 9th ed. New York: McGraw-Hill Companies.

Maughan, R., D. King, and T. Lea. 2004. Dietary supplements. *Journal of Sports Sciences* 22:95–113.

McNaughton, L., and D. Thompson. 2001. Acute versus chronic sodium bicarbonate ingestion and anaerobic work and power output. *Journal of Sports Medicine and Physical Fitness* 41:456–62.

Stephens, T. et al. 2002. Effect of sodium bicarbonate on muscle metabolism during intense endurance cycling. *Medicine and Science in Sports and Exercise* 34: 614–21.

Widmaier, E., H. Raff, and K. Strang. 2006. *Vander's Human Physiology*, 10th ed. New York: McGraw-Hill Companies.

REFERENCES

1. Adams, G., J. Foley, and R. Meyer. 1990. Muscle buffer capacity estimated from pH changes during rest-to-work transitions. *Journal of Applied Physiology* 69:968–72.

2. Aschenback, W., J. Ocel, C. Ward, E. Spangenburg, and J. Williams. 2000. Effect of oral sodium loading on high intensity arm ergometry in college wrestlers. *Medicine and Science in Sports and Exercise* 32:669–75.

3. Coombes, J. S., and L. McNaughton. 1993. The effects of bicarbonate ingestion on leg strength and power during isokinetic knee flexion and extension. *Journal of Strength and Conditioning Research* 7(4):241–49.

4. Costill, D. et al. 1984. Acid-base balance during repeated bouts of exercise: Influence of bicarbonate. *International Journal of Sports Medicine* 5:228–31.

5. Edwards, R. H. T. 1983. Biochemical bases of fatigue in exercise performance: Catastrophe theory of muscular fatigue. In *Biochemistry of Exercise*. Champaign, IL: Human Kinetics.

6. Fox, E., M. Foss, and S. Keteyian. 1998. *Fox's Physiological Basis for Exercise and Sport*. New York: McGraw-Hill Companies.

7. Fox, S. 2006. *Human Physiology*, 9th ed. New York: McGraw-Hill Companies.

8. Guyton, A., and J. E. Hall. 2000. *Textbook of Medical Physiology*. Philadelphia: W. B. Saunders.

9. Hole, J. 1995. *Human Anatomy and Physiology*. New York: McGraw-Hill Companies.

10. Hultman, E., and K. Sahlin. 1980. Acid-base balance during exercise. In *Exercise and Sport Science Reviews*, vol. 8, ed. R. Hutton and D. Miller, 41–128. Philadelphia: Franklin Institute Press.

11. Hultman, E., and J. Sjoholm. 1986. Biochemical causes of fatigue. In *Human Muscle Power*, ed. N. Jones, N. McCartney, and A. McComas. Champaign, IL: Human Kinetics.

12. Itoh, H., and T. Ohkuwa. 1991. Ammonia and lactate in the blood after short-term sprint exercise. *European Journal of Applied Physiology* 62:22–25.

13. Johnson, L. 1983. *Biology*. New York: McGraw-Hill Companies.

14. Jones, N. L. 1980. Hydrogen ion balance during exercise. *Clinical Science* 59:85–91.

15. Jones, N. et al. 1977. Effect of pH on cardiorespiratory and metabolic responses to exercise. *Journal of Applied Physiology* 43:959–64.

16. Karlsson, J. 1979. Localized muscular fatigue: Role of metabolism and substrate depletion. In *Exercise and Sport Science Reviews*, vol. 7, ed. R. Hutton and D. Miller, 1–42. Philadelphia: Franklin Institute Press.

17. Katz, A. et al. 1984. Maximal exercise tolerance after induced alkalosis. *International Journal of Sports Medicine* 5:107–10.

18. Kiil, F. 2002. Mechanisms of transjunctional transport of NaCl and water in proximal tubules of mammalian kidneys. *Acta Physiologica Scandanavia* 175:55–70.

19. Kowalchuk, J. et al. 1989. The effect of citrate loading on exercise performance, acid-base balance and metabolism. *European Journal of Applied Physiology* 58:858–64.

20. Laiken, N., and D. Fanestil. 1985. Acid-base balance and regulation of hydrogen ion excretion. In *Physiological Basis of Medical Practice*, ed. J. West. Baltimore: Lippincott Williams & Wilkins.

21. Linderman, J. et al. 1990. A comparison of blood gases and acid-base measurements in arterial, arterialized venous, and venous blood during short-term maximal exercise. *European Journal of Applied Physiology* 61: 294–301.

22. Linderman, J., and T. Fahey. 1991. Sodium bicarbonate ingestion and exercise performance: An update. *Sports Medicine* 11:71–77.

23. Marsh, G. et al. 1991. Coincident thresholds in intracellular phosphorylation potential and pH during progressive exercise. *Journal of Applied Physiology* 71:1076–81.

24. McCartney, N., G. Heigenhauser, and N. Jones. 1983. Effects of pH on maximal power output and fatigue during short-term dynamic exercise. *Journal of Applied Physiology* 55:225–29.

25. McNaughton, L. R. 1990. Sodium citrate and anaerobic performance: Implications of dosage. *European Journal of Applied Physiology* 61:392–97.

26. Meyer, R. et al. 1991. Effect of decreased pH on force and phosphocreatine in mammalian skeletal muscle. *Canadian Journal of Physiology and Pharmacology* 69:305–10.

27. Nattie, E. 1990. The alphastat hypothesis in respiratory control and acid-base balance. *Journal of Applied Physiology* 69:1201–7.

28. Nielsen, H. B. et al. 2002. Bicarbonate attenuates intracellular acidosis. *Acta Anaesthesiologica Scandinavica* 46: 579–84.

29. Poortmans, J. 1983. The intramuscular environment in peripheral fatigue. *Biochemistry of Exercise*. Champaign, IL: Human Kinetics.

30. Robertson, R. et al. 1987. Effect of induced alkalosis on physical work capacity during arm and leg exercise. *Ergonomics* 30:19–31.

31. Rogbergs, R. 1990. Effects of warm-up on blood gases, lactate and acid-base status during sprint training. *International Journal of Sports Medicine* 11:273–78.

32. Roth, D. A., and G. Brooks. 1990. Lactate transport is mediated by a membrane bound carrier in rat skeletal muscle sarcolemmal vesicles. *Archives of Biochemistry and Biophysics* 279:377–85.

33. Sahlin, K. 1983. Effects of acidosis on energy metabolism and force generation in skeletal muscle. In *Biochemistry of Exercise*. Champaign, IL: Human Kinetics.

34. Seeley, R., T. Stephens, and P. Tate. 2003. *Anatomy and Physiology*. New York: McGraw-Hill Companies.

35. Sharpo, R. et al. 1986. Effects of eight weeks of bicycle ergometer sprint training on human muscle buffer capacity. *International Journal of Sports Medicine* 7:13–17.

36. Spriet, L. 1991. Phosphofructokinase activity and acidosis during short-term tetanic contractions. *Canadian Journal of Physiology and Pharmacology* 69:298–304.

37. Stein, J. et al. 2002. *Internal Medicine.* St. Louis: Mosby Year-Book.

38. Stephens, T. J. et al. 2002. Effect of sodium bicarbonate on muscle metabolism during intense endurance cycling. *Medicine and Science in Sports and Exercise* 34: 614–21.

39. Stewart, P. A. 1983. Modern quantitative acid-base chemistry. *Canadian Journal of Physiology and Pharmacology* 61:1444–64.

40. Street, D., J. Bangsbo, and C. Juel, 2001. Interstitial pH in human skeletal muscle during and after dynamic graded exercise. *Journal of Physiology* 537:993–98.

41. Stringer, W., R. Casaburi, and K. Wasserman. 1992. Acid-base regulation during exercise and recovery in humans. *Journal of Applied Physiology* 72:954–61.

42. Vollestad, N., and O. M. Sejersted. 1988. Biochemical correlates of fatigue. *European Journal of Applied Physiology* 57:336–47.

43. Weinstein, Y. et al. 1991. Reexamination of Stewart's quantitative analysis of acid-base status. *Medicine and Science in Sports and Exercise* 23:1270–75.

44. Widmaier, E., H. Raff, and K. Strang. 2006. *Vander's Human Physiology*, 10th ed. New York: McGraw-Hill Companies.

CHAPTER 12

Temperature Regulation

■ Objectives

By studying this chapter, you should be able to do the following:

1. Define the term *homeotherm*.
2. Present an overview of heat balance during exercise.
3. Discuss the concept of "core temperature."
4. List the principal means of involuntarily increasing heat production.
5. Define the four processes by which the body can lose heat during exercise.
6. Discuss the role of the hypothalamus as the body's thermostat.
7. Explain the thermal events that occur during exercise in both a cool/moderate and hot/humid environment.
8. List the physiological adaptations that occur during acclimatization to heat.
9. Describe the physiological responses to a cold environment.
10. Discuss the physiological changes that occur in response to cold acclimatization.

■ Outline

Overview of Heat Balance During Exercise 242

Temperature Measurement During Exercise 243

Overview of Heat Production/Heat Loss 243
    Heat Production 243
    Heat Loss 244

Heat Storage in the Body During Exercise 245

Body's Thermostat—Hypothalamus 247
    Shift in the Hypothalamic Thermostat Set Point Due to Fever 248

Thermal Events During Exercise 249

Exercise in the Heat 250

Sweat Rates During Exercise 251

Exercise Performance in a Hot Environment 252
Gender and Age Differences in Thermoregulation 253
Heat Acclimatization 254
Loss of Acclimatization 256

Exercise in a Cold Environment 256
    Cold Acclimatization 256

■ Key Terms

anterior hypothalamus
conduction
convection
evaporation

homeotherms
hyperthermia
hypothermia
posterior hypothalamus

radiation
specific heat

Body core temperature regulation is critical because cellular structures and metabolic pathways are affected by temperature. For example, enzymes that regulate metabolic pathways are greatly influenced by temperature changes; an increase in body temperature above 45° C (normal core temperature is approximately 37° C) may destroy the protein structure of enzymes, resulting in death, while a decrease in body temperature below 34° C may cause a slowed metabolism and abnormal cardiac function (arrhythmias) (6, 16, 25, 28, 43). Hence, people and many animals live their entire lives only a few degrees from their thermal death point. Therefore it is clear that body temperature must be carefully regulated.

Animals that maintain a rather constant body core temperature are called **homeotherms.** The maintenance of a constant body temperature requires that heat loss must match the rate of heat production. To accomplish thermal regulation, the body is well equipped with both nervous and hormonal mechanisms that regulate metabolic rate as well as the amount of heat loss in response to body temperature changes. The temperature-maintenance strategy of homeotherms uses a "furnace" rather than a "refrigerator" to maintain body temperature at a constant level. That is, the body temperature is set near the high end of the survival range and is held constant by continuous metabolic heat production coupled with a small but continual heat loss. The rationale for this strategy seems to be that temperature regulation by heat conservation and generation is very efficient, while our cooling capacity is much more limited (31).

Because contracting skeletal muscles produce large amounts of heat, long-term exercise in a hot/humid environment presents a serious challenge to temperature homeostasis. In fact, many exercise scientists believe that overheating is the only serious threat to health that exercise presents to a healthy individual. It is the purpose of this chapter to discuss the principles of temperature regulation during exercise. The cardiovascular and pulmonary responses to exercise in a hot environment have already been discussed in chapters 9 and 10, respectively, and the influence of temperature on performance will be discussed in chapter 24.

OVERVIEW OF HEAT BALANCE DURING EXERCISE

The goal of temperature regulation is to maintain a constant deep-body temperature and thus prevent overheating or overcooling. If the core temperature is

FIGURE 12.1 During steady-state conditions, temperature homeostasis is maintained by an equal rate of body heat gain and heat loss.

to remain constant, the amount of heat lost must match the amount of heat gained (see figure 12.1). Consistent with that, if heat loss is less than heat production, there is a net gain in body heat and therefore body temperature rises; if heat loss exceeds heat production, there is a net loss in body heat and body temperature decreases.

During exercise, body temperature is regulated by making adjustments in the amount of heat that is lost. One of the important functions of the circulatory system is to transport heat. Blood is very effective in this function since it has a high capacity to store heat. When the body is attempting to lose heat, blood flow is increased to the skin as a means of promoting heat loss to the environment. In contrast, when the goal of temperature regulation is to prevent heat loss, blood is directed away from the skin and toward the interior of the body to prevent additional heat loss.

It is important to point out that within the body, temperature varies a great deal. That is, there is a gradient between deep-body temperature (i.e., deep central areas, including the heart, lungs, abdominal organs) and the "shell" (skin) temperature. In extreme circumstances (i.e., exposure to very cold temperatures), the core temperature may be 20° C higher than the shell. However, such large core-to-shell gradients are rare, and the ideal difference between core and shell temperatures is approximately 4° C (2, 58). Even within the core, temperature varies from one organ to another. Because large differences in temperature exist between one body part and another, it is important to be specific as to where body temperature is being measured. Therefore, the term *body temperature* is a misnomer and should be replaced by more descriptive terms such as *core temperature* or *skin temperature*, depending on which temperature is being discussed (2).

IN SUMMARY

- Homeotherms are animals that maintain a rather constant body core temperature. In order to maintain a constant core temperature, heat loss must match heat gain.
- Temperature varies a great deal within the body. In general, there is a thermal gradient from deep body temperature (core temperature) to the shell (skin) temperature.

TEMPERATURE MEASUREMENT DURING EXERCISE

Measurements of deep-body temperatures can be accomplished with mercury thermometers or with devices known as *thermocouples* or *thermistors*. In the laboratory setting, one of the most common sites of core temperature measurement is the rectum. Although rectal temperature is not the same as the temperature in the brain where temperature is regulated, it can be used to estimate changes in deep-body temperature during exercise. In addition, temperature measurements near the eardrum (called tympanic temperature) have been found to be a good estimate of the actual brain temperature. Another alternative is to measure the temperature of the esophagus as an indication of core temperature. Like rectal temperature, esophageal temperature is not identical to brain temperature, but it offers a measure of deep-body temperature.

While the measurements of rectal, tympanic, and esophageal temperature can easily be performed in the laboratory setting, each of these techniques has limitations in a field setting. Indeed, it would be difficult to apply these temperature measurement techniques in athletes during an American football or soccer practice session. Nonetheless, the recent development of ingestible temperature sensor telemetry systems has made on-field core temperature measurement possible and allowed the investigation of core temperature changes in athletes during practice sessions (3, 41). These ingestible temperature sensors use low-power radio frequency transmissions to communicate with a temperature monitor. These probes have been shown to be both valid and reliable in measuring core temperature in football players during practice (3).

Skin temperature can be measured by placing temperature sensors (thermistors) on the skin at various locations. The mean skin temperature can be calculated by assigning certain factors to each individual skin measurement in proportion to the fraction of the body's total surface area that each measurement represents. For example, mean skin temperature (T_s) can be estimated by the following formula (32):

$$T_s = (T_{forehead} + T_{chest} + T_{forearm} + T_{thigh} + T_{calf} + T_{abdomen} + T_{back}) \div 7$$

where $T_{forehead}$, T_{chest}, $T_{forearm}$, T_{thigh}, T_{calf}, $T_{abdomen}$, and T_{back} represent skin temperatures measured on the forehead, chest, forearm, thigh, calf, abdomen, and back, respectively.

IN SUMMARY

- Measurements of deep-body temperatures can be accomplished via mercury thermometers, or devices known as thermocouples or thermistors. Common sites of measurement include the rectum, the ear (tympanic temperature), and the esophagus.
- Skin temperature can be measured by placing temperature sensors (thermistors) on the skin at various locations.

OVERVIEW OF HEAT PRODUCTION/HEAT LOSS

As previously stated, the goal of temperature regulation is to maintain a constant core temperature. This regulation is achieved by controlling the rate of heat production and heat loss. When out of balance, the body either gains or loses heat. The temperature control center is an area in the brain called the hypothalamus. The hypothalamus works like a thermostat by initiating an increase in heat production when body temperature falls and an increase in the rate of heat loss when body temperature rises. Temperature regulation is controlled by both physical and chemical processes. Let's begin our discussion of temperature regulation by introducing those factors that govern heat production and heat loss.

Heat Production

The body produces internal heat due to normal metabolic processes. At rest or during sleep, metabolic heat production is small; however, during intense exercise, heat production is large. Heat production can be classified as (1) voluntary (exercise) or (2) involuntary (shivering or biochemical heat production caused by the secretion of hormones such as thyroxine and catecholamines) (see figure 12.2).

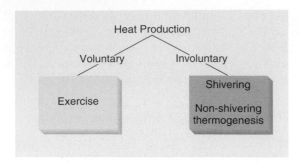

FIGURE 12.2 The body produces heat due to normal metabolic processes. Heat production can be classified as being either voluntary or involuntary.

Since the body is, at most, 20% to 30% efficient, 70% to 80% of the energy expended during exercise appears as heat. During heavy exercise, this can result in a large heat load. Indeed, work in a hot/humid environment serves as a serious test of the body's ability to lose heat.

Involuntary heat production by shivering is the primary means of increasing heat production during exposure to cold. Maximal shivering can increase the body's heat production by approximately five times the resting value (6, 17). In addition, release of thyroxine from the thyroid gland can also increase metabolic rate. Thyroxine acts by increasing the metabolic rate of all cells in the body (11, 17, 27). Finally, an increase in blood levels of catecholamines (epinephrine and norepinephrine) can cause an increase in the rate of cellular metabolism (24). The increase in heat production due to the combined influences of thyroxine and catecholamines is called *nonshivering thermogenesis.*

Heat Loss

Heat loss from the body may occur by four processes: (1) radiation, (2) conduction, (3) convection, and/or (4) evaporation. The first three of these heat loss mechanisms require a temperature gradient to exist between the skin and the environment. **Radiation** is heat loss in the form of infrared rays. This involves the transfer of heat from the surface of one object to the surface of another, with no physical contact being involved (i.e., sun transferring heat to the earth via radiation). At rest in a comfortable environment (e.g., room temperature = 21°C), 60% of the heat loss occurs via radiation. This is possible because skin temperature is greater than the temperature of surrounding objects (walls, floor, etc.), and a net loss of body heat occurs due to the thermal gradient. Note that on a hot, sunny day when surface temperatures are greater than skin temperature, the body can also

gain heat via radiation (46). Therefore, it is important to remember that radiation is heat transfer by infrared rays and can result in either heat loss or heat gain depending on the environmental conditions.

Conduction is defined as the transfer of heat from the body into the molecules of cooler objects in contact with its surface. In general, the body loses only small amounts of heat due to this process. An example of heat loss due to conduction is the transfer of heat from the body to a metal chair while a person is sitting on it. The heat loss occurs as long as the chair is cooler than the body surface in contact with it.

Convection is a form of conductive heat loss in which heat is transmitted to either air or water molecules in contact with the body. In convective heat loss, air or water molecules are warmed and move away from the source of the heat and are replaced by cooler molecules. An example of *forced convection* is a fan moving large quantities of air past the skin; this would increase the number of air molecules coming in contact with the skin and thus promote heat loss. Practically speaking, the amount of heat loss due to convection is dependent on the airflow over the skin. Therefore, under the same wind conditions, cycling at high speeds would improve convective cooling when compared to cycling at slow speeds or running. Swimming in cool water (water temperature less than skin temperature) also results in convective heat loss. In fact, water's effectiveness in cooling is about 25 times greater than that of air at the same temperature.

The final means of heat loss is **evaporation.** Evaporation accounts for approximately 25% of the heat loss at rest, but under most environmental conditions it is the most important means of heat loss during exercise (44). In evaporation, heat is transferred from the body to water on the surface of the skin. When this water gains sufficient heat (energy), it is converted to a gas (water vapor), taking the heat away from the body. Note that evaporation occurs due to a vapor pressure gradient between the skin and the air. Vapor pressure is the pressure exerted by water molecules that have been converted to gas (water vapor). Evaporative cooling during exercise occurs in the following way. When body temperature rises above normal, the nervous system stimulates sweat glands to secrete sweat onto the surface of the skin. As sweat evaporates, heat is lost to the environment, which in turn lowers skin temperature.

Evaporation of sweat from the skin is dependent on three factors: (1) the temperature and relative humidity, (2) the convective currents around the body, and (3) the amount of skin surface exposed to the environment (2, 43). At high environmental temperatures, relative humidity is the most important factor by far in determining the rate of evaporative heat loss. High relative humidity reduces the rate of evaporation. In fact, when the relative humidity is near 100%, evaporation is limited. Therefore, cooling by way of evaporation is most effective under conditions of low humidity.

Why does high relative humidity reduce the rate of evaporation? The answer is linked to the fact that high relative humidity (RH) reduces the vapor pressure gradient between the skin and the environment. On a hot/humid day (e.g., RH = 80%–90%) the vapor pressure in the air is close to the vapor pressure on moist skin. Therefore, the rate of evaporation is greatly reduced. High sweat rates during exercise in a hot/high humidity environment result in useless water loss. That is, sweating per se does not cool the skin; it is evaporation that cools the skin (40).

Let's explore in more detail those factors that regulate the rate of evaporation. The major point to keep in mind is that evaporation occurs due to a vapor pressure gradient. That is, in order for evaporative cooling to occur during exercise, the vapor pressure on the skin must be greater than the vapor pressure in the air. Vapor pressure is influenced by both temperature and relative humidity. This relationship is illustrated in table 12.1, which states that at any given temperature, a rise in relative humidity results in increased vapor pressure. Practically speaking, this means that less evaporative cooling occurs during exercise on a hot/humid day when compared to a cool/low humidity day. For example, an athlete running on a hot/humid day (e.g., air temperature = 30° C; RH = 100%) might have a mean skin temperature in the range of 33°–34° C. The vapor pressure on the skin would be approximately 35 mm Hg and the air vapor pressure would be around 32 mm Hg (table 12.1). This small vapor pressure gradient between the skin and air (3 mm Hg) would permit only limited evaporation, and therefore little cooling would occur. In contrast, the same athlete running on a cool/low humidity day (e.g., air temperature = 10° C; RH = 50%) might have a mean skin temperature of 30° C. The vapor pressure gradient between the skin and air under these conditions would be approximately 28 mm Hg (32 − 4 = 28) (table 12.1). This relatively large skin-to-air vapor pressure gradient would permit a reasonably large evaporative rate, and therefore adequate body cooling would occur under these conditions.

How much heat can be lost via evaporation during exercise? Heat loss due to evaporation can be calculated in the following manner. The body loses 0.58 kcal of heat for each ml of water that evaporates (71). Therefore, evaporation of 1 liter of sweat would result in a heat loss of 580 kcal (1,000 ml × 0.58 kcal/ml =

| TABLE 12.1 | The Relationship Between Temperature and Relative Humidity (RH) on Vapor Pressure |

50% RH Temperature °C	Vapor Pressure (mm Hg)
0	2.3
10	4.6
20	8.8
30	15.9

75% RH Temperature °C	Vapor Pressure (mm Hg)
0	3.4
10	6.9
20	13.2
30	23.9

100% RH Temperature °C	Vapor Pressure (mm Hg)
0	4.6
10	9.2
20	17.6
30	31.9

580 kcal). See A Closer Look 12.1 for additional examples of body heat loss calculations.

In summary, heat loss during exercise (other than swimming) in a cool/moderate environment occurs primarily due to evaporation. In fact, when exercise is performed in a hot environment (where air temperature is greater than skin temperature), evaporation is the only means of losing body heat. The means by which the body gains and loses heat during exercise are summarized in figure 12.3.

Heat Storage in the Body During Exercise

Now that we have discussed both heat production and heat loss, let's talk about heat storage in the body during exercise. As mentioned earlier, any heat that is produced by the working muscles during exercise and is not lost, must be stored in body tissues. Therefore, the amount of heat gain in the body during exercise is computed as the difference between heat production and heat loss:

Body heat gain during exercise = (heat produced − heat loss)

A CLOSER LOOK 12.1

Calculation of Heat Loss via Evaporation

Knowing that evaporation of 1,000 ml of sweat results in 580 kcal of heat loss permits one to calculate the sweat and evaporation rate necessary to maintain a specified body temperature during exercise. Consider the following example: John Hothead is working on a cycle ergometer at a $\dot{V}O_2$ of 2.0 liters $\cdot$ min^{-1}, (energy expenditure of 10.0 kcal $\cdot$ min^{-1}). If John exercises for twenty minutes at this metabolic rate and is 20% efficient,

how much evaporation would be necessary to prevent an increase in core temperature?[1] The total heat produced can be calculated as:

Total energy expenditure
   $= 20$ min $\times$ 10 kcal/min
   $= 200$ kcal

Total heat produced
   $= 200$ kcal $\times$ .80[1]
   $= 160$ kcal

The total evaporation necessary to prevent any heat gain would be computed as:

$$\frac{160 \text{ kcal}}{580 \text{ kcal/liter}} = .276 \text{ liters}^{[2]}$$
(evaporation necessary to prevent heat gain)

[1]If efficiency is 20%, then 80%, or .80 of the total energy expenditure, must be released as heat.
[2]Assumes no other heat-loss mechanism is active.

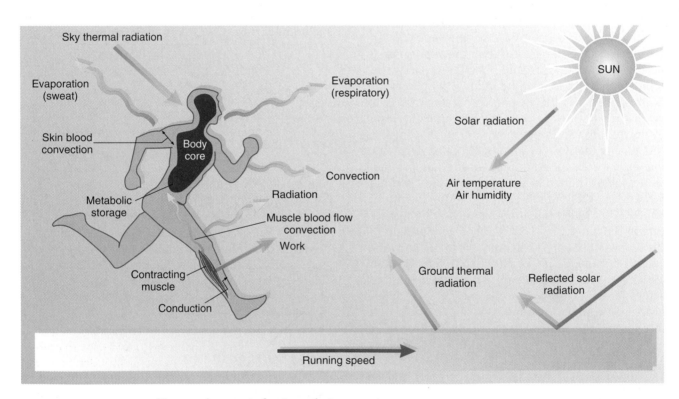

FIGURE 12.3 A summary of heat exchange mechanisms during exercise.

The amount of heat energy required to raise body temperature depends upon the size of the individual (i.e., body weight) and a characteristic of body tissue called specific heat. The term **specific heat** refers to the amount of heat energy required to raise 1 kilogram of body tissue by 1° C. The specific heat for the human body is 0.83 kilocalories (kcal) per kilogram of body mass. Therefore, the amount of heat required to ele-

vate the body temperature by 1° C can be computed as follows:

**Heat required to increase
body temperature by 1° C = (specific heat ×
body mass)**

For example, using the equation above, the amount of heat required to increase body temperature by 1° C

Calculation of Body Temperature Increase During Exercise

Knowledge of the specific heat of the human body, along with information regarding how much heat is produced and lost from the body during exercise, permits the calculation of how much body temperature will increase during an exercise session. To better understand how to perform these calculations, let's consider the following example of an athlete performing an endurance training workout. For example, a well-trained distance runner performs a training session on an outdoor track. The weather on this day is relatively hot (30° C) and humid (60% relative humidity). The runner weighs 60 kg and performs a 40-minute workout at a $\dot{V}O_2$ of 3.0 liters min^{-1} (i.e., energy expenditure of 15 kcal per minute). If this runner is 20% efficient and can lose only 60% of the heat produced during exercise, how much will her or his body temperature increase

during this exercise session? The total heat storage and body temperature increase during exercise can be calculated in the following steps:

1. **Total energy expenditure**
   = 40 min × 15 kcal/min
   = 600 kcal
2. **Total heat produced**
   = 600 kcal × 0.80[1]
   = 480 kcal
3. **Total heat stored during exercise**
   = 480 kcal × 0.40[2]
   = 192 kcal
4. **Amount of heat storage required to increase body temperature by 1° C**
   = 0.83 kcal/kg × 60 kg[3]
   = 49.8 kcal

The increase in body temperature resulting from this exercise session can now be calculated as follows:

5. **Increase in body temperature (°C) during exercise = Total heat stored during exercise (specific heat × body mass)**
   = 192 kcal/49.8 kcal/°C
   = 3.85° C

In the current example, this exercise bout would result in an increase in body temperature by 3.85° C—that is, 192 kcal/(0.83 kcal/kg × 60 kg). Therefore, if the athlete began the training session with a body temperature of 37° C, the post exercise body temperature would increase to 40.85° C (i.e., 37° C + 3.85° C).

[1] If the efficiency is 20%, then 80% or 0.80 of the total energy expenditure must be released as heat.
[2] If the athlete can only lose 60% of the heat produced during exercise, the remaining 40% or 0.40 of the heat produced, must be stored as heat energy.
[3] The amount of heat required to increase body temperature by 1° C = (specific heat × body mass)

---

in a 70-kg individual can be computed by multiplying the specific heat of the body (0.83 kcal/kg) by the individuals body weight (70 kg). Therefore, the heat required to increase body temperature by 1° C would be 58.1 kcal (i.e., 0.83 kcal/kg × 70 kg = 58.1 kcal). See A Closer Look 12.2 for more examples of body heat gain calculations.

IN SUMMARY

- Muscular exercise can result in large amounts of heat production. Since the body is at most 20% to 30% efficient, 70% to 80% of the energy expended during exercise is released as heat.
- Body heat can be lost by evaporation, convection, conduction, and radiation. During exercise in a cool environment, evaporation is the primary avenue for heat loss.
- The rate of evaporation from the skin is dependent upon three factors: (1) temperature and relative humidity, (2) convective currents around the body, and (3) the amount of skin exposed to the environment.
- Body heat storage is the difference between heat production and heat loss.

- The amount of heat required to elevate body temperature by 1° C is termed the specific heat of the body

BODY'S THERMOSTAT— HYPOTHALAMUS

Again, the body's temperature regulatory center is located in the hypothalamus. The **anterior hypothalamus** is primarily responsible for dealing with increases in body heat, while the **posterior hypothalamus** is responsible for reacting to a decrease in body temperature. In general, the hypothalamus operates much like a thermostat in your home—that is, it attempts to maintain a relatively constant core temperature around some "set point." The set-point temperature in humans is approximately 37° C.

The input to the temperature-regulating centers in the hypothalamus comes from receptors in both the skin and the core. Changes in environmental temperature are first detected by thermal receptors (both heat and cold) located in the skin. These skin temperature receptors transmit nerve impulses to the hypothalamus, which then initiates the appropriate

Physiological response to a "Heat Load"

FIGURE 12.4   A summary illustration of the physiological responses to an increase in "heat load."

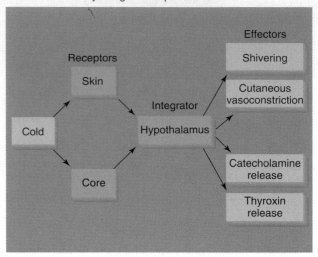

Physiological Responses to Cold

FIGURE 12.5   An illustration of the physiological responses to cold stress.

response in an effort to maintain the body's set-point temperature. Further, heat-/cold-sensitive neurons are located in both the spinal cord and the hypothalamus itself, sensing changes in the core temperature.

An increase in core temperature above the set point results in the hypothalamus initiating a series of physiological actions aimed at increasing the amount of heat loss. First, the hypothalamus stimulates the sweat glands, which results in an increase in evaporative heat loss (30, 33). In addition, the vasomotor control center withdraws the normal vasoconstrictor tone to the skin, promoting increased skin blood flow and therefore allowing increased heat loss. Figure 12.4 illustrates the physiological responses associated with an increase in core temperature. When core temperature returns to normal, the stimulus to promote both sweating and vasodilation is removed. This is an example of a control system using negative feedback (see chapter 2).

When cold receptors are stimulated in the skin or the hypothalamus, the thermoregulatory control center sets forth a plan of action to minimize heat loss and increase heat production. First, the vasomotor center directs peripheral blood vessels to vasoconstrict, which reduces heat loss (27). Second, if core temperature drops significantly, involuntary shivering begins (70). Additional responses include stimulation of the pilomotor center, which promotes piloerection (goosebumps). This piloerection reflex is an effective means of increasing the insulation space over the skin in fur-bearing animals, but is not an effective means of preventing heat loss in humans. Further, the hypothalamus indirectly increases thyroxine production and release, which increases cellular heat production (7). Finally, the posterior hypothalamus initiates the release of norepinephrine, which increases the rate of cellular metabolism (nonshivering thermogenesis). The physiological responses to a drop in core temperature are summarized in figure 12.5.

Shift in the Hypothalamic Thermostat Set Point Due to Fever

A fever is an increase in body temperature above the normal range, and it may be caused by a number of bacterial diseases or brain disorders. During a fever, certain proteins and other toxins secreted by bacteria can cause the set point of the hypothalamic thermostat to rise above the normal level. Substances that cause this effect are called *pyrogens*. When the set point of the hypothalamic thermostat is raised to a higher level than normal, all the mechanisms for raising body temperature are called into play (24). Within a few hours after the thermostat has been set to a higher level, the body core temperature reaches this new level due to heat conservation.

IN SUMMARY

- The body's thermostat is located in the hypothalamus.
- The anterior hypothalamus is responsible for reacting to increases in core temperature, while the posterior hypothalamus governs the body's responses to a decrease in temperature.
- An increase in core temperature results in the anterior hypothalamus initiating a series of physiological actions aimed at increasing heat loss. These actions include: (1) the commencement of sweating and (2) an increase in skin blood flow.
- Cold exposure results in the posterior hypothalamus promoting physiological changes that increase body heat production (shivering) and reduce heat loss (cutaneous vasoconstriction).

THERMAL EVENTS DURING EXERCISE

Now that an overview of how the hypothalamus responds to different thermal challenges has been presented, let's examine a brief scenario of the thermal events that occur during submaximal constant-load exercise in a cool/moderate environment (i.e., low humidity and room temperature). Heat production increases during exercise due to muscular contraction and is directly proportional to the exercise intensity. The venous blood draining the exercising muscle distributes the excess heat throughout the body core. As core temperature increases, thermal sensors in the hypothalamus sense the increase in blood temperature, and the thermal integration center in the hypothalamus compares this increase in temperature with the set-point temperature and finds a difference between the two (20, 43, 45). The response is to direct the nervous system to commence sweating and to increase blood flow to the skin (4, 47). These acts serve to increase body heat loss and minimize the increase in body temperature. At this point, the internal temperature reaches a new, elevated steady-state level (see figure 12.6). Note that this new steady-state core temperature does not represent a change in the set-point temperature, as occurs in fever (20, 43, 45, 73). Instead, the thermal regulatory center attempts to return the core temperature back to resting levels, but is incapable of doing so in the face of the sustained heat production associated with exercise.

Figure 12.6 also illustrates the roles of evaporation, convection, and radiation in heat loss during constant-load exercise in a moderate environment. Notice the constant but small role of convection and radiation in heat loss during this type of exercise. This is due to a constant temperature gradient between the skin and the room. In contrast, evaporation plays the most important role in heat loss during exercise in this type of environment (43, 45, 49).

During constant-load exercise, the core temperature increase is directly related to the exercise intensity and is independent of ambient temperature over a wide range of conditions (i.e., 8°–29° C with low relative humidity) (48). This point is illustrated in figure 12.7. Notice the linear rise in core temperature as the metabolic rate increases. The fact that it is the exercise intensity and not the environmental temperature that determines the rise in core temperature during exercise suggests that the method of heat loss during continuous exercise is modified according to ambient conditions (36, 48). This concept is presented in figure 12.8, which shows heat loss mechanisms during constant-intensity exercise. Note that as the ambient temperature increases, the rate of convective and radiative heat loss decreases due to a decrease in the skin-to-room temperature gradient. This decrease in convective and radiative heat loss is matched by an increase in evaporative heat loss, and core temperature remains the same (see figure 12.8).

As mentioned previously, heat production increases in proportion to the exercise intensity. This point is illustrated in figure 12.9. Notice the linear increase in energy output (expenditure), heat production, and total heat loss as a function of exercise work rate. Further, note that convective and radiative heat loss do not increase as a function of exercise work rate. This is due to a relatively constant temperature gradient between the skin and the environment. In contrast, there is a consistent rise in evaporative heat loss with increments in exercise intensity. This observation

FIGURE 12.6 Changes in metabolic energy production, evaporative heat loss, convective heat loss, and radiative heat loss during twenty-five minutes of submaximal exercise in a cool environment.

FIGURE 12.7 The relationship between metabolic rate and rectal temperature during constant load arm (●) and leg (■) exercise. From M. Nelson, 1938, "Die Regulation der Korpertemperatur bei Muskelarbeit" in *Scandinavica Archives Physiology*, 79:193. Copyright © 1938 Blackwell Scientific Publications, Ltd., Oxford, England. Reprinted by permission.

FIGURE 12.8 Heat exchange during exercise at different environmental temperatures. Notice the change in evaporative and convective/radiative heat loss as the environmental temperature increases. See text for discussion. From M. Nelson, 1938, "Die Regulation der Korpertemperatur bei Muskelarbeit" in *Scandinavica Archives Physiology*, 79:193. Copyright © 1938 Blackwell Scientific Publications, Ltd., Oxford, England. Reprinted by permission.

FIGURE 12.9 Heat exchange at rest and during cycle ergometer exercise at a variety of work rates. Note the steady increase in evaporative heat loss as a function of an increase in power output. In contrast, an increase in metabolic rate has essentially no influence on the rate of convective and radiative heat loss. From M. Nelson, 1938, "Die Regulation der Korpertemperatur bei Muskelarbeit" in *Scandinavica Archives Physiology*, 79:193. Copyright © 1938 Blackwell Scientific Publications, Ltd., Oxford, England. Reprinted by permission.

reemphasizes the point that evaporation is the primary means of losing heat during exercise.

IN SUMMARY

- During constant intensity exercise, the increase in body temperature is directly related to the exercise intensity.
- Body heat production increases in proportion to exercise intensity.

EXERCISE IN THE HEAT

Continuous exercise in a hot/humid environment poses a particularly stressful challenge to the maintenance of normal body temperature and fluid homeostasis. High heat and humidity reduce the body's ability to lose heat by radiation/convection and evaporation, respectively. This inability to lose heat during exercise in a hot/humid environment results in a greater core temperature and a higher sweat rate

FIGURE 12.10 Differences in core temperature and sweat rate during forty-five minutes of submaximal exercise in a hot/humid environment versus a cool environment.

(more fluid loss) when compared to the same exercise in a moderate environment (55–58, 60, 67). This point is illustrated in figure 12.10. Notice the marked differences in sweat rates and core temperatures during exercise between the hot/humid conditions and the moderate environment. The combined effect of fluid loss and high core temperature increases the risk of **hyperthermia** (large rise in core temperature) and heat injury (see Clinical Applications 12.1, Ask the Expert 12.1, and chapter 24).

Sweat Rates During Exercise

In an effort to increase evaporative heat loss during exercise, humans rely on their ability to increase sweat production via eccrine sweat glands (i.e., sweat glands under sympathetic cholinergic control) (35). In this regard, exercise in a hot environment greatly increases sweat rates during training or competitive conditions (3, 5, 21, 35, 63, 64). Note, however, that sweat rates may vary widely across different individuals. For example, heat acclimatized individuals have an earlier onset of sweating and a higher sweat rate during exercise. Further, large individuals (i.e., large body mass) will likely have higher sweat rates compared to smaller individuals. Finally, genetic variations in sweat rates exist such that two individuals

CLINICAL APPLICATIONS 12.1

Exercise-Related Heat Injuries Can Be Prevented

Heat injury during exercise can occur when the level of body heat production is high and environmental conditions (e.g., high ambient temperature and humidity) impede heat loss from the body. The primary cause of heat injury is hyperthermia (high body temperature). Increases in body temperature of 2° C to 3° C generally do not have ill effects (2, 7). Nonetheless, increases in body temperature above 40° C to 41° C can be associated with a variety of heat-related problems. Note that heat-related problems during exercise are not "all or none," but form a heat-injury continuum that can extend from a relatively minor problem (i.e., heat syncope) to a life-threatening, major medical emergency (i.e., heat stroke). The general symptoms of heat stress include nausea, headache, dizziness, reduced sweat rate, and the general inability to think rationally.

Each year in the United States, several heat-related problems in American football are reported (see Ask the Expert 12.1). Nonetheless, heat-related illness during exercise can be prevented. To prevent overheating during exercise, the following guidelines are useful:

■ Exercise during the coolest part of the day.
■ Minimize both the intensity and duration of exercise on hot/humid days.
■ Expose a maximal surface area of skin for evaporation (i.e., removal of clothing) during exercise.
■ When removal of clothing during exercise is not possible (e.g., American football), provide frequent rest/cool-down breaks along with intermittent clothing

shed (e.g., removal of helmet and upper clothing).
■ To avoid dehydration during exercise, workouts should permit frequent water breaks (coupled with rest/cool-down).
■ Rest/cool-down breaks during exercise should remove the athlete from radiant heat gain due to direct sunlight (e.g., sitting under a tent) and offer exposure to circulating, cool air (e.g., fans).

Once an athlete develops symptoms of heat injury, the obvious treatment is to stop exercising and immediately begin cooling the body (e.g., cold water immersion). Cold fluids with electrolytes should also be provided for rehydration. See chapter 24 for more details on the signs and symptoms of heat injury.

ASK THE EXPERT 12.1

Why Do Some Football Players Get Too Hot?
Questions and Answers with Dr. Larry Kenney

Larry Kenney, Ph.D., a professor in the Departments of Kinesiology and Physiology at the Pennsylvania State University, is an internationally known researcher in the field of temperature regulation during exercise and a leader in the American College of Sports Medicine. His research has addressed a variety of body temperature-related issues, including the effects of age and gender on thermoregulation. Indeed, Dr. Kenney's research team has performed many of the "landmark" studies that explore the effects of both age and gender on temperature regulation during exercise. Further, Dr. Kenney's laboratory has investigated the influence of different types of clothing on heat loss and gain during sports activities.

During the past 15 years in the United States, there has been an average of three heat-related deaths during football practice. These deaths often occur during the first three days of summer practice and interior linemen are commonly the victims. In this box feature, Dr. Kenney answers three questions related to "why some football players get too hot."

QUESTION 1: Why do heat-related injuries in football often occur during the first three days of summer practice?

ANSWER: Next to a history of heat stroke, a lack of acclimation to hot conditions is the single, most important predictor for heat illness. Full acclimation to the heat may require as long as two weeks, but the most important physiological changes occur during the first three days. A key event is the expansion of plasma volume occurring on days one and two that allows for cardiovascular integrity and serves as the foundation for the subsequent increase in sweating rate.

QUESTION 2: Most of the recent heat injuries in football have occurred in linemen (e.g., guards, tackles). Compared to other positions in football, why do some linemen get too hot during football practice?

ANSWER: Linemen are the most likely to report to training camp or preseason practice in a state of low heat acclimation and poor cardiovascular fitness. Because a high $\dot{V}O_2$ max accelerates acclimation and aids in thermoregulation (because more blood can be shunted to the skin), leaner, fitter players typically have an advantage during heavy exercise in hot conditions.

QUESTION 3: Recent research in your laboratory has explored the effects of exercise on body heat loss in players who wear a full football uniform versus those who wear shorts. Compared to exercise in shorts, how much of an impediment to heat loss is provided by a complete football uniform?

ANSWER: A full football uniform, depending on the configuration and type of fabric, can triple the resistance to sweat evaporation over shorts and a tee shirt alone.

For more information about heat stress in football, please see Bergeron et al. (2005) in the Suggested Readings.

---

with the same body size and level of heat acclimatization may also differ in sweat rates.

American football players, wearing full uniforms and practicing in a hot and humid environment, experience some of the largest sweat rates ever recorded for athletes. Although several reasons exist for high sweat loss in these athletes, two major contributors are that many football players possess large body masses and that football uniforms retard heat loss (see Ask the Expert 12.1 for more information). For example, a recent study revealed that the average sweat loss in football players was approximately 4 to 5 liters per hour during a practice session in a hot and humid environment (21). Further, these investigators reported that during preseason practice sessions where athletes were practicing twice a day, that the daily sweat loss ranged from 9 to 12 liters of water. Failure to replace this loss of fluid on a daily basis would result in progressive dehydration and increase the risk of heat injury (3, 63, 64). For more information

on the importance of fluid replacement during exercise see The Winning Edge 12.1.

Exercise Performance in a Hot Environment

Performance during prolonged, submaximal exercise (e.g., a marathon or long triathlon) is impaired in a hot/humid environment (42, 68). Further, athletic performance during intermittent, high-intensity exercise (e.g., soccer or rugby) is also compromised on a hot day (42). While the precise mechanisms responsible for this impaired exercise performance continue to be debated, heat stress-induced hyperthermia, along with changes in muscle blood flow and metabolism, are contributory factors (42).

Prolonged exercise in a hot environment results in increased body temperatures that can lead to hyperthermia. Hyperthermia can directly diminish exercise performance due to central nervous system

THE WINNING EDGE 12.1

Prevention of Dehydration During Exercise

Athletic performance can be impaired by sweat-induced loss of body water (i.e., dehydration). Indeed, dehydration resulting in loss of 1% to 2% of body weight is sufficient to impair exercise performance (8). Dehydration of greater than 3% of body weight further impairs physiological function and increases the risk of heat injury (8). Dehydration of greater than 3% of body weight further impairs physiological function and increases the risk of heat injury (8). Therefore, prevention of dehydration during exercise is important to both maximize athletic performance and prevent heat injuries. Dehydration can be avoided by adherence to the following guidelines:

■ Athletes should be well hydrated prior to beginning a workout or competition. This can be achieved by drinking 400 to 800 ml of fluid within three hours prior to exercise (39).

■ Athletes should consume 150 to 300 ml of fluid every fifteen to twenty minutes during exercise (39). The actual volume of fluid ingested during each drinking period should be adjusted to environmental conditions (i.e., rate of sweat loss) and individual tolerances for drinking during exercise.

■ To ensure rehydration following exercise, athletes should monitor fluid losses during exercise by recording body weight prior to the workout and then weighing immediately after the workout session. To ensure proper rehydration following exercise, the individual should consume fluids equal to approximately 150% of the weight loss. For example, if an athlete loses 1 kg of body weight during a training session, he/she should consume 1.5 liters of fluid to achieve complete rehydration (39, 63, 64).

■ Monitoring the color of urine between workouts is a practical way to judge hydration levels in athletes. For example, urine is typically clear or the color of lemonade in a well-hydrated individual. In contrast, in dehydrated individuals, urine appears as a dark-yellow fluid.

Which is the optimal rehydration fluid-water or a well-formulated sports drink? The National Athletic Trainers Association has concluded that well-designed sports drinks are superior to water for rehydration following exercise (8). The rationale for this recommendation is that these beverages increase voluntary intake by athletes and allow for more effective rehydration. For more details on fluid replacement during and following exercise please see Cheuvront and Sawka (2005) and Shirreffs (2005) in the Suggested Readings.

---

impairment. Specifically, hyperthermia can act upon the central nervous system to reduce the mental drive for motor performance (62).

Although controversial, recent research indicates that muscle blood flow is reduced during prolonged exercise in a hot environment (22). This reduction in muscle blood flow during exercise in the heat occurs due to a competition for blood between the working muscles and the skin. That is, as body temperature rises during exercise in a hot environment, blood flow moves away from the contracting muscle toward the skin to assist in cooling the body.

Compared to exercise in a cool environment, work in the heat results in a more rapid onset of muscular fatigue (18, 53). Numerous studies have investigated factors that contribute to fatigue in the heat. Collectively, these investigations reveal that heat-induced muscular fatigue is not due to a single factor but occurs because of a combination of heat-related changes in muscle metabolism (see Research Focus 12.1 for more details).

Compared to exercise in a cool environment, exercise in the heat increases muscle glycogen usage

and elevates muscle lactate production (22, 65). Collectively, these changes in muscle metabolism may also contribute to the early fatigue during prolonged exercise in a hot climate.

What strategies can athletes use to improve their exercise tolerance in a hot environment? Athletes can optimize exercise performance in the heat by becoming heat acclimatized and consuming fluid before and during exercise. The process of physiological adaptation to heat (heat acclimatization) will improve exercise tolerance and will be discussed later in this chapter (Heat Acclimatization). Guidelines for the consumption of water before and during athletic performance are presented in The Winning Edge 12.1 and are also discussed in chapter 23.

Gender and Age Differences in Thermoregulation

Although controversy exists about the issue, most women appear to be less heat tolerant than men (50). Factors contributing to women's limited heat tolerance include lower sweat rates and generally a higher

RESEARCH FOCUS 12.1

Exercise in the Heat Accelerates Muscle Fatigue

It is well established that exercise in a hot environment results in a more rapid onset of muscular fatigue compared to exercise in cool conditions (9, 18, 23). It appears that heat-related muscle fatigue is not due to a single use but results from several factors in combination (9). Indeed, high temperatures result in several bodily changes that could lead to fatigue. For example, a large increase in brain temperature may result in decreased neuromuscular drive, resulting in a decrease in motor unit recruitment and muscular fatigue.

A second potential contributor to heat-induced fatigue is the possibility that exercise in the heat may promote hypoglycemia (8) and accelerate muscle glycogen metabolism (65). This is significant because both hypoglycemia and depletion of muscle glycogen stores is associated with muscle fatigue (see chapter 4). Nonetheless, this issue remains controversial because not all studies report accelerated hypoglycemia and glycogen depletion during exercise in a hot environment (53).

Another explanation for heat-induced muscular fatigue is that free radical production is increased in skeletal muscles during exercise in the heat (75). Recall from chapter 3 that free radicals are produced in skeletal muscles during aerobic metabolism. Free radicals are molecules with an unpaired electron in their outer orbital. This is significant because molecules with unpaired electrons are highly reactive.

That is, free radicals bind quickly with other molecules, and this combination results in damage to the molecule combining with the radical. Therefore, accelerated production of free radicals during exercise in the heat could contribute to muscle fatigue because of damage to muscle contractile proteins (75).

In summary, exercise in the heat accelerates muscle fatigue. It seems likely that heat-induced fatigue is not due to a single factor but probably results from a combination of metabolic events (9). Two important factors that could contribute to heat-related muscle fatigue are decreased neuromuscular drive and an increase in muscle production of free radicals.

---

percentage of body fat than men (a high percentage of body fat reduces heat loss). However, when women and men are matched for the same degree of heat acclimatization and similar body compositions, the gender differences in the physiological responses to thermal stress are small (50).

Does aging impair one's ability to thermoregulate and exercise in the heat? This issue remains controversial, with some investigators suggesting that the ability to exercise in the heat deteriorates with old age (14) and others suggesting that age per se does not limit one's ability to thermoregulate (13, 34, 35, 52). However, two recent, well-controlled studies have concluded that exercise-conditioned old and young men show little difference in thermoregulation during exercise (52, 69). Further, a recent review of the literature on this subject has concluded that heat tolerance does not appear to be compromised by age in healthy and physically active, older subjects (34, 35). Based upon the collective evidence, it appears that deconditioning (i.e., decline in $\dot{V}O_2$ max) and a lack of heat acclimatization in older subjects may explain why some of the earlier studies reported a decrease in thermotolerance with age.

Heat Acclimatization

Regular exercise in a hot environment results in a series of physiological adjustments designed to minimize disturbances in homeostasis due to heat stress

(this is referred to as heat acclimatization). Importantly, individuals of all ages are capable of acclimating to a hot environment (34, 69). The end result of heat acclimatization is a lower heart rate and core temperature during submaximal exercise (13). Although partial heat acclimatization can occur by training in a cool environment, it is essential that athletes exercise in a hot environment to obtain maximal heat acclimatization (1). Because an elevation in core temperature is the primary stimulus to promote heat acclimatization, it is recommended that the athlete perform strenuous interval training or continuous exercise at an intensity exceeding 50% of the athlete's $\dot{V}O_2$ max in order to promote higher core temperatures (51) (see Research Focus 12.2).

The primary adaptations that occur during heat acclimatization are an increased plasma volume, earlier onset of sweating, higher sweat rate, reduced salt loss in sweat, a reduced skin blood flow, and increased synthesis of heat shock proteins (19, 38, 61). It is interesting that heat adaptation occurs rapidly, with almost complete acclimatization being achieved by seven to fourteen days after the first exposure (4, 73).

Heat acclimatization results in a 10% to 12% increase in plasma volume (6, 19). The increase in plasma volume is due to an increase in plasma proteins. This increased plasma volume maintains central blood volume, stroke volume, and sweating capacity, and allows the body to store more heat with a smaller temperature gain.

RESEARCH FOCUS 12.2

Can Exercise Training in Sweat Clothing in Cool Conditions Promote Heat Acclimatization?

Athletes who train in cool environments often travel to warmer climates to compete. Without adequate heat acclimatization, these athletes will be at a disadvantage compared to athletes who have developed a high level of heat adaptation by training in a hot/humid environment. Therefore, a key question is, "Can training in sweat clothing in a cool environment promote heat acclimatization?" The answer to this question is yes, but the magnitude of the heat acclimatization that is obtained by this method is generally less than the maximal level of acclimatization that can be achieved by daily training in a hot/humid environment (1, 12). Nonetheless, "artifi-

cial" heat training in sweat clothing in cool conditions appears to be better than attempting no heat acclimatization measures (12). See reference 12 for a review on this topic.

On a related topic, most of us have witnessed individuals exercising in a rubber suit. These exercise suits are typically made of a rubberized vinyl that covers the entire body and prevents evaporative heat loss from the skin. While exercise in these suits will promote increased body temperature and therefore will contribute to heat acclimatization, prolonged exercise in a rubber suit is a high-risk endeavor that could lead to high body temperatures and heat injury. Therefore, wear-

ing a rubber suit during exercise is not recommended because of the risk of hyperthermia associated with the prevention of evaporative heat loss. Also, note that while exercise in a rubber suit will encourage body water loss, exercise in a rubber suit does not necessarily result in the loss of body fat because in order to lose body fat, you must create an energy (i.e., caloric) deficit. Indeed, while a sweat-induced loss of body water does reduce your body weight, as soon as you replace these fluids by drinking, your body weight will return to normal. See chapter 18 for details on loss of body fat.

RESEARCH FOCUS 12.3

Heat Acclimatization and Heat Shock Proteins

Repeated bouts of prolonged exercise in a warm or hot environment result in many physiological adaptations that minimize disturbances in homeostasis due to heat stress. Collectively, these adaptations improve exercise tolerance in hot environments and reduce the risk of heat injury. Recent evidence indicates that an important part of this

adaptive process is the synthesis of heat shock proteins in numerous tissues, including skeletal muscle and the heart (54). Heat shock proteins represent a family of "stress" proteins that are synthesized in response to cellular stress (i.e., heat, acidosis, tissue injury, etc.). Although heat shock proteins perform a variety of cellular functions,

it is clear that these proteins protect cells from thermal injury by stabilizing and refolding damaged proteins. Indeed, heat shock proteins play an important role in the development of thermotolerance and protect body cells from the heat loads associated with prolonged exercise (38).

New research indicates that an important part of heat acclimatization includes the cellular production of heat shock proteins. Heat shock proteins are members of a large family of proteins called "stress proteins"; they were introduced in chapter 2. As the name implies, these stress proteins are synthesized in response to stress (e.g., heat) and are designed to prevent cellular damage due to heat or other stresses. Details of how heat shock proteins protect cells against heat stress are found in Research Focus 12.3.

As stated previously, heat adaptation results in an earlier onset of sweating. This means that sweating

begins rapidly after the commencement of exercise, which translates into less heat storage at the beginning of exercise and a lower core temperature. In addition, heat acclimatization may increase the sweating capacity almost threefold above the rate achievable prior to heat adaptation (61, 74). Therefore, much more evaporative cooling is possible, which is a major advantage in minimizing heat storage during prolonged work. Finally, sweat losses of sodium and chloride are reduced following heat acclimatization due to an increased secretion of aldosterone (73). While this adaptation results in a reduction of

TABLE 12.2	A Summary of the Primary Adaptations That Occur as a Result of Heat Acclimatization

1. Increased plasma volume
2. Earlier onset of sweating
3. Higher sweat rate
4. Reduced sodium chloride loss in sweat
5. Reduced skin blood flow
6. Increased heat shock proteins in tissues

electrolyte loss and aids in reducing electrolyte disturbances during exercise in the heat, it does not minimize the need to replace water loss, which is higher than normal (see chapters 23 and 24). A summary of heat-adaptive responses is presented in table 12.2.

Loss of Acclimatization

The rate of decay of heat acclimatization is rapid, with reductions in heat tolerance occurring within a few days of inactivity (i.e., no heat exposure) (37). In this regard, studies have shown that heat tolerance can decline significantly within seven days of no heat exposure, and complete loss of heat tolerance can occur following twenty-eight days of no heat exposure (1). Therefore, repeated exposure to heat is required to maintain heat acclimatization (72).

IN SUMMARY

- During prolonged exercise in a moderate environment, core temperature will increase gradually above the normal resting value and will reach a plateau at approximately thirty to forty-five minutes.
- During exercise in a hot/humid environment, core temperature does not reach a plateau, but will continue to rise. Long-term exercise in this type of environment increases the risk of heat injury.
- Heat acclimatization results in: (1) an increase in plasma volume, (2) an earlier onset of sweating during exercise, (3) a higher sweat rate, (4) a reduction in the amount of electrolytes lost in sweat, and (5) a reduction in skin blood flow.

EXERCISE IN A COLD ENVIRONMENT

Exercise in a cold environment enhances an athlete's ability to lose heat and therefore greatly reduces the chance of heat injury. In general, the combination of metabolic heat production and warm clothing prevents the development of **hypothermia** (large decrease in core temperature) during short-term work on a cold day. However, exercise in the cold for extended periods of time (e.g., a long triathlon), or swimming in cold water, may overpower the body's ability to prevent heat loss, and hypothermia may result. In such cases, heat production during exercise is not able to keep pace with heat loss. This is particularly true during swimming in extremely cold water (e.g., <15° C). Severe hypothermia may result in a loss of judgment, which increases the risk of further cold injury.

Individuals with a high percentage of body fat have an advantage over lean individuals when it comes to cold tolerance (27, 50). Large amounts of subcutaneous fat provide an increased layer of insulation from the cold. This additional insulation reduces the rate of heat loss and therefore improves cold tolerance. It is for this reason that women generally tolerate mild cold exposure better than men (50).

Participation in sports activities in the cold may present several other types of problems for the athlete. For example, hands exposed to cold weather become numb due to the reduction in the rate of neural transmission and reduced blood flow due to vasoconstriction. This results in a loss of dexterity and of course affects such skills as throwing and catching. In addition, exposed flesh is susceptible to frostbite, which may present a serious medical condition (6). Further details of the effects of a cold environment on performance will be presented in chapter 24.

Cold Acclimatization

In humans chronically exposed to cold (e.g., primitive societies, mountain climbers), there appear to be at least three physiological adaptations to cold exposure (15, 26, 29). First, cold adaptation results in a reduction in the mean skin temperature at which shivering begins. That is, people who are cold acclimatized begin shivering at a lower skin temperature when compared to unacclimatized individuals. The explanation for this observation is that cold-acclimatized people maintain heat production with less shivering by increasing nonshivering thermogenesis. They increase the secretion of norepinephrine, which results in an increase in metabolic heat production (6, 7, 26).

A second physiological adjustment that occurs due to cold acclimatization is that cold-adjusted individuals can maintain a higher mean hand-and-foot temperature during cold exposure when compared to unacclimatized persons. Cold acclimatization apparently results in improved intermittent peripheral vasodilation to increase blood flow (and heat flow) to both the hands and feet (66).

The third and final physiological adaptation to cold is the improved ability to sleep in cold environments. Unacclimatized people who try to sleep in cold environments will often shiver so much that sleep is impossible (6). In contrast, cold-acclimatized individuals can sleep comfortably in cold environments due to their elevated level of nonshivering thermogenesis. The exact time course of complete cold acclimatization is not clear. However, subjects placed in a cold chamber begin to show signs of cold acclimatization after one week (51).

IN SUMMARY

- Exercise in a cold environment enhances an athlete's ability to lose heat and therefore greatly reduces the chance of heat injury.
- Cold acclimatization results in three physiological adaptations: (1) improved ability to sleep in cold environments, (2) increased nonshivering thermogenesis, and (3) a higher intermittent blood flow to the hands and feet. The overall goal of these adaptations is to increase heat production and maintain core temperature, which will make the individual more comfortable during cold exposure.

STUDY QUESTIONS

1. Define the following terms: (1) *homeotherm*, (2) *hyperthermia*, and (3) *hypothermia*.
2. Why does a significant increase in core temperature represent a threat to life?
3. Explain the comment that the term *body temperature* is a misnomer.
4. How is body temperature measured during exercise?
5. Briefly discuss the role of the hypothalamus in temperature regulation. How do the anterior hypothalamus and posterior hypothalamus differ in function?
6. List and define the four mechanisms of heat loss. Which of these avenues plays the most important part during exercise in a hot/dry environment?
7. Discuss the two general categories of heat production in people.
8. What hormones are involved in biochemical heat production?
9. Briefly outline the thermal events that occur during prolonged exercise in a moderate environment. Include in your discussion information about changes in core temperature, skin blood flow, sweating, and skin temperature.
10. Calculate the amount of evaporation that must occur to remove 400 kcal of heat from the body.
11. How much heat would be removed from the skin if 520 ml of sweat evaporated during a thirty-minute period?
12. List and discuss the physiological adaptations that occur during heat acclimatization.
13. How might exercise in a cold environment affect dexterity in such skills as throwing and catching?
14. Discuss the physiological changes that occur in response to chronic exposure to cold.

SUGGESTED READINGS

Bergeron, M. et al. 2005. Youth football: Heat stress and injury risk. *Medicine and Science in Sports and Exercise* 37: 1421–30.

Brooks, G., T. Fahey, and K. Baldwin. 2005. *Exercise Physiology: Human Bioenergetics and Its Applications*, 4th ed. New York: McGraw-Hill Companies.

Cheung, S., and G. Sleivert. 2004. Multiple triggers for hyperthermic fatigue and exhaustion. *Exercise and Sport Science Reviews* 32:100–6.

Cheuvront, S., and M. Sawka. 2005. Hydration assessment in athletes. *Sports Science Exchange* 18(2):1–4.

Kenney, W. L., and T. Munce. 2003. Aging and human temperature regulation. *Journal of Applied Physiology* 95: 2598–2603.

Shirreffs, S. 2005. The importance of good hydration for work and exercise performance. *Nutrition Review* 63:S14–21.

Stocks, J., N. Taylor, M. Tipton, and J. Greenleaf. 2004. Human physiological responses to cold exposure. *Aviation and Space and Environmental Medicine* 75:444–57.

REFERENCES

1. Armstrong, L., and C. Maresh. 1991. The induction and decay of heat acclimatisation in trained athletes. *Sports Medicine* 12:302–12.
2. Åstrand, P., and K. Rodahl. 1986. *Textbook of Work Physiology*. New York: McGraw-Hill Companies.
3. Bergeron, M. et al. 2005. Youth football: Heat stress and injury risk. *Medicine and Science in Sports and Exercise* 37:1421–30.
4. Brengelmann, G. 1977. Control of sweating and skin blood flow during exercise. In *Problems with Temperature Regulation During Exercise*, ed. E. Nadel. New York: Academic Press.
5. Brooks, G., T. Fahey, and K. Baldwin. 2005. *Exercise Physiology: Human Bioenergetics and Its Applications*, 4th ed. New York: McGraw-Hill Companies.
6. Brooks, G., and T. Fahey. 1987. *Fundamentals of Human Performance*. New York: Macmillan.
7. Cabanac, M. 1975. Temperature regulation. *Annual Review of Physiology* 37:415–39.

8. Casa, D. et al. 2000. National athletic trainers association position statement: Fluid replacement for athletes. *Journal of Athletic Training* 35:212–24.

9. Cheung, S., and G. Sleivert. 2004. Multiple triggers for hyperthermic fatigue and exhaustion. *Exercise and Sport Science Reviews* 32:100–6.

10. Cheuvront, S., and M. Sawka. 2005. Hydration assessment in athletes. *Sports Science Exchange* 18(2):1–4.

11. Clausen, T., C. Van Hardeveld, and M. Everts. 1991. Significance of cation transport in control of energy metabolism and thermogenesis. *Physiological Reviews* 71:733–74.

12. Dawson, B. 1994. Exercise training in sweat clothing in cool conditions to improve heat tolerance. *Sports Medicine* 17:233–44.

13. Delamarche, P., J. Bittel, J. Lacour, and R. Flandrois. 1990. Thermoregulation at rest and during exercise in prepubertal boys. *European Journal of Applied Physiology* 60:436–40.

14. Dill D., and C. Consolazio. 1962. Responses to exercise as related to age and environmental temperature. *Journal of Applied Physiology* 17:64–69.

15. Doubt, T. 1991. Physiology of exercise in the cold. *Sports Medicine* 11:367–81.

16. Epstein, Y. 1990. Heat intolerance: Predisposing factor or residual injury? *Medicine and Science in Sports and Exercise* 22:29–35.

17. Fox, S. 2006. *Human Physiology*, 9th ed. New York: McGraw-Hill Companies.

18. Ftaiti, F. et al. 2001. Combined effect of heat stress, dehydration, and exercise on neuromuscular function in humans. *European Journal of Applied Physiology* 84:87–94.

19. Gisolfi, C., and J. Cohen. 1979. Relationships among training, heat acclimation, and heat tolerance in men and women: The controversy revisited. *Medicine and Science in Sports* 11:56–59.

20. Gisolfi, C., and C. B. Wenger. 1984. Temperature regulation during exercise: Old concepts, new ideas. In *Exercise and Sport Science Reviews*, vol. 12, ed. R. Terjung, 339–72.

21. Godek S., A. Bartolozzi, and J. Godek. 2005. Sweat rate and fluid turnover in American Football players compared to runners in a hot and humid environment. *British Journal of Sports Medicine* 39:205–11.

22. Gonzalez-Alonso, J., J. Calbet, and B. Nielsen. 1999. Metabolic and thermodynamic responses to dehydration-induced reductions in muscle blood flow in humans. *Journal of Physiology* (London) 520:577–89.

23. Gonzalez-Alonso, J. et al. 1999. Influence of body temperature on the development of fatigue during prolonged exercise in the heat. *Journal of Applied Physiology* 86:1032–9.

24 Guyton, A., and J. Hall. 2005. *Textbook of Medical Physiology*. Saunders/Elsevier.

25. Hole, J. 1995. *Human Anatomy and Physiology*. New York: McGraw-Hill Companies.

26. Hong, S., D. Rennie, and Y. Park. 1987. Humans can acclimatize to cold: A lesson from Korean divers. *News in Physiological Sciences* 2:79–82.

27. Horvath, S. 1981. Exercise in a cold environment. In *Exercise and Sport Science Reviews*, vol. 9, 221–63.

28. Hubbard, R. 1990. An introduction: The role of exercise in the etiology of exertional heatstroke. *Medicine and Science in Sports and Exercise* 22:2–5.

29. Iampietro, P., D. Bass, and E. Buskirk. 1959. Diurnal oxygen consumption and rectal temperature of men during cold exposure. *Journal of Applied Physiology* 10:398–403.

30. Johnson, J. 1992. Exercise and the cutaneous circulation. In *Exercise and Sport Science Reviews*, vol. 20, ed. J. Holloszy, 59–98.

31. Johnson, L. 1987. *Biology*. New York: McGraw-Hill Companies.

32. Kenney, W. 1988. Control of heat-induced cutaneous vasodilation in relation to age. *European Journal of Applied Physiology* 57:120–25.

33. Kenney, W., and J. Johnson. 1992. Control of skin blood flow during exercise. *Medicine and Science in Sport and Exercise* 24:303–12.

34. Kenney, W. L. 1997. Thermoregulation at rest and during exercise in healthy older adults. *Exercise and Sport Science Reviews* 25:41–76.

35. Kenney, W. L., and T. Munce. 2003. Aging and human temperature regulation. *Journal of Applied Physiology* 95:2598–2603.

36. Kruk, B. et al. 1991. Comparison in men of physiological responses to exercise of increasing intensity at low and moderate ambient temperatures. *European Journal of Applied Physiology* 62:353–57.

37. Lee, S. M. C., W. J. Williams, and S. M. Schneider. 2002. Role of skin blood flow and sweating rate in exercise thermoregulation after bed rest. *Journal of Applied Physiology* 92:2026–34.

38. Locke, M. 1997. The cellular stress response to exercise: Role of stress proteins. *Exercise and Sport Science Reviews* 25:105–36.

39. Maughan, R., and R. Murray. 2000. *Sports Drinks: Basic Science and Practical Aspects*. Boca Raton, FL: CRC Press.

40. McArdle, W., F. Katch, and V. Katch. 2001. *Exercise Physiology: Energy, Nutrition, and Human Performance*. Baltimore: Lippincott Williams & Wilkins.

41. McKenzie, J., and D. Osgood. 2004. Validation of a new telemetric core temperature monitor. *Journal of Thermal Biology* 29:605–11.

42. Morris, J., M. Nevill, H. Lakomy, C. Nicholas, and C. Williams. 1998. Effect of a hot environment on performance during prolonged, intermittent, high-intensity shuttle running. *Journal of Sports Sciences* 16:677–86.

43. Nadel, E. 1979. Temperature regulation. In *Sports Medicine and Physiology*, ed. R. Strauss. Philadelphia: W. B. Saunders.

44. Nadel, E. 1988. Temperature regulation during prolonged exercise. In *Perspectives in Exercise Science and Sports Medicine: Prolonged Exercise*, ed. D. Lamb and R. Murray, 125–52. Indianapolis: Benchmark Press.

45. Nielson, B. 1969. Thermoregulation during exercise. *Acta Physicologica Scandanavica* (Suppl.) 323:10–73.

46. Nielson, B. 1990. Solar heat load: Heat balance during exercise in clothed subjects. *European Journal of Applied Physiology* 60:452–56.

47. Nielson, B. et al. 1990. Muscle blood flow and muscle metabolism during exercise and heat stress. *Journal of Applied Physiology* 69:1040–46.

48. Nielson, M. 1938. Die Regulation der Korpertemperatur bei Muskelarbeit. *Scandanavica Archives Physiology* 79:193.

49. Noble, B. 1986. *Physiology of Exercise and Sport*. St. Louis: C. V. Mosby.

50. Nunneley, S. 1978. Physiological responses of women to thermal stress: A review. *Medicine and Science in Sports and Exercise* 10:250–55.

51. Pandolf, K. 1979. Effects of physical training and cardiorespiratory fitness on exercise-heat tolerance: Recent observations. *Medicine and Science in Sports and Exercise* 11:60–65.

52. Pandolf, K. et al. 1988. Thermoregulatory responses of middle-aged men and young men during dry-heat acclimatization. *Journal of Applied Physiology* 65:65–70.

53. Parkin, J. et al. 1999. Effect of ambient temperature on human skeletal muscle metabolism during fatiguing submaximal exercise. *Journal of Applied Physiology* 86:902–8.

54. Powers, S., H. Demirel, H. Vincent, J. Coombes, H. Naito, K. Hamilton, R. Shanely, and J. Jessup. 1998. Exercise training improves myocardial tolerance to in vivo ischemia-reperfusion injury in the rat. *American Journal of Physiology* 275:R1468–77.

55. Powers, S., E. Howley, and R. Cox. 1982. A differential catecholamine response during prolonged exercise and passive heating. *Medicine and Science in Sports and Exercise* 6:435–39.

56. Powers, S., E. Howley, and R. Cox. 1982. Ventilatory and metabolic reactions to heat stress during prolonged exercise. *Journal of Sports Medicine and Physical Fitness* 22:32–36.

57. Powers, S., E. Howley, and R. Cox. 1985. Blood lactate concentrations during submaximal work under differing environmental conditions. *Journal of Sports Medicine and Physical Fitness* 25:84–89.

58. Rasch, W. et al. 1991. Heat loss from the human head during exercise. *Journal of Applied Physiology* 71:590–95.

59. Robergs, R., and S. Roberts. 2002. *Fundamental Principles of Exercise Physiology for Fitness, Performance, and Health.* New York: McGraw-Hill Companies.

60. Robinson, S. 1963. Temperature regulation during exercise. *Pediatrics* 32:691–702.

61. Sato, F. et al. 1990. Functional and morphological changes in the eccrine sweat gland with heat acclimation. *Journal of Applied Physiology* 69:232–36.

62. Sawka, M. 1992. Physiological consequences of hypohydration: Exercise performance and thermoregulation. *Medicine and Science in Sports and Exercise* 24:657–70.

63. Shirreffs, S. 2005. The importance of good hydration for work and exercise performance. *Nutrition Review* 63:S14–21.

64. Shirreffs S., L. Armstrong, and S. Cheuvront. 2004. Fluid and electrolyte needs for preparation and recovery from training and competition. *Journal of Sports Sciences* 22:57–63.

65. Starkie, R., M. Hargreaves, D. Lambert, J. Proietto, and M. Febbraio. 1999. Effect of temperature on muscle metabolism during submaximal exercise in humans. *Experimental Physiology* 84:775–84.

66. Stocks, J., N. Taylor, M. Tipton, and J. Greenleaf. 2004. Human physiological responses to cold exposure. *Aviation and Space and Environmental Medicine* 75:444–57.

67. Stolwijk, J., B. Saltin, and A. Gagge. 1968. Physiological factors associated with sweating during exercise. *Aerospace Medicine* 39:1101–5.

68. Suzuki, Y. 1980. Human physical performance and cardiorespiratory responses to hot environments during submaximal upright cycling. *Ergonomics* 23:527–42.

69. Thomas, C., J. Pierzga, and W. Kenney. 1999. Aerobic training and cutaneous vasodilation in young and older men. *Journal of Applied Physiology* 86:1676–86.

70. Tikuisis, P., D. Bell, and I. Jacobs. 1991. Shivering onset, metabolic response, and convective heat transfer during cold air exposure. *Journal of Applied Physiology* 70:1996–2002.

71. Wenger, C. B. 1972. Heat evaporation of sweat: Thermodynamic considerations. *Journal of Applied Physiology* 32:456–59.

72. Williams, C., C. Wyndham, and J. Morrison. 1967. Rate of loss of acclimatization in summer and winter. *Journal of Applied Physiology* 22:21–26.

73. Wyndham, C. 1973. The physiology of exercise under heat stress. *Annual Review of Physiology* 35:193–220.

74. Yanagimoto, S. et al. 2002. Sweating response in physically trained men to sustained handgrip exercise in mildly hyperthermic conditions. *Acta Physiologica Scandanavia* 174:31–39.

75. Zuo, L. et al. 2000. Intra- and extracellular measurement of reactive oxygen species produced during heat stress in diaphragm muscle. *American Journal of Physiology* 279:C1058–66.

The Physiology of Training: Effect on $\dot{V}O_2$ Max, Performance, Homeostasis, and Strength

■ Objectives

By studying this chapter, you should be able to do the following:

1. Explain the basic principles of training: overload and specificity.
2. Contrast cross-sectional with longitudinal research studies.
3. Indicate the typical change in $\dot{V}O_2$ max with endurance training programs, and the effect of the initial (pretraining) value on the magnitude of the increase.
4. State typical $\dot{V}O_2$ max values for various sedentary, active, and athletic populations.
5. State the formula for $\dot{V}O_2$ max using heart rate, stroke volume, and the a-$\bar{v}$ O_2 difference; indicate which of the variables is most important in explaining the wide range of $\dot{V}O_2$ max values in the population.
6. Discuss, using the variables identified in objective 5, how the increase in $\dot{V}O_2$ max comes about for the sedentary subject who participates in an endurance training program.
7. Define *preload*, *afterload*, and *contractility*, and discuss the role of each in the increase in the maximal stroke volume that occurs with endurance training.
8. Describe the changes in muscle structure that are responsible for the increase in the

maximal a-$\bar{v}$ O_2 difference with endurance training.
9. Describe the underlying causes of the decrease in $\dot{V}O_2$ max that occurs with cessation of endurance training.
10. Describe how the capillary and mitochondrial changes that occur in muscle as a result of an endurance training program are related to the following adaptations to submaximal exercise:
    a. a lower O_2 deficit
    b. an increased utilization of FFA and a sparing of blood glucose and muscle glycogen
    c. a reduction in lactate and H^+ formation
    d. an increase in lactate removal
11. Discuss how changes in "central command" and "peripheral feedback" following an endurance training program can lower the heart rate, ventilation, and catecholamine responses to a submaximal exercise bout.
12. Contrast the role of neural adaptations with hypertrophy in the increase in strength that occurs with resistance training.

■ Outline

Principles of Training   261
  Overload   261
  Specificity   262

Research Designs to Study Training   262

Endurance Training and $\dot{V}O_2$ Max   262
  Training Programs and Changes in $\dot{V}O_2$ Max   263

$\dot{V}O_2$ Max: Cardiac Output and the Arteriovenous O_2 Difference   264
  Stroke Volume   265
  Arteriovenous O_2 Difference   267

Detraining and $\dot{V}O_2$ Max   268

Endurance Training: Effects
on Performance and
Homeostasis   269
   Biochemical Adaptations and
    the Oxygen Deficit   271
   Biochemical Adaptations
    and the Plasma Glucose
    Concentration   271

Biochemical Adaptations
  and Blood pH   273
Biochemical Adaptations and
  Lactate Removal   274

Endurance Training: Links
Between Muscle and
Systemic Physiology   275
   Peripheral Feedback   277
   Central Command   277

Physiological Effects of
Strength Training   278

Physiological Mechanisms
Causing Increased
Strength   279
   Neural Factors   279
   Muscular Enlargement   280
   Concurrent Strength and
    Endurance Training   281

■ **Key Terms**

bradycardia
ejection fraction

overload
reversibility

specificity

A theme that has been used throughout this book is that there are automatic regulatory mechanisms operating at rest and during exercise to maintain homeostasis. Figure 13.1 identifies some of the variables that are maintained within narrow limits during exercise in spite of the tremendous demands placed on various tissues and organ systems. What has become clear is that participation in regular endurance exercise increases the cardiovascular system's ability to deliver blood to the working muscles, and increases the muscle's capacity to produce energy aerobically. These parallel changes result in less disruption of the internal environment during exercise. This, of course, leads to improved performance.

The purpose of this chapter is to tie together much of what has been presented previously, since most tissues and organ systems are either directly or indirectly affected by training programs. There is a need to discuss separately those physiological changes causing an increase in $\dot{V}O_2$ max from those associated with improvements in prolonged submaximal performance. $\dot{V}O_2$ max is most closely linked to the functional capacity of the cardiovascular system to deliver blood to the working muscles during maximal and supramaximal (>100% $\dot{V}O_2$ max) work, while maintaining mean arterial blood pressure. The ability to sustain long-term, submaximal exercise is linked more to the maintenance of homeostasis due to specific structural and biochemical properties of working muscles (6, 48, 85). Finally, we will explore the physiology of strength development. Strength training causes adaptations in muscle that are potentially in conflict with those adaptations associated with running or cycling training programs. This raises questions about whether or not the effects of the two training programs actually interfere with each other. Before we begin a discussion of these topics, informa-

FIGURE 13.1 Homeostatic variables maintained within narrow limits in spite of the challenge presented by exercise.

tion about the principles of training and the design of research studies will be presented.

PRINCIPLES OF TRAINING

The three principles of training are **overload, specificity,** and **reversibility.** These principles will be applied in chapters 16 and 17 for those training for fitness, and in chapters 21 and 22 for those training for performance.

Overload

Overload refers to the observation that a system or tissue must be exercised at a level beyond which it is accustomed in order for a training effect to occur. The system or tissue gradually adapts to this overload. This pattern of progressively and systematically overloading a system or tissue as adaptations occur results in improved function over time. The typical variables that constitute the overload include the intensity, duration, and frequency (days per week) of exercise. The corollary of the overload principle, the principle of *reversibility*, simply indicates that the gains are quickly lost when the overload is removed.

Specificity

The training effect is *specific* to the muscles involved, the fiber types recruited, the principal energy system involved (aerobic versus anaerobic), the velocity of contraction, and type of muscle contraction (eccentric, concentric, or isometric). This may seem like an obvious statement in that one should not expect the arms to become trained during a ten-week jogging program. However, this also means that if an individual participates in a long, slow, distance running program that utilizes the slow-twitch muscle fibers, there is little or no training effect taking place in those fast-twitch fibers in the same muscle (48, 94). A good example of specificity is found in a study in which subjects did either cycle or run training, but had their lactate threshold (LT) evaluated before and after training on both the cycle and treadmill. Run training increased the LT 58% and 20% for the treadmill and cycle, respectively. The cycle training increased the cycle LT 39%, with no measured improvement in the treadmill LT (74). Training effects were clearly specific to the type of training.

Specificity also refers to the types of adaptations occurring in muscle as a result of training. If a muscle is engaged in endurance types of exercise, the primary adaptations are in capillary and mitochondria number, which increase the capacity of the muscle to produce energy aerobically (48, 93). If a muscle is engaged in heavy resistance training, the primary adaptation is an increase in the quantity of the contractile proteins; the mitochondrial and capillary densities may actually decrease (61). This high degree of specificity in the training effect is related to a point raised earlier, that one type of training may interfere with the adaptations to the other (see later discussion).

IN SUMMARY

- The principle of overload states that for a training effect to occur, a system or tissue must be challenged with an intensity, duration, or frequency of exercise to which it is unaccustomed. Over time the tissue or system adapts to this load. The reversibility principle is a corollary to the overload principle.
- The principle of specificity indicates that the training effect is limited to the muscle fibers involved in the activity. In addition, the muscle fiber adapts specifically to the type of activity: mitochondrial and capillary adaptations to endurance training, and contractile protein adaptations to resistive weight training.

RESEARCH DESIGNS TO STUDY TRAINING

The effect of exercise training on various physiological systems has been studied using two different designs: cross-sectional and longitudinal. In cross-sectional studies the investigator examines groups differing in physical activity (e.g., cardiac patients, sedentary students, and world-class endurance athletes) and records the differences that exist in $\dot{V}O_2$ max, cardiac output, or fiber-type distribution. These studies are relatively inexpensive to conduct and provide good descriptive information about differences that exist among various populations. They are also useful in developing questions about how these differences came about, including hypotheses about the relative role of genetics versus training. Longitudinal studies examine *changes* in $\dot{V}O_2$ max, cardiac output, or fiber-type distribution occurring over the course of a training program. These studies control for the genetic factor, since the same subject is repeatedly tested, and allow one to investigate the *rate* at which the variables respond to training or detraining. Longitudinal studies are expensive and difficult to conduct due to the potential for subjects to drop out and the demand for all equipment and procedures to be held constant at all testing points in the study. Due to these constraints, only small numbers of subjects are used in these studies. The investigator must take special care that the subjects are representative of the population, and that they do not alter other lifestyle patterns (diet, smoking, etc.) that might influence the outcome of the study (4).

As we mentioned in the introduction, the effects of training on $\dot{V}O_2$ max will be discussed separately from the effects on performance and homeostasis. The application of this information in the design of training programs for fitness and performance is found in chapters 16, 17, 21, and 22.

IN SUMMARY

- Cross-sectional training studies contrast the physiological responses of groups differing in habitual physical activity (e.g., sedentary individuals versus runners).
- Longitudinal training studies examine the changes taking place over the course of a training program.

ENDURANCE TRAINING AND $\dot{V}O_2$ MAX

Maximal aerobic power, $\dot{V}O_2$ max, is a reproducible measure of the capacity of the cardiovascular system to deliver oxygenated blood to a large muscle

TABLE 13.1	$\dot{V}O_2$ Max Values Measured in Healthy and Diseased Populations	
Population	**Males**	**Females**
Cross-country skiers	84	72
Distance runners	83	62
Sedentary: young	45	38
Sedentary: middle-aged adults	35	30
Post myocardial infarction patients	22	18
Severe pulmonary disease patients	13	13

Values are expressed in $ml \cdot kg^{-1} \cdot min^{-1}$.

Taken from Saltin and Åstrand (91), Åtrand and Rodahl (4), and Howley and Franks (51).

mass involved in dynamic work (85). Chapter 4 introduced this concept, and chapters 9 and 10 showed how specific cardiovascular and pulmonary variables respond to graded exercise up to $\dot{V}O_2$ max. The following sections discuss the effect of endurance exercise programs on the increase in $\dot{V}O_2$ max and the physiological changes bringing about that increase.

Training Programs and Changes in $\dot{V}O_2$ Max

Endurance training programs that increase $\dot{V}O_2$ max involve a large muscle mass in dynamic exercise (e.g., running, cycling, swimming, or cross-country skiing) for twenty to sixty minutes per session, three to five times per week at an intensity of about 50% to 85% $\dot{V}O_2$ max (1). Details about how to design a training program for the average individual and the athlete are presented in chapters 16 and 21, respectively. While endurance training programs of two to three months' duration cause an increase in $\dot{V}O_2$ max of about 15%, the range of improvement can be as low as 2% to 3% for those who start the program with high $\dot{V}O_2$ max values (28), and as high as 30% to 50% for those with low initial $\dot{V}O_2$ max values (28, 33, 47, 85, 90).

Table 13.1 shows that $\dot{V}O_2$ max can be less than 20 $ml \cdot kg^{-1} \cdot min^{-1}$ in patients with severe cardiovascular and pulmonary disease, and more than 80 $ml \cdot kg^{-1} \cdot min^{-1}$ in world-class distance runners and cross-country skiers. The extremely high $\dot{V}O_2$ max values measured in elite male and female endurance athletes have been ascribed to a genetic gift of a large cardiovascular capacity (4). Early work by Klissouras et al. (57) supported this idea with the observation that identical twins have very similar $\dot{V}O_2$ max values, while

fraternal twins do not. Given that identical twins have identical genes, it was suggested that 93% of the variation in $\dot{V}O_2$max values in the general population was due to genetics. On the surface, that high estimate appears to be consistent with the small changes in $\dot{V}O_2$ max that occur with the training programs just mentioned. However, questions were raised about this conclusion. It is now generally accepted that we need to revise that estimate downward to a figure somewhat closer to 40% to 66% (10, 13, 35). Although some scientists feel that these estimates are still too high (11), it is clear that a genetic predisposition for possessing a high $\dot{V}O_2$ max value is still a prerequisite for values in the range of 60 to 80 $ml \cdot kg^{-1} \cdot min^{-1}$. Further, there is evidence that the sensitivity of the individual to the effect of a training program is also genetically determined (10, 78). That is, even when one controls for a variety of pretraining measures, there will still be a great deal of variation in the degree of improvement (9). Evidence points to differences in mitochondrial DNA as being important in the individual differences in $\dot{V}O_2$ max and its response to training (13, 14, 30). See A Closer Look 13.1 for more on this exciting topic.

Consistent with these lower estimates of the genetic contribution to $\dot{V}O_2$ max are the observations that training for two to three years (33), or participation in severe interval training (47) can increase $\dot{V}O_2$ max by as much as 44%. The results of the latter study showed a linear increase in $\dot{V}O_2$ max over ten weeks of training, whereas most studies show a leveling off of the $\dot{V}O_2$ max values after only a few weeks of training. The much larger increase in $\dot{V}O_2$ max with this ten-week training program was due to a much higher intensity, frequency, and duration than are usually used in endurance exercise programs. We'll next discuss what causes the $\dot{V}O_2$ max to increase as a result of an endurance exercise program.

IN SUMMARY

- Endurance training programs that increase $\dot{V}O_2$ max involve a large muscle mass in dynamic activity for twenty to sixty minutes per session, three to five times per week, at an intensity of 50% to 85% $\dot{V}O_2$ max.
- Although $\dot{V}O_2$ max increases an average of about 15% as a result of an endurance training program, the largest increases are associated with deconditioned or patient populations having very low pretraining $\dot{V}O_2$ max values.
- Genetic predisposition accounts for 40% to 66% of one's $\dot{V}O_2$ max value. Very strenuous and/or prolonged training can increase $\dot{V}O_2$ max in normal sedentary individuals by more than 40%.

The HERITAGE Family Study

The HERITAGE Family Study was designed "to study the role of the genotype in cardiovascular, metabolic, and hormonal responses to aerobic exercise training and the contribution of regular exercise to changes in several cardiovascular disease and diabetes risk factors." Two-generational, nuclear families of Caucasian and African-American descent were recruited for the study. All participants had to be sedentary, and had to pass a variety of screening tests for inclusion (12). The results of these studies have already appeared in the literature, and will continue to appear in the literature. The following summaries relate to the role of the genotype on $\dot{V}O_2$ max, and changes in $\dot{V}O_2$ max due to endurance training.

1. The maximum heritability estimate for $\dot{V}O_2$ max among sedentary adults (adjusted for age, sex, body composition, and body mass) was found to be at least 50%, but the authors acknowledge that the value might be inflated due to inclusion of nongenetic familial factors in this estimate (13). The maternal contribution, potentially associated with mitochondrial inheritance, was about 30%.

2. The authors found considerable variation in the changes in $\dot{V}O_2$ max to a carefully controlled, twenty-week endurance exercise program, even though the average response (15%–20% increase in $\dot{V}O_2$ max) was as expected. At one extreme, some subjects showed a small *decrease* in $\dot{V}O_2$ max, while at the other, some subjects experienced an increase of more than 1 L/min. The fact that there was 2.5 times more variability between families than within families in the change in $\dot{V}O_2$ max due to training indicated the presence of a genetic factor in this response.

The maximal heritability estimate of the change in $\dot{V}O_2$ max due to training was found to be 47%, with a substantial part of that due to maternal transmission (14).

3. A follow-up study examined the regions of the genome that might be linked to the variability in $\dot{V}O_2$ max in sedentary individuals and the change in $\dot{V}O_2$ max due to a training intervention. Although none of the linkages was found to be very strong, the study did show that the genes that might be tied to the variability in $\dot{V}O_2$ max in sedentary individuals were different from those associated with the gain in $\dot{V}O_2$ max due to training (15). Given the focus on the human genome as it relates to health and disease, we are sure to hear more on this topic in the near future.

$\dot{V}O_2$ MAX: CARDIAC OUTPUT AND THE ARTERIOVENOUS O_2 DIFFERENCE

Since oxygen uptake is the product of systemic blood flow (cardiac output) and systemic oxygen extraction (arteriovenous oxygen difference), changes in $\dot{V}O_2$ max would have to be due to changes in one or more of the following variables on the right side of the equal sign:

$$\dot{V}O_2 \text{ max} = HR \text{ max} \times SV \text{ max} \times (a\text{-}\bar{v} O_2 \text{ difference}) \text{ max}$$

Cross-sectional comparisons of groups differing in their level of habitual physical activity have allowed scientists to identify the most important of these variables as the prime determinant of $\dot{V}O_2$ max. Such a comparison is presented in table 13.2, where values for $\dot{V}O_2$ max, maximal heart rate, maximal stroke volume, and the maximal a-$\bar{v}$ O_2 difference are presented for three groups of subjects: mitral stenosis patients (heart valve problem limiting stroke volume),

normally active subjects, and finally, world-class endurance athletes (85). The $\dot{V}O_2$ max is more than 100% greater for the normally active subjects compared to those with mitral stenosis, and again, almost 100% higher for the athletes as compared to the normally active subjects. What variable explains the tremendous differences in $\dot{V}O_2$ max values? Given that the maximal heart rate and the maximal a-$\bar{v}$ O_2 difference were virtually identical for the three groups, the only variable explaining the difference in $\dot{V}O_2$ max is the maximal stroke volume (43 ml versus 112 ml versus 205 ml). Consistent with this, 68% of the variation in $\dot{V}O_2$ max between men and women was ascribed to left ventricular mass, a measure of heart size (53).

Longitudinal studies provide a slightly different picture of how training causes an increase in $\dot{V}O_2$ max. Generally, maximal heart rate either remains the same or decreases with endurance training (33, 34, 85). As a result, the increase in $\dot{V}O_2$ max is shared between the increase in the stroke volume and the systemic a-$\bar{v}$ O_2 difference. Studies reported by Saltin (90) in which young sedentary subjects trained for two to three months show that the sharing is about equal, half the gain due to SV changes and half to

TABLE 13.2 Physiological Basis for Differences in $\dot{V}O_2$ Max in Different Populations

Population	$\dot{V}O_2$ max (ml · min^{-1})	=	Heart Rate (beats · min^{-1})	×	Stroke Volume (ℓ · beat^{-1})	×	a-$\bar{v}$ O$_2$ Difference (ml O$_2$ · ℓ^{-1})
Athletes	6,250	=	190	×	.205	×	160
Normally active	3,500	=	195	×	.112	×	160
Mitral stenosis	1,400	=	190	×	.043	×	170

From L. B. Rowell, *Human Circulation Regulation During Physical Stress*. Copyright © 1986 Oxford University Press, New York N.Y. Reprinted by permission.

TABLE 13.3 Longitudinal Data on Changes in Maximal Oxygen Uptake

	$\dot{V}O_2$ max (ℓ · min^{-1})	HR max (b · min^{-1})	Stroke Volume (ml · beat^{-1})	Cardiac Output (ℓ · min^{-1})	a-$\bar{v}$ O$_2$ Difference (ml · ℓ^{-1})
Subject LM					
Before training	3.58	206	124	25.5	140
Four months	4.38	210	143	28.1	142
Eighteen months	4.53	205	149	30.5	149
Subject IS					
Before training	3.07	205	122	23.9	126
Four months	3.87	205	134	26.2	131
Thirty-two months	4.36	185	151	27.6	158
Fifty-one months	4.41	186	146	26.6	166

From B. Ekblom, "Effect of Physical Training on Oxygen Transport System in Man," in *Acta Physiologica Scandinavica*. Supplement 328. Copyright © 1969 Blackwell Scientific Publications, Ltd., Oxford, England. Reprinted by permission.

an increased oxygen extraction. In older men and women, endurance training has been shown to increase $\dot{V}O_2$ max by 19% and 22%, respectively. However, while changes in stroke volume (+15%) accounted for most of the gain in $\dot{V}O_2$ max in the men, the entire increase in $\dot{V}O_2$ max in the women was due to an increase in the a-$\bar{v}$ O$_2$ difference (96). Similarly, when training is extended for years, the continued increase in $\dot{V}O_2$ max can be due to an increase in one factor more than the other. Data from Ekblom (33), shown in table 13.3, make this point. Subject LM's increase in $\dot{V}O_2$ max from the start of training was due primarily to an increase in stroke volume. The a-$\bar{v}$ O$_2$ difference changed only 9 milliliters of O$_2$ per liter of blood over the eighteen months of training. In contrast, subject IS, whose $\dot{V}O_2$ max increased 44% over fifty-one months, showed no change in maximal cardiac output from sixteen to fifty-one months; the entire increase in $\dot{V}O_2$ max was due to an expanded a-$\bar{v}$ O$_2$ difference. What causes the maximal stroke volume and the maximal arteriovenous oxygen difference to increase as a result of endurance training? The answers are provided in the next two sections.

IN SUMMARY

- In young sedentary subjects, approximately 50% of the increase in $\dot{V}O_2$ max due to training is related to an increase in maximal stroke volume (maximal heart rate remains the same), and 50% is due to an increase in the a-$\bar{v}$ O$_2$ difference.
- The large differences in $\dot{V}O_2$ max in the normal population (2 versus 6 liters/min) are due to differences in maximal stroke volume.

Stroke Volume

Stroke volume is equal to the difference between end diastolic volume (EDV) and end systolic volume (ESV). Figure 13.2 summarizes the factors increasing stroke volume: an increase in EDV due to an increase in ventricle size or an increase in venous return ("preload"), an increase in myocardial contractility (the force of contraction at a constant muscle fiber length, with other factors controlled), and a decrease in

A CLOSER LOOK 13.2

Why Do Some Individuals Have High V̇O₂ max Values, Even Though They Do Not Train?

If you test enough sedentary individuals for maximal oxygen uptake (V̇O₂ max), you will encounter some who have surprisingly high V̇O₂ max values. Researchers at York University in Toronto decided to investigate this phenomenon and determine how it was possible (65).

Over a two-year period, these investigators tested more than 1,900 individuals for V̇O₂ max. They found 6 of the 1,900 with extraordinarily high V̇O₂ max values and absolutely no history of training. These six ("high" group) were matched with six sedentary subjects ("low" group) who had normal V̇O₂ max values and no history

of training. Measurements of blood, plasma, and red blood cell volume were determined at rest, and measurements of cardiac output, heart rate, blood pressure and V̇O₂ were obtained at rest and at 25%, 50%, 75%, and 100% V̇O₂ max in all individuals.

V̇O₂ max was 65.3 ml · kg⁻¹ · min⁻¹ for the "high" group, compared to 46.2 ml · kg⁻¹ · min⁻¹ for the "low" group. The higher value (similar to what you would measure in endurance-trained athletes) was due to a higher maximal cardiac output and stroke volume, and lower total peripheral resistance (afterload). There was no difference between groups in maximal heart rate

or the arteriovenous O₂ difference. What accounted for the higher maximal stroke volume?

The authors offer two explanations. The higher stroke volume in four of the six subjects was directly linked to higher blood volume and red cell volume. The other two subjects, who also had high stroke volume and V̇O₂ max values, had blood volumes not different from the "low" group's average value. The authors hypothesized that these two subjects might have been able to redistribute a greater percentage of their total blood volume during exercise, so as to increase venous return and maximal stroke volume.

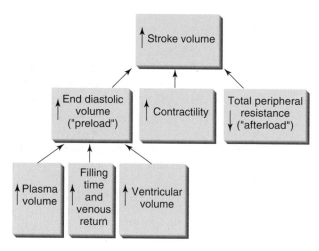

FIGURE 13.2 Factors increasing stroke volume.

resistance to blood flow out of the heart ("afterload"). Each of these will be discussed relative to the increase in the maximal stroke volume that occurs with endurance training.

End Diastolic Volume (EDV) There is evidence that left ventricle size increases as a result of endurance training with little change in ventricular wall thickness, while isometric exercises cause an increase in wall thickness with little or no change in ventricular volume (32, 71, 80). The endurance-training effect is believed to be due to the "volume loading" experienced by the heart *during exercise*. However, Rowell

(85) raises the question that the increase in stroke volume that occurs with endurance training may simply be due to the chronic stretch of the myocardium *at rest* because of the increased filling time associated with the slower resting heart rate **(bradycardia)**. Plasma volume increases with endurance training. Experimental expansion of the plasma volume (200–300 ml) causes a 4% increase in V̇O₂ max, and the loss of plasma volume is the primary reason for the decrease in V̇O₂ max in the first two weeks of detraining (23, 24). Overall, EDV increases as a result of an endurance training program, and according to the Frank-Starling mechanism (see chapter 9), an increased stretch of the ventricle leads to an increase in stroke volume (85). Have you ever wondered why some individuals have very high V̇O₂ max values, even though they do not train? See A Closer Look 13.2 for answers.

Cardiac Contractility *Cardiac contractility* refers specifically to the strength of the cardiac muscle contraction when the fiber length (EDV), afterload (peripheral resistance), and heart rate are constant (since all affect contractility). While an acute exercise bout increases cardiac contractility due to the action of the sympathetic nervous system on the ventricle, it is difficult to conclude whether or not the inherent contractility of the heart changes with endurance training. The reason for this is that the factors that directly affect contractility (EDV, heart rate, and afterload) are themselves affected by endurance training (85).

Blomqvist and Saltin (6) suggest that changes in contractility probably are not too important in explaining the increase in maximal stroke volume with endurance training. This was based on the observation that the fraction of the EDV ejected from the heart per beat **(ejection fraction)** is already so high in sedentary subjects prior to an endurance exercise program that there is not much to be gained by increasing contractility.

Afterload *Afterload* refers to the peripheral resistance against which the ventricle is contracting as it tries to push a portion of the EDV into the aorta. If the heart contracts with the same force while the peripheral resistance decreases, a greater stroke volume will be realized. What is clear is that following an endurance training program, trained muscles offer less resistance to blood flow *during maximal work*. This decrease in resistance parallels the increase in maximal cardiac output so that mean arterial blood pressure is unchanged (MAP = $\dot{Q}$ × TPR). How does endurance training cause a lower resistance in the working muscle to facilitate a higher blood flow?

One might think that the increased blood flow through the trained muscle is due to an increase in the local factors (H^+, CO_2, etc.) associated with the higher work rates achieved after an endurance training program, but it is not. This can be seen in the following example. Prior to training, a subject takes a graded exercise test while maximal values for $\dot{V}O_2$ max and $\dot{Q}$ are measured. On another day the same subject takes an exercise test set at a work rate equal to 120% of the $\dot{V}O_2$ max achieved on the previous test and, of course, measures the same value for $\dot{V}O_2$ max. This supramaximal (>100% $\dot{V}O_2$ max) test should have caused a higher concentration of local factors in the working muscles that would have facilitated vasodilation and increased muscle blood flow. However, if this vasodilation were to happen with the cardiac output already at its maximal value, mean arterial blood pressure would fall, with dire consequences (85). How is this fall in blood pressure prevented?

When an additional muscle mass is recruited to do the supramaximal work rate, other vascular beds would have to be vasoconstricted by the sympathetic nervous system to maintain blood pressure. Since the renal and splanchnic vascular beds are already maximally constricted at maximal work, the only possibility is to vasoconstrict some vascular beds in already active muscle when additional muscle groups are recruited to do the supramaximal work (85). Consequently, the increase in muscle blood flow during the maximal exercise test following an endurance training program is due to a reduction in the sympathetic vasoconstrictor activity to the arterioles of the trained muscles. This occurs simultaneously with the increase

in maximal cardiac output. This combination allows for the higher $\dot{V}O_2$ max at a constant mean arterial blood pressure, the homeostatic variable that appears to be closely regulated in maximal work (85).

Evidence supporting this explanation is found in studies in which one-legged exercise is conducted. $\dot{V}O_2$ max measured during one-legged exercise on a cycle ergometer is equal to about 75% to 80% of that measured during the regular two-legged test (22, 56). This is due to the greater arteriolar dilation and higher blood flow achieved in the working muscles during one-legged exercise. If the same degree of vasodilation were to occur in each leg when both were exercising maximally, the muscle's *capacity for blood flow* would exceed the heart's ability to provide it, and blood pressure would fall. To counter this tendency during maximal two-legged work, some of the muscle mass must be vasoconstricted to maintain blood pressure (56, 85). This is why the two-legged $\dot{V}O_2$ max value is not the sum of the $\dot{V}O_2$ max values of each leg. In conclusion, during maximal work with trained muscles following an endurance training program, there is a decrease in the resistance of that vascular bed to match the increase in maximal cardiac output to maintain blood pressure.

Arteriovenous O₂ Difference

Stroke volume causes 50% of the increase in $\dot{V}O_2$ max associated with an endurance exercise program in young, sedentary subjects; O_2 extraction is responsible for the other 50%. The increase in the arteriovenous O_2 difference could be due to an elevation of the arterial oxygen content (higher hemoglobin or PO_2), or a decrease in the mixed venous oxygen content. Given that the hemoglobin concentration does not change with training and that the arterial PO_2 is usually sufficient to maintain arterial saturation of hemoglobin (see chapter 10), the increase in the a-$\bar{v}$ O_2 difference is not due to an increase in the arterial O_2 content (85).

The increased capacity of the muscle to extract O_2 following training is believed to be due to the increase in capillary density, with the mitochondrial number being of secondary importance (6, 48, 85). The increase in capillary density in trained muscle accommodates the increase in muscle blood flow during maximal exercise, decreases the diffusion distance to the mitochondria, and slows the rate of blood flow to allow time for diffusion to take place. Changes in capillary density parallel changes in leg blood flow and $\dot{V}O_2$ max with training (85). The increases in mitochondria following endurance training favor O_2 transport from the capillary and contribute to the expanded a-$\bar{v}$ O_2 differences. However, the capacity of the mitochondria to use O_2 far exceeds the capability of the heart to deliver O_2, making mitochondrial

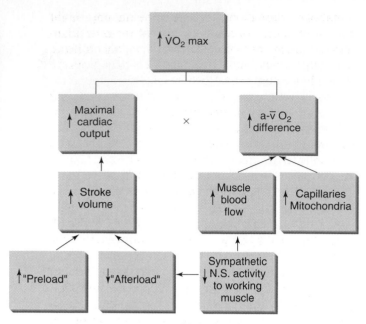

FIGURE 13.3 Summary of factors causing an increase in $\dot{V}O_2$ max with endurance training.

FIGURE 13.4 Time course of changes in $\dot{V}O_2$ max and associated cardiovascular variables with detraining. From E. F. Coyle et al., 1984, "Time Course of Loss of Adaptation after Stopping Prolonged Intense Endurance Training" in *Journal of Applied Physiology*, 57:1857–64. Copyright © 1984 American Physiological Society, Bethesda, MD. Reprinted by permission.

number *not* the factor limiting $\dot{V}O_2$ max (6, 48, 85). Figure 13.3 provides a summary of the factors causing an increase in $\dot{V}O_2$ max with an endurance training program.

IN SUMMARY

- The training-induced increase in maximal stroke volume is due to both an increase in preload and a decrease in afterload.
  a. The increased preload is primarily due to an increase in end diastolic ventricular volume and the associated increase in plasma volume.
  b. The decreased afterload is due to a decrease in the arteriolar constriction in the trained muscles, increasing maximal muscle blood flow with no change in the mean arterial blood pressure.
- In young, sedentary subjects, 50% of the increase in $\dot{V}O_2$ max is due to an increase in the systemic a-$\bar{v}$ O_2 difference. The increased a-$\bar{v}$ O_2 difference is due to an increase in the capillary density of the trained muscles that is needed to accept the increase in maximal muscle blood flow. The greater capillary density allows for a sufficiently slow red blood cell transit time through the muscle, providing enough time for oxygen diffusion, which is facilitated by the increase in the number of mitochondria.

DETRAINING AND $\dot{V}O_2$ MAX

When highly trained individuals stop training, $\dot{V}O_2$ max decreases over time. Why? Basically, because maximal cardiac output and oxygen extraction decrease. Figure 13.4 shows changes in maximal oxygen uptake, cardiac output, stroke volume, heart rate, and oxygen extraction over an eighty-four-day period of no training (26). The initial decrease (first twelve days) in $\dot{V}O_2$ max was due entirely to the decrease in stroke volume, since the heart rate and a-$\bar{v}$ O_2 difference remained the same or increased. This sudden decrease in maximal stroke volume appears to be due to the rapid loss of plasma volume with detraining (23). When plasma volume was artificially restored by infusion, $\dot{V}O_2$ max increased toward pre-detraining values (23). This was confirmed in a study in which a 200 to 300 ml expansion of plasma volume was shown to increase $\dot{V}O_2$ max, even though the hemoglobin concentration was reduced (24). Figure 13.4 shows that between the 21st and 84th days of detraining, the decrease in $\dot{V}O_2$ max is due to the decrease in the a-$\bar{v}$ O_2 difference. This was associated with a decrease in muscle mitochondria; capillary density remained the same. The overall oxidative capacity of skeletal muscle was reduced, with the percentage of type IIa fibers decreasing from 43% to 26% and the percentage of type IIx fibers increasing from 5% to 19% (25, 26). It is clear that changes in $\dot{V}O_2$ max, due to training or detraining, are caused by changes in stroke volume and the capacity of the muscle to extract oxygen. For a review of the metabolic and cardiovascular effects of detraining in humans, see Mujika and Padilla's article in the Suggested Readings.

IN SUMMARY

■ The decrease in $\dot{V}O_2$ max with cessation of training is due to both a decrease in maximal stroke volume and a decrease in oxygen extraction, the reverse of what happens with training.

ENDURANCE TRAINING: EFFECTS ON PERFORMANCE AND HOMEOSTASIS

The ability to continue prolonged, submaximal work is dependent on the maintenance of homeostasis during the activity. Endurance training results in a more rapid transition from rest to the steady-state metabolic requirement, a reduced reliance on the limited liver and muscle glycogen stores, and numerous cardiovascular and thermoregulatory adaptations that increase the chance that homeostasis will be maintained. Part of these training-induced adaptations are due to structural and biochemical changes in muscle, and we will discuss those in detail in the next few pages. However, a portion of these adaptations is related to factors external to the muscle. For example, in chapter 5 you saw how rapidly the plasma epinephrine and norepinephrine response to exercise was decreased with training. These hormones directly or indirectly affect numerous metabolic responses to exercise and may be involved in some of the adaptations to muscle associated with endurance training (77). This needs to be stated at the beginning of this section because, while we focus on the link between changes in skeletal muscle and performance, there is clear evidence that some improvements in performance occur rapidly and might precede structural or biochemical changes in skeletal muscle (41). This suggests that the initial

metabolic adaptations to endurance training might consist of neural, or neural-hormonal-receptor adaptations, which are followed by structural adaptations. If so, this would not be unlike the adaptations to strength training (see later discussion).

In the introduction to this chapter, we mentioned that the increase in performance following an endurance training program was due more to biochemical and structural changes in the trained skeletal muscle than to a small increase in $\dot{V}O_2$ max. Endurance training causes rather large changes in the biochemical and structural characteristics of the working muscles (see Hood's review of mitochondrial biogenesis due to contractile activity in the Suggested Readings). The typical changes include increases in the number of mitochondria (up to fourfold for type II fibers) and capillary density (48). The increase in mitochondria is associated with increases in the enzymes involved in oxidative metabolism: Krebs cycle, fatty-acid (β-oxidation) cycle, and the electron transport chain. Changes also occur in the "shuttle system" that is used for moving NADH from the cytoplasm, where it is produced in glycolysis, to the mitochondria, where it is used in the electron transport chain to produce ATP. Finally, changes occur in the type of LDH enzyme, which is involved in the conversion of pyruvate to lactate. It is the changes in these characteristics of muscle that "drive" or determine the overall physiological responses to a given submaximal exercise bout. Table 13.4 presents data on succinate dehydrogenase activity, a measure of the oxidative capacity of muscle, for each of the three major fiber types for people differing in fitness. An important observation is that the oxidative capacity is not different among the fibers of the endurance athlete. In contrast, these values are twice that of the type I fibers of individuals who have been exercising for months, and four times that of sedentary individuals. How long does it take for these changes to occur?

It is a common experience for most individuals who do run, swim, or cycle training that a break of only two weeks can dramatically affect performance. This is due primarily to the changes in the mitochondria's

TABLE 13.4	Succinate Dehydrogenase Activity in Thigh Muscle Fiber Types in Response to Conditioning and Deconditioning			
			Muscle Fiber Type	
			Type IIa	
Fitness Level	Range of $\dot{V}O_2$ max (ml · kg^{-1} · min^{-1})	Type I	(μmol · g^{-1} · min^{-1})	Type IIx
Deconditioned	30–40	5.0	4.0	3.5
Sedentary	40–50	9.2	5.8	4.9
Conditioning (months)	45–55	12.1	10.2	5.5
Endurance athletes	>70	23.2	22.1	22.0

Adapted from Saltin and Gollnick (94)

A CLOSER LOOK 13.3

Role of Exercise Intensity and Duration on Mitochondrial Adaptations

A muscle fiber's oxidative capacity can improve only if the muscle fiber is recruited during the exercise session. Figures 13.6a and 13.6b show changes in citrate synthase (CS) activity, a marker of mitochondrial oxidative capacity, due to exercise programs differing in duration (thirty, sixty, and ninety minutes) and intensity (~55%, ~65%, and ~75% $\dot{V}O_2$ max). Figure 13.6a shows that CS activity increased in the red gastrocnemius (primarily type IIa fibers) for all treatments, but the magnitude of the change was independent of the intensity and duration of the activity. In contrast, Figure 13.6b shows that for the white gastrocnemius (primarily type IIx fibers) CS activity increased due to both intensity and duration of activity. Why the difference? The type IIa fibers were easily recruited by the lowest exercise intensity, while very strenuous exercise was required to recruit the type IIx fibers (76). These observations support our understanding of the specificity of exercise—light to moderate exercise will improve or maintain the oxidative capacity of high oxidative fibers (type I and type IIa), while strenuous exercise is needed to change low oxidative

(type IIx) fibers (31, 97). Given the rapid loss of a muscle's oxidative capacity with cessation of training, it is no surprise that high-level endurance

performances, which require the recruitment of type IIx fibers, fall off quickly when training ceases.

FIGURE 13.6 Changes in citrate synthase activity with different intensities and durations of exercise.

FIGURE 13.5 Time-course of training/detraining adaptations in mitochondrial content of skeletal muscle. Note that about 50% of the increase in mitochondrial content was lost after one week of detraining (*a*) and that all of the adaptation was lost after five weeks of detraining. Also, it took four weeks of retraining (*b*) to regain the adaptation lost in the first week of detraining.

oxidative enzymes (50a, 63, 100). In fact, mitochondrial oxidative capacity undergoes rapid changes at the onset and termination of exercise training. Figure 13.5 shows how quickly muscle mitochondria increase at the onset of training, doubling in about five weeks of training. However, only one week of detraining (shown by the letter "a") results in a loss of about 50% of what was gained during the five weeks of training (7, 96). Three to four weeks of retraining were required to achieve the former levels (shown by the letter "b" in figure 13.5). A recent study (18) showed that only 6 sessions of 4 to 7 30-second all-out exercise bouts on a cycle ergometer resulted in a 38% increase in mitochondria activity and a 100% increase in cycle endurance capacity. The old adage, "use it or lose it" is very true for the oxidative capacity of muscle (see A Closer Look 13.3). The following sections will describe how this greater capacity for oxidative metabolism results in less disruption of physiological (e.g., plasma glucose and H^+ concentrations) variables maintained by homeostatic mechanisms.

Biochemical Adaptations and the Oxygen Deficit

At the onset of exercise, ATP is converted to ADP and P_i by the cross-bridges in order to develop tension. The increase in the ADP concentration in the cytoplasm is the immediate stimulus for ATP-producing systems to come into play to meet the ATP demands of the cross-bridges. Phosphocreatine responds immediately to this ATP need, followed by glycolysis and mitochondrial oxidative phosphorylation. The latter process provides all the ATP aerobically during the steady-state phase of the work, with the mitochondrial oxygen consumption driven by the ADP concentration. Muscle cells with few mitochondria must have a high ADP concentration to stimulate the limited number of mitochondria to consume oxygen at a given rate (48). How does endurance training affect these oxygen uptake responses at the onset of submaximal steady-state work?

The steady-state $\dot{V}O_2$ measured during a submaximal work test is not affected by endurance training. The mitochondria are still consuming the same number of O_2 molecules per minute. What is different, due to the large increase in mitochondria, oxidative enzymes, and the number of capillaries per muscle fiber, is how the ATP-producing chore is shared among the mitochondria. Figure 13.7 shows schematically that if a muscle cell has only one mitochondrion, an increase of 100 units in the ADP concentration is needed for the muscle to consume 2.0 liters of O_2 per minute. After training, when the number of mitochondria has doubled, the ADP concentration increases only half as much, since each mitochondrion needs only half the stimulation to take up 1.0 liter of O_2 per minute. The increase in the capillary density in the muscle cell after endurance training is a parallel change that supports this process. In essence, after an endurance training program, it takes less change in the ADP concentration to stimulate the mitochondria to take up the oxygen (17, 48). Since less of a change in the ADP concentration is needed to stimulate the mitochondria, the rising ADP concentration at the onset of work (due to cross-bridges causing ATP $\rightarrow$ ADP + P_i) will cause oxidative phosphorylation to be activated earlier. This translates into a faster rise in the oxygen uptake curve at the onset of work, resulting in the steady-state $\dot{V}O_2$ being achieved earlier (see figure 4.2) (45, 75). This faster rise in oxygen uptake at the onset of work means that the O_2 deficit is less: less creatine phosphate depletion and less lactate and H^+ formation (20, 43).

The reductions in lactate and H^+ formation and phosphocreatine depletion are also linked to the lower ADP concentration in the muscle cell after the endurance training program. The lower ADP concentration results in less phosphocreatine depletion

Muscle Cell: Before Training

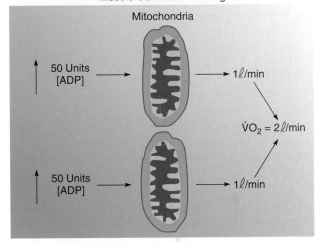

Muscle Cell: After Training

FIGURE 13.7 Influence of mitochondria number on the change in the ADP concentration needed to increase the $\dot{V}O_2$.

since the reaction for this is [ADP] + [PC] $\rightarrow$ [ATP] + [C]. The lower ADP concentration in the cell also results in less stimulation of glycolysis. Chapter 3 indicated that phosphofructokinase (PFK) is the enzyme in glycolysis that controls the rate at which glucose is metabolized, and that high levels of ADP and low levels of PC in the cell stimulate this enzyme to process glucose through the pathway. The reduced stimulation of glycolysis due to the lower ADP and higher PC concentrations following endurance training results in less reliance on anaerobic glycolysis to provide ATP at the onset of exercise (36, 43). The net result is a lower oxygen deficit, less depletion of phosphocreatine, and a reduction in lactate and H^+ formation. Figure 13.8 shows that the biochemical adaptations following endurance training result in a faster rise in the oxygen uptake curve at the onset of work, with less disruption of homeostasis.

Biochemical Adaptations and the Plasma Glucose Concentration

Plasma glucose is the primary fuel of the nervous system and, as described in chapter 5, the majority of hormonal changes associated with fasting or exercise are aimed at maintaining this important homeostatic

FIGURE 13.8 Endurance training reduces the O₂ deficit at the onset of work.

variable. How do the biochemical changes in muscle that occur as a result of endurance training help maintain the blood glucose concentration during prolonged submaximal exercise? The answer is again found in the increases in mitochondrial number and capillary density that occur with endurance training.

The increased number of mitochondria increases a muscle fiber's capacity to oxidize both carbohydrate and fat. However, the most dramatic change in muscle metabolism following training is the increased utilization of fat, and the sparing of carbohydrate. This is due to an improved capacity to take up FFA from the circulation, an increased ability to transport FFA from the cytoplasm to the mitochondria of the muscle, and an increase in the fatty-acid (β-oxidation) cycle enzymes needed to degrade the FFA to acetyl-CoA units for the Krebs cycle (48). These points will now be discussed.

Transport of FFA into Muscle Intramuscular fat provides about 50% of the lipid oxidized during exercise; plasma FFA provide the rest (50, 99). The uptake of FFA by muscle is proportional to the FFA concentration in the plasma (73). An enhanced mobilization of FFA would favor the maintenance of the plasma FFA concentration at a time when the muscle is using FFA at a faster rate. However, that does not occur, and the plasma FFA concentration is actually lower following training (16, 64). How does the endurance-trained muscle compensate for this? Plasma FFA must be transported from the capillary, across the cell membrane to the cytoplasm, and then into the mitochondria before oxidation can occur. It has been generally accepted that the first step, from capillary to cytoplasm, was accomplished by passive diffusion, and the higher the plasma FFA concentration, the greater the rate of FFA uptake by the cell. There is now evidence that the transport of FFA into the muscle cell involves a carrier molecule whose capacity to trans-

port FFA can become saturated at high plasma FFA concentrations (92). Endurance training has been shown to increase the capacity to transport FFA such that a trained individual can transport more FFA at the same plasma FFA concentration, compared to an untrained individual (55). This increased ability to transport FFA is facilitated by a greater capillary density in the trained muscle, which slows the rate of blood flow past the cell membrane, allowing more time for the FFA to be transported into the cell (92).

Transport of FFA from the Cytoplasm to the Mitochondria The FFAs are transported from the cytoplasm to the mitochondria by carnitine transferase, an enzyme associated with the mitochondrial membrane. This enzyme catalyzes the reaction of FFA and the carrier molecule, carnitine, which moves quickly across the mitochondrial membrane where the reaction is reversed, yielding the FFA for oxidation. The increase in the mitochondrial number with endurance training increases the surface area of the mitochondrial membranes and the amount of carnitine transferase such that FFA can be transported at a faster rate from the cytoplasm to the mitochondria for oxidation (94). The faster rate of transport from the cytoplasm to the mitochondria favors the movement of more FFA into the muscle cell from the plasma.

Mitochondrial Oxidation of FFA The increase in mitochondria number increases the enzymes involved in FFA oxidation, specifically, the fatty-acid (β-oxidation) cycle. This results in an increased rate at which acetyl-CoA molecules are formed from FFA for entry to the Krebs cycle, where citrate (the first molecule in the cycle) is formed. The high citrate level inhibits PFK activity in the cytoplasm and therefore reduces carbohydrate metabolism (48). The result of all of these adaptations is an increase in lipid oxidation and less reliance on carbohydrate metabolism during exercise, thus preserving the limited liver glycogen store.

IN SUMMARY

- The combination of the increase in the density of capillaries and the number of mitochondria per muscle fiber increases the capacity to transport FFA from the plasma → cytoplasm → mitochondria.
- The increase in the enzymes of the fatty acid cycle increases the rate of formation of acetyl-CoA from FFA for oxidation in the Krebs cycle. This increase in fat oxidation in endurance-trained muscle spares both muscle glycogen and plasma glucose, the latter being a focal point of homeostatic regulatory mechanisms. These points are summarized in Figure 13.9.

Biochemical Adaptations and Blood pH

The pH of blood is maintained near 7.40 ± 0.02 at rest. As described in chapter 11, acute and long-term challenges to the pH are met by responses of both the pulmonary and renal systems. How does endurance training result in less disruption of the blood pH during submaximal work? The answer relates to the reduced lactate and H^+ formation following endurance training.

Lactate formation occurs when there is an accumulation of NADH and pyruvate in the cytoplasm of the cell where lactate dehydrogenase (LDH) is present:

$$[pyruvate] + [NADH] \rightarrow [lactate] + [NAD]$$
$$LDH$$

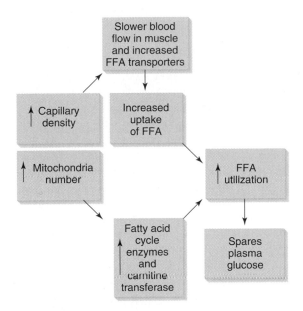

FIGURE 13.9 Increased mitochondria number and capillary density increase the rate of free-fatty-acid utilization, preserving plasma glucose.

Anything that affects the concentration of pyruvate, NADH, or the type of LDH in the cell will affect the rate of lactate formation. We have already seen that the increased number of mitochondria can have a dramatic effect on pyruvate formation: the lower ADP concentration stimulates PFK less at the onset of work, and the increased capacity to use fats reduces the need for carbohydrate oxidation during prolonged work. If less carbohydrate is used, less pyruvate is formed. In addition, the increase in mitochondria number increases the chance that pyruvate will be taken up by the mitochondria for oxidation in the Krebs cycle, rather than being bound to LDH in the cytoplasm. All of these adaptations favor a lower pyruvate concentration and a reduction in lactate formation.

There are two additional biochemical changes in muscle due to endurance training that reduce lactate and, consequently, H^+ formation. The NADH produced during glycolysis can react with pyruvate, as shown in the previous equation, or it can be transported into the mitochondrion to be oxidized in the electron transport chain to form ATP (see chapter 3). Endurance training increases the number of "shuttles" used to transport NADH from the cytoplasm into the mitochondrion (48). If the NADH formed in glycolysis is more quickly transported to the mitochondria, there will be less lactate and H^+ formation. Lastly, endurance training causes a change in the type of LDH present in the muscle cell. This enzyme exists in five forms (isozymes): M_4, M_3H, M_2H_2, MH_3, and H_4. The H_4, or heart form of LDH, has a low affinity for the available pyruvate. Endurance training shifts the LDH toward the H_4 form, making lactate and H^+ formation less likely and the uptake of pyruvate by the mitochondria more likely. Figure 13.10 summarizes the effects these biochemical changes have on lactate formation and the production of H^+ during submaximal work.

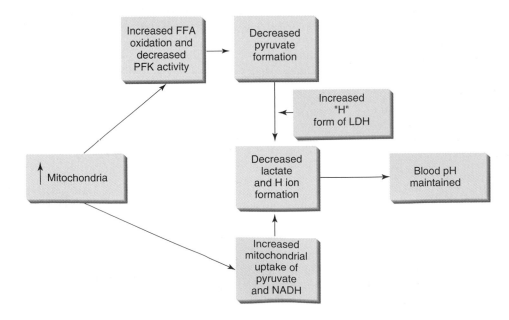

FIGURE 13.10 Increased mitochondria number decreases lactate and H^+ formation to maintain the blood pH.

A CLOSER LOOK 13.4

Exercise and Resistance to Infection

We possess considerable knowledge about the effects of exercise on metabolism, cardiovascular function, and skeletal muscle structure. In contrast, we know little about how our immune system responds to exercise. This is due, in part, to the limited number of studies that have been done in which important factors that can affect resistance to infection have been controlled. These factors include (21):

- Having a control group to account for temporal changes (circadian and seasonal) in immune function;
- Matching groups on the basis of psychological stressors that are known to affect immune function;
- Ensuring adequate dietary intake.

In addition to these concerns, it has become clear that one cannot draw broad conclusions about the relationship of exercise to overall resistance to infection from observations of a single immune response (21). In spite of these limitations there are some epidemiological and experimental studies on the effect of exercise on upper respiratory tract infections (URTI) that provide some guidance. Nieman's review (1994) of this topic suggests that the risk of URTI follows a "J"-shaped pattern relative to the amount and intensity of exercise as shown in Figure 13.11.

The model suggests that moderate exercise lowers the risk of URTI, while excessive amounts of exercise increase the risk. Evidence for this model includes the following (72, 95):

- Six times as many runners experienced URTI following a

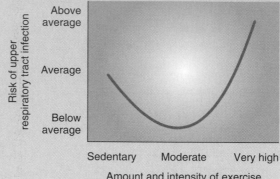

FIGURE 13.11 "J"-shaped model of relationship between varying amounts of exercise and risk of URTI. This model suggests that moderate exercise may lower the risk of respiratory infection, while excessive amounts may increase the risk (72).

marathon compared to nonparticipating runners;
- Runners training more than 96 km/wk had twice the risk of URTI as those doing only 32 km/wk;
- Races of only 5 km to 21.1 km do not seem to increase the risk of URTI in the week following the race;
- Those doing moderate exercise training (forty-five minutes of brisk walking, five days per week) experienced half as many days with URTI symptoms compared to a sedentary group;
- Elderly subjects who did 40 minutes of walking, five times per week had an incidence of URTI of only 21% compared to 50% for a sedentary control group.

It has become clear that nutrition has a major and separate impact on immune function (40):

- Dietary deficiencies of energy (calories), protein, and micronutrients (iron, zinc, and vitamins A, E, B_6, and B_{12}) contribute to depressed immune function;
- Eating a balanced diet that meets energy needs should address protein and micronutrient needs;
- If an athlete is on an energy-restricted diet, vitamin supplements are desirable. However, consuming megadoses of vitamins and minerals is not recommended;
- Consuming 30 to 60 g/hr of carbohydrate in a drink during prolonged exercise may reduce some of the immunosuppressive effects of prolonged exercise;
- There is conflicting evidence that antioxidant supplements are required or desired for athletes.

Biochemical Adaptations and Lactate Removal

Lactate accumulation in the blood is dependent on the balance between lactate production by working muscle and lactate removal by liver and other tissues. The blood lactate concentration stays at 1 mmol/liter at rest and during light exercise when there is a balance between production and removal. As the exercise intensity increases, the blood lactate could rise due to an acceleration of lactate production, or to a reduction in the rate of removal by the liver and other tissues (19). As described in chapter 9, blood flow to nonworking muscles, kidney, liver, and GI tract decreases as exercise intensity increases, reducing the rate of lactate removal. How

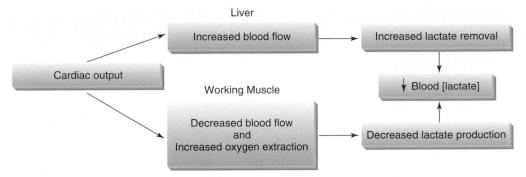

FIGURE 13.12 Effect of endurance training on the redistribution of blood flow and lactate removal during exercise at a fixed submaximal workload.

does endurance training affect blood flow to these tissues?

Endurance training causes an increase in the capillary density of the working muscles. This results in two changes favorable for oxygen transport to the mitochondria: a decrease in the distance from capillary to mitochondrion, and a decrease in the rate of blood flow through each capillary, allowing more time for the diffusion of oxygen to the mitochondria. As a result, the same submaximal work rate demands *less* blood flow to the working muscles after training. The muscle can extract more oxygen from each liter of blood (larger a-$\bar{v}$ O$_2$ difference across the muscle) to achieve the same steady-state $\dot{V}O_2$, with a lower blood flow (see A Closer Look 13.4).

Since the cardiac output for a given submaximal work rate is unchanged or only slightly decreased after training (33), where is the blood flow now distributed that was formerly going to the working muscles? Two vascular beds that receive an increase in blood flow following training are the liver and the kidneys. Since the liver is a major site for lactate removal for gluconeogenesis, the blood lactate level is lower following an endurance training program due in part to the liver's increased ability to remove lactate. Figure 13.12 summarizes these events.

IN SUMMARY

- Mitochondrial adaptations to endurance training include an increase in the enzymes involved in oxidative metabolism: Krebs cycle, fatty-acid (β-oxidation) cycle, and the electron transport chain.
- Those mitochondrial adaptations result in the following:
  a. a smaller O$_2$ deficit due to a more rapid increase in oxygen uptake at the onset of work
  b. an increase in fat metabolism that spares muscle glycogen and blood glucose
  c. a reduction in lactate and H$^+$ formation that helps to maintain the pH of the blood
  d. an increase in lactate removal

ENDURANCE TRAINING: LINKS BETWEEN MUSCLE AND SYSTEMIC PHYSIOLOGY

We have just described the importance of the local changes occurring in endurance-trained muscle on the maintenance of homeostasis during prolonged submaximal work. However, these same changes are also related to the lower heart rate, ventilation, and catecholamine responses measured during submaximal work following an endurance training program. What is the link between the changes in muscle and the improved heart rate and ventilation responses to exercise?

The following endurance training study illustrates the importance of the trained muscle in the body's overall response to a submaximal work bout. In this study, each subject's left and right legs were tested separately on a cycle ergometer at a submaximal work rate prior to and during an endurance training program. Heart rate and ventilation were measured at the end of the submaximal exercise test, and a blood sample was obtained to monitor changes in lactate, epinephrine, and norepinephrine. During the study each subject trained only one leg for thirteen sessions, fifteen minutes a session, at an exercise intensity causing a heart rate of 170 beats per minute. At the end of each week of training, the subject was tested at the same submaximal work rate used prior to starting the training program. This procedure allowed the investigator to determine how fast the "training effect" occurred. Figure 13.13 shows that heart rate, ventilation, blood lactate, and plasma epinephrine and norepinephrine responses decreased throughout the study. Results such as these have been used to support the idea that the cardiovascular, pulmonary, and sympathetic nervous systems have each adapted to the exercise. However, that may not be quite true. At the end of this training program, the "untrained" leg was trained for five consecutive days at the same

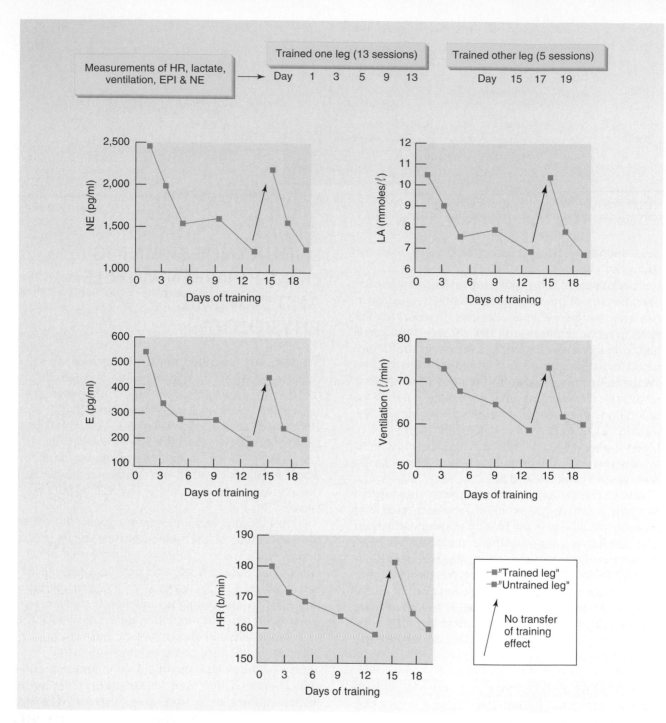

FIGURE 13.13 The lack of transfer of a training effect, indicating that the responses of the cardiovascular, pulmonary, and sympathetic nervous systems are more dependent on the trained state of the muscles involved in the activity than on some specific adaptation in those systems.

submaximal work rate used for the "trained leg." Physiological measurements were obtained during the exercise session on the first, third, and fifth days. If the cardiovascular, pulmonary, and sympathetic nervous systems had become "trained" as a result of the thirteen exercise sessions with the other leg, you might expect some "transfer" of the training effect when the

untrained leg was tested. Interestingly, figure 13.13 shows that all the systems responded as if they had never been exposed to exercise training (22). There was no transfer of the training effect from one leg to the other. This example shows that the heart rate, ventilation, and plasma catecholamine responses to prolonged submaximal exercise are determined, not by the specific adaptation of each organ or system, but by the training state of the specific muscle groups engaged in the exercise. How is this possible?

In chapter 10, the control of ventilation during exercise required a discussion of central and peripheral neural influences that could help explain the precise matching of ventilation to the increased oxygen demands of incremental exercise. This same approach will be taken here to explain how endurance training of specific muscle groups results in the decrease in cardiorespiratory and sympathetic nervous system responses to the same submaximal work rate. The output of the cardiovascular and respiratory control centers is influenced by input from higher brain centers, where the motor task originates, as well as from the muscles carrying out the task. A decrease in motor unit recruitment or a reduction in output from the receptors in the working muscles to the brain reduces these physiological responses to the work task. Following a brief summary of "peripheral" and "central" control mechanisms, an attempt will be made to show how both are involved in the reduced physiological responses to submaximal exercise.

Peripheral Feedback

Rowell (85) indicates that Zuntz and Geppert were the originators of the idea that reflexes in working muscles might control or "drive" cardiovascular or pulmonary systems in proportion to the metabolic rate. A number of receptors have been examined that respond to chemical or physical changes in muscle that might signify work rate. The involvement of the muscle spindle and Golgi tendon organ received considerable attention as possible sites for these reflexes, given their ability to monitor changes in muscle length and tension development, respectively. However, blocking the afferent nerves from these receptors did not eliminate specific cardiovascular responses to muscle tension development (70, 85). Attention has now been directed to small-diameter nerve fibers (group III and group IV fibers) that are responsive to tension, temperature, and chemical changes in muscle. These fibers increase their rate of firing action potentials in proportion to changes in metabolic rate. Figure 13.14 shows schematically the neuronal circuitry for the reflex regulation of the cardiovascular and respiratory responses to exercise by these group III and group IV fibers.

Central Command

The general idea surrounding central control of the physiological response to exercise is presented in figure 13.15. Higher brain centers (motor cortex, basal ganglia, cerebellum—see chapter 7) prepare to exe-

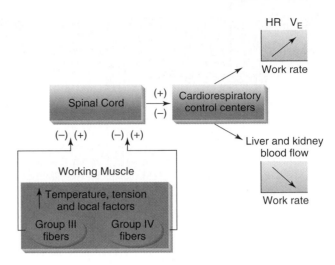

FIGURE 13.14 Peripheral control mechanisms in muscle influence the heart rate, ventilation, and kidney and liver blood flow responses to submaximal work.

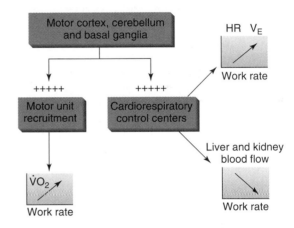

FIGURE 13.15 Central control of motor unit recruitment, heart rate, ventilation, and liver and kidney blood flow responses to submaximal work.

cute a motor task and send action potentials through lower brain centers and spinal nuclei to influence the cardiorespiratory and sympathetic nervous system responses to exercise. As more motor units are recruited to develop the greater tension needed to accomplish a work task, larger physiological responses are required to sustain the metabolic rate of the muscles (69, 85). For example, if some muscle fibers are prevented from contracting, additional muscle fibers must be recruited to maintain tension. This generates higher heart rate responses to the work task (3). How are these peripheral and central controls related to the decreases in sympathetic nervous system activity, heart rate, and ventilation observed during submaximal exercise following an endurance training program?

Aging, Strength, and Training

As we age, muscle strength declines, with most of the decline occurring after age fifty. The loss of strength is associated with the loss of muscle mass, due to a decrease in the number of both type I and type II fibers (see chapter 8). The loss of muscle fibers seems to be related to a neurological change at the level of a motor neuron, and whatever affects the motor neuron affects the fibers attached to it (29, 52). What is promising about an otherwise dismal picture is that progressive resistance training programs for the elderly result in increases in muscle hypertrophy and strength, similar to what is observed for young people (37, 38). This has major ramifications for health care given the increase in the number of people classified as elderly (8, 49, 84). For a recent review of this topic see Hunter et al. (53).

The ability to perform a fixed submaximal exercise bout for a prolonged period of time is dependent on the recruitment of a sufficient number of motor units to meet the tension (work) requirements through oxidative phosphorylation. Prior to endurance training, more mitochondria-poor motor units must be recruited to carry out a work task at a given $\dot{V}O_2$. This results in a greater "central" drive to the cardiorespiratory control centers, which causes higher sympathetic nervous system, heart rate, and ventilation responses. The feedback from chemoreceptors at the untrained muscle would also stimulate the cardiorespiratory control center. With the increase in mitochondrial number following endurance training, local factors (H^+, adenosine compounds, etc.) do not change as much. This leads to less local stimulation of blood flow and a reduced chemoreceptor input to the cardiorespiratory centers. In addition, the higher number of mitochondria allows the tension to be maintained with fewer motor units involved in the activity. This reduced "feed forward" input from the higher brain centers and reduced "feedback" from the muscle results in lower sympathetic nervous system output, heart rate, and ventilation responses to exercise (69, 85, 86).

IN SUMMARY

- The biochemical changes in muscle due to endurance training influence the physiological responses to exercise. The reduction in "feedback" from chemoreceptors in the trained muscle and a reduction in the need to recruit motor units to accomplish a work task results in reduced sympathetic nervous system, heart rate, and ventilation responses to submaximal exercise.

PHYSIOLOGICAL EFFECTS OF STRENGTH TRAINING

The basic principles of training related to improving strength have been around for thousands of years, and Morpurgo's observation that gains in strength were associated with increases in muscle size was made almost one hundred years ago (5). Despite this history, most recent research on the effects of training has focused on $\dot{V}O_2$ max and endurance performance, possibly because of their link to the prevention and treatment of heart disease. However, times and circumstances change, and in 1990 the American College of Sports Medicine (ACSM) added strength training for muscular fitness to that and subsequent position stands. In addition, the ACSM released another position stand in 2002 outlining progression models for resistance training (2). See A Closer Look 13.5 for background on why strength training is important as we age.

Before we begin, some terms need to be defined and some basic principles need to be restated. Muscular strength refers to the maximal force that a muscle or muscle group can generate and is commonly expressed as the one-repetition maximum or 1-RM, the maximum load that can be moved through a range of motion once in good form. Muscular endurance refers to the ability to make repeated contractions against a submaximal load. Consistent with our earlier discussion of training and $\dot{V}O_2$ max, large individual differences exist in the response to strength training programs, and the percent gain in strength is inversely related to the initial strength (58). These observations imply a genetic limitation to the gains that can be realized due to training, similar to what we have seen for gains in $\dot{V}O_2$ max. Finally, the basic principles of training, overload, and specificity apply here as well. For example, high-resistance training

(2–10 RM loads) results in gains in muscular strength; in contrast, low-resistance training (20+ RM loads) results in gains in muscular endurance, with less of a change in strength (58). What physiological changes occur with resistance training that result in improvements in muscular strength and endurance?

PHYSIOLOGICAL MECHANISMS CAUSING INCREASED STRENGTH

Chapter 8 described the roles that motor unit recruitment, stimulus frequency, and synchronous firing of motor units play in the development of muscle tension, as well as the fact that type II motor units develop more tension than type I motor units. In addition, we described how stimulatory (muscle spindle) and inhibitory (Golgi tendon organ) muscle reflexes affect tension development. These factors are very much involved in the improvement of strength with training.

Figure 13.16 provides a schematic to follow that will facilitate our discussion of muscular and neural factors related to gains in strength (87). In training studies of short duration (eight to twenty weeks), neural adaptations related to learning, coordination, and the ability to recruit prime movers play a major role in the gain in strength. In contrast, in long-term training

programs an increase in the size of the prime movers plays the major role in strength development. The role of anabolic steroids (see chapter 5) relates to this latter point (87). We will now consider neural and muscular factors in more detail.

Neural Factors

It has become clear that a portion of the gains in strength that occurs with training, especially early in a program, is due to neural adaptations and not an enlargement of muscle (87). Some of these observations show that neural adaptations to strength training are different from those that occur with running or cycling training. In figure 13.13 we showed that when one leg was trained on a cycle ergometer, the training effect did not "carry over" to the untrained leg. In contrast, when one arm is strength trained, a portion of the training effect is "transferred" to the other arm. In this case, the gain in strength in the trained arm was related to both muscle hypertrophy and an increased ability to activate motor units, while in the untrained arm the improvement was due solely to the latter factor—a neural adaptation (87). A study confirmed this when gains of muscular strength and endurance of a trained leg were transferred to the untrained leg (54). The neural adaptations related to strength training include an improved ability to recruit motor units to enable a person to match the strength elicited by electrical stimulation (87). Strength and conditioning specialists are

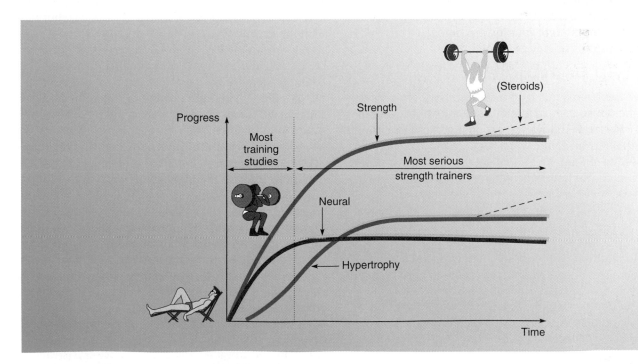

FIGURE 13.16   Relative roles of neural and muscular adaptations to resistance training.

Periodization of Strength Training

The most common resistance training workouts are structured around the exercise intensity and "sets" and "reps." Sets are the number of times a specific exercise is done, and reps refer to the number of times a movement is repeated within a set. Intensity refers to the weight lifted and may be expressed in terms of the "repetitions maximum" (RM), where 1RM is the greatest weight that can be lifted one time in good form. In chapter 16 we provide a brief summary of the debate on whether one set is as good as multiple sets in developing muscular fitness (see Clinical Applications 16.4). However, when working with athletic populations interested in performance, a strength coach may also specify the rest periods between exercises and sets, the type of muscle action (eccentric or concentric), the number of train-ing sessions per week, and possibly, the training volume (the total number of reps done in a workout). Periodized strength training uses these variables (and more) to develop workouts to achieve optimal gains in strength, power, motor performance, and/or hypertrophy over the course of a season, year, or athletic career (39, 59). Periodization describes a systematic process in which the volume and intensity of training are varied over time. For example, in "linear periodization" the individual is progressed from high volume/low intensity to low volume/high intensity over a certain time period (e.g., months). In "undulating" periodization the changes in volume and intensity occur more frequently (e.g., weekly or even daily). Are periodized programs better than nonperiodized programs?

A recent literature review (a meta-analysis) suggests that they are. Rhea and Alderman (81) found periodized programs to be more effective than nonperiodized programs for men and women, individuals with varying back-grounds in resistance training (i.e., untrained, athletes), and for all age groups. Consistent with the overload principle, additions to volume, intensity, and frequency resulted in additional adaptations. In addition, it has been shown that gradually increasing volume and decreasing intensity (reverse linear periodization) is more effective than linear or undulating peri-odization in increasing local muscle endurance (83), while daily undulat-ing programs are more effective for strength development (82).

always looking for the "best" programs to increase muscular strength. The Winning Edge 13.1 presents a recent review of how conventional programs compare to periodized strength training programs.

Muscular Enlargement

Recall that type II muscle fibers develop slightly more specific tension (i.e., force/cross-sectional area) than type I fibers (94); however, an enlargement of either fiber results in gains in strength. Strength training causes an enlargement of both type I and type II fibers, with the latter changing more than the former (58, 98). However, bodybuilders who train with low-intensity (high RM) and large-volume workouts have smaller type II fibers than powerlifters who train with heavy resistance (low RM) workouts (58, 98). It must be added that while bodybuilders have a higher percentage of slow-twitch fibers than do elite power-lifters, there are questions about whether the differ-ence is due to training or self-selection based on a genetic predisposition for success (98). Interestingly, differences between bodybuilders and powerlifters carry over to other muscular adaptations.

In contrast to the skeletal muscle adaptations that accompany running and cycling training, there is no increase in capillary density with heavy resistance training. As a result of the muscle's enlargement, cap-illary density may actually decrease (58, 98), but not without exception (66). However, bodybuilders who use low-resistance, high-volume workouts show in-creases in the capillary-to-fiber ratio such that the capillary density is similar to that of nonathletes, despite the muscle enlargement. Short-term strength training programs do not change capillary density, but mitochondrial density is decreased in proportion to the degree of hypertrophy (98). The muscle's ability to adapt is much greater than what is observed from con-ventional exercise training (see Pette's review in the Suggested Readings).

Hypertrophy and Hyperplasia During normal human development, from birth until adulthood, muscle size increases manyfold, with no change in the number of muscle fibers—a true hypertrophy. It is therefore not surprising that muscle enlargement associated with strength training is also due to a hypertrophy of existing fibers, not the generation of new fibers (hyperplasia), an observation Morpurgo made almost one hundred years ago (5, 94). However, a variety of observations have raised questions that perhaps *some* of the muscle enlargement due to training is the result of hyperplasia. Some studies report that elite bodybuilders have more fibers per motor unit than the average person, raising the point that hyperplasia might occur with long-term training (60, 62). In addition, when resistance training resulted in a 24% increase in muscle mass but only an 11% increase in fiber cross-sectional area, scientists suggested that hyperplasia might have played a role in the muscle enlargement (68). However, the vast majority of evidence favors the age-old proposition that hypertrophy is responsible for the expansion of the muscle's cross-sectional area due to resistance training (27).

Concurrent Strength and Endurance Training

At this point in the chapter it may have occurred to you that strength training might interfere with the adaptations associated with endurance training. For example, cycle training increases mitochondrial density, and strength training does the opposite. Does one type of training really interfere with the effects of the other? To date, a definite answer to this question is not available; nonetheless, let's examine studies on this issue.

In 1980, Hickson (44) showed that a ten-week combined strength and endurance training program resulted in similar gains in $\dot{V}O_2$ max compared to an endurance-only group, but there was some interference with the gains in strength. The strength-only group increased strength throughout the entire ten weeks, but the combined strength and endurance group showed a leveling off and a decrease in strength at nine and ten weeks. In contrast to this, when a ten-week (three-day-per-week) strength training program was added to a run-and-cycle training program *after* the group had leveled off in endurance performance, the group experienced a 30% gain in strength, but without hypertrophy. $\dot{V}O_2$ max was unaffected, but cycle time to exhaustion at 80% $\dot{V}O_2$ max was increased from seventy-one to eighty-five minutes. This suggests that strength training can improve the performance of prolonged heavy endurance exercise (46).

Sale et al. (89) found that relative to gains in strength (S) and endurance (E), when E-training was added to S-training (S + E), more improvements occurred in *endurance* than were generated by S-training alone. However, strength measures were unaffected. When S-training was added to E-training (E + S), more gains were made in *strength* than were generated by E-training alone; endurance measures were unaffected. The authors concluded that concurrent S- and E-training did not interfere with S- or E-development in comparison to S- or E-training alone. They suggest that the effectiveness of added training may depend on a variety of factors, such as intensity, volume, and frequency of training, status of the subjects, and how the training modes are integrated (88).

Consistent with this proposition, Putman et al (79) found that the S group, which exercised three days per week, experienced a greater gain in strength than the combined S + E group that exercised six days per week. The cross-sectional area (CSA) of type IIa fibers was increased similarly in S and S + E, but not so for the type I fibers. The S groups experienced a threefold greater change than the S + E group. In contrast, a study that required the S + E group to do only two endurance workouts and two strength workouts per week (versus three each) showed gains in strength and an increased hypertrophy is all fibers (42). Clearly the frequency of training has an impact on the potential for one type of training to interfere with the other (67).

IN SUMMARY

- Increases in strength due to short-term (eight to twenty weeks) training are the result of neural adaptations, while gains in strength in long-term training programs are due to an increase in the size of the muscle.
- There is evidence both for and against the proposition that the physiological effects of strength training interfere with the physiological effects of endurance training.

STUDY QUESTIONS

1. Define the following principles of training: *overload* and *specificity*.
2. Give one example of a cross-sectional study and a longitudinal study.
3. What are typical $\dot{V}O_2$ max values for young men and women? Cardiac patients?
4. Given the formula for $\dot{V}O_2$ max using heart rate, stroke volume, and the a-$\bar{v}$ O_2 difference, which variable is most important in explaining the differences in $\dot{V}O_2$ max in different populations? Give a quantitative example.
5. Describe how the increase in $\dot{V}O_2$ max comes about for the sedentary subject who undertakes an endurance training program.
6. Explain the importance of preload, afterload, and contractility in the increase of the maximal stroke volume that occurs with endurance training.
7. What are the most important changes in muscle structure that are responsible for the increase in the maximal a-$\bar{v}$ O_2 difference that occurs with endurance training?

8. What causes the $\dot{V}O_2$ max to decrease following termination of an endurance training program?
9. Describe how the capillary and mitochondrial changes that occur in muscle as a result of an endurance training program are related to the following adaptations to submaximal exercise:
    a. a lower O_2 deficit
    b. an increased utilization of FFA and a sparing of blood glucose and muscle glycogen
    c. a reduction in lactate and H^+ formation that helps to maintain the pH of the blood
    d. an increase in lactate removal
10. Define *central command* and *peripheral feedback* and explain how changes in muscle as a result of endurance training can be responsible for the lower heart rate, ventilation, and catecholamine responses to a submaximal exercise bout.
11. In short-term training programs, what neural factors may be responsible for the increase in strength?
12. Contrast hyperplasia with hypertrophy, and explain the role of each in the increase in muscle size that occurs with long-term strength training.
13. Does strength training interfere with the physiological effects of endurance training?

SUGGESTED READINGS

Costill, P. L. 1986. *Inside Running.* Indianapolis: Benchmark Press.

Fleck, S. J., and W. J. Kraemer. 1997. *Designing Resistance Training Programs.* Champaign, IL: Human Kinetics.

Hood, D. A. 2001. Plasticity in skeletal, cardiac, and smooth muscle. Invited review: Contractile activity-induced mitochondrial biogenesis in skeletal muscle. *Journal of Applied Physiology* 90:1137–57.

Mujika, I., and S. Padilla. 2001. Cardiorespiratory and metabolic characteristics of detraining in humans. *Medicine and Science in Sports and Exercise* 33:413–21.

Pette, D. 2002. The adaptive potential of skeletal muscle fibers. *Canadian Journal of Applied Physiology* 27(4):423–48.

REFERENCES

1. American College of Sports Medicine. 1998. The recommended quantity and quality of exercise for developing and maintaining cardiorespiratory and muscular fitness and flexibility in healthy adults. *Medicine and Science in Sports and Exercise* 30:975–91.
2. American College of Sports Medicine. 2002. Progression models in resistance training for healthy adults. *Medicine and Science in Sports and Exercise* 34:364–80.
3. Asmussen, E. et al. 1965. On the nervous factors controlling respiration and circulation during exercise. Experiments with curarization. *Acta Physiologica Scandinavica* 63:343–50.
4. Åstrand, P. O., and K. Rodahl. 1986. *Textbook of Work Physiology.* 3d ed. New York: McGraw-Hill.
5. Atha, J. 1981. Strengthening muscle. In *Exercise and Sport Science Reviews,* vol. 9, ed. D. I. Miller, 1–73. Philadelphia: The Franklin Institute Press.
6. Blomqvist, C. G., and B. Saltin. 1983. Cardiovascular adaptations to physical training. *Annual Review of Physiology* 45:169–89.
7. Booth, F. W. 1977. Effects of endurance exercise on cytochrome c turnover in skeletal muscle. *Annals of the New York Academy of Science* 301:431–39.
8. Booth, F. W., S. H. Weeden, and B. S. Tseng. 1994. Effect of aging on human skeletal muscle and motor function. *Medicine and Science in Sports and Exercise* 26:556–60.
9. Bouchard, C., M. R. Boulay, J-A. Simoneau, G. Lortie, and L. Pérusse. 1988. Heredity and trainability of aerobic and anaerobic performances: An update. *Sports Medicine* 5:69–73.
10. Bouchard, C. et al. 1986. Aerobic performance in brothers, dizygotic and monozygotic twins. *Medicine and Science in Sports and Exercise* 18:639–46.
11. Bouchard, C., F. T. Dionne, J-A. Simoneau, and M. R. Boulay. 1992. Genetics of aerobic and anaerobic performances. In *Exercise and Sport Science Reviews,* vol. 20, ed. J. O Holloszy, 27–58. Baltimore: Lippincott Williams & Wilkins.

12. Bouchard, C., A. S. Leon, D. C. Rao, J. S. Skinner, J. H. Wilmore, and J. Gagnon. 1995. The HERITAGE Family Study. Aims, design, and measurement protocol. *Medicine and Science in Sports and Exercise* 27:721–29.
13. Bouchard, C., E. W. Daw, T. Rice, L. Pérusse, J. Gagnon, M. A. Province, A. S. Leon, D. C. Rao, J. S. Skinner, and J. H. Wilmore. 1998. Family resemblance for $\dot{V}O_2$ max in the sedentary state: The HERITAGE Family Study. *Medicine and Science in Sports and Exercise* 30:252–58.
14. Bouchard, C., T. P. An, T. Rice, J. S. Skinner, J. H. Wilmore, J. Gagnon, L. Pérusse, A. S. Leon, and D. C. Rao. 1999. Family aggregation of $\dot{V}O_2$ max response to exercise: Results from the HERITAGE Family Study. *Journal of Applied Physiology* 87:1003–8.
15. Bouchard, C., T. Rankinen, Y. Chagnon, T. Rice, L. Pérusse, J. Gagnon, I. Borecki, P. An, A. S. Leon, J. S. Skinner, J. H. Wilmore, M. Province, and D. C. Rao. 2000. Genomic scan for maximal oxygen uptake and its response to training in the HERITAGE Family Study. *Journal of Applied Physiology* 88:551–59.
16. Bransford, D. R., and E. T. Howley. 1979. Effects of training on plasma FFA during exercise. *European Journal of Applied Physiology* 41:151–58.
17. Burelle, Y., and P. W. Hochachka. 2001. Endurance training induces muscle-specific changes in mitochondrial function in skinned muscle fibers. *Journal of Applied Physiology* 92:2429–38.
18. Burgomaster, K. A., S. C. Hughes, G. J. F. Heigenhauser, S. N. Bradwell, and M. J. Gibala. 2005. Six sessions of sprint interval training increases muscle oxidative potential and cycle endurance capacity in humans. *Journal of Applied Physiology* 98:1985–90.
19. Brooks, G. A. 1985. Anaerobic threshold: Review of the concept and directions for future research. *Medicine and Science in Sports and Exercise* 17:22–31.
20. Cadefau, J., H. J. Green, M. Ball-Burnett, and G. Jamieson. 1994. Coupling of muscle phosphorylation poten-

tial to glycolysis during work after short-term training. *Journal of Applied Physiology* 76:2586–93.

21. Cannon, J. G. 1993. Exercise and resistance to infection. *Journal of Applied Physiology* 74:973–81.

22. Claytor, R. P. 1985. Selected cardiovascular, sympathoadrenal, and metabolic responses to one-leg exercise training. Ph. D. diss., The University of Tennessee, Knoxville.

23. Coyle, E. F., M. K. Hemmert, and A. R. Coggan. 1986. Effects of detraining on cardiovascular responses to exercise: Role of blood volume. *Journal of Applied Physiology* 60:95–99.

24. Coyle, E. F., M. K. Hopper, and A. R. Coggan. 1990. Maximal oxygen uptake relative to plasma volume expansion. *International Journal of Sports Medicine* 11:116–19.

25. Coyle, E. F., W. H. Martin III, S. A. Bloomfield, O. H. Lowry, and J. O. Holloszy. 1985. Effects of detraining on responses to submaximal exercise. *Journal of Applied Physiology* 59:853–59.

26. Coyle, E. F., W. H. Martin III, D. R. Sinacore, M. J. Joyner, J. M. Hagberg, and J. O. Holloszy. 1984. Time course of loss of adaptations after stopping prolonged intense endurance training. *Journal of Applied Physiology: Respiratory, Environmental and Exercise Physiology* 57:1857–64.

27. Craig, B. W. 2001. Hyperplasia: Scientific fact or fiction? *National Strength & Conditioning Association* 23:42–44.

28. Cronan, T. L., and E. T. Howley. 1974. The effect of training on epinephrine and norepinephrine excretion. *Medicine and Science in Sports* 6:122–25.

29. Deschenes, M. R. 2004. Effects of aging on muscle fibre type and size. *Sports Medicine* 34(12):809–24.

30. Dionne, F. T., L. Turcotte, M-C. Thibault, M. R. Boulay, J. S. Skinner, and C. Bouchard. 1991. Mitochondrial DNA sequence polymorphism, $\dot{V}O_2$ max, and response to endurance training. *Medicine and Science in Sports and Exercise* 23:177–85.

31. Dudley, G. A., W. M. Abraham, and R. L. Terjung. 1982. Influence of exercise intensity and duration on biochemical adaptations in skeletal muscle. *Journal of Applied Physiology* 53:844–50.

32. Ehsani, A. A., J. M. Hagberg, and R. C. Hickson. 1978. Rapid changes in left ventricular dimensions and mass in response to physical conditioning. *American Journal of Cardiology* 42:52–56.

33. Ekblom, B. 1969. Effect of physical training on oxygen transport system in man. *Acta Physiologica Scandinavica* (Suppl.) 328:1–45.

34. Ekblom, B. et al. 1968. Effect of training on circulatory responses to exercise. *Journal of Applied Physiology* 24:518–28.

35. Fagard, R., E. Bielen, and A. Amery. 1991. Heritability of aerobic power and anaerobic energy generation during exercise. *Journal of Applied Physiology* 70:357–62.

36. Favier, R. J. et al. 1986. Endurance exercise training reduces lactate production. *Journal of Applied Physiology* 61:885–89.

37. Fiatarone, M. A. et al. 1990. High-intensity strength training in nonagenarians: Effects on skeletal muscle. *JAMA* 263:3029–34.

38. Fiatarone, M. A. et al. 1994. Exercise training and nutritional supplementation for physical frailty in very elderly people. *New England Journal of Medicine* 330:1769–75.

39. Fleck, S. J. 1999. Periodized strength training: A critical review. *Journal of Strength and Conditioning Research* 13:82–89.

40. Gleeson, M., D. C. Nieman, and B. K. Pedersen. 2004. Exercise, nutrition and immune function. *Journal of Sport Sciences* 22(11):115.

41. Green, H. J., S. Jones, M. E. Ball-Burnett, D. Smith, J. Livesey, and B. W. Farrance. 1991. Early muscular and metabolic adaptations to prolonged exercise training in humans. *Journal of Applied Physiology* 70:2032–38.

42. Häkkinen, K. et al. 2003. Neuromuscular adaptations during concurrent strength and endurance training versus strength training. *European Journal of Applied Physiology* 89:42–52.

43. Hagberg, J. M. et al. 1980. Faster adjustment to and recovery from submaximal exercise in the trained state. *Journal of Applied Physiology: Respiratory, Environmental and Exercise Physiology* 48:218–24.

44. Hickson, R. C. 1980. Interference of strength development by simultaneously training for strength and endurance. *European Journal of Applied Physiology* 45:255–63.

45. Hickson, R. C., H. A. Bomze, and J. O. Holloszy. 1978. Faster adjustment of O_2 uptake to the energy requirement of exercise in the trained state. *Journal of Applied Physiology: Respiratory, Environmental and Exercise Physiology* 44:877–81.

46. Hickson, R. C., B. A. Dvorak, E. M. Gorostiaga, T. T. Kurowski, and C. Foster. 1977. Linear increase in aerobic power induced by a strenuous program of endurance exercise. *Journal of Applied Physiology: Respiratory, Environmental and Exercise Physiology* 42:372–76.

47. ———. 1988. Potential for strength and endurance training to amplify endurance performance. *Journal of Applied Physiology* 65:2285–90.

48. Holloszy, J. O., and E. F. Coyle. 1984. Adaptations of skeletal muscle to endurance exercise and their metabolic consequences. *Journal of Applied Physiology: Respiratory, Environmental and Exercise Physiology* 56:831–38.

49. Hopp, J. F. 1993. Effects of age and resistance training on skeletal muscle: A review. *Physical Therapy* 73:361–73.

50. Horowitz, J. F. 2003. Fatty acid mobilization from adipose tissue during exercise. *Trends in Endrocrinology and Metabolism* 14(8):386–92.

50a. Houmard, J. A. et al. 1992. Effect of short-term training cessation on performance measures in distance runners. *International Journal of Sports Medicine* 13:572–76.

51. Howley, E. T., and B. D. Franks. 1997. *Health Fitness Instructor's Handbook*. 3rd Ed. Champaign, IL: Human Kinetics.

52. Hunter, G. R., J. P. McCarthy, and M. M. Bamman. 2004. Effects of resistance training on older adults. *Sports Medicine* 34(5):329–48.

53. Hutchinson, P. L., K. J. Cureton, H. Outz, and G. Wilson. 1991. Relationship of cardiac size to maximal oxygen uptake and body size in men and women. *International Journal of Sports Medicine* 12:369–73.

54. Kannus, P. et al. 1992. Effect of one-legged exercise on the strength, power and endurance of the contralateral leg: A randomized, controlled study using isometric and concentric isokinetic training. *European Journal of Applied Physiology* 64:117–26.

55. Kiens, B. et al. 1993. Skeletal muscle substrate utilization during submaximal exercise in man: Effect of endurance training. *Journal of Physiology* (London) 469:459–78.

56. Klausen, K. et al. 1982. Central and regional circulatory adaptations to one-leg training. *Journal of Applied Physiology: Respiratory, Environmental and Exercise Physiology* 52:976–83.

57. Klissouras, V. 1971. Heritability of adaptive variation. *Journal of Applied Physiology* 31:338–44.

58. Kraemer, W. J., M. R. Deschenes, and S. J. Fleck. 1988. Physiological adaptations to resistance exercise: Implications for athletic conditioning. *Sports Medicine* 6: 246–56.

59. Kraemer, W. J., and N. A. Ratamess. 2004. Fundamentals of resistance training: Progression and exercise prescription. *Medicine & Science in Sport & Exercise* 36(4): 674–88.

60. Larsson, L., and P. A. Tesch. 1986. Motor unit fibre density in extremely hypertrophied skeletal muscles in man: Electrophysiological signs of muscle fibre hyperplasia. *European Journal of Applied Physiology* 55:130–36.

61. MacDougall, J. D. 1986. Morphological changes in human skeletal muscle following strength training and immobilization. In *Human Muscle Power*, ed. N. L. Jones, N. McCartney, and A. J. McComas, chap. 17, 269–85. Champaign, IL: Human Kinetics.

62. MacDougall, J. D., D. G. Sale, S. E. Alway, and J. R. Sutton. 1984. Muscle fiber number in biceps brachii bodybuilders and control subjects. *Journal of Applied Physiology: Respiratory, Environmental and Exercise Physiology* 57: 1399–1403.

63. Madsen, K. et al. 1993. Effects of detraining on endurance capacity and metabolic changes during prolonged exhaustive exercise. *Journal of Applied Physiology* 75:1444–51.

64. Martin, W. H. et al. 1993. Effect of endurance training on plasma free fatty acid turnover and oxidation during exercise. *American Journal of Physiology* 265:E708–14.

65. Martino, M., N. Gledhill, and V. Jamnik. 2002. High $\dot{V}O_2$ max with no history of training is due to high blood volume. *Medicine and Science in Sports and Exercise* 34:966–71.

66. McCall, G. E., W. C. Byrnes, A. Dickinson, P. M. Pattany, and S. J. Fleck. 1996. Muscle fiber hypertrophy, hyperplasia, and capillary density in college men after resistance training. *Journal of Applied Physiology* 81(5):2004–12.

67. McCarthy, J. P., M. A. Pozniak, and J. C. Agre. 2002. Neuromuscular adaptations to concurrent strength and endurance training. *Medicine and Science in Sports and Exercise* 34:511–19.

68. Mikesky, A. E., C. J. Giddings, W. Matthews, and W. J. Gonyea. 1991. Changes in muscle fiber size and composition in response to heavy-resistance exercise. *Medicine and Science in Sports and Exercise* 23:1042–49

69. Mitchell, J. H. 1990. Neural control of the circulation during exercise. *Medicine and Science in Sports and Exercise* 22:141–54.

70. Mitchell, J. H., and R. F. Schmidt. 1983. Cardiovascular reflex control by afferent fibers from skeletal muscle receptors. In *Handbook of Physiology: The Cardiovascular System. Peripheral Circulation and Organ Blood Flow*, ed. J. T. Shepherd, F. M. Abbound, and S. R. Geiger, 623–58. Bethesda, MD: American Physiological Society.

71. Morganroth, J. et al. 1975. Comparative left ventricular dimensions in trained athletes. *Annals of Internal Medicine* 82:521–24.

72. Nieman, D. C. 1994. Exercise, infection, and immunity. *International Journal of Sports Medicine* 15:S131–S141.

73. Paul, P. 1975. Effects of long-lasting physical exercise and training on lipid metabolism. In *Metabolic Adaptation to Prolonged Physical Exercise*, ed. H. Howald and J. R. Poortmans, 156–87. Switzerland: Birkhauser Verlag Basel.

74. Pierce, E. F., A. Weltman, R. L. Seip, and D. Snead. 1990. Effects of training specificity on the lactate threshold and $\dot{V}O_2$ peak. *International Journal of Sports Medicine* 11:267–72.

75. Powers, S. K., S. Dodd, and R. E. Beadle. 1985. Oxygen uptake kinetics in trained athletes differing in $\dot{V}O_2$ max. *European Journal of Applied Physiology* 54:306–8.

76. Powers, S. K. et al. 1994. Influence of exercise and fiber type on antioxidant enzyme activity in rat skeletal muscle. *American Journal of Physiology* 266:R375–80.

77. Powers, S. K. et al. 1995. Role of beta-adrenergic mechanisms in exercise training-induced metabolic changes in respiratory and locomotor muscle. *International Journal of Sports Medicine* 16:13–18.

78. Prud'Homme, D. et al. 1984. Sensitivity of maximal aerobic power to training is genotype-dependent. *Medicine and Science in Sports and Exercise* 16:489–93.

79. Putman, C. T., X. Xu, E. Gillies, I. M. MacLean, and G. J. Bell. 2004. Effects of strength, endurance and combined training on myosin heavy chain content and fibre-type distribution in humans. *European Journal of Applied Physiology* 92:376–84.

80. Rerych, S. K. et al. 1980. Effects of exercise training on left ventricular function in normal subjects: A longitudinal study by radionuclide angiography. *American Journal of Cardiology* 45:244–52.

81. Rhea, M. R., and B. L. Alderman. 2004. A meta-analysis of periodized versus nonperiodized strength and power training programs. *Research Quarterly for Exercise and Sport* 75(4):413–22.

82. Rhea, M. R., S. D. Ball, W. T. Phillips, and L. N. Burkett. 2002. A comparison of linear and daily undulating periodized programs with equated volume and intensity for strength. *Journal of Strength and Conditioning Research* 16(2):250–55.

83. Rhea, M. R. et al. 2003. A comparison of linear and daily undulating periodized programs with equated volume and intensity for local muscular endurance. *Journal of Strength and Conditioning Research* 17(1):82–87.

84. Rogers, M. J., and W. J. Evans. 1993. Changes in skeletal muscle with aging: Effects of exercise training. In *Exercise and Sport Science Reviews*, vol. 21, ed. J. O. Holloszy, 65–102. Baltimore: Lippincott Williams & Wilkins.

85. Rowell, L. B. 1986. *Human Circulation-Regulation During Physical Stress*. New York: Oxford University Press.

86. Rowell, L. B., and D. S. O'Leary. 1990. Reflex control of the circulation during exercise: Chemoreflexes and mechanoreflexes. *Journal of Applied Physiology* 69:407–18.

87. Sale, D. G. 1988. Neural adaptation to resistance training. *Medicine and Science in Sports and Exercise* 20: S135–S145.

88. Sale, D. G., I. Jacobs, J. D. MacDougall, and S. Garner. 1990. Comparison of two regimens of concurrent strength and endurance training. *Medicine and Science in Sports and Exercise* 22:348–56.

89. Sale, D. G., J. D. MacDougall, I. Jacobs, and S. Garner. 1990. Interaction between concurrent strength and endurance training. *Journal of Applied Physiology* 68: 260–70.

90. Saltin, B. 1969. Physiological effects of physical conditioning. *Medicine and Science in Sports* 1:50–56.

91. Saltin, B., and P. O. Åstrand. 1967. Maximal oxygen uptake in athletes. *Journal of Applied Physiology* 23:353–58.

92. ———. 1993. Free fatty acids and exercise. *American Journal of Clinical Nutrition* 57 (Suppl):752S–758S.

93. Saltin, B. et al. 1977. Fiber types and metabolic potentials of skeletal muscles in sedentary man and endurance runners. *Annals of the New York Academy of Science* 301:3–29.

94. Saltin, B., and P. D. Gollnick. 1983. Skeletal muscle adaptability: Significance for metabolism and performance. In *Handbook of Physiology*, ed. L. D. Peachey, R. H.

Adrian, and S. R. Geiger, Section 10: Skeletal Muscle, chap. 19. Baltimore: Lippincott Williams & Wilkins.

95. Shephard, R. J., and P. N. Shek. 1995. Exercise, aging, and immune function. *International Journal of Sports Medicine* 16:1–6.

96. Spina, R. J. et al. 1993. Differences in cardiovascular adaptations to endurance exercise training between older men and women. *Journal of Applied Physiology* 75: 849–55.

97. Terjung, R. L. 1995. Muscle adaptations to aerobic training. *Sports Science Exchange.* vol. 8, no. 1. Barrington, IL: Gatorade Sports Science Institute.

98. Tesch, P. A. 1988. Skeletal muscle adaptations consequent to long-term heavy resistance exercise. *Medicine and Science in Sports and Exercise* 20:S132–S134.

99. Van Loon, L. J. C. 2004. Use of intramuscular triacylglycerol as a substrate source during exercise in humans. *Journal of Applied Physiology* 97:1170–87.

100. Wibom, R. et al. 1992. Adaptations of mitochondrial ATP production in human skeletal muscle to endurance training and detraining. *Journal of Applied Physiology* 73:2004–10.

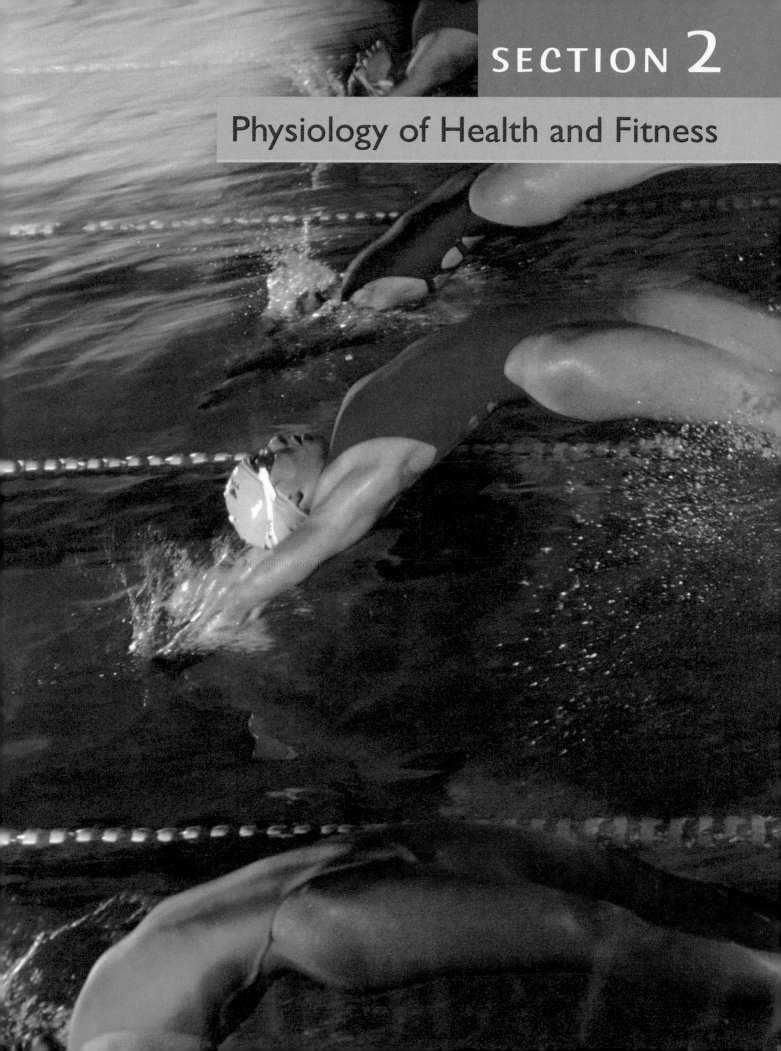

SECTION 2

Physiology of Health and Fitness

Patterns in Health and Disease: Epidemiology and Physiology

■ Objectives

By studying this chapter, you should be able to do the following:

1. Define or describe the science of epidemiology.
2. Contrast infectious with degenerative diseases as causes of death.
3. Identify the three major categories of risk factors and examples of specific risk factors in each.
4. Compare the epidemiologic triad with the web of causation as models to study infectious and degenerative diseases, respectively.
5. Describe the difference between primary and secondary risk factors for coronary heart disease (CHD).
6. Describe the steps an epidemiologist must follow to show that a risk factor is causally connected to a disease.
7. Describe the hypothesis linking resistance to insulin as a cause of hypertension.

■ Outline

Epidemiology   289

Coronary Heart Disease   291
    Physical Inactivity as a Risk
        Factor   292

Physiology   294

Synthesis   296

■ Key Terms

atherosclerosis
degenerative diseases
epidemiologic triad

epidemiology
infectious diseases
primary risk factor

secondary risk factor
web of causation

In many areas of inquiry, scientists look for connections between facts (e.g., cigarette smoking and lung cancer) and try to determine whether the linkage is a causal one or is due simply to chance. This chapter will describe the way two scientific disciplines, epidemiology and physiology, go about the business of moving from simple observations to the point of establishing that events are causally connected. Such a process allows us to understand the manner in which a disease develops and points the way toward intervention programs.

EPIDEMIOLOGY

In the mid-1850s in London there was a major outbreak of cholera, a disease characterized by vomiting and diarrhea that can lead to death (34). Although it was generally accepted in the medical community of that time that the disease was caused by "bad air" derived from decaying organic matter, Dr. John Snow thought otherwise. He systematically contacted the families of those who had died of cholera and found an association between the source of their drinking water and the death rate. People supplied by the Southwark water company experienced a cholera death rate of 5.0 per 1,000 population, compared to a rate of 0.9 per 1,000 for those supplied by other water companies (7, 34). About 100 years later, a study of British doctors showed a linear increase in lung cancer with the average number of cigarettes smoked per day. These studies are examples of the science of epidemiology in action (7, 34). In the first case, Snow looked for connections between an environmental factor (water supply) and a communicable disease (cholera) by studying subgroups of the London population. The second study built on clinical observations linking a behavior (smoking) to a chronic disease (lung cancer) to see if the two might be causally connected.

Epidemiology is defined as the "study of the distribution and determinants of health-related states or events in specified populations, and the application of this study to control of health problems" (22). Epidemiology is used in a number of different ways (7):

- To establish cause—It is important to know whether the cause of a disease is due to genetic or environmental factors, or more likely, an interaction between the two (e.g., smoking and lung cancer). This can lead to strategies to prevent the disease (e.g., don't smoke).

- To trace the natural history of a disease—Epidemiologists try to understand the normal course of a disease from a healthy state to a presymptomatic stage that leads to clinical

signs and symptoms and finally, to death or recovery. The progress of the disease can be detected and treated at any stage, but the effectiveness of the treatment can only be determined if the natural history of the disease, in the absence of treatment, is known.

- To describe the health status of populations—By knowing the total burden of disease in a population, health authorities can establish priorities in the use of health-care dollars to have the greatest benefit.

- To evaluate an intervention—Studies are done to determine the success or failure of programs established to prevent or treat a disease.

One of the major goals of epidemiology is to prevent and control diseases by understanding what causes them, but it is easier said than done, even for infectious diseases (7). Figure 14.1 describes an epidemiological model called the **epidemiologic triad** that shows connections among the environment, the agent, and the host that cause disease (15, 34). If we use the cholera example mentioned earlier, the bacteria *Vibrio cholerae* is the agent that was transmitted via a poorly treated water supply (environment) to the population (host). The model also indicates that social factors such as poor housing and malnutrition can decrease natural protective mechanisms and make the host more susceptible to disease. In the cholera example, the disease was controlled by making the drinking water safe. An important point to recognize is that disease control was achieved decades before the bacterium that causes cholera was discovered (7).

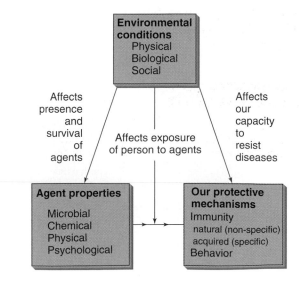

FIGURE 14.1 Epidemiologic triad: an epidemiologic model showing the interaction of the environment, host, and agent as a cause of disease.

IN SUMMARY

- Epidemiology is the study of the distribution and determinants of health states and the use of this information in the control of disease.
- Disease control can be achieved by: (1) destroying or removing the agent at its source, (2) altering the environment to reduce transmission of the agent, or improving the host's resistance to the agent, and (3) altering the host's behaviors such as improved nutrition, immunization, and exercise (15).

Over the last 100 years, attention has shifted from **infectious diseases** (e.g., tuberculosis and pneumonia) as the major causes of death to **degenerative diseases** such as cancer and cardiovascular diseases. For example, in 2002 cardiovascular diseases and cancers were responsible for about 1.5 million deaths, greatly overshadowing all other causes of death (3). The problem of establishing the cause of a disease is much more difficult when dealing with chronic, degenerative diseases such as cardiovascular disease, because genetic, environmental, and behavioral factors are involved in a very complex manner. The difficulty of establishing "cause" in these complex diseases is best described by another epidemiologic model called the **web of causation** (23, 34). Figure 14.2 shows how a combination of

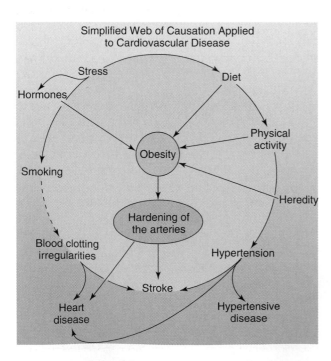

FIGURE 14.2 Web of causation: an epidemiologic model showing the complex interaction of risk factors associated with the development of chronic degenerative diseases such as cardiovascular diseases.

genetic (heredity), environmental (stress), and behavioral (diet, smoking, physical activity) factors interact to cause cardiovascular disease (34, 35). Trying to tease out the effect that one factor has on another and on the final disease process is a difficult task that makes work in epidemiology interesting and challenging. The factors in the web of causation are positively associated with the development of cardiovascular diseases, but are not sufficient in and of themselves to cause them. These factors are called "risk factors," and they play a major role in prevention programs aimed at reducing disease and premature death associated with degenerative diseases. This has led to public health programs to educate the population about risk factors and the need for each of us to take personal responsibility for our health (7, 19). See A Closer Look 14.1 for differences between leading and actual causes of death.

IN SUMMARY

- Epidemiologists show that the major causes of death in the United States are degenerative diseases such as heart disease and cancer. The development and progress of these diseases are affected by the interaction of environmental and behavioral risk factors.

In 1979, the surgeon general of the United States published a report, *Healthy People* (36), indicating that even though degenerative diseases have more complex causes than infectious diseases, the onset of these diseases can be delayed or prevented (36). Figure 14.3 shows the three major risk factor categories associated with health and disease, with specific risk factors identified under each. While some diseases (hemophilia and sickle-cell anemia) are primarily inherited, the vast majority of diseases result from an interaction of genetics and the individual's environment (36). The *inherited/biological factors* include age, gender, race, and the ease with which one might develop a disease. Nothing can be done about these risk factors; they are fixed and some people simply have a higher risk of certain degenerative diseases than others. However, what has become clear over the past fifty years is the fact that *environmental and behavioral risk factors* are most influential in the early onset of degenerative diseases or death. Fortunately, these risk factors are most susceptible to change, and this brings us back to the issue of personal responsibility as a major force determining one's well-being. Personal responsibility means more than getting sufficient exercise, or eating the proper foods. There is a need for people to speak out for clean air and water, to support community-wide blood pressure and serum cholesterol screenings, and to not drink and drive. To expand on this risk factor concept we will focus on coronary heart disease.

A CLOSER LOOK 14.1

Leading Versus Actual Causes of Death

As mentioned earlier, the leading cause of death is heart disease. This is followed by cancer (malignant neoplasm), stroke (cerebrovascular disease), chronic lung disease, unintentional injuries, and diabetes. However, such a list does not provide information about what caused the deaths. The leading actual cause of death is tobacco, accounting for 18% of all deaths. This is followed by poor diet and physical inactivity, alcohol consumption, infection (microbial agents), toxic agents, motor vehicle accidents, and firearms (24). Although these investigators had to correct their estimate of the number of deaths due to poor diet and physical inactivity (25), it did not affect the order and only slightly lowered the percent contribution—from 16.6% to 15.2%—to the death rate. In contrast to smoking and poor diet and physical inactivity, the next leading cause of death, alcohol, was only 3.5%. What is clear is the role that improved health behaviors can have on this picture—an important message for those entering the allied health professions.

FIGURE 14.3 Major categories of risk factors with examples of each.
Source: U.S. Department of Health, Education, and Welfare, 1979, *Healthy People: The Surgeon General's Report on Health Promotion and Disease Prevention*.

CORONARY HEART DISEASE

Coronary heart disease (CHD) is associated with a gradual narrowing of the arteries serving the heart due to a thickening of the inner lining of the artery. This process, **atherosclerosis,** is the leading contributor to heart attack and stroke deaths (3, 14). It is now widely accepted that some people are at a greater risk of developing CHD than others. Our understanding of the risks associated with atherosclerotic disease is based primarily on the epidemiological investigation conducted in Framingham, Massachusetts (14). When this study began in 1949, cardiovascular disease already accounted for 50% of all deaths in the United States. The Framingham Study is an observational prospective (longitudinal) study designed to determine how those who develop cardiovascular disease differ from those who do not. Approximately 5,000 men and women were examined every other year, and measures such as blood pressure, electrocardiographic abnormalities, serum cholesterol, smoking, and body weight were obtained. The investigators were then able to relate the different measures to the progression of the coronary heart disease (14). Early in the study, investigators found that about 20% of the population experienced a heart attack before sixty years of age, and of them, 20% resulted in sudden death. The natural history of this disease indicated that prevention was an important goal, and the Framingham Study is recognized for identifying the risk factors to predict subsequent disease and allow early intervention (19).

The Framingham Study found that the risk of CHD increases with the number of cigarettes smoked, the degree to which the blood pressure is elevated, and the quantity of cholesterol in the blood (19). In addition, the overall risk of CHD increases with the number of risk factors; that is, a person who has a systolic blood pressure of 160 mm Hg, a serum cholesterol of 250 mg/dl, and smokes more than a pack of cigarettes a day has about six times the risk of CHD as a person who has only one of these risk factors (13). It is important to remember that risk factors interact with each other to increase the overall risk of CHD. This has implications for prevention as well as treatment. In this regard, getting a hypertensive patient to quit smoking confers more immediate benefit than any antihypertensive drug (19). Further, regular physical activity reduces the risk of CHD, even in those who smoke and are hypertensive (see chapter 16). The Framingham Heart Study was not the only epidemiological investigation interested in these issues (see A Closer Look 14.2).

A CLOSER LOOK 14.2

Harvard Alumni Study and Aerobics Center Longitudinal Study

Two epidemiological studies that have had a major impact on our knowledge of how physical activity and cardiovascular fitness are related to the risk of heart disease and death are the Harvard Alumni Study and the Aerobics Center Longitudinal Study. The Harvard Alumni Study, initiated by Dr. Ralph S. Paffenbarger, studied undergraduates who matriculated between 1916 and 1950. These alumni filled out detailed questionnaires concerning their health status (e.g., physician-diagnosed diseases such as hypertension and diabetes),

health habits (e.g., smoking, physical activity, alcohol consumption), and physical characteristics such as height and weight. Investigators followed these alumni over time and were able to relate the subsequent appearance of a disease (e.g., coronary heart disease) or death to previously reported information on the questionnaires. You may want to read this classic article by Paffenbarger et al. on physical activity, all-cause mortality, and longevity of college alumni (29).

The Aerobic Center Longitudinal Study, directed by Steven N. Blair, examines similar relationships to that of the Harvard Alumni Study, but focuses on cardiorespiratory fitness (measured by time on a graded treadmill test) rather than self-reported physical activity. This investigation has generated several classic papers, important to our understanding of fitness and health. You may want to read this classic article by Blair et al. on physical fitness and all-cause mortality (8).

> ### IN SUMMARY
>
> - Risk factors can be divided into three categories: genetic/biological, environmental, and behavioral.
> - The risk factors of smoking, high cholesterol, and hypertension interact to magnify the risk of CHD. Similarly, elimination of one of them causes a disproportionate reduction in the risk of CHD.

After looking at the web of causation for cardiovascular disease in figure 14.2, one can understand how difficult it is to determine whether an observed association between a risk factor and a disease is a causal one or is due simply to chance. To facilitate the process of determining cause, epidemiologists apply the following guidelines (7):

- Temporal association—Does the cause precede the effect?
- Plausibility—Is the association consistent with other knowledge?
- Consistency—Have similar results been shown in other studies?
- Strength—What is the strength of the association (relative risk) between the cause and the effect? Relative risk is sometimes expressed as the ratio of the risk of disease among those exposed to the factor to the risk of those unexposed. The greater the ratio, the stronger the association.
- Dose-response relationship—Is increased exposure to the possible cause associated with increased effect?

- Reversibility—Does the removal of the possible cause lead to a reduction of the disease risk?
- Study design—Is the evidence based on strong study design?
- Judging the evidence—How many lines of evidence lead to the conclusion?

Physical Inactivity as a Risk Factor

The concern about whether a risk factor is causally related to cardiovascular disease has special significance for physical activity. For many years, physical inactivity was believed to be only weakly associated with heart disease and was not given much attention as a public health concern. However, in the late 1980s and early 1990s that view changed rather dramatically. In 1987, Powell et al. (30) did a systematic review of the literature dealing with the role of physical activity in the primary prevention of coronary heart disease, applying the just listed guidelines to establish causation. They found that the majority of studies indicated that the level of physical inactivity predated the onset of CHD, thus meeting the temporal requirement. They also found a dose-response relationship in that as physical activity increased, the risk of CHD decreased, and the association was stronger in the better studies. The latter results met the consistency and study design criteria for causality. The review found the association to be plausible given the role of physical activity in improving glucose tolerance, increasing fibrinolysis (breaking of clots), and reducing blood pressure. The investigators calculated the relative risk of CHD due to inactivity to be about 1.9, meaning that sedentary people had about twice the chance of experiencing

A CLOSER LOOK 14.3

Risk Factors for Coronary Heart Disease (CHD)

Historically, risk factors for CHD were divided into primary or major and secondary or contributing. **Primary** meant that a factor in and of itself increased the risk of CHD, and **secondary** meant that a certain factor increased the risk of CHD only if one of the primary factors was already present, or that its significance had not been precisely determined (12). Lists of risk factors have evolved over time as more epidemiological evidence has accumulated showing the association between various behaviors (e.g., physical inactivity) or characteristics (e.g., obesity) and CHD. Consequently, a practical approach used to classify risk factors is to list those that can be changed and those that can't, whether or not they are primary or secondary.

It should be noted that the American College of Sports Medicine (ACSM) (1) lists one of the subfractions of cholesterol (high-density lipoprotein cholesterol [HDL-C]) as an additional risk factor. There is good evidence that the risk of CHD is lower for those with higher concentrations of HDL-C, and the ratio of total cholesterol to HDL-C is

Can't be Changed	Can be Changed	
Heredity	Cigarette smoking	Diabetes
Gender	High serum cholesterol	Obesity
Age	High blood pressure	Stress
Race	Physical inactivity	

viewed by some as a better index of risk than total cholesterol alone (19). In fact, the ACSM considers HDL-C to be a "negative risk factor" when levels exceed 60 mg/dl. Further, over the years evidence accumulated showing that obesity may be a major risk factor (11, 20, 31), and now both the ACSM and the American Heart Association list it as such. Lastly, you may have noticed that a high-fat diet is not even cited on the list of risk factors for CHD. The reason for this is that the detrimental effect of a high-fat diet is already represented in the obesity and serum cholesterol risk factors. However, it is generally believed that controlling the type and amount of dietary fat would reduce the risk of CHD in the American population (see chapter 18).

As we have come to understand that physical inactivity, diet, and stress are risk factors for obesity, glucose intolerance (diabetes), hypertension, and high serum cholesterol, we have developed a new and potent view of how to intervene. Health promotion programs deal directly with physical inactivity, diet, and stress to prevent other risk factors from occurring. In addition, the primary nonpharmacological treatment of these primary risk factors revolves around recommendations for a low-fat diet (see chapter 18), regular physical activity (see chapter 16), and stress reduction (6, 9, 10). To estimate your or your parent's 10-year risk of having a heart attack, go to http://hin.nhlbi.nih.gov/atpiii/calculator.asp?usertype=pub.

CHD that physically active people had. The relative risk was similar to smoking (2.5), high serum cholesterol (2.4), and high blood pressure (2.1). When the authors controlled for smoking, blood pressure, cholesterol, age, and sex (all of which are associated with CHD), the association of physical activity and CHD remained, indicating that physical activity was an independent risk factor for CHD (2). See A Closer Look 14.3 for more on risk factors and heart disease.

In order to estimate the real impact a risk factor may have on a population, epidemiologists try to balance the relative risk with the number of people in the population that have the risk factor. This balancing act is summed up in the calculation of the *population attributable risk* for each risk factor (10). Figure 14.4 describes the relative risk for selected risk factors and the percent of the population affected. Given the large number of people who are inactive, changes in physical activity habits have a great potential to reduce CHD (see chapter 16). The publication of *Physical Activity and Health: A Report of the Surgeon General* emphasized the critical need to address these issues now (39).

FIGURE 14.4 Percentages of U.S. population at risk for recognized risk factors related to coronary heart disease and risk ratio for each risk factor.

- Physical inactivity is an independent risk factor for CHD.
- The relative risk of CHD due to inactivity (1.9) is similar to that of hypertension (2.1) and high cholesterol (2.4). The fact that about 59% of the population is inactive indicates the enormous impact a change in physical activity habits can have on the nation's risk for CHD.

PHYSIOLOGY

Epidemiologists are not the only scientists interested in looking at potential relationships between variables in an attempt to have a greater understanding of what causes cardiovascular disease. Physiologists study how tissues and organs function to maintain homeostasis and try to uncover the source of a problem when homeostasis is not maintained. A good example of a failure to maintain homeostasis is hypertension, a problem that affects more than 50 million Americans (3). Interestingly, investigators have found that hypertension does not generally occur in isolation. It is not uncommon for hypertensive individuals to also have multiple metabolic abnormalities such as:

- obesity—especially abdominal obesity
- insulin resistance—tissues do not take up glucose easily when stimulated with insulin, and muscle is the primary site of the insulin resistance
- dyslipidemia—abnormal levels of triglycerides

The fact that these abnormalities often occur as a group suggests a common, underlying cause that might give us a better understanding of the disease processes associated with hypertension. The coexistence of insulin resistance, dyslipidemia, and hypertension has been called Syndrome X (32) and the Metabolic Cardiovascular Syndrome (29); those who add obesity to the model call it the Deadly Quartet (21). However, Metabolic Syndrome is currently the preferred term.

Figure 14.5 shows hypothesized connections between and among these abnormalities. The central focus of the model is on insulin resistance, with skeletal muscle being the predominant tissue involved. Insulin resistance is commonly associated with obesity, especially upper body (abdominal) obesity (21, 29). However, as the arrows in figure 14.5 indicate, insulin resistance can be caused by a combination of genetic and environmental influences independent of obesity (16, 32). For example, it has been demonstrated that a high-fat, refined-sugar diet is the cause

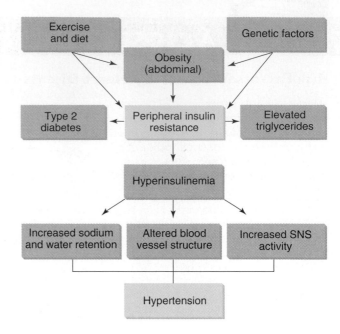

FIGURE 14.5 The insulin-resistance and hypertension hypothesis: Syndrome X.

of insulin resistance and not the obesity (4). Insulin resistance is characterized by a reduced ability to take up glucose at a given insulin concentration. In response to this resistance the pancreas secretes more insulin to promote blood glucose uptake into tissues in order to return the blood glucose concentration to normal. If the pancreas cannot secrete enough insulin, the blood glucose will remain elevated and a condition known as type 2 diabetes results. A drug may be required to stimulate the pancreas to secrete additional insulin to correct the problem (see chapter 17).

When the pancreas secretes additional insulin to deal with the insulin resistance, the plasma insulin level becomes elevated (hyperinsulinemia); this can elevate blood pressure and lead to hypertension. Figure 14.5 shows that elevated insulin levels can:

- increase sympathetic nervous system (SNS) activity leading to elevation of epinephrine and norepinephrine levels, which can increase heart rate, stroke volume, and increase blood pressure. The elevated E and NE levels can also interfere with insulin release from the pancreas and interfere with glucose uptake at the tissue, which aggravates the problem (see chapter 5),
- increase sodium and water retention, which increases plasma volume and blood pressure, and
- increase the proliferation of smooth muscle cells in small blood vessels, which can increase resistance to blood flow and drive up blood pressure.

Muscle Fiber Type and Disease Risk

Although you are familiar with the connection of muscle fiber type to performance (see chapters 8 and 19), a recent review by Dr. David Bassett, Jr., summarized potential links between fiber type and cardiovascular disease risk factors (5):

- Mean arterial blood pressure is higher in subjects with a high percentage of type II fibers, and hypertension is associated with a lower capillary density in skeletal muscle.
- Insulin resistance is related to the capillary density of skeletal

muscle; those with fewer capillaries (high percentage of type II fibers) experience greater insulin resistance.
- Obesity, especially upper body obesity, is related to a high percentage of type II fibers.

These facts suggest a strong connection between fiber type and risk factors, and when coupled with the observation that exercise training has little effect on the type I/ type II muscle fiber distribution, one may wonder about the role exercise plays in preventing or treating these risk factors.

All is not lost. As pointed out by Bassett, endurance training causes increases in both capillary density and the ability of muscle to use fat as a fuel, and type II muscle fibers take on characteristics similar to those found in type I muscle fibers. Lastly, exercise increases the sensitivity of the muscle to insulin such that less insulin is needed to control the blood glucose level. The importance of exercise in the prevention of (and as a non-pharmacological treatment for) obesity, hypertension, and insulin resistance is enhanced by such findings (see chapter 17).

Figure 14.5 also shows the connection between insulin resistance and altered blood lipids. Individuals with insulin resistance and/or abdominal obesity tend to have a higher free fatty acid (FFA) level, which can lead to an increase in plasma triglycerides. The higher FFA level could be due to the inability of insulin to suppress FFA (32), or the abdominal obesity, which is associated with an increased ability to mobilize FFA (21).

In this model, the scientists hypothesized that the cause of hypertension is the insulin resistance, with skeletal muscle being the primary tissue involved. An alternative hypothesis has been offered to what may now be viewed as the chicken-and-egg question; that is, "Which comes first?" It has been proposed that it is the hypertension that causes the insulin resistance and not the reverse. In contrast, others suggest that hypertension causes a decrease in the small blood vessels in muscle leading to a reduction in the delivery of glucose and insulin, both of which are needed to have normal glucose uptake (18). In addition, they propose that muscle fiber type is linked to hypertension (see A Closer Look 14.4). Given the seriousness of this problem, it is important to know how many people have the Metabolic Syndrome.

In order to establish the prevalence of the Metabolic Syndrome in the population, scientists first established an operational definition of the syndrome—a person had to have three or more of the following to be considered as having the syndrome (28):

- abdominal obesity: waist circumference >102 cm in men and >88 cm in women
- hypertriglyceridemia: ≥150 mg/dl
- low high-density lipoprotein (HDL) cholesterol: <40 mg/dl in men and <50 mg/dl in women

- high blood pressure: ≥130/85 mm Hg
- high fasting blood glucose: ≥110 mg/dl

The prevalence of the Metabolic Syndrome increased from 6.7% in those 20 to 29 years of age to more than 40% in those over 60 years. Adjusting for age, 23.7% of the population was identified as having this syndrome, with Mexican-Americans having the highest age-adjusted prevalence, 31.9% (17).

Independent of whether the insulin resistance precedes or follows the hypertension, there is considerable evidence that exercise can benefit people with insulin resistance. This may be due to increases in the capillary density or oxidative capacity of muscle that occurs with exercise training (see chapter 13), or an increase in glucose transporters in muscle (see chapter 5). As the model indicates, two of the most important factors related to insulin resistance are physical activity (exercise) and obesity. These latter issues will be discussed in detail in chapters 16 and 18, respectively.

IN SUMMARY

- The metabolic syndrome model describes potential causative connections between and among obesity, peripheral insulin resistance, hypertension, and dyslipidemia.
- The insulin resistance is located primarily in skeletal muscle, being greater in type II muscles with their limited capillary supply.
- Exercise can both directly and indirectly decrease the risk of CHD by influencing obesity, insulin resistance, and hypertension.

A CLOSER LOOK 14.5

Overweight and Obesity

The Body Mass Index (BMI—kg/m²) has been accepted as a standard to characterize overweight (BMI = 25.0−29.9) and obesity (BMI ≥ 30.0) (27, 41). Based on 2000 data, 65% of U.S. adults are overweight and 30% are obese (26). The concern is not just about the magnitude of the problem, but how fast obesity has increased in this country. The Centers for Disease Control and Prevention (CDC) has been tracking changes in obesity, and the news is not good (see **http://www.cdc.gov/nccdphp/dnpa/obesity/trend/maps/index.htm** for maps of the United States that trace changes in obesity since 1985). Obesity has increased dramatically—almost doubling in twenty-five years, and is continuing to increase. For the reasons mentioned earlier about the connections of obesity to other problems (see Metabolic Syndrome), an increase in the number of people with diabetes has paralleled the increase in obesity. To make matters worse, the prevalence of overweight in children has also risen during this time, and physicians are reporting cases of type 2 diabetes in middle school children—something unheard of just a few years ago.

It is no surprise that the Surgeon General has issued a "Call to Action" to prevent and decrease the problems of overweight and obesity (see Suggested Readings). *Healthy People* 2010 has released a publication, *Leading Health Indicators*, to bring additional focus on the problems of obesity and inactivity, to motivate action, and to measure progress (see **http://www.healthypeople.gov/ LHI**). The personal and economic consequences of not solving these problems are considerable.

SYNTHESIS

A common theme coming from both the web of causation for cardiovascular disease and the Metabolic Syndrome is the importance of dealing with obesity through appropriate physical activity and nutrition. Following the publication of *Healthy People* in 1979 (36), the U.S. Department of Health and Human Services published *Promoting Health/Preventing Disease: Objectives for the Nation* (37), *Healthy People* 2000 (38), and most recently, *Healthy People* 2010 (40). The health objectives listed in these reports were based on the analysis of health problems in the United States and a recognition of what can be done to reduce their magnitude. Considerable progress has been made over the years. For example, even though heart disease is still the number one killer, the death rate from cardiovascular disease has decreased 18% over the past 10 years (3). Unfortunately, it is still higher than the *Healthy People* 2010 target. These improvements are due to a wide variety of factors, including a decline in smoking, better blood pressure control, awareness of blood cholesterol, a decrease in fat intake, and better medical interventions. That is the good news. The bad news is that we have grown fatter as a society, and our level of participation in physical activity is well below the objectives set in 1990 (40) (see A Closer Look 14.5).

It is beyond the scope of this text to go into detail regarding the 2010 objectives, which are numerous and very specific (i.e., states exact percentage of people who should achieve a specific behavior or target). However, we feel that examples of a few objectives from the areas of Nutrition and Physical Activity and Fitness will point the way to later chapters. A concern in both of these areas is the need to control the growing problem of overweight and obesity that permeates our society. The nutrition objectives call for more people to:

- achieve a healthy body weight.
- eat less than 30% of total calories from fat and less than 10% from saturated fat.
- eat at least five servings of fruits and vegetables and six servings of grain products daily.

The physical activity objectives stress the need for more people to:

- engage in any leisure-time physical activity.
- participate in sustained physical activity (e.g., brisk walking) for at least thirty minutes per day.
- engage in physical activity that promotes the development and maintenance of cardiovascular fitness three or more days per week for twenty minutes or more per occasion.
- participate in physical activity to enhance and maintain muscular strength and endurance, and flexibility.

Chapter 16 provides recommendations for exercise programs to improve health (e.g., lower blood pressure) as well as improve cardiovascular fitness. Chapter 18 presents information on the proper diet needed for good health, as well as extensive detail about measuring body composition and how to achieve and maintain weight loss.

STUDY QUESTIONS

1. There is a sudden increase in the number of birth defects in one section of a large city. Describe what an epidemiologist might do to determine what is causing this problem.
2. Why is a web of causation model needed to study the causes of degenerative diseases, in contrast to infectious diseases?
3. Physical inactivity was long considered only a secondary risk factor. What "proof" did investigators have to offer to convince the scientific community otherwise?
4. What is the difference between primary and secondary risks for coronary heart disease (CHD)? Why does a high-fat diet not appear as a risk factor for CHD?
5. Draw a diagram of the hypothesized connections between and among obesity, insulin resistance, hypertension, and dyslipidemia. Indicate the primary site of insulin resistance, and explain how exercise training might reduce this problem.

SUGGESTED READINGS

U.S. Department of Health and Human Services. 1996. *Physical Activity and Health: A Report of the Surgeon General*. Atlanta, GA.: U.S. Department of Health and Human Services, Centers for Disease Control and Prevention, National Center for Chronic Disease Prevention and Health Promotion.

U.S. Department of Health and Human Services. 2000. *Healthy People* 2010: *Understanding and Improving Health*. Washington, D.C.: U.S. Government Printing Office.

U.S. Department of Health and Human Services. 2001. *The Surgeon General's Call to Action to Prevent and Decrease Overweight and Obesity*. U.S. Department of Health and Human Services, Public Health Service, Office of the Surgeon General.

REFERENCES

1. American College of Sports Medicine. 2006. *ACSM's Guidelines for Exercise Testing and Prescription*. 7th ed. Baltimore: Lippincott Williams & Wilkins.
2. American Heart Association. 1992. Statement on exercise. *Circulation* 86:340–44.
3. ———. 2005. Heart disease and stoke statistics—2005 update. Dallas: AHA.
4. Barnard, R. J., C. K. Roberts, S. M. Varon, and J. J. Berger. 1998. Diet-induced insulin resistance precedes other aspects of the metabolic syndrome *Journal of Applied Physiology*. 84:1311–15.
5. Bassett, D. R., Jr. 1994. Skeletal muscle characteristics: Relationships to cardiovascular risk factors. *Medicine and Science in Sports and Exercise* 26:957–66.
6. Bassett, D. R., Sr., and A. J. Zweifler. 1990. Risk factors and risk factor management. In *Clinical Ischemic Syndromes*, ed. G. B. Zelenock, L. D. D'Alecy, J. C. Fantone III, M. Shalfer, and J. C. Stanley, 15–46. St. Louis: Mosby.
7. Beaglehole, R., R. Bonita, and T. Kjellström. 1993. *Basic Epidemiology*. Geneva: World Health Organization.
8. Blair, S. N. et al. 1989. Physical fitness and all-cause mortality. A prospective study of men and women. *Journal of the American Medical Association* 262:2395–401.
9. Bouchard, C., R. J. Shephard, T. Stevens, J. R. Sutton, and B. D. McPherson. 1990. Exercise, fitness, and health: The consensus statement. In *Exercise, Fitness, and Health*, ed. C. Bouchard, R. J. Shephard, T. Stevens, J. R. Sutton, and B. D. McPherson, 3–28. Champaign, IL: Human Kinetics.
10. Brown, D. R. 1990. Exercise, fitness, and mental health. In *Exercise, Fitness, and Health*, ed. C. Bouchard, R. J. Shephard, T. Stevens, J. R. Sutton, and B. D. McPherson, 607–26. Champaign, IL: Human Kinetics.
11. Calle, E. E., M. J. Thun, J. M. Petrelli, C. Rodriguez, and C. W. Heath, Jr. 1999. Body-mass index and mortality in a prospective cohort of U.S. adults. *New England Journal of Medicine* 341:1097–1105.
12. Caspersen, C. J. 1989. Physical activity epidemiology: Concepts, methods, and applications to exercise science. In *Exercise and Sport Science Reviews*, vol. 17, ed. K. B. Pandolf, 423–73. Baltimore: Lippincott Williams & Wilkins.
13. Caspersen, C. J., and G. W. Heath. 1988. The risk factor concept of coronary heart disease. In *Resource Manual for Guidelines for Graded Exercise Testing and Prescription*, ed. S. N. Blair, P. Painter, R. R. Pate, L. K. Smith, and C. B. Taylor, 111–25. Philadelphia: Lea & Febiger.
14. Dawber, T. R. 1980. *The Framingham Study*. Cambridge, MA: Harvard University Press.
15. Farmer, R., and D. Miller. 1991. *Lecture Notes on Epidemiology and Public Health Medicine*. Boston: Blackwell Scientific Publications, 107–11.
16. Ferrannini, E., S. M. Haffner, and M. P. Stern. 1990. Essential hypertension: An insulin-resistant state. *Journal of Cardiovascular Pharmacology* 45 (Suppl. 5):S18–S25.
17. Ford, E. S., W. H. Giles, and W. H. Dietz. 2002. Prevalence of the Metabolic Syndrome among U.S. adults. *Journal of the American Medical Association* 287:356–59.
18. Julius, S., T. Gudbrandsson, K. Jamerson, and O. Andersson. 1992. The interconnection between sympathetics, microcirculation, and insulin resistance in hypertension. *Blood Pressure* 1:9–19.
19. Kannel, W. B. 1990. Contributions of the Framingham Study to preventive cardiology. *Journal of the American College of Cardiology* 15:206–11.
20. Kannel, W. B., and T. Gordon. 1979. Physiological and medical concomitants of obesity: The Framingham Study. In *Obesity in America*, 125–43. U.S. Department of Health, Education, and Welfare. NIH Publication No. 79–359.
21. Kaplan, N. M. 1989. The deadly quartet. *Archives of Internal Medicine* 149:1514–20.
22. Last, J. M. 1988. *A dictionary of epidemiology*, 2d ed. New York: Oxford University Press.
23. MacMahon, B., and T. F. Pugh. 1970. *Epidemiology*. Boston: Little, Brown.
24. Mokdad, A. H., J. S. Marks, D. F. Stroup, and J. L. Gerberding. 2004. Actual causes of death in the United

States, 2000. *Journal of the American Medical Association* 291:1238–45.

25. Mokdad, A. H., J. S. Marks, D. F. Stroup, and J. L. Gerberding. 2005. Correction: Actual causes of death in the United States, 2000. *Journal of the American Medical Association* 293:293–94.

26. National Health and Nutrition Examination Survey. 1999. *Prevalence of Overweight and Obesity among United States Adults, 1999–2002.* Hyattsville, MD: National Center for Health Statistics.

27. National Institutes of Health. 1998. *Clinical Guidelines on the Identification, Evaluation, and Treatment of Overweight and Obesity in Adults.* Bethesda, MD: Department of Health and Human Services, National Institutes of Health, National Heart, Lung, and Blood Institute.

28. National Heart, Blood, and Lung Institute. 2002. Third Report of the National Cholesterol Education Program (NCEP) Expert Panel. Detection, evaluation, and treatment of high blood cholesterol in adults (Adult Treatment Panel III)—Executive Summary. NIH Publication No. 02-5285. Bethesda, MD: author.

29. Paffenbarger R. S., Jr. et al. 1986. Physical activity, all-cause mortality, and longevity of college alumni. *New England Journal of Medicine* 314:605–13.

30. Powell, K. E. et al. 1987. Physical activity and the incidence of coronary heart disease. *Annual Review of Public Health* 8:253–87.

31. Rabkin, S. W., F. A. L. Mathewson, and Ping-hwa Hsu. 1977. Relation of body weight to development of ischemic heart disease in a cohort of young North American men after a 26-year observation period: The Manitoba study. *The American Journal of Cardiology* 39:452–58.

32. Reaven, G. M. 1988. Role of insulin resistance in human disease. *Diabetes* 37:1595–1607.

33. Rocchini, A. P. 1991. Insulin resistance and blood pressure regulation in obese and nonobese subjects. *Hypertension* 17:837–42.

34. Rockett, I. H. R. 1994. Population and health: An introduction to epidemiology. *Population Bulletin* 49(3), 1–48.

35. Stallones, R. A. 1966. *Public Health Monograph 76.* Washington, D.C.: U.S. Government Printing Office, p. 52.

36. U.S. Department of Health, Education, and Welfare. 1979. *Healthy People: The Surgeon General's Report on Health Promotion and Disease Prevention.* Washington, D.C.: U.S. Government Printing Office. Stock No. 017-001-00416-2.

37. U.S. Department of Health and Human Services. Fall 1980. *Promoting Health/Preventing Disease: Objectives for the Nation.* Washington, D.C.: U.S. Government Printing Office.

38. ———. 1991. *Healthy People 2000: National Health Promotion and Disease Prevention Objectives.* Washington, D.C.: U.S. Government Printing Office.

39. ———. 1996. *Physical Activity and Health: A Report of the Surgeon General.* Atlanta, GA.: U.S. Department of Health and Human Services, Centers for Disease Control and Prevention, National Center for Chronic Disease Prevention and Health Promotion.

40. ———. 2000. *Healthy People 2010: Understanding and Improving Health.* Washington, D.C.: U.S. Government Printing Office.

41. World Health Organization. 1997. *Obesity: Preventing and Managing the Global Epidemic.* Geneva: World Health Organization.

CHAPTER 15

Work Tests to Evaluate Cardiorespiratory Fitness

■ Objectives

By studying this chapter, you should be able to do the following:

1. Identify the sequence of steps in the procedures for evaluating cardiorespiratory fitness (CRF).

2. Describe one maximal and one submaximal field test used to evaluate CRF.

3. Explain the rationale underlying the use of distance runs as estimates of CRF.

4. Identify the common measures taken during a graded exercise test (GXT).

5. Describe changes in the ECG that may take place during a GXT in subjects with ischemic heart disease.

6. List three criteria for having achieved $\dot{V}O_2$ max.

7. Estimate $\dot{V}O_2$ max from the last stage of a GXT and list the concerns about the protocol that may affect that estimate.

8. Estimate $\dot{V}O_2$ max by extrapolating the HR/$\dot{V}O_2$ relationship to the person's age-adjusted maximal HR.

9. Describe the problems with the assumptions made in the extrapolation procedure used in objective 8, and name the environmental and subject variables that must be controlled to improve such estimates.

10. Identify the criteria used to terminate the GXT.

11. Explain why there are so many different GXT protocols and why the rate of progression through the test is of concern.

12. Describe the YMCA's procedure to set the rate of progression on a cycle ergometer test.

13. Estimate $\dot{V}O_2$ max with the Åstrand and Ryhming nomogram given a data set for the cycle ergometer or step.

■ Outline

Testing Procedures   300
   Screening   300
   Resting and Exercise
      Measures   302

Field Tests for Estimating
CRF   302
   Maximal Run Tests   302
   Walk Tests   304
   Canadian Home Fitness
      Test   304

Graded Exercise Tests:
Measurements   305
   Heart Rate   305
   Blood Pressure   305
   ECG   306
   Rating of Perceived
      Exertion   306
   Termination Criteria   307
$\dot{V}O_2$ Max   308

Estimation of $\dot{V}O_2$ Max from
   Last Work Rate   309
Estimation of $\dot{V}O_2$ Max
   from Submaximal HR
   Response   309

Graded Exercise Test:
Protocols   311
   Treadmill   312
   Cycle Ergometer   313
   Step Test   314

■ Key Terms

angina pectoris
arrhythmia
conduction disturbances

double product
dyspnea
field test

myocardial ischemia
ST segment depression

In chapter 14 we discussed the risk factors that limit health and contribute to coronary heart disease (CHD). One of those risk factors was a sedentary lifestyle. According to *Healthy People 2010: Understanding and Improving Health*, there is a need to increase physical activity to improve cardiorespiratory function (CRF). This implies that changes in CRF can be measured. While most scientists believe that the function of the cardiorespiratory system is represented best by the measurement of $\dot{V}O_2$ max, others feel that the monitoring of heart rate (HR) and blood pressure (BP) at several submaximal work rates provides a more sensitive indicator of changes in CRF (45). You are already familiar with the use of a graded exercise test (GXT) to measure $\dot{V}O_2$ max; this chapter picks up on that theme and discusses the types of tests used to evaluate CRF. The type of test used depends on the fitness of the person being tested, the purpose of the test (experimental or epidemiological investigation), and the facilities, equipment, and personnel available to conduct the test. The choice of the GXT would be different for a young healthy child as compared to a sixty-year-old person with coronary heart disease (CHD) risk factors. The GXT might be used as a CRF test prior to entry into a fitness program, or it could be used as a diagnostic test by a cardiologist who evaluates a twelve-lead electrocardiogram for evidence of heart disease. Clearly, the type of personnel and equipment, and of course the cost, would be very different in these two situations.

Part of the reason for such diversity in exercise testing procedures is the risk associated with exercise testing. The risk of cardiac events during exercise testing is low in previously healthy individuals, but increases as the number of risk factors increase. In general, the overall risk of severe cardiovascular complications or death is about 6/10,000 tests in a mixed population (3).

TESTING PROCEDURES

Figure 15.1 shows a sequence of steps in a "decision tree," leading to participation in a fitness program. The first step in the evaluation of CRF is to identify those who might need a physician's clearance prior to taking an exercise test or participating in an exercise program. These procedures include obtaining written informed consent from the potential participant, a review of the person's health history, the administration of selected resting physiological measures, and the use of submaximal or maximal GXTs (45). The exercise test can be stopped by the subject at any time, and the tester has the right to terminate any of the procedures if the subject displays abnormal responses or experiences symptoms suggestive of an inappropriate adaptation to the GXT (3). Depending

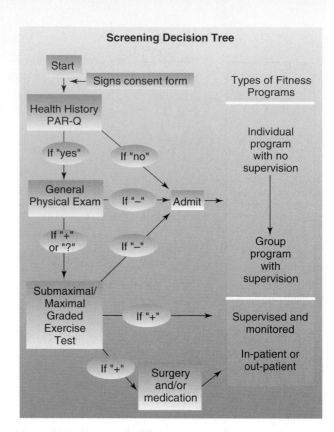

FIGURE 15.1 Decision tree in the evaluation of cardiorespiratory fitness.

on the outcome at each of these steps, the person might be admitted to a fitness program with little or no supervision, or referred for additional tests that might lead to an exercise program in which the participants are monitored and supervised.

Screening

In chapter 14 we indicated the role that risk factors play in an overall profile of health status with regard to CHD. The health histories used to screen people for GXTs or fitness programs can be as simple as the Physical Activity Readiness Questionnaire (PAR-Q) shown in figure 15.2, or a detailed form such as the $PAR_{med}-X$, which highlights absolute and relative contraindications for participating in exercise (see appendix C). An additional question added to various modifications of the PAR-Q asks about medications that might affect a person's response to exercise (e.g., an insulin-dependent diabetic or a cardiac patient taking the beta-adrenergic blocker propranolol) (32, 80). These forms are used to determine if a person needs consultation with a physician before taking a GXT, or before entering a fitness program (3). See ACSM's Guidelines for Exercise Testing and Prescription (3) for details on classifying individuals into low, moderate, or high-risk categories.

PAR-Q & YOU

Physical Activity Readiness
Questionnaire - PAR-Q
(revised 2002)

Regular physical activity is fun and healthy, and increasingly more people are starting to become more active every day. Being more active is very safe for most people. However, some people should check with their doctor before they start becoming much more physically active.

If you are planning to become much more physically active than you are now, start by answering the seven questions in the box below. If you are between the ages of 15 and 69, the PAR-Q will tell you if you should check with your doctor before you start. If you are over 69 years of age, and you are not used to being very active, check with your doctor.

Common sense is your best guide when you answer these questions. Please read the questions carefully and answer each one honestly: check YES or NO.

YES	NO		
☐	☐	1.	**Has your doctor ever said that you have a heart condition <u>and</u> that you should only do physical activity recommended by a doctor?**
☐	☐	2.	**Do you feel pain in your chest when you do physical activity?**
☐	☐	3.	**In the past month, have you had chest pain when you were not doing physical activity?**
☐	☐	4.	**Do you lose your balance because of dizziness or do you ever lose consciousness?**
☐	☐	5.	**Do you have a bone or joint problem (for example, back, knee or hip) that could be made worse by a change in your physical activity?**
☐	☐	6.	**Is your doctor currently prescribing drugs (for example, water pills) for your blood pressure or heart condition?**
☐	☐	7.	**Do you know of <u>any other reason</u> why you should not do physical activity?**

If you answered

YES to one or more questions

Talk with your doctor by phone or in person BEFORE you start becoming much more physically active or BEFORE you have a fitness appraisal. Tell your doctor about the PAR-Q and which questions you answered YES.

- You may be able to do any activity you want — as long as you start slowly and build up gradually. Or, you may need to restrict your activities to those which are safe for you. Talk with your doctor about the kinds of activities you wish to participate in and follow his/her advice.
- Find out which community programs are safe and helpful for you.

NO to all questions

If you answered NO honestly to <u>all</u> PAR-Q questions, you can be reasonably sure that you can:
- start becoming much more physically active — begin slowly and build up gradually. This is the safest and easiest way to go.
- take part in a fitness appraisal — this is an excellent way to determine your basic fitness so that you can plan the best way for you to live actively. It is also highly recommended that you have your blood pressure evaluated. If your reading is over 144/94, talk with your doctor before you start becoming much more physically active.

→

DELAY BECOMING MUCH MORE ACTIVE:
- if you are not feeling well because of a temporary illness such as a cold or a fever — wait until you feel better; or
- if you are or may be pregnant — talk to your doctor before you start becoming more active.

PLEASE NOTE: If your health changes so that you then answer YES to any of the above questions, tell your fitness or health professional. Ask whether you should change your physical activity plan.

<u>Informed Use of the PAR-Q</u>: The Canadian Society for Exercise Physiology, Health Canada, and their agents assume no liability for persons who undertake physical activity, and if in doubt after completing this questionnaire, consult your doctor prior to physical activity.

No changes permitted. You are encouraged to photocopy the PAR-Q but only if you use the entire form.

NOTE: If the PAR-Q is being given to a person before he or she participates in a physical activity program or a fitness appraisal, this section may be used for legal or administrative purposes.

"I have read, understood and completed this questionnaire. Any questions I had were answered to my full satisfaction."

NAME _____

SIGNATURE _____   DATE _____

SIGNATURE OF PARENT _____   WITNESS _____
or GUARDIAN (for participants under the age of majority)

Note: This physical activity clearance is valid for a maximum of 12 months from the date it is completed and becomes invalid if your condition changes so that you would answer YES to any of the seven questions.

 © Canadian Society for Exercise Physiology   Supported by: 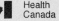 Health Canada   Santé Canada

FIGURE 15.2 Physical Activity Readiness Questionnaire (PAR-Q). A questionnaire for people aged 15 to 69. The original PAR-Q was developed by the British Columbia Ministry of Health. It has been revised by an Expert Advisory Committee assembled by the Canadian Society of Exercise Physiology and Fitness Canada (2002).

Resting and Exercise Measures

Following the screening, measurements of heart rate and blood pressure are taken at rest prior to the exercise test. Additional measurements such as a blood sample for serum cholesterol and an electrocardiogram (ECG) may also be obtained, with the latter one a necessity if the GXT is to be a diagnostic test. The exercise tests used to evaluate CRF may require a submaximal or maximal effort by the subject. They may be conducted in a lab containing sophisticated equipment, or on a running track with nothing more complicated than a stopwatch. In a submaximal GXT, HR is measured at each stage of the test that progresses from light work (~3 METs) to a predetermined end point such as 70% to 85% of predicted maximal heart rate. A treadmill, cycle ergometer, or a bench can be used to impose the work rates, and these tests will be described in detail in subsequent sections. Instead of stopping the submaximal GXT at some predetermined end point (70% to 85% maximal HR), the GXT can be taken to the point of volitional exhaustion, or to where specific signs (ECG or BP changes) or symptoms like chest pain **(angina pectoris)** or breathlessness **(dyspnea)** occur. In these cases CRF is based on the last work rate achieved. However, there are some maximal tests of CRF that are not "graded" and for which physiological measurements are not made during the test [e.g., Cooper's 12-minute or 1.5-mile run (23), and the AAHPERD's 1-mile run (2)]. These latter **field tests** will now be considered in more detail, along with the Canadian Home (Aerobic) Fitness Test (82), and a one-mile walk test (52). This will be followed by a discussion of GXTs using the treadmill, cycle ergometer, and bench step.

IN SUMMARY

- The steps to follow before conducting an exercise test to evaluate CRF include:
  a. signing of a consent form,
  b. screening, and
  c. obtaining resting HR and BP as well as cholesterol and ECG measures.

FIELD TESTS FOR ESTIMATING CRF

Maximal Run Tests

Some field tests for CRF involve a measurement of how far a person can run in a set time (twelve to fifteen minutes), or how fast a person can run a set distance (one to two miles). The advantages of such field tests include their moderately high correlation with $\dot{V}O_2$ max, the use of a natural activity, the large numbers of people who can be tested at one time, and the low cost. The disadvantages of using field tests include the difficulty of monitoring physiological responses, the importance that motivation plays in the outcome, and the fact that the test is not graded but is a maximal effort. These field tests should be used only after a person has progressed through a program of exercise at lower intensities. The most popular field test for adults is Cooper's 12-minute or 1.5-mile run (23), and for school children, the AAHPERD's one-mile walk/run (2). The aim is to determine the average velocity that can be maintained over the time or distance. These tests represent evolutionary changes from the original work of Balke (10), who showed that running tests of ten to twenty minutes provide reasonable estimates of $\dot{V}O_2$ max. The basis for the field tests is the linear relationship that exists between $\dot{V}O_2$ ($ml \cdot kg^{-1} \cdot min^{-1}$) and running speed, as shown in chapter 6. The duration of ten to twenty minutes represents a compromise that attempts to maximize the chance that the person is running at a speed demanding 90% to 95% $\dot{V}O_2$ max while minimizing the contribution of energy from anaerobic sources. In distance runs of five minutes or less, anaerobic sources would provide relatively large amounts of energy, and $\dot{V}O_2$ max would probably be overestimated. An interesting alternative to the one-mile run test for children is the PACER test (see A Closer Look 15.1.).

The method of calculating the $\dot{V}O_2$ when the running speed is known was described in detail in A Closer Look 6.2, and the formula is presented here again:

$$\dot{V}O_2 = 0.2 \ (ml \cdot kg^{-1} \cdot min^{-1} \text{ per } m \cdot min^{-1}) + 3.5 \ (ml \cdot kg^{-1} \cdot min^{-1})$$

This formula provides reasonable estimates of $\dot{V}O_2$ max for adults, but would underestimate values for young children because of their relatively poor economy of running (28). On the other hand, this formula would overestimate the value for $\dot{V}O_2$ max for those who walk, since the net cost of walking is half that of running (see A Closer Look 6.1):

$$\dot{V}O_2 = 0.1 \ (ml \cdot kg^{-1} \cdot min^{-1} \text{ per } m \cdot min^{-1}) + 3.5 \ (ml \cdot kg^{-1} \cdot min^{-1})$$

While Cooper (23) provides categories of $\dot{V}O_2$ max values by age and sex (see table 15.1), estimates of $\dot{V}O_2$ max based on distance runs are most useful when compared over time for the same individual, rather than between individuals. Variation in economy of running, motivation, and other factors makes such comparisons of estimated $\dot{V}O_2$ max values between individuals unreasonable (6, 81). In this light, distance swim and bicycle riding tests provide useful information about changes in an individual's CRF over time, even though estimates of $\dot{V}O_2$ max are not available (22, 24).

The formulas used for estimating $\dot{V}O_2$ max from a twelve-minute run are not very useful for prepubescent children, since their economy of running is less than

Progressive Aerobic Cardiovascular Endurance Run (PACER)

An alternative test of aerobic fitness for school children is the Progressive Aerobic Cardiovascular Endurance Run or PACER. This test, developed by Leger et al. (55, 56), is a 20-meter shuttle run test done to the sound of a "beep" as the student moves between the boundary lines. The time interval between beeps becomes shorter as the test progresses. The test is terminated when the student cannot keep up with the beeps, and the number of 20-meter laps completed is used to estimate aerobic fitness. Criterion-referenced standards for aerobic fitness (see A Closer Look 15.2) have been validated for this test (Chun, 2000). The PACER test is part of the fitness testing battery in the FITNESSGRAM, developed by the Cooper Institute for Aerobics (see **http://www.fitnessgram.net** for more information). This protocol has also been used as a field test to estimate $\dot{V}O_2$ max in adults (64, 88).

TABLE 15.1	Men's and Women's Aerobics Fitness Classifications

Men's

Category	AGE (YEARS)					
	13–19	20–29	30–39	40–49	50–59	60+
1. Very Poor	<35.0*	<33.0	<31.5	<30.2	<26.1	<20.5
2. Poor	35.0–38.3	33.0–36.4	31.5–35.4	30.2–33.5	26.1–30.9	20.5–26.0
3. Fair	38.4–45.1	36.5–42.4	35.5–40.9	33.6–38.9	31.0–35.7	26.1–32.2
4. Good	45.2–50.9	42.5–46.4	41.0–44.9	39.0–43.7	35.8–40.9	32.3–36.4
5. Excellent	51.0–55.9	46.5–52.4	45.0–49.4	43.8–48.0	41.0–45.3	36.5–44.2
6. Superior	>56.0	>52.5	>49.5	>48.1	>45.4	>44.3

Women's

Category	AGE (YEARS)					
	13–19	20–29	30–39	40–49	50–59	60+
1. Very Poor	<25.0*	<23.6	<22.8	<21.0	<20.2	<17.5
2. Poor	25.0–30.9	23.6–28.9	22.8–26.9	21.0–24.4	20.2–22.7	17.5–20.1
3. Fair	31.0–34.9	29.0–32.9	27.0–31.4	24.5–28.9	22.8–26.9	20.2–24.4
4. Good	35.0–38.9	33.0–36.9	31.5–35.6	29.0–32.8	27.0–31.4	24.5–30.2
5. Excellent	39.0–41.9	37.0–40.9	35.7–40.0	32.9–36.9	31.5–35.7	30.3–31.4
6. Superior	>42.0	>41.0	>40.1	>37.0	>35.8	>31.5

*Values for oxygen uptake in ml · kg^{-1} · min^{-1}

Data from Kenneth H. Cooper, 1977. *The Aerobics Way.* New York: Bantam Books, Inc.

that of an adult (28). Investigators (54) worked around this problem by testing first, second, and third grade boys and girls with 800-, 1,200-, and 1,600-meter runs, and related performance to the measured $\dot{V}O_2$ max scores. They found the 1,600-meter run was the best predictor with good test/retest reliability (r = 0.82 to 0.92) in children who were given instruction on paced running (54). While performance in a run test is obviously a function of $\dot{V}O_2$ max, both running economy and the ability to run at a high % $\dot{V}O_2$ max also play a role (12, 13). It has been shown in young children of six to eleven years of age that % $\dot{V}O_2$ max is more closely related to performance of the one-mile walk/run than is $\dot{V}O_2$ max (63). (See A Closer Look 15.2.)

$\dot{V}O_2$ max (ml · kg^{-1} · min^{-1}) estimated in an endurance run test is influenced by cardiovascular function and body fatness. It has been shown that differences in estimated $\dot{V}O_2$ max values between males and females can be explained, in part, by differences in % body fat (25, 28, 86). In a twelve-minute run test, performance was decreased 89 meters when body weight was experimentally increased to simulate an additional 5% fat (27). One should expect, then, that with a combined exercise and weight reduction program, CRF will increase due to both an increase in cardiovascular function and a decrease in % body fat. In table 15.1, categories for $\dot{V}O_2$ max values are adjusted for age due to the observation that in the general pop-

A CLOSER LOOK 15.2

Cardiovascular Fitness Standards for Children

The best way to evaluate fitness in children has been a concern for educators and scientists for most of this century (73). The most recent controversy has revolved around the question of what kind of standards to use in making judgments about a child's level of fitness. Normative standards such as percentile scores have traditionally been used to describe where a child stands relative to his or her peers. (e.g., 75th percentile). The current thinking, especially for health-related fitness tests (one-mile walk/run test and the skinfold test) is that criterion-reference standards might be more appropriate. Criterion-reference standards attempt to describe the minimum level of fitness consistent with

good health, independent of what percentile that might be in a normative data set. For example, Blair (16) showed that in adults, $\dot{V}O_2$ max values associated with a low risk of disease were not that high, e.g., ≥ 35 ml · kg^{-1} · min^{-1} for men and ≥ 30 ml · kg^{-1} · min^{-1} for women 20 to 39 years of age. This information was used in setting the criterion-reference standards for the FITNESSGRAM, the fitness evaluation program developed by the Institute for Aerobics Research. $\dot{V}O_2$ max standards were set at 42 ml · kg^{-1} · min^{-1} for boys 5 to 17 years of age. For girls, the values were set at 40 ml · kg^{-1} · min^{-1} for ages 5 to 9 years of age, with a decrease of 1 ml · kg^{-1} · min^{-1} per year until age 14, where the 35 ml · kg^{-1} ·

min^{-1} value held until age 17 years. After the criterion-reference standards were set, the designers of the test had to translate those ml · kg^{-1} · min^{-1} values into equivalent one-mile run times—the actual test the children would take. The test designers had to consider the % $\dot{V}O_2$ max the children would perform at during the run, and the fact that economy of running improves with age. These steps, while complicated, have led to standards that are now used nationwide to classify children as to whether they have a sufficient level of cardiorespiratory fitness consistent with a low risk of disease (26).

---

ulation $\dot{V}O_2$ max decreases with age. However, studies (48, 91) have shown that $\dot{V}O_2$ max does not decrease as fast in males who maintain their physical activity program and body weight. This observation provides additional rationale for a regular evaluation of CRF to keep track of small changes before they become big changes.

Walk Tests

An alternative to the maximal run tests used to evaluate CRF is a one-mile walk test in which the HR is monitored during the test (52). The equation used to predict $\dot{V}O_2$ max was based on one population of men and women, aged thirty to sixty-nine, and was then validated on another comparable population. The subject walks as fast as possible for one mile on a flat, measured track, and HR is measured at the end of the last lap. The following equation can be used to estimate $\dot{V}O_2$ max (ml · kg^{-1} · min^{-1}):

$$\dot{V}O_2 \text{ max} = 132.853 - 0.0769 \text{ (wt)}$$
$$- 0.3877 \text{ (age)} + 6.315 \text{ (sex)}$$
$$- 3.2649 \text{ (time)} - 0.1565 \text{ (HR)}$$

where (wt) is body weight in pounds, (age) is in years, (sex) equals 0 for female and 1 for male, (time) is in minutes and hundredths of minutes, and (HR) is in beats · min^{-1} measured at the end of the last quarter mile.

This test appears to fill a void in the field tests available to estimate $\dot{V}O_2$ max, since it uses a common

activity and requires the simple measurement of HR. As a participant's fitness improves, the time required for the mile and/or the HR response decreases, increasing the estimated $\dot{V}O_2$ max. A similar study using a two-kilometer walk test supports this proposition (71).

Canadian Home Fitness Test

In contrast to the Cooper 1.5-mile run test and the one-mile walk test, which require an all-out effort, the Canadian Home Fitness Test (CHFT) is a submaximal step test that uses the lowest two 8-inch steps found in a conventional staircase (82). The stepping cadence in this test is maintained by an audio tape. Prior to the test the person completes the Physical Activity Readiness Questionnaire (PAR-Q) (figure 15.2) to determine if he or she should proceed. The first stage of the test requires the individual to step for three minutes at a rate equivalent to 65% to 70% of the average $\dot{V}O_2$ max of the next oldest age group (remember $\dot{V}O_2$ max generally decreases with age). An immediate ten-second recovery pulse is counted, and if it does not exceed the maximum allowable, another three-minute step test at 65% to 70% of the average $\dot{V}O_2$ max of the person's own age group is completed. Another pulse rate is then taken. Table 15.2 shows how physical fitness can be estimated as "undesirable, minimum, or recommended" (82). $\dot{V}O_2$ max can be estimated from the CHFT results (14, 47, 83). A modified version of this test, which provides an improved estimate of $\dot{V}O_2$ max, is available (92, 93).

	TEN-SECOND PULSE RATE	
Age (yr)	**After First Three Minutes of Exercise**	**After Second Three Minutes of Exercise**
15–19	If 30 or more, stop. You have an undesirable personal fitness level.	If 27 or more, you have a minimum personal fitness level. If 26 or less, you have the recommended personal fitness level.
20–29	If 29 or more, stop. You have an undesirable personal fitness level.	If 26 or more, you have a minimum personal fitness level. If 25 or less, you have the recommended personal fitness level.
30–39	If 28 or more, stop. You have an undesirable personal fitness level.	If 25 or more, you have a minimum personal fitness level. If 24 or less, you have the recommended personal fitness level.
40–19	If 26 or more, stop. You have an undesirable personal fitness level.	If 24 or more, you have a minimum personal fitness level. If 23 or less, you have the recommended personal fitness level.
50–59	If 25 or more, stop. You have an undesirable personal fitness level.	If 23 or more, you have a minimum personal fitness level. If 22 or less, you have the recommended personal fitness level.
60–69	If 24 or more, stop. You have an undesirable personal fitness level.	If 23 or more, you have a minimum personal fitness level. If 22 or less, you have the recommended personal fitness level.

From R. J. Shephard, et al., "Development of the Canadian Home fitness Test," originally published in *Canadian Medical Association Journal*, 114:675–79, 1976. Copyright © 1976 Canadian Medical Association, Ottawa, Canada. Reprinted by permission.

IN SUMMARY

- Field tests for CRF use natural activities such as walking, running, and stepping in which large numbers of people can be tested at low cost. However, for some, physiological responses are difficult to measure, and motivation plays an important role in the outcome.
- $\dot{V}O_2$ max estimates from all-out run tests are based on the linear relationship between running speed and the oxygen cost of running.
- The Canadian Home Fitness Test is a step test that uses conventional 8-inch steps to evaluate cardiorespiratory fitness.

GRADED EXERCISE TESTS: MEASUREMENTS

Cardiorespiratory fitness is commonly measured using a treadmill, a cycle ergometer, or a stepping bench. These tests are usually incremental, in which the work rate changes every two to three minutes until the subject reaches some predetermined end point, or when some pathological sign or symptom occurs. These GXTs can be maximal or submaximal, and the variables measured during the test can be as simple as HR and BP, or as complex as $\dot{V}O_2$; it depends on the purpose of the test, and the facilities, equipment, and personnel involved (42). What follows is a brief summary of common measurements made during a GXT.

Heart Rate

Heart rate can be measured by palpation of the radial or carotid artery, using a stethoscope with the microphone on the chest wall, or by using surface electrodes that transmit the signal to an oscilloscope, electrocardiograph, or a monitor that can display heart rate directly. In palpating the carotid artery, care must be taken not to use too much pressure, since this could slow the HR by way of the baroreceptor reflex. However, when people are trained in this procedure, reliable measurements can be obtained (72, 79). Heart rate is measured over a fifteen- to thirty-second time period *during* steady-state exercise to obtain a reliable estimate of the HR. If using a *post-exercise* HR as an indication of the HR during exercise, the HR should be measured for ten seconds within the first fifteen seconds after stopping exercise, because the HR changes rapidly at this time. The ten-second count is multiplied by six to express the HR in beats $\cdot$ min^{-1} (79).

Blood Pressure

Blood pressure is measured by auscultation as described in chapter 9. It is important to use the proper cuff size and a sensitive stethoscope to obtain correct values at rest and during work. In addition, if using an aneroid sphygmomanometer, it is important to calibrate it on a regular basis against the mercury sphygmomanometer (50). During the walking or cycling exercise test (BP cannot be reliably measured during a running test), the microphone of the stethoscope is placed below the cuff and over an area where the sound is the loudest (in many cases this will be in the intramuscular space on the medial side of the arm). The subject should not be holding onto the handlebar of the cycle or treadmill during the measurement. The first Korotkoff sound is taken as systolic BP, and the fourth sound (change in tone or muffling) is taken as diastolic BP (74).

ECG

GXTs are used to diagnose CHD because exercise causes the heart to work harder and challenges the coronary arteries' ability to deliver sufficient blood to meet the oxygen demand of the myocardium. An estimate of the work (and O_2 demand) of the heart is the **double product**—the product of the HR and the systolic BP (51, 70). As you already know, HR and systolic BP increase with exercise intensity such that myocardial oxygen demand increases throughout the test. The ECG is used as an indicator of the ability of the heart to function normally during these times of imposed work. During exercise the ECG can be measured with a single bipolar lead (e.g., CM_5), but a full twelve-lead arrangement is preferred (3). The ECG is evaluated for arrhythmias, conduction disturbances, and myocardial ischemia. **Arrhythmias** are irregularities in the normal electrical rhythm of the heart that can be localized to the atria (e.g., atrial fibrillation), the AV node (e.g., premature junctional contraction), or in the ventricles (e.g., premature ventricular contractions—PVCs). **Conduction disturbances** describe a defect in which depolarization is slowed or completely blocked (e.g., first-degree AV block, or bundle branch block). **Myocardial ischemia** is defined as an inadequate perfusion of the myocardium relative to the metabolic demand of the heart. Since oxygen uptake by the myocardium is almost completely flow dependent, a flow limitation indicates an oxygen insufficiency. A *symptom* of myocardial ischemia is angina pectoris, which is pain or discomfort caused by a temporary ischemia; the pain could be located in the center of the chest, neck, jaw, or shoulders, or could radiate to the arms and hands (59). A *sign* associated with myocardial ischemia is a depression of the ST segment on the electrocardiogram (see chapter 9). Figure 15.3 shows three types of **ST segment depression.** People with upsloping or horizontal ST segment depression have similar life expectancies, but the prognosis for those with downsloping ST segment is worse (31). Interested readers are referred to Dubin's introductory text on ECG analysis (see Suggested Readings), and

FIGURE 15.3 Three types of ST segment depression. From A. D. Martin, "ECG and Medications" in E. T. Howley and B. D. Franks, *Health/Fitness Instructor's Handbook.* Copyright © 1986 Human Kinetics Publishers, Inc., Champaign, IL. Used by permission.

TABLE 15.3	Rating of Perceived Exertion Scales		
Original Rating Scale		**Revised Rating Scale**	
6		0	Nothing at all
7	Very, very light	0.5	Very, very light (just noticeable)
8		1	Very light
9	Very light	2	Light (weak)
10		3	Moderate
11	Fairly light	4	Somewhat hard
12		5	Heavy (strong)
13	Somewhat hard	6	
14		7	Very heavy
15	Hard	8	
16		9	
17	Very hard	10	Very, very heavy (almost max)
18		•	Maximal
19	Very, very hard		
20			

From: G. A. U. Borg. "Psychological Bases of Physical Exertion" in *Medicine and Science in Sports and Exercise,* 14:377–81, 1982. Copyright ©1982 American College of Sports Medicine, Indianapolis, IN. Reprinted by permission.

Ellestad's text on exercise electrocardiography (31). For individuals who cannot perform an exercise test to evaluate cardiovascular function, a pharmacologic stress test may be substituted (see Ask the Expert 15.1).

Rating of Perceived Exertion

Another common measurement made at each stage of the GXT is Borg's (17) Rating of Perceived Exertion (RPE). Table 15.3 lists his original and revised scales. The original scale used the rankings 6 to 20 to approx-

ASK THE EXPERT 15.1

Pharmacologic Testing to Diagnose Heart Disease
Questions and Answers with Dr. Barry Franklin

*Since 1985, **Barry A. Franklin, Ph.D.,** has been Director of the Cardiac Rehabilitation and Exercise Laboratories, William Beaumont Hospital, Royal Oak, Michigan. He is a past president of the American Association of Cardiovascular and Pulmonary Rehabilitation (AACVPR) and the American College of Sports Medicine (ACSM). He is the editor of the sixth edition of the ACSM's Guidelines for Exercise Testing and Prescription and is an internationally known speaker on topics related to cardiac rehabilitation.*

QUESTION 1: Could you briefly describe what a pharmacologic stress test is, what kinds of drugs are used, and likely candidates for such testing?

ANSWER: The need for noninvasive assessments of cardiac function for patients who are unable to exercise has led to the development of pharmacologic stress test for identifying coronary artery disease.

During these medically supervised tests, the patient lies quietly on a padded stretcher or table. Cardiac perfusion imaging (with technetium 99-m sestamibi [Cardiolite] or thallium chloride–201) is obtained with a gamma camera after intravenous dipyridamole or adenosine

infusion. These potent vasodilators enhance blood flow to normally perfused heart tissue, whereas heart muscle fed by obstructed coronary arteries demonstrates relative hypoperfusion.

Another popular pharmacologic test uses dobutamine, which, in contrast to dipyridamole or adenosine stress, causes cardiac ischemia by modestly increasing heart rate and myocardial contractility. Echocardiographic images, which involve a recording sensor to bounce ultrasound waves off the heart to create an image of the muscle at work, are obtained throughout the infusion. A new or worsening wall motion abnormality suggests underlying coronary artery disease.

QUESTION 2: What kinds of measurements are obtained to evaluate cardiac function?

ANSWER: Heart rate, blood pressure, and electrocardiographic measurements are routinely made every minute during these drug infusions, which generally last about six minutes. Perfusion imaging under resting conditions is then compared with imaging obtained after coronary vasodilation. Patients are also queried regarding adverse side

effects, which may include lightheadedness, chest pain or pressure, and nausea. Echocardiographic images (in contrast to perfusion images) are made during dobutamine infusions. In some cases, like exercise stress tests, pharmacologic studies may be prematurely terminated due to the development of worsening symptoms or significant heart rhythm irregularities.

QUESTION 3: Can the results of these tests be used to develop an exercise prescription?

ANSWER: It is difficult to use the results of these tests to develop an exercise prescription. This is primarily because the rises in heart rate and oxygen consumption during pharmacologic testing are far lower than those achieved with exercise stress. These tests simply suggest whether there is underlying myocardial ischemia and coronary artery disease. Consequently, many clinicians recommend an initial exercise heart rate that is twenty to thirty beats above standing rest, as the prescribed training intensity, using perceived exertion as an adjunctive intensity modulator.

---

imate the HR values from rest to maximum (60–200). The revised scale represents an attempt to provide a ratio scale of the RPE values. The RPE scores are good indicators of subjective effort and provide a quantitative way to track a person's progress through a GXT or an exercise session (19, 20, 38). This is helpful in knowing when a subject is approaching exhaustion, and the values can be used in prescribing exercise intensity (see chapter 16). However, it is important to provide clear and standardized instructions to the individual to maximize the usefulness of the RPE scale. What follows is a suggested statement from the ACSM Guidelines (3, p. 78):

> During the exercise test we want you to pay close attention to how hard you feel the exercise work rate is. This feeling should reflect your total

amount of exertion and fatigue, combining all sensations and feelings of physical stress, effort, and fatigue. Don't concern yourself with any one factor such as leg pain, shortness of breath or exercise intensity, but try to concentrate on your total, inner feeling of exertion. Try not to underestimate or overestimate your feeling of exertion; be as accurate as you can.

Termination Criteria

The reasons for stopping a GXT vary with the type of population being tested and the purpose of the test. Table 15.4, from the ACSM's *Guidelines for Exercise Testing and Prescription*, is appropriate for nondiagnostic GXTs in apparently healthy adults (3).

- Onset of angina or angina-like symptoms
- Drop in systolic blood pressure of >10 mm Hg from baseline blood pressure despite an increase in workload
- Excessive rise in blood pressure: systolic pressure >250 mm Hg or diastolic pressure >115 mm Hg
- Shortness of breath, wheezing, leg cramps, or claudication
- Signs of poor perfusion: light-headedness, confusion, ataxia, pallor, cyanosis, nausea, or cold and clammy skin
- Failure of heart rate to increase with increased exercise intensity
- Noticeable change in heart rhythm
- Subject requests to stop
- Physical or verbal manifestations of severe fatigue
- Failure of the testing equipment

*Assumes that testing is nondiagnostic and is being performed without direct physician involvement or ECG monitoring.

IN SUMMARY

- Typical measurements obtained during a graded exercise test include heart rate, blood pressure, ECG, and rating of perceived exertion.
- Specific signs (e.g., fall in systolic pressure with an increase in work rate) and symptoms (e.g., dizziness) are used to stop GXTs.

$\dot{V}O_2$ MAX

The measurement of $\dot{V}O_2$ max represents the standard against which any estimate of CRF is compared (see chapters 6 and 20 for procedures). $\dot{V}O_2$ increases with increasing loads on a GXT until the maximal capacity of the cardiorespiratory system is reached; attention to detail is crucial if one is to obtain accurate values (61). Commonly used criteria for having achieved $\dot{V}O_2$ max include a leveling off of the $\dot{V}O_2$ (<150 ml $\cdot$ kg^{-1} $\cdot$ min^{-1} or < 2.1 ml $\cdot$ kg^{-1} $\cdot$ min^{-1}) even though a higher work rate is achieved (90), a post-exercise blood lactate level of >8 mmoles $\cdot$ liter^{-1}(5), and the R exceeding 1.15 (46). Some investigators use heart rate (e.g., a value within 10 b/min of age-predicted maximal heart rate) as a criterion for having achieved $\dot{V}O_2$ max. However, due to the relatively large potential error (1 SD = 10–12 b/min) in estimating maximal heart rate with the age-predicted formulas (e.g., 220 − age), its usefulness as a criterion for having achieved $\dot{V}O_2$ max has been questioned (43). While many subjects will meet these criteria, some, especially the elderly (85), children (5), and postcoronary subjects (49), will not. In addition, one should not expect a subject to meet all of these standards (49, 85). For example, in one study (85), 20 percent of the women subjects who met the "leveling off" criterion did not even achieve an R of 1.00! The R values have been shown to vary with age and the training status of the subjects (1). In general,

these criteria are useful because they give the investigator an objective indicator of the subject's effort. However, subjects should not be expected to meet all the criteria on any single test (29, 43). (See A Closer Look 15.3.)

$\dot{V}O_2$ max is a very reproducible measure on subjects tested with the same test protocol on the same piece of equipment. The value for $\dot{V}O_2$ max does not seem to be dependent on whether the test is a continuous GXT or a discontinuous GXT as long as it is conducted with the same work instrument (29, 33, 60, 87). However, when $\dot{V}O_2$ max values are compared across protocols, some systematic differences appear (9). The highest value for $\dot{V}O_2$ max is usually measured with a running test up a grade on a treadmill, followed by a walking test up a grade on a treadmill, and then on a cycle ergometer. In American populations, walk test protocols yield values about 6% lower than those for a run test (60), while cycle test protocols yield values about 10% to 11% lower than those for a run test (29, 34, 53). Europeans show only a 5% to 7% difference in this latter comparison (9, 41). An arm ergometer test will yield values equal to about 70% of the $\dot{V}O_2$ max measured with the legs (36, 78). It is important to recognize these differences when comparing one test to another, or when comparing the same subject over time with different modes of exercise. These differences among tests have led to the convention to call $\dot{V}O_2$ *max* the value measured on a graded running test; $\dot{V}O_2$ *peak* is the term used to describe the highest $\dot{V}O_2$ achieved on walk, cycle, or arm ergometer protocol (77). However, these terms can cause confusion when applied to highly trained athletes, such as cyclists, as they have higher $\dot{V}O_2$ max values when measured on a cycle, compared to a treadmill (89). The actual measurement of $\dot{V}O_2$ max is crucial for research studies and in some clinical settings. However, it is unreasonable to expect the actual measurement of $\dot{V}O_2$ max to be used as the CRF standard in fitness programs.

A CLOSER LOOK 15.3

Lactate Criterion for Achieving $\dot{V}O_2$ Max

In P. O. Åstrand's classic study on the $\dot{V}O_2$ max of children, he was confronted with a problem—only 50 percent of the children achieved a leveling off in $\dot{V}O_2$ when the work rate was increased to maximum levels. This led Åstrand to look for an alternative indicator that the children had, in fact, achieved $\dot{V}O_2$ max. The children had completed one test per day over a period of three to four weeks, with a day or two break between tests. A blood sample was taken a few minutes after each exercise test to measure the blood lactate concentration. In the children who experienced a plateau in $\dot{V}O_2$, he found that the lactate concentration ranged from 6.7 to 10.1 mM when the $\dot{V}O_2$ curves leveled off, with the average being 8 mM. He then compared the $\dot{V}O_2$ max values of boys and girls who had experienced a leveling off in $\dot{V}O_2$ with those who had achieved a high lactate level, but not a leveling off in $\dot{V}O_2$. The average $\dot{V}O_2$ max was the same for both groups. Based on these observations, Åstrand used the elevated blood lactate value and the subjective stress of the subject to select the highest $\dot{V}O_2$ value as the subject's $\dot{V}O_2$ max when a plateau was not observed (5).

Estimation of $\dot{V}O_2$ Max from Last Work Rate

Given the complexity and cost of the procedures involved in the measurement of $\dot{V}O_2$ max, it is no surprise that in many fitness and clinical settings $\dot{V}O_2$ max is estimated with equations that allow the calculation of $\dot{V}O_2$ max from the last work rate achieved on the GXT. The equations for estimating the oxygen cost of running and walking outlined in chapter 6 allow such calculations and, in general, the estimates are reasonable (66, 67). What is important in the use of these equations is that the work test is suited to the individual. If the increments in the GXT from one stage to the next are too large relative to a person's CRF, or if the time for each stage is so short that a person might not be able to achieve the steady-state oxygen requirement for that stage, then the equations will overestimate the person's $\dot{V}O_2$ max (35, 40, 66). As described in chapter 4, poorly fit individuals take longer to achieve the steady state at moderate to heavy work rates, and this increases the chance of an overestimation of $\dot{V}O_2$ max when using these formulas. This suggests that a more conservative protocol be used for low-fit individuals to allow them to reach a steady state at each stage. A recommended procedure is to use only the last completed stage of a test. However, independent of the proper matching of the protocol with the individual, it must be remembered that these are only *estimations* (see A Closer Look 15.4).

Estimation of $\dot{V}O_2$ Max from Submaximal HR Response

Another common procedure used with GXT protocols is to estimate $\dot{V}O_2$ max on the basis of the subject's HR response to a variety of submaximal work rates (37). In these tests the HR is plotted against work rate (or estimated $\dot{V}O_2$) until the termination criterion of 70% to 85% of age-adjusted maximal HR is reached. Figure 15.4 shows the HR response for a twenty-year-old who has taken a submaximal GXT on a cycle ergometer. Heart rate was measured at each work rate until a value equal to 85% of estimated maximal HR was reached (170 b · min^{-1}). A line was drawn through the HR points and extrapolated to the estimated maximal HR, which is calculated by subtracting age from 220. Another line is dropped from that point to the x-axis, and the work rate or $\dot{V}O_2$ (in this case, 2.7 L · min^{-1}) that would have been achieved if the individual had worked until maximal HR was reached is recorded (37). While this is a simple and commonly used procedure to estimate $\dot{V}O_2$ max, it has several potential problems.

The first problem relates to the formula used for estimating the maximal HR. These estimates have a standard deviation (SD) of about 11 b · min^{-1} (57). A twenty-year-old's maximal HR might be estimated to be 200 b · min^{-1}, but if a person were out at ± 2 SD, the value would be 178 or 222 b · min^{-1}. For those who do maximal testing, one will occasionally observe subjects having *measured* maximal HRs ± 20 b · min^{-1} away from their age-adjusted estimate of maximal heart rate. Taking this as an example, what if the subject in figure 15.4 had a true maximal HR of only 180 b · min^{-1} instead of the estimated 200 b · min^{-1}? The estimated $\dot{V}O_2$ max would be an overestimation of the correct value.

Further, a submaximal end point such as 85% of estimated maximal heart rate may be very light work for one person and maximal work for another. The reason for this is related to the estimate of maximal heart rate (220 − age) mentioned earlier. If a thirty-year-old has a real maximum heart rate of 160 b · min^{-1} and the GXT takes the person to 85% of estimated maximal HR (220 − 30 = 190; 85% of 190 = 161 b · min^{-1}), then the person would be taken to maximal HR.

Another problem with submaximal GXT protocols using the HR response as the primary indicator of fitness is that any variable that affects submaximal heart rate

A CLOSER LOOK 15.4

Error in Estimating V̇O₂ max

It is important to remember that the estimation of V̇O₂ max by any of the methods described in this chapter is associated with an inherent "error" compared to the directly measured V̇O₂ max value. When investigators try to determine the validity of an exercise test to estimate V̇O₂ max, they must first test large numbers of subjects in the laboratory to actually *measure* each subject's V̇O₂ max. On another day, the investigators may have the subjects complete a distance run for time, or a standardized graded treadmill or cycle ergometer test to determine the highest percent grade/speed or work rate that the subject can achieve. That information is then used to develop an equation to predict the measured V̇O₂ max value from the time of the distance run, the last grade/speed achieved on a treadmill test, or the final work rate on the cycle ergometer test.

The predicted value will not usually equal the measured V̇O₂ max value, and a term called the *standard error* (SE) is used to describe how far off (higher or lower) the predicted value might be from the true value when using the prediction equation. One standard error (±SE) describes where 68% of the estimates are compared to the true value. If the SE were ±1 ml · kg⁻¹ · min⁻¹, then 68% of the predicted V̇O₂ max values would fall within ±1 ml · kg⁻¹ · min⁻¹ of the true value. Typically, the SE is larger than that (3, 74). For example:

- If V̇O₂ max is estimated from the last stage of a maximal test, the SE = 3 ml · kg⁻¹ · min⁻¹.

- If V̇O₂ max is estimated from heart rate values measured during a submaximal test, the SE = 4–5 ml · kg⁻¹ · min⁻¹.
- If V̇O₂ max is estimated from the one-mile walk test or the twelve-minute run test described earlier, the SE = 5 ml · kg⁻¹ · min⁻¹.

The relatively large standard errors might suggest that these tests have little value, but that is not the case. The tests are reliable, and when the same individual takes the same test over time, the change in estimated V̇O₂ max monitored by the test is a reasonable reflection of improvements in cardiorespiratory fitness. This can serve as both a motivational and educational tool when working with fitness clients.

FIGURE 15.4 Estimation of V̇O₂ max from heart rate values measured during a series of submaximal work rates on a cycle ergometer. The test was stopped when the subject reached 85% of maximal HR. A line is drawn through the HR points measured during the test and is extrapolated to the age-adjusted estimate of maximal HR. Another line is dropped from that point to the x-axis, and the V̇O₂ max is identified.

will affect the slope of the HR/V̇O₂ line and, of course, the estimate of V̇O₂ max. These variables would include: eating prior to the test, dehydration, elevated body temperature, temperature and humidity of the testing area, emotional state of the subject, medications that affect HR, and previous physical activity (7, 81). Clearly, many environmental variables must be controlled if one is to use such protocols to estimate V̇O₂ max.

Despite these problems, this estimate of V̇O₂ max is useful in providing appropriate feedback to participants in fitness programs. Following training, the HR response to any fixed submaximal work rate is lower, suggesting an increase in V̇O₂ max when the HR/V̇O₂ line is drawn through those HR points to the age-adjusted maximal HR. In this case, because the same individual is being tested over time, the 220 − age formula introduces only a constant and unknown error that will not affect the projection of the HR/V̇O₂ line. Further, the low cost, ease of measurement, and high reliability make it a good test that can be used for education and motivation (80).

IN SUMMARY

- The measurement of V̇O₂ max is the gold standard measure of cardiorespiratory fitness.
- V̇O₂ max can be estimated based on the final work rate achieved in a graded exercise test.
- V̇O₂ max can be estimated from heart rate responses to submaximal exercise by extrapolating the relationship to the subject's age-adjusted estimate of maximal heart rate. Careful attention to environmental factors that can affect the heart rate response to submaximal exercise is an important aspect of the procedures for these tests.

GRADED EXERCISE TEST: PROTOCOLS

The GXT protocols can be either submaximal or maximal, depending on the end points used to stop the test. The choice of the GXT should be based on the population (athletes, cardiac patients, children), purpose (estimate CRF, measure $\dot{V}O_2$ max, diagnose CHD), and cost (equipment and personnel) (42, 45). This section will discuss the selection of the test based on these factors and provide examples of common GXT protocols.

When choosing a GXT protocol, the population being tested must be considered, given that the last stage in a GXT for cardiac patients might not even be a warm-up for a young, athletic subject. Test protocols should vary in terms of the initial work rate, how large the increment in work rate will be between stages, and the duration of each stage. In general, the GXT for a sedentary subject might start at 2 to 3 METs (1 MET = 3.5 ml·kg^{-1}·min^{-1}), and progress at about 1 MET per stage, with each stage lasting two to three minutes to allow enough time for a steady state to be reached. For young, active subjects, the initial work rate might be 5 METs, with increments of 2 to 3 METs per stage (74). Table 15.5 shows four well-known treadmill protocols and the populations for which they are suited. The National Exercise and Heart Disease protocol (69) is usually used with poorly fit subjects, with the work rate increasing only 1 MET each three minutes. The Standard Balke protocol (11) starts at about 4 METs and progresses 1 MET each two minutes, and is suitable for most average sedentary adults. The Bruce protocol for young, active subjects (18) starts at about 5 METs and progresses at 2 to 3 METs per stage. This protocol includes walking and running up a grade, and may not be suitable for those at the low end of the fitness continuum. The last protocol shown is used by the fit and athletic populations, with the speed dependent on the fitness of the subject (7).

As mentioned earlier, one of the most common approaches used in estimating $\dot{V}O_2$ max is to take the final stage in the test and apply the formula for converting grade and speed to $\dot{V}O_2$ in ml·kg^{-1}·min^{-1}. Nagle et al. (68) and Montoye et al. (66) have shown that apparently healthy individuals reach the new steady-state requirement by approximately 1.5 minutes of each stage up to moderately heavy work. These formulas give reasonable estimates of CRF if the test has been suited to the individual (40, 66). However, if the increments in the stages are too large, or if the time at each stage is too short, then the person might not be able to reach the oxygen requirement associated with that stage of the GXT. In these cases the formulas will overestimate the subject's $\dot{V}O_2$ max. This problem is more common with low-fit individuals and suggests

TABLE 15.5   Treadmill Protocols

A—NATIONAL EXERCISE AND HEART DISEASE PROTOCOL FOR POORLY FIT SUBJECTS (69)

Stage*	METs	Speed (mph)	% Grade
1	2.5	2	0
2	3.5	2	3.5
3	4.5	2	7.0
4	5.5	2	10.5
5	6.5	2	14.0
6	7.5	2	17.5
7	8.5	3	12.5
8	9.5	3	15.0
9	10.5	3	17.5

*Stage lasts three minutes.

B—STANDARD BALKE PROTOCOL FOR NORMAL, SEDENTARY SUBJECTS (11)

Stage*	METs	Speed (mph)	% Grade
1	4.3	3	2.5
2	5.4	3	5.0
3	6.4	3	7.5
4	7.4	3	10.0
5	8.5	3	12.5
6	9.5	3	15.0
7	10.5	3	17.5
8	11.6	3	20.0
9	12.6	3	22.5

*Stage lasts two minutes.

C—BRUCE PROTOCOL FOR YOUNG, ACTIVE SUBJECTS (18)

Stage*	METs	Speed (mph)	% Grade
1	5	1.7	10
2	7	2.5	12
3	9.5	3.4	14
4	13	4.2	16
5	16	5.0	18

*Stage lasts three minutes.

D—ÅSTRAND AND RODAHL PROTOCOL FOR VERY FIT SUBJECTS (7)

Stage*	METs	Speed (mph)	% Grade
1	12.9/18	7/10	2.5
2	14.1/19.8	7/10	5.0
3	15.3/21.5	7/10	7.5
4	16.5/23.2	7/10	10.0
5	17.7/24.9	7/10	12.5

*Stage lasts two minutes; vigorous warm-up precedes test.

that the more conservative tests be used to estimate the $\dot{V}O_2$ max based on grade and speed achieved.

IN SUMMARY

■ When selecting a GXT, the population being tested must be considered. The initial work rate and the rate of change of work rate need to accommodate the capabilities of the population.

Treadmill

Treadmill GXT protocols can accommodate everyone, from those least fit to those most fit, and use the natural activities of walking and running. Treadmills set the pace for the subject and provide the greatest potential load on the cardiovascular system. However, they are expensive, not portable, and make some measurements (BP and blood sampling) difficult (81). As mentioned previously, the type of treadmill test does influence the magnitude of the measured $\dot{V}O_2$ max, with the graded running test giving the highest value, the running test at 0% grade the next highest, and the walking test protocols the lowest (9, 60). There are also some limitations in the types of measurements that can be made, depending on whether walking or running is used. For example, during running tests, the measurement of BP is not possible, and there is more potential for artifact in the ECG tracing.

In order for estimates of $\dot{V}O_2$ to be obtained from grade and speed considerations, the grade and speed settings must be correct (42). In addition, the subject must follow instructions carefully and not hold onto the treadmill railing during the test. If this is not done, estimates of $\dot{V}O_2$ max based on either the HR/$\dot{V}O_2$ extrapolation procedure or the formula that uses the last speed/grade combination achieved will not be reasonable (6, 76). For example, when a subject who was walking on a treadmill at 3.4 mph and 14% grade held onto the railing, the HR decreased 17 b · min^{-1} (6). This would result in an overestimation of the $\dot{V}O_2$ max using either of the submaximal procedures just mentioned, and special equations would have to be developed if holding onto the handrail were allowed (62). Finally, with the treadmill there is no need to make adjustments to the $\dot{V}O_2$ calculation due to differences in body weight. Treadmill tests require the subject to carry his or her own weight, and the $\dot{V}O_2$ is therefore proportional to body weight (65).

In the following example of a submaximal GXT, a forty-five-year-old male takes a Balke Standard Protocol (3 mph, 2.5% each two minutes) and the test is terminated at 85% of age-adjusted maximal HR (149 b · min^{-1}). Heart rate was measured in the last thirty seconds of each stage, and $\dot{V}O_2$ max was estimated by the

Data:		
Subject: male, age = 45 years	% grade	HR (b/min)
Estimated HR max = 175 b/min	0	100
85% HR max = 149 b/min	2.5	102
	5.0	108
	7.5	110
	10.0	123
	12.5	136
	15.0	149

% Grade	0.0	2.5	5.0	7.5	10.0	12.5	15.0	17.5	20.0
METs	3.3	4.4	5.4	6.4	7.4	8.4	9.5	10.5	11.6

FIGURE 15.5 Estimation of $\dot{V}O_2$ max from the heart rate values measured during different stages of a treadmill test. From E. T. Howley and B. D. Franks, *Health/Fitness Instructor's Handbook.* Copyright © 1986 Human Kinetics Publishers, Inc., Champaign, IL. Used by permission.

HR/$\dot{V}O_2$ extrapolation to age-adjusted maximal HR (175 b · min^{-1}). Figure 15.5 shows the plot of the HR response at each stage, and the extrapolation to the person's estimated maximal heart rate. In the early stages of the test, the HR does not increase in a predictable manner with increasing grade. This may be due to the changes in stroke volume that occur early in upright work (see chapter 9). The beginning stages also act as a warm-up and adjustment period for the subject. The HR response is usually quite linear between 110 b·min^{-1} and 85% maximal HR (8). The HR/$\dot{V}O_2$ line is extrapolated to 175 b · min^{-1}, and a vertical line is dropped to the x-axis where the estimated $\dot{V}O_2$ max is identified: 11.6 METs, or 40.6 ml · kg^{-1} · min^{-1}.

A single-stage submaximal treadmill test has been validated for use with low-risk subjects who are likely to have average values for $\dot{V}O_2$ max (30). In this test the treadmill is set at 0% grade, and a walking speed is set between 2 and 4.5 mph to elicit a heart rate between 50% and 70% of age-adjusted maximal HR. Following this four-minute warm-up, the grade is elevated to 5% for four minutes. HR is measured in the last minute and used with speed (S in mph), age (A in years), and gender (G, with female = 0 and male = 1) in the following regression equation to predict $\dot{V}O_2$ max:

$$\dot{V}O_2 \text{ max} = 15.1 + 21.8 \text{ (S)} - 0.327 \text{ (HR)} - 0.263$$
$$\text{(S} \times \text{A)} + 0.00504 \text{ (HR} \times \text{A)} + 5.98 \text{ (G)}$$

Finally, investigators have adapted the one-mile walk test mentioned earlier under "field test" so it could be done on a treadmill. Subjects completed a questionnaire to rate their level of physical activity and then walked on the treadmill at a self-selected speed that they classified as "brisk." The investigators had to develop a new prediction equation, different from the outdoor test, and it was shown to provide a valid estimate of $\dot{V}O_2$ max (75).

Cycle Ergometer

Cycle ergometers are portable, moderately priced work instruments that allow measurements to be made easily. However, they are self-paced and result in some localized fatigue (81). On mechanically braked cycle ergometers (e.g., Monark), the work rate can be increased by increasing the pedal rate or the resistance on the flywheel. Generally, the pedal rate is maintained constant during a GXT at a rate suitable to the populations being tested: 50 to 60 rpm for the low to average fit, and 70 to 100 for the high fit and competitive cyclists (39). The pedal rate is maintained by having the subject pedal to a metronome, or by providing some other source of feedback (visual analog or digital display of the rpm). The load on the wheel is increased in a sequential fashion to systematically overload the cardiovascular system. The starting work rate and the increment from one stage to the next depend on the fitness of the subject and the purpose of the test. The $\dot{V}O_2$ can be estimated from an equation that gives reasonable estimates of the $\dot{V}O_2$ up to work rates of about 1,200 kgm · min^{-1} (3):

$$\dot{V}O_2 \text{ (ml} \cdot \text{min}^{-1}) = 1.8 \text{ ml} \cdot \text{kgm}^{-1} \times \text{kgm} \cdot \text{min}^{-1}$$
$$+ (7 \text{ ml} \cdot \text{kg}^{-1} \cdot \text{min}^{-1} \times \text{kg body wt.)}$$

The cycle ergometer is different from the treadmill in that the body weight is supported by the seat, and the work rate is dependent primarily on the crank speed and the load on the wheel. This means that for a small person, the relative $\dot{V}O_2$ at any work rate is higher than that for a big person. For example, if a work rate requires a $\dot{V}O_2$ of 2,100 ml · min^{-1}, this represents a relative $\dot{V}O_2$ of 35 ml · kg^{-1} · min^{-1} for a 60-kg person, and only 23 ml · kg^{-1} · min^{-1} for a 90-kg person. In addition, the increments in the work rate, by demanding a fixed increase in the $\dot{V}O_2$ (e.g., an increment of 150 kgm · min^{-1} is equal to a $\dot{V}O_2$ change of 270 ml · min^{-1}), force a small and unfit subject to make larger cardiovascular adjustments than a large or high-fit subject. These facts have been taken into consideration by the YMCA (37) in recommending submaximal GXT protocols. The idea is to provide a means of obtaining a variety of HR responses to several submaximal work rates in a way that reduces the duration of the test.

Directions:

1. Set the first work load at 150 kgm • min^{-1} (0.5 kp).
2. If the HR in the 3rd minute is
   • less than (<) 86, set the second load at 600 kgm (2.0 kp);
   • 86 to 100, set the second load at 450 kgm (1.5 kp);
   • greater than (>) 100, set the second load at 300 kgm (1.0 kp).
3. Set the third and fourth (if required) loads according to the loads in the columns below the second loads.

FIGURE 15.6   YMCA protocol used to select work rates for submaximal cycle ergometer tests. From the YMCA *Fitness Testing and Assessment Manual*. Copyright © 2000 YMCA of the USA. Reprinted by permission.

Figure 15.6 shows the different "routes" followed in the YMCA protocol depending on the subject's HR response to a work rate of 150 kgm · min^{-1}. The YMCA protocol makes use of the observation that the relationship between $\dot{V}O_2$ and HR is a linear one between 110 and 150 b · min^{-1}. For this reason the YMCA protocol requires the subject to exercise at only one more work rate past the one that yields an HR $\geq$ 110 b · min^{-1}. As a general recommendation for all cycle ergometer tests, seat height is adjusted so that the knee is slightly bent when the foot is at the bottom of the pedal swing and parallel to the floor; the seat height is recorded for later testing. In the YMCA protocol, each stage lasts three minutes and heart rate values are obtained in the last thirty seconds of the second and third minutes. If the difference in HR is <5 b · min^{-1} between the two time periods, a steady state is assumed; if not, an additional minute is added to that stage. A line then connects the two HR values and is extrapolated to the subject's estimated maximal HR. A vertical line is dropped to the x-axis and the estimated $\dot{V}O_2$ max value is obtained as described for the submaximal treadmill protocol.

Figure 15.7 shows the YMCA protocol for a thirty-year-old female who weighs 60 kg. The first work rate

FIGURE 15.7 Example of the YMCA protocol used to estimate $\dot{V}O_2$ max. From E. T. Howley and B. D. Franks, *Health/Fitness Instructor's Handbook*. Copyright © 1986 Human Kinetics Publishers, Inc., Champaign, IL. Used by permission.

chosen was 150 kgm · min^{-1}, and a heart rate of 103 b · min^{-1} was measured. Following the YMCA protocol, the next loads were 300 and then 450 kgm · min^{-1}, and the measured HR values were 115 and 128 b · min^{-1}, respectively. A line was drawn through the two HR points greater than 110 b · min^{-1}, and extrapolated to 190 b · min^{-1}. The estimated $\dot{V}O_2$ max for this woman was approximately 2.58 liters · min^{-1} or 43 ml · kg^{-1} · min^{-1}, using the previous equation.

In addition to this extrapolation procedure for estimating $\dot{V}O_2$ max, Åstrand and Ryhming (8) provide a method that requires the subject to complete one work rate of approximately six minutes, demanding an HR between 125 and 170 b · min^{-1}. These investigators observed that at 50% $\dot{V}O_2$ max, males had an average HR of 128, and females, 138 b · min^{-1}, and at 70% $\dot{V}O_2$ max the average HRs were 154 and 164 b · min^{-1}, respectively. These data were collected on young men and women, ages eighteen to thirty. The basis for the test is that if you know from an HR response that a person is at 50% $\dot{V}O_2$ max at a work rate equal to 1.5 L · min^{-1}, then the estimated $\dot{V}O_2$ max would be twice that, or 3.0 L · min^{-1}. A nomogram (see figure 15.8) is used to estimate the $\dot{V}O_2$ max based on the subject's HR response to one six-minute work rate. Because maximal HR decreases with increasing age, and the data were collected on young subjects, Åstrand (4) established correction factors to multiply the estimated $\dot{V}O_2$ max values taken from the nomogram in order to correct for the lower maximal HR.

Siconolfi et al. (84) presented a submaximal cycle ergometer test for epidemiological investigations that is a modification of the YMCA protocol that uses the Åstrand and Ryhming (8) nomogram. It is presented here because the advantages of this test include

(1) the requirement that the subject achieve only 70% of the estimated maximal HR and (2) the procedure was validated on men and women of ages twenty to seventy years. Men over age thirty-five and all women start the test at 150 kgm · min^{-1}, and the work rate is increased that amount each two minutes until an HR ≥70% of estimated maximal HR is achieved; the subject continues for two or more minutes until a steady-state HR is measured. Men under age thirty-five begin at 300 kgm · min^{-1} and increase that amount each two minutes as above. However, when the HR is between 60% and 70% of maximal HR, the work rate is increased only 150 kgm · min^{-1}. The Åstrand and Ryhming (8) nomogram is used as before (without the age correction), and the estimated $\dot{V}O_2$ max values are used in the following equations (84):

For males:
$\dot{V}O_2$ (liters · min^{-1}) = 0.348 (X$_1$) − 0.035 (X$_2$) + 3.011

For females:
$\dot{V}O_2$ (liters · min^{-1}) = 0.302 (X$_1$) − 0.019 (X$_2$) + 1.593

where X$_1$ = $\dot{V}O_2$ max from Åstrand and Ryhming nomogram, and X$_2$ = age in years. The test yields acceptable estimates of $\dot{V}O_2$ max and puts the subject under less stress by requiring that an HR of only 70% of the age-adjusted maximal HR be achieved.

Step Test

A step-test protocol is used to estimate $\dot{V}O_2$ max in the same way that treadmill and cycle ergometer protocols are used. The step test does not require expensive equipment, the step height does not have to be calibrated, everyone is familiar with the stepping exer-

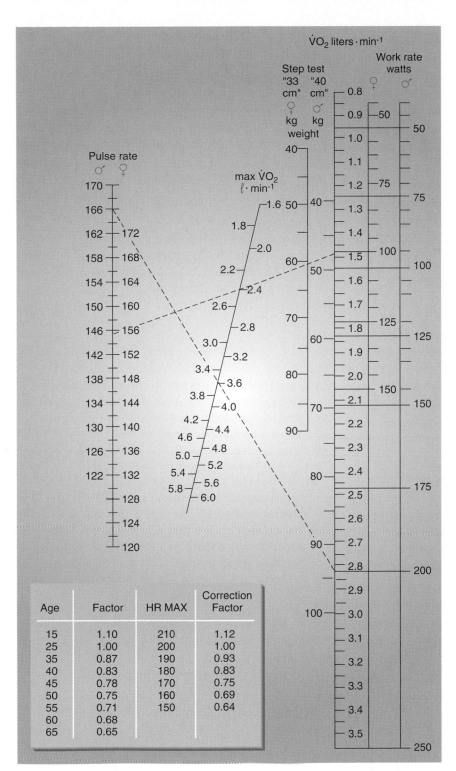

$\dot{V}O_2$ liters · min⁻¹

Step test
"33 "40
cm" cm"
♀   ♂
kg   kg
weight

Work rate
watts
♀   ♂

Pulse rate
♂   ♀

max $\dot{V}O_2$
ℓ · min⁻¹

Age	Factor	HR MAX	Correction Factor
15	1.10	210	1.12
25	1.00	200	1.00
35	0.87	190	0.93
40	0.83	180	0.83
45	0.78	170	0.75
50	0.75	160	0.69
55	0.71	150	0.64
60	0.68		
65	0.65		

FIGURE 15.8 Nomogram for the estimation of $\dot{V}O_2$ max from submaximal HR values measured on either a cycle ergometer or step test. For the cycle ergometer, the work rate in watts (1 watt = 6.1 kgm · min⁻¹) is shown on the two rightmost columns, one for men and one for women. The results of a cycle ergometer test for a man who worked at 200 watts is shown. A dashed line is drawn between the 200-watt work rate and the HR value of 166 measured during the test. The estimated $\dot{V}O_2$ max is 3.6 liters · min⁻¹. The step test uses a rate of 22.5 lifts · min⁻¹, and two different step heights, 33 cm for women and 40 cm for men. The step test scale lists body weight for the subject, and the results of a test on a 61-kg woman are shown. A dashed line is drawn between the 61 kg on the 33-cm scale and the HR value of 156 b · min⁻¹ measured during the test. The estimated $\dot{V}O_2$ max is 2.4 liters · min⁻¹. These estimates of $\dot{V}O_2$ max are influenced by the person's maximal HR, which is known to decrease with age. A correction factor chosen from the accompanying table corrects these $\dot{V}O_2$ max values when either the maximal HR or age is known. Simply multiply the $\dot{V}O_2$ value by the correction factor.

cise, and the energy requirement is proportional to body weight, as with the treadmill (58). The work rate can be increased by increasing the step height while keeping the cadence the same, or by increasing the cadence while keeping the step height the same. The step height can be varied with a hand-cranking device (68) or by using a series of wooden steps with increments in step height of 10 cm. The rate of stepping is

established with a metronome, and the stepping cadence has four counts: up, up, down, down. The subjects must step all the way up and down in time with the metronome. Figure 15.9 shows the results of a step test on a sixty-year-old female. In this step test the height of the step was kept constant at 16 centimeters and the rate of stepping increased 6 lifts · min⁻¹ each two minutes. The line drawn through the

FIGURE 15.9 Use of a step test to predict $\dot{V}O_2$ max from a series of submaximal HR responses. From E. T. Howley and B. D. Franks, *Health/Fitness Instructor's Handbook*. Copyright © 1986 Human Kinetics Publishers, Inc., Champaign, IL. Used by permission.

HR points is extrapolated to the estimated maximal HR, 160 b · min⁻¹, and a line is dropped to the horizontal axis to estimate the $\dot{V}O_2$ max using the following equation (3):

$$\dot{V}O_2 = 0.2 \text{ (step rate)} + 1.33 \times 1.8$$
$$\times \text{ (step height [m])} \times \text{ (step rate)} + 3.5$$

The equation yields values in ml · kg⁻¹ · min⁻¹, which are converted to METs by dividing by 3.5.

The Åstrand and Ryhming (8) nomogram (figure 15.8) also accommodates a step test, using a rate of 22.5 lifts per minute (metronome = 90) and step heights of 40 cm for men and 33 cm for women. The principle is the same as described for their cycle ergometer protocol.

The introduction of step ergometers (i.e., Stair-Master) allows a graded exercise test to be conducted in a manner similar to that of a treadmill. The work rates are independent of step rate, and the HR responses are slightly higher than those measured on the treadmill at any $\dot{V}O_2$ (44). Such a test has been shown to measure changes in $\dot{V}O_2$ max that result from either treadmill or step-ergometer training, indicating more commonality than specificity among step and treadmill tests (15).

In summary, there are a variety of tests that can be used to estimate CRF. The usefulness of a test is a function of both the accuracy of the measurement and the ability to repeat the test on a routine basis to evaluate changes in CRF over time. It is this latter point that decreases the need that the test be able to estimate the true $\dot{V}O_2$ max to the nearest ml · kg⁻¹ · min⁻¹. In effect, if a person is taking a submaximal GXT on a regular basis and the HR response to a fixed work rate is decreasing over time, one can reasonably conclude that the person is making progress in the intended direction, independent of how accurate the estimate of $\dot{V}O_2$ max is.

IN SUMMARY

- $\dot{V}O_2$ max can be estimated with the extrapolation procedure using the treadmill, cycle ergometer, or step.
- The subject must follow directions carefully and environmental conditions must be controlled if the estimate of $\dot{V}O_2$ max is to be reasonable and reproducible.

STUDY QUESTIONS

1. What is the sequence of steps used in evaluating cardiorespiratory fitness?
2. What is a health or cardiac risk inventory? Name one currently in use and explain its purpose.
3. A forty-year-old man runs 1.5 miles (2,415 meters) in ten minutes. What is his estimated $\dot{V}O_2$ max? Is his value "normal"?
4. Draw an example of ST segment depression and describe its significance in the diagnosis of heart disease.
5. You are monitoring a GXT in which $\dot{V}O_2$ max is measured. How would you know if a person achieved $\dot{V}O_2$ max?
6. Given the following information collected during a treadmill test on a fifty-year-old man, estimate his $\dot{V}O_2$ max.

Work Rate	Heart Rate
3 METs	110
5 METs	125
7 METs	140

7. Given the assumption that the formula, 220 − age, can be used to estimate maximal heart rate, how far off could you be in your estimate of $\dot{V}O_2$ max in question 6?
8. What information do you gain by monitoring the RPE during a GXT?
9. List five reasons for stopping a GXT.
10. Should you use the same GXT protocol on all subjects? Why or why not?

SUGGESTED READINGS

American College of Sports Medicine. 2006. *ACSM's Resource Manual for Guidelines for Exercise Testing and Prescription*, 5th ed. Baltimore: Lippincott, Williams & Wilkins.

Dubin, D. 2000. *Rapid Interpretation of EKGs: A programmed course*. 6th ed. Tampa, FL: Cover.

Heyward, V. H. 2002. *Advanced Fitness Assessment and Exercise Prescription*. 4th ed. Champaign, IL: Human Kinetics.

Scheidt, S. 1997. *Interactive electrocardiography*. Carbondale, IL: DxR Development Group; Summit, NJ: Novartis Medical Education.

REFERENCES

1. Aitken, J. C., and J. Thompson. 1988. The respiratory $\dot{V}CO_2/\dot{V}O_2$ exchange ratio during maximum exercise and its use as a predictor of maximum oxygen uptake. *European Journal of Applied Physiology* 57:714–19.
2. American Alliance for Health, Physical Education, Recreation and Dance. 1988. *Physical Best*. Reston, VA: AAHPERD.
3. American College of Sports Medicine. 2006. *ACSM's Guidelines for Exercise Testing and Prescription*. 7th ed. Baltimore: Lippincott, Williams & Wilkins.
4. Åstrand, I. 1960. Aerobic work capacity in men and women with special reference to age. *Acta Physiologica Scandinavica* 49 (Suppl.): 169.
5. Åstrand, P. O. 1952. *Experimental Studies of Physical Working Capacity in Relation to Sex and Age*. Copenhagen: Manksgaard.
6. ———. 1984. Principles of ergometry and their implications in sports practice. *International Journal of Sports Medicine* 5:102–5.
7. Åstrand, P. O., and K. Rodahl. 1986. *Textbook of Work Physiology*. New York: McGraw-Hill.
8. Åstrand, P. O., and I. Ryhming. 1954. A nomogram for calculation of aerobic capacity (physical fitness) from pulse rate during submaximal work. *Journal of Applied Physiology* 7:218–21.
9. Åstrand, P. O., and B. Saltin. 1961. Maximal oxygen uptake and heart rate in various types of muscular activity. *Journal of Applied Physiology* 16:977–81.
10. Balke, B. 1963. A simple field test for assessment of physical fitness. *Civil Aeromedical Research Institute Report* 63–66.
11. ———. 1970. Advanced exercise procedures for evaluation of the cardiovascular system. Monograph. Milton, WI: The Burdick Corporation.
12. Bassett, D. R. Jr., and E. T. Howley. 1997. Maximal oxygen uptake: Classical versus contemporary viewpoints. *Medicine and Science in Sports and Exercise* 29:591–603.
13. Bassett, D. R. Jr., and E. T. Howley. In press. Limiting factors for maximal oxygen uptake and determinants of endurance performance. *Medicine and Science in Sports and Exercise*.
14. Bell, D. G., I. Jacobs, and S. W. Lee. 1992. Blood lactate response to the Canadian Aerobic Fitness Test (CAFT). *Canadian Journal of Sport Science* 17:1, 14–18.
15. Ben-Ezra, and R. Verstraete. 1991. Step ergometry: Is it task-specific training? *European Journal of Applied Physiology* 63:261–64.
16. Blair, S. N., H. W. Kohl III, R. S. Paffenbarger, Jr., D. G. Clark, K. H. Cooper, and L. W. Gibbons. 1990. Physical fitness and all-cause mortality. *Journal of the American Medical Association* 262:2395–2401.
17. Borg, G. A. U. 1982. Psychological bases of physical exertion. *Medicine and Science in Sports and Exercise* 14:377–81.
18. Bruce, R. A. 1972. Multi-stage treadmill tests of maximal and submaximal exercise. In *Exercise Testing and Training of Apparently Healthy Individuals: A Handbook for Physicians*. 32–34. New York: American Heart Association.
19. Carton, R. L., and E. C. Rhodes. 1985. A critical review of the literature on ratings scales for perceived exertion. *Sports Medicine* 2:198–222.
20. Chow, R. J., and J. H. Wilmore. 1984. The regulation of exercise intensity by ratings of perceived exertion. *Journal of Cardiac Rehabilitation* 4:382–87.
21. Chun, D. M., C. B. Corbin, and R. P. Pangrazi. 2000. Validation of criterion-referenced standards for the mile run and progressive aerobic cardiovascular endurance tests. *Research Quarterly for Exercise and Sport* 71:125–34.
22. Conley, D. S., K. J. Cureton, D. R. Dengel, and P. G. Weyand. 1991. Validation of the 12-min swim as a field test of peak aerobic power in young men. *Medicine and Science in Sports and Exercise* 23:766–73.
23. Cooper, K. H. 1977. *The Aerobic Way*. New York: Bantam.
24. Cooper, M., and K. H. Cooper. 1972. *Aerobics for Women*. New York: Evans.
25. Cureton, K. J., L. D. Hensley, and A. Tiburzi. 1979. Body fatness and performance differences between men and women. *Research Quarterly* 50:333–40.
26. Cureton, K. J., and G. L. Warren. 1990. Criterion-referenced standards for youth health-related fitness tests: A tutorial. *Research Quarterly for Exercise and Sport* 61:7–19.
27. Cureton, K. J. et al. 1978. Effect of experimental alterations in excess weight on aerobic capacity and distance running performance. *Medicine and Science in Sports* 10:194–99.
28. Daniels, J. et al. 1978. Differences and changes in $\dot{V}O_2$ among young runners 10–18 years of age. *Medicine and Science in Sports* 10:200–3.
29. Duncan, G. E., E. T. Howley, and B. N. Johnson. 1997. Applicability of $\dot{V}O_2$ max criteria: Discontinuous versus continuous protocols. *Medicine and Science in Sports and Exercise* 29:273–78.
30. Ebbeling, C. B., A. Ward, E. M. Puleo, J. Widrick, and J. M. Rippe. 1991. Development of a single-stage submaximal treadmill walking test. *Medicine and Science in Sports and Exercise* 23:966–73.
31. Ellestad, M. 2002. *Stress Testing: Principles and Practice*. 5th ed. Philadelphia: F. A. Davis.
32. *Exercise and Your Heart*. 1981. U.S. Department of Health and Human Services. NIH Publication, No. 81–1677.
33. Falls, H., and L. D. Humphrey. 1973. A comparison of methods for eliciting maximal oxygen uptake for college women during treadmill walking. *Medicine and Science in Sports* 5:239–41.
34. Faulkner, J. A. et al. 1971. Cardiovascular responses to submaximum and maximum effort cycling and running. *Journal of Applied Physiology* 30:457–61.
35. Foster, C. et al. 1984. Prediction of oxygen uptake during exercise testing in cardiac patients and health volunteers. *Journal of Cardiac Rehabilitation* 4:537–42.
36. Franklin, B. A. 1985. Exercise testing, training and arm ergometry. *Sports Medicine* 2:100–19.
37. Golding, L. A. 2000. YMCA *Fitness Testing and Assessment Manual*. 4th ed. Champaign, IL: Human Kinetics.
38. Gutmann, M. C. et al. 1981. Perceived exertion-heart rate relationship during exercise testing and training of cardiac patients. *Journal of Cardiac Rehabilitation* 1:52–59.
39. Hagberg, J. M. et al. 1981. Effect of pedaling rate on submaximal exercise responses of competitive cyclists. *Journal of Applied Physiology* 51:447–51.
40. Haskell, W. L. et al. 1982. Factors influencing estimated oxygen uptake during exercise testing soon after myocardial infarction. *American Journal of Cardiology* 50: 299–304.

41. Hermansen, L., and B. Saltin. 1969. Oxygen uptake during maximal treadmill and bicycle exercise. *Journal of Applied Physiology* 26:31–37.

42. Howley, E. T. 1988. Exercise testing laboratory. In *Resource Manual for Guidelines for Exercise Testing and Prescription*, ed. S. N. Blair et al., chap. 47. Philadelphia: Lea & Febiger.

43. Howley, E. T., D. R. Bassett, Jr., and H. G. Welch. 1995. Criteria for maximal oxygen uptake—review and commentary. *Medicine and Science in Sports and Exercise* 27:1292–1301.

44. Howley, E. T., D. L. Colacino, and T. C. Swensen. 1992. Factors affecting the oxygen cost of stepping on an electronic stepping ergometer. *Medicine and Science in Sports and Exercise* 24:1055–58.

45. Howley, E. T., and B. D. Franks. 2003. *Health Fitness Instructor's Handbook*. 4th ed. Champaign, IL: Human Kinetics.

46. Issekutz, B., N. C. Birkhead, and K. Rodahl. 1962. The use of respiratory quotients in assessment of aerobic power capacity. *Journal of Applied Physiology* 17:47–50.

47. Jette, M. et al. 1976. The Canadian Home Fitness Test as a predictor of aerobic capacity. *Canadian Medical Association Journal* 114:680–83.

48. Kasch, F. W., J. L. Boyer, S. P. Van Camp, L. S. Verity, and J. P. Wallace. 1990. The effects of physical activity and inactivity on aerobic power in older men (a longitudinal study). *The Physician and Sportsmedicine* 18:73–83.

49. Kavanagh, T., and R. J. Shephard. 1976. Maximal exercise tests on "postcoronary" patients. *Journal of Applied Physiology* 40:611–18.

50. Kirkendall, W. M. et al. 1980. Recommendations for human blood pressure determination by sphygmomanometers. *Circulation* 62:1146A–1155A.

51. Kitamura, K. et al. 1972. Hemodynamic correlates of myocardial oxygen consumption during upright exercise. *Journal of Applied Physiology* 32:516.

52. Kline, G. M. et al. 1987. Estimation of $\dot{V}O_2$ max from a one-mile track walk, gender, age, and body weight. *Medicine and Science in Sports and Exercise* 19:253–59.

53. Kohl, H. W., L. W. Gibbons, N. F. Gordon, and S. N. Blair. 1990. An empirical evaluation of the ACSM guidelines for exercise testing. *Medicine and Science in Sports and Exercise* 22:533–39.

54. Krahenbuhl, G. S. et al. 1978. Field testing of cardiorespiratory fitness in primary school children. *Medicine and Science in Sports and Exercise* 10:208–13.

55. Leger, L. A., and J. Lambert. 1982. A maximal multistage 20-m shuttle run test to predict $\dot{V}O_2$ max. *European Journal of Applied Physiology* 49:1–12.

56. Leger, L. A., D. Mercier, C. Gadoury, and J. Lambert. 1982. The multistage 20-meter shuttle run test for aerobic fitness. *Journal of Sport Science* 6:93–101.

57. Londeree, B. R., and M. L. Moeschberger. 1984. Influence of age and other factors on maximal heart rate. *Journal of Cardiac Rehabilitation* 4:44–49.

58. Margaria, R., P. Aghemo, and E. Rovelli. 1965. Indirect determination of maximal $\dot{V}O_2$ consumption in man. *Journal of Applied Physiology* 20:1070–73.

59. Martin, A. D. 1986. ECG and medications. In *Health/Fitness Instructor's Handbook*, ed. E. T. Howley and B. D. Franks, chap. 12. Champaign, IL: Human Kinetics.

60. McArdle, W. D., F. I. Katch, and G. S. Pechar. 1973. Comparison of continuous and discontinuous treadmill and bicycle tests for max v. *Medicine and Science in Sports and Exercise* 5:156–60.

61. McConnell, T. R. 1988. Practical considerations in the testing of $\dot{V}O_2$ max in runners. *Sports Medicine* 5:57–68.

62. McConnell, T. R., and B. A. Clark. 1987. Prediction of maximal oxygen consumption during handrail-supported treadmill exercise. *Journal of Cardiopulmonary Rehabilitation* 7:324–31.

63. McCormack, W. P., K. J. Cureton, T. A. Bullock, and P. G. Weyand. 1991. Metabolic determinants of 1-mile run/walk performance in children. *Medicine and Science in Sports and Exercise* 23:611–17.

64. McNaughton, L., P. Hall, and D. Cooley. 1998. Validation of several methods of estimating maximal oxygen uptake in young men. *Perceptual and Motor Skills* 87:575–84.

65. Montoye, H. J., and T. Ayen. 1986. Body size adjustment for oxygen requirement in treadmill walking. *Research Quarterly for Exercise and Sport* 57:82–84.

66. Montoye, H. J. et al. 1985. The oxygen requirement for horizontal and grade walking on a motor-driven treadmill. *Medicine and Science in Sports and Exercise* 17:640–45.

67. Montoye, H. J., T. Ayen, and R. A. Washburn. 1986. The estimation of $\dot{V}O_2$ max from maximal and sub-maximal measurements in males, age 10–39. *Research Quarterly for Exercise and Sport* 57:250–53.

68. Nagle, F. J., B. Balke, and J. P. Naughton. 1965. Gradational step tests for assessing work capacity. *Journal of Applied Physiology* 20:745–48.

69. Naughton, J. P., and R. Haider. 1973. Methods of exercise testing. In *Exercise Testing and Exercise Training in Coronary Heart Disease*, ed. J. P. Naughton, H. K. Hellerstein, and L. C. Mohler, 79–91. New York: Academic Press.

70. Nelson, R. R. et al. 1974. Hemodynamic predictors of myocardial oxygen consumption during static and dynamic exercise. *Circulation* 50:1179–89.

71. Oja, P., R. Laukkanen, M. Pasanen, T. Tyry, and I. Vuori. 1991. A 2-km walking test for assessing the cardiorespiratory fitness of healthy adults. *International Journal of Sports Medicine* 12:356–62.

72. Oldridge, N. B., W. L. Haskell, and P. Single. 1981. Carotid palpation, coronary heart disease and exercise rehabilitation. *Medicine and Science in Sports and Exercise* 13:6–8.

73. Park, R. J. 1989. Measurement of physical fitness: A historical perspective. Washington, D.C.: U.S. Department of Health and Human Services, Public Health Service.

74. Pollock, M. L., and J. H. Wilmore. 1990. *Exercise in Health and Disease*. 2d ed. Philadelphia: W. B. Saunders.

75. Prober, D. M., P. S. Freedom, G. M. Kline, K. J. McInnis, and J. M. Rippe. 2002. Development and validation of a one-mile treadmill walk test to predict peak oxygen uptake in healthy adults. *Canadian Journal of Applied Physiology* 27(6):575–88.

76. Ragg, K. E. et al. 1980. Errors in predicting functional capacity from a treadmill exercise stress test. *American Heart Journal* 100:581–83.

77. Rowell, L. B. 1974. Human cardiovascular adjustments to exercise and thermal stress. *Physiology Reviews* 54:75–159.

78. Sawka, M. N. et al. 1983. Determination of maximal aerobic power during upper-body exercise. *Journal of Applied Physiology: Respiration, Environmental, and Exercise Physiology* 54:113–17.

79. Sedlock, D. A. et al. 1983. Accuracy of subject-palpated carotid pulse after exercise. *The Physician and Sportsmedicine* 11(4):106–16.

80. Sharkey, B. J. 1984. *Physiology of Fitness*. 2d ed. Champaign, IL: Human Kinetics.

81. Shephard, R. J. 1984. Tests of maximal oxygen uptake: A critical review. *Sports Medicine* 1:99–124.

82. Shephard, R. J., D. A. Bailey, and R. L. Mirwald. 1976. Development of the Canadian home fitness test. *Canadian Medical Association Journal* 114:675–79.

83. Shephard, R. J., S. Thomas, and I. Weller. 1991. The Canadian home fitness test: 1991 Update. *Sports Medicine* 11:358–66.

84. Siconolfi, S. F. et al. 1982. Assessing $\dot{V}O_2$ max in epidemiologic studies: Modification of the Åstrand-Ryhming test. *Medicine and Science in Sports and Exercise* 14:335–38.

85. Sidney, K. H., and R. J. Shephard. 1977. Maximum and submaximum exercise tests in men and women in the seventh, eighth, and ninth decades of life. *Journal of Applied Physiology* 43:280–87.

86. Sparling, P. B., and K. J. Cureton. 1983. Biological determinants of the sex difference in 12-minute run performance. *Medicine and Science in Sports and Exercise* 15:218–23.

87. Stamford, B. A. 1976. Step increments versus constant load tests for determination of maximal oxygen uptake. *European Journal of Applied Physiology* 35:89–93.

88. Strickland, M. K., S. R. Petersen., and M. Bouffard. 2003. Prediction of maximal aerobic power from the 20-m multi-stage shuttle run test. *Canadian Journal of Applied Physiology* 28(2):272–82.

89. Strømme, S. B., F. Ingjer, and H. D. Meen. 1977. Assessment of maximal aerobic power in specifically trained athletes. *Journal of Applied Physiology* 42:833–37.

90. Taylor, H. L., E. R. Buskirk, and A. Henschel. 1955. Maximal oxygen intake as an objective measure of cardiorespiratory performance. *Journal of Applied Physiology* 8:73–80.

91. Wallace, J. P. 1983. Physical conditioning: Intervention in aging cardiovascular function. In *Intervention in the Aging Process, Part A: Quantitation, Epidemiology, and Clinical Research*, ed. A. R. Liss, 307–23.

92. Weller, I. M. R., S. G. Thomas, P. N. Corey, and M. H. Cox. 1993. Prediction of maximal oxygen uptake from a modified Canadian aerobic fitness test. *Canadian Journal of Applied Physiology* 18(2):175–88.

93. Weller, I. M. R., S. G. Thomas, N. Gledhill, D. Paterson, and A. Quinney. 1995. A study to validate the modified Canadian aerobic fitness test. *Canadian Journal of Applied Physiology* 20(2):211–21.

CHAPTER 16

Exercise Prescriptions for Health and Fitness

■ Objectives

By studying this chapter, you should be able to do the following:

1. Characterize physical inactivity as a coronary heart disease risk factor comparable to smoking, hypertension, and high serum cholesterol.

2. Contrast *exercise* with *physical activity*; explain how both relate to a lower risk of CHD and improvement in cardiorespiratory fitness (CRF).

3. Describe the physical activity recommendation by the American College of Sports Medicine and the Centers for Disease Control and Prevention to improve the health status of sedentary U.S. adults.

4. Explain what *screening* and *progression* mean for a person wishing to initiate an exercise program.

5. Identify the optimal range of frequency, intensity, and duration of activity associated with improvements in CRF; why is more not necessarily better than less?

6. Calculate a target heart rate range by either the heart rate reserve or percent of maximal HR methods.

7. Explain why the appropriate sequence of physical activity for sedentary persons is walk → walk/jog → jog → games.

8. Explain how the target heart rate (THR) helps adjust exercise intensity in times of high heat, humidity, or while at altitude.

■ Outline

Prescription of Exercise   321
  Dose-Response   322
  Physical Activity and
    Health   323

General Guidelines for Improving
Fitness   325
  Screening   325
  Progression   325

Warm-Up, Stretch, and
  Cool-Down, Stretch   325

Exercise Prescription
for CRF   325
  Frequency   326
  Duration   326
  Intensity   326

Sequence of Physical
Activity   329
  Walking   329
  Jogging   329
  Games and Sports   330

Strength and Flexibility
Training   331

Environmental Concerns   332

■ Key Terms

dose
effect (response)

exercise
physical activity

physical fitness
target heart rate (THR) range

In chapter 14 we discussed a variety of risk factors related to cardiovascular and other diseases. Physical inactivity had long been considered only a secondary risk factor in the development of CHD—that is, an inactive lifestyle would increase a person's risk for CHD only if other primary risk factors were present. However, as explained in chapter 14, this is no longer the case. Numerous studies (41, 42, 53, 60) suggest that physical inactivity is a primary risk factor for coronary heart disease (CHD), similar to smoking, hypertension, and high serum cholesterol. These studies also show that regular vigorous physical activity is instrumental in reducing the risk of CHD in those who smoke or are hypertensive (37, 43). Based on this growing body of evidence, the American Heart Association recognized physical inactivity as a primary or major risk factor (5). Finally, epidemiological studies show that increases in physical activity (44) and fitness (9) are associated with a reduced death rate from all causes as well as from CHD. This means that physical activity should be used along with other therapies to reduce the risk of CHD in those possessing other risk factors. Consequently, there is little disagreement that regular physical activity is a necessary part of a healthy lifestyle (67). The only question is, how much?

Before we answer this question we need to distinguish among the terms physical activity, exercise, and fitness. **Physical activity** is defined as any form of muscular activity. Therefore physical activity results in the expenditure of energy proportional to muscular work, and is related to **physical fitness.** Physical fitness is defined as a set of attributes that people have or develop that relate to the ability to perform physical activity. **Exercise** represents a subset of physical activity that is planned, with a goal of improving or maintaining fitness (12). These distinctions, while subtle, are important to understand in our discussion of the role of physical activity as a part of a healthy lifestyle. For example, there is no question that a planned exercise program will improve $\dot{V}O_2$ max, and that a higher $\dot{V}O_2$ max is associated with a lower death rate (8). However, we must emphasize that physical activity, including that done at a moderate intensity, is beneficial. The reduction in the risks of CHD due to the latter types of activity may be mediated through changes in the distribution of cholesterol, or an increase in fibrinolysis (clot dissolving) activity (25). It should be no surprise that the American College of Sports Medicine, in the ACSM's *Guidelines for Exercise Testing and Prescription*, and *Physical Activity and Health: A Report of the Surgeon General*, state the need for increased participation in moderate-intensity exercise (e.g., brisk walking) throughout the life span (4, 67). Such a recommendation is consistent with exposing the general population to low-risk physical activity to achieve health-related benefits aimed at reducing cardiovas-

cular and metabolic diseases. In contrast to this general recommendation for everyone, there is a need to follow a variety of guidelines in prescribing moderate to strenuous exercise that is aimed at improving $\dot{V}O_2$ max. We will address both concerns in this chapter. For information on training for performance, see chapter 21.

IN SUMMARY

- Physical inactivity has been classified as a primary risk factor for coronary heart disease.
- Regular participation in physical activity can reduce the overall risk for those who smoke or who are hypertensive.
- Those who increase their physical activity and/or cardiorespiratory fitness have a lower death rate from all causes compared to those who remain sedentary.

PRESCRIPTION OF EXERCISE

The concern about the proper **dose** of exercise needed to bring about a desired **effect (response)** is similar to the physician's need to know the type and quantity of a drug, as well as the time frame over which it must be taken, to cure a disease. Clearly, there is a difference in what is needed to cure a headache compared to what is needed to cure tuberculosis. In the same way there is no question that the dose of physical activity needed to achieve high-level running performance is different from that required to improve a health-related outcome (e.g., lower blood pressure) or fitness (e.g., an increase in $\dot{V}O_2$ max). This dose-response relationship for medications is described in figure 16.1 (19).

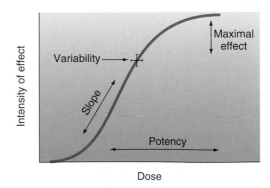

FIGURE 16.1 The relationship between the dose of a drug (expressed as the log of the dose) and the effect. Data from L. S. Goodman and A. Gilman, eds., 1975, *The Pharmacological Basis of Therapeutics*. New York: Macmillan Publishing Company.

- *Potency.* The potency of a drug is a relatively unimportant characteristic of a drug in that it makes little difference whether the effective dose of a drug is 1 μg or 100 mg as long as it can be administered in an appropriate dosage. Applied to exercise, walking four miles is as effective in expending calories as running two miles.

- *Slope.* The slope of the curve gives some information about how much of a change in effect is obtained from a change in dose. Some physiological measures change quickly for a given dose of exercise, while some health-related effects require the application of exercise over many months to see a desired outcome.

- *Maximal effect.* The maximal effect (efficacy) of a drug varies with the type of drug. For example, morphine can relieve pain of all intensities, while aspirin is effective against only mild to moderate pain. Similarly, strenuous exercise can cause an increase in $\dot{V}O_2$ max as well as modify risk factors, while light-to-moderate exercise can change risk factors with only a minimal impact on $\dot{V}O_2$ max (an important point we will return to later).

- *Variability.* The effect of a drug varies between individuals, and within individuals depending on the circumstances. The intersecting brackets in figure 16.1 indicate the variability in the dose required to bring about a particular effect, and the variability in the effect associated with a given dose. For example, gains in $\dot{V}O_2$ max due to endurance training show considerable variation, even when the initial $\dot{V}O_2$ max value is controlled for (17). See A Closer Look 13.1 for more on the issue of variability.

- *Side effect.* A last point worth mentioning that can also be applied to our discussion of exercise prescription is that no drug produces a single effect. The spectrum of effects might include adverse (side) effects that limit the usefulness of the drug (e.g., for exercise the side effects might include increased risk of injury or sudden death).

In contrast to drugs that individuals stop taking when a disease is cured, there is a need to engage in some form of physical activity throughout one's life to experience the health-related and fitness effects.

Dose-Response

The exercise dose is usually characterized by the intensity, frequency, duration, and type of activity. The intensity can be described in terms of:

- % $\dot{V}O_2$ max,
- % maximal heart rate,
- rating of perceived exertion, and
- the onset of blood lactate accumulation (the lactate threshold).

The frequency could include:

- number of days per week and
- number of times per day.

The duration of exercise for each exercise session can be given as the:

- number of minutes of exercise,
- total kilocalories (kcal) expended, and
- total kcal expended per kilogram body weight.

The type of exercise relates to whether resistance exercises or cardiovascular endurance exercises are used in the training program. For the latter, we would also distinguish among the effects of walking vs. jogging/ running vs. swimming. Although we know a considerable amount about the role that each of these variables may play in a gain in $\dot{V}O_2$ max, little is known about the minimum or optimal quantities of each variable related to health outcomes (23).

The response (effect) generated by a particular dose of exercise can include changes in $\dot{V}O_2$ max, resting blood pressure, insulin sensitivity, body weight (percent fat), and depression. Haskell (22, 23) provided an important insight into how we should rethink our understanding of cause and effect when we study how a dose of physical activity is related to the responses, physical fitness, and health. Physical activity could bring about favorable changes by:

- improving fitness (especially cardiovascular fitness) and thereby, improving health, or
- improving fitness and health simultaneously and separately, or
- improving fitness, but not a specific health outcome, or
- improving some specific health outcome, but not fitness.

It has become clear that improvements in a variety of health-related concerns are not dependent on an increase in $\dot{V}O_2$ max. This is important and provides a transition to our next section.

IN SUMMARY

- An exercise dose reflects the interaction of the intensity, frequency, and duration of exercise.
- The cause of the health-related response may be related to an improvement in $\dot{V}O_2$ max or may act through some other mechanism, making health-related outcomes and gains in $\dot{V}O_2$ max independent of each other.

CLINICAL APPLICATIONS 16.1

Dose-Response: Physical Activity and Health

A special symposium examined the links between physical activity and health using an "evidence-based approach" in which the quality of the evidence bearing on an issue was included as an important part of the analysis (36). Researchers found, in general, that higher levels of physical activity were associated with:

- lower rates of all-cause mortality, total cardiovascular disease (CVD), and coronary heart disease incidence and mortality;
- a lower incidence of obesity and type 2 diabetes, and a lower risk of CVD and all-cause mortality in those with type 2 diabetes;
- a lower risk of colon cancer and osteoporosis;

- improvement in the ability of older adults to do activities of daily living;
- a reduction in depression and anxiety in those with a mild-to-moderate condition; and
- favorable changes in cardiovascular risk factors, including blood pressure, blood lipid profile, and clotting time.

The inability to establish a clear dose-response relationship between physical activity and a number of health outcomes was linked to lack of appropriate studies; methods of measuring physical activity not being sensitive enough to accurately characterize the "dose"; the small effect of physical activity on some health outcomes; un-controlled factors such as genetic variability; and simultaneous changes in body weight, which confounded the data analysis. Clearly, there is a great need for additional, well-designed studies that use more sophisticated measurements of physical activity on a larger and more diverse population to be able to describe whether or not there is a dose-response relationship between physical activity and a specific health outcome. In that regard, some recent articles have shown a dose-response relationship for physical activity related to prostate cancer (33) and cardiovascular disease risk in women (40).

Physical Activity and Health

The issue of the proper dose of exercise to bring about a desired effect is a crucial one in the prescription of exercise for both prevention and rehabilitation. Over the past two decades we have learned that the proper dose differs greatly, depending on the outcome. For example, an improvement in some health-related variable (e.g., resting blood pressure) might be accomplished with an exercise intensity lower than that required to achieve an increase in $\dot{V}O_2$ max. In addition, the frequency with which the exercise must be taken to have the desired effect varies with the intensity and the duration of the session (see later discussion).

Certain physiological variables respond very quickly to a "dose" of exercise. For example, we have shown how rapidly the sympathetic nervous system, blood lactate, and heart rate (see chapter 13) adapt to exercise training, taking only days to see changes in response. In contrast to these rapid responses to exercise training, a variety of physiological variables such as the capillary number change more slowly (57). Similarly, when Haskell describes the potential association between physical activity and health he distinguishes between short-term (acute) and long-term (training) responses (23). The following terms are used to describe the patterns of responses in the weeks following the initiation of a dose of exercise:

- acute responses—occur with one or several exercise bouts but do not improve further

- rapid responses—benefits occur early and plateau
- linear—gains are made continuously over time
- delayed—occur only after weeks of training

The need for such distinctions can be seen in figure 16.2, which shows proposed dose-response relationships between physical activity, defined as minutes of exercise per week at 60% to 70% of maximal work capacity, and a variety of physiological responses (32): (1) blood pressure and insulin sensitivity are most responsive to exercise, (2) changes in $\dot{V}O_2$ max and resting heart rate are intermediate, and (3) serum lipid changes such as high-density lipoprotein (HDL) are delayed. For an update on dose-response issues, see Clinical Applications 16.1.

By this time it should be clear that it is difficult to provide a single exercise prescription that addresses all issues related to prevention and/or treatment of various diseases. However, in spite of this difficulty, there has been a pressing need to spell out a general exercise recommendation to improve the health status of all U.S. adults. The American College of Sports Medicine and the Centers for Disease Control and Prevention responded to this need. Their guidelines were based on a comprehensive review of the literature dealing with the health-related aspects of physical activity (45). The dose-response curve in figure 16.3 summarizes their findings. By having the most sedentary group move up to the "A" level of physical activity

CLINICAL APPLICATIONS 16.2

Achieving Health-Related Outcomes

Is Vigorous Exercise Better than Moderate Activity?

There is ongoing debate over this question, but what may be surprising to some is that moderate exercise may be vigorous! The recommendations made by the ACSM and CDC (45), and supported in *Physical Activity and Health: A Report of the Surgeon General* (67), emphasized the need to get more people active since so many Americans were totally inactive. The recommendation emphasized moderate physical activities (3–6 METs) that could be done by almost everyone, which made good sense from a public health perspective. Some fitness professionals objected to this recommendation because it appeared to back away from the fitness

guidelines advocated by the ACSM to increase $\dot{V}O_2$ max and achieve other fitness goals. However, the complete statement on the need to increase moderate physical activity also emphasized the fact that additional health gains can be achieved by participation in greater amounts of exercise. Consequently, there was no need to back away from the classic ACSM exercise prescription for health-related and fitness goals. What has become clear over the last twenty years is that a large segment of the population may be able to achieve fitness goals while doing "moderate" activity. In Haskell's keynote address at the 1999 Health and Fitness Summit (24), he emphasized that the two recommendations (moderate activity

on one hand and vigorous on the other) may not be as incompatible as they might at first appear. Given that maximal oxygen uptake ($\dot{V}O_2$ max) decreases with age, moderate activities in the range of 3 to 6 METs that require only 25% and 50% of $\dot{V}O_2$ max for someone with a 12 MET capacity require 33% and 66% of $\dot{V}O_2$ max for someone with a 9 MET capacity (30). Therefore, "moderate" activities, coupled with the lower threshold of training in deconditioned individuals, may be sufficient to elevate the metabolic rate and heart rate to the appropriate levels needed to achieve the various fitness ($\dot{V}O_2$ max) and health benefits that were a part of the original ACSM fitness recommendation.

FIGURE 16.2 Proposed dose-response relationships between amount of exercise performed per week at 60% to 70% maximum work capacity and changes in several variables. Blood pressure (BP) and insulin sensitivity (curve to the left side) appear to be most sensitive to exercise. Maximum oxygen consumption ($\dot{V}O_2$ max) and resting heart rate, which are parameters of physical fitness (middle curve), are next in sensitivity, and lipid changes such as high-density lipoprotein (HDL) (right-hand curve) are least sensitive.

shown in figure 16.3, the greatest gains in health-related benefits can be realized. Their recommendation is that *every U.S. adult should accumulate thirty minutes or more of moderate-intensity (3–6 METs) physical activity on most, preferably all, days of the week*. This recommendation

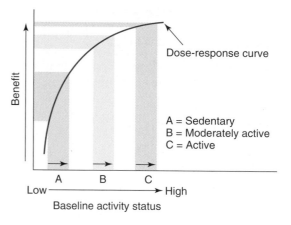

FIGURE 16.3 The dose-response curve represents the best estimate of the relationship between physical activity (dose) and health benefit (response). The lower the baseline physical activity status, the greater will be the health benefit associated with a given increase in physical activity (arrows A, B, and C). From R. R. Pate et al., 1995, "Physical Activity and Public Health" in *Journal of the American Medical Association*, 273:402–7. Chicago, IL: American Medical Association.

is based on the finding that caloric expenditure and total time of physical activity are associated with reduced cardiovascular disease and mortality. Further, doing the activity in intermittent bouts as short as ten minutes is a suitable way of meeting the thirty-minute goal (3, 45, 67). This thirty-minute recommendation can be viewed as a "minimum" physical activity recommendation for achieving health outcomes. Additional exercise, including vigorous exercise, provides additional health and fitness benefits (45). This recommendation was not greeted with joy by all, including some fitness professionals (see Clinical Applications 16.2).

IN SUMMARY

- On the basis of epidemiological and experimental evidence, the ACSM and CDC concluded that health-related benefits result from regular participation in moderate-intensity (3–6 METs) physical activity.
- They recommend that every U.S. adult should accumulate thirty minutes or more of moderate-intensity physical activity on most, preferably all, days of the week.

GENERAL GUIDELINES FOR IMPROVING FITNESS

An increase in moderate physical activity is an important goal for reducing health-related problems in sedentary individuals. These benefits occur at a point where the overall risk associated with physical activity is relatively small. However, even though the risk of cardiac arrest in habitually active men is higher *during vigorous activity*, the overall (rest + exercise) risk of cardiac arrest in vigorously active men is only 40% of the risk in sedentary men (59). Lastly, there is a growing body of evidence indicating that achievement of an average to high level of cardiorespiratory fitness ($\dot{V}O_2$ max) confers additional health benefits, as well as increasing one's ability to engage in a broad range of recreational activities. The purpose of this section is to review the general guidelines for exercise programs aimed at increasing $\dot{V}O_2$ max. In chapter 13 the concepts of overload and specificity were presented relative to the adaptations that take place with different training programs. While these principles apply here, what is important to remember is that little exercise is needed to achieve a health-related effect. This stands in marked contrast to the intensity of exercise needed to achieve performance goals (see chapter 21).

IN SUMMARY

- In previously sedentary subjects, small changes in physical activity result in large health benefits with only minimal risk.
- Strenuous exercise increases the risk of a heart attack during the activity, but reduces the overall (rest + exercise) risk of such an event.
- Moderate to high levels of cardiorespiratory fitness reduce the risk of death from all causes.

Screening

The first thing to do, if not already done in the evaluation of CRF, is to carry out some form of health status screening to decide who should begin an exercise program and who should obtain further consultation with a physician (see chapter 15 for details). The risk of cardiovascular complications during exercise is directly related to the degree of pre-existing cardiac disease. In young people the risk of sudden death is about 1/133,000 and 1/769,000 per year in men and women, respectively, due primarily to congenital or acquired heart disease. In adults the risk is one per year for every 15,000 to 18,000 individuals (4).

Progression

The emphasis in any health-related exercise program is to do too little rather than too much. By starting slowly and progressing from the easily accomplished activities to those that are more difficult, the chance of causing muscle soreness and of aggravating old injuries is reduced. The emphasis on moderate-intensity activities such as walking at 3 to 4 mph early in the fitness program is consistent with this recommendation, and the participant must be educated not to move too quickly into the more demanding activities. Once the person can walk about four miles without fatigue, the progression to a walk-jog and jogging program is a reasonable recommendation (31).

Warm-Up, Stretch, and Cool-Down, Stretch

Prior to the actual activity used in the exercise session, a variety of very light exercises and stretches are done to improve the transition from rest to the exercise state. The emphasis at the onset of an exercise session is to gradually increase the level of activity until the proper intensity is reached. Stretching exercises to increase the range of motion of the joints involved in the activity, as well as specific stretches to increase the flexibility of the lower back, are included in the warm-up. At the end of the activity session, about five minutes of cool-down activities—slow walking and stretching exercises—are recommended to gradually return HR and BP toward normal. This part of the exercise session is viewed as important in reducing the chance of a hypotensive episode after the exercise session (31).

EXERCISE PRESCRIPTION FOR CRF

The exercise program includes dynamic, large muscle activities such as walking, jogging, running, swimming, cycling, rowing, and dancing. The CRF training effect

FIGURE 16.4 Effects of increasing the frequency, duration, and intensity of exercise on the increase in $\dot{V}O_2$ max in a training program. This figure demonstrates the increasing risk of orthopedic problems due to exercise sessions that are too long, or conducted too many times per week. The probability of cardiac complications increases with exercise intensity beyond that recommended for improvements in cardiorespiratory fitness.

of exercise programs is dependent on the proper frequency, duration, and intensity of the exercise sessions. The ACSM recommends three to five sessions per week, for twenty to sixty minutes per session, at an intensity of about 40/50% to 85% heart rate reserve (HRR) or oxygen uptake reserve ($\dot{V}O_2R$) (4). The latter term, %$\dot{V}O_2R$, is being used in place of the traditional %$\dot{V}O_2$ max, but for those of average to high fitness the terms are quite similar (see later discussion). The combination of duration and intensity should result in the expenditure of about 200 to 300 kcal per session. This program is consistent with achieving weight loss goals and reducing the risk factors associated with CHD (4, 25, 47, 48, 49, 67).

Frequency

Improvements in CRF increase with the frequency of exercise sessions, with two sessions being the minimum, and the gains in CRF leveling off after three to four sessions per week (4, 68). Gains in CRF can be achieved with a two-day-per-week program, but the intensity has to be higher than the three-day-per-week program, and participants might not achieve weight loss goals (48). In addition, the high-intensity exercise associated with a two-day-per-week frequency may not be appropriate for previously sedentary individuals. The schedule of three to four days per week includes a day off between sessions and reduces the scheduling problems associated with planned exercise programs. Figure 16.4 shows that higher frequencies are associated with higher rates of injuries (16, 50).

Duration

The duration has to be viewed together with intensity, in that the total work accomplished per session (200–300 kcal) is an important variable associated with improvements in CRF once the minimal threshold of intensity is achieved (4). This is important, given that many sedentary persons could more easily accomplish an exercise session of low intensity and

long duration than the reverse, and achieve the health-related benefits of physical activity with minimal risk. For example, an 80-kg (176 lb) person walking at about 3.5 mph would consume O_2 at the rate of 1 liter per minute. Given 5 kcal per liter of O_2, the person is using 5 kcal · min^{-1}, and sixty minutes of walking would be required to expend 300 kcal. As the intensity of exercise increases, the duration needed to expend 300 kcal decreases. Figure 16.4 shows that doing strenuous exercise (75% $\dot{V}O_2$ max) for more than thirty minutes per session increases the risk of orthopedic problems.

Intensity

Intensity describes the overload on the cardiovascular system that is needed to bring about a training effect. It should be no surprise that the intensity threshold for a CRF training effect is lower for the less fit and higher for the more fit. Swain and Franklin (64) found that the threshold for an improvement in $\dot{V}O_2$ max was only 30% of oxygen uptake reserve ($\dot{V}O_2R$) for those with $\dot{V}O_2$ max values less than 40 ml · kg^{-1} min^{-1}, and only 46% $\dot{V}O_2R$ for those with a $\dot{V}O_2$ max greater than 40 ml · kg^{-1} min^{-1}. However, in general, they found that higher-intensity exercise was better for increasing $\dot{V}O_2$ max. As mentioned at the beginning of this section, the range of exercise intensities associated with an increase in $\dot{V}O_2$ max is 40/50% to 85% $\dot{V}O_2R$, which is similar to 40/50% to 85% $\dot{V}O_2$ max for people of average or better fitness (see Clinical Applications 16.3). However, for most people, 60% to 80% $\dot{V}O_2$ max seems to be a range sufficient to achieve CRF goals (31). It appears that in order for this information to be useful, the exercise leader has to know the energy requirements ($\dot{V}O_2$) of all the fitness activities so that a correct match can be made between the activity and the participant. Fortunately, because of the linear relationship between exercise intensity and HR, the exercise intensity can be set by using the HR values equivalent to 60% to 80% $\dot{V}O_2$ max. The range of heart rate values associated with the exercise intensity

Prescribing Exercise Intensity by the $\dot{V}O_2$ Reserve ($\dot{V}O_2R$) Method

Historically, the intensity portion of an exercise prescription was given as a % $\dot{V}O_2$ max, percent of maximal HR, or percent of the HR reserve (HRR). The linear relationship between HR and $\dot{V}O_2$ allowed the former to predict the latter. In this regard, some preferred the use of the HRR method because the percent values used in the calculation of the target heart rates were believed to be similar to the % $\dot{V}O_2$ max values (i.e., 60% HRR ≈ 60% $\dot{V}O_2$ max). Research by Swain and colleagues (62, 63) questioned that close association, especially for subjects at the low end of the fitness scale. They found that the % HRR was more closely linked to the % $\dot{V}O_2R$ (the difference

between maximal $\dot{V}O_2$ and resting $\dot{V}O_2$), than to % $\dot{V}O_2$ max. In the most recent version of the ACSM's position stand on the quantity and quality of exercise needed for fitness (1), this new approach was adopted. As Swain points out (61), the calculation of the %$\dot{V}O_2R$ is similar to that of the HHR. For example, the target $\dot{V}O_2$ of a person with a $\dot{V}O_2$ max of 35 ml · kg^{-1} · min^{-1} who works at 60% HRR is:

Target $\dot{V}O_2$ = (0.60)(35 ml · kg^{-1} · min^{-1}
$\qquad$ − 3.5 ml · kg^{-1} · min^{-1})
$\qquad$ + 3.5 ml · kg^{-1} · min^{-1}
Target $\dot{V}O_2$ = 18.9 ml · kg^{-1} · min^{-1}
$\qquad$ + 3.5 ml · kg^{-1} · min^{-1}
Target $\dot{V}O_2$ = 22.4 ml · kg^{-1} · min^{-1}

The advantage of this approach is that the % HRR and % $\dot{V}O_2R$ values are directly coupled over the entire range of fitness ($\dot{V}O_2$ max values) and exercise intensities, but it is most useful for those at the low end of the scale, where large discrepancies exist between % HRR and % $\dot{V}O_2$ max (61, 62, 63). On the other hand, for those with average to high fitness levels, the difference between the % $\dot{V}O_2$ max and % $\dot{V}O_2R$ is not very great. The following table gives a brief summary of the expected % $\dot{V}O_2$ max values across a broad range of $\dot{V}O_2$ max values (in METs) when exercise intensities are set at a % HRR:

Percent $\dot{V}O_2$ Max at Different Percent Heart Rate Reserve (HRR) and Cardiorespiratory Fitness ($\dot{V}O_2$ Max) Values

$\dot{V}O_2$ max (METs)	40% HRR	50% HRR	60% HRR	70% HRR	80% HRR
18	43.3	52.8	62.2	71.7	81.1
16	43.8	53.1	62.5	71.9	81.3
14	44.3	53.6	62.9	72.1	81.4
12	45.0	54.2	63.3	72.5	81.7
10	46.0	55.0	64.0	73.0	82.0
8	47.5	56.3	65.0	73.8	82.5
6	50.0	58.3	66.7	75.0	83.3

As you can see, for those at the high end of the fitness spectrum and at higher intensities of exercise, the difference between the % HRR and % $\dot{V}O_2$ max is not too great. However, for those at the low end of the fitness scale (e.g., 6 METs), there is a large (e.g., 10%) difference between the % $\dot{V}O_2$ max and % HRR at 40% HRR.

Special Notes

- When using an exercise heart rate value to estimate the % $\dot{V}O_2$ max or % $\dot{V}O_2R$ at which the individual is working, the error is about ± 6% (i.e., 60% HRR = 60 ± 6% $\dot{V}O_2$ R) for two-thirds of the population *when the measured maximal heart rate is known.*

- If we use an age-predicted maximal heart rate to set the target heart rate range, the error involved in estimating the maximal heart rate value (one standard deviation is ± 11b · min^{-1}) adds to the error in estimating % $\dot{V}O_2$ max or % $\dot{V}O_2R$.

needed to have a CRF training effect is called the **target heart rate (THR) range.** How do you determine the THR range?

Direct Method Figure 16.5 shows the HR response of a twenty-year-old subject during a maximal GXT on a treadmill. The subject's $\dot{V}O_2$ max was 12 METs, so

that 60% and 80% $\dot{V}O_2$ max is equal to about 7.2 and 9.6 METs, respectively. A line is drawn from each of these work rates up to the HR/$\dot{V}O_2$ line, and over to the y-axis where the HR values equivalent to these work rates are obtained. These HR values, 138 to 164 b · min^{-1}, represent the THR range, the proper intensity for a CRF training effect (1, 31).

FIGURE 16.5 Target heart rate range determined from the results of an exercise stress test. The heart rate values measured at work rates equal to 60% and 80% $\dot{V}O_2$ max constitute the THR range.

Indirect Methods The THR range can also be estimated by some simple calculations, knowing that the relationship between HR and $\dot{V}O_2$ is linear. The heart rate reserve, or Karvonen, method of calculating a THR range has three simple steps (34, 35):

1. Subtract resting HR from maximal HR to obtain HR reserve (HRR).
2. Take 60% and 80% of the HRR.
3. Add each HRR value to resting HR to obtain the THR range.

For example:

1. If a subject has a maximal HR of 200 b·min^{-1} and a resting HR of 60 b·min^{-1}, then the HRR is 140 b·min^{-1} (200 − 60).
2. 60% × 140 b·min^{-1} = 84 b·min^{-1} and 80% × 140 b·min^{-1} = 112 b·min^{-1}.
3. 84 b·min^{-1} + 60 b·min^{-1} = 144 b·min^{-1} 112 b·min^{-1} + 60 b·min^{-1} = 172 b·min^{-1}. The THR range is 144 to 172 b·min^{-1}.

This method gives reasonable estimates of the exercise intensity because 60% to 80% of the HRR is equal to about 60% to 80% $\dot{V}O_2$ max for those with average or high fitness (see Clinical Applications 16.3).

The other indirect method of calculating the THR range is the *percentage of maximal* HR method. In this method you simply take 70% and 85% of maximal HR to obtain the THR range. In the following example, the subject has a maximal HR of 200 b·min^{-1}. The THR range for this person is 140 to 170 b·min^{-1} (70% × 200 = 140 b·min^{-1}; 85% × 200 = 170 b·min^{-1}). Seventy percent of maximal HR is equal to about 55% $\dot{V}O_2$

max, and 85% of maximal HR is equal to about 75% $\dot{V}O_2$ max, both within the intensity range needed for CRF gains (26, 27, 28, 38).

The intensity of exercise can be prescribed by the direct method, or by either of the indirect methods. Both of the indirect methods require knowledge of the maximal HR. If the maximal HR is measured during a maximal GXT, use it in the calculations. However, if you have to use the age-adjusted estimate of maximal HR (220 − age), remember the potential error, with the standard deviation of the estimate equal to ±11 b·min^{-1}. Tanaka, Monahan, and Seals (65) evaluated the validity of the classic "220 − age" equation to estimate maximal heart rate. They carried out an analysis of 351 published studies and cross-validated the findings with a well-controlled laboratory study. They found almost identical results using both approaches: HR max = 208 − 0.7 × age. This new equation yields maximal heart rate values that are 6 b·min^{-1} lower for twenty-year-olds and 6 b·min^{-1} higher for sixty-year-olds. Although the new formula yields better estimates of HR max *on average*, the investigators emphasize the fact that the estimated HR max for a given individual is still associated with a standard deviation of 10 b·min^{-1}. Consequently, the estimated THR range is a *guideline* for exercise intensity and is meant to be used with other information (abnormal symptoms or signs) to determine if the exercise intensity is reasonable.

In this regard, Borg's RPE scale can be used as an adjunct to HR in prescribing exercise intensity for apparently healthy individuals. The RPE range of 12 to 16 on the original Borg scale covers the range of exercise intensities similar to 40/50% to 85% HRR (1, 4, 7, 15, 20, 21, 51). The RPE scale is helpful because the participant learns to associate the THR range with a certain whole-body perception of effort, decreasing the need for frequent pulse rate measurements. The RPE scale has been shown to have a high test-retest reliability (14), and it is closely linked to the % $\dot{V}O_2$ max and lactate threshold, independent of the mode of exercise and fitness of the subject (29, 56, 58). Remember, the intensity threshold needed to achieve CRF goals is lower for the less fit, and vice versa.

IN SUMMARY

- A sedentary person needs to go through a health status screening before participating in exercise.
- Exercise programs for previously sedentary persons should start with low-intensity activities (walking), and the person should not progress until he or she can walk about four miles comfortably.

- The optimal characteristics of an exercise program are: intensity = 60% to 80% $\dot{V}O_2$ max; frequency = three to four times per week; duration = minutes needed to expend about 200 to 300 kcal.
- The THR range, taken as 60% to 80% HRR, or 70% to 85% of maximal HR, is a reasonable estimate of the proper exercise intensity.
- The intensity threshold for a training effect is low (≤50% $\dot{V}O_2$ max) for the deconditioned, and high (≥85% $\dot{V}O_2$ max) for the very fit.

In order to determine if the subject is in the THR range during the activity, HR should be checked immediately after stopping, taking a ten-second pulse count within the first fifteen seconds. The pulse can be taken at the radial artery or the carotid artery; if the latter is used, the participant should use only light pressure, since heavy pressure can actually slow the HR (31, 51).

The proper intensity, frequency, and duration of exercise needed to have a CRF training effect were discussed in the previous section. It is important that sedentary individuals start slowly before exercising at the recommended intensities specified in the THR range. The next section provides some directions to make that transition.

SEQUENCE OF PHYSICAL ACTIVITY

The old adage that you should "walk before you run" is consistent with the way exercise should be recommended to sedentary persons, be they young or old. Once the person demonstrates an ability to do prolonged walking without fatigue, then controlled fitness exercises conducted at a reasonable intensity (THR) can be introduced. After that, and depending on the interest of the participant, a variety of fitness activities that are more game-like can be included. This section will deal with this sequence of activities that can lead to a fit life (31).

Walking

The primary activity to recommend to someone who has been sedentary for a long period of time is walking. This recommendation is consistent with the introductory material on health benefits, and it deals with the issue of injuries associated with more strenuous physical activity. In addition, there is good reason to believe that some subjects, especially the obese and the elderly, may use walking as their primary form of exercise. The emphasis at this stage is to simply get people active by providing an activity that can be done anywhere, anytime, and with anyone, young or old. In this way, the number of possible interfering factors that can result in the discontinuance of the exercise is reduced.

The person should choose comfortable shoes that are flexible, offer a wide base of support, and have a fitted heel cup. There are a great number of "walking" shoes available, but a special pair of shoes is not usually required. The emphasis is on getting started; if walking becomes a "serious" activity, or leads to hiking, then the investment would be reasonable. If weather is not to interfere with the activity, then proper selection of clothing is necessary. The participant should wear light, loose-fitting clothing in warm weather, and layers of wool or polypropylene in cold weather. For those who cannot bear the extremes in temperature and humidity out of doors, various shopping malls provide a controlled environment with a smooth surface. Walkers should choose the areas in which they walk with care in order to avoid damaged streets, high traffic zones, and poorly lighted areas. Safety is important in any health-related exercise program (31).

A walking program is presented in table 16.1 (31). The steps are rather simple in that progression to the next stage does not occur unless the individual feels comfortable at the current stage. The HR should be recorded as described previously, but the emphasis is not on achieving the THR. Later on in the walking program when higher walking speeds are used, the THR zone will be attained. Remember that walking, in spite of not being very strenuous by the THR zone scale, when combined with long duration is an effective part of a weight-control and CHD risk factor reduction program (42, 52). Walking is an activity that many people find they can do every day, providing many opportunities to expend calories.

Jogging

Jogging begins when a person moves at a speed and form that results in a period of flight between foot strikes; this may be 3 or 4 mph, or 6 or 7 mph, depending on the fitness of the individual. As described in chapter 6, the net energy cost of jogging/running is about twice that of walking (at slow to moderate speeds), and requires a greater cardiovascular response. This is not the only reason for the jogging program to follow a walking program; there is also more stress on joints and muscles due to the impact forces that must be tolerated during the push off and landing of jogging (13).

TABLE 16.1 Walking Program

Rules	Stage	Duration	Heart Rate	Comments
1. Start at a level that is comfortable for you.	1	15 min	_____	_____
	2	20 min	_____	_____
2. Be aware of new aches or pains.	3	25 min	_____	_____
	4	30 min	_____	_____
3. Don't progress to the next level if you are not comfortable.	5	30 min	_____	_____
	6	30 min	_____	_____
	7	35 min	_____	_____
4. Monitor your heart rate and record it.	8	40 min	_____	_____
	9	45 min	_____	_____
5. It would be healthful to walk at least every other day.	10	45 min	_____	_____
	11	45 min	_____	_____
	12	50 min	_____	_____
	13	55 min	_____	_____
	14	60 min	_____	_____
	15	60 min	_____	_____
	16	60 min	_____	_____
	17	60 min	_____	_____
	18	60 min	_____	_____
	19	60 min	_____	_____
	20	60 min	_____	_____

Reprinted, by permission, from B. D. Franks and E.T. Howley, 1989, *Fitness Leader's Handbook*, Champaign, IL: Human Kinetics Publishers, 136. This form may be copied by the fitness leader for distribution to participants.

The emphasis at the start of a jogging program is to make the transition from the walking program in such a way as to minimize the discomfort associated with the introduction of any new activity. This is accomplished by beginning with a jog-walk-jog program that eases the person into jogging by mixing in the lower energy cost and trauma associated with walking. The jogging speed is set according to the THR, with the aim to stay at the low end of the THR zone at the beginning of the program. As the participant adapts to jogging, the HR response for any jogging speed will decrease and jogging speed will have to be increased to stay in the THR zone. This is the primary marker that a training effect is taking place. Table 16.2 presents a jogging program with some simple rules to follow. Special attention is made to completing the walking program first, staying in the THR zone, and not progressing to the next level if the participant is not comfortable with the current level. Jogging is not for everyone, and for those who are obese, or have ankle, knee, or hip problems, it might be a good activity to avoid. Two activities that reduce such stress are cycling (stationary or outdoor) and swimming (31). More on exercise for special populations will be presented in chapter 17.

Games and Sports

As a person becomes accustomed to exercising in the THR range while jogging, swimming, or cycling, more uncontrolled activities can be introduced that require higher levels of energy expenditure, but do so in a more intermittent fashion. Games (paddleball, racquetball, squash), sports (basketball, soccer), and various forms of exercise to music can keep a person's interest and make it more likely that the person will maintain a physically active life. These activities should be built on a walk-and-jogging base to reduce the chance that the participant will make poor adjustments to the activity. In addition, by having the habit of walking or jogging (swimming or cycling), the participant will still be able to maintain his or her habit of physical activity when there is no one to play with or lead the class. In contrast to jogging, cycling, or swimming, it will be more difficult to stay in the THR range with these intermittent activities. It is more likely that the HR will move from below the threshold value to above the top end of the THR from time to time. This is a normal response to activities that are intermittent in nature. It must be stressed, however, that when playing games it is important that the par-

TABLE 16.2 Jogging Program

Rules

1. Complete the Walking Program before starting this program.
2. Begin each session with walking and stretching.
3. Be aware of new aches and pains.
4. Don't progress to the next level if you are not comfortable.
5. Stay at the low end of your THR zone; record your heart rate for each session.
6. Do the program on a work-a-day, rest-a-day basis.

Stage 1 Jog 10 steps, walk 10 steps. Repeat five times and take your heart rate. Stay within THR zone by increasing or decreasing walking phase. Do 20–30 minutes of activity.

Stage 2 Jog 20 steps, walk 10 steps. Repeat five times and take your heart rate. Stay within THR zone by increasing or decreasing walking phase. Do 20–30 minutes of activity.

Stage 3 Jog 30 steps, walk 10 steps. Repeat five times and take your heart rate. Stay within THR zone by increasing or decreasing walking phase. Do 20–30 minutes of activity.

Stage 4 Jog 1 minute, walk 10 steps. Repeat three times and take your heart rate. Stay within THR zone by increasing or decreasing walking phase. Do 20–30 minutes of activity.

Stage 5 Jog 2 minutes, walk 10 steps. Repeat two times and take your heart rate. Stay within THR zone by increasing or decreasing walking phase. Do 30 minutes of activity.

Stage 6 Jog 1 lap (400 meters, or 440 yards) and check heart rate. Adjust pace during run to stay within the THR zone. If heart rate is still too high, go back to the Stage 5 schedule. Do 6 laps with a brief walk between each.

Stage 7 Jog 2 laps and check heart rate. Adjust pace during run to stay within the THR zone. If heart rate is still too high, go back to Stage 6 activity. Do 6 laps with a brief walk between each.

Stage 8 Jog 1 mile and check heart rate. Adjust pace during the run to stay within THR zone. Do 2 miles.

Stage 9 Jog 2 to 3 miles continuously. Check heart rate at the end to ensure that you were within THR zone.

Reprinted, by permission, from B. D. Franks and E. T. Howley, 1989, *Fitness Leader's Handbook*, Champaign, IL: Human Kinetics Publishers, 137. This form may be copied by the fitness leader for distribution to participants.

ticipants have some degree of skill and be reasonably well matched. If one is much better than the other, neither will have a good workout (39).

STRENGTH AND FLEXIBILITY TRAINING

The focus in this chapter has been on training to improve cardiorespiratory fitness. However, the ACSM recommends both strength and flexibility exercises as part of the complete fitness program. Maintenance of the muscle mass has implications related to weight control (see chapter 18) and the integrity of the skeletal system. Further, the combination of adequate flexibility and strength allows individuals to do the activities of daily living comfortably and safely. The ACSM recommendation emphasizes dynamic exercises done on a routine basis, but there is some debate about how much is enough (see Clinical Applications 16.4).

The Activity Pyramid provides a nice summary of the overall recommendations for health and fitness (see figure 16.6). It is beyond the scope of this text to go into detail regarding strength and flexibility programs aimed at improving or maintaining these fitness components. We recommend the Suggested Readings by Faigenbaum and McInnis, for muscular strength and endurance, and by Liemohn, for flexibility and low-back function, as good starting points.

Strength Training: Single versus Multiple Sets

The ACSM recommends resistance training as a part of a well-rounded fitness program. The goals are to increase or maintain muscular strength and endurance, the fat-free mass, and bone mineral density (1). To accomplish this, the ACSM recommends:

- one set of eight to ten exercises that conditions the major muscle groups,
- eight to twelve reps per set (ten to fifteen for older people), and
- two to three sessions per week.

Although the position stand acknowledges that "multiple-set regimes may provide greater benefits," the review of literature supported the use of one set to achieve the health-related and fitness goals. This conclusion received additional support from a comprehensive review by Carpinelli and Otto (11), but not without reaction and reply to that reaction (10).

The debate was raised to a higher level when the ACSM published a second Position Stand in 2002 with a focus on progression models of resistance training for improving strength. This position stand recommended a variety of approaches to achieve strength goals, including using multiple sets. Since the appearance of that position stand, a number of systematic analyses of the research literature dealing with the issue of single set versus multiple sets have been published. They revealed the following:

- Prior to 1998 the evidence was split, and suggested that there was no difference in strength gains when a single set was compared to multiple sets. However, the use of small sample sizes, very short duration studies, and different methods for measuring strength gains complicated the interpretation of the data. After 1998 most studies showed that multiple sets were better than single sets relative to strength gains, in both short- and long-term studies (18).
- Scientists re-examined all of the literature on this topic by pooling the data from the various studies (to deal with the issues of small sample sizes and short duration studies). This analysis showed that multiple sets were better than single sets, and in the better controlled studies the differences between the two were greater (54).
- Multiple sets were shown to be more effective in increasing strength in trained individuals and over long duration training programs (69).

At this point the evidence suggests that multiple sets are better than single sets relative to gains in maximal strength. However, "when maximal strength gain is not the principal goal of the training program, a single-set protocol may be sufficient to significantly improve upper- and lower-body strength as well as being time efficient" (18). This would appear to support both the "one-set" recommendation for improving and maintaining muscular fitness in the average individual as well as the "multiple set" recommendation for those interested in achieving higher strength goals.

The issue of dose-response was discussed earlier in this chapter relative to health-related outcomes and increases in $\dot{V}O_2$ max. For strength and conditioning programs, two recent comprehensive analyses of the literature suggest the following for *maximal gains* in strength:

- For untrained subjects: do four sets at 60% 1-RM, three days a week (55).
- For trained subjects: do four sets at 80% 1-RM, two days a week (55).
- For athletes: do eight sets at 85% 1-RM, two days a week (46).

IN SUMMARY

- A logical progression of physical activities is from walking to jogging to games. The progression addresses issues of intensity, as well as the risk of injury. For many, walking may be their only aerobic activity.
- Strength and flexibility activities should be included as a regular part of an exercise program.

ENVIRONMENTAL CONCERNS

It is important that the participant be educated about the effects of extreme heat and humidity, altitude, and cold on the adaptation to exercise. The THR range acts as a guide in that it provides feedback to the participant about the interaction of the environment and the exercise intensity. As the heat and humidity increase, there is an increased need to circulate additional blood to the skin to dissipate the heat. As altitude increases, there is less oxygen bound to hemoglobin, and the person must pump more blood to the muscles to have the same oxygen delivery. In both of these situations the HR response to a fixed work bout will be higher. To counter this tendency and stay in the THR range, the subject should decrease the work rate. Exercise in most cold environments can be refreshing and safe if a person plans in advance and dresses accordingly. However, there are some

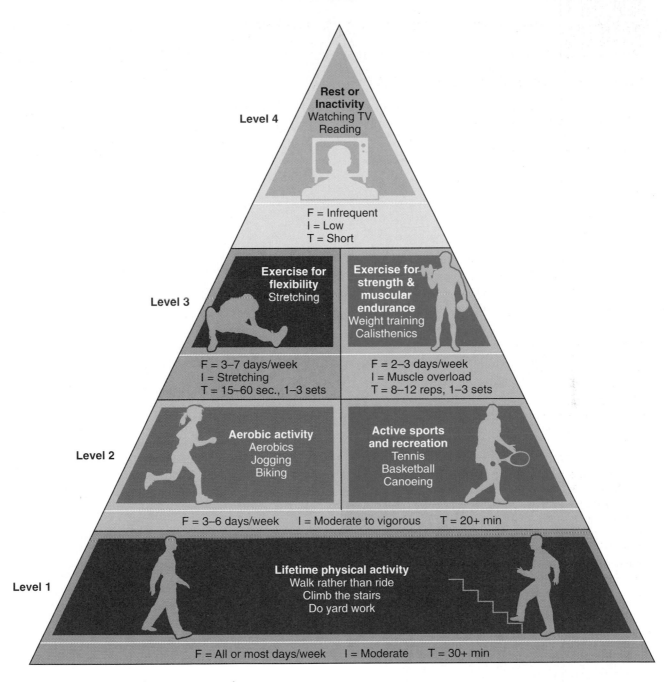

FIGURE 16.6 The physical activity pyramid.

temperature/wind combinations that should be avoided because of the inability to adapt to them. As mentioned previously, some people simply plan exercise indoors (shopping malls, health spas, home exercise) during those occasions so that their routine is not interrupted. These environmental factors will be considered in more detail in chapter 24.

IN SUMMARY

- The THR acts as a guide to adjust exercise intensity in adverse environments such as high temperature and humidity, or altitude.
- A decrease in exercise intensity will counter the effects of high environmental temperature and humidity to allow one to stay in the target HR zone.

STUDY QUESTIONS

1. What are the practical implications of classifying physical inactivity as a primary risk factor?
2. From a public health standpoint, why is there so much attention paid to increasing a sedentary person's physical activity by a small amount rather than recommending strenuous exercise?
3. What is the risk of cardiac arrest for someone who participates in a regular physical activity program?
4. What is the difference between "exercise" and "physical activity"?
5. List the optimal frequency, intensity, and duration of exercise needed to achieve an increase in cardiorespiratory function.
6. For a person with a maximal heart rate of 180 b · min^{-1} and a resting heart rate of 70 b · min^{-1}, calculate a target heart rate range by the Karvonen method and the percent of maximal HR method.
7. Recommend an appropriate progression of activities for a sedentary person wishing to become fit.
8. Why is it important to monitor heart rate frequently during exercise in heat, humidity, and at altitude?

SUGGESTED READINGS

American College of Sports Medicine. 2006. ACSM's *Resource Manual for Guidelines for Exercise Testing and Prescription*. 5th ed. Baltimore: Lippincott Williams & Wilkins.

Baechle, T. R., and R. W. Earle. 2000. *Essentials of Strength Training and Conditioning*. Champaign, IL: Human Kinetics.

Faigenbaum, A. D., and K. J. McInnis. 2003. Guidelines for muscular strength and endurance training. In *Health Fitness Instructor's Handbook*. 4th ed. E. T. Howley and B. D. Franks (eds). Champaign, IL: Human Kinetics.

Howley, E. T., and B. Don Franks. 2003. *Health Fitness Instructor's Handbook*. 4th ed. Champaign, IL: Human Kinetics.

Liemohn, W. P. 2003. Exercise prescription for flexibility and low-back function. In *Health Fitness Instructor's Handbook*. 4th ed. E. T. Howley and B. D. Franks (eds). Champaign, IL: Human Kinetics.

U.S. Department of Health and Human Services. 1996. *Physical Activity and Health: A Report of the Surgeon General*. Atlanta, GA: U.S. Department of Health and Human Services, Centers for Disease Control and Prevention, National Center for Chronic Disease Prevention and Health Promotion.

REFERENCES

1. American College of Sports Medicine. 1998. Position stand: The recommended quantity and quality of exercise for developing and maintaining cardiorespiratory and muscular fitness and flexibility in healthy adults. *Medicine and Science in Sports and Exercise* 30:975–91.
2. American College of Sports Medicine. 2002. Progression models in resistance training for healthy adults. *Medicine and Science in Sports and Exercise* 34:364–80.
3. ———. 1993. Summary statement: Workshop on physical activity and public health. *Sports Medicine Bulletin* 28:7.
4. ———. 2006. ACSM's *Guidelines for Exercise Testing and Prescription*. 7th ed. Baltimore: Lippincott Williams & Wilkins.
5. American Heart Association. 1992. Statement on exercise. *Circulation* 86:340–44.
6. Badenhop, D. T. et al. 1983. Physiologic adjustments to higher- or lower-intensity exercise in elders. *Medicine and Science in Sports and Exercise* 15:496–502.
7. Birk, T. J., and C. A. Birk. 1987. Use of ratings of perceived exertion for exercise prescription. *Sports Medicine* 4:1–8.
8. Blair, S. N., H. W. Kohl III, R. S. Paffenbarger, Jr., D. G. Clark, K. H. Cooper, and L. W. Gibbons. 1989. Physical fitness and all-cause mortality. *Journal of the American Medical Association* 262:2395–2401.
9. Blair, S. N. et al. 1995. Changes in physical fitness and all-cause mortality. *Journal of the American Medical Association* 273:1093–98.
10. Byrd, R. et al. 1999. Strength training: Single versus multiple sets. *Sports Medicine* 27:409–16.
11. Carpinelli, R. N., and R. M. Otto. 1998. Strength training: Single versus multiple sets. *Sports Medicine* 26:73–84.
12. Caspersen, C. J., K. E. Powell, and G. M. Christenson. 1985. Physical activity, exercise, and physical fitness: Definitions and distinctions for health-related research. *Public Health Reports* 100:126–31.
13. Cavanagh, P. R. 1980. *The Running Shoe Book*. Mountain View, CA: Anderson World.
14. Ceci, R., and P. Hassmen. 1991. Self-monitored exercise at three different RPE intensities in treadmill and field running. *Medicine and Science in Sports and Exercise* 23:732–38.
15. Chow, R. J., and J. H. Wilmore. 1984. The regulation of exercise intensity by ratings of perceived exertion. *Journal of Cardiac Rehabilitation* 4:382–87.
16. Dehn, M. M., and C. B. Mullins. 1977. Physiologic effects and importance of exercise in patients with coronary artery disease. *Cardiovascular Medicine* 2:365.
17. Dionne, F. T. et al. 1991. Mitochondrial DNA sequence polymorphism, $\dot{V}O_2$ max, and response to endurance training. *Medicine and Science in Sports and Exercise* 23:177–85.
18. Galvão, D. A., and D. R. Taaffe. 2004. Single- vs. multiple-set resistance training: Recent developments in the controversy. *Journal of Strength & Conditioning Research* 18:660–7.
19. Goodman, L. S., and A. Gilman (eds). 1975. *The Pharmacological Basis of Therapeutics*. New York: Macmillan Publishing Company, Inc.
20. Gutmann, M. C. et al. 1981. Perceived exertion-heart rate relationship during exercise testing and training in cardiac patients. *Journal of Cardiac Rehabilitation* 1:52–59.
21. Hage, P. 1981. Perceived exertion: One measure of exercise intensity. *The Physician and Sportsmedicine* 9(9):136–43.

22. Haskell, W. L. 1985. Physical activity and health: Need to define the required stimulus. *American Journal of Cardiology* 55:4D–9D.

23. ———. 1994. Dose-response issues from a biological perspective. In *Physical Activity, Fitness, and Health*, ed. C. Bouchard, R. J. Shephard, and T. Stevens. 1030–39. Champaign, IL: Human Kinetics.

24. ———. 1999. The issue of dose-response for physical activity and health: Getting the most out of what you put in. Keynote address presented at the ACSM Health and Fitness Summit and Exposition.

25. Haskell, W. L., H. J. Montoye, and D. Orenstein. 1985. Physical activity and exercise to achieve health-related physical fitness components. *Public Health Reports* 100:202–12.

26. Hellerstein, H. K., and R. Ader. 1971. Relationship between percent maximal oxygen uptake (% max $\dot{V}O_2$) and percent maximal heart rate (% MHR) in normals and cardiacs (ASHD). *Circulation* 43–44 (Suppl. II):76.

27. Hellerstein, H. K. et al. 1973. Principles of exercise prescription for normals and cardiac subjects. In *Exercise Training in Coronary Heart Disease*, ed. J. P. Naughton and H. K. Hellerstein., 129–67. New York: Academic Press.

28. Hellerstein, H. K., and B. A. Franklin. 1984. Exercise testing and prescription. In *Rehabilitation of the Coronary Patient*, 2d ed., N. K. Wenger and H. K. Hellerstein. 197–284. New York: Wiley.

29. Hetzler, R. K., R. L. Seip, S. H. Boutcher, E. Pierce, D. Snead, and A. Weltman. 1991. *Medicine and Science in Sports and Exercise* 23:88–92.

30. Howley, E. T. 2001. Type of activity: Resistance, aerobic and leisure versus occupational physical activity. *Medicine and Science in Sports and Exercise* 33:S364–69.

31. Howley, E. T., and B. D. Franks. 2003. *Health Fitness Instructor's Handbook*. 4th ed. Champaign, IL: Human Kinetics.

32. Jennings, G. L. et al. 1991. What is the dose-response relationship between exercise training and blood pressure? *Annals of Medicine* 23:313–18.

33. Jian, L., Z. J. Shen, A. H. Lee, and C. W. Binns. 2005. Moderate physical activity and prostate cancer risk: A case-control study in China. *European Journal of Epidemiology* 20:155–60.

34. Karvonen, J., and T. Vuorimaa. 1988. Heart rate and exercise intensity during sports activities: Practical application. *Sports Medicine* 5:303–12.

35. Karvonen, M. J., E. Kentala, and O. Mustala. 1957. The effects of training heart rate: A longitudinal study. *Annales of Medicinae Experimentalis et Biologiae Fenniae* 35:307–15.

36. Kasaniemi, Y. A., E. Danforth, Jr., M. D. Jensen, P. G. Kopelman, P. Lefebvre, and B. A. Reeder. 2001. Dose-response issues concerning physical activity and health: An evidenced-based symposium. *Medicine and Science in Sports and Exercise* 33 (Supp):S351–58.

37. Lee, I-M., C. Hsieh, and R. S. Paffenbarger. 1995. Exercise intensity and longevity in men. *Journal of the American Medical Association* 273:1179–84.

38. Londeree, B. R., and S. A. Ames. 1976. Trend analysis of the % $\dot{V}O_2$ max – HR regression. *Medicine and Science in Sports* 8:122–25.

39. Morgans, L. F. et al. 1987. Heart rate responses during singles and doubles tennis competition. *The Physician and Sportsmedicine* 15(7):67–74.

40. Oguma, Y., and T. Shinoda-Tagawa. 2004. Physical activity decreases cardiovascular disease risk in women: Review and meta-analysis. *American Journal of Preventive Medicine* 26:407–18.

41. Paffenbarger, R. S., and W. E. Hale. 1975. Work activity and coronary heart mortality. *New England Journal of Medicine* 292 (March 13):545–50.

42. Paffenbarger, R. S., R. T. Hyde, and A. L. Wing. 1986. Physical activity, all cause mortality, and longevity of college alumni. *New England Journal of Medicine* 314 (March 6):605–13.

43. ———. 1990. Physical activity and physical fitness as determinants of health and longevity. In *Exercise, Fitness and Health*, ed. C. Bouchard, R. J. Shephard, T. Stevens, J. R. Sutton, and B. D. McPherson. 33–48. Champaign, IL: Human Kinetics.

44. Paffenbarger, R. S. et al. 1993. The association of changes in physical-activity level and other lifestyle characteristics with mortality among men. *New England Journal of Medicine* 328:538–45.

45. Pate, R. R. et al. 1995. Physical activity and public health. *Journal of the American Medical Association* 273:402–7.

46. Peterson, M. D., M. R. Rhea, and B. A. Alvar. 2004. Maximizing strength development in athletes: A meta-analysis to determine the dose-response relationship. *Journal of Strength & Conditioning Research* 18:377–82.

47. Pollock, M. L. 1978. How much exercise is enough? *The Physician and Sportsmedicine* 6:50–64.

48. Pollock, M. L. et al. 1972. Effect of training two days per week at different intensities on middle-aged men. *Medicine and Science in Sports* 4:192–97.

49. Pollock, M. L. et al. 1975. Effects of mode of training on cardiovascular functions and body composition of adult men. *Medicine and Science in Sports and Exercise* 7:139–45.

50. Pollock, M. L. et al. 1977. Effects of frequency and duration of training on attrition and incidence of injury. *Medicine and Science in Sports* 9:31–36.

51. Pollock, M. L., and J. H. Wilmore. 1990. *Exercise in Health and Disease*. 2d ed. Philadelphia: W. B. Saunders.

52. Porcari, J. P., C. B. Ebbling, A. Ward, P. S. Freedson, and J. M. Rippe. 1989. Walking for exercise testing and training. *Sports Medicine* 8:189–200.

53. Powell, K. E., P. D. Thompson, and C. J. Caspersen. 1987. Physical activity and the incidence of coronary heart disease. *Annals Review of Public Health* 8:253–87.

54. Rhea, M. R., B. A. Alvar, and L. N. Burkett. 2002. Single versus multiple sets for strength: A meta-analysis to address the controversy. *Research Quarterly for Exercise and Sport* 73:485–88.

55. Rhea, M. R., B. A. Alvar, L. N. Burkett, and S. D. Ball. 2003. A meta-analysis to determine the dose response for strength development. *Medicine and Science in Sports and Exercise* 35:456–64.

56. Robertson, R. J. et al. 1990. Cross-modal exercise prescription at absolute and relative oxygen uptake using perceived exertion. *Medicine and Science in Sports and Exercise* 22:653–59.

57. Saltin, B., and P. D. Gollnick. 1983. Skeletal muscle adaptability: Significance for metabolism and performance. In *Handbook of Physiology*, ed. L. D. Peachey, R. H. Adrian, and S. R. Geiger. Section 10: Skeletal Muscle, chap. 19. Baltimore: Lippincott Williams & Wilkins.

58. Seip, R. L. et al. 1991. Perceptual responses and blood lactate concentration: Effect of training state. *Medicine and Science in Sports and Exercise* 23:80–87.

59. Siscovick, D. S. et al. 1984. The incidence of primary cardiac arrest during vigorous exercise. *New England Journal of Medicine* 311:874–77.

60. Siscovick, D. S. et al. 1984. Habitual vigorous exercise and primary cardiac arrest: Effect of other risk factors on the relationship. *Journal of Chronic Disease* 37:625–31.

61. Swain, D. P. 1999. $\dot{V}O_2$ reserve—a new method for exercise prescription. ACSM's *Health and Fitness Journal* 3: 10–14.

62. Swain, D. P., and B. C. Leutholtz. 1997. Heart rate reserve is equivalent to % $\dot{V}O_2$ reserve, not % $\dot{V}O_2$ max. *Medicine and Science in Sports and Exercise* 29:410–14.

63. Swain, D. P., B. C. Leutholtz, M. E. King, L. A. Haas, and J. D. Branch. 1998. Relationship between heart rate reserve and % $\dot{V}O_2$ reserve in treadmill exercise. *Medicine and Science in Sports and Exercise* 30:318–21.

64. Swain, D. P., and B. A. Franklin. 2002. $\dot{V}O_2$ reserve and the minimal intensity for improving cardiorespiratory fitness. *Medicine and Science in Sports and Exercise* 34:152–57.

65. Tanaka, H., K. D. Monahan, and D. R. Seals. 2001. Age-predicted maximal heart rate revisited. *Journal of the American College of Cardiology* 37:153–56.

66. U.S. Department of Health and Human Services. 1990. *Healthy People 2000: National Health Promotion and Disease Prevention Objectives*. Washington, D.C.: U.S. Government Printing Office.

67. U.S. Department of Health and Human Services. 1996. *Physical Activity and Health: A Report of the Surgeon General*. Atlanta, GA: U.S. Department of Health and Human Services, Centers for Disease Control and Prevention, National Center for Chronic Disease Prevention and Health Promotion.

68. Wenger, H. A., and G. J. Bell. 1984. The interactions of intensity, frequency and duration of exercise training in altering cardiorespiratory fitness. *Sports Medicine* 3: 346–56.

69. Wolfe, B. L., L. M. LeMura, and P. J. Cole. 2004. Quantitative analysis of single- vs. multiple-set programs in resistance training. *Journal of Strength & Conditioning Research* 18:35–47.

CHAPTER 17

Exercise for Special Populations

■ Objectives

By studying this chapter, you should be able to do the following:

1. Describe the difference between type 1 and type 2 diabetes.

2. Contrast how a diabetic responds to exercise when blood glucose is "in control," compared to when it is not.

3. Explain why exercise may complicate the life of a type 1 diabetic, while being a recommended and primary part of a type 2 diabetic's lifestyle.

4. Describe the changes in diet and insulin that might be made prior to a diabetic undertaking an exercise program.

5. Describe the sequence of events leading to an asthma attack, and how cromolyn sodium and β-adrenergic agonists act to prevent and/or relieve an attack.

6. Describe the cause of exercise-induced asthma, and how one may deal with this problem.

7. Contrast chronic obstructive pulmonary disease (COPD) with asthma in terms of causes, prognosis, and the role of rehabilitation programs in a return to "normal" function.

8. Identify the types of patient populations that one might see in a cardiac rehabilitation program, and the types of medications that these individuals may be taking.

9. Contrast the type of exercise test used for cardiac populations with the test used for the apparently healthy population.

10. Describe the physiological changes in the elderly that result from an endurance-training program.

11. Describe the guidelines for exercise programs for pregnant women.

■ Outline

Diabetes   338
   Exercise and the Diabetic   339

Asthma   342
   Diagnosis and Causes   342
   Prevention/Relief of Asthma   343

Exercise-Induced Asthma   343

Chronic Obstructive Pulmonary Disease   345
   Testing and Training   345

Hypertension   346

Cardiac Rehabilitation   347
   Population   347
   Testing   348
   Exercise Programs   348

Exercise for Older Adults   349

Exercise During Pregnancy   352

■ Key Terms

arrhythmias
beta-receptor agonist (β_2-agonist)
coronary artery bypass graft surgery (CABGS)
cromolyn sodium

diabetic coma
immunotherapy
insulin shock
ketosis
mast cell

myocardial infarction (MI)
nitroglycerin
percutaneous transluminal coronary angioplasty (PTCA)
theophylline

Chapter 16 presented some recommendations for planning an appropriate exercise program for the apparently healthy individual. Exercise has also been used as a primary nonpharmacological intervention for a variety of problems, such as obesity and mild hypertension, and as a normal part of therapy for the treatment of diabetes and coronary heart disease. This chapter will discuss the special concerns that must be addressed when exercise is used for populations with specific diseases, disabilities, or limitations. However, the student of exercise science should recognize that this information is introductory in nature. More detailed accounts are cited throughout the chapter.

DIABETES

Diabetes is a disease characterized by an absolute (type 1) or relative (type 2) insulin deficiency that results in hyperglycemia (elevated blood glucose concentration) (2, 115). Diabetes is a major health problem and leading cause of death in the United States, representing a total (direct and indirect) annual cost of $132 billion in 2002. Of the more than 18.2 million individuals with diabetes, only 13 million are diagnosed, and the disease is not evenly distributed in the population. The prevalence of diabetes is greater in older (18.3% in those over age sixty-five) than younger (8.7% in those age twenty and older) individuals, and is more common in Native Americans, African Americans, Hispanic Americans, and Asian and Pacific Island Americans (29). Diabetes injures and kills indirectly by causing blindness, kidney disease, heart disease, stroke, and peripheral vascular disease (9, 24, 25). Diabetics are divided into two distinct groups on the basis of whether or not the diabetes is caused by lack of insulin (type 1), or a resistance to insulin (type 2). Type 1, insulin-dependent diabetes, develops pri-

marily in young persons and is associated with viral (flu-like) infections. The warning signs, which develop quickly, consist of (24, 25, 118):

- frequent urination/unusual thirst,
- extreme hunger,
- rapid weight loss, weakness, and fatigue, and
- irritability, nausea, and vomiting.

Since type 1 diabetics do not produce insulin, they are dependent on exogenous (injected) insulin to maintain the blood glucose concentration within normal limits. Type 2, non-insulin-dependent, diabetes develops more slowly and later in life than does type 1 diabetes. Type 2 diabetes represents about 90% to 95% of all diabetics (11), and it is primarily linked to upper-body or android obesity. The increased mass of fat tissue results in a resistance to insulin, which is usually available in adequate amounts within the body. However, some type 2 diabetics may require injectable insulin or an oral medication that stimulates the pancreas to produce additional insulin. The treatment of type 2 diabetics includes diet (9) and exercise (10) to reduce body weight and to help control plasma glucose. Table 17.1 summarizes the differences between type 1 and type 2 diabetics (16, 26).

IN SUMMARY

- Type 1, or insulin-dependent, diabetes develops early in life and represents 5% to 10% of the diabetic population.
- Type 2, or insulin-resistant, diabetes occurs later in life and is associated with upper-body or android obesity. Diet and exercise are important parts of the treatment program for type 2 diabetes to achieve weight loss and improved insulin sensitivity.

TABLE 17.1	Summary of the Differences Between Type 1 and Type 2 Diabetes	
Characteristics	**Type 1 Insulin-Dependent**	**Type 2 Noninsulin-Dependent**
Another name	Juvenile-onset	Adult-onset
Proportion of all diabetics	~10%	~90%
Age at onset	<20	>40
Development of disease	Rapid	Slow
Family history	Uncommon	Common
Insulin required	Always	Common, but not always
Pancreatic insulin	None, or very little	Normal or higher
Ketoacidosis	Common	Rare
Body fatness	Normal/lean	Generally obese

From Berg (16) and Cantu (26).

Exercise and the Diabetic

In chapter 5 we indicated that exercise increases the rate at which glucose leaves the blood. In this way exercise has been viewed as a useful part of the treatment to regulate blood glucose in the diabetic. However, this beneficial effect of exercise is dependent on whether or not the diabetic is in reasonable "control" before exercise begins. Control means that the blood glucose concentration is close to normal. Figure 17.1 shows the effect of a prolonged exercise bout on diabetics who were in control versus those who had not taken an adequate amount of insulin. A lack of insulin causes **ketosis,** a metabolic acidosis resulting from the accumulation of too many ketone bodies (short-chain fatty acids). The type 1 diabetic who was in control shows a decrease in plasma glucose toward normal values during exercise, suggesting better control. On the other hand, those type 1 diabetics who did not inject an adequate amount of insulin before exercise show an increase in plasma glucose (10, 13). Why the difference in response? The controlled diabetic has sufficient insulin such that glucose can be taken up into muscle during exercise and can counter the normal increase in glucose release from the liver due to the action of catecholamines and glucagon (see chapter 5). In contrast, the diabetic with inadequate insulin experiences only a small increase in glucose utilization by muscle, but has the normal increase in glucose release from the liver. This, of course, causes an elevation of the plasma glucose, resulting in hyperglycemia (122).

Figure 17.2 summarizes these effects and adds one more (71). If an insulin-dependent diabetic starts exercise with too much insulin, the rate at which plasma glucose is used by muscle is accelerated, while glucose release from the liver is decreased. This causes a very dangerous hypoglycemic response. This information is crucial to understanding how to prescribe exercise for diabetics. Because the importance of exercise as a part of a treatment plan is different for type 1 and type 2 diabetics, we will discuss each type separately.

Type 1 Diabetes For many years exercise was one part of the treatment for type 1 diabetes, with insulin and diet being the other two (74). However, as mentioned earlier, if a diabetic is not in control prior to exercise, the ability to maintain a reasonable plasma glucose concentration may be compromised. Further, exercise programs, by themselves, have not been shown to improve control of blood glucose (9). The greatest concern is not the hyperglycemia and ketosis that can lead to **diabetic coma** when too little insulin is present; rather it is the possibility of hypoglycemia, which can lead to **insulin shock.** Richter and Galbo (100) and Kemmer and Berger (74) point out the difficulties a type 1 diabetic has starting an exercise

FIGURE 17.1 Effect of prolonged exercise on blood glucose and ketone body levels in normal subjects, diabetics in "control," and diabetics taking an inadequate amount of insulin (ketosis). From M. Berger et al., 1977, "Metabolic and Hormonal Effects of Muscular Exercise in Juvenile Type Diabetics" in *Diabetologia*, 13:355–65. Copyright © 1977 Springer-Verlag, New York, NY. Reprinted by permission.

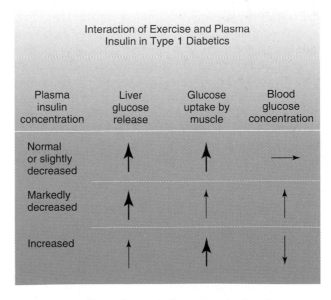

FIGURE 17.2 Effect of varied plasma insulin levels in type 1 diabetics on glucose homeostasis during exercise.

program: The person must maintain a regular exercise schedule in terms of intensity, frequency, and duration, as well as altering diet and insulin. Such regimentation is difficult for some to follow, and given the variability in how a diabetic's blood glucose might respond to exercise on a day-to-day basis, the use of exercise as a primary tool in maintaining metabolic control has been diminished (9). Because metabolic control can be achieved by altering insulin and diet based on self-monitored blood glucose, exercise complicates this picture (74, 100). However, considering the importance of physical activity in an individual's life, and the effect of regular activity on CHD risk factors, a type 1 diabetic should not be discouraged from participation in regular exercise—if there are no complications (2, 9, 24, 25, 74, 100).

The type 1 diabetic should have a careful medical exam prior to starting an exercise program. If the diabetic is over thirty, has had type 1 diabetes for more than fifteen years, has type 2 diabetes and is over 35, has one additional risk factor for coronary artery disease (CAD), known or suspected CAD, or microvascular or neurological complications due to diabetes, a graded diagnostic exercise test is recommended (2, 9, 59, 77, 118). This recommendation is based on the observation that strenuous exercise may accelerate or worsen retina, kidney, or peripheral nerve damage that is already present. The concern for the retina is related to the higher blood pressures developed during exercise, while the concern for the kidney is related to the decrease in blood flow to that organ with increasing intensities of exercise. The peripheral nerve damage may block signals coming from the foot such that serious damage may occur before it is perceived. Proper shoes for exercise, as well as the choice of the activity, are important (9, 24, 49, 77, 118).

The primary concern to address when exercise is prescribed for the type 1 diabetic is the avoidance of hypoglycemia. This is achieved through careful self-monitoring of the blood glucose concentration before, during, and after exercise, and varying carbohydrate intake and insulin depending on the exercise intensity and duration, and the fitness of the individual (9):

- Metabolic control before physical activity
  - Avoid physical activity if fasting glucose levels are >250 mg/dl and ketosis is present. Use caution if glucose levels are >300 mg/dl without ketosis.
  - Ingest added carbohydrate if glucose levels are <100 mg/dl.
- Blood glucose monitoring before and after physical activity
  - Identify when changes in insulin or food intake are needed.
  - Learn how blood glucose responds to different types of physical activity.
- Food intake
  - Consume added carbohydrate as needed to prevent hypoglycemia.
  - Carbohydrate-based foods should be readily available during and after physical activity.

The exercise prescription for the type 1 diabetic must also consider other problems associated with this disease: autonomic neuropathy, peripheral neuropathy, retinopathy, and nephropathy. Individuals with autonomic nervous system dysfunction may have abnormal heart rate and blood pressure responses to exercise. Those with peripheral nerve damage may experience pain, impaired balance, weakness, and decreased proprioception. Damage to the retina is common in diabetics and is aggravated by increased blood pressure or any jarring action directed at the head. Finally, kidney damage is also a common experience for those with type 1 diabetes. This can lead to altered blood pressure responses that can affect the retina (9, 24, 77, 118). It should be no surprise that the exercise prescription for the diabetic must address these problems, if they are present. Recommendations include (7, 9, 24, 25, 59, 77, 118):

- exercising three to four days per week (more is fine at moderate intensity); twenty to sixty minutes; 50% to 80% heart rate reserve;
- using non-weight-bearing, low-impact activities (bicycle or stationary cycle, swimming, water exercise), if weight-bearing activities are contraindicated.
- using light weights (40%–60% 1-RM) with fifteen to twenty repetitions and avoiding the Valsalva maneuver; heavy weights are acceptable for athletes with well-controlled diabetes.
- drinking more fluid and carrying a readily available form of carbohydrate and adequate identification, and
- exercising with someone who can help in an emergency.

In conclusion, although exercise may not be viewed as a primary factor in maintaining the blood glucose concentration in the normal range, the fact that type 1 diabetics who stay physically active have fewer diabetic complications is reason enough to pursue the active life (52).

IN SUMMARY

- A sedentary type 1 diabetic has to juggle diet and insulin to achieve control of the blood glucose concentration. An exercise program may complicate matters, and therefore exercise is not viewed as a primary means of achieving "control." In spite of this, the diabetic is encouraged to participate in a regular exercise program to experience its health-related benefits.
- The diabetic may have to increase carbohydrate intake and/or decrease the amount of insulin

RESEARCH FOCUS 17.1

Prevention or Delay of Type 2 Diabetes

Over the past decade, there has been an increase in the prevalence of type 2 diabetes that is linked to the increased prevalence of obesity. A great deal of activity has been under way to try and understand how to prevent or slow down the development of type 2 diabetes. One of the first things is earlier identification of people at risk of type 2 diabetes with the use of the fasting blood glucose and the oral glucose tolerance test (person drinks 75 g of glucose and blood samples are taken at thirty minutes and one, two, and three hours to track how fast glucose is taken up into tissues):

- impaired fasting glucose (IFG): if fasting blood glucose values are ≥100 mg/dl (5.6 mmol/l) but <126 mg/dl (7.0 mmol/l), and
- impaired glucose tolerance (IGT): two-hour value in an oral glucose tolerance test is ≥140 mg/dl (7.8 mmol/l) but <200 mg/dl (11.1 mmol/l).

Those with IFG or IGT are said to be "pre-diabetic" (10). Studies have shown that both drugs and lifestyle modifications can slow down or prevent the development of type 2 diabetes. However, lifestyle changes—increasing physical activity by 150 minutes per week and losing 5% to 10% of body weight seem to be a better approach than using drugs. In addition to dealing with the pre-diabetes problems, the loss of weight and increased physical activity reduce the risk of several cardiovascular risk factors. This "good news" must be balanced by the reality that we need better and cheaper ways to change the eating and physical activity behaviors of the average person.

---

prior to activity to maintain the glucose concentration close to normal *during* the exercise. The extent of these alterations is dependent on a number of factors, including the intensity and duration of the physical activity, the blood glucose concentration prior to the exercise, and the physical fitness of the individual.

Type 2 Diabetes As mentioned earlier, type 2 diabetes occurs later in life, and the patients have a variety of risk factors in addition to their diabetes: hypertension, high cholesterol, obesity, and inactivity (18, 121). Given the magnitude of this problem, more attention is being paid to identifying persons early in the disease process to delay or prevent the problem (see Research Focus 17.1). There is some epidemiological evidence that type 2 diabetes is linked to a lack of physical activity and low fitness, independent of obesity (8, 73, 75). In addition, current research supports the benefits of exercise training in the prevention and treatment of insulin resistance and type 2 diabetes (8, 11, 62, 73). In contrast to the insulin-dependent diabetic whose life may be more complicated (in terms of blood glucose control) at the start of an exercise program, exercise is a primary recommendation for the type 2 diabetic, both to help deal with the obesity that is usually present and to help control blood glucose. The combination of exercise and diet may be sufficient and may eliminate the need for insulin or the oral medication used to stimulate insulin secretion (8, 11, 26, 42, 54, 73, 115). Because type 2 diabetics represent about 90% of the whole population of diabetics, and because type 2 diabetes occurs later in life (after forty years of age), it is not uncommon to see such individuals in adult fitness programs. It is important for clear communication to exist between the participant and the exercise leader, in order to reduce the chance of a "surprise" hypoglycemic response.

Noninsulin-dependent diabetics do not experience the same fluctuations in blood glucose during exercise as do the type 1 diabetics (49); however, those taking oral medication to stimulate insulin secretion may have to decrease their dosage to maintain a normal blood glucose concentration (100). The exercise prescription for the type 2 diabetic is similar to that described in chapter 16 for improving $\dot{V}O_2$ max: dynamic aerobic activity, done at 50% to 90% maximal heart rate, for twenty to sixty minutes, four to seven times per week (2, 6, 8, 24, 25, 118, 133). Strength training with light weights is also recommended (8, 9, 24, 110, 118). However, some important distinctions need to be mentioned:

- The frequency should be as high as four to seven times per week to promote a sustained increase in insulin sensitivity and to facilitate weight loss and weight maintenance.
- Individuals should strive to achieve a *minimum* of 1,000 kcal per week from all physical activities.

As with all exercise programs for deconditioned individuals, it is more important to do too little than too much at the start of a program. By starting with moderate activity and gradually increasing the duration, exercise can be done each day. This will provide an opportunity to learn how to maintain adequate control of blood glucose while minimizing the chance of a hypoglycemic response. In addition, a "habit" of

---

exercise will develop that is crucial if one is to realize the benefits, since the exercise-induced increase in insulin sensitivity does not last long (101, 121). Further, the combination of intensity, frequency, and duration mentioned previously has been shown to directly benefit those with borderline hypertension, a condition often associated with type 2 diabetes. Consistent with the recommendations for the type 1 diabetic, clear identification and a readily available source of carbohydrate should be carried along in any exercise session. In addition, it would be much safer for a diabetic to exercise with someone who could help out if a problem occurred.

Exercise is only one part of the treatment; diet is the other. The American Diabetes Association (9) states that there are four goals related to nutrition therapy for all diabetics:

- Attain and maintain optimum metabolic outcomes, including:
  - blood glucose levels in the normal range or as close to normal as is safely possible to prevent or reduce the risk of complications of diabetes;
  - a lipid and lipoprotein profile that reduces the risk of macrovascular disease; and
  - blood pressure level that reduces the risk of vascular disease.
- Prevent and treat the chronic complications of diabetes. Modify nutrient intake and lifestyle as appropriate for the prevention and treatment of obesity, dyslipidemia, cardiovascular disease, hypertension, and nephropathy.
- Improve health through healthy food choices and physical activity.
- Address individual nutritional needs taking into consideration personal and cultural preferences and lifestyle while respecting the individual's wishes and willingness to change.

The emphasis in achieving optimal nutrition is through a high-carbohydrate diet to achieve nutrient goals for protein, vitamins, and minerals. The low-fat diet has been shown to be useful in achieving weight-loss and blood lipid goals as well as diabetic control (9). The type 2 diabetic secures a variety of benefits from proper exercise and dietary practices: lower body fat and weight (see chapter 18), increased HDL cholesterol, increased sensitivity to insulin (decreasing the need), improved capacity for work, and an improved self-concept (16, 76, 121). These changes should not only improve the prognosis of the type 2 diabetic as far as control of blood glucose is concerned, but should also reduce the overall risk of coronary heart disease (100).

IN SUMMARY

- Type 2 diabetics have a variety of risk factors in addition to their diabetes, including hypertension, high cholesterol, obesity, and inactivity.
- An exercise prescription emphasizing low-intensity, long-duration activity that is done almost every day will maximize the benefits related to insulin sensitivity and weight loss.
- The dietary recommendation is for a low-fat diet, similar to what is recommended for all Americans for good health, with the additional goals of achieving normal serum glucose and lipid levels.

ASTHMA

Asthma is a respiratory problem characterized by a shortness of breath accompanied by a wheezing sound. It is due to a contraction of the smooth muscle around the airways, a swelling of the mucosal cells, and a hypersecretion of mucus. The asthma can be caused by an allergic reaction, exercise, aspirin, dust, pollutants, and emotion (88).

Asthma is a very common disease in the United States. In 2003, 20 million persons were affected, resulting in 1.9 million emergency room visits, and more than 4,000 deaths. Estimated direct and indirect costs were $16.1 billion. The large increase in the prevalence of asthma over the past 20 years appears to be leveling off, perhaps due to better management of the problem (http://www.lungusa.org).

Diagnosis and Causes

The diagnosis of asthma is made using pulmonary-function testing. If an obstruction to airflow (e.g., low maximal expiratory flow rate) is corrected by administration of a bronchodilator, then asthma is suspected. An asthma attack is the result of an orderly sequence of events that can be initiated by a wide variety of factors. These events are important if we are to understand how certain medications prevent or relieve the asthmatic attack. Figure 17.3 summarizes these events. The focus of attention is on the **mast cell,** one of the cells that is part of tissue in the bronchial tubes. It is believed that a variety of factors such as dust, chemicals, antibodies, and exercise initiate an asthma attack by increasing Ca^{++} influx into the mast cell, causing a release of chemical mediators such as histamine, leukotrienes, and a special chemical that attracts white blood cells. The mediators, in turn, trigger the following effects:

- increase smooth muscle contraction (via an elevation of Ca^{++} in the muscle cell) leading to bronchoconstriction,

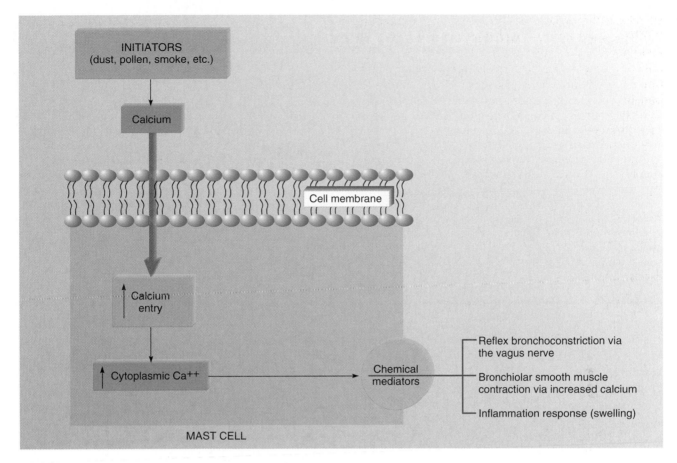

FIGURE 17.3 Proposed mechanism by which an asthma attack is initiated.

- initiate a bronchoconstrictor reflex via the vagus nerve, and
- cause an inflammation response (swelling of tissue).

Given that the vast majority of people do not experience an asthmatic attack while being exposed to these factors, a "sensitivity" or hyperirritability of the respiratory tract is a necessary prerequisite (88).

Prevention/Relief of Asthma

There are a variety of steps that can be taken to prevent the occurrence of an asthmatic attack, and to provide relief should one occur. If a person is sensitive (allergic) to something, then simple avoidance of the allergen will prevent the problem. If a person cannot avoid contact with the allergen, **immunotherapy** may be helpful in making the person less sensitive to the allergen while being treated.

Drugs have been developed to deal with the mast cell, which is a focal point in the asthmatic response, as well as the bronchiolar smooth muscle that causes the decrease in airway diameter. **Cromolyn sodium** inhibits the chemical mediator release from the mast cell, probably by interfering with Ca^{++} influx into the cell. **Beta-receptor agonists (β_2-agonist)** decrease chemical mediator release and cause the relaxation of bronchiolar smooth muscle by decreasing the Ca^{++} concentration in mast and smooth muscle cells. These effects are brought about through increased adenylate cyclase activity leading to an elevation of cytoplasmic cyclic AMP (see chapter 5). **Theophylline,** a caffeine-like drug, aids in bronchiolar smooth muscle relaxation by inhibiting phosphodiesterase, the enzyme that inactivates cyclic AMP. The result is higher cyclic AMP and lower Ca^{++} concentrations in the cell. Corticosteroids and leukotriene inhibitors are used to reduce the inflammation response, which is central to dealing with the long-term management of asthma (32, 90, 94). The net result is that both the inflammation response and the constriction of bronchiolar smooth muscle are blocked.

Exercise-Induced Asthma

A form of asthma that may be of particular interest to the reader is exercise-induced asthma (EIA). The asthmatic attack is caused by exercise and can occur five to fifteen minutes (Early Phase) or four to six hours (Late Phase) after exercise. Approximately 80% of asthmatics experience EIA, versus only 3% to 4% of

Screening for Asthma

Asthma is the leading cause of chronic illness and the most common respiratory disorder in children (36). Concern has been expressed about the need for screening programs early in life to identify those with a high risk of developing asthma. Jones and Bowen (65) measured peak expiratory flow rate before and after an all-out run in children from ten primary schools. Over a six-year follow-up period, they compared children who had a negative result with those who had a positive result (a decrease in peak expiratory flow rate of $\geq 15\%$) due to the exercise test. Of the 864 children not known to have asthma, 60 had a positive test result. A follow-up of 55 of these 60 children showed 32 had developed clinically recognizable asthma six years later. These children also had a significantly higher prevalence of respiratory illnesses. Such field tests have much to offer in gaining control over this disease. In addition to screening, there is strong support to *not* back away from physical activity for asthmatic children. Most studies show that asthmatics can exercise safely and increase their cardiorespiratory fitness. Some scientists believe that the decrease in physical activity in children may have played a role in the recent increase in the prevalence and severity of asthma (82). Finally, schoolchildren should have their medication in the gym area, rather than in a central administrator's office (90).

---

the nonallergic population (120). What is interesting is that 61% of the 1984 U.S. Olympic team members with EIA won an Olympic medal. Furthermore, if one compares 1988 Olympic athletes who experienced EIA with the athletes who did not, one finds no difference in the percentage who won medals (71, 89, 120). Clearly, if anyone wondered whether or not EIA can be controlled, those results should dispel any doubts.

Many causes of EIA have been identified over the past 100 years. These include cold air, hypocapnia (low PCO_2), respiratory alkalosis, and specific intensities and durations of exercise. The focus of attention is now on the *cooling and drying* of the respiratory tract that occurs when large volumes of dry air are breathed during the exercise session (40, 84, 107). Respiratory heat loss is related primarily to the rate of ventilation, with the humidity and the temperature of the inspired air being of secondary and tertiary importance. As you remember from chapter 10, when dry air is taken into the lungs it is moistened and warmed as it moves through the respiratory airways. In this way moisture is evaporated from the surface of the airways, which is therefore cooled.

The proposed mechanism for how EIA is initiated takes us back to the mast cell mentioned earlier. When dry air removes water from the surface of the mast cell, an increase in osmolarity occurs. This increase in osmolarity triggers the influx of Ca^{++} that leads to the increased release of chemical mediators and the narrowing of the airways (40, 70, 107). Although the temperature of the air was believed to contribute to the problem, recent evidence suggests otherwise (43). What kind of circumstances bring on EIA?

The probability of an exercise-induced bronchospasm is related to the type of exercise, the time since the previous bout of exercise, the interval since medication was taken, and the temperature and humidity of the inspired air (107). It has been known since the late 1600s that certain types of exercise cause an attack more readily than others. Running was observed to cause more attacks than cycling or walking which, in turn, caused more than swimming. Interestingly, this old observation still finds support in studies in which the temperature and the humidity of the inspired air are controlled. Running still caused more severe attacks than did swimming, even with oxygen consumption and ventilation matched (107).

Generally, EIA is precipitated more with strenuous, long-duration exercise than the reverse (70, 107). One way to deal with this is to do short-duration exercise (<5 min) at low to moderate intensities. Further, when an exercise session occurs within sixty minutes of a previous EIA attack, the degree of bronchospasm is reduced (40). This suggests that a warm-up within an hour of more strenuous exercise would reduce the severity of an attack, and there is good evidence to support that proposition (87).

There was special concern for the athletes of the 1984 Olympic Games, given the pollution in Los Angeles, which can aggravate an EIA attack (96). As mentioned before, the fact that 61% of the athletes who experienced EIA won Olympic medals suggests that procedures for preventing EIA with medication are generally established. Voy (120) reports that a simple questionnaire identified 90% of the athletes with EIA, even though only 52% were receiving treatment prior to the Olympics. Typically, a strenuous exercise challenge (e.g., running at 85%–90% of maximal heart rate on a treadmill) lasting six to eight minutes is used to evaluate the presence of EIA (7), however, field tests can also be used (see A Closer Look 17.1). In either case, a 15% or greater decrease in forced expiratory flow rate in one second (FEV_1) is classified as a positive test. The medications mentioned earlier were used to manage the condition to allow the athletes to go "all out."

In a majority of cases, EIA can be prevented with the medications mentioned earlier, used alone or in combination (22, 83, 94, 113). The asthmatic who is simply participating in a fitness program should also follow a medication plan to *prevent* the occurrence of an EIA attack. The exercise session should include the conventional warm-up, with mild to moderate activity planned in five-minute segments. Swimming is better than other types of exercise, given that air above the water contains more moisture. A scarf or face mask can be used when exercising outdoors in cold weather to help trap moisture. The participant should carry an inhaler with a β_2-agonist and use it at the first sign of wheezing (1, 51). As with the diabetic, the buddy system is a good plan to follow in case a major attack occurs.

IN SUMMARY

- An asthmatic attack is brought on when an agent causes an increased influx of Ca^{++} into a mast cell in the respiratory tract, which, in turn, triggers the release of chemical mediators. These chemical mediators cause a reflex and calcium-mediated constriction of bronchiolar smooth muscle along with an increase in secretions into the airways.
- Cromolyn sodium and β-adrenergic agonists act to prevent this by preventing the entry of Ca^{++} into the mast cell, and by increasing the level of cyclic AMP in the mast and smooth muscle cells, respectively.
- Drying of the respiratory tract leads to an increase in the osmolarity of the fluid on the surface of a mast cell. This event is believed to be the central factor in the initiation of the asthmatic attack during exercise. Exercise of short duration, preceded by a warm-up, appears to reduce the chance of an attack. Drugs should be used prior to exercise to prevent an attack, and β-adrenergic agonists should be carried along in case one occurs.

CHRONIC OBSTRUCTIVE PULMONARY DISEASE

Chronic obstructive pulmonary diseases (COPD) cause a reduction in airflow that can have a dramatic effect on daily activities. These diseases include chronic bronchitis, emphysema, and bronchial asthma, either alone or in combination. These diseases are distinct from the exercise-induced asthma discussed earlier in

that the airway obstruction remains in spite of continuous medication (34). Chronic bronchitis is characterized by a persistent production of sputum due primarily to a thickened bronchial wall with excess secretions. In emphysema, the elastic recoil of alveoli and bronchioles is reduced and those pulmonary structures are enlarged (19, 105). The patient with developing COPD cannot perform normal activities without experiencing dyspnea, but, tragically, by the time this occurs the disease is already well advanced (19). COPD is characterized by a decreased ability to exhale, and because of the narrowed airways, a "wheezing" sound is made. The person with COPD experiences a decreased capacity for work, which may influence employment, but he/she may also experience an increase in psychological problems, including anxiety (regarding the simple act of breathing) and depression (related to a loss of sense of self-worth).

It should be no surprise then that treatment of COPD includes more than simple medication and oxygen-inhalation therapy. A typical COPD rehabilitation program focuses on the goal of the patient's ability for self-care. To achieve that goal, a number of medical and support personnel are recruited to deal with the various manifestations of the disease process (89, 112). The COPD patient receives education about the different ways to deal with the disease, including breathing exercises, ways to approach the activities of daily living at home, and how to handle work-related problems. The latter can be so affected that new on-the-job responsibilities may have to be assigned, or if the person cannot meet the requirements, retirement may be the only outcome. In order to help deal with these problems, counseling by psychologists and clergy may be needed for patient and family. The extent of these problems is directly related to the severity of the disease. Those with minimal disease may require the help of only a few of the professionals just mentioned, while others with severe disease may require the assistance of all. It is therefore important to understand that the rehabilitation program is very individualized (89, 112).

Testing and Training

The consistent recommendation for anyone with known disease is to have a complete medical exam, including exercise testing, prior to beginning an exercise program (7). This is especially true for COPD patients because the severity of the disease varies greatly. Common tests used to classify COPD patients include the FEV_1, a graded exercise test to evaluate $\dot{V}O_2$ max, maximum exercise ventilation, and changes in the arterial blood gases, PO_2 and PCO_2. Table 17.2 shows a four-point scale used to grade the level of disability (66). It should be clear that there are great

TABLE 17.2 Guide to Grading Disability of COPD Patient (Based on 40-Year-Old Man)

Grade	Cause of Dyspnea	FEV$_1$ (% Predicted)	Max $\dot{V}O_2$ (ml · min^{-1} · kg^{-1})	Exercise Max $\dot{V}_E$ (ℓ · min^{-1})	Blood Gases
1	Fast walking and stair climbing	>60	>25	Not limiting	Normal PaCO$_2$, SaO$_2$
2	Walking at normal pace	<60	<25	>50	Normal PaCO$_2$; SaO$_2$ above 90% at rest and with exercise
3	Slow walking	<40	<15	<50	Normal PaCO$_2$; SaO$_2$ below 90% with exercise
4	Walking limited to less than one block	<40	<7	<30	Elevated PaCO$_2$; SaO$_2$ below 90% at rest and with exercise

From J. S. Skinner, *Exercise Testing and Exercise Prescription of Special Cases.* Copyright © 1987 Lea & Febiger. A Waverly Company, Baltimore, MD. Reprinted by permission.

differences between those with a $\dot{V}O_2$ max greater than 25 ml · kg^{-1} · min^{-1}, and those with a $\dot{V}O_2$ max less than 7 ml · kg^{-1} · min^{-1}. You might also look to the left side of the table to see how little exertion is required of those at Grade 4 to bring on the sensation of dyspnea, and to the far right to see what happens to the blood gases. It is obvious that exercise programming varies with the severity of the disease. While those with a Grade 1 disability can follow the normal exercise prescription process, those with a Grade 4 disability are probably in respiratory and cardiovascular failure. Goals for the latter group are very pragmatic: the ability to do home or work activities, to climb two flights of stairs, and so on, and these activities might require supplemental oxygen or inspiratory pressure support (19, 66, 72, 89). A wide range of exercises (e.g., walking, cycling, swimming, games, resistance training, breathing exercises) can be used to improve the patient's functional capacity (28, 34, 66), which is limited, in part, by skeletal muscle abnormalities (104). Oxygen may be needed to maintain the oxyhemoglobin saturation above 90% (33). What is clear is that the success of the program depends on a good match of the patient's limitations with the appropriate exercises (124). Generally, COPD patients achieve an increase in exercise tolerance without dyspnea and an increase in the sense of well-being, but without a reversal of the disease process (28, 66, 72, 89, 105, 127). The changes in the psychological variables are very important in the long run, given that the person's willingness to continue the exercise program is a major factor determining the rate of decline during the course of the disease (21).

IN SUMMARY

■ Chronic obstructive pulmonary disease (COPD) includes chronic asthma, emphysema, and bronchitis. These latter two diseases create changes in the lung that are irreversible and result in a gradual deterioration of function.
■ Rehabilitation is a multidisciplinary approach involving medication, breathing exercises, dietary therapy, exercise, and counseling. The programs are individually designed due to the severity of the illness, and the goals are very pragmatic in terms of the events of daily living and work.

HYPERTENSION

As mentioned in chapter 14, the risk of coronary heart disease (CHD) increases with increases in resting values of systolic and diastolic blood pressure (67). Blood pressure (BP) classifications have changed over the years, with normal BP being <120/<80 mm Hg. Prehypertension exists when either the systolic BP is 120 to 139 mm Hg or the diastolic BP is 80 to 89 mm Hg. The prehypertension category is not unlike the pre-diabetic category mentioned earlier in the chapter. The idea is to identify potential problems early and try to prevent or delay the development of hypertension. Stage 1 hypertension is a systolic BP of 140 to 159 mm Hg or a diastolic BP of 90 to 99 mm Hg. Approximately 50 million U.S. adults have hypertension (30). These stage 1 individuals represent the majority of all hypertensives, and they account for most of the morbidity and mortality associated with hypertension (53). Although there is little disagreement that medication should be used to treat hypertension, many believe that nonpharmacological approaches should be used for those with mild or borderline hypertension (4, 15, 55, 67, 68, 132). The reasons nonpharmacological approaches are recommended include the possibility of side effects due to medication, and the counterproductive behavioral changes associated with classifying a person as a "patient" (55).

Generally, the person with mild hypertension should have a physical exam to identify potential underlying problems, as well as the presence of other risk factors. Kannel (67) indicates that while medication might be used to control blood pressure when multiple risk factors (smoking, high cholesterol, inactivity, etc.) are present, the simple act of stopping smoking confers more immediate benefit against the overall risk of CHD than any medication. It is within this context that a nonpharmacological intervention program focuses on the use of exercise and diet to control blood pressure and establish behaviors that favorably influence other aspects of health (15, 55).

Dietary recommendations to control blood pressure include a reduction in sodium intake for those sensitive to excess sodium, and in caloric intake for those who are overweight (30). Kaplan's (68) review indicates that salt restriction results in an average reduction in systolic and diastolic blood pressures of 5 and 3 mm Hg, while a 1-kg weight loss is associated with a 1.6 and 1.3 mm Hg reduction, respectively. Endurance exercise is associated with a 10 mm Hg reduction in resting blood pressure in hypertensive individuals; however, the magnitude of the reduction is inversely related to the pretraining blood pressure (4, 45, 55). While not all hypertensive individuals respond to endurance exercise in this way, exercise is recommended for all, since other changes occur to reduce the risk of CHD, even if blood pressure is not reduced (55). The question is, how much exercise?

The standard American College of Sports Medicine exercise prescription for improving $\dot{V}O_2$ max (see chapter 16) is also effective in reducing blood pressure in hypertensive individuals. However, exercise in the moderate intensity range (i.e., 40%–60% of heart rate reserve) is effective and can be accomplished with lifestyle activities as well as structured exercise programs. The recommendation is to do thirty minutes on most, preferably all, days of the week (4, 7, 53, 55, 106, 123). Gordon (53) indicates that the combination of intensity, frequency, and duration should result in a weekly physical activity energy expenditure of 700 (initially) to 2,000 (goal) kcal. In addition to using exercise to lower elevated blood pressure, Gordon recommends that individuals:

- lose weight if overweight,
- limit alcohol intake (<1 ounce per day of ethanol—24 ounces of beer, 8 ounces of wine, or 2 ounces of 100-proof whiskey),
- reduce sodium intake,
- maintain adequate dietary potassium, calcium, and magnesium intake,
- stop smoking, and
- reduce dietary fat, saturated fat, and cholesterol intake.

For recreational athletes who need medication to control blood pressure, the preferred drugs are the angiotensin converting enzyme (ACE) inhibitors and calcium channel blockers (4, 123). Blood pressure should be checked frequently so that the medication regime can be altered by the physician, if necessary.

IN SUMMARY

- Exercise can be used as a nonpharmacological intervention for those with hypertension. Exercise recommendations include light to vigorous activity (40%–85% $\dot{V}O_2$ max), done three or more days per week, and for twenty to sixty minutes per session. For those on medication, blood pressure should be checked frequently.

CARDIAC REHABILITATION

Exercise training is now an accepted part of the therapy used to restore an individual who has some form of coronary heart disease (CHD). The details of how to structure such programs, from the first steps taken after being confined to a bed to the time of returning to work and beyond, are spelled out clearly in books such as ACSM's *Guidelines for Exercise Testing and Prescription* (7), Wenger and Hellerstein's *Rehabilitation of the Coronary Patient* (125), ACSM's *Exercise Management for Persons with Chronic Diseases and Disabilities*, and ACSM's *Resource Manual for Guidelines for Exercise Testing and Prescription* (see the Suggested Readings). This brief section will simply comment on various aspects of such programs.

Population

The persons served by cardiac rehabilitation programs include those who have experienced angina pectoris, myocardial infarctions (MI), coronary artery bypass graft surgery (CABGS), and angioplasty (47). Angina pectoris is the chest pain related to ischemia of the ventricle due to occlusion of one or more of the coronary arteries. The symptoms occur when the work of the heart (estimated by the double product: systolic blood pressure × HR) exceeds a certain value.

Nitroglycerin is used to prevent an attack and/or relieve the pain by relaxing the smooth muscle in veins to reduce venous return and the work of the heart (85). Angina patients may also be treated with a beta blocker like propranolol (Inderal) to reduce the HR and/or blood pressure such that the angina symptoms occur at a later stage into work. Exercise training supports this drug effect: As the person becomes trained, the HR response at any work rate is reduced. This allows the individual to take on more tasks without experiencing the chest pain.

Myocardial infarction (MI) patients have actual heart damage (loss of ventricular muscle) due to a prolonged occlusion of one or more of the coronary arteries. The degree to which left ventricular function is compromised is dependent on the mass of the ventricle permanently damaged. These patients are usually on medications to reduce the work of the heart (β-blocker), and control the irritability of the heart tissue so that dangerous **arrhythmias** (irregular heart rhythms) do not occur. Generally, these patients experience a training effect similar to those who do not have an MI (47).

Coronary artery bypass graft surgery (CABGS) patients have had surgery to bypass one or more blocked coronary arteries. In this procedure, either a saphenous vein or an internal mammary artery from the patient is sutured onto the existing coronary arteries above and below the blockage. The success of the surgery is dependent on the amount of heart damage that existed prior to surgery, as well as the success of the revascularization itself. In those who had chronic angina pectoris prior to CABGS, most find a relief of symptoms, with 70% having no more pain at five-year follow-up (48). Generally, with an increased blood flow to the ventricle there is an improvement in both left ventricular function and the capacity for work (48, 126). These patients benefit from systematic exercise training because most are deconditioned prior to surgery as a result of activity restrictions related to chest pain. In addition, exercise improves the chance that the blood vessel graft will remain open (99). Finally, the cardiac rehabilitation program helps the patient to differentiate angina pain from chest wall pain related to the surgery. The overall result is a smoother and less traumatic transition back to normal function.

Some CHD patients undergo **percutaneous transluminal coronary angioplasty (PTCA)** to open occluded arteries. In this procedure the chest is not opened; instead, a balloon-tipped catheter (a long, slender tube) is inserted into the coronary artery, where the balloon is inflated to push the plaque back toward the arterial wall (48, 116). "Stents" may be used in the PTCA procedure to help keep the artery open. These do not appear to affect the accuracy of angina or exercise test results in predicting closure of the artery (79).

Testing

The testing of patients with CHD is much more involved than that presented for the apparently healthy person in chapter 15 (41). There are classes of CHD patients for whom exercise or exercise testing is inappropriate and dangerous (7). The PAR_x screening form in appendix C lists some absolute and relative contraindications for exercise. For those who can be tested, a twelve-lead ECG is monitored at discrete intervals during the GXT, while a variety of leads are displayed continuously on an oscilloscope. Blood pressure, RPE, and various signs or symptoms are also noted. The criteria for terminating the GXT go well beyond achieving a certain percentage of maximal HR, focusing instead on various pathological signs (e.g., ST-segment depression) and symptoms, such as angina pectoris. On the basis of the response to the GXT, the person may be referred for additional testing, such as the use of radioactive molecules to evaluate perfusion ([201] thallium) and the capacity of the ventricle to eject blood ([99] technetium), or direct angiography, in which a dye that is opaque to X rays is injected into the coronary arteries to determine the blockage directly (98). The results of all the tests are used to classify the individual as a low-, intermediate-, or high-risk patient. The resulting classification has a major impact on deciding whether or not to use exercise as a part of the rehabilitation process and, if exercise is appropriate, determines the type and format of the exercise program (7).

Exercise Programs

Cardiac rehabilitation includes a "Phase I" inpatient exercise program that is used to help the patients make the transition from the cardiovascular event (e.g., a myocardial infarction that put them in the hospital) to the time of discharge from the hospital. The specific signs and symptoms exhibited by the patient are used to determine whether the patient should be placed in an exercise program, and if so, when to terminate the exercise session (7). Once the patient is discharged from the hospital, a "Phase II" program can be started. This program resembles the one mentioned earlier for apparently healthy persons in that warm-up with stretching, endurance, and strengthening exercises, and cool-down activities are included. However, the CHD patients, who are generally very deconditioned ($\dot{V}O_2$ max of ~20 ml · kg^{-1} · min^{-1}), require only light exercise to achieve their target heart rate (THR). In addition, because these patients are on a wide variety of medications that may decrease maximal heart rate, the THR zone is determined from their GXT results; the 220 − age formula cannot be used. The patients usually begin with intermittent low-intensity exercise (one minute on, one minute off) using a variety of exercises to distribute the total work output over a larger muscle mass. In time, the patient increases the duration of the work period for each exercise. The strengthening exercises emphasize a low resistance and high repetition format to involve the major muscle groups; free and machine weights can be used in a circuit program format (7, 38, 119). Given that CABGS and post-MI patients have had direct damage to their hearts, the exercise should facilitate, not interfere with, the healing process. As you might guess, given the nature of the patient and the risk involved, cardiac rehabilitation programs take place in hospitals and clinics where there is direct medical supervision and the capacity to deal with emergencies, should they occur. After a patient completes an eight- to twelve-week "Phase II" program, the person may continue in a "Phase III" program away from the hospital where there is less supervision, except for the ability to respond to an emergency (7, 98). What are the benefits of such programs to the patient with CHD?

Effects There is no question that CHD patients have improved cardiovascular function as a result of an exercise program. This is shown in higher $\dot{V}O_2$ max values, higher work rates achieved without ischemia as shown by angina pectoris or ST-segment changes, and an increased capacity for prolonged submaximal work (47, 48, 98, 103, 125). The improved lipid profile (lower total cholesterol and higher HDL cholesterol) is a function of more than the exercise alone, given that weight loss and the saturated fat content of the diet can modify these variables (13, 95). It must be mentioned that a cardiac rehabilitation program should not be viewed simply as an exercise program. It is a multi-intervention effort involving exercise, medication, diet, and counseling.

IN SUMMARY

- Cardiac rehabilitation programs include a wide variety of patients, including those having angina pectoris, bypass surgery, myocardial infarctions, and angioplasty. These patients may be taking nitroglycerin to control angina symptoms, β-blockers to reduce the work of the heart, or anti-arrhythmia medications to control dangerous heart rhythms.
- The exercise tests for CHD patients include a twelve-lead ECG and are used for referral to other tests. Exercise programs bring about large changes in functional capacity in these populations due to their low starting point. The programs are gradual and are based on their entry-level exercise tests and other clinical findings.

EXERCISE FOR OLDER ADULTS

The number of older individuals (over age sixty-five) in the United States will double between 2000 and 2030 as the "baby boom" generation comes to full maturity. Older individuals are a special challenge from the standpoint of exercise prescription due to the usual presence of chronic disease and physical activity limitations. However, participation in physical activity and exercise will go a long way in preventing the progress of diseases and in extending the years of independent living (60).

Maximal aerobic power decreases in the average population after the age of twenty at the rate of about 1% per year. A report by Kasch et al (69) shows that not only can this decline be interrupted by a physical activity program, but middle-aged men who maintain their activity and body weight show half the expected decrease in $\dot{V}O_2$ max over a twenty-year period. The same is apparently not the case for women (see A Closer Look 17.2). This is consistent with an analysis of cross-sectional and longitudinal data showing that the decrease in $\dot{V}O_2$ max with age is related to a decrease in physical activity and an increase in percent body fat (63). Unfortunately, the vast majority of people experience a steady decline in $\dot{V}O_2$ max so that by sixty years of age, their ability to engage comfortably in normal activities is reduced. This initiates a vicious cycle that leads to lower and lower levels of cardiorespiratory fitness, which may not allow them to perform daily tasks. In turn, this affects elderly people's quality of life and independence, which may necessitate reliance on others (108). A physical activity program is useful in dealing not only with this downward spiral of cardiorespiratory fitness but also with the osteoporosis that is related to the sudden hip fractures that can lead to more inactivity and death (108).

Osteoporosis is a loss of bone mass that primarily affects women over fifty years of age and is responsible for 1.5 million fractures annually (78). Type I osteoporosis is related to vertebral and distal radius fractures in fifty- to sixty-five-year-olds, and is eight times more common in women than men. Type II osteoporosis, found in those aged seventy and above, results in hip, pelvic, and distal humerus fractures and is twice as common in women (20, 64). The problem is more common in women over age fifty due to menopause and the lack of estrogen. Hormone replacement therapy (HRT) initiated early in menopause prevents bone loss and can increase bone mineral density and reduce fracture risk (20, 80). However, such treatments are not without risks. HRT has been associated with an increase in cardiovascular disease and mortality and an increased risk of certain cancers (93). Given

A CLOSER LOOK 17.2

Changes in $\dot{V}O_2$ Max with Age in Women

A recent study (46) has called into question some of our accepted wisdom about the change in $\dot{V}O_2$ max with age and the effect of fitness on that response. The authors' systematic and analytical review of the literature (a meta-analysis) showed that in endurance-trained women, $\dot{V}O_2$ max fell 6.2 ml $\cdot$ kg^{-1} $\cdot$ min^{-1} per decade, in contrast to 4.4 ml $\cdot$ kg^{-1} $\cdot$ min^{-1} and 3.5 ml $\cdot$ kg^{-1} $\cdot$ min^{-1} for active and sedentary women, respectively. This was different from what had been observed in men, and about whom most of the "accepted wisdom" had been based. It must be noted, however, that when these absolute changes (ml $\cdot$ kg^{-1} $\cdot$ min^{-1}) were expressed as a percentage of their respective $\dot{V}O_2$ max values, the percent decline was about 10% per decade for all groups, which is similar to what has been measured in sedentary men. Why did the most highly fit female subjects experience the largest change in $\dot{V}O_2$ max with age?

The investigators examined the decreases in maximal heart rate with age in these three groups to see if it might help explain why $\dot{V}O_2$ max decreased fastest in the most-fit group. Unfortunately, the decline in maximal heart rate was very similar across the three groups (7.0 to 7.9 beats $\cdot$ min^{-1} per decade) and could not explain why the most-fit group had the fastest decline in $\dot{V}O_2$ max. The authors suggested the following possibilities:

- Baseline effect. Those with the highest $\dot{V}O_2$ max values had the greatest decline. A parallel observation was found in comparisons between men and women. On average, young men have higher $\dot{V}O_2$ max values than young women; the men also have a greater decrease in $\dot{V}O_2$ max with age. However, the percent decline is about 10% per decade for both genders, similar to what has been observed for the three groups of women.
- The most-fit women were found to have a greater decrease in

their training stimulus with age, compared with sedentary women (since the sedentary women were just that, sedentary, their "change" would have been modest at best). The large reduction in training volume as they aged would help explain why the most-fit women had the greatest loss in $\dot{V}O_2$ max.
- An increase in body weight in adults with age is associated with a decline in $\dot{V}O_2$ max. (ml $\cdot$ kg^{-1} $\cdot$ min^{-1}). The authors wondered if a difference in weight gain could help explain why the most-fit (least-fat) subjects had the greatest decrease in $\dot{V}O_2$ max. Interestingly, they found no support for this in their data analysis.

The authors remind us that, in spite of these observations, men and women of any age who participate regularly in endurance training have higher $\dot{V}O_2$ max values than their less-active counterparts.

---

that prevention is better than treatment, attention is focused on adequate dietary calcium (57) and exercise throughout life (108).

Dietary calcium is important in preventing and treating osteoporosis. While the daily calcium requirement is 1,000 mg $\cdot$ d^{-1}, no group of adult women meets that standard (92). In an attempt to prevent osteoporosis, attention is directed at young women (under age twenty-five) to maximize bone growth. The calcium requirement is set to 1,200 to 1,500 mg/day to accomplish that.

Bone structure is maintained by the force of gravity (upright posture), and the lateral forces associated with muscle contraction. Weight-bearing activities (walking, jogging) are better than bicycling and swimming for maintaining spine and hip mineral, but for the low fit or those with previous fractures, these latter activities are recommended (108). Further, it may be safer to stay with a walking program rather than move to a jogging program because of the higher incidence of injuries associated with jogging (97). While we may know the exercise prescription needed to achieve cardiorespiratory fitness, we do not have the

prescription for preventing osteoporosis (109). However, two to three hours of exercise a week may reduce the expected rate of bone mineral loss with age (39, 108). In addition, there is a growing body of research supporting the need for resistance training as a part of any "bone health" program (44, 61, 78). There is also evidence that resistance training can be undertaken safely by these older adults (86). For an update on this, see Ask the Expert 17.1.

As is true for any special population, a complete medical exam is a reasonable recommendation to help discover problems or the presence of a combination of risk factors that might affect decisions about entry into an exercise program (7). There is no question that older adults, like their younger counterparts, exhibit a specificity and an adaptability to training, be it for strength or endurance (35, 55, 97). Consequently, the exercise program should provide endurance, flexibility, and strength activities within the capacity of the population being served in order to make improvements in these fitness components (117). A combination of strength training and balance training has been shown to reduce the risk of falls (128). The

Exercise and Bone Health
Questions and Answers with Dr. Susan A. Bloomfield

Dr. Susan Bloomfield is an Associate Professor in the Department of Health & Kinesiology and a member of the Intercollegiate Faculty of Nutrition at Texas A&M University. Her current research utilizes animal models to study bone adaptations to exercise and disuse and the functional relationships of muscle and bone. She also serves as Associate Lead for the Bone Loss Team of the National Space Biomedical Research Institute, whose mission is finding effective countermeasures for spaceflight-induced bone loss. She lives in College Station with her husband and two daughters, and is an avid "soccer mom" every weekend.

QUESTION 1: What are the primary factors affecting bone health?

ANSWER: Optimal bone health depends on adequate nutritional intake of calcium as well as regular exercise in the context of a normal hormonal profile. If serum levels of estrogen or testosterone are low, bone mass (usually measured by bone mineral density, or BMD) tends to decline. Interestingly, the primary effect of estrogen is to suppress activity of osteoclasts (bone-resorbing cells). Hence, estrogen deficiency, whether occurring at menopause or after prolonged amenorrhea in a young woman, "takes the brakes off" bone resorption and bone loss results. Glucocorticoids, be it endogenous cortisol or prescribed anti-inflammatory medications taken for chronic medical conditions, can directly stimulate bone resorption activity, thereby causing a loss of BMD. But if the endocrine milieu is reasonably normal, then calcium intake and physical activity patterns are the two most important determinants of bone mass and resistance to fracture.

QUESTION 2: Is exercise and good nutrition most important later in life when bone loss most often occurs?

ANSWER: Important as exercise and good nutrition are after the age of fifty, when age-related or menopause-induced bone loss becomes more apparent, the most critical years from a public health viewpoint actually fall right around puberty. We gain an incredible 30% of our eventual peak bone mass in the three years surrounding puberty; further increases in BMD occur until at least the age of twenty-five. The greatest impact of exercise on BMD and optimal bone geometry occurs during these years of rapid growth, with the result that the active child grows into an adult with a high peak bone mass before age-related loss begins. High calcium intakes (1,200–1,500 mg/d) at this age help ensure the maximal benefit. However, calcium intake is declining among American children and, ironically, most dramatically in adolescent girls who stand to benefit the most in terms of reducing their risk of osteoporotic fractures later in life. The clear public health message here is that we need to promote more consumption of calcium-rich foods (especially milk!) and more physical activity for American children and teens. In my mind this translates to the removal of soda machines from our schools' hallways and the promotion of regular physical education classes through high school. On a population-wide basis, the prevention of osteoporosis, rather than attention to treating established bone loss, is likely to be far more effective. A final caveat: It is important to encourage calcium intake of 1,200 to 1,500 mg/d and regular weight-bearing activity in older individuals, too. There is reasonably good evidence that age-related bone loss can be substantially slowed by adopting these habits.

QUESTION 3: What are the general characteristics of exercise programs that produce increments in bone mass and decrease the risk of osteoporotic fractures later in life?

ANSWER: There are important lessons to learn from key experiments done in animal models and these results are being more frequently applied to the human condition. For example, experiments by Rubin and Lanyon[1] on the ulnas of turkeys revealed the importance of the magnitude of force applied to bone (as opposed to many loading cycles) as well as a unique distribution of loading. Hence, we have the current emphasis on either weight-training or weight-bearing activities that involve impact forces to provide adequate stimulus to the skeleton. In addition, a diversified exercise program that uses a wide variety of muscle groups with frequent and varied movement patterns would be better than a monotonous signal to bone like running or cycling. The most recent findings from Robling and fellow researchers[2] using external loading of rat tibiae suggest that two to four shorter exercise bouts spread over the day might be more osteogenic (promoting gain in bone mass) than one long bout. Interestingly, this approach agrees well with the recommendations we're hearing from exercise epidemiologists that activity accumulated over the day provides significant health benefits. Incorporating more activity into our daily life (commuting by bicycle, physical work at home, more walking as well as planned exercise) holds much promise for improving bone health across the lifespan.

---

[1]Rubin, C. T., and Lanyon, L. E. 1985. Regulation of bone mass by mechanical strain magnitude. *Calcified Tissue International* 37:411–17.

[2]Robling, A. G., Burr, D. B., and Turner, C. H. 2000. Partitioning a daily mechanical stimulus into discrete loading bouts improves the osteogenic response to loading. *Journal of Bone and Mineral Research* 15:1596–1602.

A CLOSER LOOK 17.3

Exercise and Elderly People: The Training Effect

Over the past twenty years, a substantial body of knowledge has accumulated documenting the capacity of elderly people to experience a training effect similar to what has been observed in younger men and women (5). This has major ramifications when one considers the increase in the number of elderly people in our population and the need to maintain their health status and independence for as long as possible. Data on the effect of exercise on elderly people have been obtained from cross-sectional studies comparing older athletes to their sedentary counterparts and from longitudinal studies in which training programs have been carried out over many months. A brief summary of each follows (56).

Cross-sectional studies have shown that, in contrast to older sedentary individuals, endurance-trained older athletes have

- higher $\dot{V}O_2$ max values,

- higher HDL cholesterol, and lower triglycerides, total, and LDL cholesterol,
- enhanced glucose tolerance and insulin sensitivity, and
- greater strength, quicker reaction time, and a lower risk of falling.

These comparisons could be biased due to the potential for a strong genetic factor that might drive an individual to pursue an active life. In contrast, longitudinal studies compare a trained group to a control group over many months to see how each changes; this minimizes the concerns raised in the cross-sectional studies. The results from these studies parallel those mentioned previously. Endurance training:

- increases $\dot{V}O_2$ max and the kinetics of oxygen uptake in a manner similar to younger individuals, but more time may be required for the training effect

to occur (14). In men, the increase in $\dot{V}O_2$ max is due to both peripheral (skeletal muscle) and central (cardiovascular) adaptations (99). However, the increase in $\dot{V}O_2$ max in older women is due solely to peripheral adaptations (111).

- causes favorable changes in blood lipids, but the changes seem to be linked to a reduction in body fatness, rather than exercise, per se.
- lowers blood pressure to the same degree as shown for younger hypertensives.
- improves glucose tolerance and insulin sensitivity.
- increases or maintains muscular strength and bone density. It must be added that resistance training results in large increases in strength, which may play an important role in reducing the risk of falls.

potential benefits are clearly worth the time and energy invested (see A Closer Look 17.3).

In conclusion, the use of exercise programs for older adults improves cardiorespiratory fitness and helps to maintain the integrity of bone. When this is coupled with the opportunity for socialization, it is easy to see why exercise is an important part of life from youth to old age. For a more detailed presentation on this topic, see works by Spirduso and Shephard in the Suggested Readings.

IN SUMMARY

- The "normal" deterioration of physiological function with age can be attenuated or reversed with regular endurance and strength training. The benefits of participation in a regular exercise program include an improved risk factor profile (e.g., higher HDL and lower LDL cholesterol, improved insulin sensitivity, higher $\dot{V}O_2$ max, and lower blood pressure), but the training effects may take longer to realize.
- The guidelines for exercise training programs for older adults are similar to those for younger

people, emphasizing the need for a medical exam and screening for risk factors. The effort required to bring about the training effect may be less than for younger individuals.

EXERCISE DURING PREGNANCY

Pregnancy places special demands on a woman due to the developing fetus's needs for calories, protein, minerals, vitamins, and of course, the physiologically stable environment needed to process these nutrients. It is against this background that the implementation of a fitness program must be evaluated. In much the same way that a diabetic, asthmatic, or cardiac patient would initiate an exercise program, the pregnant woman should begin with a thorough medical examination by her physician to rule out complications that would make exercise inappropriate, and to provide specific information about signs or symptoms to watch for during the course of the pregnancy. Absolute contraindications for aerobic exercise during pregnancy include hemodynamically significant heart disease, restrictive lung disease, incompetent cervix/cerclage, multiple gestation at risk for premature labor, persistent second- and third-trimester bleeding, placenta previa after 26 weeks of gestation, premature labor during the current pregnancy, ruptured membranes, and preeclampsia/pregnancy-induced hypertension. Relative contraindications include severe anemia, unevaluated maternal cardiac arrhethemias, chronic bronchitis, poorly controlled type 1 diabetes, extreme morbid obesity, extreme underweight (BMI <12), history of extremely sedentary lifestyle, intrauterine growth restriction in current pregnancy, poorly controlled hypertension, orthopedic limitations, poorly controlled seizure disorder, poorly controlled hyperthyroidism, and heavy smoking (3). Clearly, to protect mother and fetus, a consultation with a physician is a reasonable recommendation prior to the initiation of an exercise program.

Interestingly, compared to our knowledge of how diabetics, asthmatics, and cardiac patients respond to exercise training, we are now only beginning to understand how the mother and fetus respond to such a program (27, 129, 131). In general, the following describe the major cardiovascular and metabolic adaptations to pregnancy compared to the nonpregnant state (129, 130):

- Blood volume increases 40% to 50%.
- Oxygen uptake is slightly higher at rest and during submaximal exercise.
- The oxygen cost of weight-bearing exercise is markedly increased.
- Heart rates are higher at rest and during submaximal exercise.
- Cardiac output is higher at rest and during submaximal exercise for the first two trimesters; in the third trimester cardiac output is lower and the potential for arterial hypotension is greater.

In spite of all these changes, moderate exercise does not appear to interfere with oxygen delivery to the fetus, and the heart rate response of the fetus shows no signs of distress. The fetal heart rate increases with the intensity and duration of exercise, and it gradually returns to normal during postexercise recovery (129, 130, 131). Cardiac output has been shown to be higher at twenty-six weeks gestation during submaximal exercise than at eight weeks following delivery. The fact that the a-$\bar{v}$ O_2 difference was lower suggests that the higher cardiac output was distributed to other vascular beds (e.g., the uterus) and muscle blood flow was maintained (102, 130, 131). Since absolute $\dot{V}O_2$ max (L/min) doesn't change much over the course of a pregnancy (81), what happens when exercise training is done during pregnancy?

In general, there is evidence that estimated $\dot{V}O_2$ max (in L/min) is increased as a result of training in previously sedentary pregnant women, while relative $\dot{V}O_2$ max (ml $\cdot$ kg^{-1} $\cdot$ min^{-1}) is maintained or increased slightly, despite the weight gain (131). What is interesting is that when well-conditioned recreational athletes trained throughout and following their pregnancy, absolute $\dot{V}O_2$ max was increased as long as thirty-six to forty-four weeks after delivery compared to a "control" group of women who maintained training and did not become pregnant (31). This suggests that the combination of pregnancy and training resulted in adaptations greater than could be achieved by training alone. What are reasonable recommendations to follow when a pregnant woman wishes to exercise?

Guidelines have been developing over the past two decades, with disagreement voiced among specialists in obstetrics and gynecology (23, 50). In an earlier set of guidelines from the American College of Obstetricians and Gynecologists, fixed criteria (e.g., don't exercise over an HR of 140 b/min) were provided, with the emphasis on taking a conservative approach to exercise prescription. Current guidelines emphasize the need to avoid doing exercise in the supine position to avoid a reduction in venous return and orthostatic hypotension (3). Weight-supported activities are encouraged due to the lower risk of injury, and attention is focused on the need for hydration to maintain body temperature in the normal range associated with exercise. Research suggests that normal exercise-induced increases in body temperatures carry little risk to the fetus (3, 27, 129).

The American College of Obstetricians and Gynecologists states that in the absence of either medical or obstetric complications, pregnant women can follow the CDC/ACSM recommendation of doing 30 minutes of moderate-intensity exercise on most, preferably all, days of the week.

- Recreational and competitive athletes with uncomplicated pregnancies can remain active during pregnancy, and modify activities as medically indicated. Pregnant women who engage in strenuous exercise require close medical supervision.
- Previously inactive women and those with medical or obstetric complications should be evaluated by a physician before exercise recommendations are made.
- A physically active woman with a history of, or at risk for, preterm labor or fetal growth restriction should reduce her activity in the second and third trimesters.

For those doing structured exercise programs, the Canadian Guidelines (37) suggest using the "talk test" (reduce intensity when conversation cannot be continued without pauses to catch one's breath) or the RPE (12–14 on the original Borg scale) to set exercise intensity. However, the following heart rate ranges were offered for additional guidance:

- less than 20 years old, 140 to 155 b/min,
- 20 to 29 years old, 135 to 150 b/min,
- 30 to 39 years old, 130 to 145 b/min, and
- 40 years or older, 125 to 140 b/min.

IN SUMMARY

- A pregnant woman should consult with her physician before starting an exercise program.
- Endurance exercise can be done during pregnancy without complication to mother or fetus.

STUDY QUESTIONS

1. What is the difference between type 1 and type 2 diabetes?
2. If a type 1 diabetic does not take an adequate amount of insulin, what happens to the blood glucose concentration during prolonged exercise? Why?
3. If exercise is helpful in controlling blood glucose, how could it complicate the life of a type 1 diabetic?
4. Provide general recommendations regarding changes in insulin and diet for diabetics who engage in exercise.
5. How is exercise-induced asthma triggered, and how do medications reduce the chance of an attack?
6. Why are exercise and diet recommended as nonpharmocological treatments for those with borderline hypertension?

7. What is COPD, and where does exercise fit in as a part of a rehabilitation program?
8. What are angina pectoris, CABGS, and angioplasty?
9. What additional measurements are made during a GXT of a cardiac patient, as compared to an apparently healthy individual?
10. How do elderly people respond to exercise training compared to younger subjects?
11. What are the concerns about exercise during pregnancy, and what are the guidelines recommended for a pregnant woman who wishes to begin an exercise program?

SUGGESTED READINGS

American College of Sports Medicine. 2003. ACSM's *Exercise Management for Persons with Chronic Diseases and Disabilities*. Champaign, IL: Human Kinetics.

American College of Sports Medicine. 2006. ACSM's *Resource Manual for Guidelines for Exercise Testing and Prescription*. 4th ed. Baltimore: Lippincott Williams & Wilkins.

Shephard, R. J. 1997. *Aging, Physical Activity, and Health*. Champaign, IL: Human Kinetics.

Spirduso, W. W. 1995. *Physical Dimensions of Aging*. Champaign, IL: Human Kinetics.

REFERENCES

1. Afrasiabi, R., and S. L. Spector. 1991. Exercise-induced asthma. *The Physician and Sportsmedicine* 19:49–62.
2. Albright, A. L. 1997. Diabetes. In ACSM's *Exercise Management for Persons with Chronic Diseases and Disabilities*, ed. J. L. Durstine. 94–100. Champaign, IL: Human Kinetics.
3. American College of Obstetricians and Gynecologists. 2002. Exercise during pregnancy and the postpartum period. (Opinion No. 267), *Obstet Gynecol*. 99:171–73.
4. American College of Sports Medicine. 2004. Position stand: Exercise and hypertension. *Medicine and Science in Sports and Exercise* 25:i–x.
5. American College of Sports Medicine. 1998. Exercise and physical activity for older adults. *Medicine and Science in Sports and Exercise*. 30:992–1008.
6. American College of Sports Medicine. (1998) The recommended quantity and quality of exercise for developing and maintaining cardiorespiratory and muscular fitness and flexibility in healthy adults. *Medicine and Science in Sports and Exercise* 30:975–91.
7. ———. 2006. ACSM's *Guidelines for Exercise Testing and Prescription*. 7th ed. Baltimore: Lippincott Williams & Wilkins.

8. American College of Sports Medicine. 2000. Position stand: Exercise and type 2 diabetes. *Medicine and Science in Sports and Exercise* 32:1345–60.
9. American Diabetes Association. 2004. Nutrition principles and recommendation in diabetes. *Diabetes Care* 27:S36–46.
10. American Diabetes Association. 2004. Physical activity/exercise and diabetes. *Diabetes Care* 27:S58–62.
11. American Diabetes Association. 2004. Diagnosis and classification of diabetes mellitus. *Diabetes Care* 27:S5–10.
12. American Diabetes Association. 2004. Prevention or delay of type 2 diabetes. *Diabetes Care* 27:S47–54.
13. American Heart Association Committee Report. 1982. Rationale of the diet-heart statement of the American Heart Association. *Nutrition Today* (Sept./Oct.):16–20; (Nov./Dec.):15–19.
14. Babcock, M., D. H. Paterson, and D. A. Cunningham. 1994. Effects of aerobic endurance training on gas exchange kinetics of older men. *Medicine and Science in Sports and Exercise* 26:447–52.
15. Bassett, D. R., and A. J. Zweifler. 1990. Risk factors and risk factor management. In *Clinical Ischemic Syndromes*, ed.

G. B. Zelenock, L. G. D'Alecy, J. C. Fantone III, M. Shlafer, and J. C. Stanley, 15–46. St. Louis: C. V. Mosby.

16. Berg, K. E. 1986. *Diabetic's Guide to Health and Fitness*. Champaign, IL.: Life Enhancement Publications.

17. Berger et al. 1977. Metabolic and hormonal effects of muscular exercise in juvenile type diabetics. *Diabetologia* 13:355–65.

18. Berger, M., and F. W. Kemmer. 1990. Discussion: Exercise, fitness, and diabetes. In *Exercise, Fitness, and Health*, ed. C. Bouchard, R. J. Shephard, T. Stephens, J. R. Sutton, and B. D. McPherson, 491–95. Champaign, IL: Human Kinetics.

19. Berman, L. B., and J. R. Sutton. 1986. Exercise and the pulmonary patient. *Journal of Cardiopulmonary Rehabilitation* 6:52–61.

20. Bloomfield, S. A., and S. S. Smith. 2003. Osteoporosis. In *ACSM's Exercise Management for Persons with Chronic Diseases and Disabilities*. 2d ed. Champaign, IL: Human Kinetics, pp. 222–29.

21. Booker, R. 2005. Care of chronic conditions. Chronic obstructive pulmonary disease: Non-pharmacological approaches. *British Journal of Nursing* 14:14–18.

22. Brysasco, V., and E. Crimi. 1994. Allergy and sports: Exercise-induced asthma. *International Journal of Sports Medicine* 15:S184–S186.

23. Caldwell, F., and T. Jopke. 1985. Questions and answers: ACSM 1985. *The Physician and Sportsmedicine* 13(8):145–51.

24. Campaigne, B. N., and R. M. Lampman. 1994. *Exercise in the Clinical Management of Diabetes*. Champaign, IL: Human Kinetics.

25. Campaign, B. N. 2001. Exercise and diabetes mellitus. In *ACSM's Resource Manual for Guidelines for Graded Exercise Testing and Prescription*. 4th ed. Baltimore: Lippincott Williams & Wilkins, pp. 277–84.

26. Cantu, D. C. 1982. *Diabetes and Exercise*. Ithaca, NY: Movement Publications.

27. Carpenter, M. W. 1994. Physical activity, fitness, and health of the pregnant mother and fetus. In *Physical Activity, Fitness, and Health*, ed. C. Bouchard, R. J. Shephard, and T. Stephens, 967–79. Champaign, IL: Human Kinetics.

28. Carter, R., J. C. Coast, and S. Idell. 1992. Exercise training in patients with chronic obstructive pulmonary disease. *Medicine and Science in Sports and Exercise* 24:281–91.

29. Centers for Disease Control and Prevention. 2004. National diabetes fact sheet: General information and national estimates on diabetes in the United States, 2003. Atlanta, GA: U.S. Department of Health and Human Services, Centers for Disease Control and Prevention.

30. Chobanian, A. V. et al. 2003. Seventh report of the joint national committee on prevention, detection, evaluation, and treatment of high blood pressure. *Hypertension* 42:1206–52.

31. Clapp, J. F. III, and E. Capeless. 1991. The $\dot{V}O_2$ max of recreational athletes before and after pregnancy. *Medicine and Science in Sports and Exercise* 23:1128–33.

32. Clark, C. J. 2003. Asthma. In *ACSM's Exercise Management for Persons with Chronic Diseases and Disabilities*. 2d ed. Champaign, IL: Human kinetics, pp. 105–10.

33. Cooper, C. B. 2003. Chronic obstructive pulmonary disease. In *ACSM's Exercise Management for Persons with Chronic Diseases and Disabilities*. 2d ed. Champaign, IL: Human Kinetics, pp. 92–98.

34. Cox, N. J. M., C.L.A. van Herwaarden, H. Folgering, and R. A. Binkhorst. 1988. Exercise and training in patients with chronic obstructive lung disease. *Sports Medicine* 6:180–92.

35. Cress, M. E., D. P. Thompson, J. Johnson, F. W. Kasch, R. G. Cassens, E. Smith, and J. C. Agre. 1991. Effect of training on $\dot{V}O_2$ max, thigh strength, and muscle morphology in septuagenarian women. *Journal of Applied Physiology* 23:752–58.

36. Cypcar, D., and R. F. Lemanske. 1994. Asthma and exercise. *Clinics in Chest Medicine* 15:351–68.

37. Davies, G. A. L., L. A. Wolfe, M. F. Mottola, and C. MacKinnon. 2003. Joint SOGC/CSEP clinical practice guideline: Exercise in pregnancy and the postpartum period. *Canadian Journal of Applied Physiology* 28:329–41.

38. DeGroot, D. W., T. J. Quinn, R. Kertzer, N. B. Vroman, and W. B. Olney. 1998. Circuit weight training in cardiac patients: Determining optimal workloads for safety and energy expenditure. *Journal of Cardiopulmonary Rehabilitation* 18:145–52.

39. Drinkwater, B. L. 1994. Physical activity, fitness, and osteoporosis. In *Physical Activity, Fitness, and Health*, ed. C. Bouchard, R. J. Shephard, and T. Stephens, 724–36. Champaign, IL: Human Kinetics.

40. Eggleston, P. A. 1986. Pathophysiology of exercise-induced asthma. *Medicine and Science in Sports and Exercise* 18:318–21.

41. Ehrman, J. K., and J. R. Schairer. 2006. Diagnostic procedures for cardiovascular disease. In *ACSM's Resource Manual for Guidelines for Exercise Testing and Prescription*. 5th ed. Baltimore: Lippincott Williams & Wilkins, pp. 277–88.

42. Ekoe, J-M. 1989. Overview of diabetes mellitus and exercise. *Medicine and Science in Sports and Exercise* 21:353–55.

43. Evans, T. M., K. W. Rundell, K. C. Beck, A. M. Levine, and J. M. Baumann. 2005. Cold air inhalation does not affect the severity of EIB after exercise or eucapnic voluntary hyperventilation. *Medicine and Science in Sports and Exercise* 37:544–49.

44. Evans, W. J. 1999. Exercise training guidelines for the elderly. *Medicine and Science in Sports and Exercise* 31:12–17.

45. Fagard, R. H., and C. M. Tipton. 1994. Physical activity, fitness, and hypertension. In *Physical Activity, Fitness, and Health*, ed. C. Bouchard, R. J. Shephard, and T. Stephens, 633–55. Champaign, IL: Human Kinetics.

46. Fitzgerald, M. D., H. Tanaka, Z. V. Tran, and D. R. Seals. 1997. Age-related declines in maximal aerobic capacity in regularly exercising vs. sedentary women: A meta-analysis. *Journal of Applied Physiology* 83:160–65.

47. Franklin, B. A. 2003. Myocardial infarction. In *ACSM's Exercise Management for Persons with Chronic Diseases and Disabilities*. 2d ed. Champaign, IL: Human Kinetics, pp. 24–31.

48. Franklin, B. A. 2003. Coronary artery bypass graft surgery and percutaneous transluminal coronary angioplasty. In *ACSM's Exercise Management for Persons with Chronic Diseases and Disabilities*. 2d ed. Champaign, IL: Human Kinetics, pp. 32–39.

49. Franz, M. J. 1987. Exercise and the management of diabetes mellitus. *Journal of the American Dietetic Association* 87:872–80.

50. Gauthier, M. M. 1986. Guidelines for exercise during pregnancy: Too little or too much. *The Physician and Sportsmedicine* 14(4):162–69.

51. Gerhard, H., and E. N. Schachter. 1980. Exercise-induced asthma. *Postgraduate Medicine* 67:91–102.

52. Giacca, A., Z. Q. Shi, E. B. Marliss, B. Zinman, and M. Vranic. 1994. Physical activity, fitness, and Type 1 diabetes. In *Physical Activity, Fitness, and Health*, ed. C. Bouchard, R. J. Shephard, and T. Stephens, 656–68. Champaign, IL: Human Kinetics.

53. Gordon, N. F. 2003. Hypertension. In *ACSM's Exercise Management for Persons with Chronic Diseases and Disabilities*. Champaign, IL: Human Kinetics, pp. 76–80.

54. Gudat, U., M. Berger, and P. J. Lefèbvre. 1994. Physical activity, fitness, and non-insulin-dependent diabetes mellitus. In *Physical Activity, Fitness, and Health*, ed. C. Bouchard, R. J. Shephard, and T. Stephens, 669–83. Champaign, IL: Human Kinetics.

55. Hagberg, J. M. 1990. Exercise, fitness, and hypertension. In *Exercise, Fitness, and Health*, ed. C. Bouchard, R. J. Shephard, T. Stephens, J. R. Sutton, and B. D. McPherson, 455–66. Champaign, IL: Human Kinetics.

56. ———. 1994. Physical activity, fitness, health, and aging. In *Physical Activity, Fitness, and Health*, ed. C. Bouchard, R. J. Shephard, and T. Stephens, 993–1005. Champaign, IL: Human Kinetics.

57. Heaney, R. P. 1987. The role of calcium in prevention and treatment of osteoporosis. *The Physician and Sportsmedicine* 15(11):83–88.

58. Hedlund, L. R., and J. C. Gallagher. 1987. The effects of fluoride on osteoporosis. *The Physician and Sportsmedicine* 15(11):111–18.

59. Hornsby, W. G., and A. L. Albright. 2003. Diabetes. In *ACSM's Exercise Management for Persons with Chronic Diseases and Disabilities*. 2d ed. Champaign, IL: Human Kinetics, pp. 133–41.

60. Howley, E. T. and B. D. Franks. 2003. Exercise for older adults. In *Health Fitness Instructor's Handbook*. 4th ed. E. T. Howley and B. D. Franks, (eds). Champaign, IL: Human Kinetics, pp. 293–303.

61. Hurley, B. F., and J. M. Hagberg. 1998. Optimizing health in older persons: Aerobic or strength training. In *Exercise and Sport Sciences Reviews*, vol. 26, ed. J. O. Holloszy, 61–89. Baltimore: Lippincott Williams & Wilkins.

62. Ivy, J. L., T. W. Zderic, and D. L. Fogt. 1999. Prevention and treatment of non-insulin-dependent diabetes mellitus. In *Exercise and Sport Sciences Reviews*, vol. 27, ed. J. O. Holloszy, 1–35. Baltimore: Lippincott Williams & Wilkins.

63. Jackson, A. et al. 1995. Changes in aerobic power of men, ages 25–70 yr. *Medicine and Science in Sports and Exercise* 27:113–20.

64. Johnston, C. C., and C. Slemenda. 1987. Osteoporosis: An overview. *The Physician and Sportsmedicine* 15(11): 65–68.

65. Jones, A., and M. Bowen. 1994. Screening for childhood asthma using an exercise test. *British Journal of General Practice* 44:127–31.

66. Jones, N. L., L. B. Berman, P. D. Bartkiewicz, and N. B. Oldridge. 1987. Chronic obstructive respiratory disorders. In *Exercise Testing and Exercise Prescription for Special Cases*, ed. J. S. Skinner, 175–87. Philadelphia: Lea & Febiger.

67. Kannel, W. B. 1990. Contribution of the Framingham study to preventive cardiology. *Journal of the American College of Cardiology* 15:206–11.

68. Kaplan, N. M. 1998. *Clinical Hypertension*. 7th ed. Baltimore: Lippincott Williams & Wilkins.

69. Kasch, F. W., J. L. Boyer, S. P. Van Camp, L. S. Verity, and J. P. Wallace. 1990. The effect of physical activity and inactivity on aerobic power in older men (a longitudinal study). *The Physician and Sportsmedicine* 18:73–83.

70. Katz, R. M. 1986. Prevention with and without the use of medications for exercise-induced asthma. *Medicine and Science in Sports and Exercise* 18:331–33.

71. Katz, R. M. 1987. Coping with exercise-induced asthma in sports. *The Physician and Sportsmedicine* 15 (July): 100–112.

72. Keilty, S. E., J. Ponte, T. A. Fleming, and J. Moxham. 1994. Effect of inspiratory pressure support on exercise tolerance and breathlessness in patients with severe stable chronic obstructive pulmonary disease. *Thorax* 49:990–94.

73. Kelley, D. E., and B. H. Goodpaster. 2001. Effects of exercise on glucose homeostasis in type 2 diabetes mellitus. *Medicine and Science in Sports and Exercise* 33: S495–501.

74. Kemmer, F. W., and M. Berger. 1983. Exercise and diabetes mellitus: Physical activity as a part of daily life and its role in the treatment of diabetic patient. *International Journal of Sports Medicine* 4:77–88.

75. Kriska, A. M., S. N. Blair, and M. A. Pereira. 1994. The potential role of physical activity in the prevention of non-insulin-dependent diabetes mellitus: The epidemiological evidence. In *Exercise and Sports Sciences Reviews*, ed. J. O. Holloszy, vol. 22, 121–43. Baltimore: Lippincott Williams & Wilkins.

76. Lampman, R. M., and D. E. Schteingart. 1991. Effects of exercise training on glucose control, lipid metabolism, and insulin sensitivity in hypertriglyceridemia and non-insulin dependent diabetes mellitus. *Medicine and Science in Sports and Exercise* 23:703–12.

77. Lampman, R. M., and B. N. Campaign. 2006. Exercise testing in patients with diabetes. In *ACSM's Resource Manual for Guidelines for Exercise Testing and Prescription*. 5th ed. Baltimore: Lippincott Williams & Wilkins, pp. 245–54.

78. Layne, J. E., and M. E. Nelson. 1999. The effect of progressive resistance training on bone density: A review. *Medicine and Science in Sports and Exercise* 31:25–30.

79. Legrand, V., R. Raskinet, G. Laarman, N. Danchin, M. A. Morel, and P. W. Serruys. 1997. Diagnostic values of exercise electrocardiography and angina after coronary artery stenting. Benestent Study Group. *American Heart Journal* 133:240–48.

80. Lindsay, R. 1987. Estrogen and osteoporosis. *The Physician and Sportsmedicine* 15(11):105–8.

81. Lotgering, F. K., M. B. van Doorn, P. C. Struijk, J. Pool, and H. C. S. Wallenburg. 1991. Maximal aerobic exercise in pregnant women: Heart rate, O_2 consumption, CO_2 production, and ventilation. *Journal of Applied Physiology* 70:1016–23.

82. Lucas, S. R., and T. A. Platts-Mills. 2005. Physical activity and exercise in asthma: Relevance to etiology and treatment. *Journal of Allergy and Clinical Immunology* 115:928–34.

83. Mahler, D. A. 1993. Exercise-induced asthma. *Medicine and Science in Sports and Exercise* 25:554–61.

84. Makker, H. K., and S. T. Holgate. 1994. Mechanisms of exercise-induced asthma. *European Journal of Clinical Investigation* 24:571–85.

85. Martin, A. D. 1986. ECG and medications. In *Health/Fitness Instructor's Handbook*, ed. E. T. Howley and B. D. Franks, 185–98. Champaign, IL: Human Kinetics.

86. McCartney, N. 1999. Acute responses to resistance training and safety. *Medicine and Science in Sports and Exercise* 31:31–37.

87. McKenzie, D. C., S. L. McLuckie, and D. R. Stirling. 1994. The protective effects of continuous and interval exercise in athletes with exercise-induced asthma. *Medicine and Science in Sports and Exercise* 26:951–56.

88. Middleton, E. 1980. A rational approach to asthma therapy. *Postgraduate Medicine* 67:107–23.

89. Miracle, V. A. 1986. Pulmonary exercise program: A model for pulmonary rehabilitation. *Journal of Cardiopulmonary Rehabilitation* 6:368–71.

90. Morton, A. R., and K. D. Fitch. 2005. In J. S. Skinner (ed) *Exercise Testing and Exercise Prescription for Special Cases*. Baltimore: Lippincott Williams & Wilkins, pp. 257–71.

91. National Institutes of Health. 1999. Data fact sheet: Asthma statistics. U.S. Department of Health and Human Services. National Heart, Lung, and Blood Institute. Washington, D.C.: author.

92. National Research Council, National Academy of Sciences. 1989. *Recommended Dietary Allowances*. Washington, D.C.: National Academy Press.

93. Nichols, D. L., and E. V. Essery. 2006. Osteoporosis and exercise. In ACSM's *Resource Manual for Guidelines for Exercise Testing and Prescription*. 5th ed. Baltimore: Lippincott Williams & Wilkins, pp. 489–99.

94. Peno-Green, L. A., and C. B. Cooper. 2006. Treatment and rehabilitation of pulmonary diseases. In ACSM's *Resource Manual for Guidelines for Exercise Testing and Prescription*. 5th ed. Baltimore: Lippincott Williams & Wilkins, pp. 452–69.

95. *Physician and Sportsmedicine*. 1987. A Roundtable: Physiological adaptations to chronic endurance exercise training in patients with coronary artery disease. *Physician and Sportsmedicine* 15(9):129–56.

96. Pierson et al. 1986. Implications of air pollution effects on athletic performance. *Medicine and Science in Sports and Exercise* 18:322–27.

97. Pollock, M. L., J. F. Carroll, J. E. Graves, S. H. Leggett, R. W. Braith, M. Limacher, and J. M. Hagberg. 1991. Injuries and adherence to walk/jog and resistance programs in the elderly. *Medicine and Science in Sports and Exercise* 23:1194–1200.

98. Pollock, M. L., and J. H. Wilmore. 1990. *Exercise in Health and Disease*. 2d ed. Philadelphia: W. B. Saunders.

99. Quaglietti, S., and V. F. Froelicher. 1994. Physical activity and cardiac rehabilitation for patients with coronary heart disease. In *Physical Activity, Fitness, and Health*, ed. C. Bouchard, R. J. Shephard, and T. Stephens, 591–608. Champaign, IL: Human Kinetics.

100. Richter, E. R., and H. Galbo. 1986. Diabetes, insulin, and exercise. *Sports Medicine* 3:275–88.

101. Rogers, M. A. 1989. Acute effects of exercise on glucose tolerance in non-insulin-dependent diabetes. *Medicine and Science in Sports and Exercise* 21:362–68.

102. Sady, S. P., M. W. Carpenter, P. D. Thompson, M. A. Sady, B. Haydon, and D. R. Coustan. 1989. Cardiovascular responses to cycle exercise during and after pregnancy. *Journal of Applied Physiology* 66:336–41.

103. Schairer, J. S., and S. J. Keteyian. 2006. Exercise testing in patients with cardiovascular disease. In ACSM's *Resource Manual for Guidelines for Exercise Testing and Prescription*. 5th ed. Baltimore: Lippincott Williams & Wilkins, pp. 439–51.

104. Serres, I., M. Hayst, C. Préfent, and J. Mercier. 1998. Skeletal muscle abnormalities in patients with COPD: p. 332. Contribution to exercise intolerance. *Medicine and Science in Sports and Exercise* 30:1019–27.

105. Shephard, R. J. 1976. Exercise and chronic obstructive lung disease. In *Exercise and Sport Sciences Reviews*, vol. 4, ed. J. Keogle and R. S. Hutton, 263–96. Los Angeles: Journal Publishing Affiliates.

106. Skinner, J. S. 2005. Hypertension. In J. S. Skinner, ed. *Exercise Testing and Exercise Prescription for Special Cases*. Baltimore: Lippincott Williams & Wilkins, pp. 305–12.

107. Sly, R. M. 1986. History of exercise-induced asthma. *Medicine and Science in Sports and Exercise* 18:314–17.

108. Smith, E. L., and C. Gilligan. 1987. Effects of inactivity and exercise on bone. *The Physician and Sportsmedicine* 15(11):91–102.

109. Snow-Harter, C., and R. Marcus. 1991. Exercise, bone mineral density, and osteoporosis. In *Exercise and Sport Sciences Reviews*, vol. 19, ed. J. O. Holloszy, 351–88. Baltimore: Lippincott Williams & Wilkins.

110. Soukup, J. T., and J. E. Kovaleski. 1993. A review of the effects of resistance training for individuals with diabetes mellitus. *Diabetes Education* 19:307–12.

111. Spina, R. J. 1999. Cardiovascular adaptations to endurance exercise training in older men and women. In *Exercise and Sport Sciences Reviews*, vol. 27, ed. J. O. Holloszy, 317–32. Baltimore: Lippincott Williams & Wilkins.

112. Stockdale-Woolley, R., M. C. Haggerty, and P. M. McMahon. 1986. The pulmonary rehabilitation program at Norwalk Hospital. *Journal of Cardiopulmonary Rehabilitation* 6:505–18.

113. Storms, W. W. 2003. Review of exercise-induced asthma. *Medicine and Science in Sports and Exercise* 35:1464–70.

114. Tate, C. A., M. F. Hyek, and G. E. Taffet. 1994. Mechanism for the responses of cardiac muscle to physical activity in old age. *Medicine and Science in Sports and Exercise* 26:561–67.

115. Thompson, D. L. 2003. Exercise and diabetes. In *Health Fitness Instructor's Handbook*. 4th ed. E. T. Howley and B. D. Franks (eds). Champaign, IL: Human Kinetics, pp. 321–27.

116. Tommaso, C. L., M. Lesch, and E. H. Sonnenblick. 1984. Alterations in cardiac function in coronary heart disease, myocardial infarction, and coronary bypass surgery. In *Rehabilitation of the Coronary Patient*, ed. N. K. Wenger and H. K. Hellerstein, 41–66. New York: Wiley.

117. Van Camp, S., and J. L. Boyer. 1989. Exercise guidelines for the elderly (part 2 of 2). *The Physician and Sportsmedicine* 17:83–88.

118. Verity, L. S. 2006. Diabetes and exercise. In ACSM's *Resource Manual for Guidelines for Exercise Testing and Prescription*. 5th ed. Baltimore: Lippincott Williams & Wilkins, pp. 470–79.

119. Verrill, D., E. Shoup, G. McElveen, K. Witt, and D. Bergey. 1992. Resistive exercise training in cardiac patients: Recommendations. *Sports Medicine* 13:171–93.

120. Voy, R. O. 1986. The U.S. Olympic Committee experience with exercise-induced bronchospasm. 1984. *Medicine and Science in Sports and Exercise* 18:328–30.

121. Vranic, M., and Wasserman, D. 1990. Exercise, fitness, and diabetes. In *Exercise, Fitness, and Health*, ed. C. Bouchard, R. J. Shephard, T. Stephens, J. R. Sutton, and B. D. McPherson, 467–90. Champaign, IL: Human Kinetics.

122. ———. 1992. Exercise and diabetes mellitus. In *Exercise and Sport Sciences Reviews*, vol. 20, ed. J. O. Holloszy, 339–68. Baltimore: Lippincott Williams & Wilkins.

123. Wallace, J. P. 2003. Exercise in hypertension—a clinical review. *Sports Medicine* 33:585–98.

124. Wedzicha, J. A., J. C. Bestall, R. Garrod, R. Garnham, E. A. Paul, and P. W. Jones. 1998. Randomized controlled trial of pulmonary rehabilitation in severe chronic obstructive pulmonary disease patients, stratified with the MRC dyspnoea scale. *European Respiration Journal* 12:363–69.

125. Wenger, N. K., and H. K. Hellerstein. 1992. *Rehabilitation of the Coronary Patient*. 3rd ed. New York: Churchill Livingstone.

126. Wenger, N. K., and J. W. Hurst. 1984. Coronary bypass surgery as a rehabilitative procedure. In *Rehabilitation of the Coronary Patient*, ed. N. K. Wenger and H. K. Hellerstein, 115–32. New York: Wiley.

127. Wilson, C. R. 2003. Evidence supporting the use of endurance exercise to decrease dyspnea in COPD. *Cardiopulmonary Physical Therapy Journal* 14:7–11.

128. Winters-Stone, K. M., and C. M. Snow. 2005. Osteoporosis. In J. S. Skinner, ed. *Exercise Testing and Exercise Prescription for Special Cases*. Baltimore: Lippincott Williams & Wilkins, pp. 171–87.

129. Wolfe, L. A., I.K.M. Brenner, and M. F. Mottola. 1994. Maternal exercise, fetal well-being and pregnancy outcome. In *Exercise and Sport Sciences Reviews*, vol. 22, ed. J. O. Holloszy, 145–94. Baltimore: Lippincott Williams & Wilkins.

130. Wolfe, L. A. 2005. Pregnancy. In J. S. Skinner, ed. *Exercise Testing and Exercise Prescription for Special Cases*. Baltimore: Lippincott Williams & Wilkins, pp. 377–91.

131. Wolfe, L. A., P. J. Ohtake, M. F. Mottola, and M. J. McGrath. 1989. Physiological interactions between pregnancy and aerobic exercise. In *Exercise and Sports Sciences Reviews*, vol. 17, ed. K. B. Pandolf, 295–351. Baltimore: Lippincott Williams & Wilkins.

132. World Hypertension League. 1991. Physical exercise in the management of hypertension: A consensus statement by the World Hypertension League. *Journal of Hypertension* 9:283–87.

133. Young, J. C. 1995. Exercise prescription for individuals with metabolic disorders. *Sports Medicine* 19:44–53.

CHAPTER 18

Body Composition and Nutrition for Health

■ Objectives

By studying this chapter, you should be able to do the following:

1. Identify the U.S. Dietary Goals relative to (a) carbohydrates and fats as a percent of energy intake, (b) salt and cholesterol, and (c) saturated and unsaturated fats.

2. Contrast the Dietary Goals with the Dietary Guidelines.

3. Describe what is meant by the terms *Recommended Dietary Allowance* (RDA) and *Dietary Reference Intakes* (DRIs), and how they relate to the Daily Value (DV) used in food labeling.

4. List the classes of nutrients.

5. Identify the fat- and water-soluble vitamins, describe what *toxicity* is, and identify which class of vitamins is more likely to cause this problem.

6. Contrast major minerals with trace minerals, and describe the role of calcium, iron, and sodium in health and disease.

7. Identify the primary role of carbohydrates, the two major classes, and the recommended changes in the American diet to improve health status.

8. Identify the primary role of fat and the recommended changes in the American diet to improve health status.

9. List the food groups represented in the MyPyramid eating plan.

10. Describe the Dietary Approaches to Stop Hypertension (DASH) eating plan, and describe similarities to the MyPyramid plan.

11. Describe the limitation of the height/weight table in determining overweight and obesity.

12. Provide a brief description of the following methods of measuring body composition: isotope dilution, photon absorptiometry, potassium-40, hydrostatic (underwater weighing), dual energy x-ray absorptiometry, near infrared interactance, radiography, ultrasound, nuclear magnetic resonance, total body electrical conductivity, bioelectrical impedance analysis, air displacement plethysmograpy, and skinfold thickness.

13. Describe the two-component model of body composition and the assumptions made about the density values for the fat-free mass and the fat mass; contrast this with the multicomponent model.

14. Explain the principle underlying the measurement of whole-body density with underwater weighing, and why one must correct for residual volume.

15. Explain why there is an error of ±2.0% in the calculation of percent body fat with the underwater weighing technique.

16. Explain how a sum of skinfolds can be used to estimate a percent body fatness value.

17. List the recommended percent body fatness values for health and fitness for males and females, and explain the concern for both high and low values.

18. Discuss the reasons why the average weight at any height (fatness) has increased while deaths from cardiovascular diseases have decreased.

19. Distinguish between obesity due to hyperplasia of fat cells and that due to hypertrophy of fat cells.

20. Describe the roles of genetics and environment in the development of obesity.

21. Explain the set point theory of obesity, and give an example of a physiological and behavioral control system.

22. Describe the pattern of change in body weight and caloric intake over the adult years.

23. Discuss the changes in body composition when weight is lost by diet alone versus diet plus exercise.

24. Describe the relationship of the fat-free mass and caloric intake to the BMR.

25. Define thermogenesis and explain how it is affected by both short- and long-term overfeeding.

26. Describe the effect of exercise on appetite and body composition.

27. Explain quantitatively why small differences in energy expenditure and dietary intake are important in weight gain over the years.

■ Outline

Nutritional Goals   360

Standards of Nutrition   362

Classes of Nutrients   363
    Water   363
    Vitamins   364
    Minerals   364
    Carbohydrates   368
    Fats   372
    Protein   373

Meeting the Guidelines and Achieving the Goals   374

Food Group Plans   374
    Evaluating the Diet   375

Body Composition   376
    Methods of Assessing Over-
        weight and Obesity   377
    Methods of Measuring Body
        Composition   378
    Two-Component System of
        Body Composition   380
    Body Fatness for Health and
        Fitness   383

Obesity and Weight Control   384
    Obesity   384

Diet, Exercise, and Weight Control   388
    Energy and Nutrient
        Balance   389
    Diet and Weight Control   390
    Energy Expenditure and
        Weight Control   391

■ Key Terms

Adequate Intake (AI)
anorexia nervosa
basal metabolic rate (BMR)
bulimia nervosa
cholesterol
Daily Value (DV)
deficiency
Dietary Guidelines for Americans
Dietary Reference Intake (DRI)
elements
energy wasteful systems
Estimated Energy Requirement (EER)

ferritin
food records
HDL cholesterol
hemosiderin
high-density lipoproteins (HDLs)
LDL cholesterol
lipoprotein
low-density lipoproteins (LDLs)
major minerals
nutrient density
osteoporosis
provitamin

Recommended Dietary Allowances (RDAs)
resting metabolic rate (RMR)
thermogenesis
toxicity
trace elements
transferrin
twenty-four-hour recall
underwater weighing
U.S. Dietary Goals
whole-body density

Chapter 14 described factors that limit health and fitness. These included hypertension, obesity, and elevated serum cholesterol. These three risk factors are linked to an excessive consumption of salt, total calories, and dietary fat, respectively. Clearly, knowledge of nutrition is essential to our understanding of health-related fitness. While chapters 3 and 4 described the metabolism of carbohydrates, fats, and proteins, this chapter will focus on the type of diet that should provide them. The first part of the chapter will present the nutritional goals for our nation, the nutrition standards and what they mean, a summary of the six classes of nutrients, and a way to evaluate our present diets and meet our nutritional goals. The second part of the chapter will discuss the role of exercise and diet in altering body composition. Nutrition related to athletic performance is covered in chapter 23.

NUTRITIONAL GOALS

The American Heart Association has focused our attention on the role of diet in the elevation of serum cholesterol, obesity, and the development of hypertension (2). Diet has also been linked to colon cancer and diabetes. In response to these problems a U.S. Senate Select Committee on Nutrition and Human Needs recruited experts to comment on and formulate **U.S. Dietary Goals** that would deal with diet-related problems (204). These goals, published in 1977, included the following:

■ Increase carbohydrate intake to represent 55% to 60% of caloric intake.

■ Decrease fat consumption to 30% of caloric intake.

■ Decrease saturated fat intake to represent only 10% of caloric intake; increase polyunsaturated and monounsaturated fats to approximately 10% of caloric intake.

■ Reduce cholesterol intake to 300 mg per day.

■ Reduce sugar consumption to account for only 15% of total calories.

■ Reduce salt consumption by about 50% to 85% to approximately 3 g per day.

In order to achieve these goals the following changes in food selection and preparation were suggested:

■ Increase the intake of fruits, vegetables, and whole grains.

■ Increase consumption of poultry and fish, and decrease intake of meat.

■ Decrease intake of foods high in fat, and partially substitute polyunsaturated fat for saturated fat.

■ Substitute nonfat milk for whole milk.

■ Decrease consumption of butter, fat, eggs, and other high-cholesterol sources.

■ Decrease consumption of sugar and foods high in sugar content.

■ Decrease consumption of salt and foods high in salt content.

Not everyone agreed with these specific quantitative goals and the strong statements that were made about the role of diet in the prevention and treatment of disease. The select committee subsequently published responses of scientists and medical doctors who disagreed with the stated dietary goals (203). The revised document encouraged weight reduction to attain "ideal weight" and recommended a reduction in the use of alcohol.

In 1980 the U.S. Department of Agriculture (200) published **Dietary Guidelines for Americans.** Rather than provide specific quantities to achieve for fat, cholesterol, salt, and carbohydrates as did the *Goals,* the *Guidelines* are more general statements aimed at people in good health. The Institute of Medicine (95) released new dietary recommendations in 2002 that provide a broader range of values for carbohydrate, fat, and protein to meet nutritional needs:

■ Adults should get 45% to 65% of their calories from carbohydrates, 20% to 35% from fat, and 10% to 35% from protein. Acceptable ranges for children are similar to those for adults, except that infants and younger children need a slightly higher proportion of fat (25%–40%).

The 2005 update of the *Dietary Guidelines for Americans* (see http://www.healthierus.gov/dietaryguidelines/) reflects the work of the Institute of Medicine and provides guidance on how to meet those nutritional standards (201). Excerpts of recommendations from this document follow:

■ Consume a variety of nutrient-dense foods and beverages within and among the basic food groups while choosing foods that limit the intake of saturated and *trans* fats, cholesterol, added sugars, salt, and alcohol.

  ● Choose a variety of fruits and vegetables each day. In particular, select from all five vegetable subgroups (dark green, orange, legumes, starchy vegetables, and other vegetables) several times a week.

  ● Consume three or more ounce-equivalents of whole-grain products per day, with the rest of the recommended grains coming from enriched or whole-grain products.

  ● Consume 3 cups per day of fat-free or low-fat milk or equivalent milk products.

  ● Keep total fat intake between 20% to 35% of calories, with most fats coming from sources of polyunsaturated and monounsaturated fatty acids, such as fish, nuts, and vegetable oils.

  ● Choose fiber-rich fruits, vegetables, and whole grains often and prepare foods and beverages with little added sugars or caloric sweeteners.

  ● Choose and prepare foods with little salt. At the same time, consume potassium-rich foods, such as fruits and vegetables.

  ● Those who choose to drink alcoholic beverages should do so sensibly and in moderation.

■ To maintain body weight in a healthy range, balance calories from foods and beverages with calories expended, engage in regular physical activity, and reduce sedentary activities.

■ Current recommendations for the distribution of calories in foods include a broad range, rather than a single goal: carbohydrates: 45% to 65%, fats: 20% to 35%, and proteins: 10% to 35%.

■ The publication, *Dietary Guidelines for Americans*, has been revised over time to reflect new science and to deal with nutrition (and physical activity) and health-related issues. The 2005 edition provides recommendations to meet the new nutritional standards with special focus on achieving energy balance.

STANDARDS OF NUTRITION

Food provides the carbohydrates, fats, protein, minerals, vitamins, and water needed for life. The quantity of each nutrient needed for proper function and health is defined in one of the **Dietary Reference Intakes (DRIs),** an umbrella term encompassing specific standards for dietary intake (95).

If you had a nutrition class, or even a few lectures dealing with nutrition, you would have been introduced to the Recommended Dietary Allowance (RDA) standards for nutrients such as protein, vitamins, and minerals. With the expansion of knowledge about the role of specific nutrients in preventing deficiency diseases and reducing the risk of chronic diseases, there was a need for a new approach to setting nutrient standards. In collaboration with Health Canada, the Food and Nutrition Board of the National Academy of Sciences has developed new nutrient standards. The term *Dietary Reference Intakes* (DRIs) is the umbrella term given to these new standards. The following descriptions will help us make the transitions from where we are to where we will be when the full implementation of the standards takes place (215).

■ **Recommended Dietary Allowance (RDA).** The average daily dietary nutrient intake level sufficient to meet the nutrient requirement of nearly all (97%–98%) healthy individuals in a particular group.

■ **Adequate Intakes (AI).** Formerly the Estimated Safe and Adequate Daily Dietary Intake, the AI describes the recommended average daily intake level based on observed or experimentally determined approximations or estimates of nutrient intake by a group (or groups) of apparently healthy people. Levels are assumed to be adequate and are used when an RDA cannot be determined. (see Appendix E)

■ **Tolerable Upper Intake Level (UL).** The highest average daily nutrient intake level that is likely to pose no risk of adverse health effects to almost all individuals in the general population. As intake increases above the UL, the potential risk of adverse effects may increase.

■ **Estimated Average Requirement (EAR).** The average daily nutrient intake level estimated to meet the requirement of half the healthy individuals in a particular group. This value is needed in order to set the RDA values.

The values for each nutrient vary due to gender, body size, whether or not long-bone growth is taking place, pregnancy, and lactation (145). Given the fact that individuals differ in their need for each nutrient, some requiring more than the average and others less, the standards were set high enough to meet the needs of almost everyone (97.5% of the population), and also account for inefficient utilization by the body (145). Previous RDA tables did not provide recommendations for carbohydrate and fat intake, but that has changed. We will provide an update from the Institute of Medicine report (95) when we discuss each.

In the past, RDA tables did not have standards for energy intake set at the same level as for the nutrients like vitamins and minerals (sufficient to meet 97% to 98% of the population). Instead, average values of energy intake were provided, which assumed an average level of physical activity. In the current recommendations, a new standard, the **Estimated Energy Requirement (EER),** is identified: the average dietary energy intake that is predicted to maintain energy balance in a healthy adult of a defined age, gender, weight, height, and level of physical activity, consistent with good health (95). The report provides energy intake recommendations for four levels of physical activity with the stated purpose of achieving a healthy body weight (see Appendix F). When it comes to the RDA for specific nutrients like vitamins and minerals, how do we know how much is contained in the food we eat?

The **Daily Value (DV)** is a standard used in nutritional labeling. For the essential nutrients (protein, vitamins, and minerals) the DVs represent the highest 1968 RDA standard for any age or gender, except for pregnant and lactating women (78). In addition, the food label contains important information about the calorie and fat content of the food. For example, if one serving of a product provides 50% of the DV for fat, it contains 50% of the total amount of fat recommended for one day (based on a 2,000-calorie diet). Figure 18.1 provides an example of a food label; the following points are highlighted:

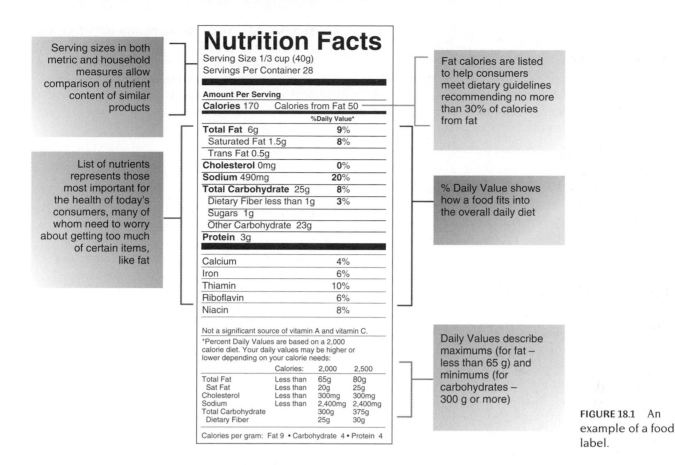

Nutrition Facts

Serving Size 1/3 cup (40g)
Servings Per Container 28

Amount Per Serving	
Calories 170	Calories from Fat 50

%Daily Value*

	%Daily Value*
Total Fat 6g	9%
Saturated Fat 1.5g	8%
Trans Fat 0.5g	
Cholesterol 0mg	0%
Sodium 490mg	20%
Total Carbohydrate 25g	8%
Dietary Fiber less than 1g	3%
Sugars 1g	
Other Carbohydrate 23g	
Protein 3g	

Calcium	4%
Iron	6%
Thiamin	10%
Riboflavin	6%
Niacin	8%

Not a significant source of vitamin A and vitamin C.

*Percent Daily Values are based on a 2,000 calorie diet. Your daily values may be higher or lower depending on your calorie needs:

		Calories:	2,000	2,500
Total Fat	Less than		65g	80g
Sat Fat	Less than		20g	25g
Cholesterol	Less than		300mg	300mg
Sodium	Less than		2,400mg	2,400mg
Total Carbohydrate			300g	375g
Dietary Fiber			25g	30g

Calories per gram: Fat 9 • Carbohydrate 4 • Protein 4

Serving sizes in both metric and household measures allow comparison of nutrient content of similar products

List of nutrients represents those most important for the health of today's consumers, many of whom need to worry about getting too much of certain items, like fat

Fat calories are listed to help consumers meet dietary guidelines recommending no more than 30% of calories from fat

% Daily Value shows how a food fits into the overall daily diet

Daily Values describe maximums (for fat – less than 65 g) and minimums (for carbohydrates – 300 g or more)

FIGURE 18.1 An example of a food label.

- serving size information,
- total calories and fat calories,
- total fat grams, saturated fat grams, trans fat grams, cholesterol, and the percent of DV for each (based on a 2,000-calorie diet),
- total carbohydrate and its sources, and
- the percent of the DV for vitamins and minerals; sodium is given special attention.

IN SUMMARY

- The Recommended Dietary Allowance (RDA) is the quantity of a nutrient that will meet the needs of almost all healthy persons.
- The Daily Value (DV) is a standard used in nutritional labeling.

CLASSES OF NUTRIENTS

There are six classes of nutrients: water, vitamins, minerals, carbohydrates, fats, and proteins. In the following sections each nutrient will be described briefly, and the primary food sources of each will be identified.

Water

Water is absolutely essential for life. While we can go without food for weeks, we would not survive long without water. The body is 50% to 75% water, depending on age and body fatness, and a loss of only 3% to 4% of body water adversely affects aerobic performance. Larger losses can lead to death (140, 222). Under normal conditions without exercise, water loss equals about 2,500 ml/day, with most lost in urine (44). However, as higher environmental temperatures and heavy exercise are added, the water loss increases dramatically to 6 to 7 liters per day (79).

Under normal conditions the 2,500 ml of water per day is replaced with beverages (1,500 ml), solid food (750 ml), and the water derived from metabolic processes (250 ml) (44). Most people are surprised by the large volume of water contributed by "solid" food until they consider the following percentages of water in "solid" food: baked potato—75%, canned peas—77%, lettuce—96% (44). A general recommendation under ordinary circumstances is to consume 1 to 1.5 ml of water per kcal of energy expenditure (145). The AI for total water intake (food + beverages) for women and men 19 to 70 years of age is set at 2.7 L/day and 3.7 L/day, respectively (96). However, to avoid potential problems associated with dehydration, one should drink water *before and during* exercise; thirst is not an adequate stimulus to achieve water balance (see chapter 23).

Water weight can fluctuate depending on the body stores of carbohydrate and protein. Water is involved in the linkage between glucose molecules in glycogen and amino acid molecules in protein. The ratio is about 2.7 of water per gram of carbohydrate, and if an individual stores 454 g (1 lb) of carbohydrate, body weight would increase by 3.7 lbs. Of course, when one diets and depletes this carbohydrate store, the reverse occurs. This results in an apparent weight loss of 3.7 lbs when only 1,816 kcal (454 g of carbohydrate times 4 kcal/g) have been lost. More on this later.

Vitamins

Vitamins were introduced in chapter 3 as organic catalysts involved in metabolic reactions. They are needed in small amounts and are not "used up" in the metabolic reactions. However, they are degraded (metabolized) like any biological molecule and must be replaced on a regular basis to maintain body stores. Several vitamins are in a precursor, or **provitamin,** form in foods, and are converted to the active form in the body. Beta-carotene, the most important of the provitamin A compounds, is a good example. A chronic lack of certain vitamins can lead to **deficiency** diseases, and an excess of others can lead to a **toxicity** condition (44). In our presentation, vitamins will be divided into the fat-soluble and water-soluble groups.

Fat-Soluble Vitamins The fat-soluble vitamins include A, D, E, and K. These vitamins can be stored in large quantities in the body; thus a deficiency state takes longer to develop than for water-soluble vitamins. However, because of their solubility, so much can be stored that a toxicity condition can occur. Vitamin D is regarded as the most toxic. It is possible to achieve a level of toxicity with only four to five times the recommended dietary allowance (44, 145). The Tolerable Upper Limit (UL) for vitamin A (3,000 μg), D (50 μg), and E (1,000 mg) have been established. Toxicity, of course, is far from a health-related goal. Table 18.1 summarizes the information on these vitamins, including the RDA/AI standards, dietary sources, function, and signs associated with deficiency or excess.

Water-Soluble Vitamins The water-soluble vitamins include vitamin C and the B vitamins: thiamin (B_1), riboflavin (B_2), niacin, pyridoxine (B_6), folic acid, B_{12}, pantothenic acid, and biotin. Most are involved in energy metabolism. You have already seen the role of niacin, as NAD, and riboflavin, as FAD, in the transfer of energy in the Krebs cycle and electron transport chain. Thiamin (as thiamine pyrophosphate) is involved in the removal of CO_2 as pyruvate enters the Krebs cycle.

Vitamin B_6, folic acid, B_{12}, pantothenic acid, and biotin are also involved as coenzymes in metabolic reactions. Vitamin C is involved in the maintenance of bone, cartilage, and connective tissue. Table 18.1 summarizes the information on these vitamins, including the RDA/AI standards, functions, dietary sources, and signs associated with deficiency or excess.

IN SUMMARY

- The fat-soluble vitamins include A, D, E, and K. These can be stored in the body in large quantities and a toxicity can develop.
- The water-soluble vitamins include thiamin, riboflavin, niacin, B_6, folic acid, B_{12}, pantothenic acid, biotin, and C. Most of these are involved in energy metabolism. Vitamin C is involved in the maintenance of bone, cartilage, and connective tissue.

Minerals

Minerals are the chemical **elements,** other than carbon, hydrogen, oxygen, and nitrogen, associated with the structure and function of the body. We have already seen the importance of calcium in bone structure and in the initiation of muscle contraction, iron in O_2 transport by hemoglobin, and phosphorus in ATP. Minerals are important inorganic nutrients and are divided into two classes: (1) **major minerals** and (2) **trace elements.** The major minerals include calcium, phosphorous, magnesium, sulfur, sodium, potassium, and chloride, with whole-body quantities ranging from 35 g for magnesium to 1,050 g for calcium in a 70-kg man (44). The trace elements include iron, iodine, fluoride, zinc, selenium, copper, cobalt, chromium, manganese, molybdenum, arsenic, nickel, and vanadium. There are only 4 g of iron and 0.0009 g of vanadium in a 70-kg man. Like vitamins, some minerals taken in excess (e.g., iron and zinc) can be toxic. The following sections will focus attention on calcium, iron, and sodium.

Calcium Calcium (Ca^{++}) and phosphorus combine with organic molecules to form the teeth and bones. The bones are a "store" of calcium that helps to maintain the plasma Ca^{++} concentration when dietary intake is inadequate (see parathyroid hormone in chapter 5). Bone is constantly turning over its calcium and phosphorus, so diet must replace what is lost. If the diet is deficient in calcium for a long period of time, loss of bone, or **osteoporosis,** can occur. This weakening of the bone due to the loss of calcium and phosphorus from its structure is more common in women than in men, is accelerated at menopause, and is directly related to the higher rate of hip fractures in women. Three major factors are implicated: dietary calcium intake, inadequate estrogen, and lack of physical activity (84, 145, 170, 171).

There is concern that the increase in osteoporosis in our society is related to an inadequate calcium intake. The adult AI for calcium is 1,000 mg/day, and while many men come close to meeting the standard, few women do (215). For example, men and women 20 to 49 years of age consume 1,025 and 797 mg/day, respectively (226). Part of the reason is the relatively low caloric intake of women compared to men. One way of dealing with this is to increase energy expenditure through exercise and, in turn, caloric intake. This should result in an increase in calcium intake. While menopause is the usual cause of a reduced secretion of estrogen, young, extremely active female athletes are experiencing this problem associated with amenorrhea (36, 43). The decrease in estrogen secretion is associated with the acceleration of osteoporosis. Estrogen therapy, with or without calcium supplementation, has been used successfully in menopausal women to reduce the rate of bone loss (142, 145). A third approach to dealing with osteoporosis is based on the observation that exercise slows the rate of bone loss (3, 28, 85, 139, 151, 170). This has been shown in runners (28), as well as tennis players (139), and is viewed as an important reason for recommending regular moderate exercise for elderly people (see Ask the Expert 17.1 in chapter 17).

Iron Iron is an important part of hemoglobin and myoglobin, as well as the cytochromes of the electron transport chain. To remain in iron balance, the RDA is set at 8 mg/day for an adult male and 18 mg/day for an adult female; the higher amount is needed to replace that which is lost in the menses. A 70-kg man has about 2,500 mg of iron in hemoglobin, 150 mg in myoglobin, 6 to 8 mg in enzymes, and about 3 mg bound to **transferrin,** the iron-transporting protein in plasma. In addition to this, iron is stored as **ferritin** or **hemosiderin** in the liver, spleen, and bone marrow. The serum ferritin concentration is a sensitive measure of iron status. Each microgram (μg) of ferritin per liter of serum indicates the presence of 10 mg of stored iron (44, 78, 82).

In spite of the higher need for iron, American women take in only 13.7 mg/day, while men take in 17.7 mg/day (226). This is due to higher caloric intakes in males than females. Since there are only 6 mg of iron per 1,000 kcal of energy in the American diet, a woman consuming 2,000 kcal/day would take in only 12 mg of iron. The male, consuming about 3,000 kcal/day, takes in 18 mg (82, 222). The diet provides iron in two forms, heme (ferrous) and nonheme (ferric). Heme iron, found primarily in meats, fish, and organ meats, is absorbed better than nonheme iron, which is found in vegetables. However, the absorption of nonheme iron can be increased by the presence of meat, fish, and vitamin C (44, 82, 222).

Anemia is a condition in which the hemoglobin concentration is low: less than 13 g/dl in men and less than 12 g/dl in women. This can be the result of blood loss (e.g., blood donation or bleeding), or a lack of vitamins or minerals in the diet. The most common cause of anemia in North America is a lack of dietary iron (44). In fact, iron deficiency is the most common nutrient deficiency. In iron deficiency anemia, more than hemoglobin is affected. The iron bound to transferrin in the plasma is reduced, and serum ferritin (an indicator of iron stores) is low (82). While children aged one to five, adolescents, young adult women, and the elderly are more apt to develop anemia, it also occurs in competitive athletes. This latter point will be discussed in detail in chapter 23.

Sodium Sodium is directly involved in the maintenance of the resting membrane potential and the generation of action potential in nerves (see chapter 7) and muscles (see chapter 8). In addition, sodium is the primary electrolyte determining the extracellular fluid volume. If sodium stores fall, the extracellular volume, including plasma, decreases. This could cause major problems with the maintenance of the mean arterial blood pressure (see chapter 9) and body temperature (see chapter 12).

The problem in our society is not with sodium stores that are too small, but just the opposite. The average sodium intakes for men and women are 4.2 and 3.1 g/day, respectively (29). The IA values of 1.5 g/day and 1.3 g/day for men and women 19 to 50 years of age are well below these values (96). The RDA is consistent with long-term concerns of both the American Heart Association and the National Research Council that excess sodium intake can contribute to hypertension in genetically susceptible individuals (2, 144). Recent reviews have confirmed the link between sodium intake and blood pressure, with evidence that reducing salt intake is feasible and will result in a reduction in cardiovascular morbidity and mortality (104, 216). This is in concert with recommendations from the *Dietary Guidelines for Americans* (201) to avoid too much sodium. The following suggestions from the Dietary Approaches to Stop Hypertension (DASH) eating plan indicates the steps that can be taken to accomplish that goal:

- Use reduced sodium or no-salt-added products. For example, choose low or reduced sodium, or no-salt-added versions of foods and condiments when available.
- Buy fresh, plain frozen, or canned with "no-salt-added" vegetables.
- Use fresh poultry, fish, and lean meat, rather than canned, smoked, or processed types.

FAT-SOLUBLE

Vitamin	Major Functions	Deficiency Symptoms	People Most at Risk
Vitamin A (retinoids) and provitamin A (carotenoids)	Promote vision: light and color Promote growth Prevent drying of skin and eyes Promote resistance to bacterial infection	Night blindness Xerophthalmia Poor growth Dry skin	People in poverty, especially preschool children (still very rare in the United States) People with alcoholism People with AIDS
D (chole- and ergocalciferol)	Facilitate absorption of calcium and phosphorus Maintain optimal calcification of bone	Rickets Osteomalacia	Breastfed infants not exposed to sunlight, elderly
E (tocopherois)	Act as an antioxidant: prevent breakdown of vitamin A and unsaturated fatty acids	Hemolysis of red blood cells Nerve destruction	People with poor fat absorption, smokers (still rare as far as we know)
K (phyilo- and menaquinone)	Help form prothrombin and other factors for blood clotting and contribute to bone metabolism	Hemorrhage	People taking antibiotics for months at a time (still quite rare)

WATER-SOLUBLE

Vitamin	Major Functions	Deficiency Symptoms	People Most at Risk
Thiamin	Coenzyme involved in carbohydrate metabolism; nerve function	Beriberi: nervous tingling, poor coordination, edema, heart changes, weakness	People with alcoholism or in poverty
Riboflavin	Coenzyme involved in energy metabolism	Inflammation of mouth and tongue, cracks at corners of the mouth, eye disorders	Possibly people on certain medications if no dairy products consumed
Niacin	Coenzyme involved in energy metabolism, fat synthesis, fat breakdown	Pellagra: diarrhea, dermatitis, dementia	Severe poverty where corn is the dominant food; people with alcoholism
Pantothenic acid	Coenzyme involved in energy metabolism, fat synthesis, fat breakdown	Tingling in hands, fatigue, headache, nausea	People with alcoholism
Biotin	Coenzyme involved in glucose production, fat synthesis	Dermatitis, tongue soreness anemia, depression	People with alcoholism
Vitamin B$_6$ pyridoxine, and other forms	Coenzyme involved in protein metabolism, neurotransmitter synthesis, hemoglobin synthesis, many other functions	Headache, anemia, convulsions, nausea, vomiting, flaky skin, sore tongue	Adolescent and adult women; people on certain medications; people with alcoholism
Folate (folic acid)	Coenzyme involved in DNA synthesis, other functions	Megaloblastic anemia, inflammation of tongue, diarrhea, poor growth, depression	People with alcoholism, pregnancy, people on certain medications
Vitamin B$_{12}$ (cobalamins)	Coenzyme involved in folate metabolism, nerve function, other functions	Macrocytic anemia, poor nerve function	Elderly people because of poor absorption; vegans, people with AIDS
Vitamin C (ascorbic acid)	Connective tissue synthesis, hormone synthesis, neurotransmitter synthesis	Scurvy: poor wound healing, pinpoint hemorrhages, bleeding gums	People with alcoholism, elderly who eat poorly

Note: Values are the Recommended Dietary Allowances (RDAs) for adults 19 to 50 years, unless marked by an asterisk (*), in which case they represent the Adequate Intakes (AIs). The Tolerable Upper Intake Levels (ULs) are listed under toxicity; intakes above these values can lead to negative health consequences.

Dietary Sources*	RDA or AI*	Toxicity Symptoms or UL

Vitamin A
  Liver
  Fortified milk
  Fortified breakfast cereals
Provitamin A
  Sweet potatoes, spinach, greens, carrots, cantaloupe, apricots, broccoli
	Women: 700 micrograms
	Men: 900 micrograms
		Fetal malformations, hair loss, skin changes, pain in bones (UL = 3,000 micrograms)

Vitamin D-fortified milk Fortified breakfast cereals Fish oils Sardines Salmon	5 micrograms	Growth retardation, kidney damage, calcium deposits in soft tissue (UL = 50 micrograms)
Vegetable oils Some greens Some fruits Fortified breakfast cereals	15 milligrams	Muscle weakness, headaches, fatigue, nausea, inhibition of vitamin K metabolism (UL = 1,000 mg)
Green vegetables Liver	Women: 90 micrograms* Men: 120 micrograms*	Anemia and jaundice (medicinal forms only)

Dietary Sources*	RDA or AI*	Toxicity Symptoms
Sunflower seeds, pork, whole and enriched grains, dried beans, peas, brewers yeast	Men: 1.2 milligrams Women: 1.1 milligrams	None possible from food
Milk, mushrooms, spinach, liver, enriched grains	Men: 1.3 milligrams Women: 1.1 milligrams	None reported
Mushrooms, bran, tuna, salmon, chicken, beef, liver, peanuts, enriched grains	Men: 16 milligrams Women: 14 milligrams	Toxicity can begin at over 35 milligrams (UL) (flushing of skin especially seen at over 100 milligrams per day)
Mushrooms, liver, broccoli, eggs; most foods have some	5 milligrams*	None
Cheese, egg yolks, cauliflower, peanut butter, liver	30 micrograms	Unknown
Animal protein foods, spinach, broccoli, bananas, salmon, sunflower seeds	1.3 milligrams	UL = 100 mg; nerve destruction at doses over 200 milligrams
Green leafy vegetables, orange juice, organ meats, sprouts, sunflower seeds	400 micrograms	UL = 1,000 micrograms
Animal foods, especially organ meats, oysters, clams (not natural in plants)	2.4 micrograms	None
Citrus fruits, strawberries, broccoli, greens	Men: 90 milligrams Women: 75 milligrams	UL = 2,000 mg

- Choose ready-to-eat breakfast cereals that are lower in sodium.
- Limit cured foods (such as bacon and ham), foods packed in brine (such as pickles, pickled vegetables, olives, and sauerkraut), and condiments (such as MSG, mustard, horseradish, catsup, and barbecue sauce). Limit even lower-sodium versions of soy sauce and teriyaki sauce—treat these condiments as you do table salt.
- Use spices instead of salt. In cooking and at the table, flavor foods with herbs, spices, lemon, lime, vinegar, or salt-free seasoning blends. Start by cutting salt in half.
- Cook rice, pasta, and hot cereals without salt. Cut back on instant or flavored rice, pasta, and cereal mixes, which usually have added salt.
- Choose "convenience" foods that are lower in sodium. Cut back on frozen dinners, mixed dishes such as pizza, packaged mixes, canned soups or broths, and salad dressing—these often have a lot of sodium.
- Rinse canned foods, such as tuna, to remove some sodium.

Those involved in athletic competition, strenuous exercise, or work in the heat must be concerned about adequate sodium replacement. Generally, because these individuals consume more kcal of food (containing more sodium), this is usually not a problem. More on this in chapter 23.

The previous sections have focused attention on three minerals—calcium, iron, and sodium—because of their relationship to current medical and health-related problems. A summary of each of the minerals, their functions, and food sources is presented in table 18.2.

IN SUMMARY

- The major minerals include calcium, phosphorus, magnesium, sulfur, sodium, potassium, and chloride. The trace elements include iron, iodine, fluoride, zinc, selenium, copper, cobalt, chromium, manganese, molybdenum, arsenic, nickel, and vanadium.
- Inadequate calcium and iron intake have been linked with osteoporosis and anemia, respectively. Those with a genetic predisposition for hypertension due to sodium retention benefit from a reduction in salt intake.

Carbohydrates

Carbohydrates and fats are the primary sources of energy in the average American diet (145) (for an update on recommendations on carbohydrates, fats, and proteins from the Institute of Medicine, see Clinical Applications 18.1). Carbohydrates suffer a bad reputation from those on diets, especially when you consider that you would have to eat over twice as much carbohydrate as fat to consume the same number of calories (4 kcal/g versus 9 kcal/g). Carbohydrates can be divided into two classes: those that can be digested and metabolized for energy (sugars and starches), and those that are undigestible (fiber). The sugars are found in jellies, jams, fruits, soft drinks, honey, syrups, and milk, while the starches are found in cereals, flour, potatoes, and other vegetables (200).

Sugars and Starches Carbohydrate is a major energy source for all tissues and a crucial source for two: red blood cells and neurons. The red blood cells depend exclusively on anaerobic glycolysis for energy, and the nervous system functions well only on carbohydrate. These two tissues can consume 180 grams of glucose per day (49). Given this need it is no surprise that the plasma glucose concentration is maintained within narrow limits by hormonal control mechanisms (see chapter 5). During strenuous exercise the muscle can use 180 grams of glucose in less than one hour. As a result of these needs, one might expect that carbohydrate would make up a large fraction of our energy intake. Currently about 50% of energy intake is derived from carbohydrate (78, 145, 226), within the range of recommended carbohydrate intakes (95). There is great interest not only in the amount of carbohydrate in the diet, but also in the type of carbohydrate as it relates to the prevention and management of diabetes (see Clinical Applications 18.2). While the goal is to increase carbohydrate intake, one of the *Dietary Guidelines for Americans* is to avoid too much sugar. Consistent with that, the recent Institute of Medicine report recommends that a *maximum* of 25% of energy come from "added sugars"—those not derived naturally from fruits. This will ensure sufficient intakes of essential nutrients that are low in the beverages and foods that are the major sources of added sugars in North American diets. The following are helpful suggestions on how to limit intake of added sugars, while meeting the overall carbohydrate goal (201):

- Choose and prepare foods and beverages with little added sugars or caloric sweeteners, such as amounts suggested in the DASH eating plan.
- Reduce the incidence of dental caries by practicing good oral hygiene and consuming sugar- and starch-containing foods and beverages less frequently.

Dietary Fiber Dietary fiber is an important part of the diet. Over the past few years, in an attempt to clar-

CLINICAL APPLICATIONS 18.1

Institute of Medicine Report

At the beginning of the chapter we indicated that a report from the Institute of Medicine (95) made a series of recommendations that will impact a wide variety of existing nutritional recommendations from both federal agencies (e.g., U.S. Department of Agriculture) and professional organizations (e.g., American Heart Association). What follows is a brief summary of information and recommendations related to the intakes of carbohydrate, fat, and protein.

- An RDA for carbohydrate was established for the first time: 130 g/day to meet the glucose needs of the brain.
- An AI for fiber was set at 38 and 25 g/day for men and women, respectively.
- No RDA, AI, or EAR standards were set for saturated fat, mono-

saturated fat, and cholesterol because they have no known beneficial role in preventing chronic disease. In addition, because they are synthesized in the body, they are not required in the diet.

- AI values were set for the omega-6 fatty acid, linoleic acid (17 and 12 g/day for young men and women, respectively) and the omega-3 fatty acid, α-linolenic acid (1.6 and 1.1 g/day for men and women, respectively).
- The long-held adult protein requirement of 0.8 g/day per kilogram of body weight was maintained.

The Institute of Medicine's report recommends a new dietary standard,

called the Acceptable Macronutrient Distribution Ranges (AMDRs). These are defined as ranges of intakes for a particular energy source that is associated with a reduced risk of chronic disease, while providing adequate intake of essential nutrients. The Institute recommends ranges of 20% to 35% fat, 45% to 65% carbohydrate, and the balance (10%–35%), protein. There is evidence that at the *extreme* end of the range, diets low in fat and high in carbohydrate reduce HDL cholesterol and increase the total cholesterol:HDL cholesterol ratio and plasma triglycerides. At the opposite end, when fat intake is high, weight gain occurs and the metabolic consequences of obesity increase, as does the plasma LDL cholesterol.

---

ify what is and is not "fiber," fiber has been divided into the following classes (95):

- *Dietary fiber* consists of nondigestible carbohydrates and lignin that are *intrinsic and intact* in plants. Examples of dietary fiber include plant nonstarch polysaccharides such as cellulose, pectin, gums, hemicellulose, β-glucans, and fibers in oat and wheat bran.

- *Functional fiber* consists of *isolated, nondigestible carbohydrates* that have beneficial physiological effects in humans. Examples of functional fiber include isolated, nondigestible plants (e.g., resistant starches, pectin, and gums) and animal (e.g., chitin and chitosan) or commercially produced (e.g., resistant starch, inulin, and indigestible dextrins) carbohydrates.

- *Total fiber* is the sum of dietary fiber and functional fiber.

Dietary fiber cannot be digested and metabolized, and consequently it provides a sense of fullness (satiation) during a meal without adding calories (59). This fact has been used by bakeries that lower the number of calories per slice of bread by adding cellulose from wood! Pectin and gum are used in food processing to thicken, stabilize, or emulsify the constituents of various food products (44).

Dietary fiber has long been linked to optimal health. Fiber acts as a hydrated sponge as it moves along the large intestine, making constipation less likely by reducing transit time (44, 59). Vegetarian diets high in soluble fiber have been linked to lower serum cholesterol due to the loss of more bile (cholesterol-containing) acids in the feces. However, the fact that vegetarian diets are also lower in the percent of calories from fat, which can also lower serum cholesterol, makes the interpretation of the data more complicated (59). While a high-fiber diet reduces the incidence of diverticulosis, a condition in which outpouchings (diverticula) occur in the colon wall, the role of fiber in preventing colon cancer is mixed (6, 44, 59). A recent review by the American Dietetic Association (ADA) indicated strong epidemiological evidence that a diet rich in fiber reduces the risk of colon cancer. In contrast, intervention studies (in which individuals received added fiber) did not confirm the epidemiological evidence. However, on balance, the ADA believes that the abundance of evidence supports the promotion of a diet high in fiber to protect against colon cancer (6).

Given the broad role of dietary fiber in normal health, it is no surprise that the *Dietary Guidelines for Americans* recommends that Americans increase their intake of fiber (201). A new AI for total fiber, based on an intake level observed to protect against coronary heart disease, has been set at 38 and 25 g/day for men

TABLE 18.2   A Summary of Minerals

		MAJOR MINERALS	
Mineral	Major Functions	Deficiency Symptoms	People Most at Risk
Sodium	Functions as a major ion of the extracellular fluid; aids nerve impulse transmission	Muscle cramps	People who severely restrict sodium to lower blood pressure (250–500 milligrams)
Potassium	Functions as a major ion of intracellular fluid; aids nerve impulse transmission	Irregular heartbeat, loss of appetite, muscle cramps	People who use potassium-wasting diuretics or have poor diets, as seen in poverty and alcoholism
Chloride	Functions as a major ion of the extracellular fluid; participates in acid production in stomach; aids nerve transmission	Convulsions in infants	No one, probably
Calcium	Provides bone and tooth strength; helps blood clotting; aids nerve impulse transmission; required for muscle contractions	Inadequate intake increases the risk for osteoporosis	Women, especially those who consume few dairy products
Phosphorus	Required for bone and tooth strength; serves as part of various metabolic compounds; functions as major ion of intracellular fluid	Poor bone maintenance is a possibility	Older people consuming very nutrient-poor diets; people with alcoholism
Magnesium	Provides bone strength; aids enzyme function; aids nerve and heart function	Weakness, muscle pain, poor heart function	Women, and people on certain diuretics

		KEY TRACE MINERALS	
Mineral	Major Functions	Deficiency Symptoms	People Most at Risk
Iron	Used for hemoglobin and other key compounds used in respiration; used for immune function	Low blood iron; small, pale red blood cells; low blood hemoglobin values	Infants, preschool children, adolescents, women in childbearing years
Zinc	Required for enzymes, involved in growth, immunity, alcohol metabolism, sexual development, and reproduction	Skin rash, diarrhea, decreased appetite and sense of taste, hair loss, poor growth and development, poor wound healing	Vegetarians, elderly people, people with alcoholism
Selenium	Aids antioxidant system	Muscle pain, muscle weakness, form of heart disease	Unknown in healthy Americans
Iodide	Aids thyroid hormone	Goiter; poor growth in infancy when mother is iodide deficient during pregnancy	None in America because salt is usually fortified
Copper	Aids in iron metabolism; works with many enzymes, such as those involved in protein metabolism and hormone synthesis	Anemia, low white blood cell count, poor growth	Infants recovering from semistarvation, people who use overzealous supplementation of zinc
Fluoride	Increases resistance of tooth enamel to dental caries	Increased risk of dental caries	Areas where water is not fluoridated and dental treatments do not make up for a lack of fluoride
Chromium	Enhances blood glucose control	High blood glucose after eating	People on intravenous nutrition, and perhaps elderly people with type 2 diabetes
Manganese	Aids action of some enzymes, such as those involved in carbohydrate metabolism	None in humans	Unknown
Molybdenum	Aids action of some enzymes	None in healthy humans	Unsupplemented intravenous nutrition

Note: Values are the Recommended Dietary Allowances (RDAs) for adults 19 to 50 years, unless marked by an asterisk (*), in which case they represent the Adequate Intakes (AIs). The Tolerable Upper Intake Levels (ULs) are listed under toxicity; intakes above these values can lead to negative health consequences.

RDA or AI*	Rich Dietary Sources	Results of Toxicity or UL
1,500 milligrams*	Table salt, processed foods, condiments, sauces, soups, chips	UL = 2,300 mg; contributes to high blood pressure in susceptible individuals; leads to increased calcium loss in urine
4,700 milligrams*	Spinach, squash, bananas, orange juice, other vegetables and fruits, milk, meat, legumes, whole grains	Results in slowing of the heartbeat; seen in kidney failure
2,300 milligrams*	Table salt, some vegetables, processed foods	UL = 3,600 mg; linked to high blood pressure in susceptible people when combined with sodium
1,000 milligrams*	Dairy products, canned fish, leafy vegetables, tofu, fortified orange juice (and other fortified foods)	UL = 2,500 mg; higher intakes may cause kidney stones and other problems in susceptible people; poor mineral absorption in general
700 milligrams (age over 18 years)	Dairy products, processed foods, fish, soft drinks, bakery products, meats	UL = 4,000 milligrams; impairs bone health in people with kidney failure; results in poor bone mineralization if calcium intakes are low
Men: 420 milligrams Women: 320 milligrams	Wheat bran, green vegetables, nuts, chocolate, legumes	UL = 350 mg, but refers only to pharmacologic agents

RDA or AI*	Rich Dietary Sources	Results of Toxicity
Men: 8 milligrams Women: 18 milligrams	Meats, spinach, seafood, broccoli, peas, bran, enriched breads	UL = 45 mg; toxicity seen when children consume 60 milligrams or more in iron pills; also in people with hemochromatosis
Men: 11 milligrams Women: 8 milligrams	Seafoods, meats, greens, whole grains	UL = 40 milligrams; reduces copper absorption; can cause diarrhea, cramps, and depressed immune function
55 micrograms	Meats, eggs, fish, seafoods, whole grains	UL = 400 micrograms; nausea, vomiting, hair loss, weakness, liver disease
150 micrograms	Iodized salt, white bread, saltwater fish, dairy products	UL = 1,100 micrograms; inhibition of function of the thyroid gland
900 micrograms	Liver, cocoa, beans, nuts, whole grains, dried fruits	UL = 10 milligrams; vomiting; nervous system disorders
Men: 4 milligrams Women: 3 milligrams	Fluoridated water, toothpaste, dental treatments, tea, seaweed	UL = 10 mg; stomach upset; mottling (staining) of teeth during development; bone pain
Men: 30–35 micrograms* Women: 20–25 micrograms*	Egg yolks, whole grains, pork, nuts, mushrooms, beer	Liver damage and lung cancer (caused by industrial contamination, not dietary excess)
Men: 2.3 milligrams* Women: 1.8 milligrams*	Nuts, oats, beans, tea	UL = 11 milligrams
45 micrograms	Beans, grains, nuts	UL = 2,000 micrograms

CLINICAL APPLICATIONS 18.2

Glycemic Index—What Is It and Is It Important?

We all know that when we eat there is an increase in insulin secretion to promote the uptake, use, and storage of carbohydrates. The degree to which the blood glucose concentration increases and remains elevated depends on the kinds and amounts of carbohydrate ingested, as well as the person's insulin response and tissue sensitivity to the insulin (178).

It is well known that certain carbohydrates elicit a more rapid blood glucose response than others. The glycemic index (GI) has been used to describe the magnitude of those differences and help those who have difficulty processing glucose make better decisions in planning meals. The GI quantifies the blood glucose response (above fasting) to an individual carbohydrate food over a two-hour period following ingestion. This response is compared to a reference food (glucose or white bread) of the same weight. Those foods with a low GI would provide less of a challenge to someone with a reduced capacity to take up and use glucose (e.g., type 2 diabetic). However, because these carbohydrates are compared on a "per gram" basis, the GI does not consider the impact that the actual amount of carbohydrate in the meal has on the response. The "glycemic load" attempts to do that by multiplying the GI by the amount of carbohydrate in the serving (178).

The simplicity of the GI and glycemic load is complicated by the fact that most meals do not contain a single carbohydrate. Factors such as the amount of protein and fat in the diet will impact the blood glucose response to the carbohydrate ingested. In spite of that, studies support the use of the GI as a tool to help shape the selection of carbohydrate-containing foods to reduce cholesterol and improve the metabolic control of diabetics (147). However, focus on the GI and glycemic load should not ignore the importance of achieving a healthy body weight in the prevention and management of diabetes (178).

---

and women, nineteen to fifty years of age, respectively (95). According to *Dietary Guidelines for Americans*, to increase the intake of fiber and complex carbohydrates, we should choose fiber-rich fruits, vegetables, and whole grains often. This can be accomplished by consuming whole fruit rather than fruit juices, eating dry beans and peas several times per week, and making sure at least half of the grain servings come from whole grains.

Fats

Dietary lipids include triglycerides, phospholipids, and **cholesterol.** If solid at room temperature, lipids are fats; if liquid, oils. Lipids contain 9 kcal/g, and represent about 33% of the American diet, slightly higher than the dietary goal of 30%, but lower than the 42% recorded in 1977 (47, 78, 145, 204, 215).

Fat not only provides fuel for energy, it is important in the absorption of fat-soluble vitamins, and for cell membrane structure, hormone synthesis (steroids), insulation, and the protection of vital organs (44). Most fat is stored in adipose tissue, for subsequent release into the bloodstream as free fatty acids (see chapter 4). Because of fat's caloric density (9 kcal/g), we are able to carry a large energy reserve, with little weight. In fact, the energy content of one pound of adipose tissue, 3,500 kcal, is sufficient to cover the cost of running a marathon. The other side of this coin is that because of this very high caloric density, it takes a long time to decrease the mass of adipose tissue when on a diet.

The focus of attention in the medical community has been on the role of dietary fat in the development of atherosclerosis, a process in which the arterial wall becomes thickened, leading to a narrowing of the lumen of the artery. This is the underlying problem associated with coronary artery disease and stroke. While the specific cause is not known, it is believed that a variety of factors can damage the protective endothelial lining of the artery, allowing substances to build up and block the artery. The factors that can accelerate this process include elevated serum cholesterol and triglycerides, high blood pressure, and cigarette smoking (52). In the section on dietary goals, two of the recommendations dealt with this problem of atherosclerosis: a reduction in salt intake (see minerals), and a reduction in fat, saturated fat, and cholesterol. A reduction in each of the last three has been shown to reduce serum cholesterol, and with it, the risk of atherosclerosis (2). See Clinical Applications 18.3 for more on the role of diet composition on risk factor development.

Usually the cholesterol concentration in the serum is divided into two classes on the basis of what type of **lipoprotein** is carrying the cholesterol. **Low-density lipoproteins (LDLs)** carry more cholesterol than do the **high-density lipoproteins (HDLs).** High levels of **LDL cholesterol** are directly related to cardiovascular risk, while high levels of **HDL cholesterol** offer protection from heart disease (2). The concentration of HDL cholesterol is influenced by heredity, gender, exercise, and diet. Diets high in saturated fats increase LDL cholesterol. A reduction in

Diet Composition and Syndrome X

In chapter 14 we introduced you to "syndrome X" ("the deadly quartet" or the "metabolic syndrome") as an example of how scientists have tried to establish links among various cardiovascular risk factors in order to better understand how one affects the other. The risk factors included elevated levels of plasma insulin (hyperinsulinemia) and lipids (hyperlipidemia), high blood pressure (hypertension), and obesity. Some suggest that obesity, especially abdominal obesity, is the underlying cause of elevated cardiovascular disease risk, while others point to insulin resistance (and the resulting elevated insulin) as the cause. In one of a series of provocative studies, Barnard et al. (9) make a case for diet composition as the underlying cause of the problem. This is an important consideration given the potential to break up the deadly quartet.

These investigators put rats on either a high-fat, refined-sugar (HFS) diet or a low-fat, complex carbohydrate (LFCC) diet for two years. Animals were taken from each group beginning at two weeks and ending at two years to evaluate changes in body fatness and fat cell size, insulin resistance (ability of a tissue to take up glucose), plasma insulin and lipid levels, and blood pressure. They found that:

- Insulin resistance and elevated levels of plasma insulin were present at two weeks in the HFS group and, therefore, preceded all other aspects of the syndrome.
- Plasma triglycerides were significantly elevated by the second month in the HFS group.
- Body fatness was not different until six months, but fat cell size was already increased in those on the HFS diet by two months.
- Blood pressure was not different until twelve months, but by eighteen months all of the rats on the HFS diet had high blood pressure.

This study showed that the composition of the diet was the cause of the insulin resistance, and that the insulin resistance preceded the other aspects of the syndrome. However, the authors acknowledged that the obesity probably contributed to the gradual worsening of the insulin resistance (demanding higher levels of insulin) over time. Blood pressure was the slowest-responding component of the syndrome and may be linked to the insulin resistance as described in chapter 14. This study confirmed the importance of diet on risk factor development and supports the recommendation of a low-fat, high-complex carbohydrate diet.

---

the sources of saturated fats, including meats, animal fat, palm oil, coconut oil, hydrogenated shortenings, whole milk, cream, butter, ice cream, and cheese would reduce LDL cholesterol. Just substituting unsaturated fats for these saturated fats will lower serum cholesterol. The American Heart Association has recommended that total fat consumption be limited to 30% of calories to reduce the risk of heart disease (2). The most recent recommendation from the Institute of Medicine provides a range of values (20%–35%); however, most of the range is consistent with the older recommendation. Dietary restriction of cholesterol has been shown to be effective in lowering serum cholesterol (2); however, this effect is influenced by the percentage of saturated fat in the diet and the initial level of serum cholesterol (i.e., those with high serum cholesterol levels benefit the most) (62). Based on currently available evidence, it is reasonable and prudent to recommend a decrease in cholesterol in the diet to 300 mg/day or less (2, 144). In addition, there is a special emphasis on eliminating trans fats from the diet. These fats rival saturated fats as a contributor to heart disease, and substituting polyunsaturated fats should reduce cholesterol levels (113). The following suggestions were provided as part of the 2005 Dietary Guidelines for Americans to have a diet low in fat, saturated fat, and cholesterol (201):

Fats and Oils

- Consume less than 10% of calories from saturated fatty acids and less than 300 mg/day of cholesterol, and keep trans fatty acid consumption as low as possible.

- Keep total fat intake between 20% and 35% of calories, with most fats coming from sources of polyunsaturated and monounsaturated fatty acids, such as fish, nuts, and vegetable oils.

- When selecting and preparing meat, poultry, dry beans, and milk or milk products, make choices that are lean, low fat, or fat free.

- Limit intake of fats and oils high in saturated and/or trans fatty acids, and choose products low in such fats and oils.

Protein

Protein, at 4 kcal/g, is not viewed as a primary energy source, as are fats and carbohydrates. Rather, it is important because it contains the nine essential (indispensable) amino acids, without which the body cannot synthesize all the proteins needed for tissues, enzymes, and hormones. The *quality of* protein in a diet is based on how well these essential amino acids are represented. In terms of quality, the best sources for protein are eggs, milk, and fish, with *good* sources being meat, poultry, cheese, and soybeans. *Fair* sources of protein include grains, vegetables, seeds and nuts, and other legumes. Given that a meal contains a variety of foods, one food of higher-quality protein tends to complement another of lower-quality protein to result in an adequate intake of essential amino acids (44).

The adult RDA protein requirement of 0.8 g/kg is easily met with diets that include a variety of the aforementioned foods. Overall, most Americans meet either of these recommendations. The protein requirement for athletes is discussed in chapter 23.

IN SUMMARY

- Carbohydrate is a primary source of energy in the American diet and is divided into two classes: that which can be metabolized (sugars and starches) and dietary fiber.
- Two recommendations to improve health status in the American population are to consume complex carbohydrates to represent about 45% to 65% of the calories, and to add more dietary fiber.
- Americans consume too much saturated fat, and the recommended change is to reduce this to no more than 10% of the total calories. Trans fat intake should be reduced as much as possible, and most fat intake should come from sources containing polyunsaturated and monounsaturated fatty acids.
- The protein requirement of 0.8 g/kg can be met with low-fat selections to minimize fat intake.

MEETING THE GUIDELINES AND ACHIEVING THE GOALS

A good diet would allow an individual to achieve the RDA/AI for protein, minerals, and vitamins, while emphasizing carbohydrates and minimizing fats. The new *Dietary Guidelines for Americans* describes a healthy diet as one that:

- emphasizes fruits, vegetables, whole grains, and fat-free or low-fat milk and milk products;
- includes lean meats, poultry, fish, beans, eggs, and nuts; and
- is low in saturated fats, trans fats, cholesterol, salt (sodium), and added sugars.

A variety of food group plans have been developed to help plan a diet consistent with these guidelines.

Food Group Plans

One of the best known plans, the Basic Four Food Group Plan, included meat and meat substitutes, milk and milk products, fruits and vegetables, and grains (breads and cereals) as the food groups. Adults chose at least two, two, four, and four servings per day from these respective groups. The emphasis was on eating a variety of items within each group in which **nutrient density** is relatively high. Nutrient density describes the nutrient content in 1,000 kcal of a food (145). Selecting foods of high nutrient density keeps the nutrients high and total kcals low. The quantity of each item within a food group in the Basic Four Food Group Plan was based on the quantity of a *specific nutrient* contained therein. For example, items on the milk list had to have the calcium content in one cup of milk, and the meat portion was based on protein content. The U.S. Department of Agriculture now uses a different approach to provide guidance in making food selections consistent with the *Dietary Guidelines for Americans*.

The Food Guide Pyramid The Food Guide Pyramid was released by the U. S. Department of Agriculture in 1992 as an approach to eating that emphasized the various food groups, as well as a broad range of intakes to satisfy a variety of caloric needs in the population. Scientists like Walter Willett (221) argued that the Food Guide Pyramid had a variety of problems (e.g., all fats are bad; no guidance on body weight and physical activity) and needed to be fixed. The Food Guide Pyramid was completely revised and released with the publication of the 2005 *Dietary Guidelines for Americans*. It is one of the two food plan approaches recommended in the *Dietary Guidelines for Americans*; the other is the DASH eating plan (see next section).

Table 18.3, adapted from a graphic on the U.S. Department of Agriculture's website (http://www.mypyramid.gov/), outlines the basic components of MyPyramid. The major food groups (grains, vegetables, fruits, milk, and meats and beans) are listed along with a tip to follow and how much is needed in each category to meet a 2,000 kcal/day energy expenditure. As you can see, special attention is focused on physical activity as one part of achieving and maintaining a healthy weight. We encourage each student to log on to this website and work your way through the menu to get a feel for the user-friendly nature of the MyPyramid plan. A major theme is that "one size does not fit all" and by providing your age, gender, and level of physical activity you can print out a dietary plan that should meet *your* energy needs as well as the various RDA/AI standards.

TABLE 18.3 MyPyramid Food Groups

Check how you did today and set a goal to aim for tomorrow

Food Group	Tip	Goal Based on a 2,000-Calorie Pattern
GRAINS	Make at least half your grains whole grains.	*6-ounce equivalents* (1-ounce equivalent is about 1 slice bread, 1 cup dry cereal, or ½ cup cooked rice, pasta, or cereal)
VEGETABLES	Try to have vegetables from several subgroups each day.	*2½ cups* Subgroups: dark green, orange, starchy, dry beans and peas, other veggies
FRUITS	Make most choices fruit, not juice.	*2 cups*
MILK	Choose fat-free or low-fat milk products most often.	*3 cups* (1½ ounces cheese = 1 cup milk)
MEAT & BEANS	Choose lean meat and poultry. Vary your choices—more fish, beans, peas, nuts, and seeds.	*5 ½-ounce equivalents* (1 ounce equivalent is 1 ounce meat, poultry, or fish, 1 egg, 1 T peanut butter, ½ ounce nuts, or ¼ cup dry beans)
PHYSICAL ACTIVITY	Build more physical activity into your daily routine at home and work.	At least *30 minutes* of moderate to vigorous activity a day, 10 minutes or more at a time.

Modified from: www.mypyramid.gov.

Dietary Approaches to Stop Hypertension (DASH) The DASH eating plan (202) was also identified in the *Dietary Guidelines for Americans* as a means to meet DRI/RDA standards and the various recommendations set forth in the document. The DASH plan was developed (as indicated in the title) to deal with hypertension, both to prevent it and to lower blood pressure in those with the problem (see **www.nhlbi.nih.gov/health/public/heart/hbp/dash/**). The DASH eating plan has been recognized for some time as an excellent approach to healthy eating consistent with reducing cardiovascular risk factors and achieving and maintaining a normal body weight. Table 18.4 shows the various food groups and serving sizes for this plan for a 2,000 kcal/day energy intake.

Evaluating the Diet

Independent of your dietary plan, the question arises as to how well you are achieving the guidelines. How do you analyze your diet? The first thing to do is to determine what you are eating, without fooling yourself. The use of the **twenty-four-hour recall** method relies on your ability to remember, from a specific time in one day, what you ate during the previous twenty-four hours. You have to judge the size of the portion you have eaten and make a judgment of whether or not that day was representative of what you normally eat. Other people use **food records,** in which a person records what is eaten throughout the day. It is recommended that a person obtain food records for three or four days per week to have a better estimate of usual dietary intake. Since the simple act of recording food intake may change our eating habits, one has to try and eat as normally as possible when recording food intake. It is important to remember that the RDA standards are to be met over the long run, and variations from those standards will exist from day to day (44).

IN SUMMARY

The 2005 *Dietary Guidelines for Americans* identified two approaches to use to meet dietary standards and achieve a healthy body weight:

- The U.S. Department of Agriculture's MyPyramid promotes a personalized approach to healthy eating and physical activity. It replaced the Food Guide Pyramid.
- The Dietary Approaches to Stop Hypertension (DASH) food plan is suitable for all to use in planning a healthy diet, whether one has hypertension or not.

TABLE 18.4 The DASH Eating Plan

The DASH eating plan shown below is based on 2,000 calories a day. The number of daily servings in a food group may vary from those listed, depending on your caloric needs. Use this chart to help you plan your menus or take it with you when you go to the store.

Food Group	Daily Servings (except as noted)	Serving Sizes	Examples and Notes
Grains and grain products	7–8	1 slice bread 1 oz dry cereal* ½ cup cooked rice, pasta, or cereal	Whole-wheat bread, English muffin, pita bread, bagel, cereals, grits, oatmeal, crackers, unsalted pretzels and popcorn
Vegetables	4–5	1 cup raw leafy vegetable ½ cup cooked vegetable 6 oz vegetable juice	Tomatoes, potatoes, carrots, green peas, squash, broccoli, turnip greens, collards, kale, spinach, artichokes, green beans, lima beans, sweet potatoes
Fruits	4–5	6 oz fruit juice 1 medium fruit ¼ cup dried fruit ½ cup fresh, frozen, or canned fruit	Apricots, bananas, dates, grapes, oranges, orange juice, grapefruit, grapefruit juice, mangoes, melons, peaches, pineapples, prunes, raisins, strawberries, tangerines
Low-fat or fat-free dairy foods	2–3	8 oz milk 1 cup yogurt 1½ oz cheese	Fat-free (skim) or low-fat (1%) milk, fat-free or low-fat buttermilk, fat-free or low-fat regular or frozen yogurt, low-fat and fat-free cheese
Meats, poultry, and fish	2 or less	3 oz cooked meats, poultry, or fish	Select only lean; trim away visible fats; broil, roast, or boil, instead of frying; remove skin from poultry
Nuts, seeds, and dry beans	4–5 per week	⅓ cup or 1½ oz nuts 2 T or ½ oz seeds ½ cup cooked dry beans	Almonds, filberts, mixed nuts, peanuts, walnuts, sunflower seeds, kidney beans, lentils, peas
Fats and oils†	2–3	1 tsp soft margarine 1 T low-fat mayonnaise 2 T light salad dressing 1 tsp vegetable oil	Soft margarine, low-fat mayonnaise, light salad dressing, vegetable oil (such as olive, corn, canola, or safflower)
Sweets	5 per week	1 T sugar 1 T jelly or jam ½ oz jelly beans 8 oz lemonade	Maple syrup, sugar, jelly, jam, fruit-flavored gelatin, jelly beans, hard candy, fruit punch, sorbet, ices

*Equals ½–1¼ cups, depending on cereal type. Check the product's Nutrition Facts Label.

†Fat content changes serving counts for fats and oils: For example. 1 T of regular salad dressing equals 1 serving; 1 T of a low-fat dressing equals ½ serving; 1 T of a fat free dressing equals 0 servings.

Modified from the DASH Eating Plan 2003. U.S. Department of Health and Human Services.

BODY COMPOSITION

Obesity is a major problem in our society, being related to hypertension, elevated serum cholesterol, and adult onset diabetes (106, 143). In addition, there is growing concern that as the incidence of childhood obesity increases, so will the pool of obese adults. In order to deal with this problem, we must be able to assess the prevalence of overweight and obesity, as well as describe in more specific terms changes in body composition. This section presents a brief overview on how to do that. For those interested in a thorough discussion of body composition assessment issues, we refer you to Heyward and Stolarczyk's *Applied Body Composition Assessment* and Roche, Heymsfield, and Lohman's *Human Body Composition* in the Selected Readings.

Methods of Assessing Overweight and Obesity

The Metropolitan Life Insurance Company's 1959 height/weight table (135) has been one of the most common methods used to make judgments about whether or not a person is overweight (table 18.5). These tables are based on that company's policyholders, and the body weights associated with the lowest rate of mortality are listed by frame size. In 1983 an updated table was published that allowed more weight at each height. It has been suggested that the lower death rates at the higher weights in the 1983 table were a result of better treatment of coronary heart disease and diabetes, which allows heavier people to live longer; a reduction in cigarette smoking; and an increase in physical activity (52).

Independent of which table is used, there are some problems associated with their use (7):

- Persons seeking and receiving insurance are not representative of the general population.

- Some persons are represented more than once in the table, since policies (not people) were tabulated.

- Heights and weights were not measured in every case (some policyholders simply stated these).

- Body frame size was not measured.

In spite of these limitations, one of the most common indices of overweight and obesity is calculated from this table. In this procedure the midpoint in the weight range for a medium frame for a given height is used as a standard against which other body weights are compared. Dividing a person's weight by the midpoint in the weight range generates a relative weight (RW) or obesity index. A person with a body weight equal to the midpoint value would have an RW = 1.00. In contrast, if we look at the 1959 table (table 18.5), a man who is 6 feet tall and weighs 200 lbs has an RW = 1.23 (200 lb ÷ 162 lb). A person who is 10% above normal (RW = 1.10) is classified as overweight, and if 20% above normal (RW = 1.20), is classified as obese. Our male subject at 23% above normal would be classified as obese.

Another measure of overweight and obesity that has been universally adopted is the Body Mass Index (BMI), which is the ratio of body weight (in kilograms) to height (in meters) squared: $BMI = wt\,[kg] \div ht\,[m^2]$. The BMI is easily calculated, and guidelines for classifying someone as overweight or obese have used percentile rankings or fixed BMI values (125). As these BMI guidelines were developed, some allowances were made for age (higher values), but some scientists felt that the higher values were too generous given their association with higher rates of morbidity and mortal-

TABLE 18.5	Desirable Weights for Men and Women, Twenty-Five Years of Age and Over		
HEIGHT* Feet Inches	Small Frame	Medium Frame	Large Frame
Men			
5 2	112–120	118–129	126–141
5 3	115–123	121–133	129–144
5 4	118–126	124–136	133–148
5 5	121–129	127–139	135–152
5 6	124–133	130–143	138–156
5 7	128–137	134–147	142–161
5 8	132–141	138–152	147–166
5 9	136–145	142–156	151–170
5 10	140–150	146–160	155–174
5 11	144–154	150–165	159–179
6 0	148–158	154–170	164–184
6 1	152–162	158–175	168–189
6 2	156–167	162–180	173–194
6 3	160–171	167–185	178–199
6 4	164–175	172–190	182–204
HEIGHT* Feet Inches	Small Frame	Medium Frame	Large Frame
Women			
4 10	92–98	96–107	104–119
4 11	94–101	98–110	106–122
5 0	96–104	101–113	109–125
5 1	99–107	104–116	112–128
5 2	102–110	107–119	115–131
5 3	105–113	110–122	118–134
5 4	108–116	113–126	121–138
5 5	111–119	116–130	125–142
5 6	114–123	120–135	129–146
5 7	118–127	124–139	133–150
5 8	122–131	128–143	137–154
5 9	126–135	132–147	141–158
5 10	130–140	136–151	145–163
5 11	134–144	140–155	149–168
6 0	138–148	144–159	153–173

*With shoes with 1-inch heels.

**With shoes with 2-inch heels.

Courtesy *Statistical Bulletin*, Metropolitan Insurance Company.

ity (25, 219, 220). Current BMI standards that have been adopted worldwide include (143):

Underweight	<18.5
Normal	18.5–24.9
Overweight	25.0–29.9
Obesity—Class I	30.0–34.9
Obesity—Class II	35.0–39.9
Extreme Obesity—Class III	≥40

The BMI standards listed above are for adults. To assess overweight and obesity in children, investigators and clinicians have relied on percentile cut offs (e.g., 85th and 95th percentile, respectively). There are ongoing attempts to identify specific BMI cut offs for ages 2 to 17 to allow easier identification of children who are overweight and obese and to take action earlier (46).

One of the major problems associated with height/weight tables and the BMI is that there is no way to know if the person is heavily muscled or simply overfat. One of the earliest uses of body composition analysis showed that with height/weight tables, "All-American" football players weighing 200 lbs would have been found unfit for military service and would not have received life insurance (218). Clearly there is a need to distinguish overweight from overfat, and that will be the purpose of the next section of this chapter.

Methods of Measuring Body Composition

The most direct way to measure body composition is to do a chemical analysis of the whole body to determine the amount of water, fat, protein, and minerals. This is a common method used in nutritional studies on rats, but it is useless in providing information for the average person. The following is a brief summary of techniques providing information about (a) the composition of the whole body and (b) the development or change in specific tissues of the body.

Isotope Dilution   Total body water (TBW) is determined by the isotope dilution method. In this method a subject drinks an isotope of water (tritiated water—^3H_2O), deuterated water (^2H_2O), or ^{18}O-labeled water ($H_2^{18}O$) that is distributed throughout the body water. After three to four hours to allow for distribution of the isotope, a sample of body fluid (serum or saliva) is obtained and the concentration of the isotope is determined. The volume of TBW is obtained by calculating how much body water would be needed to achieve that concentration. A person with a large amount of body water will dilute the isotope to a greater extent. People with large TBW volumes possess more lean tissue and less fat tissue, so TBW can be used to determine body fatness (64, 169).

Photon Absorptiometry   This method is used to determine the mineral content and density of bones. A beam of photons from iodine-125 is passed over a bone or bones, and the transmission of the photon beam through bone and soft tissue is obtained. There is a very strong positive relationship between the absorption of the photons and the mineral density of the bones (41, 125).

Potassium-40   Potassium is located primarily within the cells, along with a naturally occurring radioactive isotope of potassium: ^{40}K. The ^{40}K can be measured in a whole-body "counter" and is proportional to the mass of lean tissue (29).

Hydrostatic (Underwater) Weighing   Water has a density of about 1 g/ml, and body fat, with a density of about 0.900 g/ml, will float in water. Lean tissue has a density of about 1.100 in adults and will sink in water. Whole body density provides information about the portion of the body that is lean and fat. Underwater weighing methods are commonly used to determine body density and will be discussed in more detail (125).

Dual Energy X-Ray Absorptiometry (DEXA)   In this new technology, a single X-ray source is used to determine whole-body and regional estimates of lean tissue, bone, mineral, and fat with a high degree of accuracy. The software required for this process continues to be refined, and DEXA is expected to play a major role in the future of body composition analysis (60, 125, 131, 208).

Near Infrared Interactance (NIR)   This method is based on the absorption of light, reflectance, and near infrared spectroscopy (30). A fiber-optic probe is placed over the biceps and an infrared light beam is emitted. The light passes through subcutaneous fat and muscle and is reflected by bone back to the probe. Generally, there has been little interaction between scientists and the manufacturers in the development and validation of this type of device (125), and recent studies suggest that this technology has a way to go (33, 133).

Radiography   An X ray of a limb allows one to measure the widths of fat, muscle, and bone, and has been used extensively in tracing the growth of these tissues over time (103). Fat-width measurements can also be used to estimate total body fat (71, 107).

Ultrasound   Sound waves are transmitted through tissues and the echoes are received and analyzed. This technique has been used to measure the thickness of subcutaneous fat. Present technology allows for whole-body scans and the determination of the volumes of various organs (30).

Nuclear Magnetic Resonance (NMR)   In this method, electromagnetic waves are transmitted through tissues. Select nuclei absorb and then release energy at a particular frequency (resonance). The resonant-frequency characteristics are related to the type of tissue. Computer analysis of the signal can provide detailed images, and the volumes of specific tissues can be calculated (30).

Total Body Electrical Conductivity (TOBEC)

Body composition is analyzed by TOBEC on the basis that lean tissue and water conduct electricity better than does fat. In this method, the subject lies in a large cylindrical coil while an electric current is injected into the coil. The electromagnetic field developed in the space enclosed by the cylindrical coil is affected by the subject's body composition (158, 174, 207).

Bioelectrical Impedance Analysis (BIA)   The basis for BIA is similar to that of TOBEC, but it uses a small portable instrument. An electrical current (50 μA usually set at a frequency of 50 kHz) is applied to an extremity and resistance to that current (due to the specific resistivity and volume of the conductor—the fat-free mass) is measured (125, 174, 207). Total body water is calculated, and the value can be used to estimate percent body fatness, as was mentioned for the isotope dilution procedure. BIA devices using multiple frequencies (7, 54, and 100 kHz) show promise of improved accuracy (125, 176, 209). This technique may be an appropriate field method to use in place of or in addition to skinfolds in testing the elderly (75).

Air Displacement Plethysmography   Body density can also be calculated from body volume measurements obtained via air displacement plethysmography (in contrast to water displacement that is used in hydrostatic weighing). Small changes in pressure, due to the change in volume of air in the chamber, are used to calculate the volume of the individual sitting in the chamber. The Bod Pod uses this technology to simplify the measurement of body volume and therefore the calculation of whole body density. The information obtained is used in the same way as that collected in hydrostatic weighing (53). Although percent body fat values derived from this method may not be the same as those from hydrostatic weighing, the differences are small (136).

Skinfold Thickness   An estimate of total body fatness is made from a measure of subcutaneous fat. A number of skinfold measurements are obtained and the values used in equations to calculate body density (120, 125). Details on this technique will be presented in a later section.

Some of these procedures are expensive in terms of personnel and equipment (e.g., potassium-40, TOBEC, radiography, ultrasound, NMR, DEXA, TBW), and are not used on a routine basis for body composition analysis. BIA has gained greater acceptance in the past few years, due in part to a collaborative multi-university research project that showed it to be comparable to skinfold estimates of body fatness in men and women (125, 213). The data from these techniques can be used alone or in combination to provide an assessment of body composition. A variety of models have been proposed for this purpose (92, 125, 126, 153):

- Four-component model—this model uses information on mineral, water, protein, and fat to assess body composition. The careful measurement of each of these components allows one to account for variations in bone density (mineral) and total body water that might vary dramatically in certain populations (e.g., growing children, the elderly). These procedures would give one the best estimates of percent fat.

- Three-component model—in this model the body is divided into three components: (a) body water, protein + mineral, and fat, or (b) body water + protein, mineral, and fat. The three-component model also allows one to account for variations in either bone density or body water and improve estimates of body fatness.

- Two-component model—this, the oldest model, divides the body into two components: the fat mass and the fat-free mass. Although it is still the most commonly used approach to estimate percent fat, the assumptions underlying this model have been questioned. The limitations of the two-component model have been addressed using information collected with the three- and four-component models. The details will be provided in the following sections.

IN SUMMARY

- A height/weight table and the body mass index (BMI) can indicate "overweight" relative to an average weight, but do not provide quantitative information about the composition of that weight in terms of fat-free mass and fat mass.
- Body composition can be measured in terms of total body water (isotope dilution, bioelectric impedance analysis), bone density (photon absorptiometry), lean tissue mass (potassium-40), density (underwater weighing, air displacement plethysmography), and thickness of various tissues (ultrasound, radiography, skinfolds).
- Body composition assessment can be based on four-component (mineral, water, protein, and fat), three-component (body water, protein + mineral, and fat, or body water + protein, mineral, and fat), or two-component (fat-free mass and fat mass) models. The four-component model is the most accurate.

Two-Component System of Body Composition

Two approaches that are used extensively to estimate percent fat include the **underwater weighing** and skinfold methods. In both of these methods the investigator obtains an estimate of **whole-body density,** and from this calculates the percentage of the body that is fat and the percentage that is fat-free. This is the two-component body composition system described by Behnke that is commonly used to describe changes in body composition (10). The conversion of whole-body density values to fat and fat-free tissue components relies on "constants" used for each of those tissue components. Human fat tissue is believed to have a density of 0.900 g/ml, and fat-free tissue a density of 1.100 g/ml. Using these density values, Siri (183) derived an equation to calculate percent body fat from whole-body density:

$$\% \text{ body fat} = \frac{495}{\text{Density}} - 450$$

This equation is correct only if the density values for fat tissue and fat-free tissue are 0.900 and 1.100 g/ml, respectively. Investigators sensed that certain populations might have fat-free tissue densities different from that of 1.100 g/ml when they observed high values for body fatness for children and the elderly, and extremely low values (<0% body fat) in professional football players (75, 127, 223). Children have lower bone mineral contents, less potassium, and more water per unit fat-free mass, yielding a lower density for fat-free mass (127). Lohman (122) reports density values (g/ml) of 1.080 at age six, 1.084 at age ten, and 1.097 for boys aged fifteen-and-one-half. The lower values in the prepubescent child would overestimate percent body fat by 5%. Based on data from the multicomponent models of body composition, Lohman (124) recommends the values found in table 18.6 for Siri's equation when applied to children, youth, and young adults (see table 18.6).

In contrast to children, who have density values below 1.100 for the fat-free mass, African Americans were shown to have a density of 1.113 g/ml (173). The Siri equation would have to be modified as follows:

$$\% \text{ body fat} = \frac{437}{\text{Density}} - 393$$

While this may appear to be quite complicated, there is good reason to have the correct equation for a specific population. If judgments are to be made about the distribution of obesity in our society, it is important that estimates of body fatness be reasonably accurate. The following sections will discuss how whole-body density values are determined by under-

TABLE 18.6	Equations for Estimating % Fat from Body Density Based on Age and Gender				
AGE, YRS.	**MALE**		**FEMALE**	
	C_1	C_2	C_1	C_2
1	572	536	569	533
1–2	564	526	565	526
3–4	553	514	558	520
5–6	543	503	553	514
7–8	538	497	543	503
9–10	530	489	535	495
11–12	523	481	525	484
13–14	507	464	512	469
15–16	503	459	507	464
Young adult	495	450	505	462

Note: C_1 and C_2 are the terms in percent fat equation to substitute for the Siri equation of percent fat $= \left[\dfrac{C_1}{D_b} - C_2\right]$.

Reprinted, by permission, from T. G. Lohman, 1989, "Assessment of Body Composition in Children," in *Pediatric Exercise Science,* Vol. 1(1):22.

water weighing and skinfold procedures. Heyward and Stolarczyk's text (see the Selected Readings) provides guidance in choosing the most appropriate equation depending on age, race, gender, or other factors.

Underwater Weighing Density is equal to mass divided by volume (D = M/V). Since we already know body mass (body weight), we only have to determine body volume in order to calculate whole-body density (77). The underwater weighing method applies Archimedes' principle, which states that when an object is placed in water it is buoyed up by a counterforce equal to the water it displaces. The volume of water displaced (spilled over) would equal the *loss of weight* while the object is completely submerged. Some investigators determine body volume by measuring the actual volume of water displaced; others measure weight while the subject is underwater, and obtain body volume by subtracting the weight measured in water (M_W) from that measured in air (M_A), or ($M_A - M_W$). Both methods of determining volume are reproducible, but percent body fat values are slightly but significantly (0.7%) lower with the volume displacement method (214). The weight of water displaced is converted to a volume by dividing by the density of the water (D_W) at the time of measurement:

$$D = \frac{M}{V} = \frac{M_A}{\dfrac{(M_A - M_W)}{D_W}}$$

This denominator must now be corrected for two other volumes: the volume of air in the lungs at the

FIGURE 18.2 The underwater weighing technique illustrating two individuals with the same weight and height, but different body composition.

time of measurement [usually residual volume (V_R)], and the volume of gas in the gastrointestinal tract (V_{GI}). It is recommended that V_R be measured at the time that underwater weight is measured, but measurement on land with the subject in the same position is a suitable alternative (122). Residual volume can also be estimated with gender-specific regression equations, or by taking 24% (males) or 28% (females) of vital capacity. However, the latter two procedures introduce measurement errors of 2% to 3% fat for a given individual (141). V_{GI} can be quite variable, and while some investigators ignore this measure, others assume a 100 ml volume for all subjects (37, 125).

The density equation can now be rewritten:

$$D = \frac{M}{V} = \frac{M_A}{\dfrac{(M_A - M_W)}{D_W} - V_R - V_{GI}}$$

Figure 18.2 shows the equipment used to measure underwater weight. Water temperature is measured to obtain the correct water density. The subject is weighed on land on a scale accurate to within 100 grams. The subject puts on a diver's belt with sufficient weight to prevent floating during the weighing procedure, and sits on the chair suspended from the precision scale. The scale can be read to 10 grams and it has major divisions of 50 grams. The subject sits on the chair with the water at chin level and as a maximal exhalation is just about completed, the subject bends over and pulls the head under. When a maximal expiration is achieved, the subject holds that position for about five to ten seconds while the investigator reads the scale. This procedure is repeated six to ten times until the values stabilize. The weight of the diver's belt and chair are subtracted from this weight to obtain the true value for M_W. If V_R were to be measured at the time underwater weight is measured, the subject would have to be breathing through a mouthpiece and valve assembly that could be activated at the correct time (156).

The following data were obtained on a white male, aged thirty-six: M_A = 75.20 kg, M_W = 3.52 kg, V_R = 1.43 liters, D_W = 0.9944 at 34°C, V_{GI} = 0.1 liters.

$$D = \frac{M}{V} = \frac{75.20}{\dfrac{(75.20 - 3.52)}{0.9944} - 1.43 - 0.1} = \frac{75.20}{70.55} = 1.066$$

This density value is now used in Siri's equation to calculate percent body fat:

$$\% \text{ body fat} = \frac{495}{\text{Density}} - 450$$

$$14.3 = \frac{495}{1.066} - 450$$

The underwater weighing procedure in which RV is measured (and not estimated) has been used as the "standard" against which other methods are compared. However, remember that due to the normal biological variability in the fat-free mass in a given population, the percent body fat value is estimated to be within about ± 2.0% of the "true" value (125).

IN SUMMARY

- In the two-component system of body composition analysis, the body is divided into fat-free and fat mass, with densities of 1.100 and 0.900, respectively. The estimate of the density of the fat-free mass must account for differences that exist in various populations (i.e., children and African Americans).
- Body density is equal to mass ÷ volume. Underwater weighing is used to determine body volume using the principle of Archimedes: When an object is placed in water it is buoyed up by a counterforce equal to the water it displaces. One can measure the actual volume of water displaced, or the loss of weight while underwater. The weight of water is divided by the density of water to yield body volume, which must then be corrected for the residual volume and the volume of gas in the GI tract.
- The percent body fat value has an error of about ±2.0% due to the normal biological variation of the fat-free mass.

Sum of Skinfolds Underwater weighing, although a good way to obtain a measurement of body density, is time consuming and requires special equipment and personnel. Paralleling the development of the advanced technologies used in body composition

analysis, scientists developed equations that predicted body density from a collection of skinfold measurements. The skinfold method relies on the observation that within any population a certain fraction of the total body fat lies just under the skin (subcutaneous fat), and if one could obtain a representative sample of that fat, overall body fatness (density) could be predicted. Generally, these prediction equations were developed with the underwater weighing method used as the standard. For example, a group of college males and females would have body density measured by underwater weighing, and a variety of skinfold measures would also be obtained. The investigator would then determine what collection of skinfolds would most accurately predict the body density determined by underwater weighing.

Investigators found that subcutaneous fat represents a variable fraction of total fat (20%–70%), depending on age, sex, overall fatness, and the measurement technique used. At a specific body fatness women have less subcutaneous fat than men, and older subjects of the same sex have less than younger subjects (120). Given that these variables could influence an estimate of body density, it is no surprise that of the more than 100 equations developed, most were found to be "population specific" and could not be used for groups of different ages or sex. This obviously creates problems for exercise leaders in adult fitness programs or elementary or high school physical education teachers when they try to find the equation that works best for their particular group. Fortunately, a good deal of progress has been made to reduce these problems.

Jackson and Pollock (97) and Jackson, Pollock, and Ward (99) developed "generalized equations" for men and women—that is, equations that could be used across various age groups. In addition, these equations have been validated for athletic and nonathletic populations, including postpubescent athletes (122, 181, 182). In these equations, specific skinfold measurements are obtained and the values are used along with age to calculate body density. Here are two such equations, one for men and one for women, which can be used to predict body density (98). The body density value obtained is used in the Siri equation presented earlier to calculate percent body fat.

Men

Density = 1.1125025 − 0.0013125 (X_1) + 0.0000055 (X_1)^2
    − 0.0002440 (X_2)

Where X_1 = sum of chest, triceps, subscapular skinfolds, and X_2 = age in years.

Women

Density = 1.089733 − 0.0009245 (X_1) + 0.0000025 (X_1)^2
    − 0.0000979 (X_2)

Where X_1 = sum of triceps, suprailium, and abdominal skinfolds, and X_2 = age in years.

Jackson and Pollock (98) simplified this procedure by providing tabulated percent body fatness values for different skinfold thicknesses across age. All that is needed is the sum of skinfolds in order to obtain a percent body fatness value. Appendixes G and H show the percent body fat tables for men and women, respectively, using the sum of three skinfolds. For example, a woman, aged twenty-five, with a sum of skinfolds equal to 50 mm has a percent body fat equal to 22.9% (look to the right of the sum of skinfold column where 48–52 is shown, over to the second column—ages 23–27). Estimates of percent body fatness from skinfold measures have an error of about ±3.7% (121). Recently, concern has been expressed about the need to cross-validate the skinfold equations against the multicomponent models and to clarify the effects that age, gender, ethnicity, and fitness have on the various components of body composition, for example, the density of the fat-free mass (75, 125).

The use of skinfold measurements was extended to children in the schools for early identification of obesity. The American Alliance for Health, Physical Education, Recreation, and Dance (4, 123) developed a health-related fitness test to evaluate cardiorespiratory function, muscular strength, low back function, and body fatness. The body fatness assessment relies on a triceps and subscapular or calf skinfold(s), and percentile norms are provided. When this test was developed, the skinfold values could not be converted to percent body fatness values because the assumption that the fat-free mass had a density of 1.100 g/cc was known to be false. However, based on recent research with young populations using the four component model (188), appropriate equations are available to convert skinfolds to body fat for young African American and white girls and boys (125) (see table 18.7).

Body Fatness for Health and Fitness

The previous sections showed how to determine body density by underwater weighing and skinfold procedures. This information on body density is converted to percent body fat and can be used to make judgments about one's status relative to health and fitness. Lohman (121) recommends a range of 10% to 20% as an optimal health and fitness goal for males. He indicates that this range allows for individual differences in physical activity and preferences, and is associated with little or no health risk due to diseases associated with fatness. Values above 20% increase the risks of diabetes, heart disease, and hypertension. Values of 20% to 25% are considered moderately high, 25% to 31% high, and >31% very high. Females are generally about 3% fatter than males prior to puberty and 11% fatter after puberty. The latter is a "sex-specific" body fat difference due to the increased rate

TABLE 18.7	Prediction Equations of Percent Fat from Triceps and Calf and from Triceps and Subscapular Skinfolds in Children and Youth for Males and Females

Triceps and calf skinfolds
Males, all ages: % Fat = 0.735 ΣSF + 1.0
Females, all ages: % Fat = 0.610 ΣSF + 5.0
Triceps and subscapular skinfolds (>35 mm)
Males: % Fat = 0.783 ΣSF + I
Females: % Fat = 0.546 ΣSF + 9.7
Triceps and subscapular skinfolds (<35 mm)[a]
Males: % Fat = 1.21 (ΣSF) − 0.008 (ΣSF)^2 + I
Females: % Fat = 1.33 (ΣSF) − 0.013 (ΣSF)^2 + 2.5
(2.0 African Americans, 3.0 whites)
I = Intercept varies with maturation level and racial group for males as follows:

Age	African Americans	Whites
Prepubescent	−3.5	−1.7
Pubescent	−5.2	−3.4
Postpubescent	−6.8	−5.5
Adult	−6.8	−5.5

[a]Thus for a white pubescent male with a triceps of 15 and a subscapular of 12, the % fat would be: % Fat = 1.21 (27) − 0.008 (27)^2 − 3.4 = 23.4%

Note. Calculations were derived using Slaughter et al. (1988) equation.

Reprinted, by permission, from T. G. Lohman, 1992, *Advances in Body Composition Assessment* (Champaign, IL: Human Kinetics Publishers), 74. Calculations were derived using Slaughter et al. (1988).

of estrogen secretion at puberty. The optimal range of body fat for adult females is 15% to 25%, with 25% to 30% listed as moderately high, 30% to 35% as high, and >35% as very high (121).

Now that we know how to obtain a percent body fatness measure, and what the optimal percent body fat values are, how can we determine what the optimal body weight range is? In the following example, a female college student has 30% body fat and weighs 142 lbs. Her optimal percent fat range is 15% to 25%.

Step 1. Calculate fat-free weight:

100% − 30% fat = 70% fat free
70% × 142 lb = 99.4 lb fat-free weight

Step 2. Optimal weight = $\dfrac{\text{fat-free weight}}{(1 - \text{optimal \% fat})}$, with

optimal % fat expressed as a fraction:

For 15% = $\dfrac{99.4 \text{ lb}}{(1 - .15)}$ = 117 lb;

for 25% = $\dfrac{99.4 \text{ lb}}{(1 - .25)}$ = 132.5 lb

Her optimal weight range is 117–133 lb.

Lohman (121) also provides values for percent body fat that are below the optimal range: for boys, 6% to 10% is classified as low and <6% as very low; comparable values for girls are 12% to 15% and <12%, respectively. There is a great pressure in our society to be thin, and this can be carried to an extreme. A far-too-common problem in our high schools and colleges is an eating disorder known as **anorexia nervosa,** in which young females have an exaggerated fear of getting fat. This fear leads to food restriction and increased exercise in an attempt to stay thin, when they are, in fact, already thin (70). **Bulimia nervosa** is an eating disorder in which large quantities of food are taken in (binging), only to be followed by self-induced vomiting or the use of laxatives to rid the body of the food that was eaten (purging). While anorexia nervosa is characterized by the cessation of the menstrual cycle and the development of an emaciated state, the majority of the bingers/purgers are in the normal weight range (44).

It is clear that to stay in the optimal percent body fat range, one must balance the dietary consumption of calories with energy expenditure. We will now consider that topic.

IN SUMMARY

- Subcutaneous fat can be "sampled" as skinfold thicknesses, and a sum of skinfolds can be converted to a percent body fat with formulas derived from the relationship of the sum of skinfolds to a body composition standard based on a two-, three-, or four-component model.
- The recommended body fatness for males is 10% to 20%, and for females is 15% to 25%. There is concern about obesity and anorexia for those above and below these values, respectively.

OBESITY AND WEIGHT CONTROL

In chapter 14 we discussed the major risk factors associated with degenerative diseases. While high blood pressure, cigarette smoking, elevated serum cholesterol, and inactivity have been accepted as major risk factors (157), more and more evidence points to obesity as being a separate and independent risk factor for CHD, and one directly tied to two of the major risk factors. A wide variety of diseases are linked to obesity: hypertension, type 2 diabetes, coronary heart disease (CHD), stroke, gallbladder disease, osteoarthritis, sleep apnea and respiratory problems and some types of cancer (endometrial, breast, prostate, and colon).

In addition, obesity is also associated with complications of pregnancy, menstrual irregularities, hirsutism, stress incontinence, and psychological disorders (depression) (39, 106, 143, 159, 160).

As mentioned earlier, in spite of this information, the 1983 height/weight table of the Metropolitan Life Insurance Company listed higher weights at each height as being associated with lower death rates. In response, a twenty-six-year follow-up study of participants in the Framingham Heart Study recommended against this revision of the height/weight table with data indicating that higher relative weight was associated with increases in cardiovascular diseases (CVD) and death from CVD (94). The reason for the confusion was that the death rate was actually decreasing while the relative weight was increasing. The decrease in the death rate was believed to be due to decreases in cigarette smoking and improved health care and not the fact that people were fatter (63). It has been suggested that the better treatments available for those with diabetes and heart disease allows them to live longer at the higher body weights. It is a case of where the *average* body weight of a group is not the *optimal* weight for low risk of disease. In fact, Kannel and Gordon have stated that ". . . if everyone were at optimal weight we would have 25% less coronary heart disease and 35% less congestive heart failure and brain infarctions" (106). The recently published *Clinical Guidelines on the Identification, Evaluation, and Treatment of Overweight and Obesity in Adults* (143) points the way to reduce the disease burden associated with overweight and obesity in our society.

Obesity

If we use a BMI of ≥30 as a classification for obesity, the prevalence of obesity in U.S. adults increased from 15% in the 1976–1980 reporting period, to 23.3% in 1988–1994, and to 30.9% in 1999–2000, with little change (to 30.6%) in 2002 (83). When you include those who are classified as overweight (BMI 25.0–29.9), the prevalence of overweight and obesity was 65.7%. Consequently, we are approaching the point at which two-thirds of the U.S. adult population is overweight and one-third is obese. In addition, some ethnic groups were over-represented. More than half of non-Hispanic Black women aged forty years and older were obese and more than 80% were overweight (68, 83). However, all obesity is not the same. Studies suggest that not only is the relative body fatness related to an increased risk of CVD, but the distribution of that fatness must also be considered. Individuals with a large waist circumference compared to hip circumference have a higher risk of CVD and sudden death (185, 186). These data suggest that in addition to skinfold or underwater weighing estimates of body density, measurements of waist and hip circumferences

ASK THE EXPERT 18.1

Tracking Obesity-Related Risk:
Questions and Answers with Dr. Paul M. Ribisl.

Paul M. Ribisl, PhD, *Professor and Chair of Health and Exercise Science at Wake Forest University, is an exercise physiologist who was a co-founder of the Cardiac Rehabilitation Program at Wake Forest University. His areas of research include graded exercise testing in the diagnosis and prognosis of coronary heart disease, and exercise programming and prescription for patients with chronic degenerative diseases, including obesity and type 2 diabetes. He is currently involved in three nationally funded research trials dealing with these issues.*

QUESTION 1: Body mass index (BMI) has been accepted universally as a risk factor for cardiovascular and metabolic (e.g., type 2 diabetes) diseases. However, you have some problems with that. Please elaborate.

ANSWER: The BMI is certainly correlated with many health problems and it is generally predictive of health outcomes. Unfortunately, the BMI suffers from the fact that it only measures the ratio of body mass to an individual's height. It tells us nothing about the composition of that body mass and can lead to misinterpretation. There are individuals who are overweight and even obese who are healthy by all measures that we would want to use such as blood lipids, glucose tolerance, oxygen uptake capacity, inflammatory markers, and even percent body fat. In contrast, there are individuals who are within the normal range for BMI who are obese

and have abnormal values in these same measures. Many athletes have heavy bones and increased muscularity with low body fat percentage, which would yield a high but healthy BMI. Thus, BMI gives only part of the picture and that is why we should not rely on it as the sole measure of body composition.

QUESTION 2: What other anthropometric measurements do you recommend in addition to or in place of the BMI?

ANSWER: While the BMI has flaws, I would still use it in conjunction with other measurements. The most important single measurement is the waist circumference because it is a surrogate measure for visceral adipose tissue and is most predictive of future cardiovascular events. There is also a condition called the "hypertriglyceridemic waist" and recent research suggests that individuals with the combination of high triglycerides and large waist circumference are at higher risk for the metabolic syndrome. While it would be very informative to obtain CT scans of the abdominal region and measure visceral adipose tissue deposits, this is unrealistic. Individuals who deposit their fat in the gynoid or "pear-shape" pattern (hip and thigh) have a lower metabolic risk than those with the android or "apple" pattern (waist). Therefore, I would consider adding hip girth and a simple thigh skinfold measurement to the BMI and waist circumference. If an individual has a high

BMI and normal waist girth, but most of the excess weight is either due to greater muscle/bone mass or hip/thigh fat, then the BMI is not unhealthy. If an individual has a normal BMI and abnormal waist girth with lower muscle/bone mass and the android pattern, then even the normal BMI cannot be considered healthy.

QUESTION 3: Is there a need to measure both waist and hip circumferences?

ANSWER: The most recent research suggests that *both* the waist and the hip measurements should be measured. A large multi-country study of over 27,000 individuals from 52 countries has demonstrated that the BMI is *not* a significant predictor of the risk for myocardial infarction when the data are adjusted for waist and hip circumferences. This important study (Yusuf, S. et al. 2005. Obesity and the risk of myocardial infarction in 27,000 participants from 52 countries: A case-control study. *Lancet* 366:1640–49) revealed that waist girth was positively related, while hip girth was negatively related, to risk of myocardial infarction. This means that there was a protective influence from the deposit of excess fat around the hip/thigh region. Therefore, it appears that the best single anthropometric measure today is the waist/hip ratio and that the BMI and skinfolds can be included to provide additional information if desired. These measurements may also prove to be worthwhile to monitor change when weight loss occurs.

should also be obtained (115, 116). Ratios of waist to hip circumference >0.95 for men and >0.8 for women are associated with the CVD risk factors of insulin resistance, high cholesterol, and hypertension, and such individuals are treated even if they are only borderline obese (13, 34, 42, 185). Given that the risk of these problems is associated with abdominal obesity, the guidelines mentioned previously (143) use only waist circumference and recommend values of 102 cm

(40 in) and 88 cm (35 in) to be used for men and women, respectively, when classifying those at high risk. For more on the best measures to track obesity, see Ask the Expert 18.1.

In addition to fat tissue distribution, there is a need to determine whether the obesity is due to an increase in the amount of fat in each fat cell (hypertrophic obesity), or to an increase in the number of fat cells (hyperplastic obesity), or both (12, 14, 15). In

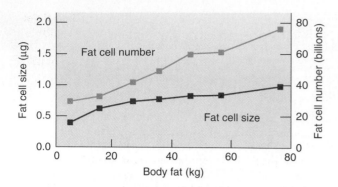

FIGURE 18.3 Relationship of fat cell size and fat cell number to total kilograms of body fat. Fat cell size is given μg of fat, and fat cell number in billions of cells. The increase in body fatness beyond about 30 kg of fat is directly related to an increasing fat cell number; fat cell size remains relatively constant.

moderate obesity where the mass of adipose tissue is less than 30 kg, the increase in fat cell size appears to be the primary means of storing the additional fat. Beyond that, the cell number is the variable most strongly related to the mass of adipose tissue (15, 90). This is shown in figure 18.3, where cell size increases up to about 30 kg of body fat, but does not significantly change thereafter. In contrast, fat cell number is strongly related to the mass of adipose tissue (184, 187).

There are about 25 billion fat cells in a normal-weight individual versus 60 to 80 billion in the extremely obese (15, 90, 187). When a person undergoes dietary restriction, the size of the fat cells decreases but the number does not (15, 90). This high fat cell number is believed to be related to the difficulty obese patients have in maintaining body weight once it has been lost (114). For example, a study was conducted to determine the pattern of weight loss, maintenance, and gain of groups classified as having obesity that is hyperplastic, hypertrophic, or both. Those with hyperplastic obesity or combined hyperplastic and hypertrophic obesity lost weight quickly, kept it off for only a short period of time, and regained it at a high rate. At this point we have seen that dieting does not change fat cell number, and that those who possess a high number of fat cells have difficulty maintaining a reduced body weight. The next question to consider is, when does the fat cell number increase?

In a longitudinal study of children during the first eighteen months of life, the fat cell number did not increase during the first twelve months, the increase in cell size being entirely responsible for the increase in body fat. In contrast, the gain in body fat from twelve to eighteen months was due entirely to an increase in fat cell number with cell size remaining stable (80). When these data were plotted along with

data from other studies, the results indicated that cell number increases throughout growth (80, 90). Given that physical activity and dietary intervention in grossly obese young children (eight years old) can slow the rate of growth in fat cell number, and that the fat cell number is tied to the inability of obese children to lose their obesity as adults, the emphasis on treatment during childhood is obvious (81, 111). Unfortunately, in spite of our understanding of the problem, the prevalence of overweight in children and adolescents (ages six to nineteen years) increased from 5% to 7% in the late 1970s to 11% in 1988–1994 and to 15% in 2000 (146), with only a small and nonsignificant increase (to 16.5%) in 2004 (83). This systematic increase over the past twenty-five years carries with it a disease burden (e.g., type 2 diabetes, formerly reserved for those over age forty and overweight). What causes obesity?

There is clearly no single cause of obesity. Obesity is related to both genetic and environmental variables. In 1965, Mayer (128) commented on the numerous studies showing that 70% to 80% of obese children had at least one obese parent, but concluded that it was difficult to interpret those data given the way cultural background interacts with genetics. In effect, the need to do hard physical work in some countries, or extreme social pressure against obesity (discussed later), might not allow a genetic predisposition to express itself. Garn and Clark (72) found a strong relationship between parental fatness and the fatness of children. They identified three categories of fatness on the basis of triceps skinfold: lean = <15th percentile; medium = 15th to 85th percentile, and obese = >85th percentile. The triceps skinfold thickness was related to parental fatness, being below average for the lean-dad/lean-mom pair and above average for the obese-dad/obese-mom pair. While this might imply that a genetic link exists, when the investigators compared husbands to wives (usually no genetic tie), the relationship was similar to that for their children, suggesting either that there was a tendency of like to mate like, or that communal living exerts a major influence.

A slightly different approach to this question was taken when the body mass index of biological and adoptive parents were compared to the values of the adopted child as an adult. On the basis of a health questionnaire they were classified as thin (≤4th percentile), median (50th percentile), overweight (92nd–96th percentile), and obese (>96th percentile). A stronger relationship existed between the BMI of the adoptee and that of the biological parent (190). However, a subsequent review of this work pointed out that while the results were consistent with a genetic effect, it was not a very strong one (21). Other observations support the importance of the environment as a cause of obesity. In American women, obesity is inversely related to socioeconomic class: 30% for lower, 18% for middle, and 5% for the upper class (76). Further, women and adolescent girls have been shown to suffer the most direct discrimination because of this obesity (212). Clearly, while we may possess a genetic predisposition for obesity, there are a variety of social factors that influence its appearance. Is there any way to determine the importance of each?

Bouchard (21) and colleagues have determined, on the basis of an analysis of the relationships between and among nine types of relatives (spouses, parent-child, siblings, uncle-nephew, etc.), that 25% of body fat and fat mass is tied to genetic factors, and 30% is due to cultural transmission. What is interesting is the components of energy expenditure that are influenced by genetic factors: (a) the amount of spontaneous physical activity, (b) resting metabolic rate, (c) thermic effect of food, and (d) relative rate of carbohydrate and fat oxidation. Further, when challenged with an excess of calories due to overeating, there is a genetic component related to the amount of weight gained, and the proportion of that weight that is stored as fat or lean tissue. Given that information, it should be no surprise that physicians and scientists who work in this area believe that genetic factors are the most important causes of obesity (26). However, as we will see, there is more to the story.

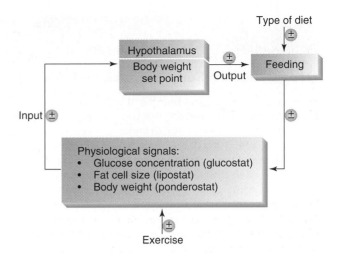

FIGURE 18.4 Physiological set point model for control of body weight by altering feeding behavior, showing the glucostatic (blood glucose), lipostatic (adipose tissue), and ponderostatic (weight) input to the hypothalamus. The signals from these latter mechanisms are compared against a "set point," and an appropriate increase or decrease in feeding behavior occurs. In this model, exercise can modify the input, and the type of diet can modify feeding behavior.

IN SUMMARY

- If everyone were at optimal weight there would be a 25% reduction in CHD, and a 35% reduction in congestive heart failure and stroke.
- Obesity associated with fat mass in excess of 30 kg is due primarily to an increase in fat cell number, with fat cell hypertrophy being related to smaller degrees of obesity. Those with hyperplasia have a more difficult time losing weight and keeping it off.
- Genetic factors account for about 25% of the transmissible variance for fat mass and percent body fat; culture accounts for 30%.

Set Point and Obesity   Obese individuals, as previously mentioned, have a great deal of difficulty maintaining a reduced weight. In fact, the tendency of a person to return to a certain weight suggests that there is a biological set point for body weight much like the set points for any negative feedback biological control system. While the hypothalamus contains centers associated with satiety and feeding behavior, we must remember that the *body weight set point is a concept, rather than a reality* (20). Figure 18.4 shows a physiological model of a body weight set point in which biological signals with regard to blood glucose (glucostatic signal), lipid stores (lipostatic signal), or

weight on feet (ponderostatic signal) provide input to the hypothalamus (20). If the collective signals indicate low energy stores, food intake is stimulated until the source of the signal is diminished and the energy stores now equal the set point. Like any biological control system, if the set point were to be increased, body weight would increase to meet this new value. Exercise can modify the signals going to the hypothalamus, and the type of diet can also influence feeding behavior. In addition, drugs can be used to directly affect the neurotransmitters in the hypothalamus to alter feeding behavior (see Clinical Applications 18.4).

In contrast to this physiological model, Booth's cognitive set-point model (20) deals with the role the environment (culture, socioeconomic class, etc.) has on body weight. Figure 18.5 shows that relative to a personally selected "ideal" body weight set point, we are constantly receiving a variety of cognitive signals about how we look, body weight, clothing size, perception of effort, and concerns about health. A mismatch between the "ideal" set point and these perceptions leads to appropriate eating behavior. Exercise can modify the signals, and the type of diet can influence the feeding behavior. This set-point model is closely related to the behavior modification approach to diet, exercise, and weight control.

In a recent review of this topic, Levitsky (118) suggests that we might want to look at this issue as a "settling-point" theory rather than a "set-point" theory. This revision suggests that biology might set a range or zone of body weights, rather than a fixed

CLINICAL APPLICATIONS 18.4

Drugs, Dietary Supplements, and Weight Loss

Obesity is such a big problem in this country that it is not surprising that people seek help wherever they can find it. In response to this need, a wide variety of nutritional supplements and drugs have been offered to help obese people lose weight. Unfortunately, there is little evidence that the dietary supplements work at all, and in the cases where some of the drugs do work, there may be unforeseen side effects that can be deadly (45). An example of the latter is "fen-phen," a combination of two drugs, dexfenfluramine (or fenfluramine) and phentermine, which keeps the serotonin and norepinephrine concentrations elevated in the hypothalamus, resulting in an appetite-suppressing effect. This drug combination was shown to be effective in weight loss for those with severe weight problems. However, when this drug combination was prescribed to millions, including to those who were only slightly overweight, problems began to appear. Following reports of pulmonary hypertension, heart valve abnormalities, and electrocardiographic irregularities, the drugs were pulled from the market (45).

As Clarkson points out (45),

- The focus of any weight loss (and maintenance) program is on long-term diet and exercise behaviors.
- Most diet drugs are approved for only a short period of time, to get a person off to a good start as the proper behaviors are put into place.
- If all the diet books, diet pills, and diet supplements worked, obesity would not be a problem.

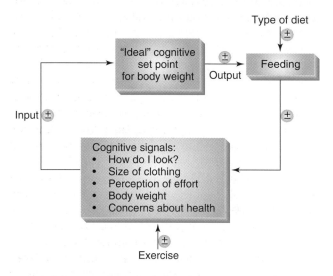

FIGURE 18.5 Cognitive set point for control of body weight by altering feeding behavior. A person's perception of "ideal" body weight is balanced against signals about how one looks, body weight, clothing, size, and so on. Exercise can modify the input, and the type of diet can modify feeding behavior.

the environmental and cognitive factors that drive eating behavior.

IN SUMMARY

- Investigators have proposed a set-point theory to explain obesity given the tendency for people who diet to return to their former weight. Theories based on weight sensors (ponderostatic), the blood glucose concentration (glucostatic), and the mass of lipid (lipostatic) have been proposed.
- A behavioral set-point theory has been proposed that relies on the person making appropriate activity and dietary judgments when body weight, size, or shape does not match up with that person's ideal.

DIET, EXERCISE, AND WEIGHT CONTROL

The Framingham Heart Study showed that body weight increases as we age. A reasonable question to ask is whether this gain in weight was due to an increase in caloric intake. Interestingly, caloric intake decreased over the same age span (23). We are forced to conclude that energy expenditure decreased faster than the decrease in caloric intake, and as a result, weight gain occurred (18). This weight gain problem can be corrected by understanding and dealing with one or both sides of the energy balance equation. We will deal with the energy balance equation first, and

weight. Within that zone, body weight may "settle" at a value determined by behaviors that are influenced by environmental and cognitive stimuli. In effect. Levitsky's "settling point" theory attempts to integrate aspects of each of the two positions just mentioned. He suggests that if the body weight zone is large enough to allow a person to move between a hypertensive condition and normal blood pressure condition or between a type 2 diabetic and nondiabetic state, then additional attention must be directed at then discuss how modifications in energy intake can affect weight loss. Finally, we will explore the variables on the energy expenditure side of the equation.

Energy and Nutrient Balance

Weight gain occurs when there is a chronic increase in caloric intake, compared to energy expenditure. A net gain of about 3,500 kcal is needed to add 1 lb (454 grams) of adipose tissue. We are all familiar with the energy balance equation:

Change in energy stores = energy intake − energy expenditure.

What is implied by this equation is that an excess energy intake of 250 kcal/day will cause body weight to increase 1 pound in 14 days (250 kcal/day × 14 day = 3,500 kcal = 1 pound). At the end of one year the person will have gained about 24 pounds. As reasonable as this equation may appear, we know that a weight gain of that magnitude will not occur. The equation is a "static" energy balance equation that does not consider the effect that the weight gain will have on energy expenditure (191).

The energy balance equation can be expressed in a manner to account for the dynamic nature of energy balance in biological systems:

Rate of change of = rate of change of − rate of change of
energy stores   energy intake   energy
                                              expenditure

When body weight increases as a result of a chronically elevated energy intake, there is a compensatory increase in the amount of energy used at rest, as well as during activity when body weight is carried about. At some point then, the additional 250 kcal/d of energy intake will be balanced by a higher rate of energy expenditure brought about by the higher body weight. Body weight will stabilize at a new and higher value, but it will be more like 3.5 pounds, rather than 24 pounds higher (191).

IN SUMMARY

- The dynamic energy balance equation correctly expresses the dynamic nature of changes in energy intake and body weight. An increase in energy intake leads to an increase in body weight; in turn, energy expenditure increases to eventually match the higher energy intake. Body weight is now stable at a new and higher value.

Nutrient Balance Investigators have taken this issue of energy balance one step further in an attempt to understand the causes of obesity. The dynamic energy balance equation can be subdivided into its components, representing the three major nutrients to generate nutrient-balance equations:

Rate of change of = rate of change of − rate of change of
protein stores   protein intake   protein oxidation

Rate of change of = rate of change of − rate of change of
carbohydrate   carbohydrate   carbohydrate
stores   intake   oxidation

Rate of change of = rate of change of − rate of change of
fat stores   fat intake   fat oxidation

If a person maintains balance for each of these nutrients—that is, what is taken in is expended—then energy balance is achieved. Nutrient balance is not a problem for protein and carbohydrate. The daily protein intake is used to maintain existing tissue protein, hormones, and enzymes. If more is taken in than is needed, the "extra" is oxidized for metabolic needs, and fat mass is not increased. The same is true for carbohydrates. Ingested carbohydrates are used to fill liver and muscle glycogen stores; the excess is oxidized and *is not* converted to fat (1, 16, 86). Carbohydrate intake promotes its own oxidation. This is a relatively new idea that has major ramifications for our understanding of nutrient and energy balance. The evidence seems to be quite convincing that *de novo* lipogenesis from carbohydrates (the making of new lipids from other nutrients) is of only minor consequence in humans. Simply, carbohydrates are either stored as carbohydrates or oxidized; they do not add *directly* to adipose tissue mass. This leaves fat.

In contrast to carbohydrate and protein, fat intake is not automatically balanced by fat oxidation. When "extra" fat is added to the diet, the same amount of carbohydrate, fat, and protein are oxidized as before; the extra fat is stored in adipose tissue. Fat intake *does not* promote its own oxidation. Fat oxidation is determined primarily by the difference between total energy expenditure and the amount of energy ingested in the form of carbohydrate and protein. Consequently, if one wishes to keep the size of the adipose tissue stores constant (i.e., maintain body weight), then one should not eat more fat than one can oxidize (65, 66, 67, 101, 102, 191). One last point. Alcohol intake is balanced by its own oxidation, but in the process, it suppresses fat oxidation. In this sense, the calories from alcohol should be included with that provided by fat (67).

In chapter 4 you were introduced to the concept of the respiratory quotient (RQ = $\dot{V}CO_2/\dot{V}O_2$) as an indicator of the fuel oxidized during exercise. An RQ of 1.0 indicates that 100% of the energy is derived from carbohydrates and an RQ of 0.7 indicates that 100% of the energy comes from fat. An RQ of 0.85 indicates that a 50%/50% mixture of carbohydrate and fat was used. This RQ concept has been extended to the foods

FIGURE 18.6 Relationship between respiratory quotient (RQ)-to-food quotient (FQ) ratio and energy balance in humans. Each point represents values for a given subject measured over a twenty-four-hour period. (From E. Jéquier. 1992. Calorie balance versus nutrient balance. In *Energy Metabolism: Tissue Determinants and Cellular Corollaries*, eds. J. M. Kinney and H. N. Tucker, p. 131. New York: Raven.)

we ingest, and it is called the Food Quotient, or FQ. The FQ is defined as the ratio of the CO_2 produced to the O_2 consumed during the oxidation of a representative sample of the diet (65). The reason for describing this is that the FQ concept can be used with the RQ concept to determine if an individual is in nutrient balance (101, 102). Figure 18.6 presents this concept, and the following comments summarize its content:

- When RQ = FQ, the person is in nutrient and energy balance; the RQ/FQ ratio is 1.0.

- When RQ > FQ, the person is not oxidizing as much fat as was consumed (positive energy balance), and some fat has been stored in adipose tissue; the RQ/FQ ratio is >1.0.

- When RQ < FQ, the person used more fat than was consumed (negative energy balance), and some of the fat stores were used; the RQ/FQ ratio is <1.0.

This concept is helpful in discussing weight control, because one could improve nutrient and energy balance with regard to fat by either reducing the amount of fat in the diet (increasing the FQ), or doing exercise to use more fat (decreasing the RQ). We will now discuss both of these options.

IN SUMMARY

- Nutrient balance exists for both protein and carbohydrate. Excess intake is oxidized and is not converted to fat.

- Excess fat intake does not drive its own oxidation; the excess is stored in adipose tissue. Achieving fat balance is an important part of weight control.
- The ratio of the Food Quotient (FQ) to the Respiratory Quotient (RQ) provides good information about the degree to which an individual is in nutrient balance.

Diet and Weight Control

A good diet provides the necessary nutrients and calories to provide for tissue growth and regeneration and to meet the daily energy requirements of work and play. In our society we are fortunate to have a wide variety of foods to meet these needs. However, we tend to consume more than the recommended amount of fat, which is believed to be related to our country's obesity problem. The focus on dietary fat is twofold:

- Fat contains more than twice the number of calories per gram as carbohydrate and can contribute to a positive energy balance.

- It is difficult to achieve nutrient balance for fat when it represents a large fraction of caloric intake.

The hypothesis that the FQ of the diet is an important aspect of weight control revolves around the factors driving energy intake. There is a mandatory need for carbohydrate oxidation by the nervous system, and we are driven to eat what is used (66, 89). If we eat a high-fat diet, we will take in a considerable amount of fat while consuming the necessary carbohydrates to refill the carbohydrate stores. This fat is stored and body weight will increase. As mentioned earlier, as body weight increases daily energy expenditure increases until an energy balance is achieved at a new and higher body weight. The fat-balance concept is consistent with this. Flatt (66) proposes that the increase in adipose tissue mass that accompanies weight gain increases the mobilization of free fatty acids, shifting the RQ to a lower value, and bringing it into balance with the FQ. In this sense, the elevation of body weight and fat mass due to a high fat/calorie diet is a compensatory mechanism that results in weight maintenance.

However, while we focus on the FQ/RQ concept, we should not forget that calories count in any weight-loss or weight-maintenance program. For example, studies in which subjects were switched from a high-fat to a low-fat diet, *while maintaining a constant caloric intake*, showed no change in energy expenditure or body weight (89, 117, 167). In addition, in conditions in which a negative caloric balance was imposed to achieve weight loss, the composition of the diet (high-fat vs. low-fat) did not matter (87). In this sense, one should not get carried away with the high-carbohydrate diet and consume calories in excess of what is needed (67). In fact, when a variety of popular diets (Atkins, Ornish, Weight Watchers, and Zone) were compared over the course of one year, each modestly reduced body weight, with no difference between diets. It should be no surprise that the best predictor of weight loss was the degree to which individuals adhered to the diet—no matter which one (51). Given these facts, why should diet composition matter in terms of weight control and obesity?

Quite simply, diets with a high fat-to-carbohydrate ratio are associated with obesity (137). When subjects are given free access to food, more calories are consumed when one eats a high-fat diet than when one eats a high-carbohydrate diet (19, 193). The high-carbohydrate content may contribute to satiety better than the high-fat diet, resulting in an earlier termination of eating (162). The nutrient balance (RQ = FQ) concept helps focus our attention on the need for a high-carbohydrate/low-fat diet to achieve and maintain a healthy level of body fatness. This diet is also consistent with what is needed to have normal cholesterol levels and sufficient carbohydrate for physical performance (see chapter 23). One of the *Dietary Guidelines for Americans* was to balance the food you eat with physical activity—maintain or improve your weight. Recommendations to accomplish this include:

- To maintain body weight in a healthy range, balance calories from foods and beverages with calories expended.
- To prevent gradual weight gain over time, make small decreases in food and beverage calories and increase physical activity.

Physical activity recommendations were presented in three stages:

- To reduce the risk of chronic disease in adulthood, engage in at least 30 minutes of moderate-intensity physical activity, above usual activity, at work or home on most days of the week.
- To help manage body weight and prevent gradual, unhealthy body weight gain in adulthood, engage in approximately 60 minutes of moderate- to vigorous-intensity activity on most days of the week while not exceeding caloric intake requirements.
- To sustain weight loss in adulthood, participate in at least 60 to 90 minutes of daily moderate-intensity physical activity while not exceeding caloric intake requirements.

One last point before leaving this topic. As we mentioned earlier in the chapter, data on energy intake is assessed by twenty-four-hour recall or food records. However, one has to be cautious when interpreting these data as part of a weight-loss program. Research suggests that these methods may result in a considerable underestimation of caloric intake, especially in obese individuals (17, 54, 119, 134, 196). This, of course, would create a misdirection in looking for the cause of the obesity problem. It should be no surprise then that careful energy balance studies are done in highly controlled laboratory situations.

In the recent Institute of Medicine (95) recommendations that set appropriate levels of energy intakes for different levels of physical activity, the experts used data from doubly labeled water (DLW) rather than dietary recall. The DLW method measures total energy expenditure in free-living individuals, without the need for the person to remember what he or she had eaten. In the DLW method, the subject ingests a drink containing two isotopes of water: $H_2^{18}O$ and ^2H_2O. Urine or blood samples are obtained over a period of seven to twenty-one days to evaluate the disappearance of ^2H_2O (relates to water flux) and $H_2^{18}O$ (reflects water flux plus the CO_2 production rate). The difference between the two rates gives information about total energy expenditure (rate of CO_2 production) and represents an improvement over earlier approaches that relied solely on dietary recall information.

IN SUMMARY

- Diets with a high fat-to-carbohydrate ratio are linked to obesity. Nutrient balance for fat can be most easily achieved with a low-fat diet (high FQ).
- Calories do count, and they must be considered in any diet aimed at achieving or maintaining a weight loss goal.

Energy Expenditure and Weight Control

The other side of the energy balance equation involves the expenditure of energy and includes the basal metabolic rate, thermogenesis (shivering and nonshivering), and exercise. We will examine each of these relative to its role in energy balance.

Basal Metabolic Rate Basal metabolic rate (BMR) is the rate of energy expenditure measured under standardized conditions (i.e., immediately after rising, twelve to eighteen hours after a meal, in a supine position in a thermoneutral environment). Because of the difficulty of achieving these conditions during routine measurements, investigators have measured **resting metabolic rate (RMR)** instead. In this latter procedure, the subject simply reports to the lab about four hours after eating a light meal, and after a period of time (thirty to sixty minutes) the metabolic rate is measured (138). Given the low level of oxygen uptake measured for BMR or RMR (200 to 400 ml · min⁻¹), a variation of only ± 20 to 40 ml · min⁻¹ represents a potential ±10% error. In the following discussion both BMR and RMR will be discussed interchangeably, except where a specific contrast must be made for clarification.

The BMR is important in the energy balance equation because it represents 60% to 75% of total energy expenditure in the average sedentary person (154). The BMR is proportional to the fat-free mass, and after age twenty it decreases approximately 2% and 3% per decade in women and men, respectively. Women have a significantly lower BMR at all ages, due primarily to their lower fat-free mass (48, 57, 152, 217). Consistent with this, when RMR is expressed per unit of fat-free mass, there is no gender difference. At any body weight the RMR decreases about 0.01 kcal/min for each 1% increase in body fatness (152). While this may appear to be insignificant, this small difference can become meaningful in the progressive increase in weight gain over time. For example, a 5% difference in body fatness at the same body weight results in a difference of 0.05 kcal · min⁻¹, or 3 kcal · hr⁻¹, which is equal to 72 kcal · d⁻¹. It must be emphasized that percent body fat makes only a small contribution to the BMR. This was confirmed in a study examining the relationship of body composition to BMR; fat mass did not improve the prediction of BMR based on the fat-free mass alone (48).

As mentioned earlier, part of the variation in BMR is due to a genetic predisposition to be higher or lower (21). The range (±3 SD) in normal BMR values is about ±21% from the average value, and such variation helps to explain the observation that some have an easier time at maintaining body weight than others. If an average adult male has a BMR of 1,500 kcal · d⁻¹, those at +3 SD can take in an additional 300 kcal · d⁻¹ (21% of 1,500 kcal) to maintain weight, while others at the low end of the range (−3 SD) would have to take in 300 fewer kcals (57, 73).

The fat-free mass is not the only factor influencing the BMR. In 1919, Benedict et al. (11) showed that prolonged dieting (reduction from about 3,100 kcal to 1,950 kcal) was associated with a 20% decrease in the BMR expressed per kilogram of body weight. This observation was confirmed in the famous Minnesota Starvation Experiment (109), and is shown in figure 18.7. In this figure the BMR is expressed as a percent of the value measured before the period of semi-starvation. The percent decrease in BMR is larger "per man" because of the loss of lean tissue (as well as fat tissue); however, when the value is expressed per kilogram of body weight or per unit of surface area (m²),

FIGURE 18.7 Decrease in basal metabolic rate during twenty-four weeks of semi-starvation.

the BMR is still shown to be reduced. A decrease in the concentration of one of the thyroid hormones (T_3) and a reduced level of sympathetic nervous system activity have been implicated in this lower BMR due to caloric restriction (22). What these data mean is that during a period of low caloric intake, the energy production of the tissues decreases in an attempt to adapt to the lower caloric intake and reduce the rate of weight loss. This is an appropriate adaptation in periods of semi-starvation, but is counterproductive in weight reduction programs. This information bears heavily on the use of low-calorie diets as a primary means of weight reduction (56, 69, 206, 210).

The BMR is also responsive to periods of overfeeding. In the dieting experiment of Benedict et al. (11) mentioned earlier, when the subjects were allowed a day of free eating, the BMR was elevated on the following day. Further, in long-term (fourteen to twenty days) overfeeding to cause obesity, increases in resting and basal metabolic rates have been recorded. In essence, during the dynamic phase of weight gain (going from a lower to a higher weight), more calories are required per kg of body weight to maintain the weight gain than to maintain normal body weight (73, 180). This increased heat production due to an excess caloric intake, called **thermogenesis,** will be discussed in the next section. However, before leaving this discussion of the BMR, we need to mention the effect of exercise.

There is no doubt that the resting metabolic rate is elevated following exercise. The questions relate to how much and how long it is elevated, and to what extent it contributes to total daily energy expenditure (27, 155). A review of this topic indicates that controversies still exist even though the questions have been studied for over one-hundred years (138). At the heart of the matter is the measure of the metabolic rate that is taken as the baseline in these experiments. Should it be the BMR? The RMR? Molé (138) suggests that we need to create a new measurement called the Standard Metabolic Rate that would take into consideration the day-to-day fluctuations in normal physical activity, dietary intake, added exercise, and body composition. In support of these concerns it has been shown that trained subjects had a higher RMR than untrained subjects only when they did heavy exercise and consumed sufficient calories to maintain energy balance (35). This suggests that the higher RMR in trained individuals is not due to chronic adaptations associated with training, but more to the higher energy flux associated with the training and diet. This is consistent with other studies showing that the RMR, expressed per kg of fat-free mass, is similar for trained and untrained individuals, and that resistance and endurance training do not affect the value (31, 32). Aside from helping to maintain or increase the lean body mass and the RMR, exercise training may favorably impact nutrient balance. Two studies, using strength training, showed a significant decrease in the twenty-four-hour (198) and sleeping (205) metabolic rate RQ values, signifying an increased use of fat. This is consistent with achieving nutrient balance and energy balance over time (227).

IN SUMMARY

- The BMR represents the largest fraction of total energy expenditure in sedentary persons. The BMR decreases with age, and women have lower BMR values than men.
- The fat-free mass is related to both the gender difference and to the decline in BMR with age. A reduction in caloric intake by dieting or fasting can reduce the BMR, while physical activity is important in maintaining it.

Thermogenesis Core temperature is maintained at about 37° C by balancing heat production with heat loss. Under thermoneutral conditions, the BMR (RMR) provides the necessary heat, but under cold environmental conditions, the process of shivering is actuated and 100% of the energy required for involuntary muscle contraction appears as heat to maintain core temperature. In addition, some animals (including newborn humans) produce heat by a process called nonshivering thermogenesis, involving brown adipose tissue. This type of adipose tissue is rich in mitochondria and increases heat production in response to norepinephrine (NE). Thyroid hormones, especially T_3, may either directly affect this process or act in a permissive manner to facilitate the action of NE (22, 23, 100). Heat production is increased by uncoupling oxidative phosphorylation; that is, oxygen is used without ATP formation, so the energy contained in NADH and FADH appears directly as heat. Those individuals with large quantities of brown adipose tissue have a greater capacity to "throw off" calories in the form of heat rather than store them in adipose tissue. It has been hypothesized that variations in brown adipose tissue might be related to the ease or difficulty with which one gains weight.

Thermogenesis involves more than brown adipose tissue. The heat generated due to the food we consume accounts for about 10% to 15% of our total daily energy expenditure; this is called the *thermic effect of food* (23, 154). Generally, this is determined by having a subject ingest a test meal (700–1,000 kcal), and the elevation in the metabolic rate is measured following the meal. This portion of our daily energy expenditure is influenced by genetic factors (21, 154), is lower in obese than lean individuals (105, 175), and is influenced by the level of spontaneous activity and the degree of insulin resistance (192). However, because it represents such a small part of the overall daily energy expenditure, it is not a good predictor of subsequent obesity.

In individuals who have been on a diet (underfeeding), just one day of overfeeding leads to an increase in the next day's BMR. The BMR then quickly returns to the level consistent with the low-caloric intake specified in the diet (11). It is as if the body is throwing off extra heat to maintain body weight during this period of relative overfeeding. This phenomenon has also been observed in the chronic overfeeding of human subjects. In Garrow's (74) and Danforth's (50) reviews of these overfeeding studies, the subjects showed an unexplained heat production associated with chronic excess caloric intakes. The elevations of the BMR have been explained on the basis of an increase in the mass of brown adipose tissue (mentioned earlier), and the involvement of other **energy wasteful systems.** These latter systems include a change in the Na^+/K^+ pump activity, or "futile cycles" in which the equivalent of one ATP is lost in each turn of the cycle (22, 23). An example of a futile cycle is when an ATP is used to convert fructose 6-phosphate to fructose 1,6-diphosphate, which, in the next step, is converted back to fructose 6-phosphate. In situations in which heat, but no ATP, is produced, the resting oxygen consumption would have to be higher to maintain the normal ATP-consuming systems. Whatever the mechanism by which this dietary thermogenesis is induced, via brown fat or by futile cycles, it must be made clear that, like the BMR, there are marked differences in how individuals respond to an increased dietary intake. Clearly, those who have a normally high BMR and are very responsive to a large caloric excess would have an easier time staying at normal weight than those who do not.

A Calorie Is a Calorie

From a weight-loss perspective, a caloric deficit that results from an increase in energy expenditure through physical activity is equivalent to that due to a decrease in caloric intake. However, as Ross et al. (165) point out, leading authorities (143) state that the addition of exercise makes only a modest contribution to weight loss. How can this be the case, given the equivalency of the caloric deficit induced by either diet or exercise? Ross et al. (165) show that in the majority of weight-loss studies in which a diet treatment was compared to an exercise treatment, the energy deficit caused by exercise was only a fraction of that caused by diet. In this situation, it is not surprising that weight loss due to diet was greater than that due to exercise; however, the weight loss due to exercise was as expected. The exercise-induced weight loss, 30% of that due to diet, was equivalent to the caloric deficit associated with the exercise (28% of that due to diet). Ross et al. (166) did a controlled experiment designed to achieve a 700 kcal/day energy deficit due to either exercise alone or diet alone. Both groups lost 16.5 lbs over twelve weeks—exactly what was expected from the 58,800 kcal deficit (700 kcal/day times eighty-four days). However, the exercise group lost more total fat, thus preserving muscle.

IN SUMMARY

- Thermogenesis (heat generation) is associated with the ingestion of meals (thermic effect of feeding), brown adipose tissue, and "futile cycles."
- The thermic effect of food represents a small part of total energy expenditure and is not predictive of obesity.

Physical Activity and Exercise Physical activity constitutes the most variable part of the energy expenditure side of the energy balance equation, being 5% to 40% of the daily energy expenditure (40, 154). There are those who have sedentary jobs and who do little physical activity during their leisure time. Others may have strenuous jobs, or expend 300 to 1,000 kcal during their leisure time every day or two. Just how important is physical activity in weight control? Epidemiological evidence suggests an inverse association between physical activity and body weight, with body fat being more favorably distributed in those who are physically active (55). One study examined the relationship of body fatness to the different components of energy expenditure. Figure 18.8 shows that body fatness was inversely related to "nonbasal" (primarily that associated with physical activity) energy expenditure. In this sense, the level of physical activity is a permissive factor for obesity (161, 172). Consistent with this, recent studies showed an inverse relationship between BMI and accumulated daily walking (measured by pedometer). Those accumulating more than 10,000 steps per day were more likely to be in the "normal" BMI range (91, 194). For those wondering if a diet calorie is the same as an exercise calorie, see Clinical Applications 18.5.

FIGURE 18.8 Relationship between body fatness and nonbasal energy expenditure is highly significant (P < 0.01); for females it is $r = -0.83$, for males $r = -0.55$.

Appetite The classic animal study describing the role of exercise on appetite was conducted by Mayer and colleagues (129). Figure 18.9 shows that when female rats exercised for twenty to sixty minutes per day (sedentary range), the caloric intake actually decreased slightly and the animals lost weight. Over the durations of one to six hours of activity the caloric intake increased proportionately and body weight was maintained, but at a level below that of the sedentary rat. Durations in excess of six hours were associated with a relative decrease in caloric intake and body weight (exhaustion). Twenty-five years after this study, Katch et al. (108) showed that in male rats accomplishing the same amount of work, those exercising at the higher intensity had a greater depression in appetite and weight gain than those at the lower intensity, with both groups being lower than the sedentary

FIGURE 18.9 Pattern of caloric intake for rats versus the durations of exercise. When rats do little or no exercise, caloric intake exceeds what is needed and body weight increases (see top-left part of figure). However, over a broad range of physical activity, caloric intake increases proportional to the activity, and body weight (top line) remains constant.

animals. In contrast, female rats tend to respond to increasing exercise intensity with an increase in appetite (150).

Mayer and colleagues (130) also studied the relationship of exercise to caloric intake on mill workers in West Bengal, India. Figure 18.10 shows a pattern of response similar to Mayer et al.'s (129) study on rats. In the activity classifications from light to very heavy work, caloric intake increased proportionately so that body weight was not different among the various groups. However, in the sedentary classification, caloric intake was as high as for the very heavy work classification, and body weight was higher than the other groups. This suggests that a minimal level of exercise is needed to help regulate appetite. This study has been cited over the years as a primary supporting piece of evidence showing exercise to be important in the regulation of appetite. However, in 1978 Garrow (73) questioned the analysis of the data at the sedentary end of the scale where the group

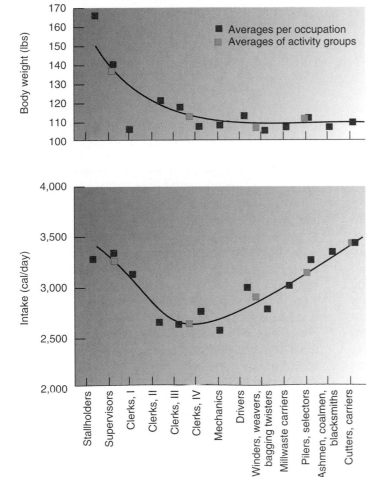

FIGURE 18.10 Pattern of caloric intake versus occupational activity in humans. For occupations ranging from light work to very heavy work, there is a balance between caloric intake and physical activity such that body weight remains constant. For sedentary occupations, caloric intake (see left side of lower figure) exceeds needs and body weight is higher than expected (see left side of top figure).

called "Clerks I" had a body weight similar to the more active groups, *but consumed about 400 kcal/day more than* those in the light work category. This analysis of the data would support a conclusion opposite that of Mayer et al. (130).

It should be clear that there would have to be some proportional increase in appetite as subjects increased physical activity, otherwise an athlete would gradually waste away during the course of a competitive season! However, when an exercise program is introduced to obese and/or sedentary individuals, appetite does not appear to increase. In Wilmore's (224) and Titchenal's (195) reviews of such exercise intervention studies, appetite did not increase in proportion to energy expenditure, suggesting a net loss of appetite. In summary, in male animals, exercise decreases appetite in proportion to exercise intensity, while in female animals, exercise stimulates appetite. Generally, in humans, caloric intake is regulated in proportion to energy expenditure over a broad range of exercise intensities and durations to help maintain body weight, but when exercise is introduced to a formerly sedentary population, a net decrease in appetite results.

Body Composition   While exercise may help regulate appetite to maintain body weight, exercise has an independent effect on the composition of that weight. This has been shown in both animal and human studies. In general, male rats that participate in regular exercise have lower body weights, less lean body mass, and very little body fat compared to their sedentary control litter mates. In contrast, female rats tend to respond to exercise training with an increase in appetite such that they are as heavy as the sedentary group, with a lower fat weight and a higher lean weight (148). Oscai et al. (149) have shown that, in addition to these general changes in body composition due to exercise, exercise or food restriction in rats results in fewer and smaller fat cells. This observation is supported by Hager et al.'s (81) finding that in a group of eight-year-old obese girls a diet/activity program was instrumental in reducing the rate of gain in fat cell number.

The advantage of using exercise compared to caloric restriction alone in weight-loss programs is that the composition of the weight that is lost is more fat tissue than lean tissue. In both animal (149) as well as human (34, 38, 58) studies using dietary restriction alone, lean body mass loss can equal 30% to 40% of the weight loss. Exercise plus diet results in less lean body mass loss and a proportionately greater fat loss (149). In addition, the preferential mobilization of fat from visceral adipose tissue results in an improved body fat distribution and risk factor profile (164, 211).

However, it must be remembered that body composition changes take place slowly in human exercise studies, and the magnitude of the change is small. Wilmore's summary (223) of exercise and body composition studies showed the average decrease in percent body fat to be only 1.6% with fitness programs ranging in duration from 6 to 104 weeks.

IN SUMMARY

- Humans increase appetite over a broad range of energy expenditure to maintain body weight; however, formerly sedentary individuals show a net loss of appetite when they undertake an exercise program.
- When weight loss occurs with an exercise and diet program, less lean body mass is lost than when the same weight loss is achieved by diet alone.

Weight Loss vs. Weight Maintenance   One point that needs to be stated at the outset is that exercise is not required to achieve weight loss. All that is necessary is a caloric deficit, the magnitude of which is easily controlled by diet (87). However, as mentioned previously, the use of exercise as a part of a weight-loss program might maintain a higher lean body mass and RMR, and result in an optimal body fatness at a higher body weight.

Although exercise might not be an essential ingredient in a weight-loss program, it is in a weight-maintenance program (189). A major, unresolved question is how much? That said, some of the general exercise recommendations for health and fitness presented in chapter 16 would be considered reasonable for weight-maintenance programs. The primary factor involved in energy expenditure is the total work accomplished, so low-intensity, long-duration exercise is as good as high-intensity, short-duration exercise in expending calories. For the sedentary, overweight person, moderate-intensity exercise is the proper choice, since it can be done for longer periods of time in each exercise session, and can be done each day. This is consistent with the physical activity recommendations from the 2005 *Dietary Guidelines for Americans* presented earlier in this chapter.

Further, at moderate intensities free fatty acids are mobilized from the periphery to provide the majority of the fuel used and help with maintaining fat balance (163). This does not mean that "fat-burning" is restricted to low-intensity activities. Individuals interested in more vigorous activity ($\sim$65% $\dot{V}O_2$ max) that can increase $\dot{V}O_2$ max can also reap the benefits of high rates of calorie and fat use (163). Finally, even

CLINICAL APPLICATIONS 18.6

Successful Losers—How Much Exercise Is Needed to Keep the Weight Off?

There is general agreement that most U.S. adults need more physical activity. The question is, how much? The systematic increase in the prevalence of obesity over the past twenty-five years has provided a strong incentive to address this issue and, to some extent, we are making progress. However, with different organizations recommending different amounts of exercise, the public is becoming confused.

In chapter 16 we presented the CDC/ACSM recommendation that all adults should do at least thirty minutes of moderate-intensity physical activity on most, preferably all, days of the week. There is clear evidence that such an increase in physical activity results in health benefits, especially for the most sedentary part of the population. This was meant to be a minimal recommendation, with clear support that "more is better." In the recent Institute of Medicine (IOM) report (95), one hour per day of moderate-intensity physical activity was recommended to help maintain weight in the normal BMI range, and for full health benefits. While on the surface the recommendations appear at odds with one another, the two are not as far apart as they may seem. The IOM report recommends thirty minutes of moderate-intensity activity for a sedentary individual to move to the "low-active" category, and sixty minutes of moderate-intensity activity to move to the "active" category. The sixty-minute recommendation is presented as what is needed to prevent weight gain. How much is needed to keep weight off once it is lost?

Dr. Rena Wing of the University of Pittsburgh and Dr. James Hill of the University of Colorado formed the National Weight Control Registry (NWCR) in 1993 to gain some insights into what made "successful losers"—individuals who lost weight and kept it off. To be included in the registry, individuals had to have lost substantial weight ($\geq$13.6 kg [30 lb]) and kept it off for at least one year. Some of the findings follow:

- The average weight loss of the registrants was 30 ± 15 kg, and they kept the weight off for an average of 5.5 ± 6.8 years.
- There was no evidence of psychological distress due to the long-term suppression of body weight (110).
- Participants used a variety of strategies to limit caloric intake (about 1,400 kcal/week, with about 25% of the calories from fat).
- Participants expended about 400 kcal/day through physical activity (132, 179)

Hill (88) and Wing's (225) most recent updates underscore the usefulness of these insights into what makes a successful loser. The six key strategies for long-term success at weight loss include: engaging in high level physical activity, eating a diet that is low in calories and fat, eating breakfast, self-monitoring weight on a regular basis, maintaining a consistent eating pattern, and catching slips before they result in larger weight regains. Clearly, these messages from those who have been successful in maintaining weight loss have great value for both the professional and the client working toward that goal.

A recent Position Stand from the American College of Sports Medicine dealing with the issues of weight loss and prevention of weight gain (5) recommends an initial goal of 150 minutes per week of moderate physical activity, pro-gressing to 200 to 300 minutes per week ($\geq$2,000 kcal/week). This recommendation is consistent with the observations from the study of "successful losers" and the earlier commentary on the ACSM/CDC and IOM recommendations. The 2005 *Dietary Guidelines for Americans* built on the IOM and other recommendations from the International Association for the Study of Obesity (168) and the International Obesity Task Force (61) to form a three-tiered recommendation:

- to reduce the risk of chronic disease in adulthood, engage in at least thirty minutes of moderate-intensity physical activity on most days of the week;
- to help manage body weight and prevent gradual, unhealthy body weight gain in adulthood, engage in approximately sixty minutes of moderate- to vigorous-intensity activity on most days of the week; and
- to sustain weight loss in adulthood, participate in at least sixty to ninety minutes of daily moderate-intensity physical activity.

There is some frustration associated with these recommendations in that a substantial percent of U.S. adults do not even meet the thirty-minute goal. Given that this segment of the population is more likely to be obese, telling them to do more when they are not doing the minimum thirty-minute recommendation may not be productive. Translating science into practice, especially in a public health context, is always a great challenge and it will be interesting to see the progress we make in the years ahead.

---

though carbohydrate makes up a large fraction of the energy supply during high-intensity exercise ($\sim$85% $\dot{V}O_2$ max) (163), training programs using intermittent high-intensity exercise have been shown to cause a greater reduction in skinfold thickness than programs conducted at the target heart rate range (197). It is clear that virtually any form of exercise contributes to fat loss and the maintenance of body weight. The important thing is to just do it. See Clinical Applications 18.6 for information on "successful losers."

TABLE 18.8 Net Caloric Cost Per Mile for Walking, Jogging, and Running

Walking

Mph	2	2.5	3	3.5	4	4.5	5
Meters/min	54	67	80	94	107	121	134
Net cost $kcal \cdot kg^{-1} \cdot mile^{-1}$	.77	.77	.77	.77	.96	1.15	1.38

Jogging/Running

Mph	3	4	5	6	7	8	9
Meters/min	80	107	134	160	188	215	241
Net cost $kcal \cdot kg^{-1} \cdot mile^{-1}$	1.53	1.53	1.53	1.53	1.53	1.53	1.53

Note: Multiply by body weight in kilograms to obtain the number of kilocalories used per mile.

From E. T. Howley and B. D. Franks, *Health/Fitness Instructor's Handbook*, 2d ed. Copyright © 1992 Human Kinetics Publishers, Inc., Champaign, IL. Used by permission.

IN SUMMARY

- Moderate-intensity exercise is an appropriate choice for most Americans to achieve health-related and weight-loss goals. Plasma free fatty acids make up a large fraction of the energy supply for that level of physical activity.
- Moderate exercise promotes the expenditure of large amounts of fat and calories, consistent with achieving weight-loss and fitness goals.
- Vigorous activity is effective in expending calories and achieving performance and fat-loss goals.

For weight-loss considerations, the caloric cost of an activity should be listed as the *net* cost (that above resting) since the *gross* cost of the activity includes energy already associated with resting metabolism. Table 18.8 shows the *net* energy cost per kg for walking and running one mile. In chapter 6, the net cost per $m \cdot min^{-1}$ of horizontal travel was 0.1 $ml \cdot kg^{-1} \cdot min^{-1}$ for walking (up to about 3.75 mph), and 0.2 $ml \cdot kg^{-1} \cdot min^{-1}$ for jogging or running. This translates to about 0.77 kcal per kg per mile for walking (0.1 $ml \cdot kg^{-1} \cdot m^{-1}$ times 1,609 $m \cdot mile^{-1}$ times .0048 kcal per ml O_2), and 1.53 kcal per kg per mile for jogging or running. If a 60-kg person wished to expend 250 kcal by walking, a distance of 5.4 miles would have to be covered (250 kcal = [60 kg × 0.77 $kcal \cdot kg^{-1} \cdot mile^{-1}$]); the distance would be only 2.7 miles if jogged. If the person walks at relatively high walking speeds, the caloric cost is higher than for the slower walking speeds, and a shorter distance would have to be walked to expend the same number of calories. As mentioned earlier, since it is the total amount of work that is important in weight loss, the total distance walked or jogged does not have to be done at any one time.

In selecting activities to achieve weight-loss goals, one must be careful not to overestimate the energy expenditure. If a table of values of the caloric cost of activities lists climbing stairs as requiring 15 $kcal \cdot min^{-1}$, one must realize that this is an impossible goal to achieve aerobically for those with a maximal oxygen uptake of less than 3 liters $\cdot min^{-1}$. Further, while an average value may be stated in such tables, some activities (e.g., swimming) have extreme variations in the energy required for the task. To deal realistically with this problem, Sharkey (177) provides a means of estimating the caloric expenditure associated with exercise for people of different fitness levels. If a person has a $\dot{V}O_2$ max equal to 10 METs, then the appropriate range of exercise intensities to be in the THR zone would be 6 to 8 METs (60% to 80% $\dot{V}O_2$ max). Since 1 MET is 1 $kcal \cdot kg^{-1} \cdot hr^{-1}$ (in addition to 3.5 $ml \cdot kg^{-1} \cdot min^{-1}$), this subject would be working in the range of 6 to 8 $kcal \cdot kg^{-1} \cdot hr^{-1}$. If the person weighs 70 kg and exercises for thirty minutes at 7 $kcal \cdot kg^{-1} \cdot hr^{-1}$, the person would expend a total of 245 kcal (70 kg × 7 $kcal \cdot kg^{-1} \cdot hr^{-1}$ × 0.5 hr). The net caloric expenditure would be about 210 kcal. Table 18.9 summarizes the estimated energy expenditure associated with exercise training for those with different $\dot{V}O_2$ max values (93). It should be clear that as the person loses weight, the num-

V̇O₂ Max (METs) $(kcal \cdot kg^{-1} \cdot hr^{-1})$	Net Energy Expenditure at 70% V̇O₂ Max $(kcal \cdot kg^{-1} \cdot min^{-1})$	Body Weight (kg)		
		50	70	90
			$(kcal \cdot hr^{-1})$	
20	13.0	650	910	1,170
18	11.6	580	812	1,044
16	10.2	510	714	918
14	8.8	440	616	792
10	6.0	300	420	540
8	4.6	230	322	414
6	3.2	160	224	287

From E. T. Howley and B. D. Franks, *Health/Fitness Instructor's Handbook*, 2d ed. Copyright © 1992 Human Kinetics Publishers, Inc., Champaign, IL. Used by permission.

ber of kcal used per fixed workout decreases, along with a decrease in the BMR. The combined effect of these two elements on the expenditure side of the weight-balance equation is that there will be a slowing of the rate of weight loss over time.

IN SUMMARY

- Participation in regular physical activity achieves a wide variety of health-related goals (e.g., increased cardiorespiratory fitness, HDL cholesterol, and fibrinolysis), and increases the chance that energy balance will be achieved.

STUDY QUESTIONS

1. Summarize the range of carbohydrate, fat, and protein intakes recommended by the Institute of Medicine.
2. What is the difference between an RDA standard and a Daily Value?
3. Is there any risk in taking fat-soluble vitamins in large quantities? Explain.
4. Which two minerals are believed to be inadequate in women's diets?
5. Relative to coronary heart disease, why is there a major focus on dietary fat?
6. Generate a one-week menu using the MyPyramid website. How do the choices compare to those in the DASH eating plan?
7. Using a height/weight table, how fat is a football player who is 74 inches tall and weighs 235 lb?
8. Identify and describe the following methods of measuring body composition: isotope dilution, potassium-40, ultrasound, bioelectrical impedance analysis, dual energy X-ray absorptiometry, skinfold thickness, and underwater weighing.
9. Contrast the four-component and two-component models of body composition assessment.
10. What is the principle of underwater weighing? Why should a different body density equation be used for children, in contrast to adults?

11. Given: a twenty-year-old college male, 180 lb, 28% fat. What is his target body weight to achieve 17% fat?
12. In terms of the resistance to weight reduction, contrast obesity due to hypertrophy with obesity due to hyperplasia of fat cells.
13. Is obesity more related to genetics or the environment?
14. If a person consumes 120 kcal per day in excess of need, what weight gain does the static energy balance equation predict compared to the dynamic energy balance equation?
15. What does *nutrient balance* mean and how is the ratio of the RQ to FQ used to determine nutrient balance?
16. Contrast a physiological set point with a behavioral set point related to obesity.
17. What happens to the BMR when a person goes on a low-calorie diet?
18. What recommendations would you give about the use of diet alone versus a combination of diet and exercise?
19. What is thermogenesis and how might it be related to a weight gain?
20. What is the effect of exercise on appetite and body composition?
21. What exercise recommendation is appropriate for someone who is sedentary and overweight and is consistent with achieving caloric-expenditure and fat-loss goals?

SUGGESTED READINGS

Clarkson, P. M. 1998. Dietary supplements and pharmacological agents for weight loss and gain. In *Exercise, Nutrition, and Weight Control; Perspectives in Exercise Science and Sport* *Medicine*, vol. 11, ed. R. D. Lamb and R. Murray. Carmel, IN: Cooper Publishing Group.

Heyward, V. H., and L. M. Stolarczyk. 2004. *Applied Body Composition Assessment.* 2d ed. Champaign, IL: Human Kinetics.

Roche, A. F., S. B. Heymsfield, and T. G. Lohman, ed. 2005. *Human Body Composition.* 2d ed. Champaign, IL: Human Kinetics.

Wardlaw, G. M. 2005. *Contemporary Nutrition.* 6th ed. New York: McGraw-Hill Companies.

REFERENCES

1. Acheson, K. J. 1987. Carbohydrate metabolism and de novo lipogenesis in human obesity. *American Journal of Clinical Nutrition* 45:78–85.

2. AHA Committee Report. 1982. Rationale of the diet-heart statement of the American Heart Association. *Nutrition Today* (Sept./Oct.):16–20, (Nov./Dec.):15–19.

3. Aloia, J. R. 1981. Exercise and skeletal health. *Journal of the American Geriatrics Society* 29:104–7.

4. American Alliance for Health, Physical Education, Recreation, and Dance. 1988. *Physical Best.* Reston, VA: AAHPERD.

5. American College of Sports Medicine. 2001. Appropriate intervention strategies for weight loss and prevention of weight gain in adults. *Medicine and Science in Sports and Exercise* 33:2145–56.

6. American Dietetic Association. 2002. Position of the American Dietetic Association: Health implications of dietary fiber. *Journal of the American Dietetic Association* 102:993–1000.

7. Andres, R. 1985. Mortality and obesity: The rationale for age-specific height-weight tables. In *Principles of Geriatric Medicine,* ed. E. L. Bierman and W. R. Hazzard, chap. 29, 311–18. New York: McGraw-Hill Companies.

8. Ballor, D. L., J. P. McCarthy, and E. J. Wilterdink. 1990. Exercise intensity does not affect the composition of diet- and exercise-induced body mass loss. *American Journal of Clinical Nutrition* 51:142–46.

9. Barnard, R. J., C. K. Roberts, S. M. Varon, and J. J. Berger. 1998. Diet induced insulin resistance precedes other aspects of the metabolic syndrome. *Journal of Applied Physiology* 84:1311–15.

10. Behnke, A. R., B. G. Feen, and W. C. Welham. 1942. The specific gravity of healthy men: Body weight ÷ volume as an index of obesity. *Journal of the American Medical Association* 118:495–98.

11. Benedict, F. G. et al. 1919. *Human Vitality and Efficiency Under Prolonged Restricted Diet.* Washington, D.C.: The Carnegie Institution of Washington.

12. Björntrop, P. 1978. The fat cell: A clinical view. In *Recent Advances in Obesity Research:* II., ed. George Bray, 153–68. Westport, CT: Technomic.

13. ———. 1985. Regional patterns of fat distribution. *Annals of Internal Medicine* 103:994–95.

14. Björntrop, P. et al. 1971. Adipose tissue fat cell size and number in relation to metabolism in randomly selected middle-aged men and women. *Metabolism* 20:927–35.

15. Björntrop, P., and L. Sjöström. 1971. Number and size of adipose tissue fat cells in relation to metabolism in human obesity. *Metabolism* 20:703–13.

16. ———. 1978. Carbohydrate storage in man: Speculations and some quantitative considerations. *Metabolism Clinical Experimental* 27:1853–65.

17. Black, A. E. et al. 1991. Critical evaluation of energy intake data using fundamental principles of energy physiology: 2. Evaluating the results of published surveys. *European Journal of Clinical Nutrition* 45:583–99.

18. Blair, S. N., and M. Z. Nichaman. 2002. Editorial: The public health problem of increasing prevalence rates of obesity and what should be done about it. *Mayo Clinic Proceedings* 17:109–13.

19. Blundell, J. E. et al. 1993. Dietary fat and the control of energy intake: Evaluating the effects of fat on meal size and postmeal satiety. *American Journal of Clinical Nutrition* (Suppl. 57):772S–778S.

20. Booth, D. A. 1980. Acquired behavior controlling energy intake and output. In *Obesity,* ed. A. J. Stunkard, 101–43. Philadelphia: W. B. Saunders.

21. Bouchard, C. 1991. Heredity and the path to overweight and obesity. *Medicine and Science in Sports and Exercise* 23:285–91.

22. Bray, G. A. 1969. Effect of caloric restriction on energy expenditure in obese patients. *The Lancet* 2:397–98.

23. ———. 1983. The energetics of obesity. *Medicine and Science in Sports and Exercise* 15:32–40.

24. ———. 1992. Pathophysiology of obesity. *American Journal of Clinical Nutrition* 55:488S–494S.

25. Bray, G. A., and R. L. Atkinson. 1992. New weight guidelines for Americans. *American Journal of Clinical Nutrition* 55:481–82.

26. Bray, G. A., B. York, and J. Delany. 1992. A survey of the opinions of obesity experts on the causes and treatment of obesity. *American Journal of Clinical Nutrition* 55:151S–154S.

27. Brehm, B. A. 1988. Elevation of metabolic rate following exercise implications for weight loss. *Sports Medicine* 6:72–78.

28. Brewer, V. 1983. Role of exercise in prevention of involutional bone loss. *Medicine and Science in Sports and Exercise* 15:445–49.

29. Brodie, D. A. 1988. Techniques of measurement of body composition Part I. *Sports Medicine* 5:11–40.

30. ———. 1988. Techniques of measurement of body composition Part II. *Sports Medicine* 5:74–98.

31. Broeder, C. E., K. A. Burrhus, L. S. Svanevik, and J. H. Wilmore. 1992. The effects of aerobic fitness on resting metabolic rate. *American Journal of Clinical Nutrition* 55:795–801.

32. ———. 1992. The effects of either high-intensity resistance or endurance training on resting metabolic rate. *American Journal of Clinical Nutrition* 55:802–10.

33. Brooke-Wavell, K. et al. 1995. Evaluation of near infra-red interactance for assessment of subcutaneous and total body fat. *European Journal of Clinical Nutrition* 49:57–65.

34. Brozek, J. et al. 1963. Densitometric analysis of body composition: Revision of some quantitative assumptions. *Annals of New York Academy of Science* 110:113–40.

35. Bullough, R. C. 1995. Interaction of acute changes in exercise energy expenditure and energy intake on resting metabolic rate. *American Journal of Clinical Nutrition* 61:473–81.

36. Bunt, J. C. 1986. Hormonal alterations due to exercise. *Sports Medicine* 3:331–45.

37. Buskirk, E. R. 1961. Underwater weighing and body density: A review of procedures. In *Techniques for Measuring Body Composition*, ed. J. Brozek and A. Henschel. Washington, D.C.: National Academy of Sciences—National Research Council.

38. Buskirk, E. R. et al. 1963. Energy balance of obese patients during weight reduction: Influence of diet restriction and exercise. *Annals of New York Academy of Science* 110 (part II):918–40.

39. Calle, E. E., M. J. Thun, J. M. Petrelli, C. Rodriguez, and C. W. Heath, Jr. 1999. Body-mass index and mortality in a prospective cohort of U.S. adults. *New England Journal of Medicine* 341:1097–1105.

40. Calles-Escandón, J., and E. S. Horton. 1992. The thermogenic role of exercise in the treatment of morbid obesity: A critical evaluation. *American Journal of Clinical Nutrition* 55:533S–537S.

41. Cameron, J. R., and J. Sorenson. 1963. Measurement of bone mineral in-vivo: An improved method. *Science* 142:230–32.

42. Campaigne, B. N. 1990. Body fat distribution in females: Metabolic consequences and implications for weight loss. *Medicine and Science in Sports and Exercise* 22:291–97.

43. Cann, C. E. et al. 1984. Decreased spinal mineral content in amenorrheic women. *Journal of the American Medical Association* 251:626–29.

44. Christian, J. L., and J. L. Greger. 1994. *Nutrition for Living*. Redwood City, CA.: Benjamin/Cummings.

45. Clarkson, P. M. 1999. The skinny on weight loss supplements & drugs. *ACSM's Health and Fitness Journal* 2:18–55.

46. Cole, T. J., M. C. Bellizzi, K. M. Flegal, and W. H. Dietz. 2000. Establishing a standard definition for childhood overweight and obesity worldwide: International survey. *British Medical Journal* 320:1240–45.

47. Coniglio, J. G. 1984. Fat. In *Nutrition Reviews' Present Knowledge in Nutrition*, 5th ed., chap. 7, 79–89. Washington, D.C.: The Nutrition Foundation.

48. Cunningham, J. J. 1991. Body composition as a determinant of energy expenditure: A synthetic review and a proposed general prediction equation. *American Journal of Clinical Nutrition* 54:963–69.

49. Dahlquist, A. 1984. Carbohydrates. In *Nutrition Reviews' Present Knowledge in Nutrition*, 5th ed., chap. 9, 116–30. Washington, D.C.: The Nutrition Foundation.

50. Danforth, E. et al. 1978. Undernutrition contrasted to overnutrition. In *Recent Advances in Obesity Research*: II, ed. G. Bray, 229–36. Westport, CT: Technomic.

51. Dansinger, M. L., J. A. Gleason, J. L. Griffith, H. P. Selker, and E. J. Schaefer. 2005. Comparison of the Atkins, Ornish, Weight Watchers, and Zone diets for weight loss and heart disease risk reduction. *Journal of the American Medical Association* 293:43–53.

52. DeBakey, M. E. et al. 1984. *The Living Heart Diet*. New York: Raven Press.

53. Dempster P., and S. Aitkens 1995. A new air displacement method for the determination of human body composition. *Medicine and Science in Sports and Exercise* 27(12):1692–97.

54. de Vries, J et al. 1994. Underestimation of energy intake by 3-d records compared with energy intake to maintain body weight in 269 nonobese adults. *American Journal of Clinical Nutrition* 60:855–60.

55. di Pietro, L. 1995. Physical activity, body weight, and adiposity: An epidemiologic perspective. In *Exercise and Sport Sciences Reviews*, vol. 23, ed. J. O. Holloszy, 275–303. Baltimore: Lippincott Williams & Wilkins.

56. Donnelly, J. E., J. Jakicic, and S. Gunderson. 1991. Diet and body composition: Effect of very low calorie diets and exercise. *Sports Medicine* 12:237–49.

57. DuBois, E. F. 1968. Basal energy, metabolism at various ages: Man. In *Metabolism*, ed. P. L. Altman and D. S. Dittmer, 345. Bethesda, MD: Federation of American Societies for Experimental Biology.

58. Durnin, J. V. G. A. 1978. Possible interaction between physical activity, body composition, and obesity in man. In *Recent Advances in Obesity Research*: II, ed. G. Bray, 237–41. Westport, CT: Technomic.

59. Eastwood, M. 1984. Dietary fiber. In *Nutrition Reviews' Present Knowledge in Nutrition*, 5th ed., chap. 12, 156–75. Washington, D.C.: The Nutrition Foundation.

60. Ellis, K. J. et al. 1994. Accuracy of dual-energy X-ray absorptiometry for body-composition measurements in children. *American Journal of Clinical Nutrition* 60:660–65.

61. Erlichman, J., A. L. Kerbey, and W. P. T. James. 2002. Physical activity and its impact on health outcomes. Paper 2: Prevention of unhealthy weight gain and obesity by physical activity: An analysis of the evidence. *Obesity Reviews*. 3:273–87.

62. Ernst, N. D., and R. I. Levy. 1984. Diet and cardiovascular disease. In *Nutrition Reviews' Present Knowledge in Nutrition*, 5th ed., chap. 50, 724–39. Washington, D.C.: The Nutrition Foundation.

63. Feinleib, M. 1985. Epidemiology of obesity in relation to health hazards. *Annals of Internal Medicine* 103:1019–24.

64. Finberg, L. 1985. Clinical assessment of total body water. In *Body-Composition Assessments in Youth and Adults*, ed. A. F. Roche, 22–23. Columbus, OH: Ross Laboratories.

65. Flatt, J. P. 1988. Importance of nutrient balance in body weight regulation. *Diabetes/Metabolism Reviews* 4:571–81.

66. Flatt, J. P. 1993. Dietary fat, carbohydrate balance, and weight maintenance. *Annals of New York Academy of Science* 683:122–40.

67. Flatt, J. P. 1995. Use and storage of carbohydrate and fat. *American Journal of Clinical Nutrition* (Suppl. 61). 952S–959S.

68. Flegal, K. M., M. D. Carroll, C. L. Ogden, and C. L. Johnson. 2002. Prevalence and trends in obesity among U.S. adults, 1999–2000. *Journal of the American Medical Association* 288:1723–27.

69. Foster, G. D. et al. 1990. Controlled trial of the metabolic effects of a very-low-calorie diet: Short- and long-term effects. *American Journal of Clinical Nutrition* 51:167–72.

70. Garfinkle, P. E., and D. M. Garner. 1982. *Anorexia Nervosa*. New York: Brunner/Mazel.

71. Garn, S. M. 1961. Radiographic analysis of body composition. In *Techniques for Measuring Body Composition*, ed. J. Brozek and H. Henschel, 36–58. Washington, D.C.: National Academy of Sciences—National Research Council.

72. Garn, S., and D. C. Clark. 1976. Trends in fatness and the origins of obesity. *Pediatrics* 57:443–56.

73. Garrow, J. S. 1978. *Energy Balance and Obesity in Man*. New York: Elsevier North-Holland.

74. Garrow, J. S. 1978. The regulation of energy expenditure in man. In *Recent Advances in Obesity Research*: II, ed. G. Bray, 200–210. Westport, CT: Technomic.

75. Going, S., D. Williams, and T. Lohman. 1995. Aging and body composition: Biological changes and methodological issues. In *Exercise and Sport Sciences Reviews* vol. 23, ed. J. O. Holloszy, 411–58. Baltimore: Lippincott Williams & Wilkins.

76. Goldblatt, P. B., M. E. Moore, and A. J. Stunkard. 1965. Social factors in obesity. *Journal of the American Medical Association* 192:1039–44.

77. Goldman, R. F., and E. R. Buskirk. 1961. Body volume measurement by underwater weighing: Description of a method. In *Techniques for Measuring Body Composition*, ed. J. Brozek and A. Henschel, 78–89. Washington, D.C.: National Academy of Sciences—National Research Council.

78. Guthrie, H. A., and M. F. Picciano. 1995. *Human Nutrition*. St. Louis: Mosby.

79. Guyton, A. G. 1977. Body fat and adipose tissue cellularity in infants: A longitudinal study. *Metabolism* 26:607–14.

80. ———. 1981. *Textbook of Medical Physiology*. 6th ed. Philadelphia: W. B. Saunders.

81. Hager, A., L. Sjöström, and B. Arvidsson. 1978. Adipose tissue cellularity in obese school girls before and after dietary treatment. *American Journal of Clinical Nutrition* 31:68–75.

82. Hallberg, L. 1984. Iron. In *Nutrition Reviews' Present Knowledge in Nutrition*. 5th ed., chap. 32, 459–78. Washington, D.C.: The Nutrition Foundation.

83. Hedley A. A. et al. 2004. Prevalence of overweight and obesity among US children, adolescents, and adults, 1999–2002. *Journal of the American Medical Association*. 291:2847–2850.

84. Heaney, R. P. 1987. The role of calcium in prevention and treatment of osteoporosis. *The Physician and Sportsmedicine* 15(11):83–88.

85. Heinrich, C. H. et al. 1990. Bone mineral content of cyclically menstruating female resistance and endurance trained athletes. *Medicine and Science in Sports and Exercise* 22:558.

86. Hellerstein, M. K. et al. 1991. Measurement of de novo hepatic lipogenesis in humans using stable isotopes. *The American Society for Clinical Investigation, Inc.* 87: 1841–52.

87. Hill, J. O. et al. 1993. Obesity treatment: Can diet composition play a role? *American College of Physicians* 119:694–97.

88. Hill, J. O., H. Wyatt, S. Phelan, and R. Wing. 2005. The National Weight Control Registry: Is it useful in helping deal with our obesity epidemic? *Journal of Nutrition Education and Behavior* 37:206–10.

89. Hirsch, J. 1995. Role and benefits of carbohydrate in the diet: Key issues for future dietary guidelines. *American Journal of Clinical Nutrition* (Suppl. 61):996S–1000S.

90. Hirsch, J., and J. L. Knittle. 1970. Cellularity of obese and nonobese human adipose tissue. *Federation Proceedings* 29:1516–21.

91. Hornbuckle, L. M., D. R. Bassett, jr., and D. L. Thompson. 2005. Pedometer-determined walking and body composition variables in African-American women. *Medicine and Science in Sports and Exercise* 37:1069–74.

92. Houtkooper, L. B., and S. B. Going. 1994. Body composition: How should it be measured? Does it affect performance? *Sports Science Exchange*, vol. 7, no. 5. Barrington, IL: Gatorade Sports Science Institute.

93. Howley, E. T., and B. Don Franks. 1992. *Health/Fitness Instructor's Handbook*. 2d ed. Champaign, IL: Human Kinetics.

94. Hubert, H. B. et al. 1983. Obesity as an independent risk factor for cardiovascular disease: A 26-year follow-up of participants in the Framingham Heart Study. *Circulation* 67:968–77.

95. Institute of Medicine. 2002. *Dietary Reference Intakes for Energy, Carbohydrate, Fiber, Fat, Fatty acids, Cholesterol, Protein, and Amino acids*. Washington, D.C.: National Academy Press.

96. Institute of Medicine. 2004. Dietary reference intakes for water, potassium, sodium, chloride, and sulfate. Washington, D.C.: National Academies Press.

97. Jackson, A. S., and M. L. Pollock. 1978. Generalized equations for predicting body density of men. *British Journal of Nutrition* 40:497–504.

98. Jackson, A. S., and M. L. Pollock. 1985. Practical assessment of body composition. *The Physician and Sportsmedicine* 13:76–90.

99. Jackson, A. S., M. L. Pollock, and A. Ward. 1980. Generalized equations for predicting body density of women. *Medicine and Science in Sports and Exercise* 12:175–82.

100. James, W. P. T., and P. Trayhurn. 1981. Thermogenesis and obesity. *British Medical Bulletin* 37:43–48.

101. Jéquier, E. 1992. Calorie balance versus nutrient balance. In *Energy Metabolism: Tissue Determinants and Cellular Corollaries*, ed. J. M. Kinney and H. N. Tucker, 123–37. New York: Raven.

102. ———. 1993. Body weight regulation in humans: The importance of nutrient balance. *News in Physiological Sciences* 8:273–76.

103. Johnston, F. E., and R. Malina. 1966. Age changes in the composition of the upper arm in Philadelphia children. *Human Biology* 38:1–21.

104. Jones, D. W. 2004. Dietary sodium and blood pressure. *Hypertension* 43:932–35.

105. Jung, R. T. et al. 1979. Reduced thermogenesis in obesity. *Nature* (London) 279:322–23.

106. Kannel, W. B., and T. Gordon. 1979. Physiological and medical concomitants of obesity: The Framingham study. In *Obesity in America*, 125–43. U.S. Department of Health, Education, and Welfare. NIH Publication No. 79–359.

107. Katch, F. I. 1985. Assessment of lean body tissues by radiography and bioelectrical impedance. In *Body-Composition Assessment in Youths and Adults*, ed. A. F. Roche, 46–51. Columbus, OH: Ross Laboratories.

108. Katch, V. L., R. Martin, and J. Martin. 1979. Effects of exercise intensity on food consumption in the male rat. *American Journal of Clinical Nutrition* 32:1401–7.

109. Keys, A. et al. 1950. *The Biology of Human Starvation*, vol. 1. Minneapolis: The University of Minnesota Press.

110. Klem, M. L., R. R. Wing, M. T. McGuire, H. M. Seagle, and J. O. Hill. 1998. Psychological symptoms in individuals successful at long-term maintenance of weight loss. *Health Psychology* 17:336–45.

111. Knittle, J. L. 1972. Obesity in childhood: A problem in adipose tissue cellular development. *Journal of Pediatrics* 81:1048–59.

112. Kolata, G. 1986. Obese children: A growing problem. *Science* 233:20–21.

113. Kris-Etherton, P. et al. 2001. Summary of the scientific conference on dietary fatty acids and cardiovascular disease. *Circulation* 103:1034–39.

114. Krotkiewski, M. et al. 1977. Adipose tissue cellularity in relation to prognosis for weight reduction. *International Journal of Obesity* 1:395–416.

115. Lapidus, L. et al. 1984. Distribution of adipose tissue and risk of cardiovascular disease and death: A 12-year follow-up of participants in the population study of women in Gothenburg, Sweden. *British Medical Journal* 289:1257–61.

116. Larsson, B. et al. 1984. Abdominal adipose tissue distribution, obesity, and risk of cardiovascular disease and death: 13-year follow-up of participants in the

study of men born in 1913. *British Medical Journal* 288:1401–4.

117. Leibel, R. L. et al. 1992. Energy intake required to maintain body weight is not affected by wide variation in diet composition. *American Journal of Clinical Nutrition* 55:350–55.

118. Levitsky, D. A. 2002. Putting behavior back into feeding behavior: A tribute to George Collier. *Appetite* 38:143–48.

119. Lightman, S. W. et al. 1992. Discrepancy between self-reported and actual caloric intake and exercise in obese subjects. *The New England Journal of Medicine* 327:1893–98.

120. Lohman, T. G. 1981. Skinfolds and body density and their relation to body fatness: A review. *Human Biology* 53:181–225.

121. ———. 1982. Body composition methodology in sports medicine. *The Physician and Sportsmedicine* 10(12):47–58.

122. ———. 1986. Applicability of body composition techniques and constants for children and youths. In *Exercise and Sport Sciences Reviews*, vol. 14, ed. K. B. Pandolf, chap. 11, 325–57. New York: Macmillan.

123. ———. 1987. The use of skinfold to estimate body fatness in children and youth. *Journal of the Alliance for Health, Physical Education, Recreation and Dance* 58 (Nov.–Dec.):98–102.

124. ———. 1989. Assessment of body composition in children. *Pediatric Exercise Science* 1:19–30.

125. ———.1992. *Advances in Body Composition Assessment*. Champaign, IL: Human Kinetics.

126. Lohman, T. G., and S. B. Going. 1993. Multicomponent models in body composition research: opportunities and pitfalls. In *Human Body Composition*, ed. K. J. Ellis and J. D. Eastman, 53–58. New York: Plenum Press.

127. Lohman, T. G. et al. 1984. Bone mineral measurements and their relation to body density in children, youth and adults. *Human Biology* 56:667–79.

128. Mayer, J. 1965. Genetic factors in human obesity. *Annals of New York Academy of Science* 131:412–21.

129. Mayer, J. et al. 1954. Exercise, food intake, and body weight in normal rats and genetically obese mice. *American Journal of Physiology* 177:544–48.

130. Mayer, J., P. Roy, and K. P. Mitra. 1956. Relation between caloric intake, body weight and physical work: Studies in an industrial male population in West Bengal. *American Journal of Clinical Nutrition* 4:169–75.

131. Mazess, R. B. et al. 1990. Dual-energy X-ray absorptiometry for total-body and regional bone-mineral and soft-tissue composition. *American Journal of Clinical Nutrition* 51:1106–12.

132. McGuire, M. T., R. R. Wing, M. L. Klem, H. M. Seagle, and J. O. Hill. 1998. Long-term maintenance of weight loss: Do people who lose weight through various weight loss methods use different behaviors to maintain their weight. *International Journal of Obesity-Related Metabolic Disorders* 22:572–77.

133. McLean, K. P., and J. S. Skinner. 1992. Validity of Futrex-5000 for body composition determination. *Medicine and Science in Sports and Exercise* 24:253–58.

134. Mertz, W. et al. 1991. What are people really eating? The relation between energy intake derived from estimated diet records and intake determined to maintain body weight. *American Journal of Clinical Nutrition* 54:291–95.

135. Metropolitan Life Insurance Company. 1959. New weight standards for men and women. *Statistical Bulletin Metropolitan Life Insurance Company* 40:1–4.

136. Millard-Stafford, M. L. et al. 2001. Use of air displacement plethysmography for estimating body fat in a four-component model. *Medicine and Science in Sports and Exercise* 33(8):1311–17.

137. Miller, W. C. 1991. Diet composition, energy intake, and nutritional status in relation to obesity in men and women. *Medicine and Science in Sports and Exercise* 23:280–84.

138. Molé, P. A. 1990. Impact of energy intake and exercise on resting metabolic rate. *Sports Medicine* 10:72–87.

139. Montoye, H. J. et al. 1980. Bone mineral in senior tennis players. *Scandinavian Journal of Sport Science* 2:26–32.

140. Moore, R., and E. R. Buskirk. 1974. Exercise and body fluids. In *Science and Medicine of Exercise and Sport*, 2d ed., ed. W. R. Johnson and E. R. Buskirk. New York: Harper & Row.

141. Morrow, J. R. et al. 1986. Accuracy of measured and predicted residual lung volume on body density measurement. *Medicine and Science in Sports and Exercise* 18:647–52.

142. Nachtigall, L. E. et al. 1979. Estrogen replacement therapy I: A 10-year prospective study in the relationship to osteoporosis. *Obstetrics and Gynecology* 53:277–81.

143. National Institutes of Health. 1998. *Clinical guidelines on the identification, evaluation, and treatment of overweight and obesity in adults*. *Obesity Research* 6 (Suppl 2).

144. National Research Council. 1989. *Diet and Health*. Washington, D.C.: National Academy Press.

145. National Research Council, National Academy of Sciences. 1989. *Recommended Dietary Allowances*. Washington, D.C.: National Academy Press.

146. Ogden, C. L., K. M. Flegal, M. D. Carroll, and C. L. Johnson. 2002. Prevalence and trends in overweight among U.S. children and adolescents, 1999–2000. *Journal of the American Medical Association* 288:1728–32.

147. Opperman, A. M. et al. 2004. Meta-analysis of the health effects of using the glycaemic index in meal planning. *British Journal of Nutrition* 92:367–81.

148. Oscai, L. B. 1973. The role of exercise in weight control. In *Exercise and Sport Sciences Reviews*, vol. 1, ed. J. H. Wilmore, 103–20. New York: Academic Press.

149. Oscai, L. B. et al. 1972. Effects of exercise and food restriction on adipose tissue cellularity. *Journal of Lipid Research* 13:588–92.

150. Oscai, L. B., P. A. Molé, and J. O. Holloszy. 1971. Effects of exercise on cardiac weight and mitochondria in male and female rats. *American Journal of Physiology* 220:1944–48.

151. Oyster, N., M. Morton, and S. Linnell. 1984. Physical activity and osteoporosis in post-menopausal women. *Medicine and Science in Sports and Exercise* 16:44–55.

152. Passmore, R. 1968. Energy metabolism at various weights: Man. Part II. Resing: Adults. In *Metabolism*, ed. P. L. Altman and D. S. Dittmer, 344–45. Bethesda, MD: Federation of American Societies for Experimental Biology.

153. Pietrobelli, A., S. B. Heymsfield, Z. M. Wang, and D. Gallagher. 2001. Multicomponent body composition models: Recent advances and future directions. *European Journal of Clinical Nutrition* 55:69–75.

154. Poehlman, E. T. 1989. A review: Exercise and its influence on resting energy metabolism in man. *Medicine and Science in Sports and Exercise* 21:515–25.

155. Poehlman, E. T., C. L. Melby, and M. I. Goran. 1991. The impact of exercise and diet restriction on daily energy expenditure. *Sports Medicine* 11:78–101.

156. Pollock, M. L., and J. H. Wilmore. 1990. *Exercise in Health and Disease*. 2d ed. Philadelphia: W. B. Saunders.

157. Pooling Project Research Group. 1978. Relationship of blood pressure, serum cholesterol, smoking habit, relative weight and ECG abnormalities to incidence of

major coronary events: Final report of the pooling project. *Journal of Chronic Diseases* 31:201–306.

158. Presta, E. et al. 1987. Body composition in adolescents: Estimation by total body electrical conductivity. *Journal of Applied Physiology* 63:937–41.

159. Rabkin, S. W., F. A. L. Mathewson, and Ping-hwa Hsu. 1977. Relation of body weight to development of ischemic heart disease in a cohort of young North American men after a 26-year observation period: The Manitoba study. *The American Journal of Cardiology* 39:452–58.

160. Rimm, A. A., and P. L. White. 1979. Obesity: Its risks and hazards. In *Obesity in America*, U.S. Department of Health, Education and Welfare. NIH Publication No. 79–359.

161. Rising, R. et al. 1994. Determinants of total daily energy expenditure: Variability in physical activity. *American Journal of Clinical Nutrition* 59:800–4.

162. Rolls, B. J. 1995. Carbohydrates, fats, and satiety. *American Journal of Clinical Nutrition* (Suppl. 61):960S–7S.

163. Romijn, J. A. et al. 1993. Regulation of endogenous fat and carbohydrate metabolism in relation to exercise intensity and duration. *American Journal of Physiology* 265:E380–E391.

164. Ross, R., and J. Rissanen. 1994. Mobilization of visceral and subcutaneous adipose tissue in response to energy restriction and exercise. *American Journal of Clinical Nutrition* 60:695–703.

165. Ross, R., J. A. Freeman, and I. Janssen. 2000. Exercise alone is an effective strategy for reducing obesity and related comorbidities. *Exercise and Sport Sciences Reviews* 28:165–70.

166. Ross, R., D. Dagnone, P.J.H. Jones, H. Smith, A. Paddags, R. Hudson, and I. Janssen. 2000. Reduction in obesity and related comorbid conditions after diet-induced weight loss or exercise-induced weight loss in men. *Annals of Internal Medicine* 133:92–103.

167. Roust, L. R., K. D. Hammel, and M. D. Jensen. 1994. Effects of isoenergetic, low-fat diets on energy metabolism in lean and obese women. *American Journal of Clinical Nutrition* 60:470–75.

168. Saris, W. H. M. et al. 2003. How much physical activity is enough to prevent unhealthy weight gain? Outcomes of the IASO 1st Stock Conference and consensus statement. *Obesity Reviews* 4:101–14.

169. Schoeller, D. A. et al. 1985. Measurement of total body water: Isotope dilution techniques. In *Body-Composition Assessment in Youths and Adults*, ed. A. F. Roche, 24–29. Columbus, OH: Ross Laboratories.

170. Schoutens, A., E. Laurent, and J. R. Poortmans. 1989. Effects of inactivity and exercise on bone. *Sports Medicine* 7:71–81.

171. Schuette, S. A., and H. M. Linkswiler. 1984. Calcium. In *Nutrition Reviews' Present Knowledge in Nutrition*, 5th ed., chap. 28, 400–412. Washington, D.C.: The Nutrition Foundation.

172. Schulz, L. O., and D. A. Schoeller. 1994. A compilation of total daily energy expenditures and body weights in healthy adults. *American Journal of Clinical Nutrition* 60: 676–81.

173. Schutte, J. E. et al. 1984. Density of lean body mass is greater in blacks than in whites. *Journal of Applied Physiology: Respiratory, Environmental, and Exercise Physiology* 56:1647–49.

174. Segal, K. R. et al. 1985. Estimation of human body composition by electrical impedance methods: A comparative study. *Journal of Applied Physiology* 58:1565–71.

175. Segal, K. R. et al. 1990. Comparison of thermic effects of constant and relative caloric loads in lean and obese men. *American Journal of Clinical Nutrition* 51:14–21.

176. Segal, K. R. et al. 1991. Estimation of extracellular and total body water by multiple-frequency bioelectrical-impedance measurement. *American Journal of Clinical Nutrition* 54:26–29.

177. Sharkey, B. 1984. *The Physiology of Fitness*. 2d ed. Champaign, IL: Human Kinetics.

178. Sheard, N. F. et al. 2004. Dietary carbohydrate (amount and type) in the prevention and management of diabetes. *Diabetes Care* 27:2266–71.

179. Shick, S. M., R. R. Wing, M. L. Klem, M. T. McGuire, and J. O. Hill. 1998. Persons successful at long-term weight loss and maintenance continue to consume a low-energy, low-fat diet. *Journal of the American Dietetic Association* 98:408–13.

180. Sims, E. A. H. et al. 1973. Endocrine and metabolic effects of experimental obesity in man. *Recent Progress in Hormonal Research* 29:457–87.

181. Sinning, W. E. et al. 1985. Validity of "generalized" equations for body composition analysis in male athletes. *Medicine and Science in Sports and Exercise* 17:124–30.

182. Sinning, W. E., and J. R. Wilson. 1984. Validity of "generalized" equations for body composition analysis in women athletes. *Research Quarterly for Exercise Sport* 55:153–60.

183. Siri, W. E. 1961. Body composition from fluid spaces and density: Analysis of methods. In *Techniques for Measuring Body Composition*, ed. J. Brozek and A. Henschel, 223–44. Washington, D.C.: National Academy of Sciences—National Research Council.

184. ———. 1980. Fat cells and body weight. In *Obesity*, ed. A. J. Stunkard, 72–100. Philadelphia: W. B. Saunders.

185. Sjöström, L. V. 1992. Morbidity of severely obese subjects. *American Journal of Clinical Nutrition* 55:508S–515S.

186. ———. 1992. Mortality of severely obese subjects. *American Journal of Clinical Nutrition* 55:516S–523S.

187. Sjöström, L., and P. Björntrop. 1974. Body composition and adipose tissue cellularity in human obesity. *Acta Media Scandinavica* 195:201–11.

188. Slaughter, M. H. et al. 1988. Skinfold equations for estimation of body fatness in children and youth. *Human Biology* 60:709–23.

189. Stefanick, M. L. 1993. Exercise and weight control. *Exercise and Sport Sciences Reviews* vol. 21, ed. J. O. Holloszy, 363–96. Baltimore: Lippincott Williams & Wilkins.

190. Stunkard, A. J. et al. 1986. An adoption study of human obesity. *The New England Journal of Medicine* 314:193–98.

191. Swinburn, B., and E. Ravussin. 1993. Energy balance or fat balance? *American Journal of Clinical Nutrition* (Suppl. 57):766S–771S.

192. Tataranni, P. et al. 1995. Thermic effect of food in humans: Methods and results from use of a respiratory chamber. *American Journal of Clinical Nutrition* 61:1013–19.

193. Thomas, C. D. et al. 1992. Nutrient balance and energy expenditure during ad libitum feeding of high-fat and high-carbohydrate diets in humans. *American Journal of Clinical Nutrition* 55:934–42.

194. Thompson, D. L., J. Rakow, and S. M. Perdue. 2004. Relationship between accumulated walking and body composition in middle-aged women. *Medicine and Science in Sports and Exercise* 36:911–14.

195. Titchenal, C. A. 1988. Exercise and food intake: What is the relationship? *Sports Medicine* 6:135–45.

196. Tremblay, A. et al. 1991. Energy requirements of a post-obese man reporting a low energy intake at weight maintenance. *American Journal of Clinical Nutrition* 54:506–8.

197. Tremblay, A., J-A Simoneau, and C. Bouchard. 1994. Impact of exercise intensity on body fatness and skeletal muscle metabolism. *Metabolism* 43:814–18.

198. Treuth, M. S. et al. 1995. Energy expenditure and substrate utilization in older women after strength training: 24-h calorimeter results. *Journal of Applied Physiology* 78:2140–46.

199. U.S. Department of Agriculture. 1992. USDA's *Food Guide Pyramid*. Washington, D.C.: Author.

200. U.S. Department of Agriculture. 1980. *Nutrition and Your Health: Dietary Guidelines for Americans*. Washington, D.C.

201. U.S. Department of Agriculture and U.S. Department of Health and Human Services. 2005. *Dietary Guidelines for Americans 2005*. Washington, D.C.: U.S. Printing Office.

202. U.S. Department of Health and Human Services. 2003. *The DASH Eating Plan*. Washington, D.C.: author.

203. U.S. Senate Select Committee on Nutrition and Human Needs. 1977. *Dietary Goals for the U.S.—Supplemental Views*. Washington, D.C.: U.S. Government Printing Office.

204. U.S. Senate Select Committee on Nutrition and Human Needs. 1977. *Eating in America: Dietary Goals for the U.S.* Cambridge, MA: The MIT Press.

205. Van Etten, L. M. L. A., K. R. Westerterp, and F. T. J. Verstappen. 1995. Effect of weight-training on energy expenditure and substrate utilization during sleep. *Medicine and Science in Sports and Exercise* 27:188–93.

206. Van Itallie, T. B. 1979. Conservative approaches to treatment. In *Obesity in America*, ed. G. Bray. Department of Health, Education, and Welfare. NIH Publication No. 79–359.

207. Van Itallie, T. B. et al. 1985. Clinical assessment of body fat content in adults: Potential role of electrical impedance methods: In *Body-Composition Assessments in Youth and Adults*, ed. A. F. Roche, 5–8. Columbus, OH: Ross Laboratories.

208. Van Loan, M. D., et al. 1995. Evaluation of body composition by dual energy X-ray absorptiometry and two different software packages. *Medicine and Science in Sports and Exercise* 27:587–91.

209. Van Marken Lichtenbelt, W. D. et al. 1994. Validation of bioelectrical-impedance measurements as a method to estimate body-water compartments. *American Journal of Clinical Nutrition* 60:159–66.

210. Vasselli, J. R., M. P. Cleary, and T. B. Van Itallie. 1984. Obesity. In *Nutrition Reviews' Present Knowledge in Nutrition*. 5th ed., chap. 4, 35–36. Washington, D.C.: The Nutrition Foundation.

211. Wabitsch, M. et al. 1994. Body-fat distribution and changes in the atherogenic risk-factor profile in obese adolescent girls during weight reduction. *American Journal of Clinical Nutrition* 60:54–60.

212. Wadden, T. A., and A. J. Stunkard. 1985. Social and psychological consequences of obesity. *Annals of Internal Medicine* 103:1062–67.

213. Wagner, D. R., and V. H. Heyward. 1999. Techniques of body composition assessment: A review of laboratory and field methods. *Research Quarterly for Exercise and Sport* 70:135–49.

214. Ward, A. et al. 1978. A comparison of body fat determined by underwater weighing and volume displacement. *American Journal of Physiology* 234:E94–E96.

215. Wardlaw, G. M. 2000. *Contemporary Nutrition*. 4th ed. New York: McGraw-Hill Companies.

216. Weinberger, M. H. 2004. Sodium and blood pressure. *Current Opinion in Cardiology* 19:353–56.

217. Weinsier, R. L., Y. Schutz, and D. Bracco. 1992. Re-examination of the relationship of resting metabolic rate to fat-free mass and to the metabolically active components of fat-free mass in humans. *American Journal of Clinical Nutrition* 55:790–94.

218. Welham, W. C., and A. R. Behnke. 1942. The specific gravity of healthy men. *Journal of the American Medical Association* 118:498–501.

219. Willett, W. C., M. Stampfer, J. Manson, and T. Van Itallie. 1991. New weight guidelines for Americans: Justified or injudicious. *American Journal of Clinical Nutrition* 53:1102–3.

220. Willett, W. C., M. Stampfer, J. Manson, and T. Van Itallie. 1992. Reply to G. A. Bray and R. L. Atlinson. *American Journal of Clinical Nutrition* 55:482–83.

221. Willett, W. C. 2001. *Eat, drink, and be healthy*. New York: Simon & Schuster.

222. Williams, M. H. 1985. *Nutritional Aspects of Human Physical and Athletic Performance*. 2d ed. Springfield, IL: Charles C. Thomas.

223. Wilmore, J. H. 1983. Body composition in sport and exercise: Directions for future research. *Medicine and Science in Sports and Exercise* 15:21–31.

224. ———. 1983. The 1983 C. H. McCloy Research Lecture. Appetite and body composition consequent to physical activity. *Research Quarterly for Exercise and Sport* 54: 415–25.

225. Wing, R. R., and S. Phelan. 2005. Long-term weight loss maintenance. *American Journal of Clinical Nutrition* 82(Suppl.): 222S–25S.

226. Wright, J. D. et al. 2003. Dietary intake of ten key nutrients for public health, United States: 1999–2000. Advance data from vital and health statistics. No. 334. Hyattsville, MD.: National Center for Health Statistics.

227. Zurlo, F. et al. 1990. Low ratio of fat to carbohydrate oxidation as predictor of weight gain: Study of 24-h RQ. *American Journal of Physiology* 259:E650–E657.

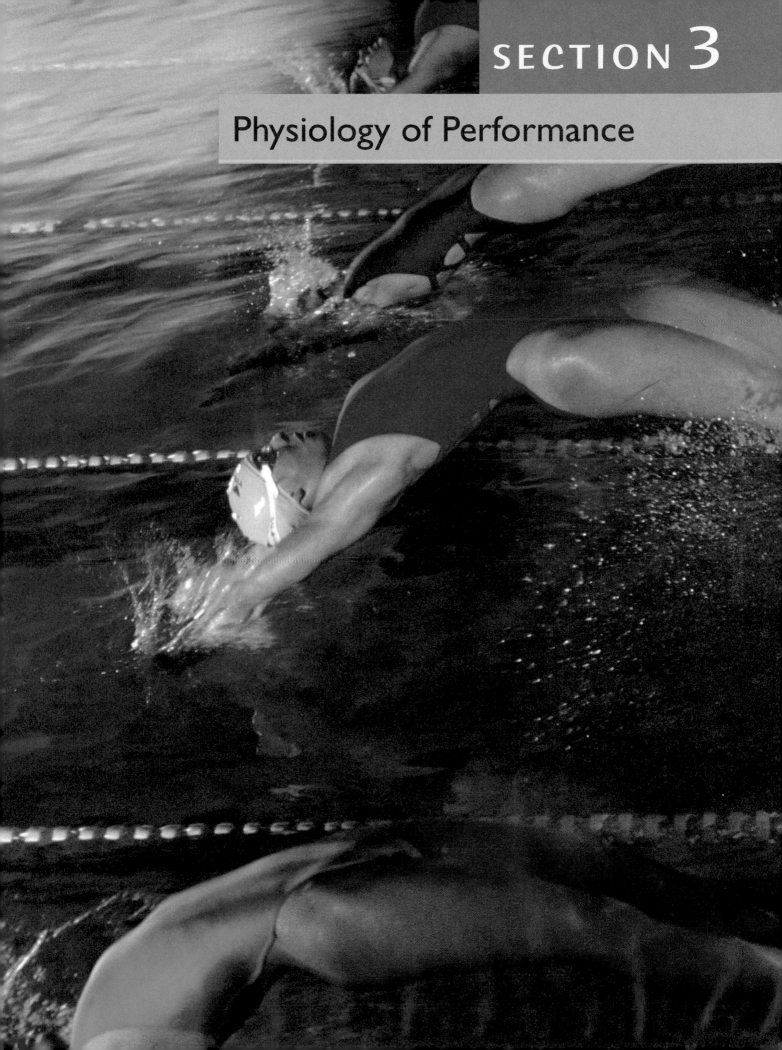

SECTION 3

Physiology of Performance

CHAPTER 19

Factors Affecting Performance

■ Objectives

By studying this chapter, you should be able to do the following:

1. Identify factors affecting maximal performance.
2. Provide evidence for and against the central nervous system being a site of fatigue.
3. Identify potential neural factors in the periphery that may be linked to fatigue.
4. Explain the role of cross-bridge cycling in fatigue.
5. Summarize the evidence on the order of recruitment of muscle fibers with increasing intensities of activity, and the type of metabolism upon which each is dependent.

6. Describe the factors limiting performance in all-out activities lasting less than ten seconds.
7. Describe the factors limiting performance in all-out activities lasting 10 to 180 seconds.
8. Discuss the subtle changes in the factors affecting optimal performance as the duration of a maximal performance increases from three minutes to four hours.

■ Outline

Sites of Fatigue   409
  Central Fatigue   409
  Peripheral Fatigue   410

Factors Limiting All-Out Anaerobic Performances   413
  Ultra Short-Term Performances (Less than Ten Seconds)   413

Short-Term Performances (10 to 180 Seconds)   415

Factors Limiting All-Out Aerobic Performances   415
  Moderate-Length Performances (Three to Twenty Minutes)   415

Intermediate-Length Performances (Twenty-One to Sixty Minutes)   416
Long-Term Performances (One to Four Hours)   417

Athlete as Machine   418

In the last few chapters we have focused on proper exercise and nutrition for health and fitness. The emphasis was on *moderation* in both in order to reduce the risk factors associated with a variety of diseases. We must now change that focus in order to discuss the factors limiting physical performance.

Performance goals require much more time, effort, and risk of injury than fitness goals. What are the requirements for optimal performance? In order to answer this question we must ask another: What kind of performance? It is clear that the requirements for the best performance in the 400-meter run are different from those associated with the marathon. Figure 19.1 shows a diagram of factors influencing performance (4). Every performance requires a certain amount of strength, as well as the "skill" to apply that strength in the best way. Further, energy must be supplied in the manner needed or performance will suffer. Different activities require differing amounts of energy from aerobic and anaerobic processes. Both the environment (altitude and heat) and diet (carbohydrate and water intake) play a role in endurance performance. Lastly, best performances require a psychological commitment to "go for the gold." The purpose of this chapter is to expand on this diagram and discuss the factors limiting performance in a variety of activities, which will point the way to the remaining chapters. However, before we discuss these factors, we will summarize the potential sites of fatigue that would clearly affect performance.

SITES OF FATIGUE

Fatigue is simply defined as an inability to maintain a power output or force during repeated muscle contractions (21). As the two examples of the 400-meter run and the marathon suggest, the causes of fatigue vary and are usually specific to the type of physical activity. Figure 19.2 provides a summary of potential sites of fatigue (21). The discussion of mechanisms starts at the brain, where a variety of factors can influence the "will to win," and continues to the cross-bridges of the muscles themselves. There is evidence to support most of the sites listed in figure 19.2 as "weak links" in the development of the muscle tension needed for optimal performance. However, there is far from perfect agreement among scientists about the exact causes of fatigue. The reasons for this include: (a) the fiber type and training state of the subject, (b) whether the muscle was stimulated voluntarily or electrically, (c) the use of both amphibian and mammalian muscle preparations, with some isolated from the body, and (d) the intensity and duration of the exercise, and whether it was continuous or intermittent activity (36, 37). Within the scope of these limitations, we will now provide a summary of the evidence about each weak link, and then apply the information to specific types of performances (see A Closer Look 19.1).

Central Fatigue

The central nervous system (CNS) would be implicated in fatigue if there were (a) a reduction in the number of functioning motor units involved in the activity or (b) a reduction in motor unit firing frequency (17). There is evidence both for and against the concept of "central fatigue"; that is, that fatigue originates in the CNS.

Merton's classic experiments showed no difference in tension development when a *voluntary* maximal contraction was compared to an *electrically induced* maximal contraction. When the muscle was

FIGURE 19.1 Factors affecting performance.

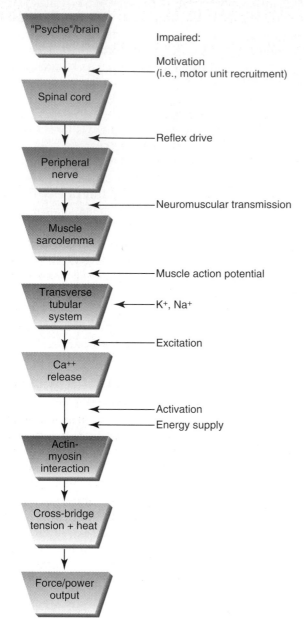

"Psyche"/brain

Impaired:

Motivation
(i.e., motor unit recruitment)

Spinal cord

Reflex drive

Peripheral
nerve

Neuromuscular transmission

Muscle
sarcolemma

Muscle action potential

Transverse
tubular
system

K^+, Na^+

Excitation

Ca^{++}
release

Activation

Energy supply

Actin-
myosin
interaction

Cross-bridge
tension + heat

Force/power
output

FIGURE 19.2 Possible sites of fatigue.

fatigued by voluntary contractions, electrical stimulation could not restore tension (29). This suggested that the CNS was not limiting performance, and that the "periphery" was the site of fatigue.

In contrast, the early work of Ikai and Steinhaus (23) showed that a simple shout during exertion could increase what was formerly believed to be "maximal" strength. Later work showed that electrical stimulation of a muscle fatigued by voluntary contractions resulted in an increase in tension development (24). These studies suggest that the upper limit of voluntary strength is "psychologically" set, given that cer-

tain motivational or arousal factors are needed to achieve a physiological limit (24). In agreement with these results (that the CNS can limit performance) are two studies by Asmussen and Mazin (4, 5). Their subjects lifted weights thirty times a minute, causing fatigue in two to three minutes. Following a two-minute pause, the lifting continued. These investigators showed that when either a physical diversion, consisting of the contraction of nonfatigued muscles, or a mental diversion, consisting of doing mental arithmetic, was used between fatiguing bouts of exercise, work output was greater than when nothing was done during the pause. They also found that if a person did a series of muscle contractions to the point of fatigue with the eyes closed, simply opening the eyes restored tension (4). These studies suggest that alterations in central nervous system "arousal" can facilitate motor unit recruitment to increase strength, and alter the state of fatigue.

Excessive endurance training (overtraining) has been associated with symptoms such as reduced performance capacity, prolonged fatigue, altered mood states, sleep disturbance, loss of appetite, and increased anxiety (14, 39, 40). Over the past decade, a considerable amount of attention has been directed at brain serotonin (5-hydroxytryptamine) as a factor in fatigue due to its links to depression, sleepiness, and mood (39, 40). There is evidence that increases and decreases in brain serotonin activity during prolonged exercise hasten and delay fatigue, respectively (15). Although regular, moderate exercise has been shown to improve the mood states of depressive patients, excessive exercise seems to have an opposite effect. Numerous experiments have been conducted over the past decade to try to understand the connection between serotonin and fatigue, but the answer remains elusive (39, 40).

The CNS is intimately involved in exercise, including the psyching-up prior to exercise (43), the recruitment of motor units, and the continual feedback from a host of receptors sensing tension, temperature, blood gases, blood pressure, and other variables. The brain integrates these various signals and generates commands that automatically reduce power output to protect the organism. In this sense, exercise begins and ends in the brain (26). Let us now look at some of the events outside the CNS that are tied to the fatigue process.

Peripheral Fatigue

While there is evidence both for and against the CNS being a site of fatigue, the vast majority of evidence points to the periphery, where neural, mechanical, or energetic events can hamper tension development (18, 46).

Free Radical Production During Exercise May Contribute to Muscle Fatigue

Free radicals are highly reactive molecules with an unpaired electron in their outer orbital. Recall that free radicals are produced in skeletal muscle during exercise as a by-product of aerobic metabolism (see chapter 3). If the production of these radicals exceeds the muscle's ability to remove the radicals via antioxidants, oxidative injury to the muscle may result in fatigue (8, 33, 34). Indeed, numerous studies demonstrate that radical production during exercise accelerates the rate of muscle fatigue (34). Of further interest is the fact that the rate of radical production in exercising skeletal muscle is accelerated during exercise in a hot environment (48). This new finding may partially explain why muscular endurance is reduced during exercise in the heat.

The precise mechanism of how free radicals produce muscle fatigue is unclear and continues to be investigated. Nonetheless, evidence indicates that free radical production in skeletal muscle during vigorous exercise can damage both the sarcoplasmic reticulum and contractile proteins (34). Damage to the sarcoplasmic reticulum can decrease muscle force production by reducing the amount of calcium released during depolarization of the muscle. Radical-mediated damage to muscle contractile proteins (e.g., actin and myosin) could impair muscle force production by limiting myosin cross-bridge binding to actin; this would reduce the number of myosin cross-bridges in the strong binding state and lower muscle force production. Because free radicals can contribute to muscle fatigue, some scientists have argued that dietary supplementation with antioxidant vitamins (e.g., vitamins E and C) may reduce the rate of muscle fatigue during exercise. However, experiments using antioxidant supplementation do not generally support the notion that dietary antioxidants improve human exercise performance (32). This issue is discussed again in chapter 25.

Neural Factors   Fatigue due to neural factors could be associated with failure at the neuromuscular junction, the sarcolemma, the transverse tubules (t-tubule), or the sarcoplasmic reticulum (SR) that is involved in calcium (Ca^{++}) storage, release, and reuptake.

Neuromuscular Junction   The action potential appears to reach the neuromuscular junction even when fatigue occurs (29). In addition, evidence based on simultaneous measurements of electrical activity at the neuromuscular junction and in the individual muscle fibers suggests that the neuromuscular junction is not the site of fatigue (11).

Sarcolemma and Transverse Tubules   It has been hypothesized that the sarcolemma might be the site of fatigue due to its inability to maintain Na^+ and K^+ concentrations during repeated stimulation. When the Na^+/K^+ pump cannot keep up, K^+ accumulates outside the membrane and decreases inside the cell. This results in a depolarization of the cell and a reduction in action potential amplitude (38). The gradual depolarization of the sarcolemma could result in altered t-tubule function, including a block of the t-tubule action potential. If the latter occurs, Ca^{++} release from the SR will be affected, as will muscle contraction (1). However, the evidence indicates that the typical reduction in the size of the action potential amplitude has little effect on force output by the muscle. In addition, the lower frequency of action potential firing with repeated stimulation of muscle seems to protect the muscle from further fatigue (rather than cause fatigue) by shifting the activation to a lower, more optimal, rate of firing (18). This does not mean that the t-tubule is not involved in the fatigue process. Under certain stimulation conditions an action potential block can occur in the t-tubule, leading to a reduction in Ca^{++} release from the SR (18, 22, 47). As a result, myosin cross-bridge activation would be adversely affected. One of the beneficial effects of training is an increase in the capacity of the Na^+/K^+ pump, which may contribute to the maintenance of the Na^+/K^+ gradient and reduce the potential for fatigue via this mechanism (22).

IN SUMMARY

- Increases in CNS arousal facilitate motor unit recruitment to increase strength and alter the state of fatigue.
- The ability of the muscle membrane to conduct an action potential may be related to fatigue in activities demanding a high frequency of stimulation.
- Repeated stimulation of the sarcolemma can result in a reduction in the size and frequency of action potentials; however, shifts in the optimal frequency needed for muscle activation preserve force output.
- Under certain conditions an action potential block can occur in the t-tubule to result in a reduction in Ca^{++} release from the SR.

Mechanical Factors   The primary mechanical factor that may be related to fatigue is cross-bridge "cycling." The action of the cross-bridge depends on (a) the functional arrangement of actin and myosin, (b) Ca^{++} being available to bind with troponin to allow the cross-bridge to bind with the active site on actin, and (c) ATP, which is needed for both the activation of the cross-bridge to cause movement, and the dissociation of the cross-bridge from actin. Exercise, especially eccentric exercise, can cause a physical disruption of the sarcomere, and reduce the capacity of the muscle to produce tension (3). A high H^+ concentration may contribute to fatigue in a variety of ways (18, 20, 36, 37):

- reduce the force per cross-bridge,
- reduce the force generated at a given Ca^{++} concentration (related to H^+ ion interference with Ca^{++} binding to troponin), and
- inhibit SR Ca^{++} release.

One sign of fatigue in isometric contractions is a longer "relaxation time"—the time from peak tension development to baseline tension. This longer relaxation time could be due to a slower cycling of the cross-bridge due to Ca^{++} not being pumped back to the sarcoplasmic reticulum fast enough, and/or inadequate ATP, which is needed for dissociation of the cross-bridge as well as for Ca^{++} pumping (25, 36, 37). It is this last factor, the availability of ATP, that has received the greatest attention.

IN SUMMARY

- The cross-bridge's ability to "cycle" is important in continued tension development. Fatigue may be related to the effect of a high H^+ concentration on the ability of troponin to bind to Ca^{++}, the inability of the sarcoplasmic reticulum to take up Ca^{++}, or the lack of ATP needed to dissociate the cross-bridge from actin.

Energetics of Contraction   Fatigue can be viewed as the result of a simple imbalance between the ATP requirements of a muscle and its ATP-generating capacity (37). As described in chapter 3, when exercise begins and the need for ATP accelerates, a series of ATP-generating reactions occur to replenish the ATP. As the cross-bridges use ATP and generate ADP, phosphocreatine provides for the immediate resynthesis of the ATP ($PC + ADP \rightarrow ATP + C$). As the phosphocreatine becomes depleted, ADP begins to accumulate and the myokinase reaction occurs to generate ATP ($ADP + ADP \rightarrow ATP + AMP$). The accumulation of all these products stimulates glycolysis to generate additional ATP, which may result in an H^+ accumulation (7). However, as ATP demand continues to exceed supply, a variety of reactions occur in the cell that limit work and

protect the cell from damage. Remember that ATP is needed to pump ions and maintain cell structure. In this sense, fatigue serves a protective function. What are the signals to the muscle cell that energy utilization must slow down? When ATP-generating mechanisms cannot keep up with ATP use, inorganic phosphate (P_i) begins to accumulate in the cell (P_i and ADP are not being converted to ATP). An increase in P_i in the muscle has been shown to inhibit maximal force, and the higher the P_i concentration, the lower the force measured during recovery from fatigue. The P_i seems to act directly on the cross-bridges to reduce its binding to actin (18, 28, 45) and also inhibits calcium release from the sarcoplasmic reticulum (2, 16). The accumulation of P_i reduces the total ATP cost per unit of force, suggesting an improvement in efficiency (31). What is interesting is that the cell does not run out of ATP, even in cases of extreme fatigue. Typically, the ATP concentration falls to only 70% of its pre-exercise level. The factors that cause fatigue reduce the rate of ATP utilization faster than ATP generation so that ATP concentration is maintained. This is believed to be a protective function aimed at minimizing changes in cellular homeostasis with continued stimulation.

IN SUMMARY

- Fatigue is directly associated with a mismatch between the rate at which the muscle uses ATP and the rate at which ATP can be supplied.
- Cellular fatigue mechanisms slow down the rate of ATP utilization faster than the rate of ATP generation to preserve the ATP concentration and cellular homeostasis.

In chapter 8 we linked the different methods of ATP production to the different muscle fiber types that are recruited during activity. We will briefly summarize this information as it relates to our discussion of fatigue. Figure 19.3 shows the pattern of recruitment of muscle fiber types with increasing intensities of exercise. Up to about 40% of $\dot{V}O_2$ max, the type I slow-twitch oxidative muscle fiber is recruited to provide tension development (37). This fiber type is dependent on a continuous supply of blood to provide the oxygen needed for the generation of ATP from carbohydrates and fats. Any factor limiting the oxygen supply to this fiber type (e.g., altitude, dehydration, blood loss, or anemia) would cause a reduction in tension development in these fibers and necessitate the recruitment of type IIa fibers to generate tension.

Type IIa fast-twitch, fatigue-resistant muscle fibers are recruited between 40% and 75% $\dot{V}O_2$ max (37). These fast-twitch fibers are rich in mitochondria, as are the type I fibers, making them dependent on oxygen delivery for tension development. They also have a

FIGURE 19.3 Order of muscle fiber type recruitment in exercise of increasing intensity. From D. G. Sale, "Influence of Exercise and Training in Motor Unit Activation" in Kent B. Pandolf, ed., *Exercise and Sport Sciences Reviews*, vol. 15. Copyright© 1987 McGraw-Hill, Inc., New York. Reprinted by permission.

great capacity to produce ATP via anaerobic glycolysis. The mitochondrial content of type IIa fibers is sensitive to endurance training, so that with detraining more of the ATP supply would be provided by glycolysis, leading to lactate production (see chapter 13). If oxygen delivery to this fiber type is decreased, or the ability of the fiber to use oxygen is decreased (due to low mitochondrial number), tension development will fall, requiring type IIx fiber recruitment to maintain tension.

Type IIx is the fast-twitch muscle fiber with a low mitochondrial content. This fiber can generate great tension via anaerobic sources of energy, but fatigues quickly. It is recruited at about 75% $\dot{V}O_2$ max, making heavy exercise dependent upon its ability to develop tension (38).

Although the primary focus of this text has been on the fitness and performance of individuals stuck (by gravity) on the earth, we are all familiar with the weakness and instability of astronauts as they emerge from the space shuttle after returning from space. With the space station now in orbit and crews rotating on a regular basis, it should be no surprise that physiologists have been studying the impact of prolonged weightlessness on muscle function (19). Ask the Expert 19.1 provides some insights into why astronauts are weaker when they return to earth.

IN SUMMARY

- Muscle fibers are recruited in the following order with increasing intensities of exercise: type I → type IIa → type IIx.

- The progression moves from the most to the least oxidative muscle fiber type. Intense exercise (>75% $\dot{V}O_2$ max) demands that type IIx fibers be recruited, resulting in an increase in lactate production.

FACTORS LIMITING ALL-OUT ANAEROBIC PERFORMANCES

As exercise intensity increases, muscle fiber recruitment progresses from type I → type IIa → type IIx. This means that the ATP supply needed for tension development becomes more and more dependent upon anaerobic metabolism (37). In this way, fatigue is specific to the type of task undertaken. If a task requires only type I fiber recruitment, then the factors limiting performance will be very different from those associated with tasks requiring type IIx fibers. With this review and summary in mind, let's now examine the factors limiting performance.

Ultra Short-Term Performances (Less than Ten Seconds)

The events that fit into this category include the shot put, high jump, long jump, and 50- and 100-meter sprints. These events require that tremendous amounts of energy be produced in a short period of time (high-power events), and type II muscle fibers must be recruited. Figure 19.4 shows that maximal performance is limited by the fiber type distribution (type I versus type II) and by the number of muscle fibers recruited, which is influenced by the level of motivation (23). Optimal performance is also affected by skill and technique, which are dependent on practice. It should be no surprise that the anaerobic sources of ATP—the ATP-PC system and glycolysis—provide the energy. Chapter 20 provides tests for anaerobic power and chapter 21 provides a detailed list of the activities dependent upon such power. There is evidence that ingestion of creatine can influence performance in high-power exercise; see chapter 25 for details.

IN SUMMARY

- In events lasting less than ten seconds, optimal performance is dependent on the recruitment of appropriate type II fibers to generate the great forces that are needed.
- Motivation or arousal is required, as well as the skill needed to direct the force.
- The primary energy sources are anaerobic, with the focus on phosphocreatine.

Muscle Adaptations to Space Travel
Questions and Answers with Dr. Robert H. Fitts

Dr. Fitts is the Wehr Distinguished Professor of Biology at Marquette University. His primary research interests include excitation contraction coupling and muscle mechanics, and the mechanism of muscle adaptation to space flight and programs of regular exercise. His research also focuses on elucidating the cellular causes of muscle fatigue. He was awarded the American College of Sports Medicine's Citation Award in 1999 for his research accomplishments and received the Researcher of the Year Award from Marquette University in 2000.

QUESTION 1: What changes occur in skeletal muscle due to space travel?

ANSWER: The primary change in skeletal muscle with space travel is fiber atrophy due to a selective loss in the myofilaments. The antigravity muscles of the legs are more affected than arm muscles, and primarily slow muscles like the soleus are more affected than fast-twitch muscles such as the gastrocnemius. Due to the loss of myofilaments, muscle fibers generate less force and power. Post-flight, the slow type I fibers show an elevated maximal shortening velocity, which is not caused by an expression of fast-type myosin. It has been hypothesized that the increased velocity results from a selective loss of the thin filament actin, which increases the space between the filaments causing the myosin cross-bridge to detach sooner at the end of the power stroke. Space flight appears to increase the muscle's reliance on carbohydrates and reduce its ability to oxidize fats. This metabolic change is not caused by a reduced activity of any of the enzymes of the β-oxidative pathway or the Krebs cycle. The loss in fiber power and increased reliance on carbohydrates cause a reduced work capacity. Additionally, post-flight crew members experience muscle soreness due to an increased susceptibility to eccentric contraction-induced fiber damage.

QUESTION 2: Do animal studies mimic the changes experienced by humans?

ANSWER: Many of the space flight induced changes in skeletal muscle are observed in rodents, nonhuman primates, and humans. Fiber atrophy caused by the selective loss of myofilaments has been observed in all species. There are species differences in the time course of the adaptive process. For example, rats flown in space show a faster rate of fiber atrophy than humans. Flights as short as two or three weeks have been shown to increase soleus muscle velocity in both rats and humans, but in rats the increase was in part due to a conversion of approximately 20% of the slow type I fibers to fast-twitch fibers containing fast myosin isozymes. In humans, short-duration space flight does not cause fiber type conversion.

QUESTION 3: Are there any intervention (training) strategies being employed to reduce the impact of space flight on skeletal muscle?

ANSWER: The primary countermeasure used to protect skeletal muscle from microgravity-induced loss has employed endurance exercise on either a bicycle or treadmill. This type of modality has not been completely successful, as crew members still lose up to 20% of their leg muscle mass following six months in space. More recently, high-intensity exercise has been incorporated into the countermeasure program. However, a reliable device for such training has not yet been installed on the international space station.

FIGURE 19.4   Factors affecting fatigue in ultra short-term events.

Short-Term Performances (10 to 180 Seconds)

Maximal performances in the ten- to sixty-second range are still predominantly (>70%) anaerobic, using the high force, fast-twitch fiber, but when a maximal performance is extended to three minutes, about 60% of the energy comes from the slower aerobic, ATP-generating processes. As a result of this transition from anaerobic to aerobic energy production, maximal running speed decreases as the length of the race increases. Given that the ATP-PC system can supply ATP for only several seconds, the vast majority of the ATP will be derived from anaerobic glycolysis (see chapter 3). Figure 19.5 shows that this will cause an accumulation of H^+ in muscle as well as blood. The elevated H^+ concentration may actually interfere with the continued production of ATP via glycolysis, or the contractile machinery itself, by interfering with troponin's ability to bind with Ca^{++}. However, it must be added that following exhausting exercise, muscle tension recovers *before* the H^+ concentration does, indicating the complex nature of the fatigue process (20, 35, 36, 43). In an effort to slow H^+ accumulation, some athletes have attempted to ingest buffers prior to a race. This procedure is discussed in detail in chapter 25, which deals with ergogenic aids and performance.

IN SUMMARY

- In short-term performances lasting 10 to 180 seconds, there is a shift from 70% of the energy supplied anaerobically at 10 seconds to 60% being supplied aerobically at 180 seconds.
- Anaerobic glycolysis provides a substantial portion of the energy, resulting in elevated lactate levels.

FACTORS LIMITING ALL-OUT AEROBIC PERFORMANCES

As the duration of an all-out performance increases, more demand is placed on the aerobic sources of energy. In addition, environmental factors such as heat and humidity, and dietary factors such as water and carbohydrate ingestion play a role in fatigue.

Moderate-Length Performances (Three to Twenty Minutes)

While 60% of ATP production is derived from aerobic processes in a three-minute maximal effort, the value jumps to 90% in a twenty-minute all-out performance. Given this dependence on oxidative energy production, the factors limiting performance include both the cardiovascular system, which delivers oxygen-rich blood to the muscles, and the mitochondrial content of the muscles involved in the activity. Since speed is a prerequisite in races lasting less than twenty minutes, type IIa fibers, which are rich in mitochondria, are involved in supplying the ATP aerobically. Races lasting less than twenty minutes are run at 90% to 100% of maximal aerobic power, so the athlete with the highest $\dot{V}O_2$ max has a distinct advantage. However, due to the fact that type IIx fibers are also recruited, high levels of blood lactic acid are also experienced, and H^+ accumulation would affect tension development as previously described (20, 35, 36, 44). Figure 19.6 summarizes the factors affecting performances requiring a high maximal oxygen uptake. The maximal stroke volume is the crucial key to a high cardiac output (see chapter 13), and is influenced by

FIGURE 19.5 Factors affecting fatigue in short-term events.

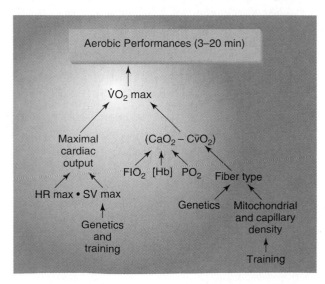

FIGURE 19.6 Factors affecting fatigue in aerobic performances lasting three to twenty minutes.

Is Maximal Oxygen Uptake Important in Distance Running Performance?

$\dot{V}O_2$ max is directly related to the rate of ATP generation that can be maintained during a distance race, even though it is not run at 100% $\dot{V}O_2$ max. The rate of ATP generation is dependent on the actual $\dot{V}O_2$ that can be maintained during the run (ml · kg⁻¹ · min⁻¹), which is a function of the runner's $\dot{V}O_2$ max and the percent $\dot{V}O_2$ max at which the runner can perform. To run a 2:15 marathon, the runner would have to maintain a $\dot{V}O_2$ of about 60 ml · kg⁻¹ · min⁻¹ throughout the race. A runner working at 80% $\dot{V}O_2$ max would need a $\dot{V}O_2$ max of 75 ml · kg⁻¹ · min⁻¹. In this way the $\dot{V}O_2$ max sets the upper limit for energy production in endurance events, but does not determine the final performance. It is clear that both the percent of $\dot{V}O_2$ max that can be maintained over the course of the run (estimated by the lactate threshold) and running economy have a dramatic impact on the speed that can be maintained over distance (9, 10). Interestingly, the progressive reduction in $\dot{V}O_2$ max with age appears to be the primary physiological mechanism associated with a reduction in the endurance performance of Master athletes, along with the reduction in the velocity at the lactate threshold (42).

both genetics and training. The arterial oxygen content (CaO_2) is influenced by the arterial hemoglobin content [Hb], the fraction of inspired oxygen (FIO_2), and PO_2 of the inspired air. Chapter 24 discusses the effect of altitude (low PO_2) on $\dot{V}O_2$ max, and chapter 25 discusses the use of blood doping (to raise the [Hb]) and oxygen breathing on aerobic performance. Training programs are discussed in chapter 21.

IN SUMMARY

- In moderate-length performances lasting three to twenty minutes, aerobic metabolism provides 60% to 90% of the ATP, respectively.
- These activities require an energy expenditure near $\dot{V}O_2$ max, with type II fibers being recruited.
- Any factor interfering with oxygen delivery (e.g., altitude or anemia) would decrease performance, since it is so dependent on aerobic energy production. High levels of lactate accompany these types of activities.

Intermediate-Length Performances (Twenty-One to Sixty Minutes)

In all-out performances lasting twenty-one to sixty minutes, the athlete will generally work at <90% $\dot{V}O_2$ max. A high $\dot{V}O_2$ max is certainly a prerequisite for success, but now other factors come into play. For example, an individual who is an "economical" runner can move at a slightly higher speed for the same amount of oxygen compared to a runner who is not economical. Differences in running economy are due to biomechanical and/or bioenergetic factors. In this case measurements of both $\dot{V}O_2$ max and running economy would be needed to predict performance (see chapter 20). However, there is another variable that must be considered. Since races of this duration are not run at $\dot{V}O_2$ max, a person who can run at a high percentage of $\dot{V}O_2$ max would have an advantage. The ability to run at a high percentage of $\dot{V}O_2$ max is related to the concentration of lactate in the blood, and one of the best predictors of race pace is the lactate threshold (9, 10). See The Winning Edge 19.1 for more on this. Interestingly, a high percentage of type I muscle fibers is associated with both a greater lactate threshold and a higher mechanical efficiency (12). Chronic severe training over many years has been linked to an improvement (+8%) in mechanical efficiency that contributed to the consecutive victories of the Tour de France champion, Lance Armstrong (13). The procedures to follow in estimating the maximal running speed for long-distance races are presented in chapter 20. Factors limiting performance in runs of twenty-one to sixty minutes are summarized in figure 19.7. Please note that we must now consider the environmental factors of heat and humidity, as well as the state of hydration of the runner. The heat load will require that a portion of the cardiac output be directed to the skin, pushing the cardiovascular system closer to maximum at any running speed. There is evidence of a critical temperature during exercise that can lead to fatigue via a reduction in the CNS drive to recruit skeletal muscle (32). See chapters 23 and 24 for information on how to deal with dehydration and environmental heat loads.

IN SUMMARY

- Intermediate-length activities lasting twenty-one to sixty minutes are usually conducted at less than 90% $\dot{V}O_2$ max, and are predominantly aerobic.
- Given the length of the activity, environmental factors such as heat, humidity, and the state of hydration of the subject play a role in the outcome.

FIGURE 19.7 Factors affecting fatigue in aerobic performances lasting twenty-one to sixty minutes.

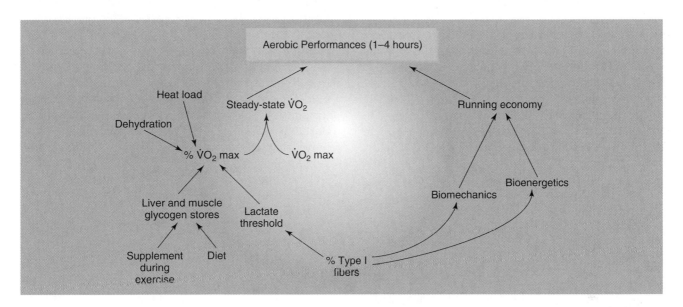

FIGURE 19.8 Factors affecting fatigue in aerobic performances lasting one to four hours.

Long-Term Performances (One to Four Hours)

Performances of one to four hours are clearly aerobic performances involving little anaerobic energy production. Using the shorter aerobic performances (less than sixty minutes) as a lead-in, the longer the performance, the greater the chance that environmental factors will play a role in the outcome. In addition, for performances greater than one hour, the ability of the muscle and liver carbohydrate stores to supply glucose may be exceeded. As pointed out in chapter 4, fatty acids can provide substantial fuel during prolonged muscular work at intensities <60% $\dot{V}O_2$ max. However, for the many endurance activities that are performed at higher exercise intensities (e.g., marathon running), muscle fibers must have carbohydrate to oxidize or performance will decline. This model may not be as useful for "ultra"-type perfor-

mances where fueling, fluid, and electrolyte imbalance issues are pushed to an extreme (27). Chapter 23 provides information about the optimal dietary strategies for performance in long-term events, including the consumption of fluids and carbohydrates during the run. Figure 19.8 summarizes the factors limiting performance in long-distance events.

IN SUMMARY

- In long-term performances of one to four hours' duration, environmental factors play a more important role as the muscle and liver glycogen stores try to keep up with the rate at which carbohydrate is used.
- Diet, fluid ingestion, and the ability of the athlete to deal with heat and humidity all influence the final outcome.

In conclusion, the factors limiting performance are specific to the type of performance. Short-term explosive performances are dependent on type IIx fibers that can generate great power through anaerobic processes. In contrast, longer-duration aerobic events require a cardiovascular system that can deliver oxygen at a high rate to muscle fibers with many mitochondria. It is clear that the testing and training of athletes must focus on the factors limiting performance for the specific event. For example, dietary carbohydrate and fluid ingestion are more crucial for the long-distance runner than the high jumper. Following chapters will explore how to appropriately test, train, and feed athletes for optimal performance.

ATHLETE AS MACHINE

One question we might keep in mind as we explore the details of how to improve performance is whether we might exceed what are regarded as reasonable and ethical boundaries for scientists, and treat the elite athlete as a machine rather than as a person. Are elite athletes being treated like racing cars in which engineers and mechanics (scientists and coaches) try to spot weaknesses that compromise performance, and then recommend solutions? Some may say yes, and indicate the worthiness of such an enterprise. Others may suggest that this has the potential to be dehumanizing if the athlete is reduced to no more than a collection of working parts that are evaluated by a variety of specialists. Much would appear to depend on the goal of the research. If we are trying to understand how we function, and we develop healthy and safe methods that allow us to overcome personal limitations, we would appear to be on the right track. In contrast, if we *use* an athlete as a tool, that would be a different story. We are all familiar with the use of athletes by some countries to advance a particular political doctrine, and the complicity of scientists who were recruited to make athletes run faster and longer, and jump higher. Fortunately, universities, hospitals, and research centers have Institutional Review Boards (IRBs) to approve research proposals so that the rights of the subject are protected. This process also forces the investigator to provide a strong rationale showing that the risk to the subject (however small) is worth the benefits that might occur. Consistent with this, research journals require authors to follow IRB guidelines if they wish their work to be considered for publication. In this way we can move forward in our understanding of the physiological mechanisms underlying fatigue, while protecting the rights of the subject.

STUDY QUESTIONS

1. List the factors influencing performance.
2. Is the limiting factor for strength development located in the CNS or out in the periphery? Support your position.
3. Tracing the path the action potential takes from the time it leaves the motor end plate, where might the "weak link" be in the mechanisms coupling excitation to contraction?
4. When fatigue occurs there is still ATP present in the cell. What is the explanation for this?
5. Describe the pattern of recruitment of muscle fiber types during activities of progressively greater intensity, and explain them.
6. As the duration of a maximal effort increases from less than ten seconds to 10 to 180 seconds, what factor becomes limiting in terms of energy production?
7. Draw a diagram of the factors limiting maximal running performances of 1,500 m to 5 km.
8. While a high $\dot{V}O_2$ max is essential to world-class performance, what role does running economy play in a winning performance?
9. Given that lactate accumulation will adversely affect endurance, what test might be an indicator of maximal sustained running (swimming, cycling) speed?
10. What is the role of environmental factors, such as altitude and heat, in very long-distance performances of one to four hours' duration?

SUGGESTED READINGS

Costill, D. L. 1986. *Inside Running.* Indianapolis: Benchmark Press.

Daniels, J. T. 2005. *Daniels' Running Formula.* 2d ed. Champaign, IL: Human Kinetics.

Jones, N. L., N. McCarney, and A. J. McComas, eds. 1986. *Human Muscle Power.* Champaign, IL: Human Kinetics.

Komi, P. V., ed. 2002. *Strength and Power in Sport.* London: Blackwell Scientific Publishers.

Porter, Ruth, ed. 1981. *Human Muscle Fatigue: Physiological Mechanisms.* London: Pitman Medical.

Simonson, E. 1971. *Physiology of Work Capacity and Fatigue.* Springfield, IL: Charles C Thomas.

REFERENCES

1. Allen, D. G., H. Westerblad, J. A. Lee, and J. Lannergren. 1992. Role of excitation-contraction coupling in muscle fatigue. *Sports Medicine* 13:116–26.

2. Allen, D. G., and H. Westerblad. 2001. Role of phosphate and calcium stores in muscle fatigue. *Journal of Physiology* 536:657–65.

3. Appell, H. J., J. M. C. Soares, and J. A. R. Duarte. 1992. Exercise, muscle damage, and fatigue. *Sports Medicine* 13:108–15.

4. Asmussen, E., and B. Mazin. 1978. A central nervous component in local muscle fatigue. *European Journal of Applied Physiology* 38:9–15.

5. ———. 1978. Recuperation after muscular fatigue by "diverting activities." *European Journal of Applied Physiology* 38:1–7.

6. Åstrand, P. O., and K. Rodahl. 1977. *Textbook of Work Physiology*. 2d ed. New York: McGraw-Hill Companies.

7. Banister, E. W., and B. J. C. Cameron. 1990. Exercise-induced hyperammonemia: Peripheral and central effects. *International Journal of Sports Medicine* 11:S129–S142.

8. Barclay, J., and M. Hansel. 1991. Free radicals may contribute to skeletal muscle fatigue. *Canadian Journal of Physiology and Pharmacology* 69:279–84.

9. Bassett, D. R., Jr., and E. T. Howley. 1997. Maximal oxygen uptake: "Classical" versus "contemporary" viewpoints. *Medicine and Science in Sports and Exercise* 29:591–603.

10. Bassett, D. R., Jr., and E. T. Howley. 2000. Limiting factors for maximal oxygen uptake and determinants of endurance performance. *Medicine and Science in Sports and Exercise*. 32:70–84.

11. Bigland-Ritchie, B. 1981. EMG and fatigue of human voluntary and stimulated contractions. In *Human Muscle Fatigue: Physiological Mechanisms*, 130–56. London: Pitman Medical.

12. Coyle, E. F. 1995. Integration of the physiological factors determining endurance performance. In *Exercise and Sport Sciences Reviews*, vol. 23, ed. J. O. Holloszy, 25–63. Baltimore: Lippincott Williams & Wilkins.

13. Coyle, E. F. 2005. Improved muscular efficiency displayed as Tour de France champion matures. *Journal of Applied Physiology* 98: 2191–96.

14. Davis, J. M., and S. P. Bailey. 1997. Possible mechanisms of central nervous system fatigue during exercise. *Medicine and Science in Sports and Exercise* 29:45–57.

15. Davis, J. M., N. L. Alderson, and R. S. Welsh. 2000. Serotonin and central nervous system fatigue: Nutritional considerations. *American Journal of Clinical Nutrition* 72 (2 Suppl):573S–78S.

16. Duke, A. M., and D. S. Steele. 2001. Mechanisms of reduced SR Ca^{+2} release induced by inorganic phosphate in rat skeletal muscle fibers. *American Journal of Cell Physiology* 281:C418–29.

17. Edwards, R. H. T. 1981. Human muscle function and fatigue. In *Human Muscle Fatigue: Physiological Mechanisms*, 1–18. London: Pitman Medical.

18. Fitts, R. H. 1994. Cellular mechanisms of muscle fatigue. *Physiological Reviews* 74:49–94.

19. Fitts, R. H., D. R. Riley, and J. J. Widrick. 2001. Functional and structural adaptation of skeletal muscle to microgravity. *Journal of Experimental Biology* 204:3201–8.

20. Fuchs, F., V. Reddy, and F. N. Briggs. 1970. The interaction of cations with the calcium-binding site of troponin. *Biochemica et Biophysica Acta.* 221:407–9.

21. Gibson, H., and R. H. T. Edwards. 1985. Muscular exercise and fatigue. *Sports Medicine* 2:120–32.

22. Green, H. J. 2004. Membrane excitability, weakness, and fatigue. *Canadian Journal of Applied Physiology* 29:291–307.

23. Ikai, M., and A. H. Steinhaus. 1961. Some factors modifying the expression of human strength. *Journal of Applied Physiology* 16:157–63.

24. Ikai, M., and K. Yabe. 1969. Training effect of muscular endurance by means of voluntary and electrical stimulation. *European Journal of Applied Physiology* 28:55–60.

25. Jones, D. A. 1981. Muscle fatigue due to changes beyond the neuromuscular junction. In *Human Muscle Fatigue: Physiological Mechanisms*, 178–96. London: Pitman Medical.

26. Kayser, B. 2003. Exercise starts and ends in the brain. *European Journal of Applied Physiology* 90:411–19.

27. Laursen, P. B., and E. C. Rhodes. 2001. Factors affecting performance in an ultraendurance triathlon. *Sports Medicine* 31(3):195–209.

28. McLester, J. R., Jr. 1997. Muscle contraction and fatigue. *Sports Medicine* 23:287–305.

29. Merton, P. A. 1954. Voluntary strength and fatigue. *Journal of Physiology* 123:553–64.

30. Myburgh, K. H. 2004. Can any metabolites partially alleviate fatigue manifestations at the cross-bridge? *Medicine and Science in Sports & Exercise* 36:20–27.

31. Nielsen, B., and L. Nybo. 2003. Cerebral changes during exercise in the heat. *Sports Medicine* 33:1–11.

32. Powers, S. K., K. C. DeRuisseau, J. Quindry, and K. L. Hamilton. 2004. Dietary antioxidants and exercise. *Journal of Sports Sciences* 22:81–94.

33. Reid, M., K. Haack, K. Franchek, P. Valberg, L. Kobzik, and M. West. 1992. Reactive oxygen in skeletal muscle. I. Intracellular oxidant kinetics and fatigue in vitro. *Journal of Applied Physiology* 73:1797–1804.

34. Reid, M., and W. Durham. 2002. Generation of reactive oxygen and nitrogen species in contracting skeletal muscle: Potential impact on aging. *Annals New York Academic Science* 959:108–16.

35. Roberts, D., and D. J. Smith. 1989. Biochemical aspects of peripheral muscle fatigue—a review. *Sports Medicine* 7:125–38.

36. Sahlin, K. 1992. Metabolic factors in fatigue. *Sports Medicine* 13:99–107.

37. Sale, D. G. 1987. Influence of exercise and training on motor unit activation. In *Exercise and Sport Sciences Reviews*, vol. 15, ed. K. B. Pandolf, 95–151. New York: Macmillan.

38. Sejersted, O. M., and G. Sjøgaard. 2000. Dynamics and consequences of potassium shifts in skeletal muscle and heart during exercise. *Physiological Reviews* 80:1411–81.

39. Strüder, H. K., and H. Weicker. 2001. Physiology and pathophysiology of the serotonergic system and its implications on mental and physical performance. Part I. *International Journal of Sports Medicine* 22:467–81.

40. ———. 2001. Physiology and pathophysiology of the serotonergic system and its implications on mental and physical performance. Part II. *International Journal of Sports Medicine* 22:482–97.

41. Tanaka, H., and D. R. Seals. 2003. Dynamic exercise performance in Masters athletes: Insight into the effects of primary human aging on physiological functional capacity. *Journal of Applied Physiology* 95:2152–62.

42. Tod, D., F. Iredale, and N. Gill. 2003. "Psyching-up" and muscular force production. *Sports Medicine* 33:47–58.

43. Trevidi, B., and W. H. Danforth. 1966. Effect of pH on the kinetics of frog muscle phosphofructokinase. *Journal of Biological Chemistry* 241:4110–12.

44. Tupling, A. R. 2004. The sarcoplasmic reticulum in muscle fatigue and disease: Role of the sarco(endo)plasmic reticulum Ca^{2+}-ATPase. *Canadian Journal of Applied Physiology* 29:308–29.

45. Vandenboom, R. 2004. The myofibrillar complex and fatigue: A review. *Canadian Journal of Applied Physiology* 29:330–56.

46. Westerblad, H. et al. 1991. Cellular mechanisms of fatigue in skeletal muscle. *American Journal of Physiology* 261:C195–C209.

47. Zuo, L. et al. 2000. Intra- and extracellular measurement of reactive oxygen species produced during heat stress in diaphragm muscle. *American Journal of Physiology* C1058–66.

CHAPTER 20

Laboratory Assessment of Human Performance

■ Objectives

By studying this chapter, you should be able to do the following:

1. Discuss the rationale for the determination of $\dot{V}O_2$ max in the evaluation of exercise performance in athletes competing in endurance events.
2. Explain the concept of "specificity of $\dot{V}O_2$ max."
3. State the rationale for the assessment of the lactate threshold in the endurance athlete.
4. Discuss the purpose and technique(s) involved in the measurement of exercise economy.
5. Provide an overview of how laboratory tests performed on the endurance athlete might be interpreted as an aid in predicting performance.
6. Describe several tests that are useful in assessing anaerobic power.
7. Discuss the techniques used to evaluate strength.

■ Outline

Laboratory Assessment of Physical Performance   422
   Physiological Testing: Theory and Ethics   422

What the Athlete Gains by Physiological Testing   422

What Physiological Testing Will Not Do   423

Components of Effective Physiological Testing   423

Direct Testing of Maximal Aerobic Power   424
   Specificity of Testing   424
   Exercise Test Protocol   425
   Determination of Peak $\dot{V}O_2$ in Paraplegic Athletes   425

Laboratory Tests to Predict Endurance Performance   426
   Use of the Lactate Threshold to Evaluate Performance   426
   Measurement of Critical Power   428

Tests to Determine Exercise Economy   429

Estimating Success in Distance Running Using the Lactate Threshold and Running Economy   429

Determination of Anaerobic Power   430
   Tests of Ultra Short-Term Maximal Anaerobic Power   431

Tests of Short-Term Anaerobic Power   433

Evaluation of Muscular Strength   434
   Criteria for Selection of a Strength-Testing Method   434
   Isometric Measurement of Strength   435
   Free-Weight Testing of Strength   435
   Isokinetic Assessment of Strength   436
   Variable-Resistance Measurement of Strength   437

critical power	muscular strength	Wingate test
dynamometer	power tests	
isokinetic	Quebec 10-second test	

In general, there have been two principal approaches to the assessment of physical performance: (1) field tests of general physical fitness, which include a variety of measurements requiring basic performance demands and (2) laboratory assessments of physiological capacities such as maximal aerobic power $\dot{V}O_2$ max), anaerobic power, and exercise economy (1, 47). It can be argued that physical fitness testing is important for an overall assessment of general conditioning, particularly in terms of evaluating student progress in a physical education conditioning class (1, 63). However, the use of these test batteries does not provide the detailed physiological information needed to assess an athlete's current level of conditioning or potential weaknesses. Therefore, more specific laboratory tests are required to provide detailed physiological information about performance in specific athletic events. It is the purpose of this chapter to discuss laboratory tests designed to measure physical work capacity. Specifically, much of the chapter will center around laboratory tests to evaluate the maximum energy transfer capacities discussed in chapters 3 and 4.

LABORATORY ASSESSMENT OF PHYSICAL PERFORMANCE

Physiological Testing: Theory and Ethics

Designing laboratory tests to assess physical performance requires an understanding of those factors that contribute to success in a particular sport or athletic event. In general, physical performance is determined by the individual's capacity for maximal energy output (i.e., maximal, aerobic, and anaerobic processes), muscular strength, coordination/economy of movement, and psychological factors (e.g., motivation and tactics) (1, 2, 8, 28). Figure 20.1 illustrates a simple model of the components that interact to determine the quality of physical performance. Many types of athletic events require a combination of several of these factors for an outstanding performance to occur. However, often one or more of these factors plays a dominating role in determining athletic success. In golf, there is little need for a high-energy output, but proper

coordination is essential. Sprinting 100 meters requires not only good technique, but a high anaerobic power output as well. In distance running, cycling, or swimming, a high capacity for aerobic energy-yielding processes is essential for success. Again, laboratory evaluation of performance requires an understanding of those factors that are important for optimal performance in a particular athletic event. Thus, a test that stresses the same physiological systems required by a particular sport or athletic event would appear to be a valid means of assessing physical performance.

A key concern in the performance of "athletic" laboratory testing is maintaining respect for the athlete's human rights. In short, laboratory testing should be performed on athletes who are volunteers and have given written consent prior to testing. Prior to testing, the exercise scientist has the responsibility of informing the athlete about the purpose of the tests and the potential risks or discomfort associated with laboratory testing.

WHAT THE ATHLETE GAINS BY PHYSIOLOGICAL TESTING

Laboratory measurement of physical performance can be expensive and time consuming. An obvious question arises: What does the athlete gain by laboratory

FIGURE 20.1 Factors that contribute to physical performance. See text for details.

Reliability of Physiological Performance Tests

In order for a physiological test of human performance to be useful, the test must be reliable. That is, the test results must be reproducible. Several factors influence the reliability of physiological performance tests. These include the caliber of athletes tested, the type of ergometer used during the test, and the specificity of the test.

It has been argued that physiological tests of performance are more reliable when highly trained and experienced athletes are tested (33). The explanation for this observation appears to be that these athletes are highly motivated

to perform and that they are better able to pace themselves in a reproducible manner during a performance test. That is, high-caliber athletes may have a better "feel" for pace, and their perceptions of fatigue are less variable than those of less experienced athletes (33).

It is clear that some ergometers are more unvarying than others in providing a constant resistance. For instance, an ergometer that maintains its calibration and delivers a constant power output during a test would result in a more reproducible test of human performance than an ergometer that

provides variable power outputs during the test.

Although controversy exists, it is believed that exercise tests with a movement pattern and exercise intensity that mimics the actual sporting event are more reliable than tests that do not imitate the event (33, 37). For example, testing racing cyclists on a cycle ergometer at an exercise intensity close to the intensity of competition should be a more reliable performance test than testing these athletes on other types of ergometers, such as treadmills.

---

testing? A testing program can benefit the athlete and coach in at least three major ways:

1. Physiological testing can provide information regarding an athlete's strengths and weaknesses in his/her sport; this information can be used as baseline data to plan individual exercise training programs. Athletic success in most sports involves the interaction of several physiological components. This is illustrated in figure 20.1. In the laboratory, the exercise scientist can often measure these physiological components separately and provide the athlete with information about which physiological components require improvement in order for the athlete to raise his/her level of athletic performance. This information becomes the foundation for an individual exercise prescription that concentrates on the identified areas of weakness (48).

2. Laboratory testing provides feedback to the athlete about the effectiveness of a training program (48). For example, comparing the results of physiological tests performed before and after a training program provides a basis for evaluating the success of the training program.

3. Laboratory testing educates the athlete about the physiology of exercise (48). By participation in laboratory testing, the athlete learns more about those physiological parameters that are important to success in his/her sport. This is important, since athletes with a basic understanding of elementary exercise physiology will likely make better

personal decisions concerning the design of both exercise training and nutritional programs.

WHAT PHYSIOLOGICAL TESTING WILL NOT DO

Laboratory testing of the athlete is not a magical aid for the identification of future Olympic gold medalists (48). Although laboratory testing can provide valuable information concerning an athlete's strengths and weaknesses, this type of testing has limitations in that it is difficult to simulate in the laboratory the physiological and psychological demands of many sports. Therefore, it is difficult to predict athletic performance from any single battery of laboratory measurements. Performance in the field is the ultimate test of athletic success, and laboratory testing should be considered primarily a training aid for coach and athlete (48). (See A Closer Look 20.1.)

COMPONENTS OF EFFECTIVE PHYSIOLOGICAL TESTING

In order for laboratory testing to be effective, several key factors need consideration (48):

1. The physiological variables to be tested should be relevant to the sport. For example, measurement of maximal handgrip strength in a distance

runner would not be relevant to the athlete's event. Therefore, only those physiological components that are important for a particular sport should be measured.

2. Physiological tests should be valid and reliable. Valid tests are tests that measure what they are supposed to measure. Reliable tests are tests that are reproducible. Based on these definitions, the need for tests that are both valid and reproducible is clear.

3. Tests should be as sport specific as possible. For instance, the distance runner should be tested while running (i.e., treadmill) and the cyclist should be tested while cycling.

4. Tests should be repeated at regular intervals. One of the main purposes of laboratory testing is to provide the athlete with systematic feedback concerning training effectiveness. In order to meet this objective, tests should be performed on a regular basis.

5. Testing procedures should be carefully controlled. The need to rigidly administer the laboratory test relates to the reliability of tests. In order for tests to be reliable, the testing protocol should be standardized. Factors to be controlled include the instructions given to the athletes prior to testing, the testing protocol itself, the calibration of instruments involved in testing, the time of the day for testing, prior exercise, diet standardization, and other factors such as sleep, illness, hydration status, or injury.

6. Test results should be interpreted to the coach and athlete in simple terms (i.e., layperson's terms). This final step is a key goal of effective laboratory testing. In order for laboratory testing to benefit the coach or athlete, the test results must be explained in language that he or she will understand.

IN SUMMARY

- Designing laboratory tests to assess physical performance requires an understanding of those factors that contribute to success in a particular sport.
- Physical performance is determined by the interaction of the following factors: (a) maximal energy output, (b) muscular strength, (c) coordination/economy of movement, and (d) psychological factors such as motivation and tactics.
- In order to be effective, physiological tests should be: (a) relevant to the sport; (b) valid and reliable; (c) sport specific; (d) repeated at regular intervals; (e) standardized; and (f) interpreted to the coach and athlete.

DIRECT TESTING OF MAXIMAL AEROBIC POWER

Let's begin our discussion of performance testing by a discussion of tests to assess the maximal aerobic energy output of an athlete. *Maximal oxygen uptake* was first mentioned in chapter 4, and is defined as the highest oxygen uptake that an individual can obtain during exercise using large muscle groups (1). By necessity, the type of exercise performed to determine $\dot{V}O_2$ max must use large muscle groups (e.g., legs). Although several tests to estimate $\dot{V}O_2$ max exist (11, 20, 81), the most accurate means of determination is by direct laboratory measurement. Direct measurement of $\dot{V}O_2$ max is generally performed in a laboratory using a motorized treadmill or cycle ergometer, and open-circuit spirometry is used to measure pulmonary gas exchange (see chapter 6). However, $\dot{V}O_2$ max has also been measured during both free and tethered swimming, cross-country skiing, bench stepping, ice skating, and during rowing (6, 11, 50, 53, 59, 87).

Historically, the measurement of $\dot{V}O_2$ max has been considered the test of choice for predicting success in endurance events such as distance running (10, 16, 22, 23, 30, 41, 48, 58, 94). For example, relative $\dot{V}O_2$ max (i.e., $\dot{V}O_2$ max expressed in $ml \cdot kg^{-1} \cdot min^{-1}$) has been shown to be the single most important factor in predicting distance running success in a heterogeneous (i.e., different $\dot{V}O_2$ max) group of athletes (14, 15, 23). The logical explanation for this finding is that since distance running is largely an aerobic event (see chapters 4 and 19), those individuals with a high $\dot{V}O_2$ max should have an advantage over individuals with lower aerobic capacities. However, as one would expect, the correlation between $\dot{V}O_2$ max and distance running performance is low in a homogeneous (i.e., similar $\dot{V}O_2$ max) group of runners (13, 70). These observations suggest that although a high $\dot{V}O_2$ max is important in determining distance running success, other variables are important as well. Therefore, measurement of $\dot{V}O_2$ max is only one in a battery of tests that should be used in evaluating physical work capacity in endurance athletes.

Specificity of Testing

As stated previously, running on a treadmill and pedaling a cycle ergometer are the two most common forms of exercise used to determine $\dot{V}O_2$ max. However, much evidence exists to suggest that a test to determine $\dot{V}O_2$ max should involve the specific movement used by the athlete in his or her event (5, 6, 64). For example, if the athlete being tested is a runner, it is important that $\dot{V}O_2$ max be assessed during running. Likewise, if the athlete being evaluated is a trained cyclist, then the exercise test should be performed on the cycle ergometer. Further, specific testing procedures have been established for cross-country skiers and swimmers as well (50, 53, 59).

Exercise Test Protocol

A test to determine $\dot{V}O_2$ max generally begins with a submaximal "warm-up" load that may last three to five minutes. After the warm-up period, the power output can be increased in several ways: (1) the work rate may be increased to a load that in preliminary experiments has been shown to represent a load near the predicted maximal load for the subject, (2) the load may be increased stepwise each minute until the subject reaches a point at which the power output cannot be maintained, or (3) the load may be increased stepwise every two to four minutes until the subject cannot maintain the desired work rate. When any one of these procedures is carefully followed, it yields approximately the same $\dot{V}O_2$ max as the others (1, 45, 69, 95), although an exercise protocol that does not exceed ten to twelve minutes seems preferable (9, 45).

The criteria to determine if $\dot{V}O_2$ max has been obtained were discussed in chapter 15. Because of the importance of this measure, some important issues will be reviewed here. The primary criterion to determine if $\dot{V}O_2$ max has been reached during an incremental exercise test is a plateau in oxygen uptake with a further increase in work rate (86). This concept is illustrated in figure 20.2. Unfortunately, when testing untrained subjects, a plateau in $\dot{V}O_2$ is rarely observed during an incremental exercise test. Does this mean that the subject did not reach his or her $\dot{V}O_2$ max? This possibility exists, but it is also possible that the subject reached his or her $\dot{V}O_2$ max at the last work rate, but could not complete another exercise stage, and

therefore a plateau in $\dot{V}O_2$ was not observed. In light of this possibility, several investigators have suggested that the validity of a $\dot{V}O_2$ max test be determined from not one but several criteria. In chapter 15 it was discussed that a blood lactate concentration of >8 mmoles $\cdot$ liter^{-1} during the last stage of exercise could be used as one of the criteria to determine if $\dot{V}O_2$ max had been obtained. However, to avoid the difficulty of taking blood samples and subsequent analysis for lactate levels, investigators have proposed additional criteria that do not involve blood sampling. For example, Williams et al. (92) and McMiken and Daniels (54) have proposed that a $\dot{V}O_2$ max test be judged as valid if any two of the following criteria are met: (1) a respiratory exchange ratio ≥ 1.15, (2) a heart rate during the last exercise stage that is ± 10 beats per minute within the subject's predicted maximum heart rate, or (3) a plateau in $\dot{V}O_2$ with an increase in work rate.

Determination of Peak $\tilde{V}O_2$ in Paraplegic Athletes

Again, by definition, $\dot{V}O_2$ max is the highest $\dot{V}O_2$ that can be attained during exercise using large muscle groups (1). However, subjects with injuries to or paralysis of their lower limbs can have their aerobic fitness evaluated through arm ergometry, which substitutes arm cranking for cycling or running. Given the aforementioned definition of $\dot{V}O_2$ max, the highest $\dot{V}O_2$ obtained during an incremental arm ergometry test is not referred to as $\dot{V}O_2$ max, but is called the peak $\dot{V}O_2$ for arm exercise.

The protocols used to determine peak $\dot{V}O_2$ during arm ergometry are similar in design to the previously mentioned treadmill and cycle ergometer protocols (76, 78). Recent evidence suggests that in subjects who are not specifically arm trained, a higher peak $\dot{V}O_2$ is obtained during arm ergometry if the test begins at some predetermined load that represents approximately 50% to 60% of peak $\dot{V}O_2$ during arm work (89). A logical explanation for these findings is that an "accelerated" incremental arm testing protocol that rapidly reaches a high power output might limit muscular fatigue early in the test, allowing the subject to reach a higher power output and therefore obtain a higher peak $\dot{V}O_2$.

In an effort to provide a more specific form of testing for paraplegics who are wheelchair racing athletes, some laboratories have modified a wheelchair by connecting the wheels to a cycle ergometer in such a way that the resistance to turn the wheels can be adjusted in the same manner as the load is altered on the cycle ergometer (73). This allows wheelchair athletes to be tested using the exact movement that they use during a race, and it is therefore superior to using arm ergometry to evaluate peak $\dot{V}O_2$ in this population.

FIGURE 20.2 Changes in oxygen uptake during an incremental cycle ergometer test designed to determine $\dot{V}O_2$ max. The observed plateau in $\dot{V}O_2$ with an increase in work rate is considered to be the "gold standard" for validation of $\dot{V}O_2$ max.

Measurement of Peak Running Velocity to Predict Performance in Distance Running

The lactate threshold and critical power measurements have generally been used to predict performance in endurance events lasting longer than twenty minutes (e.g., 10-kilometer run). In an effort to develop a laboratory or field test to predict performance in endurance events less than twenty minutes (e.g., 5-kilometer run), researchers have developed a test called "peak running velocity" (38, 61, 62, 77). The test is easy to administer and can be performed on a treadmill or track. For example, the measurement of peak running velocity on a treadmill involves a short test of progressively increasing the treadmill speed every thirty seconds (0% grade) until volitional fatigue. Peak running velocity (meters · second^{-1}) is defined as the highest speed that can be maintained for more than five seconds duration (77).

How well does peak running velocity predict performance? In a well-designed study, researchers

FIGURE 20.3 Relationship between running peak velocity and finish time of a 5-kilometer (km) race. Data from reference (77).

demonstrated that peak running velocity was an excellent predictor of success in a 5-kilometer run (77). This point is illustrated by the strong correlation between peak running velocity and 5-kilometer race time (see figure 20.3.). Surprisingly, similar findings have been reported for longer running events (e.g., 10–90 kilometer) as well

(42, 62). Although additional research is required to fully investigate the application of this test to athletic performance, peak running velocity appears to be a promising laboratory or field test to predict endurance performance.

IN SUMMARY

- The measurement of $\dot{V}O_2$ max requires the use of large muscle groups and should be specific to the movement required by the athlete in his or her event or sport.
- A $\dot{V}O_2$ max test can be judged to be valid if two of the following criteria are met: (a) respiratory exchange ratio >1:15, (b) HR during the last test stage that is ±10 beats per minute within the predicted HR max, and/or (c) plateau in $\dot{V}O_2$ with an increase in work rate.
- Arm crank ergometry and wheelchair ergometry have been used to determine the peak $\dot{V}O_2$ in paraplegic athletes.

LABORATORY TESTS TO PREDICT ENDURANCE PERFORMANCE

Exercise physiologists, coaches, and athletes have actively searched for a single laboratory test that can predict success in endurance events. Numerous tests

have been developed in an effort to predict athletic performance. In this section, we describe two well-developed laboratory tests—lactate threshold and critical power—that are useful in predicting endurance performance. Also, another laboratory test to predict performance called "peak running velocity" is introduced in Research Focus 20.1. Let's begin with a discussion of the lactate threshold.

Use of the Lactate Threshold to Evaluate Performance

Numerous studies have provided evidence that some measure of the maximal steady-state running speed is useful in predicting success in distance running events from two miles to the marathon (17, 21, 24, 44, 45, 46, 68, 83, 84). The most common laboratory measurement to estimate this maximal steady-state speed is the determination of the lactate threshold. Recall that the lactate threshold represents an exercise intensity wherein blood lactic acid levels begin to systematically increase. Since fatigue is associated with high levels of blood and muscle lactic acid, it is logical that the lactate threshold would be related to endurance performance in events lasting longer than twelve to fifteen minutes (47). Although much of the research examining the role of the lactate threshold in predicting endurance performance has centered around distance running, the same principles apply to predicting performance in endurance cycling, swimming, and cross-country skiing.

Direct Determination of Lactate Threshold Similar to the assessment of $\dot{V}O_2$ max, the determination of the lactate threshold requires athletes to be tested in a manner that simulates their competitive movements (i.e., specificity of testing). Testing protocols to determine the lactate threshold generally begin with a two- to five-minute warm-up at a low work rate followed by a stepwise increase in the power output every one to three minutes (71, 84, 87, 90, 91, 95). In general, the stepwise increases in work rate are small in order to provide better resolution in the determination of the lactate threshold (95).

To determine the blood concentration of lactic acid, blood samples are obtained at each work rate from a catheter (an indwelling tube) placed in an artery or vein in the subject's arm. After the test, these blood samples are chemically analyzed for lactic acid, and the concentration at each exercise stage is then graphed against the oxygen consumption at the time the sample is removed. This idea is illustrated in figure 20.4. How is the lactate threshold determined? Recall that the formal definition of the lactate threshold is the point after which there is a systematic and continuous rise in blood lactate concentration. Although several techniques are available, the simplest and most common procedure is to allow two independent investigators to subjectively pick the lactate "breakpoint" by visual inspection of the lactate/$\dot{V}O_2$ plot (71, 90). If the two investigators disagree as to where the threshold occurs, a third investigator is used to arbitrate.

In practice, the lactate "break point" can often be chosen by using a ruler and drawing a straight line through the lactate concentrations at the first several work rates. The last point on the line is considered the lactate threshold (figure 20.4). The obvious advantage of this technique is its simplicity. The disadvantage is that not all investigators agree that this procedure yields valid and reliable results (71). In light of this concern, several researchers have proposed that complex computer programs be used to more accurately predict the lactate threshold, or that an arbitrary lactate value (e.g., 4 mM) be used as an indication of the lactate threshold (27, 47).

Prediction of the Lactate Threshold by Ventilatory Alterations A technique to estimate the lactate threshold that does not require blood withdrawal has obvious appeal to both investigators and experimental subjects. This need for a noninvasive method to determine the lactate threshold has led to the widespread use of ventilatory and gas exchange measures to estimate the lactate threshold. Recall from chapter 10 that the rationale for the use of the "ventilatory threshold" as a "marker" of the lactate threshold is linked to the belief that the increase in blood lactic acid concentration at the lactate threshold stimulates ventilation via hydrogen ion influence on the carotid bodies. Although there are several noninvasive techniques in use today (2, 12, 79), the least complex procedure to estimate the lactate threshold by gas exchange is to perform an incremental exercise similar to the previously discussed test used to determine the lactate threshold. Upon completion of the test, the minute ventilation at each work rate during the test is graphed as a function of the oxygen uptake. Figure 20.5

FIGURE 20.5 Example of the ventilatory threshold determination. Note the linear rise in ventilation up to an oxygen uptake of 2.0 liters/minute—above which ventilation begins to increase in an alinear fashion. This break in linearity of ventilation is termed the "ventilatory threshold" and can be used as an estimate of the lactate threshold.

FIGURE 20.4 Typical graph of the changes in blood lactic acid concentrations during an incremental exercise test. The sudden rise in blood lactic acid is called the "lactate threshold."

illustrates this procedure. Similar to the determination of the lactate threshold, the usual procedure is to allow two independent researchers to visually inspect the graph and subjectively determine the point where there is a sudden increase in ventilation (figure 20.5). The point at which ventilation increases rapidly is considered the ventilatory threshold and is used as an estimate of the lactate threshold. Although some authors have criticized this technique for a lack of precision (71), it seems clear that this procedure is useful in predicting success in endurance events (25, 70).

Measurement of Critical Power

Measurement of the maximal steady-state power output is useful in predicting success in endurance events lasting 3 to 180 minutes. Another laboratory measurement that can be used to predict performance in endurance events is **critical power.** The concept of critical power is based upon the notion that athletes can maintain a specific submaximal power output without fatigue (31, 38, 42). Figure 20.6 illustrates the critical power concept for running performance. In this illustration, running speed is plotted on the y-axis and the time that the athlete can run at this speed prior to exhaustion is plotted on the x-axis. Critical power is defined as the running speed (i.e., power output) at which the running speed/time curve reaches a plateau. Therefore, in theory, the critical power is considered the power output that can be maintained indefinitely. In practice, however, this is not the case. In fact, most athletes fatigue within thirty to sixty minutes when exercising at their critical power (31).

Critical power can be determined in the laboratory by having subjects perform a series of five to seven timed exercise trials to exhaustion. This is generally accomplished over several days of testing. The results are graphed, and critical power is determined by subjective assessment of the point where the power/time curve begins to plateau or by using a mathematical technique (see references 31, 35, and 42 for details). Although figure 20.5 illustrates the critical power measurement for running, the same principle of measurement can be applied to other endurance sports (e.g., cycling, rowing, etc.) (31, 34).

How well does critical power predict performance? Several studies have shown that critical power is significantly correlated with performance in endurance events lasting 3 to 100 minutes (e.g., r = 0.67 − 0.85) (31, 34, 38, 42). Therefore, critical power is a useful laboratory predictor of success in endurance sports.

Is critical power a better predictor of success in endurance events than other laboratory measures such as the lactate threshold or $\dot{V}O_2$ max? The answer remains controversial, since many investigators report that $\dot{V}O_2$ max is the best single predictor of endurance performance success (14, 15, 23). However, in events lasting approximately thirty minutes, the lactate threshold, $\dot{V}O_2$ max, and critical power appear to be similar in their abilities to predict performance (42). This is not surprising, considering that critical power is dependent upon both $\dot{V}O_2$ max and the lactate threshold. Indeed, critical power is highly correlated to both $\dot{V}O_2$ max and the lactate threshold (42, 57). In other words, a subject with a high $\dot{V}O_2$ max and lactate threshold will also possess a high critical power.

FIGURE 20.6 Concept of critical power. **FIGURE 20.7** An oxygen cost-of-running curve for two subjects. Note the higher $\dot{V}O_2$ cost of running at any given running speed for subject A when compared to subject B. See text for details.

IN SUMMARY

- Common laboratory tests to predict endurance performance include measurement of the lactate threshold, critical power, and peak running velocity. All of these measurements have been proven useful in predicting performance in endurance events.
- The lactate threshold can be determined during an incremental exercise test using any one of several exercise modalities (e.g., treadmill, cycle ergometer, etc.). The lactate threshold represents an exercise intensity at which blood lactic acid levels begin to systematically increase.
- Critical power is defined as the running speed (i.e., power output) at which the running speed/time curve reaches a plateau.
- Peak running velocity (meters · second^{-1}) can be determined on a treadmill or track and is defined as the highest speed that can be maintained for more than five seconds.

TESTS TO DETERMINE EXERCISE ECONOMY

The topic of exercise economy was first introduced in chapter 6. The economy of a particular sport movement (e.g., running or cycling) has a major influence on the energy cost of the sport and consequently interacts with $\dot{V}O_2$ max in determining endurance performance (13, 18, 47, 56). For example, a runner who is uneconomical will expend a greater amount of energy to run at a given speed than will an economical runner. With all other variables being equal, the more economical runner would likely defeat the less economical runner in head-to-head competition. Therefore, the measurement of exercise economy would seem appropriate when performing a battery of laboratory tests to evaluate an athlete's performance potential.

How is exercise economy evaluated? Conceptually, exercise economy is assessed by graphing energy expenditure during a particular activity (e.g., running, cycling, etc.) at several speeds. In general, the energy costs of running, cycling, or swimming can be determined using similar methods. Let's use running as an example to illustrate this procedure. The economy of running is quantified by measuring the steady-state oxygen cost of running on a horizontal treadmill at several speeds. The oxygen requirement of running is then graphed as a function of running speed (7, 32). Figure 20.7 illustrates the change in $\dot{V}O_2$ in two runners at a variety of running speeds. Notice that at any given speed, runner B requires less oxygen and therefore expends less energy than runner A (i.e., runner B is more economical than runner A). A marked difference in running economy between athletes can have an important impact on performance.

FIGURE 20.7 An oxygen cost-of-running curve for two subjects. Note the higher $\dot{V}O_2$ cost of running at any given running speed for subject A when compared to subject B. See text for details.

ESTIMATING SUCCESS IN DISTANCE RUNNING USING THE LACTATE THRESHOLD AND RUNNING ECONOMY

Over the past fifteen to twenty years, many investigators have tried to apply laboratory tests to predict performance in a variety of sports (see reference (66) for examples). The sport that has received the most attention is distance running. Theoretically, the prediction of potential performance in any endurance sport involves the use of similar laboratory measurements ($\dot{V}O_2$ max, economy of movement, etc.). We will use distance running as an example of how a sport scientist or coach might use laboratory measurements to estimate an athlete's performance in a particular event. Let's begin our discussion with a brief overview of the physiological factors that contribute to distance running success. As previously mentioned, the best test for determining an endurance runner's potential is $\dot{V}O_2$ max. However, other factors modify the pace that can be maintained for races of different lengths. For example, anaerobic energy contributes significantly to the ability to maintain a specified pace during shorter distance runs (e.g., 1,500 meters) (10, 47). In longer runs (5,000 to 10,000 meters), running economy and the lactate threshold may play important roles in determining success (21, 70, 84). In order to predict endurance performance, we must determine the athlete's maximal race pace that can be maintained for a particular racing distance.

To illustrate how performance in distance running might be estimated, consider an example of predicting performance in a 10,000-meter race. We begin with an assessment of the athlete's running economy and then perform an incremental treadmill test to determine $\dot{V}O_2$ max and the lactate threshold. The test results for our runner are graphed in figure 20.8. How do we determine the maximal race pace from the laboratory data? Numerous studies have shown that a close relationship exists between the lactate or ventilatory threshold and the maximal pace that can be maintained during a 10,000-meter race (21, 70, 84). For instance, it appears that well-trained runners can run 10,000 meters at a pace that exceeds their lactate threshold by approximately 5 m $\cdot$ min^{-1} (32, 67). With this information and the data from figure 20.8, we can now predict a finish time for an athlete. First, we examine figure 20.8, part b, to determine the $\dot{V}O_2$ at the lactate threshold. The lactate threshold occurred at a $\dot{V}O_2$ of 40 ml $\cdot$ kg^{-1} $\cdot$ min^{-1}, which corresponds to a running speed of 200 m $\cdot$ min^{-1} (part a of figure 20.8). Assuming that the athlete can exceed this speed by 5 m $\cdot$ min^{-1}, the projected average race pace for a 10,000-meter run would be 205 m $\cdot$ min^{-1}. Therefore,

Exercise Physiology Applied to Sports—Can Laboratory Testing of Young Athletes Predict Future Champions?

Numerous articles in popular magazines have proclaimed the ability of laboratory testing in children to predict future athletic champions. For example, it has been argued that determination of skeletal muscle fiber type (via a muscle biopsy) in youth athletes can be used to predict the future athletic success of these individuals. The truth is that there are no laboratory measurements that accurately predict the "ultimate" athletic ability of anyone. Indeed, athletic success depends on numerous physiological and psychological factors, many of which are difficult, if not impossible, to measure in the laboratory. As mentioned earlier, the primary benefits of laboratory testing of athletes are to provide the individual with information about his or her strengths and weaknesses in a sport, to offer feedback about the effectiveness of the conditioning program, and to educate the athlete about the physiology of exercise.

(a)

(b)

FIGURE 20.8 Incremental exercise test results for a hypothetical runner. These test results can be used to predict performance in an endurance race. See text for details.

an estimate of the athlete's finish time could be obtained by dividing 10,000 meters by his predicted running speed (m · min⁻¹):

$$\text{Estimated finish time} = 10,000 \text{ m} \div 205 \text{ m} \cdot \text{min}^{-1}$$
$$= 48.78 \text{ min}$$

Although theoretical predictions of performance such as the example presented here can generally estimate performance with a reasonable degree of precision, a number of outside factors can influence racing performance. For example, motivation and race tactics play an important role in distance running success. Environmental conditions (heat/humidity, altitude, etc.) also influence an athlete's ultimate performance (see chapters 19 and 24). For information on the ability of laboratory testing to predict future champions, see The Winning Edge 20.1.

IN SUMMARY

- Success in an endurance event can be predicted by a laboratory assessment of the athlete's movement economy, $\dot{V}O_2$ max, and lactate threshold. These parameters can be used to determine the maximal race pace that an athlete can maintain for a given racing distance.

DETERMINATION OF ANAEROBIC POWER

For the assessment of anaerobic power, it is essential that the test employed use the muscle groups involved in the sport (i.e., specificity) and involve the energy pathways used in the performance of the event. Although several classification schemes have been proposed (4, 29), tests to assess maximal anaerobic power can be generally classified into (1) ultra short-term tests designed to test the maximal capacity of the "ATP-PC system," and (2) short-term tests to evaluate the maximal capacity for anaerobic glycolysis (sometimes referred to as anaerobic endurance).

FIGURE 20.9 The percent contribution of the ATP-PC system, anaerobic glycolysis, and aerobic metabolism as a function of time during a maximal effort.

Remember that events lasting less than ten seconds are believed to principally use the ATP-PC system to produce ATP, while events lasting thirty to sixty seconds utilize anaerobic glycolysis as the major bioenergetic pathway to synthesize ATP. This principle is illustrated in figure 20.9 and should be remembered when designing tests to evaluate an athlete's anaerobic power for a specific sport.

Tests of Ultra Short-Term Maximal Anaerobic Power

Several practical "field tests" have been developed to assess the maximal capacity of the ATP-PC system to produce ATP over a very short time period (e.g., one to ten seconds) (51). These tests are generally referred to as **power tests.** Recall from chapter 6 that power is defined as:

$$Power = (F \times D) \div T$$

where F is the force generated, D is the distance over which the force is applied, and T is the time required to perform the work.

Jumping Power Tests　For many years, tests such as the standing broad jump and vertical jump have been used as field tests to evaluate an individual's explosive anaerobic power. The standing broad jump is the distance covered in a horizontal leap from a crouched position, whereas the vertical jump is the distance between the standing reach height and the maximum jump-and-touch height. Both tests probably fail to adequately assess an individual's maximal ATP-PC system capacity because of their brief duration. Moreover, neither test is considered a good predictor of running success in a short dash (e.g., 40–100 yards) (72, 80). Nonetheless, the vertical jump test is considered valuable in predicting vertical leaping ability of athletes and is widely used by coaches in professional

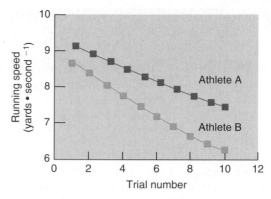

FIGURE 20.10 Illustration of the use of a series of timed 40-yard dashes to determine the anaerobic fitness of football players. In this illustration, athlete A shows a small but constant decline in running speed with each additional dash. In contrast, athlete B shows a large systematic decline in speed across dash trials. Therefore, athlete A is considered to be in better condition than athlete B. See text for details.

football, soccer, and basketball as one on the many performance tests used to evaluate athletic potential.

Running Power Tests for American Football　The 40-yard dash has been a popular test to evaluate power output in football players for many years. The athlete generally performs two to three timed 40-yard dashes with full recovery between efforts. The fastest time recorded is considered an indication of the individual's power output. Although a 40-yard dash is a rather specific test of power output for football players, there is little evidence that a 40-yard run in a straight line is a reliable predictor of an athlete's success at a particular position. Perhaps a shorter run (e.g., 10–20 yards), with several changes in direction, might provide a more specific test of power output in football players (53).

Stuart and colleagues (82) have proposed a fitness test for football players that is designed to evaluate the athlete's ability to perform repeated short bursts of power. The test is conducted in the following way. After a brief warm-up, the athlete performs a series of ten timed 40-yard dashes (maximum effort), with a twenty-five second recovery between dashes. The twenty-five second recovery period is designed to simulate the elapsed time between plays in a football game. The athletes' time for each 40-yard dash is graphed as a function of the trial number. This procedure is illustrated in figure 20.10 where line A represents data from a well-conditioned athlete and line B is data from a less-fit athlete. Notice that both lines A and B have negative slopes (fatigue slope). This demonstrates that each of the two athletes is slowing down with each succeeding 40-yard trial. Athletes who are highly conditioned will be able to

TABLE 20.1	Classification of Fitness Levels for Football Players on the Basis of a Series of 40-Yard Dash Times

Level	Category	Percentage of Maximal Velocity Maintained*
1	Superior	>90%
2	Good	85%–89%
3	Sub-par	80%–84%
4	Poor	<79%

*The "percentage of the maximal velocity maintained" is calculated by averaging the velocity of the last three trials and dividing by the average velocity over the first three trials. This ratio is then expressed as a percentage. See text for further details.

maintain faster 40-yard dash times over the ten trials when compared to less-conditioned athletes, and therefore will have a less-negative fatigue slope. In an effort to establish a set of standards for this test, Stuart and coworkers have proposed that athletes be classified into one of four groups on the basis of the maximal running velocity percentage that can be maintained over the final three 40-yard dash trials (see table 20.1). At present, levels 1 and 2 are considered acceptable levels of fitness for football players of any position, while levels 3 and 4 are labeled as subpar and poor fitness standards, respectively.

Running Tests for Soccer   Soccer (called football outside of North America) remains the most popular sport in many countries around the world. Therefore, it is not surprising that numerous performance tests have been developed for soccer players. Included in these performance tests are both tests of motor skills required for soccer and fitness tests. The design of a fitness test for soccer is complicated by the fact that soccer is a complex game requiring intermittent bursts of maximal running followed by periods of walking and/or running slowly. Therefore, soccer is a sport that utilizes both anaerobic and aerobic bioenergetic pathways to produce the required ATP. One of the most widely used field tests to determine both performance and metabolic responses of soccer athletes is the Loughborough Intermittent Shuttle Test developed at Loughborough University in England (60). This shuttle run test is designed to simulate the activity pattern of soccer players during a 90-minute match and consists of intermittent shuttle running (i.e., running back and forth) between markers placed 20 meters apart. The Loughborough intermittent shuttle test is performed with the subjects completing the following runs:

- 3 × 20 meters at walking pace
- 1 × 20 meters at maximal running speed
- 4-second recovery
- 3 × 20 meters at a running speed corresponding to 55% of individual $\dot{V}O_2$ max
- 3 × 20 meters at a running speed corresponding to 95% of individual $\dot{V}O_2$ max

This block of exercise is repeated continuously for 90 minutes. In practice, the 20-meter distance is marked on the ground (or floor), and walking and running speeds are dictated by audio signals produced from a computer. Sprint times for the maximal 20-meter runs are recorded throughout the test by infrared photoelectric cells and represent one of the measured performance variables. That is, soccer players with the highest fitness levels will be able to maintain a higher percentage of their maximal sprint speed throughout the shuttle test. Further, the total distance covered during the test is also measured as a performance variable. During this shuttle test, it is estimated that 22% of the total exercise time is spent at or above 95% $\dot{V}O_2$ max, whereas the activity level for the remainder of the test is 55% $\dot{V}O_2$ max or below (60). Complete details of the numerous tests used to evaluate soccer performance are beyond the scope of this chapter, and the reader is referred to Svensson and Drust (2005), Impellizzeri et al. (2005), Nicholas et al. (2000), and Chamari et al. (2004) in the Suggested Readings for more details about performance testing of soccer players.

Cycling Power Tests   The **Quebec 10-second test** was developed to assess ultra short-term anaerobic power in cyclists (80). The technical error of this test is small, and the procedure is highly reliable (4). The test is performed on a friction-braked cycle ergometer that contains a photocell capable of measuring flywheel revolutions; the number of flywheel revolutions and resistance against the flywheel are electrically relayed to a microcomputer for analysis. The design of the test is simple. After a brief warm-up, the subject performs two all-out 10-second cycling trials separated by a rest period. The initial resistance on the cycle flywheel is determined by the subject's weight (about 0.09 kg per kg of body weight). Upon a verbal start command by the investigator, the subject begins pedaling at 80 rpm, and the load is rapidly adjusted within two to three seconds to the desired load. The subject then pedals as fast as possible for ten seconds. Strong verbal encouragement is provided throughout the test. After a ten-minute rest period, a second test is performed and the results of the two tests averaged. The test results are reported in peak joules per kg of body weight and total joules per kg of body weight.

In addition to the evaluation of cyclists, the Quebec 10-second test has been used to test ultra short-term anaerobic power in nonathletes, runners, speed skaters, biathletes, and body builders. For complete details of these results see Bouchard et al. (4).

Tests of Short-Term Anaerobic Power

As illustrated in figure 20.9, the ATP-PC system for production of ATP during intense exercise is important for short bursts of exercise (one to ten seconds), whereas glycolysis becomes an important metabolic pathway for energy production in events lasting longer than fifteen seconds. In an effort to evaluate the maximal capacity for anaerobic glycolysis to produce ATP during exercise, several short-term anaerobic power tests have been developed. Like other performance tests, anaerobic power tests should involve the specific muscles used in a particular sport.

Cycling Anaerobic Power Tests   Researchers at the Wingate Institute in Israel have developed a thirty-second, maximal effort cycling test **(Wingate test)** designed to determine both peak anaerobic power and mean power output over the thirty-second test. This test has been shown to be highly reproducible (39) and offers an excellent means of evaluating anaerobic power output in cyclists. The test is administered in the following manner. The subject performs a short, two- to four-minute warm-up on the cycle ergometer at an exercise intensity sufficient to elevate heart rate to 150 to 160 beats $\cdot$ min^{-1}. After a three- to five-minute rest interval, the test begins with the subject pedaling the cycle ergometer as fast as possible without resistance on the flywheel. After the subject reaches full pedaling speed (e.g., two to three seconds), the test administrator quickly increases the flywheel resistance to a predetermined load. This predetermined load is an estimate (based on body weight) of a workload that would exceed the subject's $\dot{V}O_2$ max by 20% to 60% (see table 20.2). The subject continues to pedal as rapidly as possible, and the pedal rate is recorded every five seconds during the test. The highest power output over the first few seconds is considered the peak power output and is indicative of the maximum rate of the ATP-PC system to produce ATP during this type of exercise. The decline in power output during the test is used as an index of anaerobic endurance and presumably represents the maximal capacity to produce ATP via a combination of the ATP-PC system and glycolysis. The decrease in power output is expressed as the percentage of peak power decline. The peak power output obtained during a Wingate test occurs near the beginning of the test, and the lowest power output is recorded during the last five seconds of the test. The

TABLE 20.2	The Resistance Setting for the Wingate Test Is Based on the Subject's Body Weight
Subject's Body Weight (kg)	**Resistance Setting on the Flywheel (kg)**
20–24.9	1.75
25–29.9	2.0
30–34.9	2.5
35–39.9	3.0
40–44.9	3.25
45–49.9	3.5
50–54.9	4.0
55–59.9	4.25
60–64.9	4.75
65–69.9	5.0
70–74.9	5.5
75–79.9	5.75
80–84.9	6.25
>85	6.5

From B. Noble, *Physiology of Exercise and Sport.* Copyright © 1986. The C.V. Mosby Company, St. Louis MO. Reprinted by permission.

difference in these two power outputs (i.e., highest power output minus lowest power output) is then divided by the peak power output and expressed as a percentage. For instance, if the peak power output was 600 watts and the lowest power output during the test was 200 watts, then the decline in power output would be computed as:

$$(600 - 200) \div 600 = .666 \times 100\% = 67\%$$

The 67% decline in power output means that the athlete decreases his or her peak power output by 67% over the thirty-second exercise period.

Since the introduction of the Wingate test in the early 1970s, a number of modifications to the original protocol have been proposed (19, 26, 39, 65, 74). Recently, an Australian team of sport scientists (26) has developed a new test for the measurement of anaerobic power on a cycle ergometer that involves sixty seconds of maximal exercise and uses a variable resistance loading. The test design permits the measurement of both peak anaerobic power (i.e., peak ATP-PC system power) and mean (glycolytic) power output over the sixty-second maximal exercise bout. The test is designed as follows. The subject performs a five-minute warm-up at a low work rate (e.g., 120 watts). After a two-minute recovery, the subject begins pedaling as fast as possible with no load against the cycle flywheel. When peak pedaling speed is obtained (i.e., three seconds), the investigator quickly increases the load on the flywheel to 0.095 kg resistance per kg of body weight. The subject continues to pedal as fast as possible at this load for 30 seconds; at the 30-second point, the load on the flywheel is reduced to 0.075 kg resistance per kg of body weight for the remainder of the test. The subject's power output during the test is continuously monitored electronically and work output is recorded as peak power output (joules per kg) and mean power output (joules per kg) during the entire test.

The rationale for the variable load is that while a high resistance is required to elicit maximal anaerobic power, such a resistance is too great for a supramaximal test of sixty seconds' duration (26). By reducing the resistance midway through the test, the workload becomes more manageable, which enables the subject to complete a maximal effort test for the entire sixty-second period. The advantage of this test over the Wingate test is that the variable resistance design permits the measurement of peak anaerobic power and maximal anaerobic power over sixty seconds' duration. This type of test would be useful for athletes who compete in events lasting between forty-five and sixty seconds. Note that while this test maximally taxes both the ATP-PC system and glycolysis, because of the test duration, the aerobic system is also activated (see chapters 3 and 4). Therefore, while the energy required to perform sixty seconds of maximal exercise comes primarily (e.g., 70%) from anaerobic pathways, the aerobic energy contribution may reach 30%.

Running Anaerobic Power Tests   Maximal distance runs from 200 to 800 meters have been used to evaluate anaerobic power output in runners (75, 85). Because such factors as running technique and motivation influence the performance of these types of power tests, the development of appropriate norms has been difficult. Nevertheless, this type of test can be used effectively to determine improvement within individuals as a result of a training regimen.

Sport-Specific Tests   Ultra short-term and short-term sport-specific anaerobic tests can be developed to meet the needs of team sports or individual athletic events. The tests could attempt to measure the peak power output in a few seconds or measure mean power output during a period of ten to sixty seconds, depending upon the energy demands of the sport.

Tests could be developed for tennis, basketball, ice skating, swimming, and so on. In some cases, time or distance covered would be the dependent variable measured rather than a direct measurement of power output (4). This type of sport-specific test provides the coach and athlete with direct feedback about the athlete's present level of fitness; subsequent periodic

IN SUMMARY

- Anaerobic power tests are classified as:
  (a) ultra short-term tests to determine the maximal capacity of the ATP-PC system and (b) short-term tests to evaluate the maximal capacity for anaerobic glycolysis.
- Ultra short-term and short-term power tests should be sport-specific in an effort to provide the athlete and coach with feedback about the athlete's current fitness level.

testing can be used to evaluate the success of training programs.

EVALUATION OF MUSCULAR STRENGTH

Muscular strength is defined as the maximum force that can be generated by a muscle or muscle group (1). The measurement of muscular strength is a common practice in the evaluation of training programs for football players, shot putters, weight lifters, and other power athletes. Strength testing can be used to monitor training progress or the rehabilitation of injuries (52). Muscular strength can be assessed by using one of four methods: (1) isometric testing, (2) free-weight testing, (3) isokinetic testing, and (4) variable resistance testing. Before we discuss these methods of strength measurement, let's consider some general guidelines for the selection of a strength-testing method.

Criteria for Selection of a Strength-Testing Method

The criteria for selecting a method of strength testing include the following factors (72): specificity, ease of data acquisition and analysis, cost, and safety. Given the importance of proper strength-test selection, a brief discussion of each of these factors is warranted.

Specificity of strength testing considers the muscles involved in the sport movement, the movement pattern and contraction type, and the velocity of the contraction. For example, the measurement of sport-specific strength should use the muscle groups involved in the activity. Further, the testing mode should simulate the type of contraction used in the sport (isometric vs. dynamic). If the contraction used in the sport is dynamic, further consideration should be given to whether the contraction is concentric or eccentric. A final level of specificity is the velocity of shortening. There is a degree of velocity specificity in strength training; speed and power athletes perform better on high-velocity power tests than on low (88). Therefore, there is a justification for trying to make the velocity of test contractions similar to those used in the sport.

Factors such as convenience and time required for strength measurements are important considerations when measurements are made on a large number of athletes (43). Currently, a number of companies market strength measurement devices that are interfaced with computer analysis packages. These devices greatly reduce the time required for strength measurement and analysis.

Much of the commercially available computerized equipment for strength measurement is expensive. The high cost of this equipment may prevent its purchase by physical therapy, exercise science, or athletic programs with small budgets. In these cases, the physical therapist, exercise scientist, or coach must choose the best available option within his/her budget.

A final concern for the selection of a strength-testing method is the safety of the technique. Safety should be a key concern for any measurement of strength. Clearly, strength measurement techniques that put the athlete at high risk of injury should be avoided.

Isometric Measurement of Strength

Measurement of isometric strength requires a device that permits testing of the sport-specific muscle groups. These devices are commerically available from numerous sources. Most of the isometric testing devices available today are computerized instruments that are capable of measuring isometric force in a variety of muscle groups. Figure 20.11 illustrates one of these devices being used to measure leg strength during a knee extension. As the subject generates maximal isometric force, the computerized tensiometer (tension-measuring device) measures the force produced, and this information is recorded and displayed on an electronic panel on the instrument.

The measurement of isometric strength is typically performed at several joint angles. Isometric testing at each joint angle usually consists of two or more trials of maximal contractions (contraction duration of approximately 5 seconds), and the best of these trials is considered to be the measure of strength.

Advantages of isometric testing using computerized equipment include the fact that these tests are generally simple and safe to administer. For example, computerized measurement of isometric strength has been used in physical therapy to evaluate training progress in injured limbs. It has been argued that since the isometric tensiometer can be used to measure static strength at many different joint angles with a low

FIGURE 20.11 Use of a commercially available tensiometer to measure static force during a knee extension. Photo courtesy of Biodex Medical Systems, Inc.

risk of injury, this technique might be more effective in evaluating strength gains during therapeutic training than conventional weight-lifting tests (53). Disadvantages of isometric testing include the high cost of some commercial devices and the fact that many sport activities involve dynamic movements. Further, because strength differs over the full range of joint movement, isometric measurements must be made at numerous joint angles; this increases the amount of time required to perform a test.

Free-Weight Testing of Strength

The term *isotonic* means constant tension. This term is often applied to conventional weight-lifting exercise because the weight of the barbell or dumbbell remains constant as the weight is lifted over the range of movement. In a strict sense, application of the term *isotonic* to weight lifting can be criticized because the actual force or torque applied to the weight does not remain constant over the full range of movement. Acceleration and deceleration of the limbs during a weight-lifting movement often cause variation in the force applied. Nonetheless, because of the widespread usage in the literature, we will apply the term *isotonic* to conventional weight-lifting exercises. The most common measure of isotonic strength is the one-repetition maximum, but tests involving three to six repetitions have been employed.

The one-repetition maximum (1-RM) method of evaluating muscular strength involves the performance of a single, maximal lift. This refers to the maximal amount of weight that can be lifted during one complete dynamic repetition of a particular movement (e.g., bench press). To test the 1-RM for any given muscle group, the subject selects a beginning weight that is close to the anticipated 1-RM weight. If one repetition is completed, the weight is increased by a small increment and the trial repeated. This process is continued until the maximum lifting capacity is obtained. The highest weight moved during one repetition is considered the 1-RM. The 1-RM test can be performed using free weights (barbells) or an adjustable resistance exercise machine. For more details of the 1-RM test, see Powers et al. (2006) in the Suggested Readings list.

Because of safety concerns, some physical therapists and exercise scientists have recommended that an isotonic test consisting of three or six repetitions be substituted for the 1-RM test. The rationale is that the incidence of injury may be less with a weight that can be lifted a maximum of three or six times compared to the heavier weight that can be lifted during a 1-RM contraction.

In addition to the use of free weights or machines, maximal isotonic strength can be measured using dynamometers. A **dynamometer** is a device capable of measuring force. Hand-grip dynamometers have been used to evaluate grip strength for many years. Dy0 namometers operate in the following way. When force is applied to the dynamometer, a steel spring is compressed and moves a pointer along a scale. By calibrating the dynamometer with known weights, one can determine how much force is required to move the pointer a specified distance on the scale. Figure 20.12 illustrates the use of a hand-grip dynamometer to assess grip strength.

The advantages of isotonic strength testing include low cost of equipment and the fact that force is dynamically applied, which may simulate sport-specific movements. The disadvantages of free-weight testing using a 1-RM technique include the possibility of subject injury and the fact that it does not provide information concerning the force application over the full range of motion. This point will be discussed again in the next section.

Isokinetic Assessment of Strength

Over the past several years, many commercial computer-assisted devices to assess dynamic muscular force have been developed. The most common type of computerized strength measurement device on the market is an isokinetic dynamometer, which provides variable resistance. The term **isokinetic** means moving at a constant rate of speed. A variable-resistance isokinetic dynamometer is an electronic-mechanical instrument that maintains a constant speed of move-

FIGURE 20.12 Use of the typical hand-grip dynamometer. Photo courtesy of Lafayette Instrument Company.

ment while varying the resistance during a particular movement. The resistance offered by the instrument is an accommodating resistance, which is designed to match the force generated by the muscle. A force transducer inside the instrument constantly monitors the muscular force generated at a constant speed and relays this information to a computer, which calculates the average force generated over each time period and joint angle during the movement. An example of this type of instrument is pictured in figure 20.13.

A typical computer printout of data obtained during a maximum-effort leg extension on a computerized isokinetic dynamometer is illustrated in figure 20.14. This type of strength assessment provides a great deal more information than that supplied by a 1-RM test. The force curve pictured in figure 20.14 illustrates that the subject generates the smallest amount of force early in the movement pattern and the greatest amount of force during the middle portion of the movement. The 1-RM test provides only the final outcome, which is the maximum amount of weight lifted during this particular movement. That is, a 1-RM test does not provide information about the differences in

FIGURE 20.13 Use of a commercially available computer-assisted isokinetic dynamometer to measure strength during a knee extension. Photo courtesy of Biodex Medical Systems, Inc.

FIGURE 20.14 Example of a computer printout from a computer-assisted isokinetic dynamometer during a maximal-effort knee extension.

force generation over the full range of movement. Therefore, a computer-assisted isokinetic instrument appears to offer advantages over the more traditional 1-RM test. Further, isokinetic strength testing has been shown to be highly reliable (55).

Variable-Resistance Measurement of Strength

Several commercial companies market weight machines that vary the resistance (weight) during dynamic muscular contractions. The measurement of strength using a variable-resistance device is similar in principle to isotonic tests using 1-RM or three to six repetitions, with the exception that the variable-resistance machine creates a variable resistance over the range of movement. This variable resistance is typically achieved via a "cam," which in theory is designed to vary the resistance according to physiological and

mechanical factors that determine force generation by muscles over the normal range of movement.

Potential advantages of these devices include the fact that most sport movement patterns are performed using variable forces, and the design of these machines makes adjustment of weight easy, and therefore little time is required for measurement. A disadvantage of these machines is the high cost; this is compounded by the fact that several individual machines are often required to measure strength in different muscle groups.

IN SUMMARY

- Muscular strength is defined as the maximum force that can be generated by a muscle or muscle group.
- Evaluation of muscular strength is useful in assessing training programs for athletes involved in power sports or events.
- Muscular strength can be evaluated using any one of the following techniques: (a) isometric, (b) free-weight testing, (c) isokinetic, or (d) variable-resistance devices.

STUDY QUESTIONS

1. Discuss the rationale behind laboratory tests designed to assess physical performance in athletes. How do these tests differ from general physical fitness tests?
2. Define maximal oxygen uptake. Why might relative $\dot{V}O_2$ max be the single most important factor in predicting distance running success in a heterogeneous group of runners?
3. Discuss the concept of "specificity of testing" for the determination of $\dot{V}O_2$ max. Give a brief overview of the design of an incremental test to determine $\dot{V}O_2$ max. What criteria can be used to determine the validity of a $\dot{V}O_2$ max test?

4. Briefly, explain the technique employed to determine the lactate threshold and the ventilatory threshold.
5. Describe how the economy of running might be evaluated in the laboratory.
6. Discuss the theory and procedures involved in predicting success in distance running.
7. Explain how short-term maximal anaerobic power can be evaluated by field tests.
8. Describe how the Wingate test is used to assess medium-term anaerobic power.
9. Provide an overview of the 1-RM technique to evaluate muscular strength. Why might a computer-assisted

10. Discuss the advantages and disadvantages of each of the following types of strength measurement: (1) isometric, (2) free weights, (3) isokinetic, and (4) variable resistance.

SUGGESTED READINGS

Baechle, T., and R. Earle eds. 2000. *Essentials of Strength Training and Conditioning*. Champaign, IL: Human Kinetics.

Brooks, G., T. Fahey, and K. Baldwin. 2005. *Exercise Physiology: Human Bioenergetics and Its Applications*, 4th ed. New York: McGraw-Hill Companies.

Chamari et al. 2004. Field and laboratory testing in young elite soccer players. *British Journal of Sports Medicine* 38: 191–96.

Hopkins, W. et al. 2001. Reliability of power in physical performance tests. *Sports Medicine* 31:211–34.

Huggett D., D. Connelly, and T. Overend. 2005. Maximal aerobic capacity testing of older adults: A critical review. *Journal of Gerontology* 60A:57–66.

Impellizzeri, F., E. Rampinini, and S. Marcora. 2005. Physiological assessment of aerobic training in soccer. *Journal of Sports Sciences* 23:583–93.

MacDougall, J., H. Wenger, and H. Green. 1991. *Physiological Testing of the High Performance Athlete*. Champaign, IL: Human Kinetics.

Nicholas, C., F. Nuttall, and C. Williams. 2000. The Loughborough Intermittent Shuttle Test: A field test that simulates the activity pattern of soccer. *Journal of Sports Sciences* 18:97–104.

Powers, S., S. Dodd, and V. Nolan. 2006. *Total Fitness and Wellness*. San Francisco: Benjamin Cummings.

Svensson, M., and B. Drust. 2005. Testing soccer players. 23:601–18.

REFERENCES

1. Åstrand, P. O., and K. Rodahl. 1986. *Textbook of Work Physiology*. New York: McGraw-Hill Companies.
2. Beaver, W., K. Wasserman, and B. Whipp. 1986. A new method for detecting anaerobic threshold by gas exchange. *Journal of Applied Physiology* 60:2020–27.
3. Bishop, D., D. Jenkins, and A. Howard. 1998. The critical power function is dependent on the duration of the predictive exercise test chosen. *International Journal of Sports Medicine* 19:125–29.
4. Bouchard, C. et al. 1991. Testing anaerobic power and capacity. In *Physiological Testing of the High Performance Athlete*, ed. J. MacDougall, H. Wenger, and H. Green, 175–222. Champaign, IL: Human Kinetics.
5. Bouckaert, J., and J. Pannier. 1984. Specificity of $\dot{V}O_2$ max and blood lactate determinations in runners and cyclists. *International Archives of Physiology and Biochemistry* 93:30–31.
6. Bouckaert, J., J. Pannier, and J. Vrijens. 1983. Cardiorespiratory response to bicycle and rowing ergometer exercise in oarsmen. *European Journal of Applied Physiology* 51:51–59.
7. Bransford, D., and E. Howley. 1977. Oxygen cost of running in trained and untrained men and women. *Medicine and Science in Sports and Exercise* 9:41–44.
8. Brooks, G., T. Fahey, and K. Baldwin. 2005. *Exercise Physiology: Human Bioenergetics and Its Applications*, 4th ed. New York: McGraw-Hill Companies.
9. Buchfuhrer, M. et al. 1983. Optimizing the exercise protocol for cardiopulmonary assessment. *Journal of Applied Physiology* 55:1558–64.
10. Bulbulian, R., A. Wilcox, and B. Darabos. 1986. Anaerobic contribution to distance running performance of trained cross-country athletes. *Medicine and Science in Sports and Exercise* 18:107–13.
11. Burke, E. 1976. Validity of selected laboratory and field tests of physical working capacity. *Research Quarterly* 47:95–104.
12. Caiozzo, V. et al. 1982. A comparison of gas exchange indices used to detect the anaerobic threshold. *Journal of Applied Physiology* 53:1184–89.
13. Conley, D., and G. Krahenbuhl. 1980. Running economy and distance running performance of highly trained athletes. *Medicine and Science in Sports and Exercise* 12: 357–60.
14. Costill, D. 1967. The relationship between selected physiological variables and distance running performance. *Journal of Sports Medicine and Physical Fitness* 7:61–66.
15. Costill, D. 1970. Metabolic responses to distance running. *Journal of Applied Physiology* 28:251–55.
16. Costill, D. 1979. *A Scientific Approach to Distance Running*. Los Altos: Track and Field News Press.
17. Costill, D., H. Thompson, and E. Roberts. 1973. Fractional utilization of the aerobic capacity during distance running. *Medicine and Science in Sports* 5:248–52.
18. Daniels, J., and N. Daniels. 1992. Running economy of elite male and elite female distance runners. *Medicine and Science in Sports and Exercise* 24:483–89.
19. Dotan R., and O. Bar-Or. 1983. Load optimization for the Wingate anaerobic test. *European Journal of Applied Physiology* 51:409–17.
20. Ebbeling, C. et al. 1991. Development of a single-stage submaximal treadmill walking test. *Medicine and Science in Sports and Exercise* 23:966–73.
21. Farrell, P. et al. 1979. Plasma lactate accumulation and distance running performance. *Medicine and Science in Sports* 11:338–44.
22. Foster, C. 1983. $\dot{V}O_2$ max and training indices as determinants of competitive running performance. *Journal of Sports Sciences* 1:13–27.
23. Foster, C., J. Daniels, and R. Yarbough. 1977. Physiological correlates of marathon running and performance. *Australian Journal of Sports Medicine* 9:58–61.
24. Foster, C. et al. 1995. Blood lactate and respiratory measurement of the capacity for sustained exercise. In *Physiological Assessment of Human Fitness*, ed. P. Maud and C. Foster, 57–72. Champaign, IL: Human Kinetics.
25. Gaskill, S. E. et al. 2001. Validity and reliability of combining three methods to determine ventilatory threshold. *Medicine and Science in Sports and Exercise* 33:1841–48.
26. Gastin, P. et al. 1991. Variable resistance loadings in anaerobic power testing. *International Journal of Sports Medicine* 12:513–18.
27. Grant, S. et al. 2002. Reproducibility of the blood lactate threshold, 4 mmol $\cdot$ l^{-1} marker, heart rate and ratings of

perceived exertion during incremental treadmill exercise in humans. *European Journal of Applied Physiology* 87: 159–66.

28. Green, H. 1991. What do tests measure? In *Physiological Testing of the High Performance Athlete*, ed. J. MacDougall, H. Wenger, and H. Green. Champaign, IL: Human Kinetics.

29. Green, S. 1995. Measurement of anaerobic work capacities in humans. *Sports Medicine* 19:32–42.

30. Hagan, R., M. Smith, and L. Gettman. 1981. Marathon performance in relation to maximal aerobic power and training indices. *Medicine and Science in Sports and Exercise* 13:185–89.

31. Hill, D. 1993. The critical power concept. A review. *Sports Medicine* 16:237–54.

32. Hopkins, P., and S. Powers. 1982. Oxygen uptake during submaximal running in highly trained men and women. *American Corrective Therapy Journal* 36:130–32.

33. Hopkins, W., J. Hawley, and L. Burke. 1999. Design and analysis of research on sport performance enhancement. *Medicine and Science in Sports and Exercise* 31:472–85.

34. Housh, D. 1989. The accuracy of the critical power test for predicting time to exhaustion during cycle ergometry. *Ergonomics* 32:997–1004.

35. Housh, T. J. et al. 2001. The effect of mathematical modeling on critical velocity. *European Journal of Applied Physiology* 84:469–75.

36. Hoogeveen, A., G. Schep, and J. Hoogsteen. 1999. The ventilatory threshold, heart rate, and endurance cycle performance: Relationship in elite cyclists. *International Journal of Sports Medicine.* 20:114–17.

37. Hopkins, W. G., E. J. Schabort, and J. A. Hawley. 2001. Reliability of power in physical performance tests. *Sports Medicine* 31:211–34.

38. Hughson, R., C. Orok, and L. Staudt. 1984. A high-velocity treadmill running test to assess endurance running potential. *International Journal of Sports Medicine* 5:23–25.

39. Jacobs, I. 1980. The effects of thermal dehydration on performance of the Wingate anaerobic test. *International Journal of Sports Medicine* 1:21–24.

40. Katch, V. et al. 1977. Optimal test characteristics for maximal anaerobic work on the cycle ergometer. *Research Quarterly* 48:319–27.

41. Kenney, W., and J. Hodgson. 1985. Variables predictive of performance in elite middle-distance runners. *British Journal of Sports Medicine* 19:207–9.

42. Kolbe, T. et al. 1995. The relationship between critical power and running performance. *Journal of Sports Sciences* 13:265–69.

43. Kraemer, W., and A. Fry. 1995. In *Physiological Assessment of Human Fitness*, ed. P. Maud and C. Foster, 115–38. Champaign, IL: Human Kinetics.

44. LaFontaine, T., B. Londeree, and W. Spath. 1981. The maximal steady state versus selected running events. *Medicine and Science in Sports and Exercise* 13:190–92.

45. Lawler, J., S. Powers, and S. Dodd. 1987. A timesaving incremental cycle ergometer protocol to determine peak oxygen consumption. *British Journal of Sports Medicine* 21:171–73.

46. Lehmann, M. et al. 1983. Correlations between laboratory testing and distance running performance in marathoners of similar ability. *International Journal of Sports Medicine* 4:226–30.

47. Londeree, B. 1986. The use of laboratory test results with long distance runners. *Sports Medicine* 3:201–13.

48. MacDougall, J., and H. Wenger. 1991. The purpose of physiological testing. In *Physiological Testing of the High Performance Athlete*, ed. J. MacDougall, H. Wenger, and H. Green. Champaign, IL: Human Kinetics.

49. Maeder, M. et al. 2005. Impact of the exercise mode on exercise capacity: Bicycle testing revisited. *Chest* 128: 2804–11.

50. Magel, J., and J. Faulker. 1967. Maximum oxygen uptake of college swimmers. *Journal of Applied Physiology* 22:929.

51. Margaria, R. 1966. Measurement of muscular power in man. *Journal of Applied Physiology* 21:1662.

52. Mayhew, T., and J. Rothstein. 1985. Measurement of muscle performance with instruments. In *Measurement of Muscle Performance with Instruments*, ed. J. Rothstein, 57–102. New York: Churchill Livingstone.

53. McArdle, W., F. Katch, and V. Katch. 2001. *Exercise Physiology: Energy, Nutrition, and Human Performance.* Baltimore: Lippincott Williams & Wilkins.

54. McMiken, D., and J. Daniels. 1976. Aerobic requirements of maximal aerobic power in treadmill and track running. *Medicine and Science in Sports and Exercise* 8:14–17.

55. Meeteren, J., M. E. Roebroeck, and H. J. Stam. 2002. Test and retest reliability in isokinetic muscle strength measurements of the shoulder. *Journal of Rehabilitative Medicine* 34:91–95.

56. Morgan, D., and M. Craib. 1992. Physiological aspects of running economy. *Medicine and Science in Sports and Exercise* 24:456–61.

57. Moritani, T. et al. 1981. Critical power as a measure of physical work capacity and anaerobic threshold. *Ergonomics* 24:339–50.

58. Murase, Y. et al. 1981. Longitudinal study of aerobic power in superior junior athletes. *Medicine and Science in Sports and Exercise* 13:180–84.

59. Mygind, E. et al. 1991. Evaluation of a specific test in cross-country skiing. *Journal of Sports Sciences* 9:249–57.

60. Nicholas, C., F. Nuttall, and C. Williams. 2000. The Loughborough Intermittent Shuttle Test: A field test that simulates the activity pattern of soccer. *Journal of Sports Sciences* 18:97–104.

61. Noakes, T. 1988. Implications of exercise testing for prediction of athletic performance: A contemporary perspective. *Medicine and Science in Sports and Exercise* 20: 319–30.

62. Noakes, T. et al. 1990. Peak treadmill running velocity during the max test predicts running performance. *Journal of Sports Sciences* 8:35–45.

63. Noble, B. 1986. *Physiology of Exercise and Sport.* St. Louis: C. V. Mosby.

64. Pannier, J., J. Vrijens, and C. Van Cauter. 1980. Cardiorespiratory response to treadmill and bicycle exercise in runners. *European Journal of Applied Physiology* 43: 243–51.

65. Parry-Billings, M. et al. 1986. The measurement of anaerobic power and capacity: Studies on the Wingate anaerobic test. *Snipes* J9:48–58.

66. Peronnet, F., and G. Thibault. 1989. Mathematical analysis of running performance and world running records. *Journal of Applied Physiology* 67:453–65.

67. Pollock, M. 1977. Submaximal and maximal working capacity of elite distance runners: Cardiorespiratory aspects. *Annals of the New York Academy of Sciences* 301: 310–22.

68. Pollock, M., A. Jackson, and R. Pate. 1980. Discriminant analysis of physiological differences between good and elite runners. *Research Quarterly* 51:521–32.

69. Pollock, M. et al. 1976. A comparative analysis of four protocols for maximal treadmill stress testing. *American Heart Journal* 92:39–46.

70. Powers, S. et al. 1983. Ventilatory threshold, running economy, and distance running performance of trained athletes. *Research Quarterly for Exercise and Sport* 54:179–82.

71. Powers, S., S. Dodd, and R. Garner. 1984. Precision of ventilatory and gas exchange alterations as a predictor of the anaerobic threshold. *European Journal of Applied Physiology* 52:173–77.

72. Sale, D. 1991. Testing strength and power. In *Physiological Testing of the High Performance Athlete*, ed. J. MacDougall, H. Wenger, and H. Green, 21–106. Champaign, IL: Human Kinetics.

73. Sawka, M. et al. 1983. Determination of maximal aerobic power during upper body exercise. *Journal of Applied Physiology* 54:113–17.

74. Schenau, G. et al. 1991. Can cycle power output predict sprint running performance? *European Journal of Applied Physiology* 63:255–60.

75. Schnabel, A., and W. Kinderman. 1983. Assessment of anaerobic capacity in runners. *European Journal of Applied Physiology* 52:42–46.

76. Schwade, J., G. Blomquist, and W. Shapiro. 1977. A comparison of the response to arm and leg work in patients with ischemic heart disease. *American Heart Journal* 94:203–8.

77. Scott, B., and J. Houmard. 1994. Peak running velocity is highly related to distance running performance. *International Journal of Sports Medicine* 15:504–7.

78. Shaw, D. et al. 1974. Arm crank ergometer: A new method for the evaluation of coronary heart disease. *American Journal of Cardiology* 33:801–5.

79. Sherrill, D. et al. 1990. Using smoothing splines for detecting ventilatory thresholds. *Medicine and Science in Sports and Exercise* 22:684–89.

80. Simoneau, J. et al. 1983. Tests of anaerobic alactacid and lactacid capacities. *Canadian Journal of Applied Sports Sciences* 8:266–70.

81. Storer, T. et al. 1990. Accurate prediction of $\dot{V}O_2$ max in cycle ergometry. *Medicine and Science in Sports and Exercise* 22:704–12.

82. Stuart, M. K., S. Powers, and J. Nelson. Development of an anaerobic fitness test for football players. Unpublished observations.

83. Tanaka, K., and Y. Matsuura. 1984. Marathon performance, anaerobic threshold, and onset of blood lactate accumulation. *Journal of Applied Physiology* 57:640–43.

84. Tanaka, K. et al. 1983. Relationships of anaerobic threshold and onset of blood lactate accumulation with endurance performance. *European Journal of Applied Physiology* 52:51–56.

85. Taunton, J., H. Maron, and J. Wilkinson. 1981. Anaerobic performance in middle and long distance runners. *Canadian Journal of Applied Sports Sciences* 6:109–13.

86. Taylor, H., E. Buskirk, and A. Henschel. 1955. Maximal oxygen uptake as an objective measure of cardiorespiratory performance. *Journal of Applied Physiology* 8:73–80.

87. Thoden, J. 1991. Testing aerobic power. In *Physiological Testing of the High Performance Athlete*, ed. J. MacDougall, H. Wenger, and H. Green, 107–74. Champaign, IL: Human Kinetics.

88. Thorland, W. 1987. Strength and anaerobic response of elite young female sprint and distance runners. *Medicine and Science in Sports and Exercise* 19:56–61.

89. Walker, R., S. Powers, and M. Stuart. 1986. Peak oxygen uptake in arm ergometry: Effects of testing protocol. *British Journal of Sports Medicine* 20:25–26.

90. Wasserman, K. et al. 1973. Anaerobic threshold and respiratory gas exchange during exercise. *Journal of Applied Physiology* 35:236–43.

91. Weltman, A. et al. 1990. Reliability and validity of a continuous incremental treadmill protocol for the determination of lactate threshold, fixed blood lactate concentrations, and $\dot{V}O_2$ max. *International Journal of Sports Medicine* 11:26–32.

92. Williams, J., S. Powers, and S. Stuart. 1986. Hemoglobin desaturation in highly trained athletes during heavy exercise. *Medicine and Science in Sports and Exercise* 18:168–73.

93. Williams, L. 1978. Prediction of high-level rowing ability. *Journal of Sports Medicine and Physical Fitness* 18:11–15.

94. Wyndham, C. et al. 1969. Physiological requirements for world-class performances in distance running. *South African Medical Journal* 43:996–1002.

95. Zhang, Y. et al. 1991. Effect of exercise testing protocol on parameters of aerobic function. *Medicine and Science in Sports and Exercise* 23:625–30.

CHAPTER 21

Training for Performance

■ Objectives

By studying this chapter, you should be able to do the following:

1. Discuss the concept of designing a sport-specific training program based on an analysis of the energy systems utilized by the activity.

2. List and discuss the general principles of physical conditioning for improved sport performance.

3. Define the terms overload, specificity, and reversibility.

4. Outline the use of interval training and continuous training in the improvement of the maximal aerobic power in athletes.

5. Discuss the guidelines associated with planning a training program designed to improve the anaerobic power of athletes.

6. Outline the principles of training for the improvement of strength.

7. Discuss the role of gender differences in the development of strength.

8. List the factors that contribute to delayed-onset muscle soreness.

9. Discuss the use of static and ballistic stretching to improve flexibility.

10. Outline the goals of: (1) off-season conditioning, (2) preseason conditioning, and (3) in-season conditioning.

11. List and discuss several common training errors.

■ Outline

Training Principles   442
   Overload, Specificity, and Reversibility   442
   Influence of Gender, Initial Fitness Level, and Genetics   443

Components of a Training Session: Warm-Up, Workout, and Cool Down   444

Training to Improve Aerobic Power   444
   Interval Training   445
   Long, Slow-Distance Exercise   446
   High-Intensity, Continuous Exercise   446

Injuries and Endurance Training   447

Training for Improved Anaerobic Power   447
   Training to Improve the ATP-PC System   448
   Training to Improve the Glycolytic System   448

Training to Improve Muscular Strength   448
   Progressive Resistance Exercise   450
   General Strength-Training Principles   450
   Free Weights versus Machines   451

Combined Strength- and Endurance-Training Programs   451
Gender Differences in Response to Strength Training   451
Muscle Soreness   453

Training for Improved Flexibility   456

Year-Round Conditioning for Athletes   457
   Off-Season Conditioning   457
   Preseason Conditioning   457
   In-Season Conditioning   457

Common Training Mistakes   458

delayed-onset muscle soreness (DOMS)
dynamic stretching
hyperplasia
hypertrophy

progressive resistance exercise (PRE)
proprioceptive neuromuscular facilitation (PNF)
repetition
rest interval

set
static stretching
tapering
variable-resistance exercise
work interval

Traditionally, coaches and trainers have planned conditioning programs for their teams by following regimens used by teams that have successful win-loss records. This type of reasoning is not sound, since win-loss records alone do not scientifically validate the conditioning programs used by the successful teams. In fact, the successful team might be victorious by virtue of its superior athletes and not its outstanding conditioning program. Without question, the planning of an effective athletic conditioning program can best be achieved by the application of proven physiological training principles. Optimizing training programs for athletes is important, since failure to properly condition an athletic team results in a poor performance and often defeat. It is the purpose of this chapter to present an overview of how to apply scientific principles to the development of an athletic conditioning program.

TRAINING PRINCIPLES

The overall objective of a sport conditioning program is to improve performance by increasing the energy output during a particular movement (7, 78, 102). Recall that throughout this book (e.g., chapters 3, 4, and 20), emphasis has been placed on the fact that dissimilar sport activities use different metabolic pathways or "energy systems" to produce the ATP needed for movement. An understanding of exercise metabolism is important to the coach or trainer, since the design of a conditioning program to optimize athletic performance requires knowledge of the principal energy systems utilized by the sport. Consider a few examples. The performance of a 60-meter dash uses the ATP-PC system almost exclusively to produce the needed ATP. In contrast, a marathon runner depends on aerobic metabolism to provide the energy needed to complete the race. However, most sport activities use multiple energy pathways. For instance, soccer uses a combination of metabolic pathways to provide the needed ATP. Knowledge of the relative anaerobic-aerobic contributions to ATP production during an activity is the cornerstone of planning a conditioning program. A well-designed conditioning program allocates the appropriate amount of aerobic and anaerobic conditioning time to match the energy demand of

the sport. For instance, if an activity derives 40% of its ATP from anaerobic pathways and 60% from aerobic pathways (e.g., 1,500-meter run), the training program should be divided 40%/60% between anaerobic/ aerobic training (7, 78). Table 21.1 contains a list of various sports and an estimation of their predominant energy systems. The coach or trainer can use this information to allocate the appropriate amount of time to training each energy system.

This discussion does not necessarily imply that power athletes (e.g., sprinters) should not perform aerobic training. On the contrary, aerobic activity during the preseason to strengthen tendons and ligaments is generally recommended for all athletes. For a review of the effects of exercise training on the strength of tendons and ligaments, see reference 108.

Overload, Specificity, and Reversibility

The terms *overload*, *specificity*, and *reversibility* were introduced in chapters 13 and 15, and will be repeated here only briefly. Recall that an organ system (e.g., cardiovascular, skeletal muscle, etc.) increases its capacity in response to a training overload. That is, the training program must stress the system above the level to which it is accustomed. Conversely, when an athlete stops training, the training effect is quickly lost (reversibility). Studies have demonstrated that within two weeks after the cessation of training, significant reductions in $\dot{V}O_2$ max can occur (28, 29). A classic study by Saltin and colleagues (100) demonstrated that after twenty days of bed rest, a group of subjects showed a 25% reduction in $\dot{V}O_2$ max and maximal cardiac output. These rather dramatic decrements in working capacity as a result of inactivity clearly demonstrate the rapid reversibility of training.

The concept of specificity refers not only to the specific muscles involved in a particular movement, but also to the energy systems that provide the ATP required to complete the movement under competitive conditions. Therefore, training programs need to deal with specificity by using not only those muscle groups engaged during competition, but also the energy systems that will be providing the ATP. For instance, "specific training" for a sprinter would involve running high-intensity dashes. Similarly, spe-

TABLE 21.1   The Predominant Energy Systems for Selected Sports

Sport/Activity	% ATP CONTRIBUTION BY ENERGY SYSTEM		
	ATP-PC	Glycolysis	Aerobic
Baseball	80	15	5
Basketball	80	10	10
Field hockey	60	20	20
Football	90	10	—
Golf (swing)	100	—	—
Gymnastics	90	10	—
Ice hockey:			
Forwards/defense	80	20	—
Goalie	95	5	—
Rowing	20	30	50
Soccer:			
Goalie/wings/strikers	80	20	—
Halfbacks	60	20	20
Swimming:			
Diving	98	2	—
50 meters	95	5	—
100 meters	80	15	—
200 meters	30	65	5
400 meters	20	40	40
1,500 meters	10	20	70
Tennis	70	20	10
Track and field:			
100/200 meters	98	2	—
Field events	90	10	—
400 meters	40	55	5
800 meters	10	60	30
1,500 meters	5	35	60
5,000 meters	2	28	70
Marathon	—	2	98
Volleyball	90	10	—
Wrestling	45	55	—

From E. L. Fox and D. K. Mathews, *Interval Training: Conditioning for Sports and General Fitness.* Copyright © 1974 Saunders College Publishing, Orlando FL. Reprinted by permission of the author.

cific training for a marathoner would involve long, slow-paced runs in which virtually all of the ATP needed by the working muscles would be derived from aerobic metabolism.

Influence of Gender, Initial Fitness Level, and Genetics

At one time, it was believed that conditioning programs for women had special requirements that differed from those used to train men. Today, however, much evidence exists to demonstrate that men and women respond to training programs in a similar fashion (15, 17, 63, 86, 91, 107). Therefore, the same general approach to physiological conditioning can be used in planning programs for men and women. This does not mean that men and women should perform identical exercise training sessions (e.g., same volume and intensity). Indeed, individual training programs should be designed appropriately to match the level of fitness and maturation of the athlete, regardless of gender. Individual "exercise prescriptions" is an important concern in the design of training programs and will be discussed in further detail in the next several paragraphs.

It is a common observation that individuals differ greatly in the degree to which their performance benefits from training programs. Many factors contribute to the observed individual variations in the training response. One of the most important influences is the athlete's beginning level of fitness. In general, the amount of training improvement is always greater in those who are less conditioned at the beginning of the training program (101). It has been demonstrated that sedentary, middle-aged men with heart disease may improve their $\dot{V}O_2$ max by as much as 50%, whereas the same training program in normal, active adults improves $\dot{V}O_2$ max by only 10% to 15% (61, 78). Similarly, conditioned athletes may improve their level of conditioning by only 3% to 5% following an increase in training intensity. However, this 3% to 5% improvement in the trained athlete may be the difference between winning an Olympic gold medal and failing to place in the event.

Additionally, it seems likely that genetics plays an important role in how an individual responds to a training program (7). For instance, a person with a high genetic endowment for endurance sports is likely to respond differently to endurance training than one with a markedly different genetic profile. It is for this reason, and the fact that athletes begin conditioning programs at different levels of fitness, that training programs should be individualized. It is unrealistic to expect each athlete on the team to perform the same amount of work or to exercise at the same work rate during training sessions.

Note that while training can greatly improve performance, there is no substitute for genetically inherited athletic talent if the individual is to compete at a world-class level. For example, there is a limit to how much training can improve aerobic power. Therefore, those individuals with a low genetic endowment for aerobic power cannot, under any training program, increase their $\dot{V}O_2$ max to world-class levels. Åstrand and Rodahl (7) have commented that if you want to become a world-class athlete you must choose your parents wisely.

IN SUMMARY

- The general objective of sport conditioning is to improve performance by increasing the maximum energy output during a particular movement. A conditioning program should allocate the appropriate amount of training time to match the aerobic and anaerobic energy demands of the sport.
- Muscles respond to training as a result of a progressive overload. When an athlete stops training, there is a rapid decline in fitness due to detraining (reversibility).
- In general, men and women respond to conditioning in a similar fashion. The amount of training improvement is always greater in those individuals who are less conditioned at the onset of the training program.

COMPONENTS OF A TRAINING SESSION: WARM-UP, WORKOUT, AND COOL DOWN

Every training session should consist of three components: (1) warm-up, (2) workout, and (3) cool down. This idea was first introduced in chapter 16 and will be mentioned only briefly here. The warm-up prior to a training workout has several important objectives. First, warm-up exercises increase cardiac output and blood flow to the skeletal muscles to be used during the training session. Secondly, the warm-up activity results in an increase in muscle temperature, which elevates muscle enzyme activity (76). Finally, preliminary exercise affords the athlete an opportunity to perform stretching exercises. The duration of the warm-up may be from five to twenty minutes, depending on environmental conditions and the nature of the training activity (30, 116). Although limited data exist, it is commonly believed that a proper warm-up may reduce the possibility of muscle injury due to pulls or strains (14, 43, 95, 97). Additional research is needed to definitively answer this question.

Immediately following the training session, a period of low-intensity, "cool-down" exercises should be performed. The principal objective of a cool down is to return "pooled" blood from the exercised skeletal muscles back to the central circulation. Similar to the warm-up, the length of the cool down may vary from ten to thirty minutes, depending on environmental conditions, the age and fitness level of the individual, and the nature of the training session.

IN SUMMARY

- Every training session should consist of a warm-up period, a workout session, and a cool-down period.
- Although limited data exist, it is believed that a warm-up reduces the risk of muscle and/or tendon injury during exercise.

TRAINING TO IMPROVE AEROBIC POWER

Recall from chapter 13 that endurance training improves $\dot{V}O_2$ max by increasing both maximal cardiac output and increasing the a-$\bar{v}$ O_2 difference (i.e., increasing the muscle's ability to extract O_2). Therefore, a training program designed to improve maximal aerobic power must overload the circulatory system and stress the oxidative capacities of skeletal muscles

TABLE 21.2 Guidelines for Determining the Intensity or Work Rate During Interval Training for Running and Swimming Different Distances

Interval Training Distances (Yards) Running	Swimming	Work Rate for Each Interval
100	25	One to five seconds slower than best time
220	50	Three seconds slower than best time
440	100	One to four seconds faster than average 440-yard run or 100-yard swim times recorded during a mile run or 440-yard swim
880–1,320	165–320	Three to four seconds slower than the average 440-yard run or 100-yard swim times recorded during a mile run or 440-yard swim

From E. L. Fox and D. K. Mathews, *Interval Training: Conditioning for Sports and General Fitness.* Copyright © 1974 Saunders College Publishing, Orlando FL. Reprinted by permission of the author.

as well (7, 25, 30). As in all training regimens, specificity is critical. The athlete should stress the specific muscles to be used in his or her sport (113). In other words, runners should train by running, cyclists should train on the bicycle, swimmers should swim, and so forth.

There are three principal aerobic training methods used by athletes: (1) interval training, (2) long, slow distance (low-intensity), and (3) high-intensity, continuous exercise. Controversy exists as to which of these training methods results in the greatest improvement in $\dot{V}O_2$ max. Indeed, there does not appear to be a magic training formula for all athletes to follow. However, there is evidence that it is training intensity and not duration that is the most important factor in improving $\dot{V}O_2$ max (16, 31, 36, 39, 49, 60, 93). Nonetheless, from a psychological standpoint, it would appear that a mixing of all three methods would provide the needed variety to prevent the athlete from becoming bored with a single and rather monotonous training program.

Note that improvement of $\dot{V}O_2$ max is only one variable related to endurance. Recall from chapter 20 that although a high $\dot{V}O_2$ max is important for success in endurance events, both movement economy and the lactate threshold are also important variables. Therefore, training to improve endurance performance should not only be geared toward the improvement of $\dot{V}O_2$ max, but should increase the lactate threshold and improve running economy. A brief discussion of various training methods used to improve endurance performance follows.

Interval Training

Interval training involves the performance of repeated exercise bouts, with brief recovery periods in between. The length and intensity of the work interval depends on what the athlete is trying to accomplish. For instance, a longer work interval requires a greater involvement of aerobic energy production, while a shorter, more intense interval provides greater participation of anaerobic metabolism. Therefore, interval training that is designed to improve $\dot{V}O_2$ max should generally utilize intervals longer than sixty seconds to maximize the involvement of aerobic ATP production. Further, it is generally believed that high-intensity intervals are more effective in improving aerobic power, and perhaps the lactate threshold, than low-intensity intervals (40, 42, 68). These improvements may be due to the recruitment of fast-twitch (types IIa and IIb) fibers during this type of high-intensity exercise.

One obvious advantage of interval training over continuous running is that this method of training provides a means of performing large amounts of high-intensity exercise in a short time. Further, this training method offers two ways of providing a training overload. For example, the interval training prescription can be modified to provide "overload" in terms of increasing either the total number of exercise intervals performed or the intensity of the work interval. Adjustments to either of these factors allow the coach or athlete to alter the workout plan to accomplish specific training goals.

How does one design an interval workout? A complete discussion of the theory and rationale of designing an interval training program to improve athletic performance is beyond the scope of this chapter. For a detailed discussion of interval training, the reader is referred to Fox and Mathews (42). Additionally, table 21.2 provides some general guidelines for determining the intensity for running or swimming intervals.

In planning an interval training session, the following variables need to be considered: (1) length of the work interval, (2) intensity of the effort, (3) duration of the rest interval, (4) number of interval sets, and (5) the number of work repetitions. The length of the **work interval** refers to the distance to be covered during the work effort. In training to improve aerobic power, the work interval should generally last longer than sixty seconds. The intensity of the work effort during interval training can be monitored from a ten-second HR count upon completion of the interval (i.e., 10 sec HR count × 6 = HR per min). In general, exercise HRs should reach 85% to 100% of the maximal HR during interval training. The time between work efforts is termed the **rest interval** and consists of light activity such as walking. The length of the rest interval is generally expressed as a ratio of the duration of the work interval. For example, if the work interval for running 400 meters was seventy-five seconds, a rest interval of seventy-five seconds would result in a 1:1 ratio of work to rest. Generally, the rest interval should be at least as long as the work interval (7). In planning an interval training program for athletes who are not already highly trained, a work:rest ratio of 1:3 or 1:2 seems preferable. As a rule of thumb, the HR should drop to approximately 120 beats · min^{-1} near the end of the recovery interval (7).

A **set** is a specified number of work efforts performed as a unit. For instance, a set may consist of 8 × 400-meter runs with a prescribed rest interval between each run. The term **repetition** is the number of work efforts within one set. In the example just given, 8 × 400-meter run repetitions constituted one set. The number of repetitions and sets performed per workout depends on the purpose of the particular training session and the fitness levels of the athletes involved. For more details on interval training, see reference 71.

Long, Slow-Distance Exercise

The use of long, slow-distance (LSD) runs (or cycle rides, long swims, etc.) became a popular means of training for endurance events in the 1970s (24). In general, this method of training involves performing exercise at a low intensity (i.e., 57% $\dot{V}O_2$ max or approximately 70% of max HR) for durations that are generally greater in length than the normal competition distance. Although it seems reasonable that this type of training is a useful means of preparing an athlete to compete in long, endurance competitions (marathon running), recent evidence suggests that short-term, high-intensity exercise is superior to long-term, low-intensity exercise in improving $\dot{V}O_2$ max (60, 61).

One of the historical reasons researchers have used training sessions of long duration is the common belief that improvements in endurance are proportional to the volume of training performed. Indeed, many coaches and athletes believe that improvements in athletic performance are directly related to how much work was performed during training, and that athletes can reach their potential only by doing long-duration exercise bouts. Evidence by Costill and colleagues (27) contradicts this belief. These workers demonstrated that athletes training 1.5 hours per day performed as well as athletes training 3 hours per day. In fact, the athletes who trained 3 hours per day performed more poorly in some events than the group training 1.5 hours per day. This study illustrates the point that "more" is not always better in endurance training. Therefore, coaches and athletes should carefully consider the volume of training required to reach maximal benefits from long, slow-distance exercise.

High-Intensity, Continuous Exercise

Again, there is a growing volume of evidence to suggest that continuous, high-intensity exercise is an outstanding means of improving $\dot{V}O_2$ max and the lactate threshold in athletes (31, 36, 39, 49, 60). Although the exercise intensity that promotes the greatest improvement in $\dot{V}O_2$ max may vary from athlete to athlete, it is believed that exercise intensities between 80% and 90% $\dot{V}O_2$ max are optimal (see figure 21.1). Further, it seems likely that a work rate that is equal to or slightly above the lactate threshold provides excellent improvement in maximum aerobic power and thus is a useful guideline for planning training programs (93).

Recall from chapter 20 that the lactate threshold can be determined in the laboratory during an incremental exercise test. Additionally, the lactate threshold can be estimated noninvasively using the ventilatory threshold (see chapters 10 and 20). In the field, it is not practical to take repeated blood samples to determine the training speed that equals the lactate threshold during each training session, nor is it practical to continuously monitor ventilation during

FIGURE 21.1 Relationship between training intensity and percent improvement in $\dot{V}O_2$ max. Data from references 31, 36, and 60.

training. Therefore, the athlete needs a simple, non-invasive means of evaluating exercise intensity. Exercise heart rate appears to be the most practical means of evaluating exercise intensity during training. During the laboratory assessment of the lactate threshold or ventilatory threshold, it is standard practice to record heart rate stage-by-stage. The heart rate that corresponds to the metabolic rate at which the lactate threshold occurred can then be used by the athlete during training sessions as a guide to optimize training intensity. An alternative to direct laboratory testing to determine the lactate threshold is to have the athletes train at a fixed percentage of their maximal heart rates. Weltman and colleagues (114) have developed exercise prescription guidelines for male endurance runners. These authors suggest that if the lactate threshold is to be used as the exercise training intensity, then athletes should exercise at ≥90% heart rate max or 95% of heart rate reserve. At present, it is unknown if these guidelines apply to women athletes or to athletes in sports other than distance running.

The objective during high-intensity, continuous training is to exercise at a heart rate near the lactate threshold for approximately twenty-five to fifty minutes, with the duration of the training session being dependent on the fitness level of the athlete. As the athlete improves, it may become necessary to repeat the laboratory testing and alter the training intensity accordingly.

For more information about specific approaches to endurance training, see Kubukeli et al. (2002) in the Suggested Readings.

IN SUMMARY

- Historically, training to improve maximal aerobic power has used three methods: (1) interval training, (2) long, slow-distance, and (3) high-intensity, continuous exercise.
- Although controversy exists as to which of the training methods results in the greatest improvement in $\dot{V}O_2$ max, there is growing evidence that it is intensity and not duration that is the most important factor in improving $\dot{V}O_2$ max.

INJURIES AND ENDURANCE TRAINING

An important question associated with any type of endurance training is what type of training program presents the lowest risk of injury to the athlete. At present, a clear answer to this question is not available. However, a recent review of exercise-training-induced injuries suggests that the majority of training injuries are a result of overtraining (e.g., overuse injuries) (82). The overuse injury can come from either short-term, high-intensity exercise or long-term, low-intensity exercise (82). A commonsense guideline to avoid overuse injuries is to avoid large increases in training volume or intensity. Perhaps the most useful rule of thumb for increasing the training load is the "ten percent rule" (82). In short, the ten percent rule suggests that training intensity or duration should not be increased more than 10% per week to avoid an overtraining injury. For example, a runner running 50 miles per week could increase his/her weekly distance to 55 miles (10% of 50 = 5) the following week.

In addition to overtraining, several other exercise-induced injury risk factors have been identified (82). Among these factors are musculotendonous imbalance of strength and/or flexibility, footwear problems (i.e., excessive wear), anatomical malalignment, poor running surface, and disease (e.g., arthritis, old fracture, etc.).

Note that gender is not an injury risk factor for endurance training (82). While some evidence exists that the female runner may sustain a higher incidence of overuse injuries than males of the same age, this may be due to cultural differences, the result of less running by teenage girls (83). Micheli (82) has suggested that many of the leg injuries in female runners appear to be the result of overtraining. This may be especially true for poorly conditioned women beginning training programs designed for well-trained men.

IN SUMMARY

- The majority of training injuries are a result of overtraining (e.g., overuse injuries) and can come from either short-term, high-intensity exercise or prolonged, low-intensity exercise.
- A useful rule of thumb for increasing the training load is the "ten percent rule." The ten percent rule states that training intensity or duration should not be increased more than 10% per week to avoid an overtraining injury.

TRAINING FOR IMPROVED ANAEROBIC POWER

Athletic events lasting less than sixty seconds depend largely on anaerobic production of the necessary energy. In general, training to improve anaerobic power centers around the need to enhance either the ATP-PC system or anaerobic glycolysis (lactic acid system) (81). However, some activities require major contributions of both of these anaerobic metabolic pathways to provide the necessary ATP for competition (see table 21.1). Again, it is critical that the training program use the specific muscle groups that are required by the athlete during competition.

Training to Improve the ATP-PC System

Sports such as football, weight lifting, and short dashes in track (100 meters) depend on the ATP-PC system to provide the bulk of the energy needed for competition. Therefore, optimal performance requires a training program that will maximize ATP production via the ATP-PC pathway.

Training to improve the ATP-PC system involves a special type of interval training. In order to maximally stress the ATP-PC metabolic pathway, short, high-intensity intervals (five to ten seconds' duration) using the muscles utilized in competition are ideal. Because of the short durations of this type of interval, little lactic acid is produced and recovery is rapid. The rest interval may range between thirty and sixty seconds, depending on the fitness levels of the athletes. For example, a training program for football players might involve repeated 30-yard dashes (with several directional changes), with a thirty-second rest period between efforts. The number of repetitions per set would be determined by the athletes' fitness levels, environmental factors, and perhaps other considerations.

Training to Improve the Glycolytic System

After approximately ten seconds of a maximal effort, there is a growing dependence on energy production from anaerobic glycolysis (7, 12, 41). In order to improve the capacity of this energy pathway, the athlete must overload the "system" via short-term, high-intensity efforts. In general, high-intensity intervals of twenty to sixty seconds' duration are useful in overloading this metabolic pathway.

This type of anaerobic training is both physically and psychologically demanding and thus requires a high commitment on the part of the athlete. Further, this type of training may drastically reduce muscle glycogen stores. It is for these reasons that athletes often alternate hard-interval training days and light training sessions. For more details on training for improved anaerobic performance, see Ask the Expert 21.1.

IN SUMMARY

- Training to improve anaerobic power involves a special type of interval training. In general, the intervals are of short duration and consist of high-intensity exercise (near-maximal effort).

TRAINING TO IMPROVE MUSCULAR STRENGTH

The goal of a strength-training program is to increase the maximum amount of force that can be generated by a particular muscle group. In general, any muscle that is regularly exercised at a high intensity (i.e., intensity near its maximum force-generating capacity) will become stronger (59). Strength-training exercises can be classified into three categories: (1) isometric or static, (2) dynamic or isotonic (includes **variable-resistance exercise**), and (3) isokinetic. Recall that isometric exercise is the application of force without joint movement, and that dynamic exercise involves force application with joint movement (see chapters 8 and 20). Variable-resistance exercise is the term used to describe exercise performed on machines such as Nautilus equipment, which provide a variable amount of resistance during the course of an isotonic contraction. Isokinetic exercise is the exertion of force at a constant speed. Although isometric exercise has been shown to improve strength, isotonic and isokinetic strength training are generally preferred in the preparation of athletes because isometric training does not increase strength over the full range of motion—only at the specific joint angle maintained during training (12, 35, 59, 116).

What physiological adaptations occur as a result of strength training? This issue was discussed in chapter 13 and will be addressed only briefly here. One of the obvious and perhaps most important physiological changes that occurs following a strength-training program is the increase in muscle mass. Recall from chapter 8 that the amount of force that can be generated by a muscle group is proportional to the cross-sectional area of the muscle (66). Therefore, larger muscles exert greater force than smaller muscles. Many investigators believe that the increase in muscle size via resistance training is due to **hypertrophy** (an increase in muscle fiber diameter due to an increase in myofibrils) (1, 2, 25, 51–53, 107). However, Gonyea and associates argue that muscles also increase their size in response to strength training by **hyperplasia** (increase in the number of muscle fibers) (51–56, 84, 103, 105). Although this issue remains controversial, it appears that most (if not all) of the increase in muscle size due to strength training occurs via hypertrophy (25, 51–53).

Of further interest is the finding that strength training may result in fast-fiber-type conversions in humans (107). Staron and colleagues (107) demonstrated that twenty weeks (two training sessions per week) of high-intensity strength training resulted in a conversion of type IIb fibers to type IIa in college-age females. The physiological significance of this type of fiber conversion is unclear. However, these results

Training to Improve Anaerobic Performance
Questions and Answers with Dr. Michael Hogan

Michael Hogan, Ph.D., *Professor in the Department of Medicine at the University of California–San Diego, is an internationally known exercise physiologist whose research focuses on delivery and utilization of oxygen in skeletal muscle. Dr. Hogan has published more than 100 research articles and his work is widely cited in the scientific literature. Further, he has been a leader in numerous scientific organizations including the American College of Sports Medicine and the American Physiological Society. In addition to being an internationally known scientist, Dr. Hogan continues to be an active competitor in the pole vault. As a collegiate athlete, Dr. Hogan was a four-year letterman in track and field and a school record holder in the pole vault at the University of Notre Dame. In the years following his graduation from college, Dr. Hogan has continued to train and compete in the pole vault and has recently excelled in both national and international age-group championships in this event. In this box feature, Dr. Hogan answers questions related to training to improve anaerobic power.*

QUESTION 1: It Is well known that genetics plays a significant role in determining the maximal aerobic power in athletes. How important is genetics in determining the maximal anaerobic power in athletes?

ANSWER: Surprisingly, few studies have examined the importance of genetics in determining anaerobic capacity. Unfortunately, similar to the data on aerobic exercise, research suggests that training can only improve anaerobic capacity a relatively small amount above that which was genetically determined. This is primarily due to the fact that the type of muscle fiber best for anaerobic performance, the type IIb fiber, is determined early in development and the percentage of muscle mass that is type IIb does not vary to a large extent over a lifetime. Indeed, the number of fibers contained within a muscle cannot increase, nor can the percentage of a muscle fiber type within the muscle be altered to a large degree. Therefore, anaerobic capacity appears to be largely genetically determined since the percentage of type IIb fibers that the muscle contains is relatively fixed and this factor is a primary determinant of anaerobic capacity.

QUESTION 2: In designing a training program to improve anaerobic power, should weekly training sessions be planned on a "hard-easy" cycle?

ANSWER: Absolutely! This is possibly even more critical in anaerobic power training versus aerobic training. The reason for this is that to improve anaerobic capacity, extremely high-intensity exercise needs to be conducted to totally activate all of the type IIb fibers within the muscle (which are the last fibers recruited during the muscle activation process). An important component of anaerobic training is to work during the "hard" cycle at an extremely high intensity that subsequently results in minor muscle damage. Then, during the "easy" cycle, repair of injured fibers will result in fibers that have a higher capacity to perform anaerobic exercise. This will usually occur by regenerating fibers with larger cross-sectional areas, so that muscle power is increased. A key concern is the duration of the "hard-easy" cycles, as each individual athlete will be very different in how much high-intensity exercise can be endured before the athlete "breaks down" and injury ensues. Knowing the proper balance of "hard-easy" is the difference between an Olympic gold medal and an injured athlete.

QUESTION 3: In sports or athletic events (e.g., 200-meter dash) that require energy from both the ATP-PC system and glycolysis, is it possible to design a training program to improve energy production from each of these bioenergetic systems?

ANSWER: Yes, these bioenergetic systems can be altered to some degree, although not nearly to the degree that adaptation to endurance training (i.e., cardiovascular and oxidative enzyme changes) can be accomplished with aerobic training. The key to anaerobic performance that requires high ATP turnover rates for a short period of time (thirty to sixty seconds) is to have as much capacity in the glycolytic and ATP-PC systems and to minimize the factors that lead to fatigue in these short, high intensity exercise bouts. Studies have demonstrated that glycolytic enzymes can be increased in all fiber types by high-intensity training, so that more ATP can be generated anaerobically when necessary. Anaerobic training will also slightly improve aerobic capacity of the muscle, which can be important in that any aerobic generation of ATP will result in "sparing" of the ATP-PC and reduced lactic acid prduction. Anaerobic training will also improve the speed at which PC can be degraded, so that a faster ATP turnover is possible. This translates into improved anaerobic performance.

reflect the dynamic nature of skeletal muscles to adapt to various workloads.

Strength training may also induce central nervous system changes, which can increase the number of motor units recruited, alter motor neuron firing rates, enhance motor unit synchronization during a particular movement pattern, and result in the removal of neural inhibition (85, 96). These four processes result in an improvement in the amount of muscular force generated and appear to occur within

Exercise Physiology Applied to Sports

Strength Training: Single Sets versus Multiple Sets for Maximal Strength Gains

A widely discussed issue in strength training continues to be the number of sets required to provide maximal muscle hypertrophy and strength gains. Historically, it has been believed that multiple sets (i.e., three or more) produced maximal strength gains. However, reports published in the late 1990s argued that a resistance-training program comprised of only one set of exercises provided strength gains equal to a training program using three sets (18, 106). These reports triggered much discussion among exercise sci-

entists, and numerous studies investigating this important topic have been completed in recent years. Collectively, these studies provide several new insights into the dose-response effect of weight training (47, 92, 117). First, the number of sets required to provide maximal strength gains differs between subject populations. For example, highly trained athletes require multiple sets (e.g., four to eight sets) per muscle group for maximal strength gains (47, 92). In contrast, compared to highly trained athletes, recreationally trained nonathletes can achieve maximal strength gains with a fewer number of sets (e.g., three to eight sets)

per muscle group (47, 92). Further, it appears that nontrained individuals can achieve large strength gains during the early phase of a strength-training program by as few as one to four sets per muscle group (47, 92). However, as training progression occurs and higher strength gains are desired, multiple-set training programs produce greater strength gains in this population (47). Therefore, a consensus of the literature suggests that multiple sets of weight lifting is required to provide maximal strength gains for all individuals other than untrained, beginning weight trainers.

---

a few weeks after starting a strength-training program (67, 85, 87).

Progressive Resistance Exercise

The most common form of strength training is weight lifting using free weights or various types of weight machines (i.e., isotonic or isokinetic training). In order to improve strength, weight training must employ the overload principle by periodically increasing the amount of weight (resistance) used in a particular exercise. This method of strength training was first described in 1948 by Delorme and Watkins (32) and is called **progressive resistance exercise (PRE).** Since this early work, numerous other systems of training to improve muscular strength have been proposed, but the concept of PRE is the basis for most weight-training programs.

General Strength-Training Principles

Muscles increase in strength by being forced to contract at relatively high tensions. If muscles are not overloaded, then there is no improvement in strength. The first application of the overload principle was used by the famous Olympic wrestler, *Milo of Crotona* (500 B.C.). Milo incorporated overload in his training routine by carrying a bull calf on his back each day until the animal reached maturity. Since the days of

Milo, athletes have applied the principle of overload to training by lifting heavy objects.

The perfect training regimen for optimum improvement of strength remains controversial. Indeed, there does not appear to be a magic formula for strength training that meets the needs of everyone (3, 35). This is not surprising, given that subjects vary in their responses to training loads due to differences in the initial fitness level and their response to training (74). Therefore, as with endurance training, the exercise prescription for strength training should be tailored to the individual. However, a general guideline for a strength-training prescription is as follows: In general, the recommended intensity of training is four to twelve repetitions maximum (RM) and practiced in multiple sets (10, 11, 18, 47, 92, 106, 110, 111). Clearly, strength gains are less when the number of repetitions is more than fifteen. Rest days between workouts seem critical for optimal strength improvement (11, 110). Therefore, a training schedule of three days per week is often recommended.

A common belief among coaches and athletes is that strength increases in direct proportion to the volume of training (i.e., number of sets performed). Although there is a physiological link between training volume and strength gains, the optimal number of sets to improve strength remains a controversial issue (see The Winning Edge 21.1). It is likely that the optimal number of sets for maximal improvement of muscular strength may vary among subjects of different ages and fitness levels. Further, it is clear that weight-training programs incorporating extremely high training volumes (e.g., >10 sets) are not required for optimal strength gains (47, 92, 111).

Similar to other training methods, strength training should involve those muscles used in competition. Indeed, strength-training exercises should stress the muscles in the same movement pattern used during the athletic competition. For instance, a shot putter should perform exercises that strengthen the specific muscles of the arm, chest, back, and legs that are involved in "putting the shot."

A final concern in the design of strength-training programs for sport performance is that the speed of muscle shortening during training should be similar to those speeds used during the event. For example, many sports require a high velocity of movement. Several studies have shown that strength-training programs using high-velocity movements in a sport-specific movement pattern produce superior gains in strength/power-oriented sports (33, 38, 70, 98). These findings reinforce the notion that specificity of training dictates specific adaptations to specific stresses (108). For a review of strength-training research, see Galvao and Taafee (2004), Wolfe et al. (2004), and Peterson et al. (2005) in the Suggested Readings.

Free Weights versus Machines

Over the past several years, much controversy has centered around the question of whether training with free weights (barbells) or various types of weight machines (Nautilus, Universal, etc.) produces the greater strength gains in athletes. At present, a definitive answer to this question is not available. When comparing strength gains obtained on various types of weight machines, no differences exist between variable-resistance machines and constant-resistance machines (75). However, Stone and O'Bryant (110) argue that strength training using free weights is superior to training with many commercial weight machines (both constant and variable resistance) for the following reasons: (1) data exist to support the notion that free weights produce greater strength gains during short-term training periods than the gains produced by many types of weight machines (109, 112), (2) the use of free weights provides movement versatility and allows a greater specificity of training than weight machines, and (3) training with free weights (unlike many weight machines) involves large muscle mass and multi-segment exercise, which forces the athlete to control both balance and stabilizing factors. This type of training is useful, since most sports require the athlete to maintain balance and body stability during competition (110). Although free weights offer some advantages over commercial

weight machines, disadvantages also exist. Possible disadvantages include the potential for injury (dropping weights), extra people required for spotting, and the amount of time required to learn proper lifting technique. Table 21.3 summarizes some of the advantages and disadvantages of strength training using isometric, isotonic (free weights, Nautilus, etc.), and isokinetic machines.

Combined Strength- and Endurance-Training Programs

Strength and endurance training are often done concurrently by athletes and fitness enthusiasts. Some investigators have argued that performing combined strength- and endurance-training programs may antagonize the strength gains achieved by weight training alone (37, 59, 99). For example, two studies have demonstrated that untrained subjects who perform a combination of endurance and strength training achieve lower strength gains than subjects performing weight training alone (37, 59). However, whether the combination of weight and endurance training impedes strength gains probably depends on several factors, including the training state of the subjects, the volume and frequency of training, and the way the two training methods are integrated (99). In this regard, Sale (99) has recently demonstrated that athletes who perform concurrent strength- and endurance-training programs on the same day show a reduction in strength gains compared to athletes performing strength training alone. In contrast, these authors reported that athletes who perform concurrent strength- and endurance-training programs on separate days gain strength as rapidly as athletes performing strength training only. Similar findings have been reported by others (19, 79). What is the explanation for these findings? A possible explanation is that same-day, endurance-plus-strength training may result in a reduced strength-training effort, particularly when endurance training is performed first. Indeed, fatigue or anticipation may reduce the amount of effort that subjects apply to strength training when the two programs are performed on the same day. Therefore, although more research in this area is required, a current recommendation for the training of power athletes would be for the athlete to perform strength- and endurance-training programs on separate days.

Gender Differences in Response to Strength Training

It is well established that when absolute strength (i.e., total amount of force applied) is compared in untrained men and women, men are typically stronger.

TABLE 21.3 Summary of Potential Advantages and Disadvantages of Weight-Training Programs Using Various Types of Equipment

Program	Equipment	Advantages	Disadvantages
Isometric	Variety of home-designed devices	Minimal cost; less time required	Not directly applicable to most sport activities; may become boring; progress is difficult to monitor
Isotonic	Free weights	Low cost; specialized exercises may be designed to simulate a particular sport movement; progress easy to monitor	Injury potential due to dropping weights; increase workout time due to time required to change weights
Isotonic	Commercial weight machines (i.e., Universal®)	Generally safe; progress easy to monitor; small amount of time required to change weight	Does not permit specialized exercise; high cost
Variable resistance	Commercial devices (e.g., Nautilus®)	Has a cam system that provides a variable resistance that changes to match the joint's ability to produce force over the range of motion; progress easy to monitor; safety	High cost; limited specialized exercises
Isokinetic	Commercial isokinetic devices (e.g., Cybex®)	Allows development of maximal resistance over full range of motion; exercises can be performed at a variety of speeds	High cost; limited specialized exercises

Modified from reference 9.

FIGURE 21.2 Arm flexor strength of men and women graphed as a function of muscle cross-sectional area.

This difference is greatest in the upper body, where men are approximately 50% stronger than women, whereas men are only 30% stronger than women in the lower body (86). This apparent sex difference in strength is eliminated when force production in men and women is compared on the basis of the cross-sectional area of muscle. Figure 21.2 illustrates this point.

Notice that as the cross-sectional area of muscle increases (x-axis), the arm flexor strength (y-axis) increases in a linear fashion and is independent of sex. That is, human muscle can generate 3 to 4 kg of force per cm^2 of muscle cross-section regardless of whether the muscle belongs to a male or a female (66).

An often-asked question is "Do women gain strength as rapidly as men when training with weights?" In an effort to answer this question, Wilmore (115) compared the strength change between a group of untrained men and women before and after ten weeks of isotonic weight training. The results revealed that no differences existed between sexes in the percentage of strength gained during the training period (see figure 21.3). Similar findings have been reported in other studies, and they demonstrate that untrained men and women respond similarly to weight training (63, 71, 91). However, the aforementioned studies are considered short-term training periods and may not reflect what occurs over long-term training. For instance, it is generally believed that men exhibit a greater degree of muscular hypertrophy than women as a result of long-term weight training. This gender difference in muscular hypertrophy appears to be related to the fact that men have

FIGURE 21.3 Strength changes in men and women as a result of a ten-week strength-training program.

twenty to thirty times higher blood levels of testosterone. For a review of strength training for female athletes, see reference 63.

Muscle Soreness

It is a common experience for novice weight trainers and sometimes even veteran strength athletes to notice a **delayed-onset muscle soreness (DOMS)** that appears twenty-four to forty-eight hours after strenuous exercise. The search for an answer to the question of "What causes DOMS?" has extended over many years. A number of possible explanations have been proposed, including a buildup of lactic acid in muscle, muscle spasms, and torn muscle and connective tissue. It is clear that lactic acid does not cause this type of soreness. Based on present evidence, it appears that DOMS is due to tissue injury caused by excessive mechanical force exerted upon muscle and connective tissue (5, 20, 21, 44, 45, 104). Perhaps the strongest data to support this viewpoint come from electron microscopy studies in which electron micrographs taken of muscles suffering from DOMS reveal microscopic tears in these muscle fibers (45).

How does DOMS occur, and what is the physiological explanation for DOMS? Complete answers to these questions are not currently available (for reviews, see references 5, 22, and 94). However, current evidence suggests that DOMS occurs in the following manner (5, 94): (1) strenuous muscular contractions (especially eccentric contractions) result in structural damage in muscle (i.e., disruption of sarcomeres); (2) membrane damage occurs, including damage to the membranes of the sarcoplasmic reticulum; (3) calcium leaks out of the sarcoplasmic reticulum and collects in the mitochondria, which inhibits ATP production; (4) the buildup of calcium also activates enzymes (proteases), which degrade cellular proteins, including contractile proteins (50); (5) membrane damage combined with a breakdown of muscle

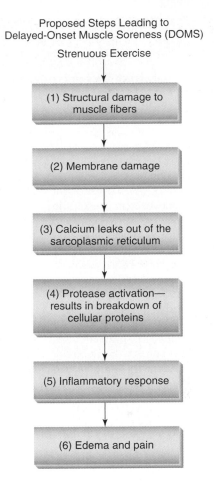

FIGURE 21.4 Proposed model to explain the occurrence of delayed-onset muscle soreness (DOMS) resulting from strenuous muscular exercise.

proteins and results in an inflammatory process, which includes an increase in prostaglandins/histamine production and production of free radicals (23); and finally (6) the accumulation of histamines and edema surrounding muscle fibers stimulates free nerve endings (pain receptors), which results in the sensation of pain the muscle (see figure 21.4).

How does one avoid being a victim of DOMS following exercise? It appears that DOMS occurs most frequently following intense exercise using muscles that are unaccustomed to being worked (22). Further, eccentric exercise (i.e., lengthening contractions) appears to cause greater suffering from DOMS than does concentric work. Therefore, a general recommendation for the avoidance of DOMS is to slowly begin a specific exercise during the first five to ten training sessions. This pattern of slow progression allows the exercised muscles to "adapt" to the exercise stress and therefore reduces the incidence or severity of DOMS (see Research Focus 21.1). For more information on DOMS, see Ask the Expert 21.2 and Proske and Allen (2005) in the Suggested Readings.

Protection Against Exercise-Induced Muscle Soreness: The Repeated Bout Effect

Performing a bout of unfamiliar exercise often results in muscle injury and delayed-onset muscle soreness (DOMS). This is particularly true when the bout of unfamiliar exercise involves eccentric actions. Interestingly, following recovery from DOMS, a subsequent bout of the same exercise results in minimal symptoms of muscle injury and soreness; this is called the "repeated bout effect" (80). This protective effect of prior exercise has been recognized for over forty years. Although many theories have been proposed to explain the repeated bout effect, the specific mechanism responsible for this exercise-induced protection is unknown and continues to be debated. In general, three primary theories have been proposed to explain the repeated bout effect: (1) neural theory; (2) connective tissue theory; and (3) cellular theory (80).

The neural theory proposes that the exercise-induced muscle injury occurs in a relatively small number of active type II (fast) fibers. In the subsequent exercise bout, there is a change in the pattern of recruitment of muscle fibers to increase motor unit activation to recruit a larger number of muscle fibers. This results in the contractile stress being distributed over a larger number of fibers. Hence, there is a reduction in stress within individual fibers, and no muscle injury occurs during subsequent exercise bouts.

The connective tissue theory argues that muscle damage due to the initial exercise bout results in an increase in connective tissue to provide more protection to the muscle during the stress of exercise. This increased connective tissue is postulated to be responsible for the repeated bout effect.

Finally, the cellular theory predicts that exercise-induced muscle damage results in the synthesis of new proteins (e.g., stress proteins, cytoskeletal proteins, etc.) that improve the integrity of the muscle fiber. The synthesis of these "protective proteins" reduces the strain on the muscle fiber and protects the muscle from exercise-induced injury.

Which of these theories best explains the repeated bout effect is unknown. It seems unlikely that one theory can explain all of the various observations associated with the repeated bout effect. Thus, it is possible that the repeated bout effect occurs through the interaction of various neural, connective tissue, and cellular factors that respond to the specific type of exercise-induced muscle injury (80). This idea is summarized in figure 21.5.

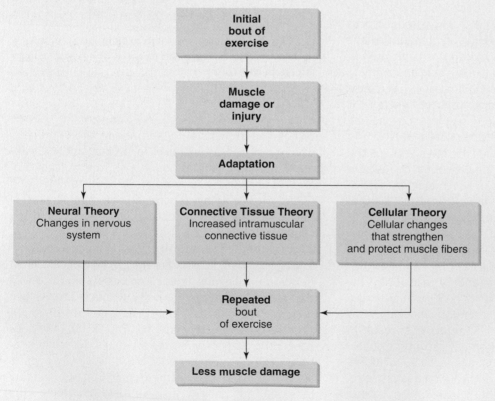

FIGURE 21.5 Proposed theories to explain the "repeated bout effect." Briefly, an initial bout of exercise results in muscle injury. This muscular injury results in a physiological adaptation, which occurs via changes in the nervous system, muscle connective tissue, and/or cellular changes within muscle fibers. One or all of these adaptations serve to protect the muscle from injury during a subsequent bout of exercise. Figure redrawn from McHugh et al. (80).

ASK THE EXPERT 21.2

Exercise-Induced Muscle Soreness
Questions and Answers with Dr. Priscilla Clarkson

Priscilla M. Clarkson is a Professor of Exercise Science and Associate Dean for the School of Public Health and Health Sciences at the University of Massachusetts–Amherst. She has served as President of the American College of Sports Medicine (ACSM) and has received numerous academic awards including the National ACSM Citation Award, the New England ACSM Honor Award, the Excellence in Education Award from the Gatorade Sport Science Institute, and the University of Massachusetts Chancellor's Medal.

Professor Clarkson has published over 100 scientific research articles and has given numerous national and international scientific presentations. The major focus of her research is exercise-induced muscle soreness and damage. In this box feature, she responds to three applied questions related to exercise and muscle soreness.

QUESTION 1: Several popular fitness publications have suggested that the use of nonsteroidal anti-inflammatory drugs (e.g., ibuprofen) following an intense exercise bout will reduce exercise-induced muscle soreness. Is this concept supported by the research literature?

ANSWER: Studies that examined the effects of nonsteroidal anti-inflammatory drugs (NSAIDs) on the reduction of muscle soreness after exercise have produced inconsistent results. There are many reasons to explain these inconsistent findings including the different types and intensities of exercises used to induce soreness, different types of NSAIDs used, and different doses of the NSAID. Another important reason for the lack of consistent results is that the amount of reduction in soreness by the NSAIDs is small, generally less than 15%. On a scale of 1–10 (with 10 being very, very sore), a person who scores an 8 would be expected to see a reduction of soreness to about a 7. This is a small reduction relative to the large intersubject variability in the

soreness response to the exercise. In other words, some individuals will experience a high degree of soreness while others experience little soreness in response to the same exercise stimulus. Therefore, to detect small differences in soreness due to a treatment, a large population of subjects needs to be tested. Published studies on the effects of NSAIDs on muscle soreness have used sample sizes that are likely too small to provide conclusive evidence.

A key question is whether NSAIDs should even be considered as a treatment to reduce muscle soreness. NSAIDs, like all drugs, have side effects. Given that NSAIDs will only reduce muscle soreness by a small amount and the long-term consequences of NSAID use on muscle recovery are not known, it may be unwise to risk experiencing side effects for so little benefit. Moreover, soreness will dissipate in a couple of days anyway with no intervention. Unless the muscle pain is unbearable, NSAIDs should be used with discretion.

QUESTION 2: Animal studies suggest that estrogen may protect skeletal muscle from stress-induced injury. This has led to the speculation that women may be protected from exercise-induced muscle injury. Do the studies performed in your laboratory suggest that compared to men, women are less susceptible to exercise-induced muscle damage?

ANSWER: The data from animal models clearly show that estrogen serves a protective role against contraction-induced muscle injury. When these data were first published, it was assumed that women would show less injury in response to eccentric exercise compared with men, because of the higher estrogen levels in women. However, our laboratory examined differences in the development of muscle soreness and

losses in muscle force and range of motion (common indirect indicators of muscle damage) in a large group of men and women both immediately after and during several days following exercise. We found that the men and women experienced a similar degree of soreness and strength loss. However, women actually showed a greater loss in range of motion. Clearly, estrogen does not play the same role in women as has been seen in the animal models of exercise-induced muscle injury.

QUESTION 3: Some authors have postulated that supplementation with oral creatine could reduce exercise-induced muscle injury by protecting muscle membranes. Research in your laboratory has directly addressed this issue in humans. Based on your data, does creatine supplementation protect skeletal muscle against exercise-induced injury?

ANSWER: To determine whether creatine supplementation would protect against eccentric contraction-induced injury, we had subjects ingest either 20 g creatine or a placebo for five days. This dosage has been shown to increase creatine levels in skeletal muscle. After the five-day supplementation period, subjects performed fifty maximal, eccentric contractions of the elbow flexors. The results indicated that the development of soreness and muscle injury did not differ between the groups. Therefore, these results indicate that creatine supplementation offers no obvious protection against this type of exercise damage to muscle. Any protection offered by an increased amount of creatine in the muscle may be no match for the strain induced by the severe exercise that the subjects performed. Whether using a less-strenuous exercise would have shown any benefits of creatine awaits further study.

- Improvement in muscular strength can be achieved via progressive overload by using either isometric, isotonic, or isokinetic exercise. Isotonic or isokinetic training seems preferable to isometric exercise in developing strength gains in athletes, since isometric strength gains occur only at the specific joint angles that are held during isometric training.

- Although untrained men exhibit greater absolute strength than untrained females, there do not appear to be gender differences in strength gains during a short-term weight-training program.

- Delayed-onset muscle soreness (DOMS) is thought to occur due to microscopic tears in muscle fibers or connective tissue. This results in cellular degradation and an inflammatory response, which results in pain within twenty-four to forty-eight hours after strenuous exercise.

TRAINING FOR IMPROVED FLEXIBILITY

Historically, it has been believed that improvement of flexibility via stretching reduces the risk of exercise-induced injury. Nonetheless, at present, limited evidence exists to support the concept that stretching prevents injuries during exercise and participation in many sports (4, 58). Further, it is possible that a high degree of flexibility in all joints may not be desirable in all sports. For instance, excessive flexibility is often indicative of proneness to injury in contact sports. For example, the shoulder joint is structurally weak when compared to the hip joint. This is because the glenoid fossa of the scapula (socket where the head of the humerus fits) is very shallow. Therefore, the main stability of the shoulder joint is provided by the surrounding musculature. Hence, an increase in shoulder muscle mass might reduce flexibility, but it would also lower the chance of shoulder injury in contact sports by increasing shoulder stability.

Although improved flexibility may not reduce the risk of exercise-induced injury, the ability to move joints through a full range of motion is important in many sports. Indeed, loss of flexibility can result in a reduction of movement efficiency. Therefore, many athletic trainers and coaches recommend regular stretching exercises to improve flexibility and perhaps optimize the efficiency of movement.

There are two general stretching techniques in use today: (1) **static stretching** (continuously holding a stretch position), and (2) **dynamic stretching** (sometimes referred to as *ballistic stretching* if movements are not controlled). Although both techniques result in an improvement in flexibility, static stretching is considered to be superior to dynamic stretching because: (1) there is less chance of injury (11), (2) static stretching causes less muscle spindle activity when compared to dynamic stretching, and (3) there is less chance of muscle soreness. Stimulation of muscle spindles during dynamic stretching can produce a stretch reflex and therefore result in muscular contraction. This type of muscular contraction counteracts the desired lengthening of the muscle and may increase the chance of injury.

Research has shown that thirty minutes of static stretching exercises performed twice per week will improve flexibility within five weeks (34). It is recommended that the stretch position be held for ten seconds at the beginning of a flexibility program and increased to sixty seconds after several training sessions. Each stretch position should be repeated three to five times, with the number increased up to ten repetitions. Overload is applied by increasing the range of motion during the stretch position and increasing the amount of time the stretch position is held.

Preceding a static stretch with an isometric contraction of the muscle group to be stretched is an effective means of improving muscle relaxation and may enhance the development of flexibility (14, 34, 116). This stretching technique is called **proprioceptive neuromuscular facilitation (PNF).** The procedure generally requires two people and is performed as follows (72): A training partner moves the target limb passively through its range of motion; after reaching the end point of the range of motion, the target muscle is isometrically contracted (against the partner) for six to ten seconds. The target muscle then relaxes and is again stretched by the partner to a greater range of motion. The physiological rationale for the use of PNF stretching is that muscular relaxation follows an isometric contraction because the contraction stimulates Golgi tendon organs, which inhibit contraction during the subsequent stretching exercise.

- Limited evidence exists to support the notion that improved joint mobility (flexibility) reduces the incidence of exercise-induced injury.
- Stretching exercises are often recommended to improve flexibility and optimize the efficiency of movement.
- Improvement in flexibility can be achieved via static or dynamic stretching, with static stretching being the preferred technique.

YEAR-ROUND CONDITIONING FOR ATHLETES

It is common for today's athletes to engage in year-round conditioning exercises. This is necessary to prevent gain of excessive body fat and to prevent extreme physical detraining between competitive seasons. The training periods of athletes can be divided into three phases: (1) off-season training, (2) preseason training, and (3) in-season training. A brief description of each training period follows.

Off-Season Conditioning

In general, the objectives of off-season conditioning programs are to: (1) prevent excessive fat weight gain, (2) maintain muscular strength or endurance, (3) maintain ligament and bone integrity, and (4) maintain a reasonable skill level in the athlete's specific sport. Obviously, the exact nature of the off-season conditioning program will vary from sport to sport. For example, a football player would spend considerably more time performing strength-training exercises than would a distance runner. Conversely, the runner would incorporate more running into an off-season conditioning program than would the football player. Hence, specific exercises should be selected on the basis of the sport's demands (12).

No matter what the sport, it is critical that an off-season conditioning program provide variety for the athlete. Further, off-season conditioning programs generally use a training regimen that is composed of low-intensity, high-volume work. This combination of low-intensity training and variety may prevent the occurrence of "overtraining syndromes" and the development of psychological staleness. Figure 21.6 contains a list of some recommended training activities for off-season conditioning.

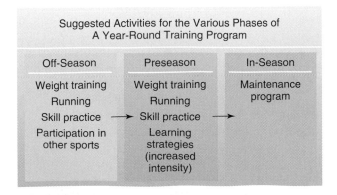

Suggested Activities for the Various Phases of A Year-Round Training Program

Off-Season	Preseason	In-Season
Weight training	Weight training	Maintenance program
Running	Running	
Skill practice →	Skill practice →	
Participation in other sports	Learning strategies (increased intensity)	

FIGURE 21.6 Recommended activities for the various phases of year-round training.

Off-season conditioning allows athletes to concentrate on fitness areas where they may be weak. Therefore, it is important that off-season programs be designed for the individual. For instance, a basketball player may lack leg strength and power and therefore have a limited vertical jump. An off-season conditioning program allows this athlete to engage in specific strength-training activities that will improve leg power and enhance vertical jumping capacity.

Preseason Conditioning

The principal objective of preseason conditioning (e.g., eight to twelve weeks prior to competition) is to increase to a maximum the capacities of the predominant energy systems used in a particular sport (12). In the transition from off-season conditioning to preseason conditioning there is a gradual shift from low-intensity, high-volume exercise to high-intensity, low-volume exercise. As in all phases of a training cycle, the program should be sport specific.

In general, the types of exercise performed during preseason conditioning are similar to those used during off-season conditioning (figure 21.6). The principal difference between off-season and preseason conditioning is the intensity of the conditioning effort. During preseason conditioning, the athlete applies a progressive overload by increasing the intensity of workouts, whereas off-season conditioning involves high-volume, low-intensity workouts.

In-Season Conditioning

The general goal of in-season conditioning for most sports is to maintain the fitness level achieved during the preseason training program. For instance, in a sport such as football, in which there is a relatively long competitive season, the athlete must be able to maintain strength and endurance during the entire season. A complicating factor in planning an in-season conditioning program for many team sports is that the season may not have a clear-cut ending. That is, at the end of the regular season, playoff games may extend the season an additional several weeks. Therefore, it is difficult in these types of sports to plan a climax in the conditioning program, and so there is the need for a maintenance training program.

In planning an in-season conditioning program, the goal is to design a program that is of sufficient volume and intensity to maintain strength and endurance during the entire playing season. Note that strength can be maintained during the competitive season by as little as one workout every seven to ten days (110). However, maintenance of cardiovascular fitness appears to require a minimum of two to three training days per week (62).

A CLOSER LOOK 21.1

Overtraining and the Immune System

The human immune system is a complex array of cells and hormones charged with the responsibility of preventing infections and cancer. There is growing evidence that moderate levels of exercise training improve immune function and decrease the risk of infection (73, 88, 89). However, it is now clear that heavy training regimens coupled with a lack of rest (i.e., overtraining) result in a weakened immune system and an increased risk of disease. The relationship between various levels of exercise training and the risk of infection is described by a "J"-shaped curve (see chapter 13, figure 13.13) (89). Close inspection of figure 13.13 illustrates that movement from a sedentary lifestyle to an active lifestyle involving a moderate level of exercise training reduces the risk of infection. However, overtraining, due to a very high training intensity or volume, increases the risk of infection. Therefore, athletes should be able to recognize the symptoms of overtraining. When overtraining symptoms appear, the athlete must be prepared to reduce his/her training load to avoid a reduction in immune function.

IN SUMMARY

- Year-round conditioning programs for athletes include an off-season program, a preseason program, and an in-season program.
- The general objectives of an off-season conditioning program are to prevent excessive fat weight gain, maintain muscular strength and endurance, maintain bone and ligament strength, and preserve a reasonable skill level in the athlete's specific sport.

COMMON TRAINING MISTAKES

Some of the most common training errors include: (1) overtraining, (2) undertraining, (3) using exercises and work-rate intensities that are not sport specific, (4) failure to plan long-term training schedules to achieve specific goals, and (5) failure to taper training prior to a competition. Let's discuss each of these training errors briefly.

Overtraining may be a more significant problem than undertraining for several reasons. First, overtraining (workouts that are too long or too strenuous) may result in injury or reduce the athlete's resistance to disease (see A Closer Look 21.1). Further, overtraining may result in a psychological staleness, which can be identified by a general lack of enthusiasm on the part of the athlete (80). The general symptoms of overtraining include: (1) elevated heart rate and blood lactate levels at a fixed submaximal work rate, (2) loss in body weight due to a reduction in appetite, (3) chronic fatigue, (4) psychological staleness, (5) multiple colds

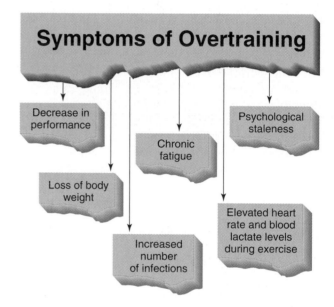

FIGURE 21.7 Common symptoms of overtraining.

or sore throats, and/or (6) a decrease in performance (see figure 21.7). An overtrained athlete may exhibit one or all of these symptoms (12, 14, 46, 64, 116). Therefore, it is critical that coaches and trainers recognize the classic symptoms of overtraining and be prepared to reduce their athletes' workloads when overtraining symptoms appear. Recall that specific training programs should be planned for athletes when possible to compensate for individual differences in genetic potential and fitness levels. This is an important point to remember when planning training programs for athletic conditioning.

For more details on overtraining, see Halson and Jeukendrup (2004) and Urhausen and Kindermann (2002) in the Suggested Readings.

Another common mistake in the training of athletes is the failure to plan sport-specific training exercises. Often coaches or trainers fail to understand the importance of the law of specificity, and develop training exercises that do not enhance the energy capacities of the skeletal muscles used in competition. This error can be avoided by achieving a broad understanding of the training principles discussed earlier in this chapter.

Further, coaches, trainers, and athletes should plan and record training schedules designed to achieve specific fitness objectives at various times during the year. Failure to plan a training strategy may result in the misuse of training time and ultimately result in inferior performance.

Finally, failure to reduce the intensity and volume of training prior to competition is also a common training error. Achieving a peak athletic performance requires a healthy blend of proper nutrition, training, and rest. Failure to reduce the training volume and/or intensity prior to competition results in inadequate rest and compromises performance. Therefore, in an effort to achieve peak performance, athletes should reduce their training load for several days prior to competition; this practice is called **tapering.** The goal of tapering is to provide time for muscles to resynthesize glycogen to maximal levels and to allow muscles to heal from training-induced damage. While the optimum length of a taper period continues to be debated, a reduced training load of three to twenty-one days has been used successfully in both strength and endurance sports (26, 48, 62, 65, 77). Indeed, runners and swimmers can reduce their training load by approximately 60% for up to twenty-one days without a reduction in performance (26, 48, 65).

IN SUMMARY

- Common mistakes in training include undertraining, overtraining, performing nonspecific exercises during training sessions, failure to carefully schedule a long-term training plan, and failure to taper training prior to a competition.
- Symptoms of overtraining include: (1) elevated heart rate and blood lactate levels at a fixed submaximal work rate, (2) loss in body weight due to a reduction in appetite, (3) chronic fatigue, (4) psychological staleness, (5) increased number of infections, and/or (6) a decrease in performance.
- *Tapering* is the term applied to short-term reduction in training load prior to competition. Research has shown that tapering prior to a competition is useful in improving performance in both strength and endurance events.

STUDY QUESTIONS

1. Explain how knowledge of the energy systems used in a particular activity or sport might be useful in designing a sport-specific training program.
2. Provide an outline of the general principles of designing a training program for the following sports: (1) football, (2) soccer, (3) basketball, (4) volleyball, (5) distance running (5,000 meters), and (6) 200-meter dash (track).
3. Define the following terms as they relate to interval training: (1) *work interval*, (2) *rest interval*, (3) *work-to-rest ratio*, and (4) *set*.
4. How can interval training be used to improve both aerobic and anaerobic power?
5. List and discuss the three most common types of training programs used to improve $\dot{V}O_2$ max.
6. Discuss the practical and theoretical differences between an interval training program used to improve the ATP-PC system and a program designed to improve the lactic acid system.
7. List the general principles of strength development.
8. Define the terms *isometric*, *isotonic*, and *isokinetic*.
9. Outline the model to explain delayed-onset muscle soreness proposed by Armstrong.
10. Discuss the use of static and dynamic stretching to improve flexibility. Why is a high degree of flexibility not desired in all sports?
11. List and discuss the objectives of: (1) off-season conditioning, (2) preseason conditioning, and (3) in-season conditioning.
12. What are some of the more common errors made in the training of athletes?

SUGGESTED READINGS

American College of Sports Medicine Position Stand. 2002. Progression models in resistance training for adults. *Medicine and Science in Sports and Exercise* 34:364–80.

Angeli, A. et al. 2004. The overtraining syndrome in athletes: A stress related disorder. *Journal of Endocrinological Investigation* 27:603–12.

Baechle, T., and R. Earle, eds. 2000. *Essentials of Strength Training and Conditioning*. Champaign-Urbana, IL: Human Kinetics.

Brooks, G., T. Fahey, and K. Baldwin. 2005. *Exercise Physiology: Human Bioenergetics and Its Applications*, 4th ed. New York: McGraw-Hill Companies.

Galvao, D., and D. Taafee. 2004. Single- vs. multiple-set resistance training: Recent developments in the controversy. *Journal of Strength and Conditioning Research*. 18:660–67.

Halson, S., and A. Jeukendrup. 2004. Does overtraining exist? An analysis of overreaching and overtraining research. *Sports Medicine* 34:967–81.

Hart, L. 2005. Effect of stretching on sport injury risk: A review. *Clinical Journal of Sports Medicine* 15:371–78.

Kamen, F. 2004. Neural issues in the control of muscular strength. *Research Quarterly for Exercise and Sport* 75:3–8.

Kubukeli, Z., T. Noakes, and S. Dennis. 2002. Training techniques to improve endurance exercise performance. *Sports Medicine* 32:489–509.

Munn, J. et al. 2005. Training with unilateral resistance exercise increases contralateral strength. *Journal of Applied Physiology* 99:1880–84.

Peterson, M., M. Rhea, and B. Alvar. 2005. Alterations of the dose-response for muscular strength development: A review of meta-analytic efficacy and reliability for designing training prescription. *Journal of Strength and Conditioning Research* 19:950–58.

Proske, U., and T. Allen. 2005. Damage to skeletal muscle from eccentric exercise. *Exercise and Sport Science Reviews* 33:98–104.

Seiler, S., and K. Hetlelid. 2005. The impact of rest duration on work intensity and RPE during interval training. *Medicine and Science in Sports and Exercise* 37:1601–07.

Urhausen A., and W. Kindermann. 2002. Diagnosis of overtraining: What tools do we have? *Sports Medicine* 32:95–102.

Wolfe, B., L. LeMura, and P. Cole. 2004. Quantitative analysis of single-vs. multiple set programs in resistance training. *Journal of Strength and Conditioning Research* 18:35–47.

REFERENCES

1. Alway, S. 1990. Muscle cross sectional area and torque in resistance-trained subjects. *European Journal of Applied Physiology* 60:86–90.

2. ———. 1990. Twitch contractile adaptations are not dependent on the intensity of isometric exercise in human triceps surae. *European Journal of Applied Physiology* 60:346–52.

3. American College of Sports Medicine. 2002. Progression models in resistance training for healthy adults. *Medicine and Science in Sports and Exercise* 34:364–80.

4. Andersen, J. 2005. Stretching before and after exercise: Effect on muscle soreness and injury risk. *Journal of Athletic Training* 40:218–20.

5. Armstrong, R. 1984. Mechanisms of exercise-induced delayed onset of muscular soreness: A brief review. *Medicine and Science in Sports and Exercise* 16:529–38.

6. Angeli, A. et al. 2004. The overtraining syndrome in athletes: A stress related disorder. *Journal of Endocrinological Investigation* 27:603–12.

7. Åstrand, P. O., and K. Rodahl. 1986. *Textbook of Work Physiology*. New York: McGraw-Hill Companies.

8. Baechle, T., and R. Earle, eds. 2000. Essentials of strength training and conditioning. Champaign-Urbana, IL: Human Kinetics.

9. Bell, G. J. et al. 2000. Effect of concurrent strength and endurance training on skeletal muscle properties and hormone concentrations in humans. *European Journal of Applied Physiology* 81:418–27.

10. Berger, R. A. 1962. Optimum repetitions for the development of strength. *Research Quarterly* 33:334–38.

11. ———. 1982. *Applied Exercise Physiology*. Philadelphia: Lea & Febiger.

12. Bowers, R., and E. Fox. 1992. *Sports Physiology*. New York: McGraw-Hill Companies.

13. Brooks, G., T. Fahey, and K. Baldwin. 2005. *Exercise Physiology: Human Bioenergetics and Its Applications, 4th ed*. New York: McGraw-Hill Companies.

14. Brooks, G. A., T. Fahey, T. White, and K. Baldwin. 2000. *Exercise Physiology: Human Bioenergetics and Its Applications*. Mountain View, CA: Mayfield.

15. Burke, E. 1977. Physiological similar effects of similar training programs in males and females. *Research Quarterly* 48:510–17.

16. Burke, E., and B. D. Franks. 1975. Changes in $\dot{V}O_2$ max resulting from bicycle training at different intensities holding total mechanical work constant. *Research Quarterly* 46:31–37.

17. Burke, E. J., ed. 1980. *Toward an Understanding of Human Performance*. Ithaca, NY: Mouvement Publications.

18. Carpinelli, R., and R. Otto. 1998. Strength training: Single versus multiple sets. *Sports Medicine* 26:73–84.

19. Chilibeck, P. D., D. G. Syrotuik, and G. J. Bell. 2002. The effect of concurrent endurance and strength training on quantitative estimates of subsarcolemmal and intermyofibrillar mitochondria. *International Journal of Sports Medicine* 23:33–39.

20. Clarkson, P., and S. Sayers. 1999. Etiology of exercise-induced muscle damage. *Canadian Journal of Applied Physiology* 24:234–48.

21. Clarkson, P. et al. 1986. Muscle soreness and serum creatine kinase activity following isometric, eccentric, and concentric exercise. *International Journal of Sports Medicine* 7:152–55.

22. Clarkson, P. et al. 1992. Muscle function after exercise-induced muscle damage and rapid adaptation. *Medicine and Science in Sports and Exercise* 24:512–20.

23. Close, G. et al. 2005. The emerging role of free radicals in delayed onset muscle soreness and contraction-induced injury. *Comparative Biochemistry and Physiology* 142:257–66.

24. Costill, D. 1979. *A Scientific Approach to Distance Running*. Los Altos: Track and Field News.

25. Costill, D. et al. 1979. Adaptations in skeletal muscle following strength training. *Journal of Applied Physiology* 46:96–99.

26. Costill, D. et al. 1985. Effects of reduced training on muscular power in swimmers. *Physician and Sports Medicine* 13:94–101.

27. Costill, D. et al. 1991. Adaptations to swimming training: Influence of training volume. *Medicine and Science in Sports and Exercise* 23:371–77.

28. Coyle, E. et al. 1984. Time course of loss of adaptations after stopping prolonged intense endurance training. *Journal of Applied Physiology* 57:1857–64.

29. Coyle, E. et al. 1985. Effects of detraining on responses to submaximal exercise. *Journal of Applied Physiology* 59:853–59.

30. Daniels, J., R. Fitts, and G. Sheehan. 1978. *Conditioning for Distance Running*. New York: Wiley.

31. Davies, C. T. M., and A. Knibbs. 1971. The training stimulus: The effects of intensity, duration, and frequency of effort on maximum aerobic power output. *Int. Z. Angew* 20:299–305.

32. Delorme, T., and A. Watkins. 1948. Techniques of progressive resistance exercise. *Archives of Physical and Rehabilitative Medicine* 29:263–66.

33. Deschenes, M. 1989. Short review: Motor coding and motor unit recruitment pattern. *Journal of Applied Sport Science Research* 3:33–39.

34. DeVries, H. 1962. Evaluation of static stretching procedures for improvement of flexibility. *Research Quarterly* 33:222–29.

35. DiNubile, N. 1991. Strength training. *Clinics in Sports Medicine* 10:33–63.

36. Dudley, G., W. Abraham, and R. Terjung. 1982. Influence of exercise intensity and duration on biochemical adaptations in skeletal muscle. *Journal of Applied Physiology* 53:844–50.

37. Dudley, G., and R. Djamil. 1985. Incompatibility of strength and endurance training. *Journal of Applied Physiology* 59:1446–51.

38. Ewing, J. et al. 1990. Effects of velocity of isokinetic training on strength, power, and quadriceps muscle fiber characteristics. *European Journal of Applied Physiology* 61:159–62.

39. Fox, E. et al. 1973. Intensity and distance of interval training programs and changes in maximal aerobic power. *Medicine and Science in Sports* 5:18–22.

40. Fox, E. et al. 1975. Frequency and duration of interval training programs and changes in aerobic power. *Journal of Applied Physiology* 38:481–84.

41. Fox, E., S. Robinson, and D. Wiegman. 1969. Metabolic energy sources during continuous and interval running. *Journal of Applied Physiology* 27:174–78.

42. Fox, E. L., and D. Mathews. 1974. *Interval Training: Conditioning for Sports and General Fitness.* Philadelphia: W. B. Saunders.

43. Franks, B. 1983. Physical warm-up. In *Ergogenic Aids in Sports*, ed. M. Williams, 340. Champaign, IL: Human Kinetics.

44. Friden, J., and R. Lieber. 1992. Structural and mechanical basis of exercise-induced injury. *Medicine and Science in Sports* 24:521–30.

45. Friden, J., M. Sjöström, and B. Ekblom. 1983. Myofibrillar damage following eccentric exercise in man. *International Journal of Sports Medicine* 4:170–76.

46. Fry, R. et al. 1994. Psychological and immunological correlates of acute overtraining. *British Journal of Sports Medicine* 28:241–46.

47. Galvao, D., and D. Taafee. 2004. Single- vs. multiple-set resistance training: Recent developments in the controversy. *Journal of Strength and Conditioning Research* 18: 660–67.

48. Gibala, M. et al. 1994. The effects of tapering on strength performance in trained athletes. *International Journal of Sports Medicine* 15:492–97.

49. Gibbons, E. et al. 1983. Effects of various training intensity levels on anaerobic threshold and aerobic capacity in females. *Journal of Sports Medicine and Physical Fitness* 23:315–18.

50. Gissel, H., and T. Clausen. 2001. Excitation-induced Ca^{2+} influx and skeletal muscle cell damage. *Acta Physiologica Scandanavia* 171:327–34.

51. Goldberg, A. 1965. Muscle hypertrophy in hypophysectomized rats. *Physiologist* 8:175–78.

52. Gollnick, P. et al. 1981. Muscular enlargement and number of fibers in skeletal muscles of rats. *Journal of Applied Physiology* 50:936–43.

53. Gollnick, P. et al. 1983. Fiber number and size in overloaded chicken anterior latissimus dorsi muscle. *Journal of Applied Physiology* 54:1292–97.

54. Gonyea, W. 1980. The role of exercise in inducing skeletal muscle fiber splitting. *Journal of Applied Physiology* 48:421–26.

55. Gonyea, W. et al. 1986. Exercise induced increases in muscle fiber number. *European Journal of Applied Physiology* 55:137–41.

56. Gonyea, W., G. Ericson, and F. Bonde-Peterson. 1977. Skeletal muscle fiber splitting induced weight lifting exercise in cats. *Acta Physiologica Scandanavica* 99:105–9.

57. Halson, S., and A. Jeukendrup. 2004. Does overtraining exist? An analysis of overreaching and overtraining research. *Sports Medicine* 34:967–81.

58. Hart, L. 2005. Effect of stretching on sport injury risk: A review. *Clinical Journal of Sports Medicine* 15:371–78.

59. Hickson, R. 1980. Interference of strength development by simultaneously training for strength and endurance. *European Journal of Applied Physiology* 45:255–63.

60. Hickson, R., H. Bomze, and J. Holloszy. 1977. Linear increase in aerobic power induced by a strenuous program of endurance exercise. *Journal of Applied Physiology* 42:372–76.

61. Hickson, R. et al. 1981. Time course of the adaptive responses of aerobic power and heart rate to training. *Medicine and Science in Sports and Exercise* 13:17–20.

62. Hickson, R., and M. Rosenkoetter. 1981. Reduced training frequencies and maintenance of increased aerobic power. *Medicine and Science in Sports and Exercise* 13:13–16.

63. Holloway, J., and T. Baeche. 1990. Strength training for female athletes: A review of selected aspects. *Sports Medicine* 9:216–28.

64. Hooper, S. 1995. Markers for monitoring overtraining and recovery. *Medicine and Science in Sports and Exercise* 27:106–12.

65. Houmard, J. 1990. Reduced training maintains performance in distance runners. *International Journal of Sports Medicine* 11:46–51.

66. Ikai, M., and T. Fukunaga. 1968. Calculation of muscle strength per unit of cross-sectional area of a human muscle by means of ultrasonic measurements. *Int. Z. Angew. Physiol.* 26:26–31.

67. Kamen, F. 2004. Neural issues in the control of muscular strength. *Research Quarterly for Exercise and Sport* 75:3–8.

68. Knuttgen, H. et al. 1973. Physical conditioning through interval training with young male adults. *Medicine and Science in Sports* 5:220–26.

69. Kraemer, W. J. et al. 2001. Effect of resistance training on women's strength/power and occupational performances. *Medicine and Science in Sports and Exercise* 33: 1011–25.

70. Kraemer, W., N. Duncan, and J. Volek. 1998. Resistance training and elite athletes: Adaptations and program considerations. *Journal of Orthopedics and Sports Physical Therapy* 28:110–19.

71. Laursen, P. B., and D. G. Jenkins. 2002. The scientific basis for high-intensity interval training optimising training programmes and maximising performance in highly trained endurance athletes. *Sports Medicine* 32: 53–73.

72. Liemohn, W., and G. Sharpe. 1992. Muscular strength and endurance, flexibility, and low-back function. In *Health/Fitness Instructor's Handbook*, ed. E. Howley and D. Frank, 179–96. Champaign, IL: Human Kinetics.

73. MacKinnon, L. 1998. *Advances in Exercise Immunology.* Champaign, IL: Human Kinetics.

74. Malina, R., and C. Bouchard. 1986. Sport and human genetics. *Proceedings of the 1984 Olympic Scientific Congress*, vol. 4. Champaign, IL: Human Kinetics.

75. Manning, R. et al. 1990. Constant vs. variable resistance knee extension training. *Medicine and Science in Sports and Exercise* 22:397–401.

76. Martin, B. et al. 1975. Effect of warm-up on metabolic responses to strenuous exercise. *Medicine and Science in Sports* 7:146–49.

77. Martin, D. 1994. Effects of interval training and a taper on cycling performance and isokinetic leg strength. *International Journal of Sports Medicine* 15:485–91.

78. McArdle, W., F. Katch, and V. Katch. 1996. *Exercise Physiology: Energy, Nutrition, and Human Performance*. Baltimore: Lippincott Williams & Wilkins.

79. McCarthy, J. P., M. A. Pozniak, and J. C. Agre. 2002. Neuromuscular adaptations to concurrent strength and endurance training. *Medicine and Science in Sports and Exercise* 34:511–19.

80. McHugh, M., D. Connolly, R. Eston, and G. Gleim. 1999. Exercise-induced muscle damage and potential mechanisms for the repeated bout effect. *Sports Medicine* 27:157–70.

81. Medbo, J., and S. Burgers. 1990. Effect of training on the anaerobic capacity. *Medicine and Science in Sports and Exercise* 22:501–7.

82. Micheli, L. 1988. Injuries and prolonged exercise. In *Prolonged Exercise*, ed. D. Lamb and R. Murray, 393–407. Indianapolis: Benchmark Press.

83. Micheli, L. et al. 1980. Etiological assessment of overuse stress fractures in athletes. *Nova Scotia Medical Bulletin* 43–47.

84. Mikesky, A. et al. 1991. Changes in muscle fiber size and composition in response to heavy-resistance exercise. *Medicine and Science in Sports and Exercise* 23:1042–49.

85. Moritani, T., and H. DeVries. 1979. Neural factors versus hypertrophy in the time course of muscle strength gain. *American Journal of Physical Medicine* 58:115–19.

86. Morrow, J., and W. Hosler. 1981. Strength comparisons in untrained men and trained women. *Medicine and Science in Sports and Exercise* 13:194–98.

87. Munn, J. et al. 2005. Training with unilateral resistance exercise increases contralateral strength. *Journal of Applied Physiology* 99:1880–84.

88. Nash, M. 1994. Exercise and immunology. *Medicine and Science in Sports and Exercise* 26:125–27.

89. Nieman, D. 1994. Exercise, infection, and immunity. *International Journal of Sports Medicine* 15:S131–S141.

90. Nieman, D., and B. Pedersen. 1999. Exercise and immune function: Recent developments. *Sports Medicine* 27:73–80.

91. O'Shea, J., and J. Wegner. 1981. Power weight training in the female athlete. *Physician and Sports Medicine* 9:109–14.

92. Peterson, M., M. Rhea, and B. Alvar. 2005. Alterations of the dose-response for muscular strength development: A review of meta-analytic efficacy and reliability for designing training prescription. *Journal of Strength and Conditioning Research* 19:950–58.

93. Priest, J., and R. Hagan. 1987. The effects of maximum steady-state pace on running performance. *British Journal of Sports Medicine* 21:18–21.

94. Proske, U., and T. Allen. 2005. Damage to skeletal muscle from eccentric exercise. *Exercise and Sport Science Reviews* 33:98–104.

95. Rodenburg, J. et al. 1994. Warm-up, stretching and massage diminish harmful effects of eccentric exercise. *International Journal of Sports Medicine* 15:414–19.

96. Rube, N., and N. Secher. 1990. Effect of central factors on fatigue following two- and one-leg static exercise in man. *Acta Physiologica Scandanavica* 141:87–95.

97. Safran, M. et al. 1989. Warm-up and muscular injury prevention. *Sports Medicine* 4:239–49.

98. Sale, D. 1988. Neural adaptation to resistance training. *Medicine and Science in Sports and Exercise* 20 (Suppl.): S135–45.

99. Sale, D. et al. 1990. Comparison of two regimens of concurrent strength and endurance training. *Medicine and Science in Sports and Exercise* 22:348–56.

100. Saltin, B. et al. 1968. Response to exercise after bed rest and after training. *Circulation* 38 (Suppl. 7):1–78.

101. Sharkey, B. 1970. Intensity and duration of training and the development of cardiorespiratory endurance. *Medicine and Science in Sports* 2:197–202.

102. ———. 1990. *Physiology of Fitness*. Champaign, IL: Human Kinetics.

103. Sjöström, M. et al. 1991. Evidence of fiber hyperplasia in human skeletal muscles from healthy young men. *European Journal of Applied Physiology* 62:301–4.

104. Smith, L. 1991. Acute inflammation: The underlying mechanism in delayed onset muscle soreness. *Medicine and Science in Sports and Exercise* 23:542–51.

105. Sola, O., D. Christensen, and A. Martin. 1973. Hypertrophy and hyperplasia of adult chicken anterior latissimus dorsi muscle following stretch with and without denervation. *Experimental Neurology* 41:76–100.

106. Starkey, D., M. Pollock, Y. Ishida, M. Welsch, W. Brechue, J. Graves, and M. Fiegenbaum. 1996. Effect of resistance exercise training volume on strength and muscle thickness. *Medicine and Science in Sports and Exercise* 28:1311–20.

107. Staron, R. et al. 1989. Muscle hypertrophy and fast fiber type conversions in heavy resistance-trained women. *European Journal of Applied Physiology* 60:71–79.

108. Stone, M. 1990. Muscle conditioning and muscle injuries. *Medicine and Science in Sports and Exercise* 22:457–62.

109. Stone, M., R. Johnson, and D. R. Carter. 1979. A short-term comparison of two different methods of resistance training on leg strength and power. *Athletic Training* 14:158–60.

110. Stone, M., and H. O'Bryant. 1986. *Weight Training: A Scientific Approach*. Minneapolis: Burgess.

111. Trzaskoma, Z. et al. 1992. Investigation of an experimental weight-training programme. *Journal of Sports Sciences* 10:109–17.

112. Wathen, D. 1980. A comparison of the effects of selected isotonic and isokinetic exercises, modalities, and programs on the vertical jump in college football players. *National Strength Coaches Association Journal* 2:47–48.

113. Wells, C., and R. Pate. 1988. Training for performance of prolonged exercise. In *Prolonged Exercise*, ed. D. Lamb and R. Murray, 357–88. Indianapolis: Benchmark Press.

114. Weltman, A. et al. 1990. Percentages of maximal heart rate, heart rate reserve, and $\dot{V}O_2$ max for determining endurance training intensity for male runners. *International Journal of Sports Medicine* 11:218–22.

115. Wilmore, J. 1974. Alterations in strength, body composition, and anthrometric measurements consequent to a 10-week weight training program. *Medicine and Science in Sports* 6:133–39.

116. Wilmore, J., and D. Costill. 1993. *Training for Sport and Activity*. New York: McGraw-Hill Companies.

117. Wolfe, B., L. LeMura, and P. Cole. 2004. Quantitative analysis of single-vs. multiple set programs in resistance training. *Journal of Strength and Conditioning Research* 18:35–47.

CHAPTER 22

Training for the Female Athlete, Children, and Special Populations

By studying this chapter, you should be able to do the following:

1. Describe the incidence of amenorrhea in female athletes versus the general population.
2. List those factors thought to contribute to "athletic" amenorrhea.
3. Discuss the general recommendations for training during menstruation.
4. List the general guidelines for exercise during pregnancy.
5. Define the term *female athlete triad*.
6. Discuss the possibility that chronic exercise presents a danger to: (1) the cardiopulmonary system or (2) the musculoskeletal system of children.
7. List those conditions in type 1 diabetics that might limit their participation in a vigorous training program.
8. Explain the rationale for the selection of an insulin injection site for type 1 diabetics prior to a training session.
9. List the precautions that asthmatics should take during a training session.
10. Discuss the question "Does exercise promote seizures in epileptics?"

Outline

Factors Important to Women Involved in Vigorous Training   464
   Exercise and Menstrual Disorders   464
   Training and Menstruation   465
   The Female Athlete and Eating Disorders   465
   Bone Mineral Disorders and the Female Athlete   466
   Training During Pregnancy   466

Risk of Knee Injury in Female Athletes   466

Sports Conditioning for Children   469
   Training and the Cardiopulmonary System   469
   Training and the Musculoskeletal System   469

Competitive Training for Diabetics   470

Training for Asthmatics   472

Epilepsy and Physical Training   472
   Does Exercise Promote Seizures?   473
   Risk of Injury Due to Seizures   473

Key Terms

amenorrhea
anorexia nervosa
articular cartilage
bulimia
dysmenorrhea
epilepsy
epiphyseal plate (growth plate)

Certainly the general physiological principles of exercise training to improve performance apply to anyone interested in improving athletic performance (see chapter 21). However, when planning competitive training programs for special populations, there are several specific issues that require individual consideration. For instance, there are special training concerns for both the female athlete and children. Also, there are specific guidelines for the training of diabetics, asthmatics, and epileptics. It is the purpose of this chapter to address each of these issues. Let's begin our discussion with the topic of exercise training for the female athlete.

FACTORS IMPORTANT TO WOMEN INVOLVED IN VIGOROUS TRAINING

The involvement of large numbers of women in competitive athletics has been a recent phenomenon. Over the past three decades, the number of women actively engaged in competitive athletics has increased exponentially. Unfortunately, many of the decisions regarding the participation of women in sports and exercise programs have been made on the basis of limited, or absent, physiological information. Research concerning women and exercise was scarce until recent years. Although many questions concerning the female athlete remain to be answered, current research indicates that there is no reason to limit the healthy female athlete from active participation in endurance or power sports (37). In fact, the general responses of females to exercise and training are essentially the same as those described for males (54), with the exception that exercise thermoregulation is moderately impaired in female athletes during the luteal phase of the menstrual cycle (61). The fact that men and women respond to exercise training in a similar manner is logical, since the cellular mechanisms that regulate most physiological and biochemical responses to exercise are the same for both sexes. However, there are several specific concerns related to female participation in vigorous training. In this section we will discuss four key issues related to the female athlete: (1) exercise and the menstrual cycle, (2) eating disorders, (3) bone mineral disorders, and (4) exercise during pregnancy.

Exercise and Menstrual Disorders

Over the past several years there have been increasing reports concerning the influence of intense exercise training on the length of the menstrual cycle (18, 19, 29, 32, 36, 51, 71). Indeed, there are numerous reports in the literature of female athletes who experience

"athletic" amenorrhea. The term **amenorrhea** refers to a cessation of menstruation; it is generally defined as less than four menses per year (49).

How common is athletic amenorrhea? It appears that the incidence of amenorrhea is higher in some activities than in others. For example, the occurrence of irregular menses is rather high in distance running and ballet dancing, while much lower incidences are reported for swimming and cycling (3, 49). For example, the incidence of amenorrhea in the general population is approximately 3%, while the incidence in distance runners is 24% (18).

What causes menstrual cycle dysfunction in athletes? The current belief is that the cause may vary among individual athletes and is probably due to multiple factors. Although some studies linked a low percentage of body fat with athletic amenorrhea (49), recent evidence does not fully support the notion that low body fat is the principal cause of amenorrhea (32, 71). Whatever the cause of amenorrhea in athletes, it appears to be related to the total amount of training (12, 29, 50). Figure 22.1 illustrates this point. As the weekly training distance increases, the incidence of athletic amenorrhea increases in proportion to the increase in training stress. This finding can be interpreted to mean that too much training either directly or indirectly influences the incidence of amenorrhea. There are at least two ways in which training might influence normal reproductive function. First, exercise alters blood concentrations of numerous hormones (42, 71), which may result in a modification of feedback to the hypothalamus (see chapter 5). This, in turn, may influence the release of female reproductive hormones and therefore modify the menstrual cycle (49). A second possibility is that high training mileage may result in increased psychological stress. Psychological stress may disrupt the menstrual cycle by increasing blood levels of catecholamines or endoge-

FIGURE 22.1 The relationship between training distance and the incidence of amenorrhea. Notice that as the training distance increases, there is a direct increase in the incidence of amenorrhea.

nous opiates, which play a role in regulating the reproductive system (49). For a review of the reproductive system and exercise in women, see Loucks et al. (1992) in the Suggested Readings.

Training and Menstruation

The consensus opinion among physicians is that there is little reason for the healthy female athlete to avoid training or competition during menses (37). Indeed, evidence exists that outstanding performances and world records have been established during all phases of the menstrual cycle (21). Therefore, it is not recommended that the female athlete alter her training or competitive schedule because of menses.

Dysmenorrhea (painful menstruation) can be problematic for female athletes. Several reports show that the incidence of dysmenorrhea is higher in athletic populations than in nonathletic groups (37). The explanation for this observation is unknown. However, it is possible that prostaglandins (a type of naturally occurring fatty acid) are responsible for dysmenorrhea in both athletes and nonathletes. The release of prostaglandins begins just prior to the onset of menstrual flow, and may last for two to three days after menses begins. These prostaglandins cause the smooth muscle in the uterus to contract, which in turn causes ischemia (reduced blood flow) and pain (37).

Although athletes who experience dysmenorrhea can continue to train, this is often difficult, since physical activity may increase the discomfort. Athletes who experience severe dysmenorrhea should see a physician for treatment. Hale (37) reports that athletes often experience a reduction in dysmenorrhea pain with the use of antiprostaglandin drugs. These drugs are considered safe and can be taken without interrupting training schedules.

The Female Athlete and Eating Disorders

The low social acceptance for individuals with a high percentage of body fat and an emphasis on having the "perfect" body have increased the incidence of eating disorders. Two of the more common eating disorders that affect both female and male athletes are anorexia nervosa and bulimia (76). Because of the relatively high occurrence of these eating disorders in female athletes, we discuss both the symptoms and health consequences of these abnormal eating behaviors.

Anorexia Nervosa **Anorexia nervosa** is a common eating disorder that is unrelated to any specific physical disease. The end result of extreme anorexia nervosa is a state of starvation in which the individual becomes emaciated due to a refusal to eat. The psychological cause of anorexia nervosa is unclear, but it

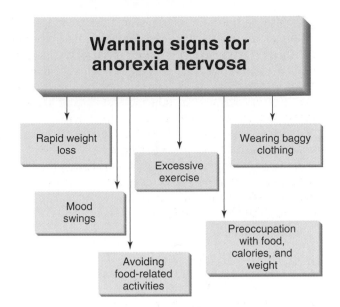

FIGURE 22.2 Warning signs for anorexia nervosa.

seems to be linked to an unfounded fear of fatness that may be related to family or societal pressures to be thin (74). The incidence of this eating disorder has grown in recent years. It appears that individuals with the highest probability of developing anorexia nervosa are upper-middle-class, young females who are extremely self critical. Currently, it is estimated that the incidence of anorexia nervosa is as high as one out of every 200 adolescent girls (3, 9).

The anorexic may use a variety of techniques to remain thin, including starvation, exercise, and laxatives (60, 76). The effects of anorexia include excessive weight loss, cessation of menstruation, and, in extreme cases, death. Since anorexia is a serious mental and physical disorder, medical treatment by a team of professionals (physician, psychologist, nutritionist) is necessary to correct the problem. Treatment may require years of psychological counseling and nutritional guidance. The first step in seeking professional treatment for anorexia nervosa is the recognition that a problem exists. Figure 22.2 illustrates the common symptoms of anorexia.

Bulimia **Bulimia** is overeating (called binge eating) followed by vomiting (called purging). The bulimic repeatedly ingests large quantities of food and then forces himself or herself to vomit in order to prevent weight gain. Bulimia may result in damage to the teeth and the esophagus due to vomiting of stomach acids. Like anorexia nervosa, bulimia is most common in female athletes, has a psychological origin, and requires professional treatment when diagnosed. Several authors indicate that the incidence of bulimia may be as low as 1% or as high as 20% among U.S. females aged thirteen to twenty-three (3, 9).

Warning signs for bulimia

- Noticeable weight loss
- Depressive moods
- Strict dieting followed by eating binges
- Excessive concern about weight
- Increasing criticism of one's body
- Bathroom visits after meals

FIGURE 22.3 Warning signs for bulimia.

Most bulimics look normal and are of normal weight. Even when their bodies are slender, their abdomens may protrude due to being stretched by frequent eating binges. Common symptoms of bulimia are illustrated in figure 22.3.

Eating Disorders: A Final Comment Eating disorders have become a major problem in female athletes. Some experts have estimated that as many as 50% of elite female athletes experience some type of eating disorder. The sports with the highest incidence of eating disorders are distance running, swimming, diving, figure skating, gymnastics, body building, and ballet. Although maintaining an optimal body composition for competition is important to achieve athletic success, eating disorders are not an appropriate means of weight loss. Therefore, trainers, athletes, and coaches need to recognize the warning signals of eating disorders and be prepared to assist the athlete in obtaining the appropriate help. For more details, see Penas-Lledo et al. (2002), Sundot-Borgen et al. (2002), and Yager and Andersen (2005) in the Suggested Readings.

Bone Mineral Disorders and the Female Athlete

A growing concern for the female athlete is the loss of bone mineral content (osteoporosis). In general, there are two major causes of bone loss in the female athlete (24, 25):

1. estrogen deficiency due to amenorrhea and
2. inadequate calcium intake due to eating disorders.

Unfortunately, many female athletes suffer a bone loss due to both amenorrhea and the inadequate calcium intake associated with an eating disorder (24, 25). Although exercise training has been shown to reduce the rate of bone loss due to estrogen deficiency and low calcium intake, exercise cannot completely reverse this process (53). Therefore, the only solution to the problem of bone mineral loss in the female athlete is to correct the estrogen deficiency and/or increase the calcium intake to normal levels. In both cases, a physician should be involved in prescribing the correct treatment for the individual athlete (see A Closer Look 22.1).

Training During Pregnancy

Chapter 17 provided a brief overview of what is currently known about exercising for fitness during pregnancy. While it is generally agreed that women who are physically fit prior to becoming pregnant may continue to perform moderate-intensity (short-duration) exercise during pregnancy (6, 11, 15, 23, 44, 48, 53, 66), controversy exists concerning the wisdom of high-intensity training for pregnant women. Although controversial, some animal studies have demonstrated that long-duration exercise (more than thirty minutes) during pregnancy results in a reduction in both uterine blood flow and fetal weight at term (16, 34, 56, 68). For example, one study reported that placental diffusion capacity decreases as a direct function of both the duration and intensity of exercise during pregnancy (34). At present it is unclear if these results can be extrapolated to humans, since pregnant women have performed maximal exercise with no apparent adverse effects on fetal or maternal outcome (6, 14). However, because of the limited number of studies examining the effect of heavy exercise on the health of mother and baby, more research is needed before firm exercise guidelines can be established. Until a definitive answer to this question is available, Hale (37) has recommended that the pregnant female be discouraged from engaging in prolonged or high-intensity training. For those athletes wishing to maintain fitness during pregnancy, Hale recommends aquatic programs, since swimming or other forms of aquatic exercise allow cardiovascular training in a medium that offers the body support and accelerated heat transfer. Specific guidelines for exercise to maintain fitness during pregnancy were listed in chapter 17 (see table 17.3).

Risk of Knee Injury in Female Athletes

Knee injuries are common in many sports. Although the risk of knee injuries varies across sports, studies reveal that compared to males, female athletes are at

A CLOSER LOOK 22.1

The Female Athlete Triad

It generally accepted that three of the most common health problems facing the young female athlete are (1) amenorrhea, (2) eating disorders, and (3) bone mineral loss. Collectively, these problems are interrelated and are called the female athlete triad (8, 59, 72). Growing evidence indicates that these problems are linked and that one problem can promote another (8, 10, 59, 71, 72). For example, an eating disorder can lead to inadequate nutrient intake resulting in a diminished intake of calcium and vitamin D. Further, eating disorders are known to contribute to amenorrhea, and long-term amenorrhea is associated with low blood levels of estrogen (71). Importantly, the combination of inadequate calcium/vitamin D intake and low estrogen levels can result in a loss of bone mineral content.

At present, researchers do not completely understand the cause of the female athlete triad. However, evidence indicates that the three corners of the female athlete triad are interrelated through both psychological and physiological mechanisms. These interactions are illustrated in figure 22.4. For example, psychological pressures to perform well in athletic competition, coupled with the physiological stress of intense exercise training, can lead to eating disorders and an energy imbalance. Although the causes of menstrual disorders are multiple, it seems that the amenorrhea observed in many female athletes is due a negative energy balance due to both an eating disorder and intense exercise training (8). Collectively, this stress results in disturbances in the hormones that regulate the menstrual cycle, and if energy availability continues to be low over a prolonged period of time, the menstrual cycle is temporarily "switched

FIGURE 22.4 Interrelationships between the three components that comprise the female athlete triad. It is believed that a combination of both psychological and physiological stress can lead to eating disorders and energy imbalance in female athletes. This energy imbalance, coupled with other stresses (psychological and physiological), can promote menstrual problems such as amenorrhea. Amenorrhea is associated with lowered blood levels of estrogen, which increases the risk of bone mineral loss. Further, decreased energy intake may lead to deficiencies in both calcium and vitamin D consumption and also contribute to a loss of bone minerals.

off" to conserve energy (8). The ensuing amenorrhea results in reduced production of estrogen by the ovaries and low blood levels of estrogen. Since estrogen protects the skeleton from bone resorption, reduced estrogen increases the risk of bone mineral loss (8, 71). Collectively, low estrogen levels and deficiencies of calcium and vitamin D (due to eating disorders) places the female athlete at great risk for osteopenia (loss of bone mineral density) (8).

What is the incidence of the female athlete triad among athletic women? A recent study involving female athletes from a variety of sports concluded that approximately 4% of all female athletes meet the criteria for the female athlete triad by exhibiting an eating disorder, amenorrhea, and bone mineral loss (69). Further, as many as 26% of these female athletes possessed at least two of the components of the female ath-

lete triad. Interestingly, this study also revealed that as many as 3% of nonathletic women (ages 13–29) may also suffer from all three components of the triad (69). Therefore, the health problems associated with the female athlete triad are not limited to athletes alone.

Growing evidence indicates that each component of the female athlete triad develops on a continuum and the triad may occur in stages (22). If early stages are not treated properly, they can progress toward the extremes of the triad. Therefore, protection of the female athlete's health from the triad is dependent upon early detection of symptoms of one or more of the components of the triad and successful treatment of the problem. For more details on the female athlete triad, please see Birch (2005) and Waldrop (2005) in the Suggested Readings.

higher risk for knee injury in jumping and cutting sports (e.g., basketball, volleyball, soccer, etc.) (26). In particular, knee injuries such as anterior cruciate ligament (ACL) injuries occur at a higher rate in female athletes compared to male athletes at a similar level of competition (26, 77). For example, in a study of male and female professional basketball players, female athletes suffered 60% more ACL injuries than males (77). This increased risk of knee injury in female athletes is not limited to professional athletes and impacts both collegiate and high school athletes as well (26, 55, 78). For example, National Collegiate Athletic Association statistics reveal that women sustain ACL injuries at a rate that is almost four times higher than men in basketball and 2.4 times higher than men in soccer (26).

Why are females at a greater risk for ACL injuries? Unfortunately, a definitive answer to this question is not available. However, it has been speculated that several factors may play a role in placing women at higher risk for knee injuries; these include fluctuation in sex hormones during the menstrual cycle, gender differences in knee anatomy, and dynamic neuromuscular imbalances (26). A discussion of the evidence to support each of these potential risk factors follows.

In reference to sex hormones and knee injuries, studies reveal that the risk of ACL injury is increased in female athletes during the follicular and ovulatory phase of the menstrual cycle (26). However, the direct link between sex hormones and the increased risk of tear of the ACL remains unclear. In this regard, some investigators propose that sex hormones influence the structure of the ACL, perhaps compromising both the strength of the ligament and/or proprioceptive feedback (26). Nonetheless, direct evidence to support this concept is limited.

Studies investigating gender differences in knee anatomy as a determinant of the risk of knee injuries have failed to provide definitive evidence that anatomical explanations are responsible for gender differences in the rate of knee injuries. For example, although women are more likely to have knee joint laxity (loose joint) than men, this fact has not been correlated to the higher rate of knee injury in women (26). Therefore, it does not appear that gender differences in knee anatomy can explain why females are at higher risk for ACL injuries.

Dynamic neuromuscular imbalance in the knee is an area of research related to ACL tears in women that continues to grow. Dynamic neuromuscular imbalance refers to a combination of imbalanced factors including muscular strength, proprioception, and landing biomechanics. In regard to muscle strength, women have less quadriceps and hamstring strength than men, even when normalizing for body weight (43). This is significant because exercises that strengthen both the quadriceps and hamstring mus-

cles provide protection against knee injury (39). Evidence also exists that the higher incidence of knee injury in women compared to men may be linked to an imbalance in knee proprioceptive and neuromuscular control in female athletes (26). Nonetheless, more detailed studies are required before a firm conclusion can be reached on the role that proprioception plays in gender differences in knee injury. Finally, published reports reveal that women run, jump, and land differently than men when playing sports (26). This is important because the usual mechanism for noncontact ACL injury involves a deceleration in limb speed before changing directions or landing with the knee between full extension and 20 degrees of flexion (26). In this regard, compared to males, female athletes have been shown to land with knee angles that pose a greater risk of ACL injury (26). Therefore, a neuromuscular difference between males and females that impacts landing or other movement strategies may partly explain why female athletes are at greater risk for knee injuries in sports compared to male athletes.

In summary, compared to men, female athletes are at high risk for certain types of knee injuries (e.g., ACL injury). Current evidence suggests that male/female differences in dynamic neuromuscular imbalance (e.g., leg muscle strength, jumping and landing strategies) may contribute to gender differences in the risk of knee injuries. For a detailed discussion of this topic, please see Dugan (2005) in the Suggested Readings.

IN SUMMARY

- The incidence of amenorrhea in female athletes appears to be highest in distance runners and ballet dancers when compared to other sports. Although the cause of amenorrhea in female athletes is not clear, it appears likely that multiple factors (e.g., the amount of training and psychological stress) are involved.
- There appears to be little reason for female athletes to avoid training during menstruation unless they experience severe discomfort due to dysmenorrhea. Athletes who experience severe dysmenorrhea should see a physician for treatment.
- Some experts have estimated that as many as 50% of elite female athletes experience some type of eating disorder. Two of the more common eating disorders are anorexia nervosa and bulimia.
- The three most common health problems facing the young female athlete are amenorrhea, eating disorders, and bone mineral loss; collectively, these problems have been called the "female athlete triad."

Risk of Sudden Cardiac Death in Young Athletes

In healthy young athletes, the risk of sudden cardiac injury or death during participation in sports or exercise is very small. In the United States, approximately ten to thirteen cases of sudden cardiac death are reported each year (64). Given that approximately four million young people are involved in competitive sports in the United States, this places the statistical chance of an apparently healthy adolescent dying from unexpected cardiac death at 1 in 250,000 (64).

Four cardiovascular abnormalities account for the majority of sudden cardiac deaths in young athletes: (1) hypertrophic cardiomyopathy (pathologically enlarged heart); (2) congenital (inherited) abnormalities of the coronary arteries; (3) aortic aneurysms; and (4) congenital stenosis (narrowing) of the aortic valve (64).

Can a medical exam identify athletes at risk for sudden death? In many cases, yes. A medical history and a physical exam from a qualified physician are excellent tools for detecting heart disease that could pose a risk for the young athlete participating in sports. However, some cardiac abnormalities that can cause death during sports participation are difficult to detect during routine medical examination (64). Nonetheless, a medical exam along with a cardiac evaluation can potentially reduce the risk of sudden cardiac death by identifying those young athletes who are predisposed to cardiac injury (31).

- Short-term, low-intensity exercise does not appear to have negative consequences during pregnancy. However, data suggest that long-duration or high-intensity training should be avoided during pregnancy.
- Female athletes are at greater risk for knee injuries compared to males. Evidence suggests that male/female differences in dynamic neuromuscular imbalance (e.g., differences in leg muscle strength and/or jumping and landing strategies) may contribute to gender differences in the risk of knee injuries.

SPORTS CONDITIONING FOR CHILDREN

There are many unanswered questions about the physiologic responses of the healthy child to various types of exercise. This is due to the limited number of investigators studying children and exercise, and because of ethical considerations in studying children. For instance, few investigators would puncture a child's artery, take a muscle biopsy, or expose a child to harsh environments (e.g., heat, cold, high altitudes) to satisfy scientific curiosity. Because of these ethical constraints, current knowledge concerning training for children is limited primarily to the cardiopulmonary system, with a growing body of information concerning the possibility of musculoskeletal injury as a result of specific types of sports training. The following discussion addresses some of the important issues concerning child participation in vigorous conditioning programs.

Training and the Cardiopulmonary System

As youth sports teams increase in popularity, one of the first questions asked is "Are the hearts of children strong enough for intensive sports conditioning?" In other words, is there a possibility of "overtraining" young athletes, with the end result being permanent damage to the cardiovascular system? The answer to this question is no. Children involved in endurance sports such as running or swimming improve their maximal aerobic power comparable to adults and show no indices of damage to the cardiopulmonary system (27, 28, 40, 58, 63). Over the past several years, children have safely trained and completed marathon runs in less than four hours. If proper techniques of physical training are employed, with a progressive increase in cardiopulmonary stress, children appear to adapt to endurance training in a fashion similar to adults (27, 28, 52, 63). (See Clinical Applications 22.1.)

Training and the Musculoskeletal System

Organized vigorous training in some types of sports (e.g., swimming, basketball, volleyball, track and field) does not appear to adversely affect growth and development in children (52). This is true for both boys (28) and girls (4). In fact, moderate physical training has been shown to augment or optimize growth in children (1, 4, 27, 28). Therefore, many investigators have concluded that a certain amount of physical activity is necessary for normal growth and development (1, 4, 52). However, is there danger of overtraining? Can children perform heavy endurance training or strength training without long-term musculoskeletal problems? This

FIGURE 22.5 Location of the growth plate (epiphyseal plate) associated with the long bones in the leg.

issue remains controversial. There is evidence that the growing bones of a child are more susceptible to certain types of mechanical injury than those of the adult, primarily because of the presence of growth cartilage (52). Growth cartilage is present at the growth plate **(epiphyseal plate), articular cartilage** (cartilage at joints), and the sites of major muscle-tendon insertion in the child (52). The location of the growth plate for the knee joint is illustrated in figure 22.5. The growth plate is the site of bone growth in long bones. The time at which bone growth ceases varies from bone to bone, but growth is generally complete by eighteen to twenty years of age (52). Upon completion of growth, growth plates ossify (harden with calcium) and disappear, and growth cartilage is replaced by a permanent "adult" cartilage.

Is there an optimal level of training for children, above which musculoskeletal injuries may occur? The apparent answer to this question is yes. Clinical evidence suggests that excessive throwing in organized youth league baseball may result in injury to the elbow (Little League elbow) (52). This same problem is not observed in free-play situations (52). Indeed, new injury patterns are developing in children as the number of children participating in organized sports increases (2). A statement from the American College of Sports Medicine indicated that up to 50% of all injuries sustained by children while playing organized sports could be avoided by attention to proper train-

ing techniques, safety procedures, and proper use of safety equipment (2).

A major concern for children participating in endurance training (e.g., running) or strength training (e.g., weight lifting) is that the constant microtrauma of repetitive training can cause premature closure of the growth plate and therefore retard normal long bone growth. Experimental literature on training and specific bone lengths indicates reduced bone lengths in rats and mice exposed to forced swimming and running (52). Corresponding data on humans do not exist. However, given the evidence available on the influence of physical activity on bone growth and development, it appears that the advice Steinhaus (65) offered over seventy years ago is sound. That is, the pressure effects of regular physical activity may stimulate bone growth to an optimal length, but excessive pressure (overtraining) can retard linear growth. The practical problem in dealing with young athletes is that it is difficult to define excessive pressure. In other words, how much training is optimal to bring about the desired physiological training responses without causing musculoskeletal problems? At present, a simple answer to this question is not available. There is an obvious need for detailed research in this area to produce guidelines for youth coaches and trainers in the development of conditioning programs for children engaged in competitive athletics. For more information about children and exercise, see Ask the Expert 22.1.

IN SUMMARY

- Although physical activity has been shown to optimize growth in children, questions remain as to the possibility of overtraining with resultant injuries to the musculoskeletal system. In particular, there is evidence that the growing bones of children are more susceptible to certain types of mechanical injury due to the presence of growth cartilage.

COMPETITIVE TRAINING FOR DIABETICS

As discussed in chapter 17, there is a beneficial effect of exercise on diabetes, and physicians often recommend regular exercise for diabetics as a part of their therapeutic regimen (i.e., to help maintain control of blood glucose levels) (30). We will limit our discussion to type 1 diabetics, since type 2 diabetics are less likely to engage in training for performance purposes. Can type 1 diabetics train vigorously and take part in competitive athletics? The answer to this question is a qualified yes. In long-term diabetic patients

Children and Exercise
Questions and Answers with Dr. Oded Bar-Or

Oded Bar-Or, M.D., *professor in the Department of Pediatrics at McMaster University in Hamilton, Ontario, Canada, is an internationally known pediatric physician and scientist in the field of pediatric exercise physiology. Further, Dr. Bar-Or has been a professional leader in numerous scientific organizations including the American College of Sports Medicine. A significant portion of Dr. Bar-Or's research has focused on issues related to pediatric exercise. Without question, Dr. Bar-Or's research team has performed many of the "pioneering" studies that explore the physiological responses of children during exercise. In this box feature, Dr. Bar-Or answers questions related to a variety of topics linked to pediatric exercise.*

QUESTION 1: Based on the current medical evidence, what is your advice about the wisdom of children and adolescents participating in strength-training programs?

ANSWER: The short answer to this question is that strength training is both effective and safe for adolescents. For example, there is strong evidence that even before puberty, resistance training results in strength gains in children. In fact, relative to their strength prior to beginning a training program, prepubescents have a similar, or often greater, percentage improvement in strength, compared with adolescents or young adults.

Regarding safety, recent studies suggest that strength training in children causes no damage to bones, joints, or tendons. While not backed by scientific evidence, it is commonly recommended that children should not use weights (or other resistance devices) that are extremely heavy. Practically speaking, this translates to a weight that can be lifted at least seven to ten repetitions in each set of exercises. Unfortunately, there is insufficient information about the safety of weight lifting (e.g., Olympic style) for children.

QUESTION 2: Do sweat rates and body temperatures differ between adults and children during prolonged exercise?

ANSWER: Compared with adults, children's heat dissipation during prolonged exercise relies more on convection and radiation (through increased blood flow to the skin) and less on evaporation of sweat. While children often have more sweat glands per square centimeter of body surface area, the amount of sweat produced by each gland is only 40% that of adults. In spite of their low evaporative capacity, children are effective temperature regulators when exercise is performed in cool, neutral, or even warm environments. It is only when air temperature exceeds skin temperature by 7° to 10° C (e.g., air temperature more than 40° C), that children have a lower tolerance to prolonged exercise, compared with adults.

QUESTION 3: Given that children lose fluid via sweating and/or urine formation during exercise, what are your recommendations about providing fluids and/or sports drinks to children during active sports participation?

ANSWER: Like adults, children who perform prolonged exercise, particularly on hot or humid days, can lose large amounts of body water resulting in "involuntary dehydration." Consuming adequate amounts of fluid following exercise can counteract this type of dehydration. Enhanced drinking in children following exercise can be achieved through three means: (1) an increase in a drink's palatability (which depends on temperature, color, and flavor), (2) stimulation of osmoreceptors in the hypothalamus and gastrointestinal tract, and (3) education about the importance of drinking fluids.

During exercise, people prefer cool beverages (e.g., 15° C or lower). Preferred flavors vary among children. Flavor is important, as adding flavor to tap water can increase voluntary drinking by 40% to 50%. Addition of salt (NaCl) will stimulate osmoreceptors and further enhance drinking. In one study, addition of flavor, sodium chloride (18 mmol/L NaCl), and carbohydrate (e.g., similar to a sport drink) increased the voluntary drinking by 90% in boys who exercised intermittently in the heat for three hours.

"Education" denotes teaching a child to drink every fifteen to twenty minutes during and following a prolonged exercise event. A practical guideline for quantity is: "drink until you are no longer thirsty and then add a few extra gulps." A child who weighs 40 kg or less should add approximately 100 ml beyond thirst. A larger child should drink another 200 ml of fluid.

---

with microvascular complications (damage to small blood vessels) or neuropathy (nerve damage), exercise should be limited and extensive training is not generally recommended (52). However, in individuals who maintain good blood glucose control and are free from other medical complications, diabetes in itself should not limit the type of exercise or sporting event (67).

What precautions should the diabetic athlete take to allow safe participation in training programs? An overview of exercise training for fitness in diabetic populations was presented in chapter 17 and will be reviewed here only briefly. The key to safe participation in sport conditioning for the diabetic athlete is to learn to avoid hypoglycemic episodes during training. Since diabetics vary in their response to insulin, each diabetic athlete, in cooperation with his or her personal physician, must determine the appropriate combination of exercise, diet, and insulin for optimal control of blood glucose concentrations. In general, exercise should take place after a meal and should be part of regular routine. It is often recommended that a reduction in the amount of insulin injected be considered on days in which the athlete is engaged in strenuous training (30, 62, 67). A major concern for the diabetic athlete is the site of the insulin injection prior to exercise. Insulin injected subcutaneously in the leg prior to running (or other forms of leg exercise) results in an increased rate of insulin uptake due to elevated leg blood flow. This could result in exercise-induced hypoglycemia and may be avoided by using an insulin injection site in the abdomen or the arm (69). Conversely, if the training regimen requires arm exercise (e.g., rowing), the site of insulin injection should be away from the working muscle (e.g., abdomen). Having a glucose solution or carbohydrate snack available during training sessions may help avoid hypoglycemic incidents during workouts.

Can diabetics obtain the same benefits from training as nondiabetics? The consensus answer to this question is yes. Although untrained, diabetic children tend to be less fit than normal children (45), young diabetics respond to a conditioning program in a manner similar to healthy children (52). Empirical observations suggest that when the diabetic athlete's blood glucose is carefully regulated, he or she can compete and excel in a variety of competitive sports.

IN SUMMARY

- Type 1 diabetics who are free of diabetic complications should not be limited in the type or quantity of exercise.
- The key for safe sports participation for the type 1 diabetic is for the athlete to learn to avoid hypoglycemic episodes.

TRAINING FOR ASTHMATICS

It is generally agreed that most children, adolescents, and adults with asthma can safely participate in all sports with the exception of SCUBA diving, provided they are able to control exercise-induced bronchospasms via medication or careful monitoring of activity levels (17, 52). A prerequisite for planning

training programs for asthmatics is that the proper therapeutic regimen for managing the athlete's particular type of asthma be worked out prior to commencement of a vigorous training program (see chapter 17). Once the asthma is under control, planning the training schedule for asthmatic athletes is identical to planning for athletes without asthma (see chapter 21). However, as mentioned in chapter 17, it is often recommended that the asthmatic athlete keep an inhaler (containing a bronchodilator) handy during training sessions, and that workouts be conducted with other athletes in case a major attack occurs.

The issue of the safety of an asthmatic participating in SCUBA diving continues to be debated. The controversy centers around the fact that divers who experience an asthma attack while diving are at high risk for pulmonary barotrauma (damage to the lung due to high pressure) (17). However, a recent review on the subject suggests that asthmatics with normal airway function at rest who do not exhibit exercise-induced asthma have a risk of barotrauma during diving similar to that of healthy individuals (17).

IN SUMMARY

- Asthmatics can safely participate in all sports with the possible exception of SCUBA diving, provided they are able to control exercise-induced bronchospasms via medication or careful monitoring of activity levels.
- The question of the safety of an asthmatic participating in SCUBA diving continues to be unanswered. Nonetheless, recent evidence suggests that asthmatics who do not exhibit exercise-induced asthma and have normal airways at rest are at no greater risk during diving than are healthy individuals.

EPILEPSY AND PHYSICAL TRAINING

The term **epilepsy** refers to a transient disturbance of brain function, which may be characterized by a loss of consciousness, muscle tremor, and sensory disturbances. Since the occurrence of epileptic seizures is not easily predicted, should epileptics engage in vigorous training programs? Unfortunately, there is little information available to answer this question. Before a clear-cut recommendation for the participation of epileptics in athletics can be made, two fundamental questions must be answered. First, does intense physical activity increase the risk of an epileptic seizure? Second, does the occurrence of a seizure during a particular sports activity expose the athlete to unnecessary risk? Let's examine the available evidence concerning each of these questions.

Does Exercise Promote Seizures?

There is one rare type of epileptic seizure that has been shown to be induced by exercise per se (13). These are tonic (continuous motor activity) seizures, which have been reported to occur during a variety of sports activities. Fortunately, this type of seizure can be controlled in most instances by anticonvulsant drugs.

As for other types of seizure disorders, physicians remain divided in their opinions as to whether exercise increases the risk of seizure occurrence. A report by Gotze et al. (35) suggests that exercise does not increase the risk of seizures in epileptic children or adolescents. In fact, Gotze (35) argues that exercise appears to reduce the incidence of seizures in epileptics by increasing the threshold for seizures. In support of these claims, a review (70) on epilepsy and sports has concluded that there is a reduction in the number of seizures during exercise. In contrast, Kuijer (46) has suggested that the epileptic is at an increased risk of experiencing a seizure during exercise and during recovery from exercise. In this regard, several factors related to exercise have been hypothesized to increase the risk of seizures (70): (1) physical fatigue, (2) hyperventilation, (3) hypoxia, (4) hyperthermia, (5) hypoglycemia, and (6) electrolyte imbalance. In conclusion, division exists in the medical community concerning the risk of exercise and seizures. It seems logical that generalizations about exercise and the epileptic patient cannot be made. Each patient is unique concerning the type, frequency, and severity of epileptic seizures. Therefore, physicians, parents, and coaches must make case-by-case decisions on the wisdom of competitive sports for individual patients.

Another specific concern for the participation of epileptics in contact sports is whether a blow to the head might mediate a seizure. Again, physicians remain divided in their opinions. Some authors believe the risks are high (41), while Livingston (47) argues that no studies exist to prove that repeated head trauma in epileptics causes a recurrence of seizures. Livingston's argument is based on thirty-six years of personal experience with hundreds of seizure patients who have participated in a variety of contact sports such as football, wrestling, and even boxing. While all of these contact sports predispose the athlete to head trauma, Livingston (47) states that he has not observed a single case wherein recurrent seizures occurred due to head trauma.

Risk of Injury Due to Seizures

Clearly, there are many competitive sports activities (e.g., football, boxing) during which the occurrence of a seizure would expose the athlete to a risk of harm. However, the occurrence of a seizure during many types of daily routine activities (e.g., climbing stairs) or recreational sports (e.g., SCUBA diving, mountain climbing) could also pose a threat to the epileptic. Whether or not the epileptic should participate in physical training or sports must be determined on an individual basis by the use of common sense and advice from a sports physician. The benefit-risk ratio of sports participation may vary greatly from case to case and is dependent on the exact nature of the patient's epilepsy and the sport being considered. A child with only a minor seizure problem may, with the aid of medication, experience only a rare seizure with little visible alteration in behavior or consciousness due to the seizure. This type of epileptic could likely participate in most training activities without harm (7, 35). In contrast, an epileptic who experiences frequent and major seizures would not be a candidate for many types of sports. For a detailed discussion of epilepsy and exercise, see van Linschoten et al. (70).

IN SUMMARY

- Questions about safe participation for epileptics in training programs must be answered on an individual basis. The benefit-risk ratio of sports participation may vary greatly from case to case and depends on the type of epilepsy involved and the sport being considered.

STUDY QUESTIONS

1. Outline several possible causes of "athletic" amenorrhea.
2. What is the current recommendation for training and competition during menstruation?
3. Discuss the role of prostaglandins in mediating dysmenorrhea.
4. Based on present information, what are reasonable guidelines for advising the pregnant athlete concerning the intensity and duration of training?
5. Define the *female athlete triad*.
6. What factors contribute to bone mineral loss in the female athlete?
7. Discuss the notion that intense exercise might result in permanent damage to (a) the cardiovascular system or (b) the musculoskeletal system in children.
8. What is the recommendation for type 1 diabetics with no physical complications for entering a competitive training program?
9. What factors should be considered when advising the diabetic athlete concerning safe participation in

athletic conditioning? Include in your discussion suggestions concerning meal timing, injection sites for insulin, and the availability of glucose drinks during training sessions.

10. What is the current opinion concerning the safe participation of asthmatics in competitive athletics?

11. Define the term *epilepsy*.
12. Discuss the possibility that exercise increases the risk of seizures for epileptics.
13. What factors should be considered in assessing the risk-to-benefit ratio of sports participation for epileptics?

SUGGESTED READINGS

Birch, K. 2005. Female athlete triad. *British Journal of Sports Medicine* 330:244–46.

Brooks, G., T. Fahey, and K. Baldwin. 2005. *Exercise Physiology: Human Bioenergetics and Its Applications*, 4th ed. New York: McGraw-Hill Companies.

Dugan, S. 2005. Sports-related knee injuries in female athletes. *American Journal of Physical Medicine and Rehabilitation* 84:122–31.

Fahey, P. et al. 1996. The athlete with type 1 diabetes: Managing insulin, diet, and exercise. *American Family Physician* 55:1611–17.

Otis, C. et al. 1997. American College of Sports Medicine position stand. The female athlete triad. *Medicine in Science in Sports and Medicine* 29:I–ix.

Penas-Lledo, E. et al. 2002. Excessive exercise in anorexia nervosa and bulimia nervosa: Relationship to eating characteristics and general psycholopathology. *International Journal of Eating Disorders* 31:370–75.

Sundgot-Borgen, J. et al. 2002. The effect of exercise, cognitive therapy and nutritional counseling in treating bulimia nervosa. *Medicine and Science in Sports and Exercise* 34:190–95.

Yager J., and A. Andersen. 2005. Anorexia nervosa. *New England Journal of Medicine* 353:1481–88.

Waldrop, J. 2005. Early indentification and interventions for female athlete triad. *Journal of Pediatric Health Care* 19:213–20.

Warren, M., and L. Goodman. 2003. Exercise-induced endocrine pathologies. *Journal of Endocrinological Investigation* 26:873–78.

REFERENCES

1. Adams, E. 1938. A comparative anthropometric study of hard labor during youth as a stimulator of physical growth of young colored women. *Research Quarterly* 9:102–8.

2. American College of Sports Medicine. 1993. Current comment on the prevention of sport injuries of children and adolescents. *Medicine and Science in Sports and Exercise* 25 (Suppl.):1–7.

3. Andersen, A. 1983. Anorexia nervosa and bulimia. *Journal of Adolescent Health Care* 4:15–21.

4. Åstrand, P. O. et al. 1963. Girl swimmers. *Acta Paediatric Scandanavica* 147(Suppl.):1–75.

5. Baker, E. 1981. Menstrual dysfunction and hormonal status in athletic women: A review. *Fertility and Sterility* 36:691–96.

6. Beilock, S. L., D. L. Feltz, and J. M. Pivarnik. 2001. Training patterns of athletes during pregnancy and postpartum. *Research Quarterly for Exercise and Sport* 72:39–46.

7. Bennett, D. 1981. Sports and epilepsy: To play or not to play. *Seminars in Neurology* 1:345–57.

8. Birch, K. 2005. Female athlete triad. *British Journal of Sports Medicine* 330:244–46.

9. Borgen, J., and C. Corbin. 1987. Eating disorders among female athletes. *Physician and Sportsmedicine* 15:89–95.

10. Brooks, G., T. Fahey, and K. Baldwin. 2005. *Exercise Physiology: Human Bioenergetics and Its Applications*, 4th ed. New York. McGraw-Hill Companies.

11. Bullard, J. 1981. Exercise and pregnancy. *Canadian Family Physician* 27:977–82.

12. Bullen, B. et al. 1985. Induction of menstrual disorders by strenuous exercise in untrained women. *New England Journal of Medicine* 312:1349–53.

13. Burger, L., R. Lopez, and F. Elliot. 1972. Tonic seizures induced by movement. *Neurology* 22:656–59.

14. Carpenter, M. et al. 1988. Fetal heart rate response to maternal exertion. *Journal of the American Medical Association* 259:3006.

15. Clapp, J. et al. 1992. Exercise in pregnancy. *Medicine and Science in Sports and Exercise* 24:S294–S300.

16. Curet, L. et al. 1976. Effect of exercise on cardiac output and distribution of uterine blood flow in pregnant ewes. *Journal of Applied Physiology* 40:725–28.

17. Cypcar, D., and R. Lemanske. 1994. Asthma and exercise. *Clinics in Chest Medicine* 15:351–68.

18. Dale, E., D. Gerlach, and A. Wilhute. 1979. Menstrual dysfunction in distance runners. *Obstetrics and Gynecology* 54:47–53.

19. Dale, E. et al. 1979. Physical fitness profiles and reproductive physiology of the female distance runner. *Physician and Sportsmedicine* 7:83–95.

20. Davies, B., D. Bailey, R. Budgett, D. Sanderson, and D. Griffin. 1999. Intensive training during a twin pregnancy. A case report. *International Journal of Sports Medicine* 20:415–18.

21. De Souza, M., and D. Metzger. 1991. Reproductive dysfunction in amenorrheic athletes and anorexic patients: A review. *Medicine and Science in Sports and Exercise* 23:995–1007.

22. De Souza. 2003. Menstrual disturbances in athletes: A focus on luteal phase defects. *Medicine and Science in Sports and Exercise* 35:1553–63.

23. Dressendorfer, R. 1978. Physical training during pregnancy and lactation. *Physician and Sportsmedicine* 6:74–80.

24. Drinkwater, B. 1990. Menstrual history as a determinant of current bone density in young athletes. *Journal of the American Medical Association* 263:545–48.

25. Drinkwater, B. et al. 1984. Bone mineral content of amenorrheic and eumenorrheic athletes. *New England Journal of Medicine* 311:277–81.

26. Dugan, S. 2005. Sports-related knee injuries in female athletes. *American Journal of Physical Medicine and Rehabilitation* 84:122–31.

27. Ekblom, B. 1969. Effect of physical training on oxygen transport system in man. *Acta Physiologica Scandanavica* 328(Suppl.):1–45.

28. Eriksson, B. 1972. Physical training, oxygen supply and muscle metabolism in 11–13 year-old boys. *Acta Physiologica Scandanavica* 384(Suppl.):1–48.

29. Feicht, C. et al. 1978. Secondary amenorrhea in athletes. *Lancet* 2:1145–46.

30. Felig, P., and V. Koivisto. 1979. The metabolic response to exercise: Implications for diabetes. In *Therapeutics through Exercise*, ed. D. Lowenthal, K. Bharadwaja, and W. Oaks. New York: Grune & Stratton.

31. Franklin, B., G. Fletcher, N. Gordon, T. Noakes, P. Ades, and G. Balady. 1997. Cardiovascular evaluation of the athlete. *Sports Medicine* 24:97–119.

32. Galle, P. et al. 1983. Physiologic and psychologic profiles in a survey of women runners. *Fertility and Sterility* 39:633–39.

33. Gidwani, G. 1999. Amenorrhea in the athlete. *Adolescent Medicine* 10:275–90.

34. Gilbert, R. et al. 1979. Placental diffusing capacity and fetal development in exercising or hypoxic guinea pigs. *Journal of Applied Physiology* 46:828–34.

35. Gotze, W., S. Kubicki, and M. Munter. 1967. Effect of physical activity on seizure threshold investigated by electroencephalographic telemetry. *Diseases of the Nervous System* 28:664–67.

36. Gray, D., and E. Dale. 1983. Variables associated with secondary amenorrhea in women runners. *Journal of Sports Sciences* 1:55–67.

37. Hale, R. 1984. Factors important to women engaged in vigorous physical activity. In *Sports Medicine*, ed. R. Strauss. Philadelphia: W. B. Saunders.

38. Hartmann, S., and P. Bung. 1999. Physical exercise during pregnancy—physiological considerations and recommendations. *Journal of Perinatal Medicine* 27:204–15.

39. Hewett, T. et al. 1999. The effect of neuromuscular training on the incidence of knee injury in female athletes. A prospective study. *American Journal of Sports Medicine* 27:699–706.

40. Ingjer, F. 1992. Development of maximal oxygen uptake in young elite cross-country skiers: A longitudinal study. *Journal of Sports Sciences* 10:49–63.

41. Jennett, B. 1974. Early traumatic epilepsy: Incidence and significance after non-muscle injuries. *Archives of Neurology* 30:394–98.

42. Jurkowski, J. et al. 1978. Ovarian hormonal responses to exercise. *Journal of Applied Physiology* 44:109–14.

43. Kanehisa, H. et al. 1996. Sex difference in force generation capacity during repeated maximal knee extensions. *European Journal of Applied Physiology* 73:557–62.

44. Kolata, G. 1983. Exercise during pregnancy reassessed. *Science* 219:832–33.

45. Komatsu, W. et al. 2005. Aerobic exercise capacity in normal adolescents and those with type 1 diabetes mellitus. *Pediatric Diabetes* 6:145–49.

46. Kuijer, A. 1980. Epilepsy and exercise, electroencephalographical and biochemical studies. In *Advances in Epileptology: The X Epilepsy International Symposium*, ed. J. Wada and J. Penry. New York: Raven Press.

47. Livingston, S., and W. Berman. 1973. Participation of epileptic patients in sports. *Journal of the American Medical Association* 224:236–38.

48. Lokey, E. et al. 1991. Effects of physical exercise on pregnancy outcomes: A meta-analytic review. *Medicine and Science in Sports and Exercise* 23:1234–39.

49. Loucks, A., and S. Horvath. 1985. Athletic amenorrhea: A review. *Medicine and Science in Sports and Exercise* 17:56–72.

50. Loucks, A. et al. 1992. The reproductive system and exercise in women. *Medicine and Science in Sports and Exercise* 24:S288–93.

51. Lutter, J., and S. Cushman. 1982. Menstrual patterns in female runners. *Physician and Sportsmedicine* 10:60–72.

52. Micheli, L. 1984. *Pediatric and Adolescent Sports Medicine*. Philadelphia: W. B. Saunders.

53. Micklesfield, L. et al. 1995. Bone mineral density in mature, premenopausal ultramarathon runners. *Medicine and Science in Sports and Exercise* 27:688–96.

54. Mitchell, J. et al. 1992. Acute response and chronic adaptation to exercise in women. *Medicine and Science in Sports and Exercise* 24:S258–S265.

55. National Federation of High School Associations. 2002. High school participation survey. Indianapolis.

56. Nelson, P., R. Gilbert, and L. Longo. 1983. Fetal growth and placental diffusing capacity in guinea pigs following long-term maternal exercise. *Journal of Developmental Physiology* 5:1–10.

57. Neuman, T. et al. 1994. Asthma and diving. *Annals of Allergy* 73:344–50.

58. Nottin, S. et al. 2002. Central and peripheral cardiovascular adaptations to exercise in endurance-trained children. *Acta Physiologica Scandanavia* 175:85–92.

59. Otis, C. et al. 1997. American College of Sports Medicine position stand. The female athlete triad. *Medicine in Science in Sports and Medicine* 29:i–ix.

60. Penas-Lledo, F. J., V. Leal, and G. Waller. 2002. Excessive exercise in anorexia nervosa and bulimia nervosa: Relation to eating characteristics and general psychopathology. *International Journal of Eating Disorders* 31:370–75.

61. Pivarnik, J. et al. 1992. Menstrual cycle phase affects temperature regulation during endurance exercise. *Journal of Applied Physiology* 72:543–48.

62. Pruett, E. 1985. Insulin and exercise in the non-diabetic man. In *Exercise Physiology*, ed. K. Fotherly and S. Pal. New York: Walter de Gruyter.

63. Rowland, T. 1992. Trainability of the cardiorespiratory system during childhood. *Canadian Journal of Sports Sciences* 17:259–63.

64. Rowland, T. 1999. Screening for risk of cardiac death in young athletes. *Sports Science Exchange* 12(3):1–5.

65. Steinhaus, A. 1933. Chronic effects of exercise. *Physiological Review* 13:103–47.

66. Sternfeld, B. et al. 1995. Exercise during pregnancy and pregnancy outcome. *Medicine and Science in Sports and Exercise* 27:634–40.

67. Sutton, J. 1984. Metabolic responses to exercise in normal and diabetic individuals. In *Sports Medicine*, ed. R. Strauss. Philadelphia: W. B. Saunders.

68. Terada, J. 1974. Effect of physical activity before pregnancy on fetuses of mice exercised forcibly during pregnancy. *Teratology* 10:141–44.

69. Torstveit, M., and J. Sundgot-Boggen. 2005. The female athlete triad exists in both elite athletes and controls. *Medicine and Science in Sports and Exercise* 37:1449–59.

70. van Linschoten, R. et al. 1990. Epilepsy and sports. *Sports Medicine* 10:9–19.

71. Warren, M. 1980. The effects of exercise on pubertal progression and reproductive function in girls. *Journal of Clinical Endocrinology and Metabolism* 51:1150–57.

72. Weimann, E. 2002. Gender-related differences in elite gymnasts: The female athlete triad. *Journal of Applied Physiology* 92:2146–52.

73. West, R. 1998. The female athlete: The triad of disordered eating, amenorrhea, and osteoporosis. *Sports Medicine* 26:63–71.

74. Williams, M. *Lifetime Fitness and Wellness.* 1998. New York: McGraw-Hill Companies.

75. Wilmore, J. 1991. Eating and weight disorders in the female athlete. *International Journal of Sports Medicine* 1:104–17.

76. Yager J., and A. Andersen. 2005. Anorexia nervosa. *New England Journal of Medicine* 353:1481–88.

77. Zelisko, J. et al. 1982. A comparison of men's and women's professional basketball injuries. *American Journal of Sports Medicine* 10:297–99.

78. Zilmer, D. et al. 1992. Gender specific injury patterns in high school varsity basketball. *Journal of Women's Health* 1:69–76.

CHAPTER 23

Nutrition, Body Composition, and Performance

■ Objectives

By studying this chapter, you should be able to do the following:

1. Describe the effect of various carbohydrate diets on muscle glycogen and on endurance performance during heavy exercise.

2. Contrast the "classic" method of achieving a supercompensation of the muscle glycogen stores with the "modified" method.

3. Describe some potential problems when glucose is ingested immediately prior to exercise.

4. Describe the importance of blood glucose as a fuel in prolonged exercise, and the role of carbohydrate supplementation during the performance.

5. Contrast the evidence that protein is oxidized at a faster rate during exercise with the evidence that the use of labeled amino acids may be an inappropriate methodology to study this issue.

6. Describe the need for protein *during* the adaptation to a new, more strenuous exercise level with the protein need when the adaptation is complete.

7. Defend the recommendation that a protein intake that is 12% to 15% of energy intake is sufficient to meet an athlete's need.

8. Describe the recommended fluid replacement strategies for athletic events of different intensities and durations, citing evidence to support your position.

9. Describe the salt requirement of the athlete compared to that of the sedentary individual, and the recommended means of maintaining sodium balance.

10. List the steps leading to iron deficiency anemia and the special problem that athletes have in maintaining iron balance.

11. Provide a brief summary of the effects of vitamin supplementation on performance.

12. Characterize the role of the pregame meal on performance and the rationale for limiting fats and proteins.

13. Describe the various components of the somatotype and what the following ratings signify: 171, 711, and 117.

14. Describe what the endomorphic and mesomorphic components in the Heath-Carter method of somatotyping represent in conventional body composition analysis.

15. Explain why one must be careful in recommending specific body fatness values for individual athletes.

■ Outline

Nutrition and Performance   478
  Carbohydrate   478
  Protein   482
  Water and Electrolytes   486
  Minerals   489

Vitamins   490
  Precompetition Diet   491

Body Composition and Performance   492

Somatotype   492
  Body Fatness and Performance   492

ectomorphy   glucose polymer   somatotype
endomorphy   mesomorphy   supercompensation

This chapter on nutrition, body composition, and performance is an extension of chapter 18, since the primary emphasis must be on achieving health-related goals before performance-related goals are examined. In fact, the information presented here must be examined in light of what the average person needs. Does an athlete need additional protein? What percent body fat is a reasonable goal for an athlete? We will address these questions in that order.

NUTRITION AND PERFORMANCE

In Chapter 18 we indicated the recommended range of nutrient intakes:

- Adults should get 45% to 65% of their calories from carbohydrates, 20% to 35% from fat, and 10% to 35% from protein.

This simple statement is important because it sets the stage for a discussion of what athletes should and do eat to support vigorous training programs and provide the fuel for the diverse performances that make up competitive athletics.

Carbohydrate

The recommended range for carbohydrate intake is quite broad to meet the needs of the whole population and allow one to address special needs linked to a reduced capacity for using carbohydrates (e.g., type 2 diabetics). Because carbohydrate oxidation makes up a larger percent of total energy production as exercise intensity increases, it should be no surprise that most athletes need more carbohydrate than the average person. Both Brotherhood (8) and Sherman (97) report that the average percent of carbohydrate in an athlete's diet is only about 50%, which is surprisingly low given the importance of carbohydrate in prolonged moderate to heavy exercise (see chapter 4). This section will consider the use of carbohydrates in the days prior to a performance and, secondly, during the performance itself.

Carbohydrate Diets and Performance   In 1967, three studies were published from the same Swedish laboratory that set the stage for our understanding of the role of muscle glycogen in performance (1, 7, 61).

Hermansen et al. (61) showed muscle glycogen to be systematically depleted during heavy (77% $\dot{V}O_2$ max) exercise, and when exhaustion occurred, glycogen content was near zero. Ahlborg et al. (1) found that work time to exhaustion was directly related to the initial glycogen store in the working muscles. Bergstrom et al. (7) confirmed and extended this by showing that by manipulating the quantity of carbohydrate in the diet, the concentration of glycogen in muscle could be altered and, along with it, the time to exhaustion. In their study, subjects consumed 2,800 kcal/d using either a low-CHO (fat and protein) diet, a mixed diet, or a high-carbohydrate diet in which 2,300 kcal came from carbohydrate. Glycogen contents of the quadriceps femoris muscle were, respectively, 0.63 (low), 1.75 (average), and 3.31 (high) g/100 g muscle, and performance time for exercise at 75% $\dot{V}O_2$ max averaged 57, 114, and 167 minutes. Figure 23.1 shows these results. In brief, the muscle glycogen content and performance time could be varied with diet. These laboratory findings were confirmed by Karlsson and Saltin (69), who had trained subjects run a 30-km race twice, once following a high-carbohydrate diet and the other time after a mixed diet. The initial muscle glycogen level was 3.5 g/100 g muscle following the CHO diet and 1.7 g/100 g muscle following the

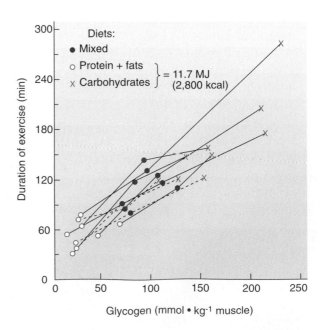

FIGURE 23.1   Effect of different diets on the muscle glycogen concentration and work time to exhaustion.

mixed diet. The best performance of all subjects occurred during the high-CHO diet. Interestingly, the pace at the start of the race was not faster; instead, the additional CHO allowed subjects to maintain the pace for a longer period of time. An important finding in this study was that compared to those on the high-CHO diet, pace did not fall off for those on the mixed diet until about halfway through the race (about one hour or so). This suggests that the normal mixed diet used in the study would be suitable for run or cycle races lasting less than one hour.

Given the importance of muscle glycogen in prolonged endurance performance, it is no surprise that investigators have tried to determine what conditions will yield the highest muscle glycogen content. In 1966, Bergstrom and Hultman (6) had subjects do one-legged exercise to exhaust the glycogen store in the exercised leg while not affecting the resting leg's glycogen store. When this procedure was followed with a high-carbohydrate diet, the glycogen content was more than twice as high in the previously exercised leg, compared to the control leg. Further, they found that in subjects who had the high-carbohydrate diet following the protein/fat diet (plus doing exhausting exercise), the muscle glycogen stores were higher than when the mixed diet preceded the high-carbohydrate treatment (6). This combination of information led to the following *classical method* of achieving a muscle glycogen **supercompensation:**

- prolonged, strenuous exercise to exhaust muscle glycogen store,
- a fat/protein diet for three days while continuing to train, and
- a high-carbohydrate diet (90% CHO) for three days, with inactivity.

There were some practical problems with this approach to achieving a high muscle glycogen content given that it required seven days to prepare for a race. Further, some subjects could not tolerate either the extremely low- (high fat and protein) or high- (90%) carbohydrate diets. Sherman (96) proposed a *modified plan* that causes supercompensation. The plan requires a tapering of the workout from ninety minutes to forty minutes while eating a 50% CHO diet (350 g/d). This is followed by two days of twenty-minute workouts while eating a 70% CHO diet (500–600 g/d) and, finally, a day of rest prior to the competition with the 70% CHO diet (or 500–600 g/d). This regimen was shown to be effective in increasing the glycogen stores to *high values* consistent with good performance (see figure 23.2). Two recent studies showed that with a carbohydrate intake of about 10g/kg body weight using foods with a high glycemic index (see chapter 18), only one day was needed to achieve very high muscle glycogen levels in all muscle fiber types (10, 42). However, what should

FIGURE 23.2 Modification of the classic glycogen loading technique to achieve high muscle glycogen levels with minimal changes in a training or diet routine. Glycogen levels are in glucose units (gu) per kilogram (kg).

you do if you need to replenish the glycogen stores quickly following heavy exercise?

The limiting factor in muscle glycogen synthesis is glucose transport across the cell membrane. Following a bout of heavy exercise there is an increase in the muscle cell's permeability to glucose, an increase in glycogen synthase activity, and an increase in the muscle's sensitivity to insulin (65). The glucose ingestion needs to be initiated immediately after exercise, and should be repeated each two hours for six hours; a delay of only two hours slows the rate of synthesis (68). Glucose or **glucose polymers** are better than fructose for synthesizing muscle glycogen, but some fructose should be ingested, since it may be better for replenishing liver glycogen (47, 65, 97). Finally, the addition of a small amount of protein as part of post-exercise carbohydrate supplementation may assist in the rapid uptake of glucose, especially if the quantity of carbohydrate taken in is less than optimal (9, 68). Such procedures can replenish muscle glycogen in twenty-four hours (42). What is needed for the day-to-day replenishment of muscle glycogen?

It takes about twenty-four hours to replenish muscle glycogen following prolonged, strenuous exercise, provided that about 500 to 700 g of carbohydrate are ingested (26, 47, 65). The point that must be

The Zone Diet

The proper diet for health and performance that has been emphasized in this text is one high in complex carbohydrates (55%–60%), low in fat (≤30%), and moderate in protein. The Zone Diet, developed by Dr. Barry Sears, argues otherwise, suggesting that its special balance of nutrients favorably influences endurance performance. The diet revolves around the consumption of food in the exact proportions of 40% carbohydrate, 30% protein, and 30% fat for all meals and snacks. These proportions are believed to trigger a better insulin-to-glucagon response, which, in turn, produces "good" eico-sanoids. Eicosanoids are hormone-like molecules derived from essential fatty acids; they include the prostaglandins, thromboxanes, and leukotrienes. The eicosanoid that is the primary focus of this diet is the protagladin PGE_1, a vasodilator and stimulator of lipolysis.

The diet uses an individual's fat-free mass (FFM) to establish the protein intake for the day (1.8–2.2 g per kg FFM), and this value is used to set the caloric intake values for fat and carbohydrate following the prescribed proportions.

Cheuvront's critical review of the Zone Diet points out some shortcomings relative to any purported gains in endurance performance that might be derived from this diet (17):

- It is a low-carbohydrate diet, the kind that has been shown to lead to poor performances in endurance events.
- The protein guidelines used to establish the caloric intake result in a calorie-deficient diet for endurance athletes, something that is inconsistent with athletic performance.

- Although the lipid biochemistry is factual, the links made among nutrition, endocrinology, lipid metabolism, and exercise physiology are oversimplified and sometimes paradoxical.
- The eicosanoid that is the primary focus of this diet (PGE_1) and is believed to be responsible for improved muscle oxygenation is not found in skeletal muscle.

A recent study by Jarvis et al. (67) confirmed many of these shortcomings of the Zone Diet (decreased caloric intake, loss of body weight, reduction in time to exhaustion for exercise done at 80% $\dot{V}O_2$ max) and supported Cheuvront's conclusion. Cheuvront (17) concludes that the diet should be considered "ergolytic" rather than "ergogenic."

---

emphasized is that a person who is eating 55% to 60% of calories from carbohydrate is already consuming what is needed to replace muscle glycogen on a day-to-day basis. If an athlete requires 4,000 kcal per day for caloric balance and 55% to 60% is derived from carbohydrates, then 2,200 to 2,400 kcal (55%–60% of 4,000 kcal) or 550 to 600 g of carbohydrate will be consumed. This quantity is consistent with what is needed to restore muscle glycogen to normal levels twenty-four hours after strenuous exercise (3a). This is important for training considerations, and this "regular" diet would require little or no change to meet the carbohydrate load (500–600 g/d) described by Sherman to achieve supercompensation (96). In contrast to the high-carbohydrate diet recommendation, the Zone Diet has been promoted as the best way to improve performance (see The Winning Edge 23.1).

IN SUMMARY

- Performance in endurance events is improved by a diet high in carbohydrates due primarily to the increase in muscle glycogen.
- When workouts are tapered over several days while additional CHO (70% of dietary intake) is consumed, a "supercompensation" of the glycogen store can be achieved.

Carbohydrates Prior to or During a Performance

The focus on muscle glycogen as the primary carbohydrate source in heavy exercise has always diminished the role that blood glucose plays in maintaining carbohydrate oxidation in muscle. In Coggan and Coyle's review (22), they correct this perception for exercises that last three to four hours, in which blood glucose and muscle glycogen share equally in contributing to carbohydrate oxidation. In fact, as muscle glycogen decreases, the role that blood glucose plays increases until, at the end of three to four hours of exercise, it may be the sole source of carbohydrate. This is what makes blood glucose an important fuel in prolonged work, and why so much attention has been directed at trying to maintain the blood glucose concentration.

Unfortunately, the liver glycogen supply also decreases with time during prolonged exercise, and because gluconeogenesis can supply glucose at a rate of only 0.2 to 0.4 g/min when the muscles may be consuming it at a rate of 1 to 2 g/min, hypoglycemia is a real possibility. Hypoglycemia (blood glucose concentration <2.5 mmoles/liter) results when the rate of blood glucose uptake is not matched by release from the liver and/or small intestine. Hypoglycemia has been shown to occur during exercise at 58% $\dot{V}O_2$ max for 3.5 hours (5) and at 74% $\dot{V}O_2$ max for 2.5 hours (31). However, the number of subjects who demonstrate central nervous system dysfunction varied from none

(43) to only 25% of the subjects (31). While there is no absolutely clear association between hypoglycemia and fatigue, the availability of blood glucose as an energy source is, without question, linked to the performance of prolonged (three to four hours) strenuous exercise (22). How should carbohydrate be taken in before and during exercise to maintain the high rate of carbohydrate oxidation needed for performance?

The timing and the type of carbohydrate taken in to slow down the depletion of the body's carbohydrate stores are important factors. One of the earliest studies showed that when 75 g of glucose were ingested thirty to forty-five minutes before exercise requiring 70% to 75% $\dot{V}O_2$ max, plasma glucose and insulin were elevated at the start of exercise, and muscle glycogen was used at a *faster rate* during the exercise (25). This is counter to the goal of sparing muscle glycogen, and performance has been shown to decrease 19% with such a treatment (45). In contrast to this early study, a review of this topic indicated that the blood glucose and plasma insulin responses to pre-exercise glucose feedings are quite variable (some will experience a lowering of blood glucose, most will not), and that, in general, performance in prolonged exercise is either improved or not affected (3, 97). Finally, the composition (% fat and % carbohydrate) of the pre-exercise meal appears to have little or no effect on metabolism or performance (87, 93). The pre-exercise carbohydrate feeding is viewed as a means of topping off both muscle and liver glycogen stores. Generally, such procedures result in carbohydrates being used at a higher rate, but because of the large amount of carbohydrate ingested, the plasma glucose concentration is maintained for a longer period of time. The following observations and recommendations are offered relative to pre-exercise feedings (97):

- the pre-exercise feeding should contain between 1 and 5 g of carbohydrate per kilogram of body weight, and should be taken one to four hours before exercise;

- the carbohydrate source should be an easily digestible, solid, high-carbohydrate food, but if it is taken one hour before exercise, it should be in liquid form;

- the athlete should test the procedure in training before using it in competition; and

- the athlete should be aware of any sensations (e.g., fatigue) that might indicate a sensitivity to the carbohydrate load, which would not be beneficial to performance.

These recommendations were supported, in general, by a recent statement on nutrition and athletic performance (3). While ingesting carbohydrates prior to exercise seems to be an appropriate procedure, the most potent effect is when this is combined with carbohydrate feeding during exercise (107, 117).

In contrast to the pre-exercise feeding studies in which there was some variability in the outcome, there is a great deal of consensus that feeding carbohydrate during exercise delays fatigue and improves performance. Interestingly, the improved performance appears to have nothing to do with sparing the muscle glycogen store. Muscle glycogen is depleted at the same rate during prolonged moderate (70%–75% $\dot{V}O_2$ max) exercise, with or without carbohydrate ingestion; however, liver glycogen is not (18, 22). The ingestion of carbohydrate appears to spare the liver glycogen store by directly contributing carbohydrate for oxidation. If additional carbohydrate is not ingested during prolonged exercise, the blood glucose concentration decreases as the liver stores are depleted, resulting in an inadequate rate of carbohydrate oxidation by muscle. Central nervous system activation of muscle is diminished by hypoglycemia, resulting in a reduced power output (85). Consistent with that, the rating of perceived exertion (RPE) is lower with carbohydrate supplementation during prolonged exercise (14, 104). Figure 23.3 shows Coggan and Coyle's model of how carbohydrate is supplied to muscle during prolonged

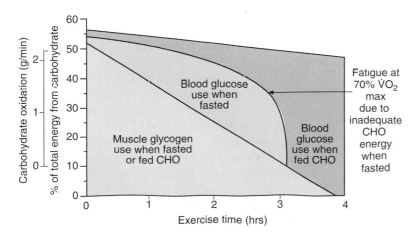

FIGURE 23.3 Blood glucose and muscle glycogen use when subjects fasted or were fed carbohydrates (CHO) during prolonged exercise.

exercise under fasted and fed conditions. The rate of muscle glycogen depletion is not different; however, when fed carbohydrates, the subjects last longer due to the increased availability of blood glucose. When is the best time to consume carbohydrates during exercise?

Coggan and Coyle indicate that carbohydrates can be ingested throughout exercise, or can be taken thirty minutes before the anticipated time of fatigue, with no difference in the outcome (22). This is consistent with their contention that it is the increased availability of glucose late in exercise that delays fatigue. In exercise tests at 75% $\dot{V}O_2$ max, the time to fatigue was extended by about forty-five minutes with carbohydrate ingestion. Since muscles use blood glucose at the rate of about 1 to 1.3 g/min late in exercise, sufficient carbohydrate should be ingested to provide an additional 45 to 60 g (45 min × 1 to 1.3 g/min) of carbohydrate. There is general agreement that this can be achieved when carbohydrates are taken in at the rate of about 30 to 60 g/hr during exercise (22). The 120 to 240 g of glucose consumed (4 hrs × 30 to 60 g/hr) provides for the 45 to 60 g needed at the end of exercise, but also supports the elevated carbohydrate metabolism throughout exercise. Glucose, sucrose, or glucose polymer solutions are all successful in maintaining the blood glucose concentration during exercise, but the palatability of the solution is improved if glucose polymer solutions are used for concentrations above 10%. The addition of caffeine to a carbohydrate supplement increases the oxidation of carbohydrates during exercise (119). Further, adding protein to a carbohydrate supplement increases performance beyond that of carbohydrate alone (66). Carbohydrate delivery from the stomach to the small intestine increases with the concentration of glucose, but fluid delivery slows down when the carbohydrate concentration exceeds 8%. This trade-off in glucose versus fluid delivery can be balanced by drinking 375 to 750 ml/hr of an 8% solution of carbohydrate, which would deliver 30 to 60 grams of glucose per hour to the blood (3, 29). One final point. Even when the blood glucose concentration is maintained by either glucose infusion or ingestion during exercise, the subject will eventually stop; this indicates that fatigue is related to more than the delivery of fuel to muscles (22). For an update on carbohydrate drinks and performance, see Ask the Expert 23.1.

IN SUMMARY

- Pre-exercise feedings should contain 1 to 5 g of carbohydrate per kilogram of body weight and should be taken one to four hours before exercise.

- Muscle glycogen is depleted at the same rate, whether or not glucose is ingested during prolonged performance.
- The ingestion of glucose solutions during exercise extends performance by providing carbohydrate to the muscle at a time when muscle glycogen is being depleted.

Protein

The adult RDA for protein is 0.8 gm · kg⁻¹ · d⁻¹ and is easily met by a diet having 12% of its energy (kcal) as protein. For example, if the daily energy requirement for an adult male weighing 72 kg is 2,900 kcal/day, then about 348 kcal are taken in as protein (12% of 2,900 kcal). At 4 kcal/g, this person would consume approximately 87 g protein per day, representing 1.2 g · kg⁻¹ · d⁻¹ (87 g/70 kg), or 50% more than the RDA standard. Does an athlete have to take in more protein than specified in the RDA, or is the normal diet adequate? Confusing as it may seem, the answer to *both* questions appears to be yes.

Protein Requirement During Exercise Adequacy of protein intake has been based primarily on nitrogen(N)-balance studies. Protein is about 16% N by weight, and when N-intake (dietary protein) equals N-excretion, the person is in N-balance. Excretion of less N than one consumes is called positive N-balance, and the excretion of more N than one consumes is called negative N-balance. This latter condition, if maintained, is inconsistent with good health due to the potential loss of lean body mass. Based on these N-balance studies it was generally believed that the 0.8 g · kg⁻¹ · d⁻¹ RDA standard was adequate for those engaged in prolonged exercise. In these studies, urinary N excretion was usually used as an index of N-excretion, since about 85% of N is excreted this way (72). However, some experiments suggest this method of measurement may underestimate amino acid utilization in exercise. Lemon and Mullin (76) found that while there was no difference in urinary N excretion compared to rest, the loss of N in sweat increased 60- to 150-fold during exercise, suggesting that as much as 10% of the energy requirement of the exercise was met by the oxidation of amino acids.

Other studies, using different techniques, supported these observations. Muscle has been shown to release the amino acid alanine in proportion to exercise intensity (44), and the alanine is used in gluconeogenesis in the liver to generate new plasma glucose. Several investigators have infused a stable isotope (^{13}C-label) of the amino acid leucine to study the rate at which amino acids are mobilized and oxidized during exercise. In general, the rate of oxidation

Carbohydrate Drinks and Performance
Questions and Answers with Dr. Ronald J. Maughan

Ron Maughan obtained his B.Sc. (Physiology) and Ph.D. from the University of Aberdeen, and held a lecturing position in Liverpool before returning to Aberdeen where he stayed for more than 20 years. He is now located at the School of Sport & Exercise Sciences, Loughborough University, Loughborough, England.. He chaired the British Olympic Association nutrition group for eight years and now chairs the Nutrition Working Group of the International Olympic Committee. His research interests are in the physiology, biochemistry, and nutrition of exercise performance, with an interest in both the basic science of exercise and the applied aspects that relate to health and to performance in sport.

QUESTION 1: Athletes use carbohydrate drinks to improve performance. What type of athlete would benefit most from this strategy?

ANSWER: All athletes will find these drinks useful in some training and competition situations. During exercise, they are especially important when the exercise time exceeds about thirty to forty minutes. They provide carbohydrate as an energy source and this is especially important if there has not been an opportunity for complete recovery of the body's carbohydrate stores since the last training session or competition. These drinks also promote water absorption and supply some electrolytes, so they are particularly important when sweat losses are high. Athletes should get into the habit of using these drinks in training as well as in competition. Training sessions feel easier, the risks of heat illness are greatly reduced, and the quality of training is better maintained. This is a message particularly for strength and power athletes who may train for long periods, but who often do not have the awareness of the need for rehydration that exists in endurance sports.

QUESTION 2: Given the existing research support for this strategy, what are the most important questions remaining to be answered?

ANSWER: Many questions remain to be answered, but these relate mostly to the application of the basic science in practical situations. The basic formulation of carbohydrate-electrolyte drinks is not likely to change substantially, but we need to have a better understanding of the optimum formulation for use in different situations. There are almost certainly situations in which a higher or a lower carbohydrate content would be better. There is also some debate about the need for electrolyte replacement in different situations. We also need to learn how to communicate more effectively with athletes and coaches, and this is perhaps the biggest challenge we face at present.

QUESTION 3: Are there any differences between these traditional carbohydrate drinks and the new "energy drinks" being advertised to improve performance?

ANSWER: The new energy drinks are mostly very high in sugar; hence, the energy, and also usually contain caffeine to give a feeling of more energy. These can have disadvantages in some situations. Because the osmolality of these drinks is very high, the body actually secretes water into the small intestine after they have been ingested. This exacerbates any dehydration and can cause gastrointestinal discomfort. The amount of caffeine in these drinks varies, but there must be a concern that some might cause problems for athletes called for drug testing in competition. Caffeine is not banned in training but ingestion of large amounts in competition can lead to a positive test.

(measured by the appearance of $^{13}CO_2$) is higher during exercise than at rest in rats and humans (33, 62, 108). Taken as a group, these studies suggest that amino acids are used as a fuel during exercise to a greater extent than previously believed. They also suggest that the protein requirement for those involved in prolonged exercise is higher than the RDA (72). However, there is more to the story.

Oxidation of Amino Acids   Part of the justification for a greater protein requirement in those who exercise is based on work using isotopes of amino acids whose metabolism could be traced during exercise. That is, if an amino acid is metabolized, the "labeled" $^{13}CO_2$ is exhaled and can be used as a marker of its rate of use. The essential amino acid leucine has been used as being representative of the amino acid pool. The previously mentioned work showed that leucine oxidation is increased with exercise (33, 62, 108). This implies that the catabolism of protein is higher during exercise compared to rest. Wolfe et al. (116) confirmed this greater rate of leucine oxidation during exercise but failed to show an increase in urea production, a primary index of protein catabolism. It was concluded that the N contained in leucine does not find its way to plasma urea N as a result of exercise (114, 115); instead, the N in leucine is transferred to intermediates (pyruvate) to form alanine, which is later used in the liver in gluconeogenesis.

These results raised additional questions, so another experiment was conducted to see if leucine was, in fact, representative of the amino acid pool.

FIGURE 23.4   Effect of exercise on nitrogen balance.

The investigators used the amino acid lysine and found different results for the same experimental procedures. On the basis of their experiments, Wolfe et al. (115, 116) concluded that leucine cannot be used as a model of whole-body protein metabolism during exercise, that changes in (or lack of) urea production during exercise may not reflect an accurate picture of protein breakdown, and finally, that *the data provide no rationale for increasing protein intake when exercising* (115, 116). A review supports this proposition, and indicates that even if the leucine requirement is three times the RDA in individuals who exercise, the mixed diet of a typical athlete is sufficient to meet those needs (11). This takes us back to nitrogen-balance studies as a focal point of determining the protein requirements for athletes.

Whole-Body Nitrogen Balance Studies   The ability to maintain N-balance during exercise appears to be dependent on the:

- training state of the subject,
- quality and quantity of protein consumed,
- total calories consumed,
- body's carbohydrate store, and
- intensity, duration, and type (resistance versus endurance) of exercise (11, 13, 72, 73, 74).

If measurements of protein utilization are made during the first few days of an exercise program, formerly sedentary subjects show a negative N-balance (figure 23.4). However, after about twelve to fourteen days of training, this condition disappears and the person can maintain N-balance (52). So, depending on the point into the training program where the measurements are made, one could conclude that either more protein is needed (during the adaptation to exercise) or that protein needs can be met by the RDA (after the adaptation is complete) (13). Butterfield indicates that in N-balance studies the length of time needed to achieve a new steady state depends on the magnitude of the change in the level of N-intake, and the absolute amount of N consumed, and that the recommended minimum of a ten-day adaptation period may be inadequate when N-intake is very large (11).

Another factor influencing the conclusion one would reach about protein needs during exercise is whether the person is in caloric balance—that is, taking in enough kcal to cover the cost of the added exercise. For example, it has been shown that by increasing the energy intake 15% *more* than that needed to maintain weight, an increase in N-retention occurred during exercise when these subjects consumed only 0.57 $g \cdot kg^{-1} \cdot d^{-1}$ of egg white protein (13). In a parallel study by the same group (103), a 15% *deficit* in energy intake was created while subjects consumed either 0.57 or 0.8 $g \cdot kg^{-1} \cdot d^{-1}$ egg white protein. When taking in 15% fewer calories than needed, the 0.8 $g \cdot kg^{-1} \cdot d^{-1}$ protein intake was associated with a negative N-balance of 1 $g \cdot d^{-1}$. However, when the subjects did one or two hours of exercise, the negative N-balance improved to a loss of only 0.51, or 0.27 g/d, respectively. During the treatment in which the subjects were in caloric balance, the RDA of 0.8 $g \cdot kg^{-1} \cdot d^{-1}$ was sufficient to achieve a positive N-balance for both durations of exercise. It is clear, then, that in order to make proper judgments about the adequacy of the protein intake, the person must be in energy balance.

A final nutritional factor that can influence the rate of amino-acid metabolism during exercise is the availability of carbohydrate. Lemon and Mullin (76) showed that the quantity of urea found in sweat was cut in half when subjects were carbohydrate loaded as opposed to carbohydrate depleted (see figure 23.5). Further, as figure 23.6 shows, the ingestion of glucose during the latter half of a three-hour exercise test at 50% $\dot{V}O_2$ max reduces the rate of oxidation of the amino acid leucine (33). So, not only is caloric balance important in protein metabolism, but the ability of the diet to provide adequate carbohydrate must also be considered.

Dietary Goals for Athletes   So, how much protein does an athlete need? To answer that question one needs to consider the fact that the RDA for protein

FIGURE 23.5 Effect of initial muscle glycogen levels on sweat urea nitrogen excretion during exercise. A high muscle glycogen level decreases the excretion of urea nitrogen in sweat during exercise.

FIGURE 23.6 Effect of glucose ingestion on the rate of metabolism of the amino acid leucine. Glucose ingestion decreases the rate of amino acid oxidation.

varies from country to country (0.8 to 1.2 $g \cdot kg^{-1} \cdot d^{-1}$), and that most of these standards do not consider vigorous exercise. The Dutch did, and offered 1.5 $g \cdot kg^{-1} \cdot d^{-1}$ as the standard for athletes (74). So, again, how much protein is needed? It depends on the type and intensity of the exercise. For low-intensity exercise (35%–50% $\dot{V}O_2$ max), the RDA of 0.8 $g \cdot kg^{-1} \cdot d^{-1}$ appears to be sufficient. For high-intensity endurance exercise, the requirement appears to be around 1.2 to 1.4 $g \cdot kg^{-1} \cdot d^{-1}$ (11, 73, 74, 75), but for strength training there is less agreement. Butterfield (11) feels that 0.9 $g \cdot kg^{-1} \cdot d^{-1}$, close to the RDA, is sufficient for "maintenance" of existing body protein stores in strength trainers. For those strength-training athletes who are adding muscle mass, the requirement may be as high as 1.6 to 1.7 $g \cdot kg^{-1} \cdot d^{-1}$ (3). This conclusion has been consistently supported over the past fifteen years and is unlikely to change in the near future (11,

75, 89, 102). Scientists express the need for the athlete to maintain caloric balance because of the consequences a negative caloric balance can have on N-balance (see earlier discussion).

Another way to approach this question is to consider the protein requirement of a human from childhood to adulthood. The RDA for protein is 1.5 $g \cdot kg^{-1} \cdot d^{-1}$ during the second six months of life, decreasing to 0.95 $g \cdot kg^{-1} \cdot d^{-1}$ by ages four to eight, and reaching the adult value of 0.8 $g \cdot kg^{-1} \cdot d^{-1}$ by age eighteen (see appendix D). During this period of time an individual increases body weight by a factor of ten (15 lb to 150 lb). This is not unlike what was previously mentioned about the adaptation to exercise. During the initial days of an exercise training program when the muscles are adapting to the new exercise, the protein requirement might be higher than the RDA, and data of Gontzea (51, 52) support this proposition. However, once the person has adapted to the exercise, the requirement would revert to the RDA.

At the beginning of this section on the protein requirements for athletes, a question was raised: Does an athlete have to take in more protein than the RDA, or is the normal diet adequate? During intense endurance training or strength training, the requirement of protein may be higher than the RDA. So the answer is yes to that part of the question. It is also yes to the second part, in that the average person typically takes in 50% more than the RDA for protein. While the dietary goal for protein is 12% of total kcal, Brotherhood (8) reports that an average athlete's diet is about 16% protein, exceeding 1.5 $g \cdot kg^{-1} \cdot d^{-1}$ (88% more than RDA!). These values exceed the RDA of young children who are in a chronic state of positive nitrogen-balance, and approach the upper limit of the recommendations of Lemon (11, 73, 74). It would appear that while scientists deal with questions of the effect of exercise on the oxidation of amino acids, and to what extent the RDA for athletes is greater than 0.8 $g \cdot kg^{-1} \cdot d^{-1}$, the athlete following a normal dietary pattern will consume more than enough protein to meet the needs associated with exercise, assuming that caloric intake is adequate.

Some concern has been raised about consuming too much dietary protein, especially with regard to amenorrheic athletes (12). High-protein diets lead to an increase in Ca^{++} excretion, and for many years it was believed that the Ca^{++} was of bone origin and of real concern for the amenorrheic athlete (40, 59). Recent studies suggest otherwise. Short-term diets high in protein have been shown to simultaneously increase Ca^{++} absorption from the intestine, and there is no evidence of an impact on net stores of bone Ca^{++}. In contrast, those on a low-protein diet show a reduction in Ca^{++} absorption from the intestine, and long-term use of such diets could seriously compromise skeletal health (70, 71).

- The protein requirement for those engaged in light-to-moderate endurance exercise is equal to the RDA of $0.8 \text{ g} \cdot \text{kg}^{-1} \cdot \text{d}^{-1}$; however, it is $1.2–1.4 \text{ g} \cdot \text{kg}^{-1} \cdot \text{d}^{-1}$ for athletes who participate in high-intensity endurance exercise.
- For resistance training, there is more dispute about the requirement. It may be only $0.9 \text{ g} \cdot \text{kg}^{-1} \cdot \text{d}^{-1}$ for those maintaining strength or as high as $1.6–1.7 \text{ g} \cdot \text{kg}^{-1} \cdot \text{d}^{-1}$ for those adding lean mass and strength.
- Bottom line: The average protein intake of an athlete exceeds $1.5 \text{ g} \cdot \text{kg}^{-1} \cdot \text{d}^{-1}$, more than enough to cover the higher protein requirement.

Water and Electrolytes

Chapter 12 described in some detail the need to dissipate heat during exercise in order to minimize the increase in core temperature. The primary mechanism for heat loss at high work rates in a comfortable environment, and at all work rates in a hot environment, is the evaporation of sweat. Sweat rates increase linearly with exercise intensity, and in hot weather sweat rates can reach 2.8 liters per hour (23). In spite of attempts to replace water during marathon races, some runners lose 8% of their body weight (23). Given that water losses in excess of 3% are regarded as potentially harmful (110), there is a clear need to maintain water balance. Of course, more than water is lost in sweat. An increased sweat rate means that a wide variety of electrolytes, such as Na^+, K^+, Cl^-, and Mg^{++}, are lost as well (23). These electrolytes are needed for normal functioning of excitable tissues, enzymes, and hormones. It should be no surprise then that investigators have been concerned about the optimal way to replace water and electrolytes to reduce the chance of health-related problems and increase the chance of optimal performance (80).

Water Replacement—Before Exercise Knowing that one is going to lose body water during exercise, some investigators have tried to anticipate this by providing a volume of water or electrolyte beverage prior to the start of exercise. In these studies the subjects drank 1 to 3 liters of water and/or dilute saline prior to exercise. Williams (110) and Herbert (60) report that subjects generally had lower heart rate and body temperature responses to exercise in the hyperhydrated state than in the control condition. However, it is unlikely that an athlete would choose to consume such large volumes prior to exercise. Based on an analysis of the needs of athletes in different types of performances, Gisolfi and Duchman (49) suggest the following guidelines for pre-event drinks:

- for exercise of less than one hour (80%–130% $\dot{V}O_2$ max), drink 300 to 500 ml containing 30 to 50 g of carbohydrate, and
- for exercise durations of more than one hour (30%–90% $\dot{V}O_2$ max), drink 300 to 500 ml of water.

Water Replacement—During Exercise If an athlete doesn't "replace" water before it is lost, then water replacement during an activity is the next step. Fortunately, for some sports in which play is intermittent (football, tennis, golf), water replacement during the activity is possible. However, in athletic events like marathon running, there are no formal breaks in the activity to allow for replacement. It is in these latter activities, in which a high rate of heat production is coupled with the potential problems of environmental heat and humidity, that the athlete is at great risk. Studies confirm the need to replace fluids as they are lost during exercise in order to maintain moderate heart rate and body temperature responses (54, 90). Figure 23.7 shows changes in esophageal temperature, heart rate, and rating of perceived exertion during two hours of exercise at 62% to 67% $\dot{V}O_2$ max under four conditions of fluid replacement: (a) no fluid, (b) small fluid (300 ml/hr), (c) moderate fluid (700 ml/hr), and (d) large fluid (1,200 ml/hr). The fluid was a "sport drink" containing 6% carbohydrate and electrolyte. As you can see, there were marked differences in the responses over time. The lowest heart rate, body temperature, and rating of perceived exertion were associated with the highest rates of fluid replacement (27, 30). It must be added that while most of the attention on fluid replacement is directed at those who participate in prolonged endurance exercise, it is clear that the same message must reach those who participate in intermittent exercise (98). Given that fluid replacement during exercise is clearly beneficial, how much fluid should be taken at one time? Should it be warm or cold? Should it contain electrolytes and glucose?

Costill and colleagues (24, 28) provided some of the original answers to these questions. One study examined the effects of fluid volume, temperature, glucose concentration, and the intensity of exercise on the rate at which fluid leaves the stomach to the small intestine. They determined this by giving the subject the fluid in question, and then fifteen minutes later aspirating the contents of the stomach. Figure 23.8 summarizes the results of that study. A glucose concentration above 139 mM (2.5%) slowed gastric emptying (i.e., increased residue; figure 23.8a). The optimal volume to ingest was 600 ml (figure 23.8b),

FIGURE 23.7 Core temperature (esophageal temperature), heart rate, and perceived exertion during 120 min of exercise when subjects ingested no fluid, or small (300 ml/hr), moderate (700 ml/hr) and large (1,200 ml/hr) volumes of fluid. A rating of 17 for perceived exertion corresponds to "Very Hard," 15 is "Hard," and 13 is "Somewhat Hard." Values are means ± SE.
*Significantly lower than no fluid, $P < 0.05$.
† Significantly lower than small fluid, $P < 0.05$.
§ Significantly lower than moderate fluid, $P < 0.05$.

and colder drinks appeared to be emptied faster (i.e., decreased residue; figure 23.8c). Finally, exercise had no effect on gastric emptying until the intensity exceeded 65% to 70% $\dot{V}O_2$ max (figure 23.8d). Using the same technique, which has been shown to be valid (46), studies have confirmed that intensities below 75% $\dot{V}O_2$ max do not affect the rate of gastric emptying (82), and that there is no difference between running and cycling in the rate of gastric emptying for exercise intensities of 70% to 75% $\dot{V}O_2$ max (63, 82, 92). However, dehydration and/or high body temperature have

been shown to delay gastric emptying (81, 91). While most of the later work supports the findings shown in figure 23.8, the one exception is with regard to the carbohydrate content of the drink.

In the original study (24), the effectiveness of a drink was evaluated fifteen minutes after ingestion by aspirating the contents of the stomach. Davis and colleagues (36, 37) questioned the use of the aspiration technique, since it simply measures how much fluid leaves the stomach, not how much is actually absorbed into the blood from the small intestine. They used heavy water (D_2O) as a tracer of fluid absorption from the gastrointestinal tract to the blood and found that a 6% glucose-electrolyte solution was absorbed as fast or faster than water at rest (36) or during exercise (37). Two additional studies that used the aspiration technique (77, 86) found that when either a 10% glucose solution or glucose polymer solutions containing 5% to 10% carbohydrate were ingested at fifteen- to twenty-minute intervals during prolonged exercise at 65% to 70% $\dot{V}O_2$ max, there was no difference in the gastric emptying rate of either solution compared to water. The improved performance of the carbohydrate drinks in the most recent studies may be related to the experimental procedures, which included the ingestion of small volumes ($\sim$200 ml) at regular intervals (fifteen to twenty minutes) during prolonged exercise, with the aspiration occurring at the end of the entire exercise session (not fifteen minutes after ingestion). An additional benefit of these glucose solutions is that the extra carbohydrate helps to maintain the blood glucose during exercise (see earlier discussion). It must be added, however, that drinks containing 12% glucose remained in the stomach longer, with subjects complaining of gastrointestinal distress (37, 78, 79). If fluid intake is most important and carbohydrate is secondary, a drink should be fashioned accordingly.

In addition to the guidelines for pre-event drinks, Gisolfi and Duchman (49) also provide guidelines for drinks during exercise:

- during exercise lasting less than one hour (80%–130% $\dot{V}O_2$ max), the athlete should drink 500 to 1,000 ml of water;
- for exercise durations between one and three hours (60%–90% $\dot{V}O_2$ max), the drink should contain 10 to 20 mEq of Na^+, and Cl^-, and 6% to 8% carbohydrate, with 500 to 1,000 ml/hr meeting the carbohydrate need, and 800 to 1,600 ml/hr meeting the fluid need; and
- for events of more than three hours' duration, the drink should contain 20 to 30 mEq of Na^+, and Cl^-, and 6% to 8% carbohydrate, with 500 to 1,000 ml/hr meeting the carbohydrate and fluid needs of most athletes.

FIGURE 23.8 Effect of fluid volume, glucose concentration, solute temperature, and the intensity of exercise on the rate of fluid absorption from the gastrointestinal tract.

Allowances must be made for the individual differences in the frequency and volume of ingestion. These authors also provided a drink for recovery that is consistent with the need to replenish electrolytes and muscle glycogen: the drink should contain 30 to 40 mEq of Na^+, and Cl^-, and deliver 50 g of carbohydrate per hour. The addition of salt to the drink enhances its palatability, promotes fluid and carbohydrate absorption, and replenishes some of the electrolytes lost during the activity. An additional reason sodium has been added to the drinks is related to concerns that have been raised about the potential for hyponatremia, a dangerously low Na^+ concentration that can occur when a person hydrates only with water or hypotonic drinks during extremely long (four+ hours), ultra-endurance athletic events (3, 83, 106). (See The Winning Edge 23.2).

Salt (NaCl) One of the Dietary Guidelines for Americans presented in chapter 18 was to decrease the intake of sodium. While the point was made that Americans consume two to three times the amount needed for optimal health, is the dietary intake sufficient for an athlete who participates in regular vigorous physical activity? The mass of sodium in the body determines the water content, given the way water is reabsorbed at the kidney. If a person becomes sodium depleted, body water decreases, and the risk of heat injury increases. An untrained and unacclimatized individual (see chapter 24) loses more Na^+ in sweat than a trained and acclimatized person. If the unacclimatized person has 1.9 g Na^+ per liter of sweat and loses 5 liters of sweat (11 pounds), the person would lose 9.5 grams of Na^+ per day. As the person becomes

acclimatized to heat, the sodium content in sweat decreases to about half that and Na^+ loss is about 5 g/day. Given that Na is 40% of NaCl by weight, a person would have to consume 12.5 g of salt per day to meet that demand. Interestingly, that is about what an average American, eating an average diet, now consumes (118). It is generally believed that an individual with a high Na^+ loss can stay in sodium/water balance by simply adding salt to food at mealtime, rather than by consuming salt tablets (110). *The best single test of the success of the salt/water replacement procedures is to have an athlete weigh in each day.* The general dietary routine followed by athletes must be successful, since early morning body weight remains relatively constant despite large daily sweat losses (8).

Hyponatremia

A primary driving force shaping fluid replacement recommendations over the past 60 years was the potential for dehydration during athletic events due to inadequate consumption of fluids. Over the past decade, a different problem has surfaced—that associated with drinking too much fluid during a long-term athletic event and diluting the body's sodium level (3, 83, 84). A study of runners in the 2002 Boston Marathon found that 13% had hyponatremia (sodium concentration of $\leq$135 mM), and 0.6% had critical hyponatremia (sodium concentration of $\leq$120 mM). The latter is a potential deadly issue. Hyponatremia was associated with those who took more than four hours to complete the marathon and gained weight during the run due to the consumption of large amounts of hypotonic fluids (2). In response to this, track-and-field organizations attempted to educate participants to drink no more fluids than they lose, and to practice this strategy during their practice runs. In the 2005 Boston Marathon, the number of cases of hyonatremia was markedly reduced, with dehydration again being the typical fluid replacement issue. In that same year, the ACSM released recommendations resulting from their Rountable Series on the topic: hydration and physical activity (14):

- **Work to minimize risk of both hyponatremia and dehydration.** Hyponatremia is a rare condition (~1/1,000 finishers) that affects primarily slow-paced athletes in marathons (>4 hours) and triathlons (>9 to 13 hours). Athletes are encouraged to neither under- nor overhydrate as each has significant consequences. Dehydration, especially during warm/hot weather conditions occurs more frequently and is also life threatening. The message is to drink intelligently, not maximally.
- **Drink to match fluid loss and on a schedule.** Athletes should determine their typical sweat rate during practice runs (weight lost per hour + fluid consumed per hour) and aim to replace what is lost. The fluid should be consumed over a set period of time, rather than rapidly in a "catch-up" fashion. If athletes are not sweating much and are not thirsty, fluid replacement should be modest.
- **Consume salty foods and beverages.** Foods and beverages with sodium help promote fluid retention and stimulate thirst. Those performing long-duration exercise should consume snacks and fluids containing sodium to help prevent hyponatremia.

TABLE 23.1	Stages of Iron Deficiency	
Stages	**Description**	**Test**
Iron depletion	Lack of iron stores in the bone and liver due to long-term dietary iron deficiency	Bone marrow biopsy; serum ferritin $<12\ \mu g \cdot \ell^{-1}$
Iron-deficient erythropoieses	Red blood cell production decreases due to inadequate hemoglobin formation	Unbound protoporphyrin (used in the formation of hemoglobin) increases due to low iron stores
Iron deficiency anemia	Hemoglobin falls to low levels	Men: $<13\ g \cdot dl^{-1}$ Women: $<12\ g \cdot dl^{-1}$; *with* evidence that first two stages exist

From Haymes (55).

Minerals

Iron   As mentioned in chapter 18, iron deficiency is the most common nutritional deficiency. The stages of iron deficiency are spelled out in table 23.1, as well as the tests used to detect deficiencies (55). An analysis of the literature suggests that both male and female athletes have higher rates of depleted iron stores and/or iron deficiency anemia (8, 21, 55). Given that hemoglobin is a necessary part of the oxygen-transport process, it is not surprising that in individuals with very low hemoglobin values (<11 g/d), endurance and work performance are decreased (48, 50). Interestingly, when the low-hemoglobin condition is corrected in iron-deficient animals by transfusion, $\dot{V}O_2$ max is brought back to normal but not endurance time. This suggests that while hemoglobin levels may

FIGURE 23.9 Recovery of various physiological capacities with iron repletion. Note that recovery of endurance lagged behind $\dot{V}O_2$ max.

be high enough to achieve a normal $\dot{V}O_2$ max, iron deficiency affects the iron-containing cytochromes (electron transport chain) that are involved in oxidative phosphorylation, and endurance performance is adversely affected (35). In a similar study (34), iron supplementation brought the $\dot{V}O_2$ max back to normal values faster than that of mitochondrial activity (measured by pyruvate oxidase activity) and endurance performance (see figure 23.9).

What causes iron deficiency in athletes? Inadequate intake of dietary iron, as in the general population, has been cited as a primary cause of iron deficiency in women athletes (20). In addition, exercise has been associated with increased hemoglobin loss in feces, sweat, and urine (57, 88, 100). When this is combined with evidence showing a greater hemolysis of red blood cells due to simple "pounding" of the feet on the pavement during running, and a reduced level of haptoglobin in the plasma, which is needed to take the hemoglobin to the liver, one can understand why more hemoglobin is lost in the urine and some athletes are at risk of iron deficiency anemia (32, 57). Consistent with this, Diehl et al. (39) have shown decreases in serum ferritin over the course of a field hockey season, and from one hockey season to the next, in female athletes. The average value at the end of the season on third-year players was $10.5 \ \mu g \cdot \ell^{-1}$ (below the $12 \ \mu g \cdot \ell^{-1}$ standard), indicating iron depletion (55).

Generally, when a person has a deficiency in iron stores there is an increased uptake of dietary iron. Unfortunately, athletes do not appear to follow that pattern; studies show that athletes absorb less than half the dietary iron absorbed by a comparable group of sedentary anemic individuals (41). This absorption problem increases the difficulty of returning to normal iron status: athletes may have a higher need and yet, when deficient, do not absorb the iron as well as do sedentary individuals. Given that the total kcal intake of some athletes (especially women) will be inadequate in terms of iron intake (6 mg iron per 1,000 kcal in the average American diet), supplementation may be needed (20). Women runners lose about 1.7 to 2.3 mg of iron per day while absorbing only about 1.0 mg; this leaves them in negative iron balance. Athletes who are at risk need to be educated about increasing iron intake in their diets by making wise food choices. Some may choose to take an iron supplement each day as an ounce of prevention, but such a practice is not without problems (e.g., intolerance, overdose, drug interactions), and should not be done indiscriminately (3, 16, 112).

Vitamins

Chapter 18 provided the details about the RDA for each vitamin. Many of these vitamins are directly involved in energy production, acting as coenzymes in mitochondrial reactions associated with aerobic metabolism. Unfortunately, the old adage that "if a little is good, more will be better" has been applied to the question of whether or not the RDA for athletes is higher than that for sedentary people, rather than a factual research base. In general, the major reviews of this issue over the past *thirty years* have systematically concluded that, in general:

- vitamin supplementation is unnecessary for the athlete on a well-balanced diet,
- people who are *clearly deficient* in certain vitamins have improved performance when values return to normal, and
- individuals taking large doses of fat-soluble vitamins or vitamin C should be concerned about toxicity (5, 19, 105, 109).

The central concern raised by these reviewers is for the small athlete on a low-energy diet who may not make wise food selections, a point reinforced in a recent set of recommendations (3). In fact, some adolescent and adult female athletes have dietary intakes of vitamin E, B_6, B_{12}, and folate below the RDA standards (56). In these situations a single RDA multivitamin/mineral pill might be appropriate (3, 5). For those who believe the adage and want to take a high-potency multivitamin, one study showed that ninety days on such a pill had no effect on maximal aerobic power, endurance running performance, or strength (99). Additional information on the use of nutritional supplements to improve athletic performance is presented in chapter 25, where ergogenic aids are discussed.

TABLE 23.2 Suggested Pregame Meals

Breakfast	Calories	Lunch	Calories
4 ounces orange juice	60	4 ounces tomato juice	25
8 ounces skim milk	80	2 ounces turkey	100
2 slices toast	140	2 slices bread	140
2 tablespoons preserves	110	8 ounces skim milk	80
1 poached egg	80	1 orange	60
		2 plain cookies	120
Total calories	470		525

From M. H. Williams, *Nutritional Aspects of Human Physical and Athletic Performance*, 2d ed. Copyright © 1985. Charles C Thomas, Publisher, Springfield IL. Reprinted by permission.

IN SUMMARY

■ Iron deficiency in American athletes may be related to an inadequate intake of dietary iron as well as a potentially greater loss in sweat and feces. In spite of this deficiency, athletes may absorb less than half of what a sedentary group of anemic individuals absorbs. Iron supplementation may be recommended for female athletes as a result of an annual clinical assessment of iron status.

■ Vitamin supplementation is unnecessary for an athlete on a well-balanced diet. However, for those with a clear deficiency, supplementation is warranted.

Precompetition Diet

The two most important nutritional practices associated with optimal performance in endurance exercise are (a) to eat a high-carbohydrate diet in the *days preceding* competition when the intensity and duration of workouts are reduced, and (b) to drink liquids at regular intervals *during* the competition. Consistent with our previous discussion, the purposes of the pregame meal are the following (3, 53, 110):

■ to provide adequate hydration,

■ to provide carbohydrate to "top off" already high carbohydrate stores in the liver,

■ to avoid the sensation of hunger on a relatively empty stomach, and

■ to minimize GI tract problems (gas, diarrhea).

Unfortunately, the type of pregame meal served at various universities throughout this country may rely more on tradition than nutrition. The standard rare steak before a boxing match or football game to bring out the animal instinct, or careful planning to make sure that the color of the Jell-O is the same as it was when the team won last year's championship, are less than rational, but may be useful in pulling the team together to get ready for competition. Problems arise when the pregame meal is responsible for poor performance because of its own characteristics (high fat and protein) or the inability of the athlete to tolerate the meal without vomiting or experiencing diarrhea due to the emotion associated with competition. These latter conditions would cause a dehydration inconsistent with optimal performance. It is clear that beyond what is recommended in the nutrient makeup of a pregame meal, the ability of the athlete to tolerate it must be considered (3, 110).

Nutrients in Pregame Meal The number of kcal in a pregame meal should be 500 to 1,000, and the primary nutrient should be complex carbohydrates because they are easily digested and provide glucose to increase liver glycogen. It is generally recommended that large amounts of simple sugars should not be consumed immediately prior to competition (110). The fat content of the pregame meal should be kept to a minimum because fat is more slowly digested and is not needed as a fuel for exercise. Body stores are more than adequate. The protein content of the pregame meal should be small. The digestion and metabolism of protein increases the quantity of acids in the blood that must be buffered and finally excreted by the kidneys (53, 110). Table 23.2 presents two pregame meals that meet these considerations (110). These meals should be eaten about three hours prior to competition.

Some coaches and athletes prefer one of the commercially available liquid meals as the pregame meal because of convenience. These liquid meals can also be consumed throughout the day (along with

Jell-O is a registered trademark of General Foods, Inc.

additional water) when events or games are scheduled over long periods of time. Given that some people may not react favorably to any new "food," these liquid meals should be tried on practice days rather than on game day to make sure they are suitable.

IN SUMMARY

- The pregame meal should provide for hydration and adequate carbohydrate to "top off" stores while minimizing hunger symptoms, gas, and diarrhea. Varieties of commercially available liquid meals are consistent with these goals.

BODY COMPOSITION AND PERFORMANCE

A simple observation of the track-and-field events at the Olympic Games suggests that the physical characteristics of those successful in the shot put are different from those successful in the marathon. The purpose of this section is to reinforce that observation by providing a brief review of **somatotype** and body fatness related to performance.

SOMATOTYPE

In 1940, Sheldon (94) published *The Varieties of Human Physique*, in which he introduced the concept of the somatotype. In his scheme each person could be characterized as possessing a certain amount of the following three components of body form:

Endomorphy—relative predominance of soft roundness and large digestive viscera. He used the prefix *endo* as it relates to the *endo*dermal embryonic layers from which the digestive track is derived.

Mesomorphy—relative predominance of muscle, bone, and connective tissue ultimately derived from the *meso*dermal embryonic layer.

Ectomorphy—relative predominance of linearity and fragility with a great surface area-to-mass ratio giving great sensory exposure to the environment. The nervous system is derived from the *ecto*dermal embryonic layer.

Sheldon photographed 4,000 college men and ranked each of these three components on a scale of 1 to 7, with 1 representing the least amount of a component and 7 representing the greatest amount. A somatotype is a three-number sequence (e.g., 171 is one-seven-one) characterizing the endomorphic, mesomorphic, and ectomorphic components, respectively. Figure 23.10 shows the extremes of each somatotype. It must be remembered that somatotype considers only body form or shape and does not consider size. Tanner (101) used a two-dimensional plot of the original somatotypes of Sheldon's 4,000 college students on whom the 1 to 7 scale was based. This distribution of somatotypes is shown in figure 23.11 where a contrasting distribution is also presented, showing the somatotypes of 137 Olympic track-and-field athletes. Not surprisingly, the body form or type associated with world-class performance is different from that of the average population and differs by sport and event.

The values used in these figures were based on the Sheldon photographs (95), but according to the somatotyping method of Heath-Carter (58), Sheldon's 1 to 7 scale was too confining in that there are components in certain body types that exceed that given the value of 7. Using their method of somatotyping, Heath-Carter (58) cite the following examples of extremes in somatotypes: (a) extremely obese individuals having endomorphy values as high as 12, (b) members of the Manu tribe of the Admirality Islands with values of 9.5 for mesomorphy, and (c) members of the Nilote tribe in Africa having ectomorphic values of 8 and 9. When Olympic athletes were rated with this Heath-Carter scale, weight lifters and throwers were outside the normal distribution of Sheldon's mesomorphy scale. As one moves from these weight lifters and throwers to the distance runners and basketball players, the somatotype becomes progressively more ectomorphic. The distribution of somatotypes for the women athletes was shifted down and to the left, indicating smaller mesomorphic and larger endomorphic components (38).

Further, the Heath-Carter scale views the somatotype, especially the endomorphic and mesomorphic components, to be dynamic with the potential to change over time. Sheldon had viewed the somatotype as more of a permanent form for a given individual. The Heath-Carter method sees the endomorphic component as being equivalent to relative fatness or leanness and is closely tied to the sum of skinfolds. The mesomorphic component is viewed as being an estimate of the relative musculoskeletal development and similar to lean body mass. This latter translation of somatotype values into body composition values is a good lead into our next section.

Body Fatness and Performance

The somatotypes of the athletes involved in the Olympic Games represent low relative fatness (low endomorphy) and high relative fat-free mass (high mesomorphy). This two-component system of body composition was described in detail in chapter 18,

FIGURE 23.10 Extremes of somatotypes: endomorphy (top), mesomorphy (middle), and ectomorphy (bottom). Photo courtesy of W. H. Sheldon Trust.

where optimal body fatness goals were presented for health and fitness:

Males: 10%–20% fat

Females: 15%–25% fat

The question is, are these values optimal for athletic performance?

Table 23.3 lists a summary of body fatness values by sport (111). Many are average values and do not represent the range that might be observed in a study. For example, a study might find an average value of 12% body fat for a group of football players, but the range might be 5% to 19%. In a sport or activity in which body weight must be carried along (e.g., running

American College Students

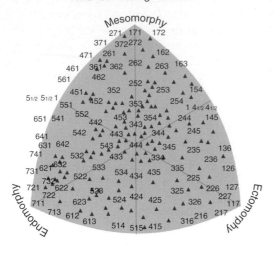

Somatotype distribution of 4,000 American
college students redrawn from Sheldon (1940).
Each dot represents 20 students

Olympic track-and-field athletes

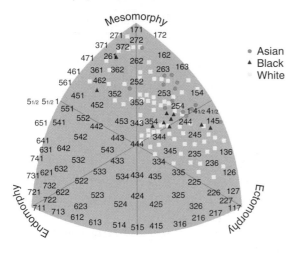

• Asian
▲ Black
□ White

Somatotype distribution of
137 Olympic track-and-field athletes

FIGURE 23.11 Contrast of the distribution of somatotypes of American college students and Olympic track-and-field athletes.

Athletic Group or Sport	Male	Female
Baseball	11.8–14.2	—
Basketball	7.1–10.6	20.8–26.9
Canoeing	12.4	—
Football		
Backs	9.4–12.4	—
Linebackers	13.7	—
Linemen	15.5–19.1	—
Quarterbacks, kickers	14.1	—
Gymnastics	4.6	9.6–23.8
Ice hockey	13–15.1	—
Jockeys	14.1	—
Orienteering	16.3	18.7
Pentathlon	—	11.0
Racquetball	8.3	14.0
Skiing		
Alpine	7.4–14.1	20.6
Cross-country	7.9–12.5	15.7–21.8
Nordic combined	8.9–11.2	—
Ski jumping	14.3	—
Soccer	9.6	—
Speed skating	11.4	—
Swimming	5.0–8.5	20.3
Tennis	15.2–16.3	20.3
Track and field		
Distance runners	3.7–18.0	15.2–19.2
Middle distance runners	12.4	—
Sprinters	16.5	19.3
Discus	16.3	25.0
Jumpers/hurdlers	—	20.7
Shot put	16.5–19.6	28.0
Volleyball	—	21.3–25.3
Wrestling	4.0–14.4	

TABLE 23.3 Percent Body Fat Values for Male and Female Athletes

From J. H. Wilmore, "Body Composition in Sport Medicine: Directions for Future Research," in *Medicine and Science in Sports Medicine* 15:21–31, 1983. Copyright © 1983 American College of Sports Medicine, Indianapolis IN. Reprinted by permission.

or jumping), there is a negative correlation between body fatness and performance (111, 113).

There is little question that regular measurements of body composition are useful for athletes in order to monitor changes during the season as well as over the off-season. In this way the athlete will know whether changes in body weight represent gains or losses of body fatness. What is more difficult is providing a fixed absolute recommendation about what body fatness should be for optimal performance for each individual.

One of the main reasons one must be careful in making absolute recommendations, such as "This ath-

lete should reduce her percent body fat from 15.6% to 14.0%," is that the athlete may already be 14% body fat. Each *individual estimate* of body fatness, even done by the underwater weighing technique, has an error in measurement that cannot be ignored. With appropriate methods and careful measurement, percent fat can be estimated with an error of about 3% to 4% fat. So when an athlete is measured as being 15.0% body fat, the true value may be as high as 19% and as low as 11% (64).

Another reason caution must be used in making an absolute recommendation for each athlete is that it ignores the normal variation in body fatness found in elite athletes in any particular sport. An elite group of volleyball players may have an average value of 12%, but the range among the team members might be 6% to 16%. No one would think of telling the athlete with 6% body fat to increase body fatness to reach the team average, and the same advice holds true for the one at 16% body fatness who is playing with world-class skill. A recommendation to alter body composition to achieve better performance must be made against the background of present performance and general health status as seen in sleeping patterns, adequate diet, mental outlook, and so on. The implementation of longer workouts or a reduction in caloric intake might change the percent body fat in the appropriate direction, but either one could adversely affect the athlete's ability to tolerate a workout or to study for exams. Wilmore's (113) observation of one of the best female distance runners who held most of the American middle distance records should be remembered when making such recommendations: The champion was 17% body fat when most of the elite female runners were <12%.

Monitoring body fatness in athletes by skinfold or underwater weighing is a reasonable procedure to follow because it allows a coach or trainer to observe *changes* in body fatness over the course of a season and from one year to the next. The information is also useful to the athletes who, when they finish their competitive careers, must attend to what is a reasonable body weight in order to be within the optimal body fatness range for health and fitness.

IN SUMMARY

- A somatotype is a numerical representation on a 1 to 7 scale of the degree to which a person possesses a high level of endomorphy, mesomorphy, or ectomorphy. Athletes are clearly different from the ordinary population, indicating a natural predisposition needed for success.
- The body fat percentage consistent with excellence in performance is different for men and women, and varies within gender from sport to sport. Average values for a team should not be applied to any single individual without regard to overall health status as seen in diet, sleep, and mental outlook. Further, it is "natural" for some athletes to have a higher body fatness than others in order to perform optimally.

STUDY QUESTIONS

1. What procedures would you follow to cause a supercompensation of muscle glycogen?
2. How much of a change in carbohydrate intake would be required for an individual who already achieves the dietary goal for carbohydrate?
3. How could glucose ingestion prior to exercise actually increase the rate of glycogen depletion?
4. Does carbohydrate ingestion during exercise slow down muscle glycogen depletion? Does it improve performance?
5. Is the protein requirement of an athlete higher than that of a sedentary person? Should protein intake be increased?
6. How would you recommend that a person replace water loss due to exercise?
7. How does the fluid replacement strategy differ for short and long races?
8. How would you recommend that a potential iron deficiency anemia condition be dealt with?
9. Does an athlete need additional vitamins for optimal performance? Why?
10. What are the primary considerations for a pregame meal?
11. What is a somatotype and how is it different for athletes compared to the average college population?
12. Given a female distance runner with 17% body fat, what should you consider before making a recommendation for change?

SUGGESTED READINGS

American College of Sports Medicine. 2000. Nutrition and athletic performance. *Medicine and Science in Sports and Exercise* 32:2130–45.

Williams, M. H. 2004. *Nutrition for Health, Fitness, & Sport*, 7th ed. New York. McGraw-Hill Companies.

REFERENCES

1. Ahlborg, B. et al. 1967. Muscle glycogen and muscle electrolytes during prolonged physical exercise. *Acta Physiologica Scandinavica* 70:129–42.
2. Almond, C. S. et al. 2005. Hyponatremia among runners in the Boston Marathon. *New England Journal of Medicine* 352:1550–56.
3. American College of Sports Medicine. 2000. Nutrition and athletic performance. *Medicine and Science in Sports and Exercise* 32:2130–45.
4. Barr, S. I., D. L. Costill, and W. J. Fink. 1991. Fluid replacement during prolonged exercise: Effects of water, saline, or no fluid. *Medicine and Science in Sports and Exercise* 23:811–17.

5. Belko, A. Z. 1987. Vitamins and exercise—an update. *Medicine and Science in Sports and Exercise* 19:S191–S196.

6. Bergstrom, J., and E. Hultman. 1966. Muscle glycogen synthesis after exercise: An enhancing factor localized to the muscle cells in man. *Nature* 210:309.

7. Bergstrom, J. et al. 1967. Diet, muscle glycogen and physical performance. *Acta Physiologica Scandinavica* 71:140–50.

8. Brotherhood, J. R. 1984. Nutrition and sports performance. *Sports Medicine* 1:350–89.

9. Burke, L. M., B. Kiens, and J. L. Ivy. 2004. Carbohydrates and fat for training and recovery. *Journal of Sports Sciences* 22:15–30.

10. Bussau, V. A., T. J. Fairchild, A. Rao, P. Steele, and P. A. Fournier. 2002. Carbohydrate loading in human muscle: An improved 1 day protocol. *European Journal of Applied Physiology* 87:290–95.

11. Butterfield, G. 1991. Amino acids and high protein diets. In *Ergogenics: Enhancement of Performance in Exercise and Sport*, ed. D. R. Lamb and M. H. Williams, 87–117. Carmel, IN: Brown & Benchmark.

12. Butterfield, G. E. 1987. Whole-body protein utilization in humans. *Medicine and Science in Sports and Exercise* 19:S157–S165.

13. Butterfield, G. E., and D. H. Calloway. 1984. Physical activity improves protein utilization in young men. *British Journal of Nutrition* 51:171–84.

14. Carter, J., A. E. Jeukendrup, T. Mundel, and D. A. Jones. 2003. Carbohydrate supplementation improves moderate and high-intensity exercise in the heat. *Pflugers Archiv-European Journal of Physiology* 446:211–19.

15. Casa, D. J., P. M. Clarkson, and W. O. Roberts. 2005. American College of Sports Medicine Roundtable on hydration and physical activity: Consensus statement. *Current Sports Medicine Reports* 4:115–27.

16. Chatard, J. C., I. Mujika, C. Guy, and J. R. Lacour. 1999. Anemia and iron deficiency in athletes. *Sports Medicine* 27:229–40.

17. Cheuvront, S. N. 1999. The Zone Diet and athletic performance. *Sport Medicine* 27:213–28.

18. Chryssanthopoulos, C., C. Williams, and A. Nowitz. 2002. Influence of a carbohydrate-electrolyte solution ingested during running on muscle glycogen utilisation in fed humans. *International Journal of Sports Medicine* 23:279–84.

19. Clarkson, P. M. 1991. Vitamins and trace minerals. In *Ergogenics: Enhancement of Performance in Exercise and Sport*, ed. D. R. Lamb and M. H. Williams, 123–82. Carmel, IN: Brown & Benchmark.

20. Clement, D. B., and R. C. Asmundson. 1982. Nutritional intake and hematological parameters in endurance runners. *Physician and Sportsmedicine* 10:37–43.

21. Clement, D. B., and L. L. Sawchuk. 1984. Iron status and sports performance. *Sports Medicine* 1:65–74.

22. Coggan, A. R., and E. F. Coyle. 1991. Carbohydrate ingestion during prolonged exercise: Effects on metabolism and performance. In *Exercise and Sport Sciences Reviews*, vol. 19, ed. J. O. Holloszy, 1–40. Philadelphia: Lippincott Williams & Wilkins.

23. Costill, D. L. 1977. Sweating: Its composition and effects on body fluids. *Annals of the New York Academy of Sciences* 301:160–74.

24. Costill, D. L., and B. Saltin. 1974. Factors limiting gastric emptying during rest and exercise. *Journal of Applied Physiology* 37:679–83.

25. Costill, D. L. et al. 1977. Effects of elevated plasma FFA and insulin on muscle glycogen usage during exercise. *Journal of Applied Physiology* 43:695–99.

26. Costill, D. L. et al. 1981. The role of dietary carbohydrates in muscle glycogen resynthesis after strenuous running. *American Journal of Clinical Nutrition* 34:1831–36.

27. Coyle, E. F. 1994. Fluid and carbohydrate replacement during exercise: How much and why? *Sports Science Exchange* vol. 7, no. 3. Barrington, IL: Gatorade Sports Science Institute.

28. Coyle, E. F. et al. 1978. Gastric-emptying rates of selected athletic drinks. *Research Quarterly* 49:119–24.

29. Coyle, E. F., and S. J. Montain. 1992. Carbohydrate and fluid ingestion during exercise: Are there trade-offs? *Medicine and Science in Sports and Exercise* 24:671–78.

30. Coyle, E. F., and S. J. Montain. 1992. Benefits of fluid replacement with carbohydrate during exercise. *Medicine and Science in Sports and Exercise* 24:S324–S330.

31. Coyle, E. F. et al. 1983. Carbohydrate feeding during prolonged strenuous exercise can delay fatigue. *Journal of Applied Physiology* 55:230–35.

32. Davidson, R. J. L. 1969. March or exertional haemoglobinuria. *Seminars in Hematology* 6:150–61.

33. Davies, C. T. M. et al. 1982. Glucose inhibits CO_2 production from leucine during whole body exercise in man. *Journal of Physiology* 332:40–41.

34. Davies, K. J. A. et al. 1982. Muscle mitochondrial bioenergetics, oxygen supply, and work capacity during dietary iron deficiency and repletion. *American Journal of Physiology* 242:E418–E427.

35. Davies, K. J. A. et al. 1984. Distinguishing effects of anemic and muscle iron deficiency on exercise bioenergetics in the rat. *American Journal of Physiology* 246:E535–E543.

36. Davis, J. M. et al. 1987. Accumulation of deuterium oxide in body fluids after ingestion of D_2O-labeled beverages. *Journal of Applied Physiology* 63:2060–66.

37. Davis, J. M. et al. 1988. Effects of ingesting 6% and 12% glucose/electrolyte beverages during prolonged intermittent cycling in the heat. *European Journal of Applied Physiology* 57:563–69.

38. de Garay, A., L. Levine, and J. Carter. 1974. *Genetic and Anthropological Studies of Olympic Athletes*. New York: Academic Press.

39. Diehl, D. M. et al. 1986. Effects of physical training and competition on the iron status of female hockey players. *International Journal of Sports Medicine* 6:264–70.

40. Drinkwater, B. L. et al. 1984. Bone mineral content of amenorrheic and eumenorrheic athletes. *New England Journal of Medicine* 311:277–81.

41. Ehn, L., B. Carlwark, and S. Hoglund. 1980. Iron status in athletes involved in intense physical activity. *Medicine and Science in Sports and Exercise* 12:61–64.

42. Fairchild, T. J., S. Fletcher, P. Steele, C. Goodman, B. Dawson, and P. A. Fournier, 2002. Rapid carbohydrate loading after a short bout of near maximal-intensity exercise. *Medicine and Science in Sports and Exercise* 34:980–86.

43. Felig, P. et al. 1982. Hypoglycemia during prolonged exercise in normal men. *New England Journal of Medicine* 306:895–900.

44. Felig, P., and J. Wahren. 1971. Amino acid metabolism in exercising man. *Journal of Clinical Investigation* 50:2703–14.

45. Foster, C., D. L. Costill, and W. J. Fink. 1979. Effects of preexercise feedings on endurance performance. *Medicine and Science in Sports* 11:1–5.

46. Foster, C., and N. N. Thompson. 1990. Serial gastric emptying studies: Effect of preceding drinks. *Medicine and Science in Sports and Exercise* 22:484–87.

47. Friedman, J. E., P. D. Neufer, and G. L. Dohm. 1991. Regulation of glycogen resynthesis following exercise: Dietary considerations. *Sports Medicine* 11:232–43.

48. Gardner, G. W. et al. 1977. Physical work capacity and metabolic stress in subjects with iron deficiency anemia. *American Journal of Clinical Nutrition* 30:910–17.

49. Gisolfi, C. V., and S. M. Duchman. 1992. Guidelines for optimal replacement of beverages for different athletic events. *Medicine and Science in Sports and Exercise* 24:679–87.

50. Gledhill, N. 1985. The influence of altered blood volume and oxygen transport capacity on aerobic performance. In *Exercise and Sport Sciences Reviews*, vol. 13, ed. R. L. Terjung, 75–93.

51. Gontzea, I., P. Sutzescu, and S. Dumitrache. 1974. The influence of muscular activity on nitrogen balance, and on the need of man for protein. *Nutrition Reports International* 10:35–43.

52. ———. 1975. The influence of adaptation of physical effort on nitrogen balance in man. *Nutrition Reports International* 11:231–36.

53. Guild, W. R. 1960. Pre-event nutrition, with some implications for endurance athletes. In *Exercise and Fitness*. Chicago: The Athletic Institute.

54. Hamilton, M. T., J. Gonzalez-Alonso, S. J. Montain, and E. F. Coyle. 1991. Fluid replacement and glucose infusion during exercise prevent cardiovascular drift. *Journal of Applied Physiology* 71:871–77.

55. Haymes, E. M. 1987. Nutritional concerns: Need for iron. *Medicine and Science in Sports and Exercise* 19:S197–S200.

56. ———. 1991. Vitamin and mineral supplementation to athletes. *International Journal of Sports Nutrition* 1:146–69.

57. Haymes, E. M., and J. J. Lamanca. 1989. Iron loss in runners during exercise: Implications and recommendations. *Sports Medicine* 7:277–85.

58. Heath, B. H., and J. E. L. Carter. 1967. A modified somatotype method. *American Journal of Physical Anthropology* 27:57–74.

59. Hegsted, M. et al. 1981. Urinary calcium and calcium balance in young men affected by level of protein and inorganic phosphate intake. *Journal of Nutrition* 111:553–62.

60. Herbert, W. 1983. Water and electrolytes. In *Ergogenic Aids in Sports*, ed. M. A. Williams. Champaign, IL: Human Kinetics.

61. Hermansen, L., E. Hultman, and B. Saltin. 1967. Muscle glycogen during prolonged severe exercise. *Acta Physiologica Scandinavica* 71:129–39.

62. Hood, D. A., and R. L. Terjung. 1990. Amino acid metabolism during exercise and following endurance training. *Sports Medicine* 9:23–35.

63. Houmard, J. A., P. C. Egan, R. A. Johns, P. D. Neufer, T. C. Chenier, and R. G. Israel. 1991. Gastric emptying during 1 h of cycling and running at 75% $\dot{V}O_2$ max. *Medicine and Science in Sports and Exercise* 23:320–25.

64. Houtkooper, L. B., and S. B. Going. 1994. Body composition: How should it be measured? Does it affect performance? *Sports Science Exchange* vol. 7, no. 5. Barrington, IL: Gatorade Sports Science Institute.

65. Ivy, J. L. 1991. Muscle glycogen synthesis before and after exercise. *Sports Medicine* 11:6–19.

66. Ivy, J. L., P. T. Res, R. C. Sprague, and M. O. Widzer. 2003. Effect of a carbohydrate-protein supplement on endurance performance during exercise of varying intensity. *International Journal of Sport Nutrition & Exercise Metabolism* 13:382–95.

67. Jarvis, M., L. McNaughton, A. Seddon, and D. Thompson. 2002. The acute 1-week effects of the Zone Diet on body composition, blood lipid levels, and performance in recreational endurance athletes. *Journal of Strength and Conditioning Research* 16:50–57.

68. Jentjens, R., and A. Jeukendrup. 2003. Determinants of post-exercise glycogen synthesis during short-term recovery. *Sports Medicine* 33:117–44.

69. Karlsson, J., and B. Saltin. 1971. Diet, muscle glycogen, and endurance performance. *Journal of Applied Physiology* 31:203–6.

70. Kerstetter, J. E., K. O. O'Brien, D. M. Caseria, D. E. Wall, and K. L. Insogna. 2005. The impact of dietary protein on calcium absorption and kinetic measures of bone turnover in women. *Journal of Clinical Endocrinology & Metabolism* 90:26–31.

71. Kerstetter, J. E., K. O. O'Brien, and K. L. Insogna. 2003. Dietary protein, calcium metabolism, and skeletal homeostasis revisited. *American Journal of Clinical Nutrition* 78:584S–92S.

72. Lemon, P. W. R. 1987. Protein and exercise: Update 1987. *Medicine and Science in Sports and Exercise* 19:S179–S190.

73. ———. 1991a. Protein and amino acid needs of the strength athlete. *International Journal of Sport Nutrition* 1:127–45.

74. ———. 1991b. Effect of exercise on protein requirements. *Journal of Sport Sciences* 9:53–70.

75. ———. 1995. Do athletes need more dietary protein and amino acids? *International Journal of Sport Nutrition* 5:S39–S61.

76. Lemon, P. W. R., and J. P. Mullin. 1980. Effect of initial muscle glycogen levels on protein catabolism during exercise. *Journal of Applied Physiology* 48:624–29.

77. Mitchell, J. B. et al. 1988. Effects of carbohydrate ingestion on gastric emptying and exercise. *Medicine and Science in Sports and Exercise* 20:110–15.

78. Mitchell, J. B., D. L. Costill, J. A. Houmard, W. J. Fink, R. A. Robergs, and J. A. Davis. 1989. Gastric emptying: Influence of prolonged exercise and carbohydrate concentration. *Medicine and Science in Sports and Exercise* 21:269–74.

79. Mitchell, J. B., and K. W. Voss. 1991. The influence of volume on gastric emptying and fluid balance during prolonged exercise. *Medicine and Science in Sports and Exercise* 23:314–19.

80. Murray, R. 1995. Fluid needs in hot and cold environments. *International Journal of Sport Nutrition* 5:S62–S73.

81. Neufer, P. D., A. J. Young, and M. N. Sawka. 1989a. Gastric emptying during exercise: Effects of heat stress and hypohydration. *European Journal of Applied Physiology* 58:433–39.

82. ———. 1989b. Gastric emptying during exercise: Effects of heat stress and hypohydration. *European Journal of Applied Physiology* 58:440–45.

83. Noakes, T. D., R. J. Norman, R. H. Buck, J. Godlonton, K. Stevenson, and D. Pittaway. 1990. The incidence of hyponatremia during prolonged ultraendurance exercise. *Medicine and Science in Sports and Exercise* 22:165–70.

84. Noakes, T. 2002. Hyponatremia in distance runners: fluid and sodium balance during exercise. *Current Sports Medicine Reports* 1:197–207.

85. Nybo, L. 2003. CNS fatigue and prolonged exercise: Effect of glucose supplementation. *Medicine & Science in Sports & Exercise* 35:589–94.

86. Owen, M. D. et al. 1986. Effects of ingesting carbohydrate beverages during exercise in the heat. *Medicine and Science in Sports and Exercise* 18:568–75.

87. Paul, D., K. A. Jacobs, R. J. Geor, and K. W. Hinchcliff. 2003. No effect of pre-exercise meal on substrate metabolism and time trial performance during intense endurance exercise. *International Journal of Sport Nutrition & Exercise Metabolism* 13(4):489–503.

88. Paulev, P. E., R. Jordal, and N. S. Pedersen. 1983. Dermal excretion of iron in intensely trained athletes. *Clinical Chimica Acta* 127:19–27.

89. Phillips, S. M. 2004. Protein requirements and supplementation in strength sports. *Nutrition* 20:689–95.

90. Pitts, G., R. Johnson, and F. Consolazio. 1944. Work in the heat as affected by intake of water, salt and glucose. *American Journal of Physiology* 142:353–59.

91. Rehrer, N. J., E. J. Beckers, F. Brouns, F. T. Hoor, and W. H. M. Saris. 1990. Effects of dehydration on gastric emptying and gastrointestinal distress while running. *Medicine and Science in Sports and Exercise* 22:790–95.

92. Rehrer, N. J., F. Brouns, E. J. Beckers, F. T. Hoor, and W. H. M. Saris. 1990. Gastric emptying with repeated drinking during running and bicycling. *International Journal of Sports Medicine* 11:238–43.

93. Rowlands, D. S., and W. G. Hopkins. 2002. Effect of high-fat, high-carbohydrate, and high-protein meals on metabolism and performance during endurance cycling. *International Journal of Sport Nutrition & Exercise Metabolism* 12:318–35.

94. Sheldon, W. H. 1940. *The Varieties of Human Physique*. New York: Harper & Brothers.

95. Sheldon, W. H., C. W. Dupertuis, and E. McDermott. 1954. *Atlas of Men*. New York: Harper & Brothers.

96. Sherman, W. M. 1983. Carbohydrates, muscle glycogen, and muscle glycogen supercompensation. In *Ergogenic Aids in Sports*, ed. M. H. Williams, chap. 1, 3–26. Champaign, IL: Human Kinetics.

97. ———. 1991. Carbohydrate feedings before and after exercise. In *Perspectives in Exercise Science and Sports Medicine Volume 4: Ergogenics—Enhancement of Performance in Exercise and Sport*, ed. D. R. Lamb and M. R. Williams. New York: McGraw-Hill Companies.

98. Shi, X. C., and C. V. Gisolfi. 1998. Fluid and carbohydrate replacement during intermittent exercise. *Sports Medicine* 25:157–72.

99. Singh, A., F. M. Moses, and P. A. Deuster. 1992. Chronic multivitamin-mineral supplementation does not enhance physical performance. *Medicine and Science in Sports and Exercise* 24:726–32.

100. Stewart, J. G. et al. 1984. Gastrointestinal blood loss and anemia in runners. *Annals of Internal Medicine* 100:843–45.

101. Tanner, J. M., S. S. Stevens, and W. B. Tucker. 1964. *The Physique of the Olympic Athlete*. London: George Allen and Unwin.

102. Tarnopolsky, M. 2004. Protein requirements for endurance athletes. *Nutrition* 20:662–68.

103. Todd, K. S., G. Butterfield, and D. H. Calloway. 1984. Nitrogen balance in men with adequate and deficit energy intake at 3 levels of work. *Journal of Nutrition* 114:2107–18.

104. Utter, A. C. et al. 2004. Carbohydrate supplementation and perceived exertion during prolonged running. *Medicine & Science in Sports & Exercise* 36:1036–41.

105. Van der Beek, E. J. 1985. Vitamins and endurance training: Food for running or faddish claims? *Sports Medicine* 2:175–97.

106. Vrijens, D. M. J., and N. J. Rehrer. 1999. Sodium-free fluid ingestion decreases plasma sodium during exercise in the heat. *Journal of Applied Physiology* 86:1847–51.

107. Walberg-Rankin, J. 1995. Dietary carbohydrate as an ergogenic aid for prolonged and brief competitions in sport. *International Journal of Sport Nutrition* 5:S13–S27.

108. White, T. P., and G. A. Brooks. 1981. [U-^{14}C] glucose, -alanine, and -leucine oxidation in rats at rest and two intensities of running. *American Journal of Physiology* 241:E155–E165.

109. Williams, M. H. 1985. *Nutritional Aspects of Human Physical and Athletic Performance*. Springfield, IL: Charles C Thomas.

110. ———. 1985. *The Nutrition for Fitness Answer Book*. New York: McGraw-Hill Companies.

111. ———. 1983. Body composition in sport and exercise: Directions for future research. *Medicine and Science in Sports and Exercise* 15:21–31.

112. ———. 1999. Pumping dietary iron. *ACSM's Health & Fitness Journal* 3:15–22.

113. Wilmore, J. H. 1984. Body composition and sports medicine: Research considerations. In *Report of the Sixth Ross Conference on Medical Research*, 78–82. Columbus, OH: Ross Laboratories.

114. Wolfe, R. R. 1987. Does exercise stimulate protein breakdown in humans?: Isotopic approaches to the problem. *Medicine and Science in Sports and Exercise* 19: S172–S178.

115. Wolfe, R. R. et al. 1982. Isotopic analysis of leucine and urea metabolism in exercising humans. *Journal of Applied Physiology: Respiration, Environmental, and Exercise Physiology* 52:458–66.

116. Wolfe, R. R. et al. 1984. Isotopic determination of amino acid-urea interactions in exercise in humans. *Journal of Applied Physiology* 56:221–29.

117. Wright, D. A., W. M. Sherman, and A. R. Dernbach. 1991. Carbohydrate feedings before, during, or in combination improve cycling endurance performance. *Journal of Applied Physiology* 71:1082–88.

118. Wright, J. D. et al. 2003. Dietary intake of ten key nutrients for public health, United States: 1999–2000. Advance data from vital and health statistics, no. 334. Hyattsville, MD: National Center for Health Statistics.

119. Yeo, S. E., R. L. P. G. Jentjens, G. A. Wallis, and A. E. Jeukendrup. 2005. Caffeine increases exogenous carbohydrate oxidation during exercise. *Journal of Applied Physiology* 99:844–50.

CHAPTER 24

Exercise and the Environment

By studying this chapter, you should be able to do the following:

1. Describe the changes in atmospheric pressure, air temperature, and air density with increasing altitude.
2. Describe how altitude affects sprint performances and explain why that is the case.
3. Explain why distance running performance decreases at altitude.
4. Draw a graph to show the effect of altitude on $\dot{V}O_2$ max and list the reasons for this response.
5. Graphically describe the effect of altitude on the heart rate and ventilation responses to submaximal work, and explain why these changes are appropriate.
6. Describe the process of adaptation to altitude, and the degree to which this adaptation can be complete.
7. Explain why such variability exists among athletes in the decrease in $\dot{V}O_2$max upon exposure to altitude, the degree of improvement in $\dot{V}O_2$ max at altitude, and the gains made upon return to sea level.
8. Describe the potential problems associated with training at high altitude and how one might deal with them.
9. Explain the circumstances that caused physiologists to reevaluate their conclusions that humans could not climb Mount Everest without oxygen.
10. Explain the role that hyperventilation plays in helping to maintain a high oxygen-hemoglobin saturation at extreme altitudes.
11. List and describe the factors influencing the risk of heat injury.
12. Provide suggestions for the fitness participant to follow to minimize the likelihood of heat injury.
13. Describe in general terms the guidelines suggested for running road races in the heat.
14. Describe the three elements in the heat stress index, and explain why one is more important than the other two.
15. List the factors influencing hypothermia.
16. Explain what the wind chill index is relative to heat loss.
17. Explain why exposure to cold water is more dangerous than exposure to air of the same temperature.
18. Describe what the "clo" unit is and how recommendations for insulation change when one does exercise.
19. Describe the role of subcutaneous fat and energy production in the development of hypothermia.
20. List the steps to follow to deal with hypothermia.
21. Explain how carbon monoxide can influence performance, and list the steps that should be taken to reduce the impact of pollution on performance.

■ Outline

Altitude 500
   Atmospheric Pressure 500
   Short-Term Anaerobic
     Performance 500
   Long-Term Aerobic
     Performance 501
   Maximal Aerobic Power and
     Altitude 501
   Adaptation to High
     Altitude 503

Training for Competition
   at Altitude 504
   The Quest for Everest 506

Heat 509
   Hyperthermia 509

Cold 512
   Environmental Factors 512
   Insulating Factors 513
   Energy Production 515

Dealing with
   Hypothermia 516

Air Pollution 516
   Particulate Matter 517
   Ozone 517
   Sulfur Dioxide 517
   Carbon Monoxide 517

■ Key Terms

clo
hyperoxia

hypoxia
normoxia

By now it should be clear that performance is dependent on more than simply having a high $\dot{V}O_2$ max. In chapter 23, we saw the role of diet and body composition on performance, and in chapter 25 we will formally consider "ergogenic" or work-enhancing aids and performance. Sandwiched between these chapters will be a discussion of how the environmental factors of altitude, heat, cold, and pollution can influence performance.

ALTITUDE

In the late 1960s, when the Olympic Games were scheduled to be held in Mexico City, our attention was directed at the question of how altitude (2,300 meters at Mexico City) would affect performance. Previous experience at altitude suggested that many performances would not equal former Olympic standards or, for that matter, the athlete's own personal record (PR) at sea level. On the other hand, some performances were actually expected to be better because they were conducted at altitude. Why? What happens to $\dot{V}O_2$ max with altitude? Can a sea-level resident ever completely adapt to altitude? We will address these and other questions after a brief review of the environmental factors that change with increasing altitude.

Atmospheric Pressure

The atmospheric pressure at any spot on earth is a measure of the weight of a column of air directly over that spot. At sea level the weight (and height) of that column of air is greatest. As one climbs to higher and higher altitudes the height and, of course, the weight

of the column are reduced. Consequently, atmospheric pressure decreases with increasing altitude, the air is less dense, and each liter of air contains fewer molecules of gas. Since the *percentages* of O_2, CO_2, and N_2 are the same at altitude as at sea level, any change in the *partial pressure* of each gas is due solely to the change in the atmospheric or barometric pressure (see chapter 10). The decrease in the partial pressure of O_2 (PO_2) with increasing altitude has a direct effect on the saturation of hemoglobin and, consequently, oxygen transport. This lower PO_2 is called **hypoxia,** with **normoxia** being the term to describe the PO_2 under sea-level conditions. The term **hyperoxia** describes a condition in which the inspired PO_2 is greater than that at sea level (see chapter 25). In addition to the hypoxic condition at altitude, the air temperature and humidity are lower, adding potential temperature regulation problems to the hypoxic stress of altitude. How do these changes affect performance? In order to answer that question we will divide performances into short-term anaerobic performances and long-term aerobic performances.

Short-Term Anaerobic Performance

In chapters 3 and 19 we described the importance of the anaerobic sources of ATP in maximal performances lasting two minutes or less. If this information is correct, and we think it is, then the short-term anaerobic races shouldn't be affected by the low PO_2 at altitude, since O_2 transport to the muscles is not limiting performance. Table 24.1 shows this to be the case when the sprint performances of the 1968 Mexico City Olympic Games were compared to those in the 1964 Tokyo Olympic Games (51). The performances

A CLOSER LOOK 24.1

Jumping Through Thin Air

In the 1968 Olympic Games in Mexico City, Bob Beamon shattered the world record in the long jump with a leap of 29 feet, 2.5 inches. Due to the fact that the record was achieved at altitude where air density is less than that at sea level, some questions were raised about the true magnitude of the achievement. Recent progress in biomechanics has made it possible to determine just how much would have been gained by doing the long jump at altitude (109). The calculations had to consider the mass of the jumper, a drag coefficient based on the frontal area exposed to the air while jumping, and the difference in the air density between sea level and Mexico City. The result indicated that approximately 2.4 cm (less than an inch) would have been gained by doing the jump at altitude where the air density is less. Recently, scientists have tried to predict the effect of altitude on running performances by considering the opposing factors of lower air density and the reduced availability of oxygen (82). The latter factor is discussed relative to long-distance races.

Olympic Games	Short Races: Men				Short Races: Women			
	100 m	*200 m*	*400 m*	*800 m*	*100 m*	*200 m*	*400 m*	*800 m*
1964 (Tokyo)	10.0 s	20.3 s	45.1 s	1 m 45.1 s	11.4 s	23.0 s	52.0 s	2 m 1.1 s
1968 (Mexico City)	9.9 s	19.8 s	43.8 s	1 m 44.3 s	11.0 s	22.5 s	52.0 s	2 m 0.9 s
% change*	+1.0	+2.5	+2.9	+0.8	+3.5	+2.2	0	+0.2

TABLE 24.1 Comparison of Performances in Short Races in the 1964 and 1968 Olympic Games

*+ sign indicates improvement over 1964 performance.

From E. T. Howley, "Effect of Altitude on Physical Performance," in G. A. Stull and T. K. Cureton, *Encyclopedia of Physical Education, Fitness and Sports: Training, Environment, Nutrition, and Fitness.* Copyright © 1980 American Alliance for Health, Physical Education, Recreation and Dance, Reston VA. Reprinted by permission.

improved in all but one case, in which the time for the 400-meter run for the women was the same. The reasons for the improvements in performance include the "normal" gains made over time from one Olympic Games to the next and the fact that the density of the air at altitude offers less resistance to movements at high speeds. Improvements in the 100-meter and 400-meter races for each increase of 1,000 meters in altitude have been estimated to be about 0.08 s and 0.06 s, respectively (4, 87). The issue of lower air resistance sparked controversy over Bob Beamon's fantastic performance in the long jump in the Mexico City Games (see A Closer Look 24.1).

Long-Term Aerobic Performance

Maximal performances in excess of two minutes are primarily dependent on oxygen delivery, and, in contrast to the short-term performances, are clearly affected by the lower PO_2 at altitude. Table 24.2 shows the results of the distance running events from 1,500 meters up through the marathon and the 50,000-meter walk, and as you can see, performance was diminished at all distances but the 1,500-meter run (51). This performance is worthy of special note, given that it was expected to be affected as were the others. It is more than just of passing interest that the record setter was Kipchoge Keino, who was born and raised in Kenya at an altitude similar to that of Mexico City. Did he possess a special adaptation due to his birthplace? We will come back to this question in a later section. We would like to continue our discussion of the effect of altitude on performance by asking, "Why did the performance fall off by as much as 6.2% in the long-distance races?"

IN SUMMARY

- The atmospheric pressure, PO_2, air temperature, and air density decrease with altitude.
- The lower air density at altitude offers less resistance to high-speed movement, and sprint performances are either not affected or are improved.

Maximal Aerobic Power and Altitude

The decrease in distance running performance at altitude is similar to what occurs when a trained runner becomes untrained—it would clearly take longer to

Olympic Games	Long Races: Men					
	1,500 m	*3,000 m*	*5,000 m*	*10,000 m*	*Marathon*	*50,000 m Walk*
1964 (Tokyo)	3 m 38.1 s	8 m 30.8 s	13 m 48.8 s	28 m 24.4 s	2 h 12 m 11.2 s	4 h 11 m 11.2 s
1968 (Mexico City)	3 m 34.9 s	8 m 51.0 s	14 m 05.0 s	29 m 27.4 s	2 h 20 m 26.4 s	4 h 20 m 13.6 s
% change*	+1.5	−3.9	−1.9	−3.7	−6.2	−3.6

*+ sign indicates improvement over 1964 performance.

From E. T. Howley, "Effect of Altitude on Physical Performance," in G. A. Stull and T. K. Cureton, *Encyclopedia of Physical Education, Fitness and Sports: Training, Environment, Nutrition, and Fitness.* Copyright © 1980 American Alliance for Health, Physical Education, Recreation and Dance, Reston VA. Reprinted by permission.

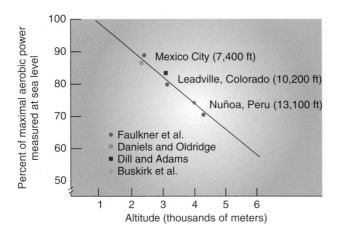

FIGURE 24.1 Changes in maximal aerobic power with increasing altitude. The sea-level value for maximal aerobic power is set to 100%. From E. T. Howley, "Effect of Altitude on Physical Performance," in G. A. Stull and T. K. Cureton, E*ncyclopedia of Physical Education, Fitness and Sports: Training, Environment, Nutrition, and Fitness.* Copyright © 1980 American Alliance for Health, Physical Education, Recreation and Dance, Reston VA. Reprinted by permission.

run a marathon! The similarity in the effect is related to a decrease in maximal aerobic power that occurs with detraining and with increasing altitude. Figure 24.1 shows that $\dot{V}O_2$ max decreases in a linear fashion, being about 12% lower at 2,400 meters (7,400 feet), 20% lower at 3,100 meters (10,200 feet), and 27% lower at about 4,000 meters (13,100 feet) (10, 19, 22, 28). While it should be no surprise that endurance performance decreases with such changes in $\dot{V}O_2$ max, why does $\dot{V}O_2$ max decrease?

Cardiovascular Function at Altitude Maximal oxygen uptake is equal to the product of the maximal cardiac output and the maximal arteriovenous oxygen difference, $\dot{V}O_2 = CO \times (CaO_2 - C\bar{v}O_2)$. Given this relationship, the decrease in $\dot{V}O_2$ max with increasing

altitude could be due to a decrease in cardiac output and/or a decrease in oxygen extraction.

Maximal cardiac output is equal to the product of maximal heart rate and maximal stroke volume. In several studies the maximal heart rate was unchanged at altitudes of 2,300 meters (25, 85), 3,100 meters (37), and 4,000 meters (10), while changes in maximal stroke volume were somewhat inconsistent (56). If these two variables, maximal stroke volume and maximal heart rate, do not change with increasing altitude, then the decrease in $\dot{V}O_2$ max must be due to a difference in oxygen extraction.

While oxygen extraction $(CaO_2 - C\bar{v}O_2)$ could decrease due to a decrease in the arterial oxygen content (CaO_2) or an increase in the mixed venous oxygen content $(C\bar{v}O_2)$, the primary cause is the desaturation of the arterial blood due to the low PO_2 at altitude. As you recall from chapter 10, as the arterial PO_2 falls there is a reduction in the volume of oxygen bound to hemoglobin. At sea level, hemoglobin is about 96% to 98% saturated with oxygen. However, at 2,300 meters and 4,000 meters, saturation falls to 88% and 71%, respectively. These decreases in the oxygen saturation of hemoglobin are similar to the reductions in $\dot{V}O_2$ max at these altitudes described earlier. Since maximal oxygen transport is the product of the maximal cardiac output and the arterial oxygen content, the capacity to transport oxygen to the working muscles at altitude is reduced due to desaturation, even though maximal cardiac output may be unchanged up to altitudes of 4,000 meters (56). However, it must be added that a variety of studies have shown a decrease in maximal heart rate at altitude. While some of these decreases have been observed at altitudes of 3,100 meters (22) and 4,300 meters (25), it is more common to find lower maximal heart rates above altitudes of 4,300 meters. For example, compared to maximal HR at sea level, maximal HR was observed to be 24 to 33 beats/minute lower at 4,650 meters (15,300 feet) and

FIGURE 24.2 The effect of altitude on the heart-rate response to submaximal exercise.

FIGURE 24.3 The effect of altitude on the ventilation response to submaximal exercise.

47 beats/minute lower at about 6,100 meters (20,000 feet) (40, 86). This depression in maximal heart rate is reversed by acute restoration of normoxia, or the use of atropine (40). This altitude-induced bradycardia suggests that myocardial hypoxia may trigger the slower heart rate to decrease the work and, therefore, the oxygen demand of the heart muscle. Given this lower maximal HR, it means that $\dot{V}O_2$ max may decrease at a faster rate at the higher altitudes due to the combined effects of the desaturation of hemoglobin and the decrease in maximal cardiac output.

This desaturation of arterial blood at altitude affects more than $\dot{V}O_2$ max. The cardiovascular responses to submaximal work are also influenced. Due to the fact that each liter of blood is carrying less oxygen, more liters of blood must be pumped per minute in order to compensate. This is accomplished through an increase in the HR response, since the stroke volume response is at its highest point already, or it is actually lower at altitude due to the hypoxia (2). This elevated HR response is shown in figure 24.2 (37). This has implications for more than the performance-based athlete. The average person who participates in an exercise program will have to decrease the intensity of exercise at altitude in order to stay in the target heart rate zone. Remember, the exercise prescription needed for a cardiovascular training effect includes a proper duration of exercise to achieve a total caloric expenditure of about 200 to 300 kcal, and if the intensity is too high the person will have more difficulty completing the workout.

Respiratory Function at Altitude In the introduction to this section we mentioned that the air is less dense at altitude. This means that there are fewer O_2 molecules per liter of air, and if a person wished to consume the same number of liters of O_2, pulmonary ventilation would have to increase. At 5,600 meters (18,400 feet), the atmospheric pressure is one-half that at sea level and the number of molecules of O_2

per liter of air is reduced by one-half; therefore, a person would have to breathe twice as much air to take in the same amount of O_2. The consequences of this are shown in figure 24.3, which presents the ventilation responses of a subject who exercised at work rates demanding about a $\dot{V}O_2$ of 1 to 2 L · min⁻¹ at sea level and at three altitudes exceeding 4,000 meters. The pulmonary ventilation is elevated at all altitudes, reaching values of almost 180 L · min⁻¹ at 6,400 meters (21,000 feet) (86). This extreme ventilatory response requires the respiratory muscles, primarily the diaphragm, to work so hard that fatigue may occur. We will see more on this in a later section dealing with the assault on Mount Everest.

IN SUMMARY

- Distance-running performances are adversely affected at altitude due to the reduction in the PO_2, which causes a decrease in hemoglobin saturation and $\dot{V}O_2$ max.
- Up to moderate altitudes (~4,000 meters) the decrease in $\dot{V}O_2$ max is due primarily to the decrease in the arterial oxygen content brought about by the decrease in atmospheric PO_2. At higher altitudes, the rate at which $\dot{V}O_2$ max falls may be increased due to a reduction in maximal cardiac output.
- Submaximal performances conducted at altitude require higher heart rate and ventilation responses due to the lower oxygen content of arterial blood and the reduction in the number of oxygen molecules per liter of air, respectively.

Adaptation to High Altitude

The body's response to the low PO_2 at altitude is to produce additional red blood cells to compensate for the desaturation of hemoglobin. In the mining community of Morococha, Peru, where people reside at altitudes above 4,540 meters, hemoglobin levels of 211 g · L^{-1} have been measured, in contrast to the normal 156 g · L^{-1} of the sea-level residents in Lima. This higher hemoglobin compensates rather completely for the low PO$_2$ at those altitudes (54):

Sea level: 156 g · L^{-1} times 1.34 ml O$_2$ · g^{-1} at 98% saturation = 206 ml · L^{-1}

4,540 m: 211 g · L^{-1} times 1.34 ml O$_2$ · g^{-1} at 81% saturation = 224 ml · L^{-1}

Probably the best test of the degree to which these high-altitude residents have adapted is found in the $\dot{V}O_2$ max values measured at altitude. Average values of 46 to 50 ml · kg^{-1} · min^{-1} were measured on the altitude natives (57, 69, 70, 71), which compares favorably with sea-level natives in that country and in ours. In addition, recreational runners at 3,600 meters have been shown to have $\dot{V}O_2$ max values similar to those of their sea-level counterparts (36).

There is no question that any sea-level resident who makes a journey to altitude and stays a while will experience an increase in red blood cell number. However, the adaptation will probably never be complete. This conclusion is drawn from a study that compared $\dot{V}O_2$ max values of several different groups: (a) Peruvian lowlanders and Peace Corps volunteers who came to altitude as adults, (b) lowlanders who came to altitude as children and spent their growing years at altitude, and (c) permanent altitude residents (28). The $\dot{V}O_2$ max values were 46 ml · kg^{-1} · min^{-1} for the altitude residents and those who arrived there as children. In contrast, the lowlanders who arrived as adults and spent only one to four years at altitude had values of 38 ml · kg^{-1} · min^{-1}. This indicates that in order to have complete adaptation one must spend the developmental years at high altitude. This may help explain the surprisingly good performance of Kipchoge Keino's performance in the 1,500-meter run at the Mexico City Olympic Games mentioned earlier, since he spent his childhood at an altitude similar to that of Mexico City. This proposition has been supported in a review of how humans adapt to high altitude (93, 97). However, another explanation for the faster adaptation of those who were born and raised at altitude is a genetic predisposition acquired over thousands of years by those who have lived at high altitude. Support for this comes from studies done on those living in the both the Andes region (93) and Tibet (67).

IN SUMMARY

- Persons adapt to altitude by producing more red blood cells to counter the desaturation caused by the lower PO$_2$. Altitude residents who spent their growing years at altitude show a rather complete adaptation as seen in their arterial oxygen content and $\dot{V}O_2$ max values. Lowlanders who arrive as adults show only a modest adaptation.

Training for Competition at Altitude

It was clear to many of the middle- and long-distance runners who competed in the Olympic Trials or Games in 1968 that the altitude was going to have a detrimental effect on performance. Using $\dot{V}O_2$ max as an indicator of the impact on performance, scientists studied the effect of immediate exposure to altitude, the rate of recovery in $\dot{V}O_2$ max as the individual stayed at altitude, and whether or not $\dot{V}O_2$ max was higher than the prealtitude value upon return to sea level. The results were interesting, not due to the general trends that were expected, but to the extreme variability in response among the athletes. For example, the decrease in $\dot{V}O_2$ max upon ascent to a 2,300-meter altitude ranged from 8.8% to 22.3% (85), at 3,090 meters it ranged from 13.9% to 24.4% (22), and at 4,000 meters the decrease ranged from 24.8% to 34.3% (10). One of the major conclusions that could be drawn from these data is that the best runner at sea level might not be the best at altitude if that person had the largest drop in $\dot{V}O_2$ max. Why such variability? Studies of this phenomenon suggest that the variability in the decrease in $\dot{V}O_2$ max across individuals relates to the degree to which athletes experience desaturation of arterial blood during maximal work (58, 62, 79). Chapter 10 described the effect that arterial desaturation has on $\dot{V}O_2$ max of superior athletes *at sea level*. If such desaturation can occur under sea-level conditions, then the altitude condition should have an additional impact, with the magnitude of the impact being greater on those who suffer some desaturation at sea level. Consistent with that, exposure to a simulated altitude of 3,000 meters resulted in a 20.8% decrease in $\dot{V}O_2$ max for trained subjects and only a 9.8% decrease for untrained subjects (58).

The decrease in $\dot{V}O_2$ max upon exposure to altitude was not the only physiological response that varied among the athletes. There was also a variable response in the size of the increase in $\dot{V}O_2$ max as the subjects stayed at altitude and continued to train. One study, lasting twenty-eight days at 2,300 meters, found the $\dot{V}O_2$ max to increase from 1% to 8% over that time (85). Some found the $\dot{V}O_2$ max to gradually improve over a period of ten to twenty-eight days (5, 20, 22, 85), while others (25, 37) did not. In addition,

Live High, Train Low

The observations mentioned earlier have led some to recommend the "live high, train low" strategy as a way of improving endurance performance. However, support for this is mixed due to the influence of a wide variety of factors: subjects, length of study, intensity and volume of training, the altitude (be it simulated or real), and the length of stay at altitude (115). However, one study tried to shed some light on why there is such variability in response to this training strategy (16). Thirty-nine collegiate runners were divided into "responders" and "nonresponders" on the basis of changes in their 5,000-meter run time following training at a high-altitude training camp. All of the runners had lived "high" (2,500 m), but some had trained at 2,500 to 3,000 m (high-high group), some at 1,200 to 1,400 m (high-low group), and some had done low-intensity training at 2,500 to 3,000 m and interval work at low altitude (high-high-low). The responders were found to have an increase in

plasma erythropoietin (EPO), red blood cell volume, and $\dot{V}O_2$ max, which provides a strong physiological connection to the increased performance in the 5,000-m run after altitude training. Interestingly, while the nonresponders had an increase in EPO, they did not have an increase in either red blood cell mass or $\dot{V}O_2$ max. Another difference between the responders and nonresponders was in their ability to maintain the quality of their workouts at altitude: nonresponders demonstrated a 9% reduction in interval-training velocity and a significantly lower $\dot{V}O_2$ during the intervals. There were two take-home messages from this study:

■ live at high enough an altitude to elicit an increase in red blood cell mass (due to an acute increase in EPO), and
■ train low enough to maintain interval-training velocity. For runners who experience a signif-

icant desaturation of hemoglobin at sea level, even low-altitude training may be inconsistent with maintaining interval-training velocity.

The same researchers reinforced these points in a recent study that showed that elite male and female runners who lived for twenty-seven days at 2,500 m and did high-intensity training at 1,250 m improved both $\dot{V}O_2$ max (by 3%) and sea-level performance (103). These findings are consistent with the approach recommended by Daniels and Oldridge some thirty-five years ago (20).

As is the case for all of science, there is more than one way to look at the issue of how altitude exposure can improve performance. The interested reader is directed to a debate between the developers of the "living high, training low" approach (59) and the "training high, living low" approach (46).

---

when the subjects returned to sea level and were retested, some found the $\dot{V}O_2$ max to be higher than before they left (5, 20, 22), while others found no improvements (10, 28, 34). Why was there such variability in response?

There are several possibilities. If an athlete was not in peak condition before ascending to altitude, then the combined stress of the exercise and altitude could increase the $\dot{V}O_2$ max over time while at altitude and show an additional gain upon return to sea level. There is evidence both for (92) and against (1, 24) the idea that the combination of altitude and exercise stress leads to greater changes in $\dot{V}O_2$ max than exercise stress alone. Another reason for the variability is related to the altitude at which the training was conducted. When runners trained at high (4,000 meters) altitude, the intensity of the runs (relative to sustained sea-level speeds) had to be reduced in order to complete a workout, due to the reduction in $\dot{V}O_2$ max that occurs at altitude. As a result, the runner might actually "detrain" while at altitude, and subsequent performance at sea level might not be as good as it was before going to altitude (10). Daniels

and Oldridge (20) provided a way around this problem by having runners alternate training at altitude (seven to fourteen days) and sea level (five to eleven days). Using an altitude of only 2,300 meters, the runners were still able to train at "race pace" and detraining did not occur. In fact, thirteen personal records were achieved by the athletes when they raced at sea level. A recent study using the one-leg training model supports this approach. Subjects trained one leg under hypoxic conditions equivalent to 2,300 meters altitude, while the control leg was exercised under normoxic (sea level) conditions at the same work rate. The subjects exercised three to four times per week for four weeks. The combination of exercise and hypoxia resulted in higher mitochondrial enzyme activity and myoglobin concentration compared to the control leg (105). See The Winning Edge 24.1 for more on this topic. In contrast, but consistent with our previous discussion, those exposed to extreme altitude (e.g., Mount Everest) experienced decreases in muscle fiber area and mitochondria volume (34, 45, 50, 61). See the following discussion for additional details.

FIGURE 24.4 The highest altitudes attained by climbers in the twentieth century. In 1924 the climbers ascended within 300 meters of the summit without oxygen. It took another fifty-four years to climb those last 300 meters.

IN SUMMARY

- When athletes train at altitude, some experience a greater decline in $\dot{V}O_2$ max than others. This may be due to differences in the degree to which each athlete experiences a desaturation of hemoglobin. Remember, some athletes experience desaturation during maximal work at sea level.

- Some athletes show an increase in $\dot{V}O_2$ max while training at altitude while others do not. This may be due to the degree to which the athlete was trained before going to altitude.

- In addition, some athletes show an improved $\dot{V}O_2$ max upon return to sea level, while others do not. Part of the reason may be the altitude at which they train. Those who train at high altitudes may actually "detrain" due to the fact that the quality of their workouts suffers at the high altitudes. To get around this problem, one can alternate low-altitude and sea-level exposures.

The Quest for Everest

The most obvious tie between exercise and altitude is mountain climbing. The climber faces the stress of altitude, cold, radiation, and, of course, the work of climbing up steep slopes or sheer rock walls. A goal of some mountaineers has been to climb Mount Everest, at 8,848 meters, the highest mountain on earth. Figure 24.4 shows various attempts to climb Everest during the twentieth century (110). Special note should be made of Hillary and Tensing, who were the first to do it, and Messner and Habeler, who, to the amazement of all, did it without supplementary oxygen in 1978. This achievement brought scientists back to Everest in 1981 asking how this was possible. This section provides some background to this fascinating story.

In 1924, Norton's climbing team attempted to scale Everest without O_2, and almost succeeded—they stopped only 300 meters from the summit (76). This 1924 expedition was noteworthy because data were collected on the climbers and porters by physicians and scientists associated with the attempt. In addition, new questions have been raised about two of the climbers who died in their attempt to reach the summit (see A Closer Look 24.2). The story of this assault is good reading for those interested in mountain climbing and provides evidence of the keen powers of observation of the scientists. Major Hingston noted the respiratory distress associated with climbing to such heights, stating that at 5,800 meters (19,000 feet) "the very slightest exertion, such as the tying of a bootlace, the opening of a ration box, the getting into a sleeping bag, was associated with marked respiratory distress." At 8,200 meters (27,000 feet) one climber "had to take seven, eight, or ten complete respirations for every single step forward. And even at that slow rate of progress he had to rest for a minute or two every twenty or thirty yards" (76). Pugh, who made observations during a 1960–61 expedition to Everest, believed that fatigue of the respiratory muscles may be the primary factor limiting such endeavors at extreme altitudes (86). Further, Pugh's observations of the decreases in $\dot{V}O_2$ max at the extreme altitudes suggested that $\dot{V}O_2$ max would be just above basal metabolism at the summit, making the task an unlikely one at best. How then did Messner and Habeler climb Everest without O_2?

This was one of the primary questions addressed by the 1981 expedition to Everest. As mentioned earlier, $\dot{V}O_2$ max decreases with altitude due to the lower barometric pressure, which causes a lower PO_2 and a

Mallory and Irvine—Did They Reach the Summit?

In the 1924 Everest expedition, two of the climbers, Norton and Somervell, left camp at 8,220 m (27,000 feet) to challenge the summit without supplemental oxygen. Somervell had to stop due to the cold air aggravating his frostbitten throat, but Norton continued on until he reached 8,580 m (28,314 feet)—a record for those not using supplemental oxygen that lasted for fifty-four years. A few days later, George L. Mallory and Andrew C. Irvine made an attempt with oxygen, but they never returned. Given that they were last seen on the way to the summit; questions were raised about whether they had made it, and died on the way down. The 1999 Mallory and Irvine Research Expedition attempted to answer this question by finding their remains, and perhaps, some evidence that they might have achieved their goal. They knew that both climbers had cameras, and they were hoping to find photographic evidence to put this question to rest. The team did find Mallory's body at 27,000 feet, but unfortunately, could not find a camera. After burying Mallory, they looked for additional evidence to try and determine where he fell from, to land where he did. One of his oxygen bottles placed him in a position consistent with a move to the summit; however, there was not enough evidence to conclude that the two climbers had achieved their goal. Nor was there enough to prove that they had not. The mystery continues (42).

desaturation of hemoglobin. In effect, the $\dot{V}O_2$ max at the summit of Everest was predicated on the observed rate of decrease in $\dot{V}O_2$ max at lower altitudes and then extrapolated to the barometric pressure at the top of the mountain. One of the first major findings of the 1981 expedition was that the barometric pressure at the summit was 17 mm Hg higher than previously believed (112, 113). This higher barometric pressure increased the estimated inspired PO_2 and made a big difference in the predicted $\dot{V}O_2$ max. Figure 24.5 shows that the $\dot{V}O_2$ max predicted from the 1960–61 expedition was near the basal metabolic rate, while the value predicted from the 1981 expedition was closer to 15 ml · kg^{-1} · min^{-1} (112, 113). This $\dot{V}O_2$ max value was confirmed in the Operation Everest II project in which subjects did a simulated ascent of Mount Everest over a forty-day period in a decompression chamber (19, 104). This $\dot{V}O_2$ max value of 15 ml · kg^{-1} · min^{-1} helps to explain how the climbers were able to reach the summit without the aid of supplementary oxygen. However, it was not the only reason.

The arterial saturation of hemoglobin is dependent upon the arterial PO_2, PCO_2, and pH (see chapter 10). A low PCO_2 and a high pH cause the oxygen hemoglobin curve to shift to the left, so that hemoglobin is more saturated under these conditions than under normal conditions. A person who can ventilate great volumes in response to hypoxia can exhale more CO_2 and cause the pH to become elevated. It has been shown that those who successfully deal with altitude have strong hypoxic ventilatory drives, allowing them to have a higher arterial PO_2 and oxygen saturation (98). In fact, when alveolar PCO_2 values were obtained at the top of Mount Everest in the 1981 expedition, the climbers had values much lower than expected (111). This ability to hyperventilate, coupled with the baro-

FIGURE 24.5   Plot of maximal oxygen uptake measured at a variety of altitudes, expressed as inspired PO_2 values. The 1964 data of Pugh et al. predicted the $\dot{V}O_2$ max to be equal to basal metabolic rate. The estimation based on the finding that the barometric pressure (and PO_2) was higher than expected as the summit shifts the estimate to about 15 ml · kg^{-1} · min^{-1}.

metric pressure being higher than expected, resulted in higher arterial PO_2, and of course, $\dot{V}O_2$ max values. How high must your $\dot{V}O_2$ max be in order to climb Mount Everest?

Figure 24.5 shows that the climbers in the 1981 expedition had $\dot{V}O_2$ max values at sea level that were higher than those of the 1960–61 expedition. In fact, several of the climbers had been competitive marathon runners (113), and, given the need to transport oxygen at these high altitudes in order to do work, having such a high $\dot{V}O_2$ max would appear to be a prerequisite to success in climbing without oxygen. Subsequent measurements on other mountaineers who had scaled 8,500 meters or more without oxygen

The Lactate Paradox

When a submaximal test is conducted at altitude, the heart rate, ventilation, and lactate responses are higher than what are measured at sea level. This is no surprise for the heart rate and ventilation responses, since there is less oxygen per liter of blood and air, respectively. The elevated lactate response is also not unexpected; the assumption being that the hypoxia of altitude provides additional stimulation of glycolysis. What is surprising is that when the same exercise is done after the subject has been acclimatized to altitude for three or four weeks (chronic hypoxia), the lactate response is substantially reduced. This is the lactate paradox—that the same hypoxic stimulus in chronic hypoxia gives rise to a lower lactate response than observed when the subject is first exposed (acute hypoxia) to altitude (90).

A wide variety of studies have been done to try and uncover the causes of the reduced lactate response to exercise during chronic exposure to altitude. The results from some of these studies have shown that the lower lactate is not due to a greater oxidative capacity of the muscle, an improved capillary-to-fiber ratio, or an improvement in oxygen delivery (35, 90). Instead, the reduction in lactate seems to be associated with a lower plasma epinephrine concentration which, as we know from chapter 5, would provide less stimulation of glycogenolysis via β-adrenergic receptor stimulation (72, 90). Evidence supporting this proposition comes from a study in which propranolol (a β-adrenergic receptor blocking drug) was shown to reduce the lactate response to acute hypoxia to a level seen only after chronic hypoxia (90). However, the changes in epinephrine with acclimatization to altitude cannot entirely explain the lower lactate response (72). The lower lactate response may also be due to muscular adaptations resulting in tighter metabolic control such that the ADP concentration does not increase as much during exercise; this results in less stimulation of glycolysis (see chapter 13) (35). Consequently, the lactate paradox may be the result of both hormonal (epinephrine) and intracellular (lower [ADP]) adaptations that occur with chronic exposure to hypoxia.

A study by van Hall et al (107), published in 2001, suggested that the lactate paradox was simply a time-dependent phenomenon, being present during the early weeks of acclimatization and disappearing thereafter. A recent study by Pronk et al. (80) challenged this conclusion. They measured the lactate response to the same absolute work load on ascent to altitude and at two, four, six, and eight weeks to track changes in the response over time at altitude. They observed the expected increase in the blood lactate response to exercise upon ascent to altitude, and the now classic decrease in the blood lactate response with continued exposure to altitude. They also confirmed the link of the lactate response to changes in plasma catecholamines. They concluded that there was no evidence of a reversal of the lactate paradox with continued altitude exposure. Lundby and van Hall's response (60) to this study, and Pronk's counterresponse, (81) make interesting reading and point the way for a collaboration that may resolve their differences.

---

confirmed this by showing them to possess primarily type I muscle fibers and to have an average $\dot{V}O_2$ max of 60 ± 6 ml $\cdot$ kg^{-1} $\cdot$ min^{-1} (77). However, there was one notable exception: One of the subjects in this study was Messner, who had climbed Mount Everest without oxygen; his $\dot{V}O_2$ max was 48.8 ml $\cdot$ kg^{-1} $\cdot$ min^{-1} (77). West et al. (114) provide food for thought in this regard: "It remains for someone to elucidate the evolutionary processes responsible for man being just able to reach the highest point on Earth while breathing ambient air." However, there is more to consider in climbing Mount Everest than a person's $\dot{V}O_2$ max.

It has been a common experience in mountain climbing, especially with prolonged exposure to high altitudes, for climbers to lose weight, secondary to a loss of appetite (55). Clearly, if a large portion of this weight loss were muscle, it would have a potential impact in the climber's ability to scale the mountain. Some recent work from both simulated and real ascents of Mount Everest provide some insight into what changes are taking place in muscle and what may be responsible for those changes. In the Operation Everest II forty-day simulation of an ascent to Mount Everest, the subjects experienced a 25% reduction in the cross-sectional area of type I and type II muscle fibers, and a 14% reduction in muscle area (34, 61). These observations were supported by data from a real ascent that combined both heavy exercise and severe hypoxia (45, 50). What could have caused these changes? The Operation Everest II data on nutrition and body composition showed that caloric intake decreased 43% from 3,136 to 1,789 kcal/day over the course of the forty-day exposure to hypoxia. The subjects lost an average of 7.4 kg, with most of the weight from lean body mass, despite the availability of palatable food (91). The hypoxia itself was a sufficient stimulus to suppress the appetite and alter body composition. Whether or not such changes in muscle mass are linked directly to changes in $\dot{V}O_2$ max, they would clearly affect performance. (See A Closer Look 24.3 for how acute, versus chronic, exposure to altitude can affect the lactate response to exercise.)

- Climbers reached the summit of Mount Everest without oxygen in 1978. This surprised scientists who thought $\dot{V}O_2$ max would be just above resting $\dot{V}O_2$ at that altitude. They later found that the barometric pressure was higher than they previously had thought and that the estimated $\dot{V}O_2$ max was about $15 \ ml \cdot kg^{-1} \cdot min^{-1}$ at this altitude.
- Those who are successful at these high altitudes have a great capacity to hyperventilate. This drives down the PCO_2 and the $[H^+]$ in blood, and allows more oxygen to bind with hemoglobin at the same arterial PO_2.
- Finally, those who are successful at climbing to extreme altitudes must contend with the loss of appetite that results in a reduction in body weight and in the cross-sectional area of type I and type II muscle fibers.

HEAT

Chapter 12 described the changes in body temperature with exercise, how heat loss mechanisms are activated, and the benefits of acclimatization. This section will extend that discussion by considering the prevention of thermal injuries during exercise.

Hyperthermia

Our core temperature (37° C) is within a few degrees of a value (45° C) that could lead to death (see chapter 12). Given that, and the fact that distance running races, triathlons, fitness programs, and football games occur during the warmer part of the year, the potential for heat injury is increased (11, 38, 53). Heat injury is not an all-or-none affair, but includes a series of stages that need to be recognized and attended to in order to prevent a progression from the least to the most serious (52). Table 24.3 summarizes each stage,

TABLE 24.3	Heat-Related Problems	
Heat Illness	**Signs and Symptoms**	**Immediate Care**
Heat syncope	Headache Nausea	Normal intake of fluids
Heat cramps	Muscle cramping (calf is very common)	Isolated cramps: Direct pressure to cramp and release, stretch muscle slowly and gently, gentle massage, ice
	Multiple cramping (very serious)	Multiple cramps: Danger of heat stroke, *treat as heat exhaustion*
Heat exhaustion	Profuse sweating Cold, clammy skin	Move individual out of sun to a well-ventilated area
	Normal temperature or slightly elevated	Place in shock position (feet elevated 12–18 in); prevent heat loss or gain
	Pale	Gentle massage of extremities
	Dizzy	Gentle range of motion of the extremities
	Weak, rapid pulse	Force fluids
	Shallow breathing	Reassure
	Nausea	Monitor body temperature and other vital signs
	Loss of consciousness	Refer to physician
Heat stroke	Generally, no perspiration	This is an *extreme medical emergency*
	Dry skin	Transport to hospital quickly
	Very hot	Remove as much clothing as possible without exposing the individual
	Temperature as high as 106° F	
	Skin color bright red or flushed (blacks—ashen)	Cool quickly starting at the head and continuing down the body; use any means possible (fan, hose down, pack in ice)
	Rapid and strong pulse	Wrap in cold, wet sheets for transport
	Labored breathing—semi-reclining position	Treat for shock; if breathing is labored, place in a semi-reclining position

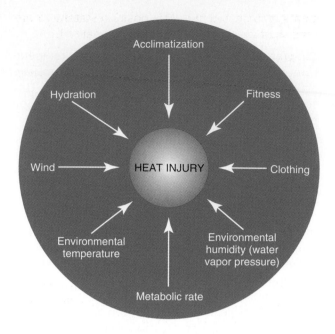

FIGURE 24.6   Factors affecting heat injury.

FIGURE 24.7   The effect of different types of uniforms on the body temperature response to treadmill running.

identifying signs, symptoms, and the immediate care that should be provided (15). While it is important to recognize and deal with these problems, it is better to prevent them from happening.

Figure 24.6 shows the major factors related to heat injury. Each one independently influences susceptibility to heat injury:

Fitness   A high level of fitness is related to a lower risk of heat injury (31). Fit subjects can tolerate more work in the heat (23), acclimatize faster (11), and sweat more (8).

Acclimatization   Exercise in the heat, either low intensity (<50% $\dot{V}O_2$ max) and long duration (60–100 min), or moderate intensity (75% $\dot{V}O_2$ max) and short duration (30–35 min), increases the capacity to sweat, and reduces salt loss (49). Acclimatization leads to lower body temperature and HR responses during exercise and a reduced chance of salt depletion (11). Interestingly, although acclimatization increases work tolerance in the heat, exhaustion is experienced at similar core temperatures (75).

Hydration   Inadequate hydration reduces sweat rate and increases the chance of heat injury (11, 94, 95, 96). Chapter 23 discussed the procedures for fluid replacement. Generally, there are no differences among water, electrolyte drinks, or carbohydrate-electrolyte drinks in replacing body water during exercise (14, 18, 116).

Environmental Temperature   Convection and radiation heat loss mechanisms are dependent on a temperature gradient from skin to environment. Exercising in temperatures greater than

skin temperatures results in a heat *gain*. Evaporation of sweat must then compensate if body temperature is to remain at a safe value.

Clothing   Expose as much skin surface as possible to encourage evaporation. Choose materials, such as cotton, that will "wick" sweat to the surface for evaporation. Materials impermeable to water will increase the risk of heat injury. Figure 24.7 shows the influence of different uniforms on the body temperature response to treadmill running (68).

Humidity (water vapor pressure)   Evaporation of sweat is dependent on the water vapor pressure gradient between skin and environment. In warm/hot environments, the relative humidity is a good index of the water vapor pressure, with a lower relative humidity facilitating evaporation.

Metabolic Rate   Given that core temperature is proportional to work rate, metabolic heat production plays an important role in the overall heat load the body experiences during exercise. Decreasing the work rate decreases this heat load, as well as the strain on the physiological systems that must deal with it. Carbohydrate and fat metabolism are not affected when moderate exercise is done in a hot environment, compared to a thermoneutral one (117).

Wind   Wind places more air molecules into contact with the skin and can influence heat loss in two ways. If a temperature gradient for heat loss exists between the skin and the air, wind will increase the rate of heat loss by convection. In a similar manner, wind increases the rate of evaporation, assuming the air can accept moisture.

Implications for Fitness   The person exercising for fitness needs to be educated about all of the previously listed factors. Suggestions might include:

- providing information on heat illness symptoms: cramps, lightheadedness, and so on,
- exercising in the cooler part of the day to avoid heat gain from the sun or structures heated by the sun,
- gradually increasing exposure to high heat/humidity to safely acclimatize,
- drinking water before, during, and after exercise and weighing in each day to monitor hydration,
- wearing only shorts and a tank top to expose as much skin as possible,
- taking heart rate measurements several times during the activity and reducing exercise intensity to stay in the target heart rate (THR) zone.

The latter recommendation is most important. The heart rate is a sensitive indicator of dehydration, environmental heat load, and acclimatization. Variation in any of these factors will modify the heart rate response to any fixed, submaximal exercise. It is therefore important for fitness participants to monitor heart rate on a regular basis and to slow down to stay within the THR zone. Age is sometimes raised as a predisposing factor related to heat injury, but that may not be the case once you account for the factors mentioned above. We would like to direct the interested reader to a brief and clearly written review of this topic by Kenney and Munce in the Suggested Readings.

Implications for Performance Heat injury has been a concern in athletics for decades. Initially, the vast majority of attention was focused on football because of the large number of heat-related deaths associated with that sport (12). Emphasis on preseason conditioning to improve fitness and promote acclimatization, replacing water during practice and games, and weighing in each day to monitor hydration resulted in a steady reduction of heat-related deaths throughout the early 1990s. However, since that time there has been an increase in the number of heat-related deaths in football, especially at the high school level. In fact, among U.S. high school athletes, heat illness is the third leading cause of death (17). There is a need to return to the vigilance and practices that resulted in the low death rates of the early1990s. It might be added that during the time that the number of heat-related deaths in football players was decreasing, there was an increase in another athletic activity—long-distance road races (38, 53). In response to this problem, and on the basis of sound research, the American College of Sports Medicine developed a Position Stand on the Prevention of Thermal Injuries During Distance Running (3). The elements recommended in this position statement are consistent with what we previously presented:

Medical Director

- A sports medicine physician should work with the race director to enhance safety and coordinate first-aid measures.

Race Organization

- Minimize environmental heat load by planning races for the cooler months, and at a time of day (before 8:00 A.M. or after 6:00 P.M.) to reduce solar heat gain.
- Use an environmental heat stress index (see next section, Environmental Heat Stress) to help make decisions about whether or not to run a race.
- Have a water station every 2 to 3 km; encourage runners to drink 150 to 300 milliliters of water every fifteen minutes.
- Clearly identify the race monitors and have them look for those who might be in trouble due to heat injury.
- Have traffic control for safety.
- Use radio communication throughout the race course.

Medical Support

- Medical director coordinates ambulance service with local hospitals and has the authority to evaluate or stop runners who appear to be in trouble.
- Medical director coordinates medical facilities at race site to provide first aid.

Competitor Education

- Provide information about factors related to heat illness that were discussed previously.
- Encourage the "buddy system" (see chapter 17).

The primary focus in these recommendations is on safety.

Environmental Heat Stress The previous discussion mentioned high temperature and relative humidity as factors increasing the risk of heat injuries. In order to quantify the overall heat stress associated with any environment, a Wet Bulb Globe Temperature (WBGT) guide was developed (3). This overall heat stress index is composed of the following measurements:

Dry Bulb Temperature (T_{db})

- ordinary measure of air temperature taken in the shade

Black Globe Temperature (T_g)

- measure of the radiant heat load measured in direct sunlight

Wet Bulb Temperature (T_{wb})

- measurement of air temperature with a thermometer whose mercury bulb is covered with a wet cotton wick. This measure is sensitive to the relative humidity (water vapor pressure) and provides an index of the ability to evaporate sweat.

The formula used to calculate the WBGT temperature shows the importance of this latter wet bulb temperature in determining heat stress (3):

$$WBGT = 0.7\ T_{wb} + 0.2\ T_g + 0.1\ T_{db}$$

The risk of heat stress is catagorized as follows:

- WBGT >28° C (>82° F)   Very high risk

- WBGT = 23–28° C (73–82° F)   High risk

- WBGT = 18–23° C (65–73° F)   Moderate risk

- WBGT <18° C (<65° F)   Low risk of heat injury

- WBGT <10° C (<50° F)   Low risk of hyperthermia, but possibility of hypothermia

---

IN SUMMARY

- Heat injury is influenced by environmental factors such as temperature, water vapor pressure, acclimatization, hydration, clothing, and metabolic rate. The fitness participant should be educated about the signs and symptoms of heat injury, the importance of drinking water before, during, and after the activity, gradually becoming acclimated to the heat, exercising in the cooler part of the day, dressing appropriately, and checking the HR on a regular basis.

- Road races conducted in times of elevated heat and humidity need to reflect the coordinated wisdom of the race director and medical director to minimize heat and other injuries. Concerns include running the race at the correct time of the day and season of the year, frequent water stops, traffic control, race monitors to identify and stop those in trouble, and communication between race monitors, medical director, ambulance services, and hospitals.

- The heat stress index includes dry bulb, wet bulb, and globe temperatures. The wet bulb temperature, which is a good indicator of the water vapor pressure, is more important than the other two in determining overall heat stress.

COLD

Altitude and heat stress are not the only environmental factors having an impact on performance. A WBGT of 10° C or less is associated with hypothermia. Hypothermia results when heat loss from the body exceeds heat production. Cold air facilitates this process in more ways than are readily apparent. First, and most obvious, when air temperature is less than skin temperature, a gradient for heat loss exists for convection, and physiological mechanisms involving peripheral vasoconstriction and shivering come into play to counter this gradient. Second, and less obvious, cold air has a low water vapor pressure, which encourages the evaporation of moisture from the skin to further cool the body. The combined effects can be deadly, as witnessed in Pugh's report of three deaths during a "walking" competition over a forty-five-mile distance (83).

Figure 24.8 shows the factors related to hypothermia. These include environmental factors such as temperature, water vapor pressure, wind, and whether air or water are involved; insulating factors such as clothing and subcutaneous fat; and the capacity for sustained energy production. We will now comment on each of these relative to hypothermia. For recent reviews on the physiological responses to cold, and how to prevent frostbite see the Suggested Readings by Stocks et al. and Rintamaki, respectively.

Environmental Factors

Heat loss mechanisms introduced in chapter 12 included conduction, convection, radiation, and evaporation. Given that hypothermia is the result of higher heat loss than heat production, understanding how these mechanisms are involved will facilitate a discussion of how to deal with this problem.

Conduction, convection, and radiation are dependent on a temperature gradient between skin and environment; the larger the gradient, the greater the

FIGURE 24.8 Factors affecting hypothermia.

rate of heat loss. What is surprising is that the environmental temperature does not have to be below freezing in order to cause hypothermia. In effect, there are other environmental factors that interact with temperature to create the dangerous condition by facilitating heat loss, namely, wind and water.

Wind Chill Index The rate of heat loss at any given temperature is directly influenced by the wind speed. Wind increases the number of cold air molecules coming into contact with the skin so that heat loss is accelerated. The wind chill index indicates what the "effective" temperature is for any combination of temperature and wind speed. Siple and Passel (101) developed a formula for predicting how fast heat would be lost at different wind speeds and temperatures:

Wind chill (kcal $\cdot$ m^{-2} $\cdot$ h^{-1}) =
$$\left[\sqrt{WV \times 100} + 10.45 - WV \right] \times (33 - T_A)$$

Where: WV = wind velocity (m $\cdot$ sec^{-1}); 10.45 is a constant; 33 is 33° C, which is taken as the skin temperature; and T_A = ambient dry bulb temperature in °C. Siple and Passel estimated how long it would take for exposed flesh to freeze and tabulated the levels of "danger" associated with combinations of wind speed and temperature.

This formula (30), which had been used for many years, was thought to overestimate the effect of increasing wind speed on tissue freezing and underestimated the effect of decreasing temperature (21). The following wind chill formula has been adopted by the National Weather Service (http://www.crh.noaa.gov/dtx/New_Wind_Chill.htm):

$$\text{Wind chill (°F)} = 35.74 + 0.6215 \, (T) - 35.75 \, (V^{0.16}) + 0.4275T \, (V^{0.16})$$

Where: wind speed (V) is in mph, and temperature (T) is in ° F.

Table 24.4 provides the calculated wind chill temperatures for a variety of wind speeds and temperatures, along with estimates of the time it would take for frostbite to occur. Keep in mind that if you are running, riding, or cross-country skiing into the wind, you must add your speed to the wind speed to evaluate the full impact of the wind chill. For example, cycling at 20 mph into calm air at 0° F is equivalent to a wind chill temperature of −22° F. However, it is clear that wind is not the only factor that can increase the rate of heat loss at any given temperature.

Water The thermal conductivity of water is about twenty-five times greater than that of air, so you can lose heat twenty-five times faster in water compared to air of the same temperature (47). Figure 24.9 shows death can occur in only a few hours when a person is shipwrecked in cold water. Unlike air, water offers little or no insulation at the skin-water interface, so heat is rapidly lost from the body. Given that movement in such cold water would increase heat loss from the arms and legs, the recommendation is to stay as still as possible in long-term immersions (47).

IN SUMMARY

- Hypothermia is influenced by natural and added insulation, environmental temperature, vapor pressure, wind, water immersion, and energy production.
- The wind chill index describes how wind lowers the effective temperature at the skin such that convective heat loss is greater than what it would be in calm air at that same temperature.
- Water causes heat to be lost by convection twenty-five times faster than it would be by exposure to air of the same temperature.

Insulating Factors

The rate at which heat is lost from the body is inversely related to the insulation between the body and the environment. The insulating quality is related to the thickness of subcutaneous fat, the ability of clothing to trap air, and whether or not the clothing is wet or dry.

Subcutaneous Fat An excellent indicator of total body insulation per unit surface area (through which heat is lost) is the average subcutaneous fat thickness (41). Pugh and Edholm's (84) observation that a "fat" man was able to swim for seven hours in 16° C water with no change in body temperature while a "thin" man had to leave the water in thirty minutes with a core temperature of 34.5° C, supports this statement. Long-distance swimmers tend to be fatter than short-course swimmers. The higher body fatness does more than help maintain body temperature; fatter swimmers are more buoyant, requiring less energy to swim at any set speed (44). In addition, body fatness plays a role in the onset and magnitude of the shivering response to cold exposure (see later discussion in the Energy Production section).

Clothing Clothing can extend our natural subcutaneous fat insulation to allow us to sustain very cold environments. The insulation quality of clothing is given in **clo** units, where 1 clo is the insulation needed at rest (1 MET) to maintain core temperature when the environment is 21° C, the RH = 50%, and the air movement is 6 m $\cdot$ min^{-1} (9). Still air next to the body has a clo rating of 0.8. As the air temperature falls, clothing with a higher clo value must be

TABLE 24.4 **Wind Chill Chart**

									Temperature (°F)									
Calm	**40**	**35**	**30**	**25**	**20**	**15**	**10**	**5**	**0**	**−5**	**−10**	**−15**	**−20**	**−25**	**−30**	**−35**	**−40**	**−45**
5	36	31	25	19	13	7	1	−5	−11	−16	−22	−28	−34	−40	−46	−52	−57	−63
10	34	27	21	15	9	3	−4	−10	−16	−22	−28	−35	−41	−47	−53	−59	−66	−72
15	32	25	19	13	6	0	−7	−13	−19	−26	−32	−39	−45	−51	−58	−64	−71	−77
20	30	24	17	11	4	−2	−9	−15	−22	−29	−35	−42	−48	−55	−61	−68	−74	−81
25	29	23	16	9	3	−4	−11	−17	−24	−31	−37	−44	−51	−58	−64	−71	−78	−84
30	28	22	15	8	1	−5	−12	−19	−26	−33	−39	−46	−53	−60	−67	−73	−80	−87
35	28	21	14	7	0	−7	−14	−21	−27	−34	−41	−48	−55	−62	−69	−76	−82	−89
40	27	20	13	6	−1	−8	−15	−22	−29	−36	−43	−50	−57	−64	−71	−78	−84	−91
45	26	19	12	5	−2	−9	−16	−23	−30	−37	−44	−51	−58	−65	−72	−79	−86	−93
50	26	19	12	4	−3	−10	−17	−24	−31	−38	−45	−52	−60	−67	−74	−81	−88	−95
55	25	18	11	4	−3	−11	−18	−25	−32	−39	−46	−54	−61	−68	−75	−82	−89	−97
60	25	17	10	3	−4	−11	−19	−26	−33	−40	−48	−55	−62	−69	−76	−84	−91	−98

Wind (MPH) (row axis label)

Frostbite Times ▇ 30 minutes ▇ 10 minutes ▇ 5 minutes

Wind Chill (°F) = $35.74 + 0.6215T - 35.75 (V^{0.16}) + 0.4275 (V^{0.16})$

Where T = Air Temperature (°F)   V = Wind Speed (mph)

(Effective 11/01/01)

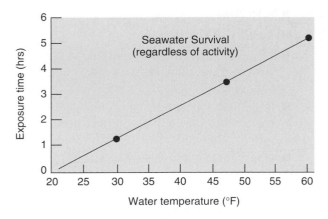

FIGURE 24.9 The effect of different water temperatures on survival of shipwrecked individuals.

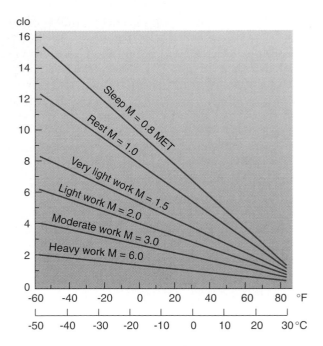

FIGURE 24.10 Changes in the insulation requirement of clothing (plus air) with increasing rates of energy expenditure over environmental temperatures of −50 to +30° C.

worn to maintain core temperature, since the gradient between skin and environment increases (78). Figure 24.10 shows the insulation needed at different energy expenditures across a broad range of temperatures from −60 to +80° F (9). It is clear that as energy production increases, insulation must decrease to maintain core temperature. By wearing clothing in layers, insulation can be removed piece by piece, since less insulation is needed to maintain core temperature. By following these steps, sweating, which can rob the clothing of its insulating value, will be minimized. A practical example of how clothing helps maintain body temperature (and comfort) can be seen in the following study. Heat loss from the head increases linearly from +32° C to −21° C, with about *half* of the entire heat production being lost through the head when the temperature is −4° C. Wearing a simple "helmet" with a clo rating of 3.5 allows an individual to stay out indefinitely at 0° C (29).

Clothing offers insulation by trapping air, a poor conductor of heat. If the clothing becomes wet, the insulating quality decreases, since the water can now conduct heat away from the body at a faster rate (47). A primary goal, then, is to avoid wetness, due either to sweat or to weather. This problem is exacerbated by the cold environment's very low water vapor pressure. Recall from chapter 12 that the water vapor pressure in the environment is the primary factor influencing evaporation and that at low environmental temperatures the water vapor pressure is low even when the relative humidity is high. Think of a time when you finished playing a game indoors and stepped outside into cold, damp weather to cool off. You noticed "steam" coming off your body; how is this possible when the RH is near 100%? The water vapor pressure is high at the skin surface, since the skin temperature is elevated; so, a gradient for water vapor pressure exists. You will cool off very fast under these

circumstances. This is why *cold, wet, windy* environments carry an extra risk of hypothermia. The wind not only provides for greater convective heat loss as described in the wind chill chart, but it also accelerates evaporation (39).

Energy Production

Figure 24.10 shows that the amount of insulation needed to maintain core temperature decreases as energy expenditure increases. This is also true for our "natural" insulation, subcutaneous fat. McArdle et al. (74) showed that when fat men (27.6% fat) were immersed for one hour in 20° C, 24° C, and 28° C water, the resting $\dot{V}O_2$ and core temperature did not change compared to values measured in air. In thinner men (<16.8% fat), the $\dot{V}O_2$ increased to counter the rapid loss of heat; however, the core temperature still decreased. When these same subjects did exercise in the cold water, requiring a $\dot{V}O_2$ of 1.7 $\ell \cdot min^{-1}$, the fall in body temperature was either prevented or retarded (73), showing the importance of high rates of energy production in preventing hypothermia. More recent studies support these observations, showing an earlier onset and greater magnitude of shivering in lean subjects when exposed to cold air (106). Similar findings have been reported for fit subjects (6). Given the importance of body fatness in the metabolic response to cold exposure, are there differences due to gender?

A review of this topic indicated that women cool faster than men upon exposure to cold water and, despite the greater stimulus to shiver, do not respond with a greater $\dot{V}O_2$. However, when a prescribed amount of exercise is done, men and women respond similarly. In contrast, when the exercise intensity is chosen voluntarily, women exercise at a relatively lower $\dot{V}O_2$ and body temperature falls to a greater extent than in men (32). Interestingly, amenorrheic women exhibit a greater delay (60 min) in activating metabolism when exposed to cold, compared to eumenorrheic women (20 min) and men (10 min). These differences between men and women cannot be explained by differences in body fatness or body surface area (33). In addition, the availability of fuel (muscle glycogen and plasma FFA) seems to have little effect on adaptations to the cold (63, 64, 65, 66, 118).

IN SUMMARY

- Subcutaneous fat is the primary "natural" insulation and is very effective in preventing rapid heat loss when a person is exposed to cold water.
- Clothing extends this insulation, and the insulation value of clothing is described in clo units, where a value of 1 describes what is needed to maintain core temperature while sitting in a room set at 21° C and 50% RH with an air movement of $6 \text{ m} \cdot \text{sec}^{-1}$.
- The amount of insulation needed to maintain core temperature is less when one exercises because the metabolic heat production helps maintain the core temperature. Clothing should be worn in layers when exercising so one can shed one insulating layer at a time as body temperature increases.
- Energy production increases on exposure to cold, with an inverse relationship between the increase in $\dot{V}O_2$ and body fatness. Women cool faster than men when exposed to cold water, exhibiting a longer delay in the onset of shivering and a lower $\dot{V}O_2$, despite a greater stimulus to shiver.

Dealing with Hypothermia

As body temperature falls, the person's ability to carry out coordinated movements is reduced, speech is slurred, and judgment is impaired (99). People can die from hypothermia, and the condition must be dealt with when it occurs. The following steps on how to do this are taken from Sharkey (99):

- Get person out of the cold, wind, and rain.
- Remove all wet clothing.
- Provide warm drinks, dry clothing, and a warm, dry sleeping bag for a mildly impaired person.
- If semiconscious, keep the person awake, remove clothing, and put into a sleeping bag with another person.
- Find a source of heat (e.g., camp fire).

IN SUMMARY

- If a person becomes hypothermic, get the person out of the wind, rain, and cold; remove wet clothing and put on dry clothing; use a sleeping bag for warmth; and if it is a severe case, remove clothing from the person and have another person in the sleeping bag to provide warmth; finally, provide some source of heat.

AIR POLLUTION

Air pollution includes a variety of gases and particulates that are products of the combustion of fossil fuels. The "smog" that results when these pollutants are in high concentration can have a detrimental effect on health and performance. The gases can affect performance by decreasing the capacity to transport oxygen, increasing airway resistance, and altering the perception of effort required when the eyes "burn" and the chest "hurts." A study on traffic policemen, who are routinely exposed to a full range of pollutants throughout their workday, makes the point. Although their physiological responses were normal at rest, during an exercise test about one-third of the policemen experienced ECG changes and elevated blood pressure responses, with the vast majority of those individuals also experiencing a desaturation of hemoglobin (<80 mm Hg) (108). In addition, children living in an air-polluted environment had significantly lower $\dot{V}O_2$ max values compared to those living in areas with better air quality (119).

The physiological responses to these pollutants are related to the amount or "dose" received. The major factors determining the dose are the concentration of the pollutant, the duration of the exposure to the pollutant, and the volume of air inhaled. This last factor increases during exercise and is one reason why physical activity should be curtailed during times of peak pollution levels (26). The following discussion focuses on the major air pollutants: particulate matter, ozone, sulfur dioxide, and carbon monoxide.

Particulate Matter

The air is full of microscopic and submicroscopic particles, many of which can be tied to motor vehicles (especially diesels) and industrial sources. Over the past ten years, more attention has been focused on the very small particles because of their potential to promote pulmonary infection and actually cross the epithelium to enter the circulation (27). Fine particle pollution causes an elevation in blood pressure in those with pre-existing cardiovascular disease, and may contribute to an increased risk of cardiac mortality and morbidity (100, 120).

Ozone

The ozone we breathe is generated by the reaction of UV light and emissions from internal combustion engines. While a single, two-hour exposure to a high ozone concentration, 0.75 parts per million (ppm), decreases $\dot{V}O_2$ max, recent studies show that a six- to twelve-hour exposure to a concentration of only 0.12 ppm (the U.S. air quality standard) decreases lung function and increases respiratory symptoms. Further, in amateur cyclists who practiced and raced in air containing varying concentrations of ozone, the decrease in pulmonary function following activity was directly related to the ozone concentration (7). Interestingly, an adaptation to ozone exposure can occur, with subjects showing a diminished response to subsequent exposures during the "ozone season." However, concern about long-term lung health suggests that it would be prudent to avoid heavy exercise during the time of day when ozone and other pollutants are elevated (26).

Sulfur Dioxide

Sulfur dioxide (SO_2) is produced by smelters, refineries, and electrical utilities that use fossil fuel for energy generation. SO_2 does not affect lung function in normal subjects, but it causes bronchoconstriction in asthmatics. These latter responses are influenced by the temperature and humidity of the inspired air, as mentioned in chapter 17. Nose breathing is encouraged to "scrub" the SO_2, and drugs like cromolyn sodium and β_2-agonists can partially block the asthmatic's response to SO_2 (26).

Carbon Monoxide

Carbon monoxide (CO) is derived from the burning of fossil fuel, coal, oil, gasoline, and wood, as well as from cigarette smoke. Carbon monoxide can bind to hemoglobin to form carboxyhemoglobin (HbCO) and

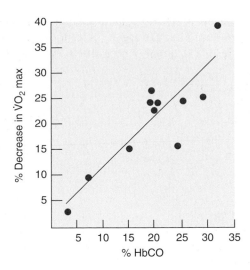

FIGURE 24.11 The effect of the concentration of carbon monoxide in the blood on the change in $\dot{V}O_2$ max.

decrease the capacity for oxygen transport. This has the potential to affect the physiological responses to submaximal exercise (43) and $\dot{V}O_2$ max, as does altitude. The carbon monoxide concentration [HbCO] in blood is generally less than 1% in nonsmokers, but may be as high as 10% in smokers (88). Horvath et al. (48) found that the critical concentration of HbCO needed to decrease $\dot{V}O_2$ max was 4.3%. Figure 24.11 shows the relationship between the blood HbCO concentration and the decrease in $\dot{V}O_2$ max; beyond 4.3% HbCO, $\dot{V}O_2$ max decreases 1% for each 1% increase in HbCO (89).

In contrast, when one performs light work, at about 40% $\dot{V}O_2$ max, the [HbCO] can be as high as 15% before endurance is affected. The cardiovascular system has the capacity to compensate with a larger cardiac output when the HbO_2 concentration is reduced during submaximal work (48, 88, 89). Since it takes two to four hours to remove half the CO from the blood once the exposure has been removed, CO can have a lasting effect on performances (26).

Unfortunately, it is difficult to predict what the actual [HbCO] will be in any given environment. One must consider the previous exposure to the pollutant, as well as the length of time and rate of ventilation associated with the current exposure. As a result, Raven (88) provides the following guidelines for exercising in an area with air pollution:

- Reduce exposure to the pollutant prior to exercise, since the physiological effects are time- and dose-dependent.
- Stay away from areas where you might receive a "bolus" dose of CO: smoking areas, high-traffic areas, urban environments.

- Do not schedule activities around the times when pollutants are at their highest levels (7–10 A.M. and 4–7 P.M.) due to traffic.

The Air Quality Index (AQI) is a measure of the quality of the air for five major air pollutants regulated by the Clean Air Act: ground-level ozone, particulate matter, carbon monoxide, sulfur dioxide, and nitrogen dioxide. The AQI scale runs from zero to 500, with values of zero to 50 being "good," 51 to 100 "moderate," 101 to 150 "unhealthy for sensitive groups," and 151 to 200 "unhealthy." This information is generally provided in a local community's weather forecast and should be suited to the individual—some will experience symptoms at lower levels of pollution than others (13).

IN SUMMARY

- Air pollution can affect performance. Exposure to ozone decreases $\dot{V}O_2$ max and respiratory function, while sulfur dioxide causes bronchoconstriction in asthmatics.
- Carbon monoxide binds to hemoglobin and reduces oxygen transport in much the same way that altitude does.
- To prevent problems associated with pollution of any type, reduce exposure time; stay away from "bolus" amounts of the pollutant; and schedule activity at the least polluted part of the day.
- The Air Quality Index should be monitored to determine if conditions are safe for exercising outdoors.

STUDY QUESTIONS

1. Describe the changes in barometric pressure, PO_2, and air density with increasing altitude.
2. Why is sprint performance not affected by altitude?
3. Explain why maximal aerobic power decreases at altitude and what effect this has on performance in long-distance races.
4. Graphically describe the effect of altitude on the HR and ventilation responses to submaximal work and provide recommendations for fitness participants who occasionally exercise at altitude.
5. Describe the process by which an individual adapts to altitude, and contrast the adaptation of the permanent residents of high altitude with that of the lowlander who arrives there as an adult.
6. While training at altitude can be beneficial, how could someone "detrain"? How can you work around this problem?
7. It was formerly believed that a person could not climb Mount Everest without oxygen because the estimated

$\dot{V}O_2$ max at altitude was close to basal metabolic rate. When two climbers accomplished the feat in 1978, scientists had to determine how this was possible. What were the primary reasons allowing the climb to take place without oxygen?
8. List and describe the factors related to heat injury.
9. What is the heat stress index and why is the wet bulb temperature weighed so heavily in the formula?
10. List the factors related to hypothermia.
11. Explain what the wind chill index is relative to convective heat loss.
12. What is a clo unit, and why is the insulation requirement less when you exercise?
13. What would you do if a person had hypothermia?
14. Explain how carbon monoxide can influence $\dot{V}O_2$ max and endurance performance.
15. What steps would you follow to minimize the effect of pollution on performance?

SUGGESTED READINGS

Houston, C. 1994. High adventure: The romance between medicine and mountaineering. *Exercise and Sport Science Reviews* 22:1–22.

Kenney, W. L., and T. A. Munce. 2003. Invited review: aging and human temperature regulation. *Journal of Applied Physiology* 95:2598–603.

Johnson, L., J. Hemmleb, and E. Simonson. 1999. *The Ghosts of Everest*. Seattle, WA: Mountaineers Books. (Detailed account of the expedition that found Mallory's body.)

Messner, R. 1999. *Everest: Expedition to the Ultimate*. Seattle, WA: Mountaineers Books. (A story of the first trip to the summit by Messner and Habeler without oxygen.)

Reeves, J. T. et al. 1992. Oxygen transport during exercise at altitude and the lactate paradox: Lessons from Operation Everest II and Pikes Peak. In *Exercise and Sport Sciences Reviews*, vol. 20, ed. J. O. Holloszy, 275–96. Baltimore: Lippincott Williams & Wilkins.

Rintamaki, H. 2000. Predisposing factors and prevention of frostbite. *International Journal of Circumpolar Health* 59:114–21.

Stocks, J. M., N. A. Taylor, M. J. Tipton, and J. E. Greenleaf. 2004. Human physiological responses to cold exposure. *Aviation Space & Environmental Medicine* 75:444–57.

REFERENCES

1. Adams, W. C. et al. 1975. Effects of equivalent sea-level and altitude training on $\dot{V}O_2$ max and running performance. *Journal of Applied Physiology* 39:262–66.

2. Alexander, J. K. et al. 1967. Reduction of stroke volume during exercise in man following ascent to 3,100 m altitude. *Journal of Applied Physiology* 23:849–58.

3. American College of Sports Medicine. 1996. Heat and cold illnesses during distance running. *Medicine and Science in Sports and Exercise* 28:139–48.

4. Arsac, L. M. 2002. Effects of altitude on the energetics of human best performances in 100 m running: A theoretical analysis. *European Journal of Applied Physiology* 87:78–84.

5. Balke, B., F. J. Nagle, and J. Daniels. 1965. Altitude and maximum performance in work and sports activity. *Journal of the American Medical Association* 194:646–49.

6. Bittel, J. H. M. et al. 1988. Physical fitness and thermoregulatory reactions in a cold environment in men. *Journal of Applied Physiology* 65:1984–89.

7. Brunekreef, B., G. Hoek, O. Breugelmans, and M. Leentvaar. 1994. Respiratory effects of low-level photochemical air pollution in amateur cyclists. *American Journal of Respiratory, Critical Care Medicine* 150:962–66.

8. Buono, M. J., and N. T. Sjoholm. 1988. Effect of physical training on peripheral sweat production. *Journal of Applied Physiology* 65:811–14.

9. Burton, A. C., and O. G. Edholm. 1955. *Man in a Cold Environment*. London: Edward Arnold.

10. Buskirk, E. R. et al. 1967. Maximal performance at altitude and on return from altitude in conditioned runners. *Journal of Applied Physiology* 23:259–66.

11. Buskirk, E. R., and D. E. Bass. 1974. Climate and exercise. In *Science and Medicine of Exercise and Sport*, ed. W. R. Johnson and E. R. Buskirk, 190–205. New York: Harper & Row.

12. Buskirk, E. R., and W. C. Grasley. 1974. Heat injury and conduct of athletics. In *Science and Medicine of Exercise and Sport*, ed. W. R. Johnson and E. R. Buskirk, 206–10. New York: Harper & Row.

13. Campbell, M. E., Q. Li, S. E. Gingrich, R.G. Macfarlane, and S. Cheng. 2005. Should people be physically active outdoors on smog alert days? *Canadian Journal of Public Health. Revue Canadienne de Sante Publique* 96:24–28.

14. Carter, J. E., and C. V. Gisolfi. 1989. Fluid replacement during and after exercise in the heat. *Medicine and Science in Sports and Exercise* 21:532–39.

15. Carver, S. 1986. Injury prevention and treatment. In *Health/Fitness Instructor's Handbook*, ed. E. T. Howley and B. Don Franks, 211–32. Champaign, IL: Human Kinetics.

16. Chapman, R. F., J. Stray-Gundersen, and B. D. Levine. 1998. Individual variation in response to altitude training. *Journal of Applied Physiology* 85:1448–56.

17. Coris, E. E., A. M. Ramirez, and D. J. Van Durme. 2004. Heat illness in athletes: The dangerous combination of heat, humidity and exercise. *Sports Medicine* 34:9–16.

18. Costill, D. L. et al. 1975. Water and electrolyte replacement during repeated days of work in the heat. *Aviation, Space and Environmental Medicine* 46 (6):795–800.

19. Cymerman, A. et al. 1989. Operation Everest II: Maximal oxygen uptake at extreme altitude. *Journal of Applied Physiology* 66:2446–53.

20. Daniels, J., and N. Oldridge. 1970. The effects of alternate exposure to altitude and sea level on world-class middle-distance runners. *Medicine and Science in Sports* 2:107–12.

21. Danielsson, U. 1996. Windchill and the risk of tissue freezing. *Journal of Applied Physiology* 81:2666–73.

22. Dill, D. B., and W. C. Adams. 1971. Maximal oxygen uptake at sea level and at 3,090-m altitude in high school champion runners. *Journal of Applied Physiology* 30:854–59.

23. Drinkwater, B. L. et al. 1976. Aerobic power as a factor in women's response to work within hot environments. *Journal of Applied Physiology* 41:815–21.

24. Engfred, K. et al. 1994. Hypoxia and training-induced adaptation of hormonal responses to exercise in humans. *European Journal of Applied Physiology* 68:303–9.

25. Faulkner, J. A. et al. 1968. Maximum aerobic capacity and running performance at altitude. *Journal of Applied Physiology* 24:685–91.

26. Folinsbee, L. J. 1990. Discussion: Exercise and the environment. In *Exercise, Fitness, and Health*, ed. C. Bouchard, R. J. Shephard, T. Stevens, J. R. Sutton, and B. D. McPherson, 179–83. Champaign, IL: Human Kinetics.

27. Frampton, M. W. et al. 2004. Effects of exposure to ultrafine carbon particles in healthy subjects and subjects with asthma. *Research Report—Health Effects Institute* 126:1–63.

28. Frisancho, A. R. et al. 1973. Influence of developmental adaptation on aerobic capacity at high altitude. *Journal of Applied Physiology* 34:176–80.

29. Froese, G., and A. C. Burton. 1957. Heat loss from the human head. *Journal of Applied Physiology* 10:235–41.

30. Gates, D. M. 1972. *Man and His Environment: Climate*. New York: Harper & Row.

31. Gisolfi, G. V., and J. Cohen. 1979. Relationships among training, heat acclimation, and heat tolerance in men and women: The controversy revisited. *Medicine and Science in Sports* 11:56–59.

32. Graham, T. E. 1988. Thermal, metabolic, and cardiovascular changes in men and women during cold stress. *Medicine and Science in Sports and Exercise* 20 (Suppl.): S185–S192.

33. Graham, T. E., M. Viswanathan, J. P. van Dijk, and J. C. George. 1989. Thermal and metabolic responses to cold by men and by eumenorrheic and amenorrheic women. *Journal of Applied Physiology* 67:282–90.

34. Green, H. J., J. R. Sutton, A. Cymerman, P. M. Young, and C. S. Houston. 1989. Operation Everest II: Adaptations in human skeletal muscle. *Journal of Applied Physiology* 66:2454–61.

35. Green, H. J. et al. 1992. Altitude acclimatization and energy metabolic adaptations in skeletal muscle during exercise. *Journal of Applied Physiology* 73:2701–8.

36. Greksa, L. P., H. Spielvogel, and L. Paredes-Fernandez. 1993. Maximal aerobic power in high altitude runners. *Annals of Human Biology* 20:395–400.

37. Grover, R. et al. 1967. Muscular exercise in young men native to 3,100 m altitude. *Journal of Applied Physiology* 22:555–64.

38. Hanson, P. G., and S. W. Zimmerman. 1979. Exertional heatstroke in novice runners. *Journal of the American Medical Association* 242:154–57.

39. Hardy, J. D., and P. Bard. 1974. Body temperature regulation. In *Medical Physiology*, 13th ed., vol. 2, ed. V. B. Mountcastle, 1305–42. St. Louis: C. V. Mosby.

40. Hartley, L. H., J. A. Vogel, and J. C. Cruz. 1974. Reduction of maximal exercise heart rate at altitude and its reversal with atropine. *Journal of Applied Physiology* 36:362–65.

41. Hayward, M. G., and W. R. Keatinge. 1981. Roles of subcutaneous fat and thermoregulatory reflexes in determining ability to stabilize body temperature in water. *Journal of Physiology* (London) 320:229–51.

42. Hemmleb, J. and L. Johnson. 1999. Discovery on Everest. *Climbing* 188:98–190.

43. Hirsch, G. L. et al. 1985. Immediate effects of cigarette smoking on cardiorespiratory responses to exercise. *Journal of Applied Physiology* 58:1975–81.

44. Holmer, I. 1979. Physiology of swimming man. In *Exercise and Sport Sciences Reviews*, vol. 7, ed. R. S. Hutton and D. I. Miller. Salt Lake City: Franklin Institute.

45. Hoppeler, H., E. Kleinert, C. Schleger, H. Classon, H. Howald, S. R. Kayar, and P. Cerretelli. 1990. II. Morphological adaptations of human skeletal muscle to

chronic hypoxia. *International Journal of Sports Medicine* 11:S3–S9.

46. Hoppeler, H., and M. Vogt. 2001. Hypoxia training for sea-level performance. Training high–living low. *Advances in Experimental Medicine & Biology* 502:61–73.

47. Horvath, S. M. 1981. Exercise in a cold environment. In *Exercise and Sport Sciences Reviews*, vol. 9, ed. D. I. Miller, 221–63. Salt Lake City: Franklin Institute.

48. Horvath, S. M. et al. 1975. Maximal aerobic capacity of different levels of carboxyhemoglobin. *Journal of Applied Physiology* 38:300–303.

49. Houmard, J. A., D. L. Costill, J. A. Davis, J. B. Mitchell, D. D. Pascoe, and R. A. Robergs. 1990. The influence of exercise intensity on heat acclimation in trained subjects. *Medicine and Science in Sports and Exercise* 22:615–20.

50. Howald, H., D. Pette, J. A. Simoneau, A. Uber, H. Hoppeler, and P. Cerretelli. 1990. III. Effects of chronic hypoxia on muscle enzyme activities. *International Journal of Sports Medicine* 11:S10–S14.

51. Howley, E. T. 1980. Effect of altitude on physical performance. In *Encyclopedia of Physical Education, Fitness, and Sports: Training, Environment, Nutrition, and Fitness*, ed. G. A. Stull and T. K. Cureton, 177–87. Salt Lake City: Brighton.

52. Hubbard, R. W., and L. E. Armstrong. 1989. Hyperthermia: New thoughts on an old problem. *The Physician and Sportsmedicine* 17:97–113.

53. Hughson, R. L. et al. 1980. Heat injuries in Canadian mass participation runs. *Canadian Medicine Medical Association Journal* 122:1141–44.

54. Hurtado, A. 1964. Animals in high altitudes: Resident man. In *Handbook of Physiology: Section 4—Adaptation to the Environment*, ed. D. B. Dill. Washington, D.C.: American Physiological Society.

55. Kayser, B. 1994. Nutrition and energetics of exercise at altitude. *Sports Medicine* 17:309–23.

56. Kollias, J., and E. Buskirk. 1974. Exercise and altitude. In *Science and Medicine of Exercise and Sport*, 2d ed., ed. W. R. Johnson and E. R. Buskirk. New York: Harper & Row.

57. Kollias, J. et al. 1968. Work capacity of long-time residents and newcomers to altitude. *Journal of Applied Physiology* 24:792–99.

58. Lawler, J., S. K. Powers, and D. Thompson. 1988. Linear relationship between $\dot{V}O_2$ max and $\dot{V}O_2$ max decrement during exposure to acute hypoxia. *Journal of Applied Physiology* 64:1486–92.

59. Levine, B. D., and J. Stray-Gundersen. 2001. The effects of altitude training are mediated primarily by acclimatization, rather than by hypoxic exercise. *Advances in Experimental Medicine & Biology* 502:75–88.

60. Lundby, C., and G. van Hall. 2004. Lactate metabolism at high altitude. *High Altitude Medicine and Biology* 5:195–96.

61. MacDougall, J. D., H. J. Green, J. R. Sutton, G. Coates, A. Cymerman, P. Young, and C. S. Houston. 1991. Operation Everest II: Structural adaptations in skeletal muscle in response to extreme simulated altitude. *Acta Physiologica Scandinavica* 142:421–27.

62. Martin, D., and J. O'Kroy. 1993. Effects of acute hypoxia on the $\dot{V}O_2$ max of trained and untrained subjects. *Journal of Sports Science* 11:37–42.

63. Martineau, L., and I. Jacobs. 1988. Muscle glycogen utilization during shivering thermogenesis in humans. *Journal of Applied Physiology* 65:2046–50.

64. ———. 1989. Muscle glycogen availability and temperature regulation in humans. *Journal of Applied Physiology* 66:72–78.

65. ———. 1989. Free fatty acid availability and temperature regulation in cold water. *Journal of Applied Physiology* 67:2466–72.

66. ———. 1991. Effects of muscle glycogen and plasma FFA availability on human metabolic responses in cold water. *Journal of Applied Physiology* 71:1331–39.

67. Marconi, C. et al. 2004. Second generation Tibetan lowlanders acclimatize to high altitude more quickly than Caucasians. *Journal of Physiology* 556(Pt 2):661–71.

68. Mathews, D. K., E. L. Fox, and D. Tanzi. 1969. Physiological responses during exercise and recovery in a football uniform. *Journal of Applied Physiology* 26:611–15.

69. Mazess, R. B. 1969. Exercise performance at high altitude in Peru. *Federation Proceedings* 28:1301–6.

70. ———. 1969. Exercise performance of Indian and white high-altitude residents. *Human Biology* 41:494–518.

71. ———. 1970. Cardiorespiratory characteristics and adaptations to high altitudes. *American Journal of Physical Anthropology* 32:267–78.

72. Mazzeo, R. S. et al. 1994. Beta-adrenergic blockade does not prevent the lactate response to exercise after acclimatization to high altitude. *Journal of Applied Physiology* 76:610–15.

73. McArdle, W. D. et al. 1984. Thermal adjustment to cold-water exposure in exercising men and women. *Journal of Applied Physiology: Respiratory, Environmental, and Exercise Physiology* 56:1572–77.

74. McArdle, W. D. et al. 1984. Thermal adjustment to cold-water exposure in resting men and women. *Journal of Physiology: Respiratory, Environmental, and Exercise Physiology* 56:1565–71.

75. Nielsen, B. et al. 1993. Human circulatory and thermoregulatory adaptations with heat acclimation and exercise in a hot, dry environment. *Journal of Physiology (London)* 460:467–85.

76. Norton, E. F. 1925. *The Fight for Everest: 1924.* New York: Longmans, Green.

77. Oelz, O. et al. 1986. Physiological profile of world-class high-altitude climbers. *Journal of Applied Physiology* 60:1734–42.

78. Pascoe, D. D., L. A. Shanley, and E. W. Smith. 1994. Clothing and exercise. I. Biophysics of heat transfer between the individual, clothing, and environment. *Sports Medicine* 18:38–54.

79. Powers, S. K., D. Martin, and S. Dodd. 1993. Exercise-induced hypoxaemia in elite athletes. *Sports Medicine* 16:14–22.

80. Pronk, M. et al. 2003. Persistence of the lactate paradox over 8 weeks at 3,800 m. *High Altitude Medicine and Biology* 4:431–43.

81. Pronk, M. et al. 2004. Lactate metabolism at high altitude: A reply. *High Altitude Medicine and Biology* 5:197–98.

82. Pronnet, F., G. Thibault, and D. L. Cousineau. 1991. A theoretical analysis of the effect of altitude on running performance. *Journal of Applied Physiology* 70:399–404.

83. Pugh, L. G. C. 1964. Deaths from exposure in Four Inns Walking Competition. *Lancet* 1(March 14–15): 1210–12.

84. Pugh, L. G. C., and O. G. Edholm. 1955. The physiology of Channel swimmers. *Lancet* 2:761–68.

85. Pugh, L. G. C. E. 1967. Athletes at altitude. *Journal of Physiology (London)* 192:619–46.

86. Pugh, L. G. C. E. et al. 1964. Muscular exercise at great altitudes. *Journal of Applied Physiology* 19:431–40.

87. Quinn, M. D. 2004. The effects of wind and altitude in the 400-m sprint. *Journal of Sports Sciences* 22:1073–81.

88. Raven, P. B. 1980. Effects of air pollution on physical performance. In *Encyclopedia of Physical Education, Fitness, and Sports: Training, Environment, Nutrition, and Fitness*, vol. 2, ed. G. A. Stull and T. K. Cureton, 201–16. Salt Lake City: Brighton.

89. Raven, P. B. et al. 1974. Effect of carbon monoxide and peroxyacetyl nitrate on man's maximal aerobic capacity. *Journal of Applied Physiology* 36:288–93.

90. Reeves, J. T. et al. 1992. Oxygen transport during exercise at altitude and the lactate paradox: Lessons from Operation Everest II and Pikes Peak. In *Exercise and Sport Sciences Reviews*, vol. 20, ed. J. O. Holloszy, 275–96. Baltimore: Lippincott Williams & Wilkins.

91. Rose, M. S., C. S. Houston, C. S. Fulco, G. Coates, J. R. Sutton, and A. Cymerman. 1988. Operation Everest II: Nutrition and body composition. *Journal of Applied Physiology* 65:2545–51.

92. Roskamm, H. et al. 1969. Effects of a standardized ergometer training program at three different altitudes. *Journal of Applied Physiology* 27:840–47.

93. Rupert, J. L., and P. W. Hochachka. 2001. Genetic approaches to understanding human adaptation to altitude in the Andes. *Journal of Experimental Biology* 204(Pt 18):3151–60.

94. Saltin, B. 1964. Circulatory response to submaximal and maximal exercise after thermal dehydration. *Journal of Applied Physiology* 19:1125–32.

95. Sawka, M. N. et al. 1984. Influence of hydration level and body fluids on exercise performance in the heat. *Journal of the American Medical Association* 252(9):1165–69.

96. Sawka, M. N. et al. 1985. Thermoregulatory and blood responses during exercise at graded hypohydration levels. *Journal of Applied Physiology* 59:1394–1401.

97. Schmidt, W. et al. 2002. Blood volume and hemoglobin mass in endurance athletes from moderate altitude. *Medicine & Science in Sports & Exercise* 34:1934–40.

98. Schoene, R. B. et al. 1984. Relationship of hypoxic ventilatory response to exercise performance on Mount Everest. *Journal of Applied Physiology: Respiratory, Environmental, and Exercise Physiology* 56:1478–83.

99. Sharkey, B. J. 1984. *Physiology of Fitness*. 2d ed. Champaign, IL: Human Kinetics.

100. Sharman, J. E., J. R. Cockcroft, and J. S. Coombes. 2004. Cardiovascular implications of exposure to traffic air pollution during exercise. *Quarterly Journal of Medicine* 97:637–43.

101. Siple, P. A., and C. F. Passel. 1945. Measurements of dry atmospheric cooling in subfreezing temperatures. *Proceedings of the American Philosophical Society* 89:177–99.

103. Stray-Gundersen, J., R. F. Chapman, and B. E. Levine. 2001. "Living high–training low" altitude training improves sea level performance in male and female elite runners. *Journal of Applied Physiology* 91:1113–20.

104. Sutton, J. R. et al. 1988. Operation Everest II: Oxygen transport during exercise at extreme simulated altitude. *Journal of Applied Physiology* 64:1309–21.

105. Terrados, N., E. Jansson, C. Sylven, and L. Kaijser. 1990. Is hypoxia a stimulus for synthesis of oxidative enzymes and myoglobin? *Journal of Applied Physiology* 68:2369–72.

106. Tikuisis, P., D. G. Bell, and I. Jacobs. 1991. Shivering onset, metabolic response, and convective heat transfer during cold air exposure. *Journal of Applied Physiology* 70:1996–2002.

107. Van Hall, G., J. A. L. Calbet, H. Søndergaard, and B. Saltin. 2001. The re-establishment of the normal blood lactate response to exercise in humans after prolonged acclimatization to altitude. *Journal of Physiology* 536:963–75.

108. Volpino, P. et al. 2004. Respiratory and cardiovascular function at rest and during exercise testing in a healthy working population: effects of outdoor traffic air pollution. *Occupational Medicine (Oxford)* 54:475–82.

109. Ward-Smith, A. J. 1983. The influence of aerodynamic and biomechanic factors on long jump performance. *Journal of Biomechanics* 16:655–58.

110. West, J. B., and P. D. Wagner. 1980. Predicted gas exchange on the summit of Mt. Everest. *Respiration Physiology* 42:1–16.

111. West, J. B. et al. 1983. Pulmonary gas exchange on the summit of Mount Everest. *Journal of Applied Physiology: Respiratory, Environmental, and Exercise Physiology* 55:678–87.

112. West, J. B. et al. 1983. Barometric pressures at extreme altitudes on Mt. Everest: Physiological significance. *Journal of Applied Physiology* 54:1188–94.

113. West, J. B. et al. 1983. Maximal exercise at extreme altitudes on Mt. Everest. *Journal of Applied Physiology* 55:688–98.

114. West, J. B. et al. 1962. Arterial oxygen saturation during exercise at high altitude. *Journal of Applied Physiology* 17:617–21.

115. Wolski, L. A., D. C. McKenzie, and H. A. Wenger. 1996. Altitude training for improvements in sea level performance. *Sports Medicine* 22:251–63.

116. Yaspelkis, B. B., and J. L. Ivy. 1991. Effect of carbohydrate supplements and water on exercise metabolism in the heat. *Journal of Applied Physiology* 71:680–87.

117. Yaspelkis, B. B. et al. 1993. Carbohydrate metabolism during exercise in hot and thermoneutral environments. *International Journal of Sports Medicine* 14:13–19.

118. Young, A. J., M. Sawka, P. D. Neufer, S. R. Muza, E. W. Askew, and K. B. Pandolf. 1989. Thermoregulation during cold water immersion is unimpaired by low muscle glycogen levels. *Journal of Applied Physiology* 66:1809–16.

119. Yu, I. T., T. W. Wong, and H. J. Liu. 2004. Impact of air pollution on cardiopulmonary fitness in schoolchildren. *Journal of Occupational & Environmental Medicine* 46:946–52.

120. Zanobetti, A. et al. 2004. Ambient pollution and blood pressure in cardiac rehabilitation patients. *Circulation* 110:2184–89.

CHAPTER 25

Ergogenic Aids

■ Objectives

By studying this chapter, you should be able to do the following:

1. Define *ergogenic aid*.
2. Explain why a "placebo" treatment in a "double-blind design" is used in research studies involving ergogenic aids.
3. Describe, in general, the effectiveness of nutritional supplements on performance.
4. Describe the effect of additional oxygen on performance; distinguish between hyperbaric oxygenation and that accomplished by breathing oxygen-enriched gas mixtures.
5. Describe blood doping and its potential for improving endurance performance.
6. Explain the mechanism by which ingested buffers might improve anaerobic performances.
7. Explain how amphetamines might improve exercise performance.
8. Describe the various mechanisms by which caffeine might improve performance.
9. Identify the risks associated with using chewing tobacco to obtain a nicotine "high."
10. Describe the risks of cocaine use and how it can cause death.
11. Describe the physiological and psychological effects of different types of warm-ups.

■ Outline

Research Design Concerns 523

Dietary Supplements 524

Aerobic Performance 524
   Oxygen 524

Blood Doping 527

Anaerobic Performance 529
   Blood Buffers 529

Drugs 530

Amphetamines 530
Caffeine 531
Cocaine 534
Nicotine 535

Physical Warm-Up 536

■ Key Terms

autologous transfusion
blood boosting
blood doping
blood packing
dental caries
double-blind research design

ergogenic aid
erythrocythemia
erythropoietin (EPO)
homologous transfusion
hyperbaric chamber
induced erythrocythemia

normocythemia
placebo
sham reinfusion
sham withdrawal
sympathomimetic

The preceding chapters have described exercise and dietary plans related to performance. However, no presentation of factors affecting performance would be complete without a discussion of **ergogenic aids.** Ergogenic aids are defined as work-producing substances or phenomena believed to increase performance (65).

Ergogenic aids include nutrients, drugs, warm-up exercises, hypnosis, stress management, blood doping, oxygen breathing, music, and extrinsic biomechanical aids. Although we discussed nutritional issues related to performance in chapter 23, we will provide additional detail about the role of dietary supplements as ergogenic aids in this chapter. In addition, we will discuss ergogenic aids related to aerobic performance (oxygen inhalation and blood doping) and anaerobic performance (blood buffers), as well as various drugs (amphetamines, caffeine, cocaine, and nicotine) and physical warm-up. Please note that anabolic steroids and growth hormone were discussed in chapter 5.

While the attention of the reader will be focused on athletic performance, where an improvement of less than 1% would alter world records, it must be noted that industrial physiologists have long been concerned about the relationship of lighting, environmental temperature, and background noise (music) to performance in the workplace (68). Research work in this area must be done carefully, with special attention to the research design due to the number of factors that can influence the outcome of the study.

RESEARCH DESIGN CONCERNS

It is sometimes difficult to compare the results of one research study on ergogenic aids with another. The reason for this is that the effect of an ergogenic aid depends on a number of variables (56):

- Amount—too little or too much may show no effect
- Subject—the ergogenic aid may be effective in "untrained" subjects but not "trained" subjects, or vice versa
    —the "value" of an ergogenic aid is determined by the subject
- Task—may work in short-term, power-related tasks, but not in endurance tasks, or vice versa
    —may work for gross-motor, large-muscle activities and not with fine-motor activities, or vice versa
- Use—an ergogenic aid used on an acute (short-term) basis may show a positive effect, but in the long run may compromise performance, or vice versa

Given these variables, scientists are careful in designing experiments in order not to be "fooled" by the result. For example, an *athlete* may improve performance because he or she believes the substance improves performance, so the "belief" is more important than the substance in determining the outcome. Further, an *investigator* may "believe" in the ergogenic aid and inadvertently offer different levels of encouragement during the testing of athletes under the influence of the ergogenic aid. These problems are controlled for by using a **placebo** as a treatment condition, and using a **double-blind research design,** respectively.

A placebo is a "look-alike" substance relative to the ergogenic aid under consideration, but it contains nothing that will influence performance. The need for such a control is seen in figure 25.1, which describes the gain in strength by a group that was taking a placebo but was *told* it was an anabolic steroid. It is contrasted with the group's performance prior to taking the placebo. The rate of strength gain was higher with the placebo, indicating the need for such a control if one is to isolate the true effect of a substance (2).

A double-blind research design is one in which neither the subject nor the investigator knows who is receiving the placebo or the substance under investigation. The subjects are randomly assigned to receive pill x or pill y. After all data are collected, the "code" is broken to find out which pill (x or y) was the placebo and which was the substance under investigation. These designs are very complex and difficult to carry out, but they reduce the chance of subject or investigator bias (68).

The scientist must also be careful in the selection of subjects. If a substance is tested as a potential aid

FIGURE 25.1 Changes in performance when subjects were told they were taking an anabolic steroid, but were really taking a placebo.

to sprinters, it would be reasonable to select subjects from that population so the results can be generalized to that group. Further, the tests used by the investigator should be as close as, or actually be, the performance task (e.g., 100-meter dash). In short, results obtained on a proper subject population but under controlled laboratory conditions using conventional physiological tests may not be useful when taken to the "field" (68).

IN SUMMARY

- Ergogenic aids are defined as substances or phenomena that are work-producing and are believed to increase performance.
- Due to the fact that an athlete's *belief* in a substance may influence performance, scientists use a placebo or look-alike substance to control for this effect. In addition, scientists use a double-blind research design in which the investigator and subject are both unaware of the treatment.

DIETARY SUPPLEMENTS

We discussed issues related to basic nutrition in chapter 18, and provided additional detail about the role of nutrition in performance in chapter 23. In this section we go a step further and discuss the role that dietary supplements may play in athletic performance—a point of interest to many athletes. A survey of athletes indicated that 46% used dietary supplements. Elite athletes used supplements more than college or high school athletes, and women used them more than men (90). For recent reviews on dietary supplements and performance, see Maughn et al. (63) and Juhn (53) in references, and texts by Fink, Burgoon, and Milesky (2006), and Jeukendrup and Gleeson (2004) in the Suggested Readings.

One has only to open a strength-training magazine to become aware of the incredible number of dietary supplements promoted as improving the effects of a workout, be it size or strength. Table 25.1 provides a summary of a number of dietary supplements used by strength-training athletes to increase strength, muscle mass, and athletic performance. The columns provide information about the claim made for each substance and the evidence for or against that claim. A quick reading of table 25.1 indicates that little or no support exists for any of the supplements, with the exception of creatine. We all know of the role of phosphocreatine (PC) in high-power events, or at the onset of endurance exercise (see chapters 3 and 4). Numerous studies show that creatine supplementation can increase the muscle's creatine concentration. Does it affect performance? (See The Winning Edge 25.1 for more on this rapidly changing story.)

Carnitine, another dietary supplement listed in table 25.1, is associated with the transport of fatty acids from the cytoplasm into the mitochondria. Table 25.1 indicates that there was no support for its proported claim to promote fat loss. However, endurance athletes are also interested in carnitine because of its putative effect on fat use, which may spare carbohydrates and reduce the lactate concentration during exercise. However, Heinonen's review (46) suggests that carnitine supplementation does not enhance fat oxidation nor spare glycogen, reduce body fat, affect lactate accumulation, or affect maximal oxygen uptake.

For an update on the effect of herbs on athletic performance, see a review by Kundrat (2005) in the Suggested Readings.

IN SUMMARY

- For the most part, there is little evidence that dietary supplements provide a performance advantage to athletes, with the possible exception of creatine.

AEROBIC PERFORMANCE

Chapter 20 detailed the various tests used to evaluate the physiological factors related to endurance performance. Clearly, an increased ability to transport O_2 to the muscles and a delay in the onset of lactate production are related to improved performance. Two ergogenic aids have been used to try to influence O_2 delivery: the breathing of O_2-enriched mixtures and blood doping.

Oxygen

Given the importance of aerobic metabolism in the production of ATP for muscular work, it is not surprising that scientists have been interested in the effect of additional oxygen (hyperoxia) on performance. But in order to discuss this issue we must ask the following question: How and when was the O_2 administered to achieve a higher PO_2 in the blood? In his insightful review of this topic, Welch (103) stressed the difficulty of comparing results from studies in which hyperoxia is achieved by increasing the percent of O_2 in the inspired air with those that use a **hyperbaric** (high-pressure) **chamber** with 21% or higher O_2 mixtures. Figure 25.2 shows that performance improves throughout the range of inspired oxygen pressures when O_2-enriched mixtures are used at a normal pressure of 1 atmosphere ("constant pressure"), compared to the use of a hyperbaric chamber ("increasing pressure"). The second part of the question is related to the time of administration of the supplemental O_2. Results vary depending on whether the O_2 is administered

TABLE 25.1 Dietary Supplements for Strength Trainers

Supplement	Description	Claim	Evidence	Comment
Antioxidants (e.g., vitamins A, C, and E)	Chemicals that protect cells from oxidative damage caused by free radicals	Reduce muscle damage resulting from severe or eccentric exercise	Little evidence that performance is enhanced, but some evidence that oxidative damage caused by exercise may be lessened	With continued training, antioxidants produced by the body may be sufficient; if diet is inadequate, supplement
Proteins or branched-chain amino acids	High-protein diets or unique amino acid supplements	Meet greater protein needs associated with training	Dietary intake already exceeds upper limit of known protein requirements	Diet adequate
Lysine, arginine, and ornithine	Amino acids	Increase growth hormone secretion; promote muscle growth	May increase growth hormone, but of very limited magnitude; no effect on muscle mass	Costly and ineffective
β-hydroxy–β-methylbutyrate	Metabolite of amino acid leucine	Anti-catabolic—decreases muscle protein breakdown	Might be useful in those beginning a training program; does not increase strength or fat-free mass in trained individuals	Expensive and of little benefit
Chromium	Plays role in insulin action	Enhances amino acid uptake	No effect on muscle mass or strength	If taken as picolinate salt, may be dangerous
Vanadium	Plays a role in insulin action	Enhances amino acid uptake	No effect on muscle mass or strength	High doses have serious side effects
Boron	Trace element	Enhances testosterone concentration	No effect	Diet adequate for normally nourished individuals
Creatine	Amino acid	Increases anaerobic power	Improves performance in selected tasks (e.g., repeated sprint bouts)	See The Winning Edge 25.1
Dehydroepiandrosterone (DHEA)	Precursor to testosterone	Enhances testosterone concentration and muscle mass	No effect on testosterone, strength, or muscle mass	Increases estrogen levels and decreases HDL cholesterol; could result in a positive drug test for testosterone
Androstenedione (andro)	Precursor to testosterone	Enhances testosterone concentration and muscle mass	No effect on testosterone, strength, or muscle mass	Increases estrogen levels and decreases HDL cholesterol; could result in a positive drug test for testosterone
Carnitine	Used in fat metabolism	Enhances fat use, decreases body fat	No deficiency in athletes; no effect on metabolic response to exercise	Diet adequate

From Juhn (52) and Maughan, King, and Lea (64).

THE WINNING EDGE 25.1

Creatine Monohydrate

We are all familiar with the importance of phosphocreatine (PC) as an energy source during short-term, explosive exercise, and as the energy source that helps us to make the transition to the steady state of oxygen uptake during submaximal aerobic exercise (see chapters 3 and 4). Because of PC's importance in explosive exercise, there has been a great deal of interest in the potential of the dietary supplement creatine monohydrate to increase the muscle's concentration of PC and, hopefully, performance.

The total creatine concentration in muscle is about 120 mmol · kg^{-1}, and 2 grams are excreted per day. These 2 grams are replaced by diet (1 gram) and by synthesis (1 gram) from amino acids (22, 103). The first step in a typical creatine monohydrate "loading" plan consists of adding 20 to 25 g to the diet per day for five to seven days. This results in a ~20% increase in muscle creatine, which approaches what is thought to be the upper limit of the muscle's capacity to store creatine. There is evidence that this elevated level can be achieved with doses as low as 3 g per day—given time. Independent of the means used to achieve the higher levels of creatine in muscle, there is great variability among subjects (22, 103):

- Individuals with lower initial values (e.g., vegetarians) have greater increases, and some

individuals with high presupplement values may not respond to the increased creatine. This has led to the terms *responders* and *nonresponders*.

- The ingestion of glucose with the creatine reduces this variation and enhances uptake.

In general, the short-term loading scheme appears to improve the ability to maintain muscular force and power output during various exhaustive bouts of exercise, including in older individuals (42), but not without exception (103, 110). However, since caffeine has been shown to counteract the ergogenic effect of creatine loading (100), one would have to be very careful with one's diet.

In contrast to scientists using a five- to seven-day loading regime to determine the effect of an elevated muscle creatine concentration, athletes take the creatine supplement for long periods of time to improve performance. The elevated level of creatine in muscle achieved in the loading phase can be maintained by consuming 2 to 5 grams of creatine monohydrate per day. Interestingly, the "mechanism" for any increase in performance may be only indirectly related to the creatine. For example, greater gains

in strength achieved in a weight-training program may be mediated by the athlete's ability to increase the intensity of training, which would, in turn, allow for a greater physiological adaptation (i.e., strength gain) to the training (103). What about the down side of creatine supplementation?

Creatine supplementation appears to increase body mass, but this is probably due more to water retention than protein synthesis. Consequently, athletes who must "carry" their own body weight (e.g., runners) might have to be careful not to negatively affect performance (22, 110). There are reports of gastrointestinal distress, nausea, and muscle cramping associated with the use of this dietary supplement; however, recent reports suggest that at least out to 21 months, there are no long-term adverse effects (11, 80). Should it be banned? Volek (42) provides an interesting analogy: Creatine supplementation is linked to enhanced performance of high-intensity, repetitive bouts of exercise in the same way that carbohydrate supplementation is linked to improvements in endurance performance (see chapter 23).

---

prior to, during, or following exercise. For that latter reason, this section on oxygen will be organized by those conditions.

Prior to Exercise The rationale for the use of supplemental oxygen prior to exercise is to try to "store" additional oxygen in the blood so that more will be available at the onset of exercise. It has been estimated that the hemoglobin in arterial blood is about 97% saturated with O_2 at rest (200 ml O_2/L blood). Breathing 100% O_2 would increase the O_2 bound to hemoglobin by only 3%, or 6 milliliters. However, the amount of oxygen physically dissolved in solution is proportional to the arterial PO_2, and when the PO_2

increases from about 100 mm Hg (breathing 21% O_2 at sea level) to about 700 mm Hg (breathing 100% O_2), the dissolved oxygen increases from 3 ml/L to 21 ml/L. If a person has a total blood volume of 5 liters, approximately 100 milliliters of additional O_2 can be "stored" prior to exercise. However, if the person takes a few breaths between the time the O_2 breathing stops and the event begins, the O_2 store will return to that associated with air breathing (110).

The focus of attention on the use of oxygen prior to exercise has been on short-term exercise. In general, in runs of 880 yards or less, weight lifting, stair climbing, and swims of 200 yards or less, the O_2 breathing seemed to be beneficial (69, 110). In addi-

FIGURE 25.2 The effect of PO_2 on performance. Constant pressure experiments used oxygen-enriched gas mixtures at sea-level pressure, while the increasing pressure experiments used a hyperbaric chamber to increase the PO_2. From H.W. Welch, "Effects of Hypoxia and Hyperpoxia on Human Performance" in Kent B. Pandolf, ed., *Exercise and Sport Sciences Reviews*, vol. 15. Copyright © 1987 McGraw-Hill, Inc., New York. Reprinted by permission.

tion, evidence suggested that the O_2 breathing needed to take place within two minutes of the task (110). Some concern has been expressed about these findings due to the fact that in some cases the subjects knew they were breathing O_2, a factor that could have affected the results (110). Overall, considering the fact that O_2 cannot be breathed up to the start of a sprint event in swimming or track, any effect would be lost before the starter's gun is fired. Therefore, unless one participates in a breath-holding event, oxygen breathing prior to exercise will have little effect on performance.

During Exercise The rationale for the use of oxygen during exercise to improve performance is based on the proposition that muscle is hypoxic during exercise and additional O_2 delivery will alleviate the problem (104). If this is the case, then the additional O_2 in the blood during O_2 breathing should increase the delivery of O_2 to the muscle and improve performance. However, Welch et al. (104) showed that when one breathes hyperoxic gas mixtures, the increase in the O_2 content of arterial blood (CaO_2) is balanced by a *decrease* in blood flow to the working muscles such that O_2 delivery ($CaO_2 \times$ flow) is not different from normoxic (21% O_2) conditions. $\dot{V}O_2$ max is increased by only 2% to 5% with hyperoxia, which is about what would be expected, since maximal cardiac output doesn't change and the a-$\bar{v}$ O_2 difference does not increase more than 5% to 6% (84) [$\dot{V}O_2$ max $= \dot{Q}$ max $\times$ ($CaO_2 - C\bar{v}O_2$)].

In spite of similarities in O_2 delivery during hyperoxia and normoxia, *performance* has been shown to

increase dramatically as a result of an increase in inspired O_2. Figure 25.2, presented in the introduction to this section, showed a performance increase of 40% while breathing 100% O_2. How could this be if O_2 delivery to muscles is not substantially different? The increased availability of O_2 has been shown to decrease pulmonary ventilation and reduce the work of breathing, a change that should lead to an increase in performance (103, 111, 112). In addition, those athletes who experience "desaturation" of hemoglobin during maximal work (see chapters 9 and 24) while breathing 21% O_2 could benefit by breathing oxygen-enriched gas mixtures (77). One study found that when sprinters did three repeat 300-meter sprints at different speeds on a treadmill while breathing 40% oxygen (compared to 21%), hemoglobin saturation was maintained and the fall in blood pH was less (73). Finally, the high PO_2 slows glycolysis during heavy exercise, resulting in a slower accumulation of lactate and H^+ in the plasma and extending the time to exhaustion (48, 103). The reduction in lactate formation in hyperoxia appears to be due to a reduction in the rate of glycogen breakdown so that it is better matched with its subsequent oxidation in the Krebs cycle (93). Given the impracticality of trying to provide O_2 mixtures to athletes *during* performance, this research on hyperoxia is more useful as a tool to answer questions related to the age-old question of what factor, O_2 delivery or the muscle's capacity to consume O_2, limits aerobic performance (103).

After Exercise The rationale for the use of supplemental oxygen after exercise is that the subject might recover more quickly following exercise and be ready to go again. Some of the early work showed just that, but because the subjects knew what gas they were breathing, the results have to be interpreted with caution (69, 110). Wilmore (110) summarized the effects of several studies and concluded that there was no benefit of O_2 breathing during recovery on heart rate, ventilation, and post-exercise oxygen uptake. This conclusion was supported by studies showing no effect of O_2 breathing on subsequent performance in all-out exercise (80).

| IN SUMMARY |

- Oxygen breathing before or after exercise seems to have little or no effect on performance, while oxygen breathing during exercise improves endurance performance.

Blood Doping

In chapter 13 we described how $\dot{V}O_2$ max is limited by maximal cardiac output, given the constraint that blood pressure had to be maintained by vasoconstriction of the active muscle mass. Since maximal O_2 transport is equal to the product of maximal cardiac output ($\dot{Q}$ max) and the O_2 content of arterial blood (CaO_2), one way to improve O_2 delivery to tissue when $\dot{Q}$ max cannot change is to increase the quantity of hemoglobin in each liter of blood. **Blood doping** refers to the infusion of red blood cells (RBCs) in an attempt to increase the hemoglobin concentration ([Hb]) and, consequently, O_2 transport (CaO_2 is equal to the [Hb] $\times$ 1.34 ml O_2/gm Hb). Other terms to describe this are **blood boosting** and **blood packing,** with **induced erythrocythemia** being the proper medical term. However, before we get into this topic it must be remembered that an increase in blood volume (independent of an increase in the hemoglobin concentration) would also favorably affect $\dot{V}O_2$ max and aerobic performance (40).

In blood doping, a subject receives a transfusion of blood, which may be his or her own **(autologous transfusion)** or blood from a matched donor **(homologous transfusion).** The latter procedure is acceptable in times of medical emergencies, but carries the risk of infection and blood-type incompatibility (39); it is therefore not recommended in blood-doping procedures. The need to use your own blood in order to achieve the goal of a higher [Hb] creates some interesting problems that led to confusion in the early days of research in this area. The primary problem was related to the mismatch between the maximum time blood could be refrigerated and the time period needed for the subject to produce new RBCs and bring the [Hb] back to normal before the reinfusion. Maximum storage time with refrigeration is three weeks, during which time about 1% of the RBCs are lost per day. In addition, some RBCs adhere to the storage containers or become so fragile that they will not function upon reinfusion. Due to these problems only about 60% of the removed RBCs could be reinfused (39). The normal time period for replacement of the RBCs following a 400-milliliter donation is three to four weeks, and following a 900-milliliter donation, five to six weeks or more are required. If the blood were reinfused at the end of the three-week maximal storage time, the investigator might not have been able to achieve the condition of an increased [Hb] due to RBC loss (decreased 40%) and the below-normal (anemic) values in the subjects. Gledhill (39) makes a strong case for this as a primary reason why studies prior to 1978 showed inconsistent changes in $\dot{V}O_2$ max and performance with blood doping. Another major problem encountered in these early studies was the lack of an adequate research design. There was a need to have a group undergoing a **"sham" withdrawal** (needle placed in the arm but no blood is removed) and a **"sham" reinfusion** (needle placed in the arm but blood is not returned) to act as placebo controls.

FIGURE 25.3 Changes in hemoglobin levels in blood following removal (phlebotomy) and reinfusion.

The central factor allowing a more careful study of blood doping was the introduction of the freezer preservation technique, which allows the blood to be stored frozen for years with only a 15% RBC loss. This allows plenty of time for the subject to become **normocythemic** (achieve normal [Hb]), so that any effect of the reinfusion can be correctly evaluated (39).

The general findings were that reinfusions of single units (~450 milliliters) of blood showed small but insignificant increases in [Hb], $\dot{V}O_2$ max, and performance, while the infusion of two units (900 milliliters) significantly increased the [Hb] (8%–9%), $\dot{V}O_2$ max (4%–5%), and performance (3%–34%). The infusion of three units (1,350 milliliters) of blood caused slightly greater increases in [Hb] (10.8%) and $\dot{V}O_2$ max (6.6%). This large reinfusion caused borderline **erythrocythemia** to be approached, so a 1,350-milliliter infusion probably represents the upper limit that can be used. Figure 25.3 shows a gradual reduction in [Hb] toward the normal value following reinfusion, indicating that increased O_2 transport is maintained for ten to twelve weeks. This is an important point as far as performance gains are concerned (37).

The improvements in performance (3%–34%) were much more variable than the changes in [Hb] or $\dot{V}O_2$ max. Part of the reason for this variation was the type of performance test used. The greatest change was observed in a running test to exhaustion that lasted less than ten minutes, while the smallest change was observed in a five-mile time trial, with the improvement being fifty-one seconds compared to a preinfusion run time of 30:17 (109). Given that the laboratory results show consistent gains, the question raised by Eichner, "Does it work in the field?," still needs to be answered (28). Until the answer is known, blood doping will continue to be a useful laboratory tool to study the factors limiting $\dot{V}O_2$ max (91).

While the blood doping issue will always raise a question of ethics, Gledhill presents what amounts to a moral dilemma in the use of blood doping in getting athletes ready for performance at altitude. In chapter 24 we discussed the changes in $\dot{V}O_2$ max and performance at altitude. Those athletes who stay at altitude experience a natural increase in RBC production to deal with the hypoxia. As Gledhill (39) points out, those athletes who can afford to train at altitude accomplish what blood doping does in a manner that is acceptable to the International Olympic Committee. The availability of a recombinant DNA analog of **erythropoietin (EPO),** the hormone that stimulates red blood cell production, has complicated the picture.

Erythropoietin is used as a part of therapy for those who undergo chemotherapy or dialysis (due to kidney disease). The hormone stimulates red blood cell production to reduce the chance of anemia. This is crucial for a wide variety of patients, and investigators are trying to optimize the use of EPO (59). While normal cross-country training does not seem to increase plasma levels of naturally occurring erythropoietin (6), acute exposure to 3,000 and 4,000 meters of simulated altitude has been shown to increase the concentration 1.8- and 3.0-fold, respectively (26). The real concern, of course, is the potential abuse of the DNA-derived analog of this hormone to generate the effects of blood doping, without having to undergo the blood withdrawals and reinfusions. Such abuse is not without its risks, in that RBC production can get out of hand. This could lead to extremely high RBC levels, which would impair blood flow to the heart and brain, resulting in a myocardial infarction or a stroke. However, if an athlete were to use the drug and experience the desired increase in RBC production, the RBC effect would last for some weeks, while the level of erythropoietin would return quickly to resting values, making detection of this blood-doping procedure difficult to trace (87). With the emergence of artificial oxygen carriers, the situation is becoming even more complicated (86). An organization composed of scientists, pharmaceutical companies, and hematologists has been formed to work systematically to prevent the abuse of these products by unethical athletes (3). We refer the interested reader to two recent reviews on this topic by Fisher (2003) and Gaudard et al. (2003) in the Suggested Readings.

IN SUMMARY

- Blood doping refers to the reinfusion of red blood cells in order to increase the hemoglobin concentration and oxygen-carrying capacity of the blood.
- Due to improvements in blood storage techniques, blood doping has been shown to be effective in improving $\dot{V}O_2$ max and endurance performance.

ANAEROBIC PERFORMANCE

Improvements in endurance performance focus on the supply of carbohydrate and oxygen to muscle (see previous sections on oxygen and blood doping in this chapter and on carbohydrate in chapter 24). However, in short-term, all-out performances in which anaerobic energy sources provide the vast majority of energy for muscle contraction, the focus of attention shifts to the buffering of the H^+ released from muscle. This section will consider a means by which investigators have tried to buffer the H^+ and improve performance.

Blood Buffers

Elevations in the $[H^+]$ in muscle can decrease the activity of phosphofructokinase (PFK) (98), which may slow glycolysis, interfere with excitation-contraction coupling events by reducing Ca^{++} efflux from the terminal cisternae of the sarcoplasmic reticulum (35), and reduce the binding of Ca^{++} to troponin (70). Decreases in muscle force development have been shown to be linked to increases in muscle $[H^+]$ in both frog muscle (32) and human muscle (96). Finally, when Adams and Welch (1) showed that performance times in heavy exercise (90% $\dot{V}O_2$ max) could be altered by breathing 60% O_2 compared to 21% or 17% O_2, the point of exhaustion was associated with the same arterial $[H^+]$. The mechanisms involved in the regulation of the plasma $[H^+]$ were described in detail in chapter 11. Briefly, the primary means by which H^+ is buffered *during* exercise is through its reaction with the plasma bicarbonate reserve to form carbonic acid, which subsequently yields CO_2 that is exhaled (respiratory compensation). As the bicarbonate buffer store decreases, the ability to buffer H^+ is reduced and the plasma $[H^+]$ will increase. Knowing this, scientists have explored ways of increasing the plasma buffer store to slow down the rate of H^+ increase during strenuous exercise.

As early as 1932 (23), induced alkalosis (means unknown) was shown to extend run time to exhaustion from (min:sec) 5:22 to 6:04. Since that time a wide variety of studies have supported these findings. On the basis of several reviews (10, 49, 55, 74, 78, 107) there appears to be agreement that:

- the optimal dose of bicarbonate used to improve performance was 0.3 g per kilogram of body weight (along with 1 liter of water),
- tasks of a minute or less in duration, even at extremes of intensity, did not seem to benefit from the induced alkalosis, and
- performance gains were shown for tasks of high intensity that lasted about one to ten

minutes, or involved repeated bouts of high-intensity exercise with short recovery periods.

The positive impact of the buffers may be related to maintaining the oxygen saturation of hemoglobin during maximal exercise, as well as any improvements at the level of the muscle (72). Sodium citrate has also been shown to be an effective buffer for anaerobic performances of two to four minutes when taken at 0.5 g/kg (49, 67). However, a recent study comparing the relative benefits of a variety of buffers recommended bicarbonate as the better choice to enhance sprint performance (101). The variability in the effectiveness of the sodium bicarbonate treatment suggests that some short-term anaerobic activities are more dependent on the muscle or plasma $[H^+]$ as a primary cause of fatigue than others. Welch (103) indicates that while subjects may stop at the same $[H^+]$ within any exercise protocol, the differences that exist among studies in the "terminal" $[H^+]$ suggest the other factors are more limiting as far as performance is concerned. The use of these agents to cause an alkalosis is not without risks. Large doses of sodium bicarbonate can cause diarrhea and vomiting, both of which are sure to affect performance (38, 55, 107).

IN SUMMARY

■ The ingestion of sodium bicarbonate improves performances of one to ten minutes' duration or repeated bouts of high-intensity exercise.

DRUGS

A variety of drugs have been used to aid performance. Some drugs are as common and "legal" as caffeine and nicotine, while others, like amphetamines and cocaine, are banned from use. We will briefly examine each of these drugs, exploring how they might work to improve performance, as well as the evidence about whether or not they do.

Amphetamines

Amphetamines are stimulants that have been used primarily to recover from fatigue and improve endurance. In 1972, Golding (41) indicated that it was the most abused group of drugs at that time. Amphetamines are readily absorbed in the small intestine, and while the effects reach a peak two to three hours after ingestion, they persist for twelve to twenty-four hours (50, 56). Amphetamines are both a **sympathomimetic** drug (simulates catecholamine effects) and a central nervous system stimulant. The drug produces its effects by altering the metabolism and synthesis of catecholamines, or receptor affinity for catecholamines (50, 56).

The most consistent effect of amphetamines is to increase one's arousal or wakefulness, leading to a perception of increased energy and self-confidence (50). The drug affects the redistribution of blood flow, driving it away from the skin and splanchnic areas and delivering more to muscle or brain. This could lead to problems related to a decrease in lactic acid removal (see chapter 3) and an increase in body temperature (see chapter 12). Animal studies show that amphetamines can increase endurance-type performances. However, the dose of the drug was shown to be important, in that smaller doses (1–2 mg/kg) did not have an effect different from control, and large doses (16 mg/kg) appeared to reduce the ability of the rat to swim. Data collected using run tests on rats indicate the same detrimental effect of high doses (7.5–10 mg/kg) of amphetamines (50).

Ivy (50) concluded from an analysis of studies on human subjects that amphetamines extend endurance and hasten recovery from fatigue. Time to exhaustion was increased in spite of no effect on submaximal or maximal $\dot{V}O_2$ (14, 50). Two explanations have been offered. Ivy (50) feels that the endurance aspect of performance can be improved due to amphetamines' catecholamine-like effect in mobilizing FFA and sparing muscle glycogen, similar to that of caffeine (see the caffeine section, this chapter). Chandler and Blair (14) believe that the amphetamines may simply mask fatigue and interfere with the perception of the normal biological signals that fatigue has occurred. It is this latter conclusion that has raised the most concern about the safety of the athlete, in that during prolonged submaximal work, especially in a hot and/or humid environment, the decreased blood flow to the skin could cause hyperthermia, leading to death (16, 50, 56).

As mentioned at the beginning of this section, amphetamines' major effect is in increasing wakefulness and producing a state of arousal. However, while amphetamines have restored reaction time in fatigued subjects, the drug does not affect reaction time in alert, motivated, and nonfatigued subjects (18). Given that athletes are usually alert and motivated prior to competition, Golding (41) suggests that amphetamines would be counterproductive, making users hyperirritable and interfering with their sleep. Finally, it is risky to extrapolate from data collected under tightly controlled laboratory conditions using discrete measures related to performance ($\dot{V}O_2$ max, endurance time, reaction time) to the actual performance in a skilled sport in front of a hostile audience for a national championship. That might be excitement enough. Sometimes a drug used for one purpose finds its way into the sporting world because of its unique impact on muscle. See A Closer Look 25.1 for such an example.

A CLOSER LOOK 25.1

Clenbuterol—A Drug with Special Ergogenic Effects

Clenbuterol is a drug that was developed to treat airway diseases such as asthma. Its chemical action in the body is to activate beta-2 receptors in tissue (see chapter 5). Although the drug is useful in the treatment of airway diseases, in the early 1980s it was discovered that clenbuterol is a powerful anabolic agent in skeletal muscles. Indeed, a fourteen-day treatment of animals with clenbuterol (2 mg/kg/day) results in a 10% to 20% increase in muscle mass [see Yang (116) for a review]. The changes include a transition in fiber type from type I to type II, and a selective hypertrophy of type II fibers (21). Further, the time course of

clenbuterol-induced muscular hypertrophy is rapid, with muscle growth beginning within two days after commencement of treatment.

Since the discovery that clenbuterol is a powerful anabolic agent in skeletal muscle, scientific interest in the clinical use of this drug has grown. For example, this compound is potentially useful in the treatment of conditions that result in muscle wasting (i.e., aging, spinal cord injury, etc.) (62). Unfortunately, some athletes now use clenbuterol in an effort to increase muscle size and improve performance in power events (e.g., sprinting, football, etc.).

Although there is evidence that oral administration of this drug increases muscle strength/mass in some populations, there is no evidence that this is the case for trained athletes. Further:

- Even when muscle size is increased, resistance to fatigue may be worsened.
- Some athletes who tried the drug stopped because of an increase in tremors.
- Serious side effects include cardiac arrhythmias.

It sounds like the use of this drug would push risk-taking to a new level (16, 116).

IN SUMMARY

- Amphetamines have a catecholamine-like effect that leads to an increased arousal and a perception of increased energy and self-confidence.
- While amphetamines improve the performance of fatigued subjects, they do not have this effect on alert, motivated, and nonfatigued subjects.

Caffeine

Caffeine is a stimulant that is found in a wide variety of common foods, drinks, and over-the-counter drugs (see table 25.2). Caffeine has been viewed as an on-again, off-again ergogenic aid. Caffeine was banned by the International Olympic Committee (IOC) in 1962, then removed from the list of banned drugs in 1972. In 1984, the IOC again banned "high levels" in the urine that might have been the result of caffeine injections or suppositories; the standard was set at 12 μg/ml (100, 106). Caffeine is again off the list of banned substances. Part of the reason is the availability of caffeine in food and drinks, which makes it very difficult thing to track and control in an athlete's diet. Caffeine is absorbed rapidly from the GI tract, and is significantly elevated in the blood at fifteen minutes, with the peak concentration achieved at sixty minutes. Caffeine is diluted by body water, and the physiological response is proportional to the concentration in the body water. There is a natural variability in how peo-

ple respond to caffeine, with evidence that chronic users are less responsive than abstainers (5, 100).

While caffeine can affect a wide variety of tissues, figure 25.4 shows that its role as an ergogenic aid is based on its effects on skeletal muscle and the central nervous system, and in the mobilization of fuels for muscular work. The evidence for the enhanced function of skeletal muscle is based primarily on *in vitro* and *in situ* muscle preparations and shows that caffeine can increase tension development (76, 100). This was shown most clearly in fatigued muscle and was believed to be due to enhanced Ca^{++} availability (61). In one human study, caffeine had no effect on maximum voluntary contraction or the maximal tension elicited by electrical stimulation. However, there was greater tension development at lower levels of electrical stimulation in both rested and fatigued muscles. The change in endurance measured by time at 50% of maximal voluntary contraction tension was variable and nonsignificant (58).

Caffeine has long been recognized as a stimulator of the CNS. Caffeine can pass the blood-brain barrier and affect a variety of brain centers, which usually leads to an increased alertness and decreased drowsiness (76, 100). The best evidence supporting caffeine as a CNS stimulant is in the decreased perception of fatigue during prolonged exercise in subjects who took caffeine (19). A recent systematic review of the literature supports this proposition with findings that the rating of perceived exertion (RPE) is lower during exercise with caffeine ingestion, accounting for some of the improvement in performance (25).

CAFFEINE CONTENT OF POPULAR BEVERAGES AND FOOD		CAFFEINE CONTENT OF VARIOUS SOFT DRINKS	
Item	**Caffeine (mg)[a]**	**Soft Drinks**	**Caffeine (mg per 12-oz Serving)[b]**
Coffee (5-oz Cup)		Sugar-Free Mr. PIBB	58
Drip method	110–150	Mountain Dew	54
Percolated	64–124	Mello Yello	52
Instant	40–108	TAB	46
Decaffeinated	2–5	Coca-Cola	46
Instant decaffeinated	2	Diet Coke	46
Tea (Loose or Bags)		Shasta Cola	44
(5-oz Cup)		Shasta Diet Cola	44
One-minute brew	9–33	Mr. PIBB	40
Three-minute brew	20–46	Dr Pepper	40
Five-minute brew	20–50	Sugar-Free Dr Pepper	40
Tea Products		Pepsi Cola	38.4
Instant tea (5-oz cup)	12–28	Diet Pepsi	36
Iced tea (12-oz cup)	22–36	Pepsi Light	36
Cocoa		RC Cola	36
Made from mix	6	Diet Rite	0
Milk chocolate (1 oz)	6	Canada Dry Diet Cola	0
Baking chocolate (1 oz)	35		

CAFFEINE IN DRUG PREPARATIONS[c]		CAFFEINE IN DRUG PREPARATIONS[c]	
Classification	**Caffeine (mg per Tablet or Capsule)**	**Classification**	**Caffeine (mg per Tablet or Capsule)**
Over-the-Counter Stimulants		**Cold Remedies**	
No Doz tablets	100	Coryban-D	30
Vivarin tablets	200	Dristan	0
Pain Relievers		Triaminicin	30
Anacin	32	**Weight-Control Aids**	
Excedrin	65	Dexatrim	200
Midol	32	Prolamine	140
Plain aspirin, any brand	0	**Prescription Pain Relievers**	
Vanquish	33	Cafergot	100
Diuretics		Darvon Compound	32.4
Aqua Ban	100	Fiorinal	40
		Migralam	100

[a]Data from Consumers Union, Food and Drug Administration, National Coffee Association, and National Soft Drink Association.

[b]Data from National Soft Drink Association.

[c]Values taken from *The Physicians' Desk Reference for Nonprescription Drugs*, 1983.

From J. L. Slavin and D. J. Joensen, "Caffeine and Sport Performance" in *The Physician and Sportsmedicine* 13:191, 193, May 1985. Copyright © 1985. McGraw-Hill Healthcare Group, Minneapolis, MN. Reprinted by permission. (68)

The role of caffeine in the mobilization of fuel has received considerable attention as the primary means by which it exerts its ergogenic effect. Caffeine has been shown to cause an elevation of glucose and an increase in fatty acid utilization. The elevated glucose could be due to the stimulation of the sympathetic nervous system and the resulting increase in catecholamines, which would increase the mobilization of glucose from the liver. On the other hand, the glucose concentration could be elevated due to a decreased rate of removal related to the suppression of insulin release by catecholamines (see chapter 5) (100). However, some of these metabolic effects are not dependent on catecholamines; instead, they may be related to the products of caffeine breakdown (e.g., theophylline), which are metabolic stimuli in their own right (44).

Lipid mobilization has been shown to be increased as a result of caffeine ingestion. Figure 25.5 shows that the mechanism of action could be related either to the elevated catecholamines increasing the level of cyclic AMP in the adipose cell or to caffeine's blocking of phosphodiesterase activity, which is responsible for breaking down cyclic AMP. Van Handel (100) feels that the latter mechanism is less likely, given the dose of

caffeine needed. Plasma free fatty acids increase quickly *at rest* after ingestion of caffeine (fifteen minutes) and continue to increase over the next several hours (100). However, *during exercise*, plasma FFA may (24, 94) or may not (19, 24, 29, 43, 51) be significantly elevated as a result of caffeine ingestion. In addition, while the respiratory exchange ratio may (13, 29, 51) or may not (43, 95) be reduced, both glucose kinetics (85) and the lactate threshold (7, 24, 36) have been shown not to be affected by caffeine ingestion. In addition, there is also variability in the effect of caffeine on improvements in work output or total work time, making it an "ergogenic aid" for some and not for others (24, 25, 29, 36, 43, 51, 92, 106). However, in the better-controlled studies, caffeine enhanced performance in intense cycling lasting about five minutes, and in simulated 1,500-meter race time (44). In contrast, no ergogenic effect has been seen for power output in repeated bouts of short-term intense exercise (45). What causes such variability?

The ergogenic effect appears to be dose dependent and may vary with the type of subject (17); however, gender and menstrual cycle status do not appear to affect the pharmacokinetics of how caffeine is handled (64). While some studies show physiological changes with doses as low as 5 to 7 mg/kg (19, 29), others find a 10 mg/kg dose to be inadequate (51). In fact, in other studies (65), a dose of 15 mg/kg was

FIGURE 25.4 Factors influenced by caffeine that might cause an improvement in performance.

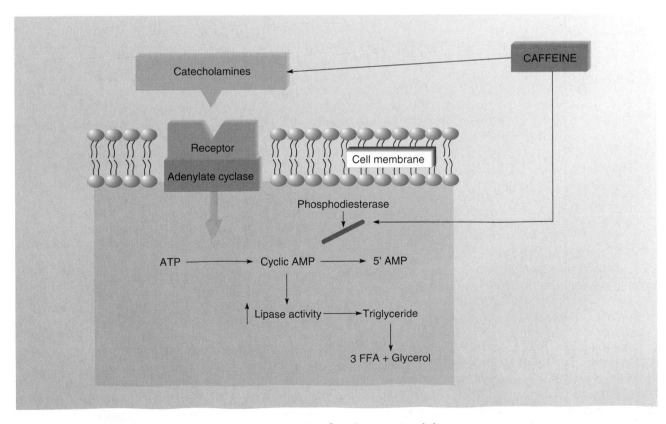

FIGURE 25.5 Mechanisms by which caffeine might increase free-fatty-acid mobilization.

needed to see an increase in fat metabolism (65, 66). There is also evidence that patterns of caffeine use affect the response to exercise. For example, habitual caffeine users who abstain from caffeine for four days are more responsive to caffeine during exercise than in their normal mode of daily caffeine use (31). Further, heavy caffeine users (>300 mg per day) respond differently than those consuming little caffeine (24). Van Handel (100) makes the point that what an investigator observes in a controlled laboratory setting may be masked by a normal sympathetic nervous system response to competition. Given the potential side effects such as insomnia, diarrhea, anxiety, tremulousness, and irritability (100) and the variability among subjects in response to caffeine, one might not see much of an improvement in performance (27, 92, 43). Although caffeine has a diuretic effect, a recent study indicated that rehydration with caffeine containing beverages during nonexercise periods of two-a-day practices did not hinder hydration status (30).

In the past few years, there has been a dramatic increase in research dealing with caffeine-ephedrine mixtures. Ephedrine is a drug similar to amphetamines and is widely available in over-the-counter medications—purchases of which are controlled in many states to reduce the manufacture of methamphetamine. For a recent review of the impact of these combined caffeine-ephedrine mixtures on performance, see the review by Magkos and Kavouras (2004) in the Suggested Readings.

IN SUMMARY

- Caffeine can potentially improve performance at the muscle or in the central nervous system, or in the delivery of fuel for muscular work. Caffeine can elevate blood glucose and simultaneously increase the utilization of fat.
- Caffeine's ergogenic effect on performance is variable, and appears to be dose-related and less pronounced in subjects who are daily users of caffeine.

Cocaine

Cocaine is presented in this section on ergogenic aids because of the publicity surrounding its use by professional athletes. While this is meant to provide information about the drug rather than to describe cocaine's role in athletic performance, the little experimental evidence available shows the drug to have a detrimental effect on endurance performance (12, 16, 18). Cocaine acts as a local anesthetic and a powerful stimulator of the cardiovascular and central nervous systems. Peruvian natives used it as an ergogenic aid in the sixth century to improve work performance at altitude (57). Cocaine can be taken in a

variety of ways:

- Sniffing—inhaled through the nose to be absorbed through the nasal mucosa. The "high" is rapid and peaks in about twenty minutes.
- Smoking—coca paste: rapid onset, short-acting
  —free-basing: onset is rapid, intense "rush," short-acting
- Intravenous injection—rapid onset, peaks in three to five minutes
- "Crack"—almost pure cocaine smoked in pipe or cigarette. The effects are similar to those of the intravenous injection method (57)

Cocaine gives a person a sense of euphoria and feelings of increased mental and physical power. However, the drug is psychologically addictive, becoming the focal point in a user's life. The dark side of this drug's effects occurs when euphoria leads to paranoia, anxiety, insomnia, hallucinations, and delusions (57). An overdose of cocaine can lead to arrhythmias, coma, seizures, hyperthermia, and death (57). Figure 25.6 presents an outline of the mechanism by which cocaine may have caused the death of two professional athletes (13).

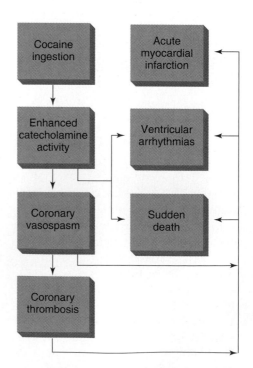

FIGURE 25.6 Mechanisms by which cocaine can kill. From John D. Cantwell, "Cocaine and Cardiovascular Events," in *The Physician and Sportsmedicine* 14(11):77–82. Copyright © 1986 McGraw-Hill Healthcare, Minneapolis, MN. Reprinted by permission.

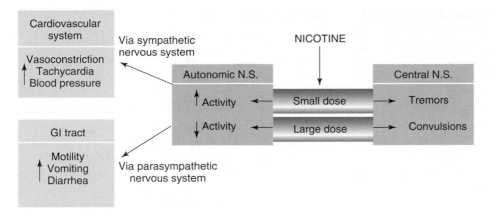

FIGURE 25.7 Schematic representation of how nicotine can have both relaxing and stimulating effects.

Nicotine

Nicotine is a drug with no therapeutic application. However, the fact that it is a part of cigarette and chewing tobacco makes it one of the most abused substances. Nicotine has unpredictable effects due to the fact that it can simultaneously increase sympathetic, parasympathetic, and central nervous system activities (see figure 25.7). Small doses of nicotine increase autonomic activity, while large doses lead to a blocking of the response. The cardiovascular system responds with increases in heart rate and blood pressure due to increased sympathetic nerve activity, and the GI tract responds with an increase in activity via parasympathetic nerve stimulation. There is evidence that both resting metabolic rate and cardiovascular responses to light exercise are increased following nicotine administration (62, 75). Nicotine is easily absorbed through the lungs, mucous membranes, and the skin, and the half-life of nicotine is about thirty to sixty minutes (95).

Nicotine is primarily taken in by either smoking or chewing tobacco. Independent of whether it has a calming or a stimulating effect on an individual, the smoking and chewing of tobacco are associated with major health problems. We already know from chapter 14 that cigarette smoking is linked directly to a variety of cancers and heart and lung diseases. That alone is motivation enough to discourage smoking, independent of the fact that it increases the work of breathing (82), decreases $\dot{V}O_2$ max (54), and lengthens the time needed for $\dot{V}O_2$ to achieve a steady state during submaximal exercise (83). The point is, of course, that cigarette smoke contains more than nicotine, specifically, carbon monoxide and various carcinogens. But what if the nicotine could be obtained without the cigarette smoke?

Smokeless tobacco has become a part of the American sport scene. Smokeless tobacco includes (a) loose leaf tobacco that is placed between the cheek and lower gum and is "chewed," (b) snuff, moist or dry powdered tobacco, that is "dipped" and placed between the cheek or lip and lower gum, and (c) compressed tobacco, a "plug," that is used as loose leaf tobacco.

In the 1990s, the focus of attention was on the use of these products by athletes and the impact that might have on children. Despite media and educational campaigns to inform the public about the risks involved, we have not been as successful as we might like in curbing use of smokeless tobacco. About 7.8 million people over the age of twelve use smokeless tobacco. Unfortunately the percentage of high school senior boys using these products (11.8%) is higher than that of adult males (9.5%) (71).

While one might be worried about a young person becoming addicted to nicotine through the use of smokeless tobacco, the greatest concern is with regard to damage to teeth **(dental caries)** and gums (periodontal disease), including oral cancer. The increase in dental caries (2.4 times more than nonusers) is related, in part, to the sugar content in the pouch (35%) and plug (24%) tobacco. However, it is more important to focus attention on periodontal disease and cancer. The withdrawal of the gum from a tooth's surface exposes the tooth to greater damage that can lead to the loss of the tooth and potentially to bone loss. The loss of the gum occurs in the area where the tobacco is held in the mouth, indicating a clear link. Further, lesions of the mucosa can develop, which can ultimately lead to cancer. While it is known that regular smoking can cause oral cancer, smokeless tobacco users are actually at a greater risk. Independent of any potential beneficial effect of nicotine on performance, the use of smokeless tobacco should be discouraged. Once "hooked," the habit is more difficult to break than that associated with cigarette smoking.

IN SUMMARY

- Cocaine is a powerful stimulator of the cardio-vascular and central nervous systems. It provides a sense of euphoria and feelings of increased mental and physical power. However, it is psychologically addictive and potentially deadly.
- Nicotine has varied effects depending on whether the parasympathetic or sympathetic nervous system is stimulated. The use of smokeless tobacco can cause dental caries, gum disease, and oral cancer.

PHYSICAL WARM-UP

Warming up prior to moderate or strenuous activity is a general recommendation made for those involved in fitness programs or athletes involved in various types of performance. While most of us accept this as a reasonable recommendation, is there good scientific support for it? In Franks's original 1972 review (33), he found that 53% of the studies supported the proposition that warm-up was better than no warm-up, 7% the opposite, and 40% found no difference between the two. Concerns were raised about the wide variety of tasks and the methods used to evaluate the effectiveness of warm-up. In his 1983 review, Franks (34) analyzed the role of the participant (trained or untrained), the duration and intensity of the warm-up, and the type of performance as the variables involved in a determination of the effectiveness of warm-up. Before we summarize these findings a few definitions must be presented.

Warm-up refers to exercise conducted prior to a performance, whether or not muscle or body temperature is elevated. Warm-up activities can be *identical to the performance* (baseball pitcher throwing with normal form and high speed to a catcher prior to the batter stepping up), *directly related to the performance* (shot putter practicing at 75% of normal effort prior to a competition), or *indirectly related to a performance* (general activities to increase body temperature or arousal) (34). Generally all three are used in a typical warm-up prior to performance, in the reverse order of the above descriptions.

The theoretical benefits of warm-up are physiological, psychological, and safety-related. Physiological benefits would include less muscle resistance and faster enzymatic reactions at high body temperatures. This might lower the oxygen deficit at the onset of work (52, 82), decrease the RER during the subsequent activity (47), or cause a favorable shift in the lactate threshold (15). A recent review supported most of these effects, but questioned the impact of the warm-up on speeding up rate-limiting enzyme reactions (8). Increases in body temperature as a result of warm-up have been linked to improved performance (34). Skilled performances benefit from identical and direct warm-up, with indirect warm-up sometimes acting in a facilitatory manner. The warm-up procedures can increase arousal, which is good up to a point, and provide the optimal "mental set" for improved performance (8, 34).

Stretching, as a part of warming up, has been recommended as a way to reduce the risk of soft tissue injury. There is no question that such a practice improves joint flexibility, but the most recent reviews on this topic provide little support that injury risk is reduced. Weldon and Hill (105) found that most of the available studies were of poor quality, and it was not possible to draw a definitive conclusion regarding stretching and exercise-related injuries. A group of researchers at the Centers for Disease Control and Prevention drew the same conclusion from their review of the literature, and indicated that there was not enough evidence to either endorse or discontinue routine stretching before or after exercise to prevent injuries (97). Witvrouw and colleagues (113) agreed with these general conclusions when applied to most sports. However, for those sports demanding high-intensity stretch-shortening cycles (e.g., soccer, basketball), stretching was viewed as important to keep the muscle-tendon unit compliant enough to store and release energy during explosive movements. Finally, Shrier's comment on the CDC article indicated that there was a need to separate out the effects of stretching outside of periods of exercise from the stretching that precedes exercise. There is evidence that the former approach is associated with injury prevention. Clearly, more research is needed (88). From a safety standpoint, apart from the potential for soft tissue injuries, there is some evidence that warm-up reduces the "stress" experienced when doing strenuous work. In Barnard et al.'s (4) classic study, six of ten fire fighters who did not warm up experienced an ischemic response (reduced myocardial blood flow) as shown by a depressed ST segment on the ECG during strenuous exercise (see chapter 17). All had normal ECG responses when a gradual warm-up preceded the strenuous exercise.

Warming up obviously affects a wide variety of factors, but is there evidence that it favorably affects performance? The answer is "yes," but with some caveats (9).

- In short-term performances (max effort of ≤ 10 s) a three- to five-minute warm-up improves performance. However, an intense warm-up may result in a decrement in performance due, in part, to a reduction in high-energy phosphates.

- Warm-up improves intermediate-term performances (>10 s, but ≤ 5 min), but not if the intensity is too low ($\leq 40\%$ $\dot{V}O_2$ max) or the recovery time is too long (5–10 minutes). The goal is to begin the performance with a slightly elevated baseline $\dot{V}O_2$, and be sufficiently recovered.

- For long-term performances (fatiguing effort for $\geq$ 5mintes), an elevated baseline $\dot{V}O_2$ also improves performance. However, if the warm-up depletes muscle glycogen or increases thermal strain (by elevating body temperature too much), performance may suffer.

So, what is the recommended warm-up? For short-term performances, a warm-up at $\sim 40\%$ to 60% $\dot{V}O_2$ max for 5 to 10 minutes, followed by a five-minute recovery is recommended. For intermediate- or long-term performances, the warm-up at $\sim 60\%$ to 70% $\dot{V}O_2$ max for 5 to 10 minutes, with a ≤ 5 minute recovery (9). This is very similar to what Franks reported some 20 years ago (34).

IN SUMMARY

- Warm-up activities can be identical to performance, directly related to performance, or indirectly related to performance (general warm-up). Warm-up causes both physiological and psychological changes that are beneficial to performance.

STUDY QUESTIONS

1. What is an ergogenic aid?
2. Why must an investigator use a "placebo" treatment to evaluate the effectiveness of an ergogenic aid?
3. Provide a brief summary of the role that dietary supplements play in improving performance.
4. What is a double-blind research design?
5. Does breathing 100% O_2 improve performance? Recovery?
6. Breathing hyperoxic gas mixtures improves performance without changing O_2 delivery to tissue. How is this possible?
7. What is blood doping and why does it appear to improve performance now when it did not in the earliest investigations?
8. How might ingested buffers improve short-term performances?
9. While amphetamines improve performance in fatigued individuals, they might not have this effect on motivated subjects. Why?
10. How might caffeine improve long-term performances? Can the results be extrapolated to "real" performances in the field?
11. Chewing tobacco may provide a nicotine "high," but not without risks. What are they?
12. Describe the different types of warm-up activities and the mechanisms by which they may improve performance.

SUGGESTED READINGS

Fink, H. H., L. A. Burgoon, and A. E. Mikesky. 2006. *Practical Applications in Sports Nutrition*. Sudbury, MA: Jones and Bartlett Publishers.

Fisher, J. W. 2003. Erythropoietin: Physiology and pharmacology update. *Experimental Biology & Medicine* 228:1–14.

Gaudard, A., E. Varlet-Marie, F. Bressolle, and M. Audran. 2003. Drugs for increasing oxygen and their potential use in doping: A review. *Sports Medicine* 33:187–212.

Jeukendrup, A., and M. Gleeson. 2004. *Sports Nutrition: An introduction to energy production and performance*. Champaign, IL: Human Kinetics Publishers, Inc.

Kundrat, Susan. 2005. Herbs and athletes. *Sport Science Exchange*, no. 96. Gatorade Sport Science Institute.

Magkos, F., and S. A. Kavouras. 2004. Caffeine and ephedrine: Physiological, metabolic and performance-enhancing effects. *Sports Medicine* 34:871–89.

REFERENCES

1. Adams, R. P., and H. G. Welch. 1980. Oxygen uptake, acid-base status, and performance with varied inspired oxygen fractions. *Journal of Applied Physiology: Respiratory, Environmental, and Exercise Physiology* 49:863–68.
2. Ariel, G., and W. Saville. 1972. Anabolic steroids: The physiological effects of placebos. *Medicine and Science in Sports* 4:124–26.
3. Ashenden, M. J. 2002. A strategy to deter blood doping in sport. *Haematologica* 87:225–32.
4. Barnard, R. J. et al. 1973. Cardiovascular responses to sudden strenuous exercise—heart rate, blood pressure and ECG. *Journal of Applied Physiology* 34:833–37.
5. Bell, D. G., and T. M. McLellan. 2002. Exercise endurance 1, 3, and 6 h after caffeine ingestion in caffeine users and nonusers. *Journal of Applied Psychology* 93:1227–34.
6. Berglund, B., G. Birgegard, and P. Hemmingsson. 1988. Serum erythropoietin in cross-country skiers. *Medicine and Science in Sports and Exercise* 20:208–9.

7. Berry, M. J., J. V. Stoneman, A. S. Weyrich, and B. Burney. 1991. Dissociation of the ventilatory and lactate thresholds following caffeine ingestion. *Medicine and Science in Sports and Exercise* 23:463–69.

8. Bishop, D. 2003. Warm up I: Potential mechanisms and the effects of passive warm up on exercise performance. *Sports Medicine* 33:439–54.

9. Bishop, D. 2003. Warm up II: Performance changes following active warm up and how to structure the warm up. *Sports Medicine* 33:483–98.

10. Bishop, D., J. Edge, C. Davis, and C. Goodman. 2004. Induced metabolic alkalosis affects muscle metabolism and repeated-sprint ability. *Medicine & Science in Sports & Exercise* 36:807–13.

11. Bizzarini, E., and L. De Angelis. 2004. Is the use of oral creatine supplementation safe? *Journal of Sports Medicine & Physical Fitness* 44:411–16.

12. Bracken, M. E., D. R. Bracken, A. R. Nelson, and R. K. Conlee. 1988. Effect of cocaine on exercise endurance and glycogen use in rats. *Journal of Applied Physiology* 64:884–87.

13. Cantwell, John D. 1986. Cocaine and cardiovascular events. *The Physician and Sportsmedicine* 14(11):77–82.

14. Chandler, J. V., and S. N. Blair. 1980. The effect of amphetamines on selected physiological components related to athletic success. *Medicine and Science in Sports and Exercise* 12:65–69.

15. Chwalbinska-Moneta, J., and O. Hanninen. 1989. Effect of active warming up on thermoregulatory, circulatory, and metabolic responses to incremental exercise in endurance-trained athletes. *International Journal of Sports Medicine* 10:25–29.

16. Clarkson, P. M., and H. S. Thompson. 1997. Drugs and sports: Research findings and limitations. *Sports Medicine* 24:366–84.

17. Conlee, R. K. 1991. Amphetamine, caffeine, and cocaine. In *Perspectives in Exercise Science and Sports Medicine. Vol. 4: Ergogenics—Enhancement of Performance in Exercise and Sports*, ed. D. R. Lamb and M. H. Williams, 285–330. New York: McGraw-Hill Companies.

18. Conlee, R. K., D. R. Barnett, K. P. Kelly, and D. H. Han. 1991. Effects of cocaine on plasma catecholamine and muscle glycogen concentrations during exercise in the rat. *Journal of Applied Physiology* 70:1323–27.

19. Costill, D. L., G. Dalsky, and W. Fink. 1978. Effects of caffeine ingestion on metabolism and exercise performance. *Medicine and Science in Sports* 10:155–58.

20. Cox, G. R., B. Desbrow, P. G. Montgomery, M. E. Anderson, C. R. Bruce, T. A. Macrides, D. T. Martin, A. Moquin, A. Roberts, J. A. Hawley, and L. M. Bruce. 2002. Effect of different protocols of caffeine intake on metabolism and endurance performance. *Journal of Applied Physiology* 93:990–09.

21. Criswell, D. S., S. K. Powers, and R. A. Herb. 1996. Clenbuterol-induced fiber type transition in the soleus of adult rats. *European Journal of Applied Physiology* 74:391–96.

22. Dement, T. W., and E. C. Rhodes. 1999. Effects of creatine supplementation on exercise performance. *Sports Medicine* 28:49–60.

23. Dill, D. B., H. T. Edwards, and J. H. Talbot. 1932. Alkalosis and the capacity for work. *Journal of Biological Chemistry* 97:LVII–LIX.

24. Dodd, S. L., E. Brooks, S. K. Powers, and R. Tulley. 1991. The effect of caffeine on graded exercise performance in caffeine naive versus habituated subjects. *European Journal of Applied Physiology* 62:424–29.

25. Doherty, M., and P. M. Smith. 2005. Effects of caffeine ingestion on rating of perceived exertion during and after exercise: A meta-analysis. *Scandinavian Journal of Medicine & Science in Sports* 15:69–78.

26. Eckardt, K., U. Boutellier, A. Kurtz, M. Schopen, E. A. Koller, and C. Bauer. 1989. Rate of erythropoietin formation in humans in response to acute hypobaric hypoxia. *Journal of Applied Physiology* 66:1785–88.

27. Eichner, E. R. 1986. The caffeine controversy: Effects on endurance and cholesterol. *The Physician and Sportsmedicine* 14:124–32.

28. ———. 1987. Blood doping results and consequences from the laboratory and the field. *The Physician and Sportsmedicine* 15(1):121–29.

29. Essig, D., D. L. Costill, and P. J. Van Handel. 1980. Effect of caffeine ingestion on utilization of muscle glycogen and lipid during leg ergometer cycling. *International Journal of Sports Medicine* 1:86–90.

30. Fiala, K. A., D. J. Casa, and M. W. Roti. 2004. Rehydration with a caffeinated beverage during the nonexercise periods of 3 consecutive days of 2-a-day practices. *International Journal of Sport Nutrition & Exercise Metabolism* 14:419–29.

31. Fisher, S. M. et al. 1986. Influence of caffeine on exercise performance in habitual caffeine users. *International Journal of Sports Medicine* 7:276–80.

32. Fitts, R. H., and J. O. Holloszy. 1976. Lactate and contractile force in frog muscle during development of fatigue and recovery. *American Journal of Physiology* 231:430–33.

33. Franks, B. D. 1972. Physical warm-up. In *Ergogenic Aids and Muscular Performance*, ed. W. P. Morgan, chap. 6, 160–91. New York: Academic Press.

34. ———. 1983. Physical warm-up. In *Ergogenic Aids in Sport*, ed. M. H. Williams, chap. 13, 340–75. Champaign, IL: Human Kinetics.

35. Fuchs, F., V. Reddy, and F. N. Briggs. 1970. The interaction of cations with the calcium-binding site of troponin. *Biochemistry Biophysics Acta* 221:407–9.

36. Gastin, P. B., J. E. Misner, R. A. Boileau, and M. H. Slaughter. 1990. Failure of caffeine to enhance exercise performance in incremental treadmill running. *The Australian Journal of Science and Medicine in Sport* 22:23–27.

37. Gledhill, N. 1982. Blood doping and related issues: A brief review. *Medicine and Science in Sports and Exercise* 14:183–89.

38. ———. 1984. Bicarbonate ingestion and anaerobic performance. *Sports Medicine* 1:177–80.

39. ———. 1985. The influence of altered blood volume and oxygen transport capacity on aerobic performance. In *Exercise and Sport Sciences Reviews*, vol. 13, ed. R. L. Terjung, 75–94. New York: Macmillan.

40. Gledhill, N., D. Warburton, and V. Jamnik. 1999. Hemoglobin, blood volume, cardiac function and aerobic power. *Canadian Journal of Applied Physiology* 24:54–65.

41. Golding, L. A. 1972. Drugs and hormones. In *Ergogenic Aids and Muscular Performance*, ed. W. P. Morgan. New York: Academic Press.

42. Gotshalk, L. A., J. S. Volek, R. S. Staron, C. R. Denegar, F. C. Hagerman, and W. J. Kraemer. 2002. Creatine supplementation improves muscular performance in older men. *Medicine and Science in Sports and Exercise* 34:537–43.

43. Graham, T. E., and L. L. Spriet. 1991. Performance and metabolic responses to a high caffeine dose during prolonged exercise. *Journal of Applied Physiology* 71:2292–98.

44. ———. 1996. Caffeine and exercise performance. *Sports Science Exchange*, vol. 9, no. 1. Chicago, IL: Gatorade Sports Science Institute.

45. Greer, F., C. McLean, and T. E. Graham. 1998. Caffeine, performance, and metabolism during repeated Wingate exercise tests. *Journal of Applied Physiology* 85:1502–8

46. Heinonen, O. J. 1996. Carnitine and physical exercise. *Sports Medicine* 22:109–32.

47. Hetzler, R. K. et al. 1986. Effect of warm-up on plasma free fatty acid responses and substrate utilization during submaximal exercise. *Research Quarterly for Exercise and Sport* 57:223–28.

48. Hogan, M. C., R. H. Cox, and H. G. Welch. 1983. Lactate accumulation during incremental exercise with varied inspired oxygen fractions. *Journal of Applied Physiology* 55:1134–40.

49. Horswill, C. A. 1995. Effects of bicarbonate, citrate, and phosphate loading on performance. *International Journal of Sport Nutrition* 5:S111–S119.

50. Ivy, John L. 1983. Amphetamines. In *Ergogenic Aids in Sport*. Champaign, IL: Human Kinetics.

51. Ivy, J. L. et al. 1979. Influence of caffeine and carbohydrate feedings on endurance performance. *Medicine and Science in Sports and Exercise* 11:6–11.

52. Jones, A. M., K. Koppo, and M. Burnley. 2003. Effects of prior exercise on metabolic and gas exchange responses to exercise. *Sports Medicine* 33(13):949–71.

53. Juhn, M. S. 2003. Popular sports supplements and ergogenic aids. *Sports Medicine* 33:921–39.

54. Klausen, K., S. Andersen, and S. Nandrup. 1983. Acute effects of cigarette smoking and inhalation of carbon monoxide during maximal exercise. *European Journal of Applied Physiology* 51:371–79.

55. Linderman, J., and T. Fahey. 1991. Sodium bicarbonate ingestion and exercise performance. *Sports Medicine* 11:71–77.

56. Lombardo, J. A. 1986. Stimulants and athletic performance (part 1 of 2): Amphetamines and caffeine. *The Physician and Sportsmedicine* 14(11):128–42.

57. ———. 1986. Stimulants and athletic performance (part 2): Cocaine and nicotine. *The Physician and Sportsmedicine* 14(12):85–89.

58. Lopes, J. M. et al. 1983. Effect of caffeine on skeletal muscle function before and after fatigue. *Journal of Applied Physiology: Respiratory, Environmental, and Exercise Physiology* 54:1303–5.

59. Macdougall, I. C. 1998. Meeting the challenges of the new millennium: Optimizing the use of recombinant human erythropoietin. *Nephrology, Dialysis, Transplantation* 13(Supp. 2):23–27.

60. MacIntosh, B. R., R. W. Barbee, and W. N. Stainsby. 1981. Contractile response to caffeine of rested and fatigued skeletal muscle. *Medicine and Science in Sports and Exercise* 13:95.

61. Maltin, C., and M. Delray. 1992. Satellite cells in innervated and denervated muscles treated with Clenbuterol. *Muscle and Nerve* 15:919–25.

62. Marks, B. L., and K. A. Perkins. 1990. The effects of nicotine on metabolic rate. *Sports Medicine* 10:277–85.

63. Maughan, R. J., D. S. King, and T. Lea. 2004. Dietary supplements. *Journal of Sports Sciences* 22:95–113.

64. McLean, C., and T. E. Graham. 2002. Effects of exercise and thermal stress on caffeine pharmacokinetics in men and eumenorrheic women. *Journal of Applied Physiology* 93:1471–78.

65. McNaughton, L. 1987. Two levels of caffeine ingestion on blood lactate and free fatty acid responses during incremental exercise. *Research Quarterly for Exercise and Sport* 58:255–59.

66. McNaughton, L. R. 1986. The influence of caffeine ingestion on incremental treadmill running. *British Journal of Sports Medicine* 20:109–12.

67. McNaughton, L., and R. Cedaro. 1992. Sodium citrate ingestion and its effects on maximal anaerobic exercise of different durations. *European Journal of Applied Physiology* 64:36–41.

68. Morgan, W. P. 1972. Basic considerations. In *Ergogenic Aids and Muscular Performance*, ed. W. P. Morgan. New York: Academic Press.

69. Morris, A. F. 1983. Oxygen. In *Ergogenic Aids in Sports*. Champaign, IL: Human Kinetics.

70. Nakamura, Y., and S. Schwartz. 1972. The influence of hydrogen ion concentration on calcium binding and release by skeletal muscle sarcoplasmic reticulum. *Journal of General Physiology* 59:22–32.

71. National Cancer Institute. Web address: http://dccps.nci.nih.gov/tcrb/less_facts.html.

72. Nielsen, H. B., P. P. Bredmose, M. Strømstad, S. Volianitis, B. Quistorff, and N. H. Secher. 2002. Bicarbonate attenuates arterial desaturation during maximal exercise in humans. *Journal of Applied Physiology* 93:724–31.

73. Nummela, A., I. Hamalainen, and H. Rusko. 2002. Effect of hyperoxia on metabolic responses and recovery in intermittent exercise. *Scandinavian Journal of Medicine & Science in Sports* 12:309–15.

74. Oopik, V., I. Saaremets, L. Medijainen, K. Karelson, T. Janson, and S. Timpmann. 2003. Effects of sodium citrate ingestion before exercise on endurance performance in well trained college runners. *British Journal of Sports Medicine* 37:485–89.

75. Perkins, K. A., J. E. Sexton, R. D. Solberg-Kassel, and L. H. Epstein. 1991. Effects of nicotine on perceived exertion during low intensity activity. *Medicine and Science in Sports and Exercise* 23:1283–88.

76. Powers, S. K., and S. Dodd. 1985. Caffeine and endurance performance. *Sports Medicine* 2:165–74.

77. Powers, S. K. et al. 1989. Effects of incomplete pulmonary gas exchange on V̇O₂ max. *Journal of Applied Physiology* 66:2491–95.

78. Price, M., P. Moss, and S. Rance. 2003. Effects of sodium bicarbonate ingestion on prolonged intermittent exercise. *Medicine & Science in Sports & Exercise.* 35:1303–8.

79. Rawson, E. S., and P. M. Clarkson. 2003. Scientifically debatable: is creatine worth its weight? *Sports Science Exchange—Number 91* 16:1–6.

80. Robbins, M. K., K. Gleeson, and C. W. Zwillich. 1992. Effect of oxygen breathing following submaximal and maximal exercise on recovery and performance. *Medicine and Science in Sports and Exercise* 24:720–25.

81. Robergs, R. A., D. D. Pascoe, D. L. Costill, W. J. Fink, J. Chwalbinska-Moneta, J. A. Davis, and R. Hickner. 1991. Effects of warm-up on muscle glycogenolysis during intense exercise. *Medicine and Science in Sports and Exercise* 23:37–43.

82. Rode, A., and R. J. Shepard. 1971. The influence of cigarette smoking on the oxygen cost of breathing in near maximal exercise. *Medicine and Science in Sports* 3:51–55.

83. Rotstein, A., M. Sagiv, A. Yaniv-Tamir, N. Fisher, and R. Dotan. 1991. Smoking effect on exercise response kinetics of oxygen uptake and related variables. *International Journal of Sports Medicine* 12:281–84.

84. Roy, B. D., M. J. Bosman, and M. A. Tarnopolsky. 2001. An acute oral dose of caffeine does not alter glucose kinetics during prolonged dynamic exercise in trained endurance athletes. *European Journal of Applied Physiology* 85:280–86.

85. Safran, M. R., A. V. Seaber, and W. E. Garrett. 1989. Warm-up and muscular injury prevention—an update. *Sports Medicine* 8:239–49.

86. Schumacher, Y. O., and M.J. Ashenden. 2004. Doping with artificial oxygen carriers—an update. *Sports Medicine* 34:141–50.

87. Scott, W. C. 1990. The abuse of erythropoietin to enhance athletic performance (letter). *Journal of the American Medical Association* 264:1660.

88. Shrier, I. 2004. Special communications—letters to the editor-in-chief. *Medicine & Science in Sports & Exercise* 36:1832–33.

89. Slavin, J. L., and D. J. Joensen. 1985. Caffeine and sport performance. *The Physician and Sportsmedicine* 13:191–93.

90. Sobal, J., and L. F. Marquart. 1994. Vitamin/mineral supplement use among athletes: A review of the literature. *International Journal of Sport Nutrition* 4:320–34.

91. Spriet, L. L. 1991. Blood doping and oxygen transport. In *Perspectives in Exercise Science and Sports Medicine. Vol. 4: Ergogenics—Enhancement of Performance in Exercise and Sport*, ed. D. R. Lamb and M. H. Williams, 213–48. New York: McGraw-Hill Companies.

92. ———. 1995. Caffeine and performance. *International Journal of Sport Nutrition* 5:S84–S99.

93. Stellingwerff, T., L. Glazier, M. J. Watt, P. J. LeBlanc, G. J. Heigenhauser, and L. L. Spriet. 2005. Effects of hyperoxia on skeletal muscle carbohydrate metabolism during transient and steady-state exercise. *Journal of Applied Physiology* 98:250–56.

94. Tarnopolsky, M. A., S. A. Atkinson, J. D. MacDougall, D. G. Sale, and J. R. Sutton. 1989. Physiological responses to caffeine during endurance running in habitual caffeine users. *Medicine and Science in Sports and Exercise* 21:418–24.

95. Taylor, P. 1980. Ganglionic stimulating and blocking agents. In *Goodman and Gilman's The Pharmacological Basis of Therapeutics*, 6th ed., ed. A. G. Gilman, L. S. Goodman, and A. Gilman. New York: Macmillan.

96. Tesch, P. et al. 1978. Muscle fatigue and its relation to lactate accumulation and LDH activity in man. *Acta Physiologica Scandinavia* 103:413–20.

97. Thacker, S. B., J. Gilchrist, D. F. Stroup, and C. D. Kimsey Jr. 2004. The impact of stretching on sports injury risk: A systematic review of the literature. *Medicine & Science in Sports & Exercise* 36:371–78.

98. Trevedi, B., and W. H. Danforth. 1966. Effect of pH on the kinetics of frog muscle phosphofructokinase. *Journal of Biological Chemistry* 241:4110–12.

99. Vandenberghe, K., N. Gillis, M. Van-Leemputte, P. Van-Hecke, F. Vanstaple, and P. Hespel. 1996. Caffeine counteracts the ergogenic action of muscle creatine loading. *Journal of Applied Physiology* 80:452–57.

100. Van Handel, P. 1983. Caffeine. In *Ergogenic Aids in Sports*, ed. M. H. Williams. Champaign, IL: Human Kinetics.

101. Van Montfoort, M. C., L. Van Dieren, W. G. Hopkins, and J. P. Shearman. 2004. Effects of ingestion of bicarbonate, citrate, lactate, and chloride on sprint running. *Medicine & Science in Sports & Exercise* 36:1239–43.

102. Volek, J. S. 1999. What we now know about creatine. *ACSM's Health & Fitness Journal* 3:27–33.

103. Welch, H. G. 1987. Effects of hypoxia and hyperoxia on human performance. In *Exercise and Sports Sciences Reviews*, vol. 15, ed. K. B. Pandolf, 191–222. New York: Macmillan.

104. Welch, H. G. et al. 1977. Effects of hyperoxia on leg blood flow and metabolism during exercise. *Journal of Applied Physiology* 42:385–90.

105. Weldon, S. M., and R. H. Hill. 2003. The efficacy of stretching for prevention of exercise-related injury: A systematic review of the literature. *Manual Therapy* 8:141–50.

106. Wilcox, A. R. 1990. Caffeine and endurance performance. *Sports Science Exchange*, vol. 3, no. 26. Chicago, IL: Gatorade Sports Science Institute.

107. ———. 1992. Bicarbonate loading. *Sports Science Exchange*, vol. 4, no. 36. Chicago, IL: Gatorade Sports Science Institute.

108. ———. 1998. Nutritional ergogenics and sport performance. In *The President's Council on Physical Fitness and Sports Research Digest*, ed. C. Corbin and B. Pangrazi. Series 3, no. 2.

109. Williams, M. H. et al. 1981. The effect of induced erythrocythemia upon 5-mile treadmill run time. *Medicine and Science in Sports and Exercise* 13:169–75.

110. Wilmore, J. H. 1972. Oxygen. In *Ergogenic Aids and Muscular Performance*, ed. W. P. Morgan, 321–42. New York: Academic Press.

111. Wilson, G. D., and H. G. Welch. 1975. Effects of hyperoxic gas mixtures on exercise tolerance in man. *Medicine and Science in Sports* 7:48–52.

112. Wilson, G. D., and H. G. Welch. 1980. Effects of varying concentrations of N_2/O_2 and He/O_2 on exercise tolerance in man. *Medicine and Science in Sports and Exercise* 12:380–84.

113. Witvrouw, E., N. Mahieu, L. Danneels, and P. McNair. 2004. Stretching and injury prevention—an obscure relationship. *Sports Medicine* 34:443–49.

114. Yang, Y., and M. McElligott. 1989. Multiple actions of beta-2-agonists on skeletal muscle and adipose tissue. *Biochemical Journal* 261:1–10.

Calculation of Oxygen Uptake and Carbon Dioxide Production

Calculation of Oxygen Consumption

Calculation of oxygen consumption is a relatively simple process that involves subtracting the amount of oxygen exhaled from the amount of oxygen inhaled:

(1) Oxygen consumption $(\dot{V}O_2) =$ [volume of O_2 inspired] − [volume of O_2 expired]

The volume of O_2 inspired (I) is computed by multiplying the volume of air inhaled per minute $(\dot{V}_I)$ by the fraction (F) of air that is made up of oxygen. Room air is 20.93% O_2. Expressed as a fraction, 20.93% becomes .2093 and is symbolized as F_IO_2. When we exhale, the fraction of O_2 is lowered (i.e., O_2 diffuses from the lung to the blood) and the fraction of O_2 in the expired (E) gas is represented by F_EO_2. The volume of expired O_2 is the product of the volume of expired gas $(\dot{V}_E)$ and F_EO_2. Equation (1) can now be symbolized as:

(2) $\dot{V}O_2 = (\dot{V}_I \cdot F_IO_2) - (\dot{V}_E \cdot F_EO_2)$

The exercise values for F_IO_2, F_EO_2, $\dot{V}_I$, and $\dot{V}_E$ for a subject are easily measured in most exercise physiology laboratories. In practice, F_IO_2 is not generally measured but is assumed to be a constant value of .2093 if the subject is breathing room air. F_EO_2 will be determined by a gas analyzer, and $\dot{V}_I$ and $\dot{V}_E$ can be measured by a number of different laboratory devices capable of measuring airflow. Note that it is not necessary to measure both $\dot{V}_I$ and $\dot{V}_E$. This is true because if $\dot{V}_I$ is measured, $\dot{V}_E$ can be calculated (and vice versa). The formula used to calculate $\dot{V}_E$ from the measurement of $\dot{V}_I$ is called the "Haldane transformation" and is based on the fact that nitrogen (N_2) is neither used nor produced in the body. Therefore, the volume of N_2 inhaled must equal the volume of N_2 exhaled:

(3) $[\dot{V}_I \cdot F_IN_2] = [\dot{V}_E \cdot F_EN_2]$

Therefore, $\dot{V}_I$ can be computed if $\dot{V}_E$, F_IO_2, and F_EO_2 are known. For example, to solve for $\dot{V}_I$:

(4) $\dot{V}_I = \dfrac{(\dot{V}_E \cdot F_EN_2)}{F_IN_2}$

Likewise, if $\dot{V}_I$ was measured, $\dot{V}_E$ can be computed as:

(5) $\dot{V}_E = \dfrac{(\dot{V}_I \cdot F_IN_2)}{F_EN_2}$

The values for F_IN_2 and F_EN_2 are obtained in the following manner. If the subject is breathing room air, F_IN_2 is considered to be a constant .7904. The final remaining piece to the puzzle is F_EN_2. Recall that the three principal gases in air are N_2, O_2, and CO_2 and the sum of their fractions must add up to 1.0 (i.e., $F_ECO_2 + F_EO_2 + F_EN_2 = 1.0$). Therefore, F_EN_2 can be computed by subtracting the sum of F_ECO_2 and F_EO_2 from 1 (i.e., $F_EN_2 = 1 - (F_ECO_2 + F_EO_2)$. Since the expired fractions of O_2 and CO_2 will be determined by gas analyzers, F_EN_2 can then be calculated.

Calculation of Carbon Dioxide Production

The volume of carbon dioxide produced $(\dot{V}CO_2)$ can be calculated in a manner similar to $\dot{V}O_2$. That is, the volume of CO_2 produced is equal to:

(6) $\dot{V}CO_2 =$ [Volume of CO_2 expired] − [Volume of CO_2 inspired]
or
(7) $\dot{V}CO_2 = (\dot{V}_E \cdot F_ECO_2) - (\dot{V}_I \cdot F_ICO_2)$

The steps in performing this calculation are the same as in the computation of $\dot{V}O_2$. That is, $\dot{V}_E$ and $\dot{V}_I$ must be measured (or calculated) and the fraction of expired carbon dioxide (F_ECO_2) must be determined by a gas analyzer. Similar to F_IO_2, the fraction of inspired carbon dioxide (F_ICO_2) is considered to be a constant value of .0003.

Standardization of Gas Volumes

By convention, $\dot{V}O_2$ or $\dot{V}CO_2$ are expressed in liters $\cdot$ min^{-1} and standardized to a reference condition called "STPD." STPD is an acronym for "standard temperature pressure dry." In a similar manner, pulmonary ventilation is expressed in liters $\cdot$ min^{-1} and standardized to a reference standard called BTPS, an acronym for "body temperature pressure saturated." The purpose of these reference standards is to allow comparison of gas volumes measured in laboratories throughout the world, which may vary in ambient temperature and barometric pressures. Standardization of gas volumes to a specified temperature and pressure is necessary because gas volume is dependent upon both temperature and pressure. For instance, a given number of gas molecules will occupy a greater volume at a higher temperature and lower pressure than at a lower temperature and higher pressure. This means that a fixed number of gas molecules would change volume as a function of the ambient temperature and barometric pressure. This poses a serious problem to researchers trying to make comparisons of respiratory gas exchange since temperature and pressures vary day by day and vary from one laboratory to another. By standardizing temperature and pressure conditions for gases, the scientist or technician knows that two equal volumes of gas contain the same number of molecules. It is for these reasons that respiratory gases must be corrected to a reference temperature and volume.

CORRECTION OF GAS VOLUMES TO REFERENCE CONDITIONS

Before we begin a discussion of "how to" calculate gas volume corrections, it is necessary to introduce two important gas laws. The first, called "Charles's Law," states that the relationship between temperature and gas volume is directly proportional. That is, the gas volume is directly related to temperature, so that increasing or decreasing the temperature of a gas (at a constant pressure) causes a proportional volume increase or decrease, respectively. This relationship is expressed mathematically in the following way:

$$(8)\ \frac{T_1}{T_2} = \frac{V_1}{V_2}$$

The units for temperature in equation (8) are the Kelvin (K) or Absolute (A) scale, where $0°$ C $= 273°$ K [i.e., $20°$ C $= (273° + 20°) = 293°$ K]. In using Charles's Law for gas temperature corrections, we rearrange equation (8) to solve for V_2:

$$(9)\ V_2 = \frac{V_1 \cdot T_2}{T_1}$$

Let's leave Charles's Law for the moment and introduce a second gas law known as Boyle's Law. Boyle's Law states that at a constant temperature, the number of gas molecules in a given volume varies inversely with the pressure and is represented mathematically in the following equation:

$$(10)\ P_1 V_1 = P_2 V_2$$

Again, rearranging equation (10) to solve for V_2:

$$(11)\ V_2 = \frac{P_1 \cdot V_1}{P_2}$$

Pressure in equations (10) and (11) is expressed in mm Hg or Torr. Note that when respiratory gases are corrected for pressure differences that a correction is often made for water vapor, even though water vapor pressure is dependent only upon temperature (since respiratory gas is saturated with water vapor). When the gas volume is to be corrected to "0" water vapor pressure or "dried" as in STPD, the vapor pressure of water (PH_2O) at the ambient temperature is subtracted from the ambient or initial pressure (P_1) in Boyle's Law as follows:

$$(12)\ V_2 = \frac{V_1(P_1 - PH_2O)}{P_2}$$

COMBINED CORRECTION FACTORS

We can now combine Charles's Law and Boyle's Law (complete with water vapor correction) into one equation for STPD and BTPS conditions. Let's consider the STPD correction first.

STPD Correction

Gas volumes measured in the laboratory under room conditions of temperature and pressure are expressed as "ambient temperature pressure and saturated" (ATPS). This means that the gas volume is not a standardized volume but rather a volume that is subject to the ambient conditions of temperature and pressure. As previously stated, since ATPS conditions may vary from laboratory to laboratory, there is a need to correct $\dot{V}O_2$ and $\dot{V}CO_2$ volumes to the reference volume, STPD. Correcting a volume to STPD requires the standardization of temperature to $0°$ C ($273°$ K), pressure to 760 mm Hg (sea level), and a correction for vapor pressure. For simplicity we will divide the gas correction procedure into two parts: (1) temperature and (2) pressure correction.

Step 1: Temperature Correction Let's consider the temperature correction first. For this correction, we use equation (9) (Charles's Law):

$$V_2 = \frac{V_1 \cdot T_2}{T_1}$$

where:

V_2 = volume corrected to standard temperature (V_{ST})
V_1 = ATPS volume (V_{ATPS})
T_1 = absolute temperature in ambient surroundings
     ($273°$ K + $T_a°$ C)
where: T_a = ambient temperature
T_2 = absolute standard temperature ($273°$ K)

Therefore, correcting an ATPS gas volume to V_{ST} is performed using the following equation:

$$(13)\ V_{ST} = V_{ATPS}\left[\frac{273°}{(273° + T_a)}\right]$$

Step 2: Barometric Pressure and Water Vapor Pressure Correction To correct for barometric pressure and vapor pressure, we use equation (12), where:

V_1 = volume ATPS
V_2 = volume corrected to standard pressure and
     dry (V_{SPD})
P_1 = ambient barometric pressure in mm Hg
P_2 = standard barometric pressure (760 mm Hg)
PH_2O = partial pressure of water vapor at ambient
       temperature (see table A.1 for a list of vapor
       pressures at various ambient temperatures)

Therefore, when correcting V_{SPD} from ATPS volumes, the following equation is used:

$$(14)\ V_{SPD} = V_{ATPS}\left[\frac{P_1 - PH_2O}{760\ mm\ Hg}\right]$$

At this point we are ready to combine both the temperature correction factor equation (13) and the pressure and vapor pressure correction factor equation (14) into one equation and compute one single STPD correction factor. Combining equations (13) and (14) we arrive at:

$$(15)\ V_{STPD} = V_{ATPS}\left[\frac{273°}{(273° + T_a)}\right]\left[\frac{(P_1 - PH_2O)}{760\ mm\ Hg}\right]$$

Let's consider a sample problem to illustrate correction of ATPS volumes to STPD volumes.

Given:

V_{ATPS} = 90.0 liters
Laboratory temperature = 21° C
Ambient barometric pressure = 742 mm Hg
H_2O vapor pressure at 21° C (from table A.1)
    = 18.7 mm Hg

TABLE A.1 Water Vapor Pressure as a Function of Ambient Temperature

Temperature (°C)	Saturation Water Vapor Pressure (PH_2O), mm Hg
18	15.5
19	16.5
20	17.5
21	18.7
22	19.8
23	21.1
24	22.4
25	23.8
26	25.2
27	26.7

Using the above sample conditions and equation (15), the STPD correction would be as follows:

$$V_{STPD} = 90\left[\frac{273°}{(273° + 21°)}\right]\left[\frac{742 - 18.7}{760}\right]$$
$$= 79.5\ liters\ STPD$$

It is important to point out that if inspired gas volumes are measured and the relative humidity of the inspired gas is not 100%, then equation (15) must be modified by multiplying the relative humidity (RH) of the inspired gas (expressed as a fraction) by the partial pressure of water vapor at ambient temperature (e.g., if RH = 80%, then use .8 × PH_2O).

BTPS Correction

As previously mentioned, all ventilatory volumes are corrected to BTPS conditions. This correction procedure is similar to the STPD correction procedure with two exceptions: (1) Standard temperature is 310° K instead of 273° K (e.g., 310° = 273° K + 37° C [normal core temperature]). This correction is necessary because body temperature is usually greater than ambient temperature and results in an increase in gas volume. (2) The partial pressure of vapor pressure at body temperature is subtracted from P_1 in equation (14). This correction is necessary because the partial pressure of water vapor at body temperature is generally greater than PH_2O at ambient conditions (i.e., at 37° the PH_2O = 47 mm Hg).

Therefore, correcting from ATPS to BTPS would involve the following equation:

$$(16)\ V_{BTPS} = V_{ATPS}\left[\frac{310°}{273° + T_a}\right]\left[\frac{P_1 - PH_2O}{P_1 - 47}\right]$$

Let's consider a sample calculation of converting V_{ATPS} to V_{BTPS} using the following conditions:

Laboratory temperature = 20° C
Ambient barometric pressure = 752 mm Hg
PH_2O at 20° C = 17.5 mm Hg
V_{ATPS} = 60 liters

Therefore:

$$V_{BTPS} = 60 \left[\frac{310°}{273° + 20°} \right] \left[\frac{752 - 17.5}{752 - 47} \right]$$
$$= 65.4 \text{ liters BTPS}$$

Problems

1. Calculate $\dot{V}O_2$ and $\dot{V}CO_2$ given:

   $\dot{V}_E$ (ATPS) = 100 liters · min^{-1}
   F_EO_2 = .1768
   F_ECO_2 = .0351
   Assume F_IO_2 = .2093 and F_ICO_2 = .0003
   Ambient temperature = 21° C
   Barometric pressure = 749 mm Hg

2. Calculate the respiratory exchange ratio (R) from $\dot{V}O_2$ and $\dot{V}CO_2$ values computed in question number 1.

3. Calculate V_{BTPS} and V_{STPD} given:

   V_{ATPS} = 45.3 liters
   Laboratory temperature = 19° C
   Ambient barometric temperature = 746 mm Hg
   Body temperature = 37° C

Answers

1. $\dot{V}O_2$ = 2.73 ℓ · min^{-1}
   $\dot{V}CO_2$ = 3.54 ℓ · min^{-1}

2. R = 1.15

3. V_{BTPS} = 50.19 liters
   V_{STPD} = 40.65 liters

Estimated Energy Expenditure During Selected Activities

It is often desirable to estimate energy expenditure during various types of physical activities. The following table provides a means of computing an estimated energy expenditure (per minute) using both the individual's body weight and the number of metabolic equivalents (METS) required to perform the activity. Specifically, one MET is equal to 0.0175 kcal · kg^{-1} · min^{-1}. Therefore, the formula to compute caloric expenditure during physical activity is:

Energy expenditure (kcal per min) = 0.0175 kcal · kg^{-1} · min^{-1} · MET^{-1} × METS × body weight (kg)

For example, the energy cost of bicycling (leisure, less than 10 mph) is 4.0 METS (see table below). The caloric expenditure for a 70 kg person cycling at this speed can be computed as follows:

Energy expenditure (kcal per min) = 0.0175 kcal · kg^{-1} · min^{-1} · MET^{-1} × 4.0 METS × 70 (kg) = 4.9 kcal per min

FIGURE I   Appendix 1. Updated Compendium of Physical Activities

METS	Specific Activity	Examples
8.5	bicycling,	bicycling, BMX or mountain
4.0	bicycling,	bicycling, <10 mph, leisure, to work or for pleasure (Taylor Code 115)
8.0	bicycling,	bicycling, general
6.0	bicycling,	bicycling, 10–11.9 mph, leisure, slow, light effort
8.0	bicycling,	bicycling, 12–13.9 mph, leisure, moderate effort
10.0	bicycling,	bicycling, 14–15.9 mph, racing or leisure, fast, vigorous effort
12.0	bicycling,	bicycling, 16–19 mph, racing/not drafting or >19 mph drafting, very fast, racing general
16.0	bicycling,	bicycling, >20 mph, racing, not drafting
5.0	bicycling,	unicycling
7.0	conditioning exercise,	bicycling, stationary, general
3.0	conditioning exercise,	bicycling, stationary, 50 watts, very light effort
5.5	conditioning exercise,	bicycling, stationary, 100 watts, light effort
7.0	conditioning exercise,	bicycling, stationary, 150 watts, moderate effort
10.5	conditioning exercise,	bicycling, stationary, 200 watts, vigorous effort
12.5	conditioning exercise,	bicycling, stationary, 250 watts, very vigorous effort
8.0	conditioning exercise,	calisthenics (e.g. pushups, situps, pullups, jumping jacks), heavy, vigorous effort

Data compiled from Ainsworth, et al. 2000. "Compendium of Physical Activities: An Update of Activity Codes and MET Intensities." *Medicine and Science in Sports and Exercise*: S498–S516.

FIGURE 1 (Continued)

METS	Specific Activity	Examples
3.5	conditioning exercise,	calisthenics, home exercise, light or moderate effort, general (example: back exercises), going up & down from floor (Taylor Code 150)
8.0	conditioning exercise,	circuit training, including some aerobic movement with minimal rest, general
6.0	conditioning exercise,	weight lifting (free weight, nautilus or universal-type), power lifting or body building, vigorous effort (Taylor Code 210)
5.5	conditioning exercise,	health club exercise, general (Taylor Code 160)
9.0	conditioning exercise,	stair-treadmill ergometer, general
7.0	conditioning exercise,	rowing, stationary ergometer, general
3.5	conditioning exercise,	rowing, stationary, 50 watts, light effort
7.0	conditioning exercise,	rowing, stationary, 100 watts, moderate effort
8.5	conditioning exercise,	rowing, stationary, 150 watts, vigorous effort
12.0	conditioning exercise,	rowing, stationary, 200 watts, very vigorous effort
7.0	conditioning exercise,	ski machine, general
6.0	conditioning exercise,	slimnastics, jazzercise
2.5	conditioning exercise,	stretching, hatha yoga
2.5	conditioning exercise,	mild stretching
6.0	conditioning exercise,	teaching aerobic exercise class
4.0	conditioning exercise,	water aerobics, water calisthenics
3.0	conditioning exercise,	weight lifting (free, nautilus or universal-type), light or moderate effort, light workout, general
1.0	conditioning exercise,	whirlpool, sitting
4.8	dancing,	ballet or modern, twist, jazz, tap, jitterbug
6.5	dancing,	aerobic, general
8.5	dancing,	aerobic, step, with 6–8 inch step
10.0	dancing,	aerobic, step, with 10–12 inch step
5.0	dancing,	aerobic, low impact
7.0	dancing,	aerobic, high impact
4.5	dancing,	general, Greek, Middle Eastern, hula, flamenco, belly, swing
5.5	dancing,	ballroom, fast (Taylor Code 125)
4.5	dancing,	ballroom, fast (disco, folk, square), line dancing, Irish step dancing, polka, contra, country
3.0	dancing,	ballroom, slow (e.g. waltz, foxtrot, slow dancing), samba, tango, 19th C, mambo, chacha
5.5	dancing,	Anishinaabe Jingle Dancing or other traditional American Indian dancing
3.0	fishing and hunting,	fishing, general
4.0	fishing and hunting,	digging worms, with shovel
4.0	fishing and hunting,	fishing from river bank and walking
2.5	fishing and hunting,	fishing from boat, sitting
3.5	fishing and hunting,	fishing from river bank, standing (Taylor Code 660)
6.0	fishing and hunting,	fishing in stream, in waders (Taylor Code 670)
2.0	fishing and hunting,	fishing, ice, sitting
2.5	fishing and hunting,	hunting, bow and arrow or crossbow
6.0	fishing and hunting,	hunting, deer, elk, large game (Taylor Code 170)
2.5	fishing and hunting,	hunting, duck, wading
5.0	fishing and hunting,	hunting, general
6.0	fishing and hunting,	hunting, pheasants or grouse (Taylor Code 680)
5.0	fishing and hunting,	hunting, rabbit, squirrel, prairie chick, raccoon, small game (Taylor Code 690)
2.5	fishing and hunting,	pistol shooting or trap shooting, standing
3.3	home activities,	carpet sweeping, sweeping floors
3.0	home activities,	cleaning, heavy or major (e.g. wash car, wash windows, clean garage), vigorous effort
3.5	home activities,	mopping
2.5	home activities,	multiple household tasks all at once, light effort
3.5	home activities,	multiple household tasks all at once, moderate effort
4.0	home activities,	multiple household tasks all at once, vigorous effort
3.0	home activities,	cleaning, house or cabin, general
2.5	home activities,	cleaning, light (dusting, straightening up, changing linen, carrying out trash)
2.3	home activities,	wash dishes—standing or in general (not broken into stand/walk components)
2.5	home activities,	wash dishes; clearing dishes from table—walking
3.5	home activities,	vacuuming

FIGURE 1 (Continued)

METS	Specific Activity	Examples
6.0	home activities,	butchering animals
2.0	home activities,	cooking or food preparation—standing or sitting or in general (not broken into stand/walk components), manual appliances
2.5	home activities,	serving food, setting table—implied walking or standing
2.5	home activities,	cooking or food preparation—walking
2.5	home activities,	feeding animals
2.5	home activities,	putting away groceries (e.g. carrying groceries, shopping without a grocery cart), carrying packages
7.5	home activities,	carrying groceries upstairs
3.0	home activities,	cooking Indian bread on an outside stove
2.3	home activities,	food shopping with or without a grocery cart, standing or walking
2.3	home activities,	non-food shopping, standing or walking
2.3	home activities,	ironing
1.5	home activities,	sitting—knitting, sewing, lt. wrapping (presents)
2.0	home activities,	implied standing—laundry, fold or hang clothes, put clothes in washer or dryer, packing suitcase
2.3	home activities,	implied walking—putting away clothes, gathering clothes to pack, putting away laundry
2.0	home activities,	making bed
5.0	home activities,	maple syruping/sugar bushing (including carrying buckets, carrying wood)
6.0	home activities,	moving furniture, household items, carrying boxes
3.8	home activities,	scrubbing floors, on hands and knees, scrubbing bathroom, bathtub
4.0	home activities,	sweeping garage, sidewalk or outside of house
3.5	home activities,	standing—packing/unpacking boxes, occasional lifting of household items light—moderate effort
3.0	home activities,	implied walking—putting away household items—moderate effort
2.5	home activities,	watering plants
2.5	home activities,	building a fire inside
9.0	home activities,	moving household items upstairs, carrying boxes or furniture
2.0	home activities,	standing—light (pump gas, change light bulb, etc.)
3.0	home activities,	walking—light, non-cleaning (readying to leave, shut/lock doors, close windows, etc.)
2.5	home activities,	sitting—playing with child(ren)—light, only active periods
2.8	home activities,	standing—playing with child(ren)—light, only active periods
4.0	home activities,	walk/run—playing with child(ren)—moderate, only active periods
5.0	home activities,	walk/run—playing with child(ren)—vigorous, only active periods
3.0	home activities,	carrying small children
2.5	home activities,	child care: sitting/kneeling—dressing, bathing, grooming, feeding, occasional lifting of child—light effort, general
3.0	home activities,	child care: standing—dressing, bathing, grooming, feeding, occasional lifting of child—light effort
4.0	home activities,	elder care, disabled adult, only active periods
1.5	home activities,	reclining with baby
2.5	home activities,	sit, playing with animals, light, only active periods
2.8	home activities,	stand, playing with animals, light, only active periods
2.8	home activities,	walk/run, playing with animals, light, only active periods
4.0	home activities,	walk/run, playing with animals, moderate, only active periods
5.0	home activities,	walk/run, playing with animals, vigorous, only active periods
3.5	home activities,	standing—bathing dog
3.0	home repair,	airplane repair
4.0	home repair,	automobile body work
3.0	home repair,	automobile repair
3.0	home repair,	carpentry, general, workshop (Taylor Code 620)
6.0	home repair,	carpentry, outside house, installing rain gutters, building a fence, (Taylor Code 640)
4.5	home repair,	carpentry, finishing or refinishing cabinets or furniture
7.5	home repair,	carpentry, sawing hardwood
5.0	home repair,	caulking, chinking log cabin
4.5	home repair,	caulking, except log cabin
5.0	home repair,	cleaning gutters
5.0	home repair,	excavating garage
5.0	home repair,	hanging storm windows
4.5	home repair,	laying or removing carpet

FIGURE I (Continued)

METS	Specific Activity	Examples
4.5	home repair,	laying tile or linoleum, repairing appliances
5.0	home repair,	painting, outside home (Taylor Code 650)
3.0	home repair,	painting, papering, plastering, scraping, inside house, hanging sheet rock, remodeling
4.5	home repair,	painting, (Taylor Code 630)
3.0	home repair,	put on and removal of tarp—sailboat
6.0	home repair,	roofing
4.5	home repair,	sanding floors with a power sander
4.5	home repair,	scraping and painting sailboat or powerboat
5.0	home repair,	spreading dirt with a shovel
4.5	home repair,	washing and waxing hull of sailboat, car, powerboat, airplane
4.5	home repair,	washing fence, painting fence
3.0	home repair,	wiring, plumbing
1.0	inactivity, quiet	lying quietly and watching television
1.0	inactivity, quiet	lying quietly, doing nothing, lying in bed awake, listening to music (not talking or reading)
1.0	inactivity, quiet	sitting quietly and watching television
1.0	inactivity, quiet	sitting quietly, sitting smoking, listening to music (not talking or reading), watching a movie in a theater
0.9	inactivity, quiet	sleeping
1.2	inactivity, quiet	standing quietly (standing in a line)
1.0	inactivity, light	reclining—writing
1.0	inactivity, light	reclining—talking or talking on phone
1.0	inactivity, light	reclining—reading
1.0	inactivity, light	meditating
5.0	lawn and garden,	carrying, loading or stacking wood, loading/unloading or carrying lumber
6.0	lawn and garden,	chopping wood, splitting logs
5.0	lawn and garden,	clearing land, hauling branches, wheelbarrow chores
5.0	lawn and garden,	digging sandbox
5.0	lawn and garden,	digging, spading, filling garden, composting, (Taylor Code 590)
6.0	lawn and garden,	gardening with heavy power tools, tilling a garden, chain saw
5.0	lawn and garden,	laying crushed rock
5.0	lawn and garden,	laying sod
5.5	lawn and garden,	mowing lawn, general
2.5	lawn and garden,	mowing lawn, riding mower (Taylor Code 550)
6.0	lawn and garden,	mowing lawn, walk, hand mower (Taylor Code 570)
5.5	lawn and garden,	mowing lawn, walk, power mower
4.5	lawn and garden,	mowing lawn, power mower (Taylor Code 590)
4.5	lawn and garden,	operating snow blower, walking
4.5	lawn and garden,	planting seedlings, shrubs
4.5	lawn and garden,	planting trees
4.3	lawn and garden,	raking lawn
4.0	lawn and garden,	raking lawn (Taylor Code 600)
4.0	lawn and garden,	raking roof with snow rake
3.0	lawn and garden,	riding snow blower
4.0	lawn and garden,	sacking grass, leaves
6.0	lawn and garden,	shoveling snow, by hand (Taylor Code 610)
4.5	lawn and garden,	trimming shrubs or trees, manual cutter
3.5	lawn and garden,	trimming shrubs or trees, power cutter, using leaf blower, edger
2.5	lawn and garden,	walking, applying fertilizer or seeding a lawn
1.5	lawn and garden,	watering lawn or garden, standing or walking
4.5	lawn and garden,	weeding, cultivating garden (Taylor Code 580)
4.0	lawn and garden,	gardening, general
3.0	lawn and garden,	picking fruit off trees, picking fruits/vegetables, moderate effort
3.0	lawn and garden,	implied walking/standing—picking up yard, light, picking flowers or vegetables
3.0	lawn and garden,	walking, gathering gardening tools
1.5	miscellaneous,	sitting—card playing, playing board games
2.3	miscellaneous,	standing—drawing (writing), casino gambling, duplicating machine

FIGURE 1 (Continued)

A-9

METS	Specific Activity	Examples
1.3	miscellaneous,	sitting—reading, book, newspaper, etc.
1.8	miscellaneous,	sitting—writing, desk work, typing
1.8	miscellaneous,	standing—talking or talking on the phone
1.5	miscellaneous,	sitting—talking or talking on the phone
1.8	miscellaneous,	sitting—studying, general, including reading and/or writing
1.8	miscellaneous,	sitting—in class, general, including note-taking or class discussion
1.8	miscellaneous,	standing, reading
2.0	miscellaneous,	standing—miscellaneous
1.5	miscellaneous,	sitting—arts and crafts, light effort
2.0	miscellaneous,	sitting—arts and crafts, moderate effort
1.8	miscellaneous,	standing—arts and crafts, light effort
3.0	miscellaneous,	standing—arts and crafts, moderate effort
3.5	miscellaneous,	standing—arts and crafts, vigorous effort
1.5	miscellaneous,	retreat/family reunion activities involving sitting, relaxing, talking, eating
2.0	miscellaneous,	touring/traveling/vacation involving walking and riding
2.5	miscellaneous,	camping involving standing, walking, sitting, light-to-moderate effort
1.5	miscellaneous,	sitting at a sporting event, spectator
1.8	music playing,	accordion
2.0	music playing,	cello
2.5	music playing,	conducting
4.0	music playing,	drums
2.0	music playing,	flute (sitting)
2.0	music playing,	horn
2.5	music playing,	piano or organ
3.5	music playing,	trombone
2.5	music playing,	trumpet
2.5	music playing,	violin
2.0	music playing,	woodwind
2.0	music playing,	guitar, classical, folk (sitting)
3.0	music playing,	guitar, rock and roll band (standing)
4.0	music playing,	marching band, playing an instrument, baton twirling (walking)
3.5	music playing,	marching band, drum major (walking)
4.0	occupation,	bakery, general, moderate effort
2.5	occupation,	bakery, light effort
2.3	occupation,	bookbinding
6.0	occupation,	building road (including hauling debris, driving heavy machinery)
2.0	occupation,	building road, directing traffic (standing)
3.5	occupation,	carpentry, general
8.0	occupation,	carrying heavy loads, such as bricks
8.0	occupation,	carrying moderate loads upstairs, moving boxes (16–40 pounds)
2.5	occupation,	chambermaid, making bed (nursing)
6.5	occupation,	coal mining, drilling coal, rock
6.5	occupation,	coal mining, erecting supports
6.0	occupation,	coal mining, general
7.0	occupation,	coal mining, shoveling coal
5.5	occupation,	construction, outside, remodeling
3.0	occupation,	custodial work—buffing the floor with electric buffer
2.5	occupation,	custodial work—cleaning sink and toilet, light effort
2.5	occupation,	custodial work—dusting, light effort
4.0	occupation,	custodial work—feathering arena floor, moderate effort
3.5	occupation,	custodial work—general cleaning, moderate effort
3.5	occupation,	custodial work—mopping, moderate effort
3.0	occupation,	custodial work—take out trash, moderate effort
2.5	occupation,	custodial work—vacuuming, light effort
3.0	occupation,	custodial work—vacuuming, moderate effort
3.5	occupation,	electrical work, plumbing

FIGURE 1 (Continued)

METS	Specific Activity	Examples
8.0	occupation,	farming, baling hay, cleaning barn, poultry work, vigorous effort
3.5	occupation,	farming, chasing cattle, non-strenuous (walking), moderate effort
4.0	occupation,	farming, chasing cattle or other livestock on horseback, moderate effort
2.0	occupation,	farming, chasing cattle or other livestock, driving, light effort
2.5	occupation,	farming, driving harvester, cutting hay, irrigation work
2.5	occupation,	farming, driving tractor
4.0	occupation,	farming, feeding small animals
4.5	occupation,	farming, feeding cattle, horses
4.5	occupation,	farming, hauling water for animals, general hauling water
6.0	occupation,	farming, taking care of animals (grooming, brushing, shearing sheep, assisting with birthing, medical care, branding)
8.0	occupation,	farming, forking straw bales, cleaning corral or barn, vigorous effort
3.0	occupation,	farming, milking by hand, moderate effort
1.5	occupation,	farming, milking by machine, light effort
5.5	occupation,	farming, shoveling grain, moderate effort
12.0	occupation,	fire fighter, general
11.0	occupation,	fire fighter, climbing ladder with full gear
8.0	occupation,	fire fighter, hauling hoses on ground
17.0	occupation,	forestry, ax chopping, fast
5.3	occupation,	forestry, ax chopping, slow
7.0	occupation,	forestry, barking trees
11.0	occupation,	forestry, carrying logs
8.0	occupation,	forestry, felling trees
8.0	occupation,	forestry, general
5.0	occupation,	forestry, hoeing
6.0	occupation,	forestry, planting by hand
7.0	occupation,	forestry, sawing by hand
4.5	occupation,	forestry, sawing, power
9.0	occupation,	forestry, trimming trees
4.0	occupation,	forestry, weeding
4.5	occupation,	furriery
6.0	occupation,	horse grooming
8.0	occupation,	horse racing, galloping
6.5	occupation,	horse racing, trotting
2.6	occupation,	horse racing, walking
3.5	occupation,	locksmith
2.5	occupation,	machine tooling, machining, working sheet metal
3.0	occupation,	machine tooling, operating lathe
5.0	occupation,	machine tooling, operating punch press
4.0	occupation,	machine tooling, tapping and drilling
3.0	occupation,	machine tooling, welding
7.0	occupation,	masonry, concrete
4.0	occupation,	masseur, masseuse (standing)
7.5	occupation,	moving, pushing heavy objects, 75 lbs or more (desks, moving van work)
12.0	occupation,	skindiving or SCUBA diving as a frogman (Navy Seal)
2.5	occupation,	operating heavy duty equipment/automated, not driving
4.5	occupation,	orange grove work
2.3	occupation,	printing (standing)
2.5	occupation,	police, directing traffic (standing)
2.0	occupation,	police, driving a squad car (sitting)
1.3	occupation,	police, riding in a squad car (sitting)
4.0	occupation,	police, making an arrest (standing)
2.5	occupation,	shoe repair, general
8.5	occupation,	shoveling, digging ditches
9.0	occupation,	shoveling, heavy (more than 16 pounds/minute)
6.0	occupation,	shoveling, light (less than 10 pounds/minute)

FIGURE I (Continued)

METS	Specific Activity	Examples
7.0	occupation,	shoveling, moderate (10 to 15 pounds/minute)
1.5	occupation,	sitting—light office work, general (chemistry lab work, light use of hand tools, watch repair or micro-assembly, light assembly/repair), sitting, reading, driving at work
1.5	occupation,	sitting—meetings, general, and/or with talking involved, eating at a business meeting
2.5	occupation,	sitting; moderate (heavy levers, riding mower/forklift, crane operation), teaching stretching or yoga
2.3	occupation,	standing; light (bartending, store clerk, assembling, filing, duplicating, putting up a Christmas tree), standing and talking at work, changing clothes when teaching physical education
3.0	occupation,	standing; light/moderate (assemble/repair heavy parts, welding, stocking, auto repair, pack boxes for moving, etc.), patient care (as in nursing)
4.0	occupation,	lifting items continuously, 10–20 lbs, with limited walking or resting
3.5	occupation,	standing; moderate (assembling at fast rate, intermittent, lifting 50 lbs, hitch/twisting ropes)
4.0	occupation,	standing; moderate/heavy (lifting more than 50 lbs, masonry, painting, paper hanging)
5.0	occupation,	steel mill, fettling
5.5	occupation,	steel mill, forging
8.0	occupation,	steel mill, hand rolling
8.0	occupation,	steel mill, merchant mill rolling
11.0	occupation,	steel mill, removing slag
7.5	occupation,	steel mill, tending furnace
5.5	occupation,	steel mill, tipping molds
8.0	occupation,	steel mill, working in general
2.5	occupation,	tailoring, cutting
2.5	occupation,	tailoring, general
2.0	occupation,	tailoring, hand sewing
2.5	occupation,	tailoring, machine sewing
4.0	occupation,	tailoring, pressing
3.5	occupation,	tailoring, weaving
6.5	occupation,	truck driving, loading and unloading truck (standing)
1.5	occupation,	typing, electric, manual or computer
6.0	occupation,	using heavy power tools such as pneumatic tools (jackhammers, drills, etc.)
8.0	occupation,	using heavy tools (not power) such as shovel, pick, tunnel bar, spade
2.0	occupation,	walking on job, less than 2.0 mph (in office or lab area), very slow
3.3	occupation,	walking on job, 3.0 mph, in office, moderate speed, not carrying anything
3.9	occupation,	walking on job, 3.5 mph, in office, brisk speed, not carrying anything
3.0	occupation,	walking, 2.5 mph, slowly and carrying light objects less than 25 pounds
3.0	occupation,	walking, gathering things at work, ready to leave
4.0	occupation,	walking, 3.0 mph, moderately and carrying light objects less than 25 lbs
4.0	occupation,	walking, pushing a wheelchair
4.5	occupation,	walking, 3.5 mph, briskly and carrying objects less than 25 pounds
5.0	occupation,	walking or walk downstairs or standing, carrying objects about 25 to 49 pounds
6.5	occupation,	walking or walk downstairs or standing, carrying objects about 50 to 74 pounds
7.5	occupation,	walking or walk downstairs or standing, carrying objects about 75 to 99 pounds
8.5	occupation,	walking or walk downstairs or standing, carrying objects about 100 pounds or over
3.0	occupation,	working in scene shop, theater actor, backstage employee
4.0	occupation,	teach physical education, exercise, sports classes (non-sport play)
6.5	occupation,	teach physical education, exercise, sports classes (participate in the class)
6.0	running,	jog/walk combination (jogging component of less than 10 minutes) (Taylor Code 180)
7.0	running,	jogging, general
8.0	running,	jogging, in place
4.5	running	jogging on a mini-tramp
8.0	running,	running, 5 mph (12 min/mile)
9.0	running,	running, 5.2 mph (11.5 min/mile)
10.0	running,	running, 6 mph (10 min/mile)
11.0	running,	running, 6.7 mph (9 min/mile)
11.5	running,	running, 7 mph (8.5 min/mile)
12.5	running,	running, 7.5 mph (8 min/mile)
13.5	running,	running, 8 mph (7.5 min/mile)

FIGURE I (Continued)

METS	Specific Activity	Examples
14.0	running,	running, 8.6 mph (7 min/mile)
15.0	running,	running, 9 mph (6.5 min/mile)
16.0	running,	running, 10 mph (6 min/mile)
18.0	running,	running, 10.9 mph (5.5 min/mile)
9.0	running,	running, cross country
8.0	running,	running (Taylor Code 200)
15.0	running,	running, stairs, up
10.0	running,	running, on a track, team practice
8.0	running,	running, training, pushing a wheelchair
2.0	self care,	standing—getting ready for bed, in general
1.0	self care,	sitting on toilet
1.5	self care,	bathing (sitting)
2.0	self care,	dressing, undressing (standing or sitting)
1.5	self care,	eating (sitting)
2.0	self care,	talking and eating or eating only (standing)
1.0	self care,	taking medication, sitting or standing
2.0	self care,	grooming (washing, shaving, brushing teeth, urinating, washing hands, putting on make-up), sitting or standing
2.5	self care,	hairstyling
1.0	self care,	having hair or nails done by someone else, sitting
2.0	self care,	showering, toweling off (standing)
1.5	sexual activity,	active, vigorous effort
1.3	sexual activity,	general, moderate effort
1.0	sexual activity,	passive, light effort, kissing, hugging
3.5	sports,	archery (non-hunting)
7.0	sports,	badminton, competitive (Taylor Code 450)
4.5	sports,	badminton, social singles and doubles, general
8.0	sports,	basketball, game (Taylor Code 490)
6.0	sports,	basketball, non-game, general (Taylor Code 480)
7.0	sports,	basketball, officiating (Taylor Code 500)
4.5	sports,	basketball, shooting baskets
6.5	sports,	basketball, wheelchair
2.5	sports,	billiards
3.0	sports,	bowling (Taylor Code 390)
12.0	sports,	boxing, in ring, general
6.0	sports,	boxing, punching bag
9.0	sports,	boxing, sparring
7.0	sports,	broomball
5.0	sports,	children's games (hopscotch, 4-square, dodge ball, playground apparatus, t-ball, tetherball, marbles, jacks, acrace games)
4.0	sports,	coaching: football, soccer, basketball, baseball, swimming, etc.
5.0	sports,	cricket (batting, bowling)
2.5	sports,	croquet
4.0	sports,	curling
2.5	sports,	darts, wall or lawn
6.0	sports,	drag racing, pushing or driving a car
6.0	sports,	fencing
9.0	sports,	football, competitive
8.0	sports,	football, touch, flag, general (Taylor Code 510)
2.5	sports,	football or baseball, playing catch
3.0	sports,	frisbee playing, general
8.0	sports,	frisbee, ultimate
4.5	sports,	golf, general
4.5	sports,	golf, walking and carrying clubs (See footnote at end of the Compendium)
3.0	sports,	golf, miniature, driving range
4.3	sports,	golf, walking and pulling clubs (See footnote at end of the Compendium)

FIGURE 1 (Continued)

METS	Specific Activity	Examples
3.5	sports,	golf, using power cart (Taylor Code 070)
4.0	sports,	gymnastics, general
4.0	sports,	hacky sack
12.0	sports,	handball, general (Taylor Code 520)
8.0	sports,	handball, team
3.5	sports,	hand gliding
8.0	sports,	hockey, field
8.0	sports,	hockey, ice
4.0	sports,	horseback riding, general
3.5	sports,	horseback riding, saddling horse, grooming horse
6.5	sports,	horseback riding, trotting
2.5	sports,	horseback riding, walking
3.0	sports,	horseshoe pitching, quoits
12.0	sports,	jai alai
10.0	sports,	judo, jujitsu, karate, kick boxing, tae kwan do
4.0	sports,	juggling
7.0	sports,	kickball
8.0	sports,	lacrosse
4.0	sports,	motor-cross
9.0	sports,	orienteering
10.0	sports,	paddleball, competitive
6.0	sports,	paddleball, casual, general (Taylor Code 460)
8.0	sports,	polo
10.0	sports,	racquetball, competitive
7.0	sports,	racquetball, casual, general (Taylor Code 470)
11.0	sports,	rock climbing, ascending rock
8.0	sports,	rock climbing, rappelling
12.0	sports,	rope jumping, fast
10.0	sports,	rope jumping, moderate, general
8.0	sports,	rope jumping, slow
10.0	sports,	rugby
3.0	sports,	shuffleboard, lawn bowling
5.0	sports,	skateboarding
7.0	sports,	skating, roller (Taylor Code 360)
12.5	sports,	roller blading (in-line skating)
3.5	sports,	sky diving
10.0	sports,	soccer, competitive
7.0	sports,	soccer, casual, general (Taylor Code 540)
5.0	sports,	softball or baseball, fast or slow pitch, general (Taylor Code 440)
4.0	sports,	softball, officiating
6.0	sports,	softball, pitching
12.0	sports,	squash (Taylor Code 530)
4.0	sports,	table tennis, ping pong (Taylor Code 410)
4.0	sports,	tai chi
7.0	sports,	tennis, general
6.0	sports,	tennis, doubles (Taylor Code 430)
5.0	sports,	tennis, doubles
8.0	sports,	tennis, singles (Taylor Code 420)
3.5	sports,	trampoline
4.0	sports,	volleyball (Taylor Code 400)
8.0	sports,	volleyball, competitive, in gymnasium
3.0	sports,	volleyball, non-competitive, 6–9 member team, general
8.0	sports,	volleyball, beach
6.0	sports,	wrestling (one match = 5 minutes)
7.0	sports,	wallyball, general
4.0	sports,	track and field (shot, discus, hammer throw)

FIGURE I (Continued)

METS	Specific Activity	Examples
6.0	sports,	track and field (high jump, long jump, triple jump, javelin, pole vault)
10.0	sports,	track and field (steeplechase, hurdles)
2.0	transportation,	automobile or light track (not a semi) driving
1.0	transportation,	riding in a car or truck
1.0	transportation,	riding in a bus
2.0	transportation,	flying airplane
2.5	transportation,	motor scooter, motorcycle
6.0	transportation,	pushing plane in and out of hangar
3.0	transportation,	driving heavy truck, tractor, bus
7.0	walking,	backpacking (Taylor Code 050)
3.5	walking,	carrying infant or 15 pound load (e.g. suitcase), level ground or downstairs
9.0	walking,	carrying load upstairs, general
5.0	walking,	carrying 1 to 15 lb load, upstairs
6.0	walking,	carrying 16 to 24 lb load, upstairs
8.0	walking,	carrying 25 to 49 lb load, upstairs
10.0	walking,	carrying 50 to 74 lb load, upstairs
12.0	walking,	carrying 74+ lb load, upstairs
3.0	walking,	loading/unloading a car
7.0	walking,	climbing hills with 0 to 9 pound load
7.5	walking,	climbing hills with 10 to 20 pound load
8.0	walking,	climbing hills with 21 to 42 pound load
9.0	walking,	climbing hills with 42+ pound load
3.0	walking,	downstairs
6.0	walking,	hiking, cross country (Taylor Code 040)
2.5	walking,	bird watching
6.5	walking,	marching, rapidly, military
2.5	walking,	pushing or pulling stroller with child or walking with children
4.0	walking,	pushing a wheelchair, non-occupational setting
6.5	walking,	race walking
8.0	walking,	rock or mountain climbing (Taylor Code 060)
8.0	walking,	up stairs, using or climbing up ladder (Taylor Code 030)
5.0	walking,	using crutches
2.0	walking,	walking, household
2.0	walking,	walking, less than 2.0 mph, level ground, strolling, very slow
2.5	walking,	walking, 2.0 mph, level, slow pace, firm surface
3.5	walking,	walking for pleasure (Taylor Code 010)
2.5	walking,	walking from house to car or bus, from car or bus to go places, from car or bus to and from the worksite
2.5	walking,	walking to neighbor's house or family's house for social reasons
3.0	walking,	walking the dog
3.0	walking,	walking, 2.5 mph, firm surface
2.8	walking,	walking, 2.5 mph, downhill
3.3	walking,	walking, 3.0 mph, level, moderate pace, firm surface
3.8	walking,	walking, 3.5 mph, level, brisk, firm surface, walking for exercise
6.0	walking,	walking, 3.5 mph, uphill
5.0	walking,	walking, 4.0 mph, level, firm surface, very brisk pace
6.3	walking,	walking, 4.5 mph, level, firm surface, very, very brisk
8.0	walking,	walking, 5.0 mph
3.5	walking,	walking, for pleasure, work break
5.0	walking,	walking, grass track
4.0	walking,	walking, to work or class (Taylor Code 015)
2.5	walking,	walking to and from an outhouse
2.5	water activities,	boating, power
4.0	water activities,	canoeing, on camping trip (Taylor Code 270)
3.3	water activities,	canoeing, harvesting wild rice, knocking rice off the stalks
7.0	water activities,	canoeing, portaging

FIGURE 1 (Continued)

METS	Specific Activity	Examples
3.0	water activities,	canoeing, rowing, 2.0–3.9 mph, light effort
7.0	water activities,	canoeing, rowing, 4.0–5.9 mph, moderate effort
12.0	water activities,	canoeing, rowing, >6 mph, vigorous effort
3.5	water activities,	canoeing, rowing, for pleasure, general (Taylor Code 250)
12.0	water activities,	canoeing, rowing, in competition, or crew or sculling (Taylor Code 260)
3.0	water activities,	diving, springboard or platform
5.0	water activities,	kayaking
4.0	water activities,	paddle boat
3.0	water activities,	sailing, boat and board sailing, windsurfing, ice sailing, general (Taylor Code 235)
5.0	water activities,	sailing, in competition
3.0	water activities,	sailing, Sunfish/Laser/Hobby Cat, Keel boats, ocean sailing, yachting
6.0	water activities,	skiing, water (Taylor Code 220)
7.0	water activities,	skimobiling
16.0	water activities,	skindiving, fast
12.5	water activities,	skindiving, moderate
7.0	water activities,	skindiving, scuba diving, general (Taylor Code 310)
5.0	water activities,	snorkeling (Taylor Code 320)
3.0	water activities,	surfing, body or board
10.0	water activities,	swimming laps, freestyle, fast, vigorous effort
7.0	water activities,	swimming laps, freestyle, slow, moderate or tight effort
7.0	water activities,	swimming, backstroke, general
10.0	water activities,	swimming, breaststroke, general
11.0	water activities,	swimming, butterfly, general
11.0	water activities,	swimming, crawl, fast (75 yards/minute), vigorous effort
8.0	water activities,	swimming, crawl, slow (50 yards/minute), moderate or light effort
6.0	water activities,	swimming, lake, ocean, river (Taylor Codes 280, 295)
6.0	water activities,	swimming, leisurely, not lap swimming, general
8.0	water activities,	swimming, sidestroke, general
8.0	water activities,	swimming, synchronized
10.0	water activities,	swimming, treading water, fast vigorous effort
4.0	water activities,	swimming, treading water, moderate effort, general
4.0	water activities,	water aerobics, water calisthenics
10.0	water activities,	water polo
3.0	water activities,	water volleyball
8.0	water activities,	water jogging
5.0	water activities,	whitewater rafting, kayaking, or canoeing
6.0	winter activities,	moving ice house (set up/drill holes, etc.)
5.5	winter activities,	skating, ice, 9 mph or less
7.0	winter activities,	skating, ice, general (Taylor Code 360)
9.0	winter activities,	skating, ice, rapidly, more than 9 mph
15.0	winter activities,	skating, speed, competitive
7.0	winter activities,	ski jumping (climb up carrying skis)
7.0	winter activities	skiing, general
7.0	winter activities,	skiing, cross country, 2.5 mph, slow or light effort, ski walking
8.0	winter activities,	skiing, cross country, 4.0–4.9 mph, moderate speed and effort, general
9.0	winter activities,	skiing, cross country, 5.0–7.9 mph, brisk speed, vigorous effort
14.0	winter activities,	skiing, cross country, >8.0 mph, racing
16.5	winter activities,	skiing, cross country, hard snow, uphill, maximum, snow mountaineering
5.0	winter activities,	skiing, downhill, light effort
6.0	winter activities,	skiing, downhill, moderate effort, general
8.0	winter activities,	skiing, downhill, vigorous effort, racing
7.0	winter activities,	sledding, tobogganing, bobsledding, luge (Taylor Code 370)
8.0	winter activities,	snow shoeing
3.5	winter activities,	snowmobiling
1.0	religious activities,	sitting in church, in service, attending a ceremony, sitting quietly
2.5	religious activities,	sitting, playing an instrument at church

FIGURE 1 (Continued)

METS	Specific Activity	Examples
1.5	religious activities,	sitting in church, talking or singing, attending a ceremony, sitting, active participation
1.3	religious activities,	sitting, reading religious materials at home
1.2	religious activities,	standing in church (quietly), attending a ceremony, standing quietly
2.0	religious activities,	standing, singing in church, attending a ceremony, standing, active participation
1.0	religious activities,	kneeling in church/at home (praying)
1.8	religious activities,	standing, talking in church
2.0	religious activities,	walking in church
2.0	religious activities,	walking, less than 2.0 mph—very slow
3.3	religious activities,	walking, 3.0 mph, moderate speed, not carrying anything
3.8	religious activities,	walking, 3.5 mph, brisk speed, not carrying anything
2.0	religious activities,	walk/stand combination for religious purposes, usher
5.0	religious activities,	praise with dance or run, spiritual dancing in church
2.5	religious activities,	serving food at church
2.0	religious activities,	preparing food at church
2.3	religious activities,	washing dishes/cleaning kitchen at church
1.5	religious activities,	eating at church
2.0	religious activities,	eating/talking at church or standing eating, American Indian Feast days
3.0	religious activities,	cleaning church
5.0	religious activities,	general yard work at church
2.5	religious activities,	standing—moderate (lifting 50 lbs., assembling at fast rate)
4.0	religious activities,	standing—moderate/heavy work
1.5	religious activities,	typing, electric, manual, or computer
1.5	volunteer activities,	sitting—meeting, general, and/or with talking involved
1.5	volunteer activities,	sitting—light office work, in general
2.5	volunteer activities,	sitting—moderate work
2.3	volunteer activities,	standing—light work (filing, talking, assembling)
2.5	volunteer activities,	sitting, child care, only active periods
3.0	volunteer activities,	standing, child care, only active periods
4.0	volunteer activities,	walk/run play with children, moderate, only active periods
5.0	volunteer activities,	walk/run play with children, vigorous, only active periods
3.0	volunteer activities,	standing—light/moderate work (pack boxes, assemble/repair, set up chairs/furniture)
3.5	volunteer activities,	standing—moderate (lifting 50 lbs., assembling at fast rate)
4.0	volunteer activities,	standing—moderate/heavy work
1.5	volunteer activities,	typing, electric, manual, or computer
2.0	volunteer activities,	walking, less than 2.0 mph, very slow
3.3	volunteer activities,	walking, 3.0 mph, moderate speed, not carrying anything
3.8	volunteer activities,	walking, 3.5 mph, brisk speed, not carrying anything
3.0	volunteer activities,	walking, 2.5 mph slowly and carrying objects less than 25 pounds
4.0	volunteer activities,	walking, 3.0 mph moderately and carrying objects less than 25 pounds, pushing something
4.5	volunteer activities,	walking, 3.5 mph, briskly and carrying objects less than 25 pounds
3.0	volunteer activities,	walk/stand combination, for volunteer purposes

Physical Activity Prescriptions

PARmed-X — PHYSICAL ACTIVITY READINESS MEDICAL EXAMINATION

The PARmed-X is a physical activity-specific checklist to be used by a physician with patients who have had positive responses to the Physical Activity Readiness Questionnaire (PAR-Q). In addition, the Conveyance/Referral Form in the PARmed-X can be used to convey clearance for physical activity participation, or to make a referral to a medically-supervised exercise program.

Regular physical activity is fun and healthy, and increasingly more people are starting to become more active every day. Being more active is very safe for most people. The PAR-Q by itself provides adequate screening for the majority of people. However, some individuals may require a medical evaluation and specific advice (exercise prescription) due to one or more positive responses to the PAR-Q.

Following the participant's evaluation by a physician, a physical activity plan should be devised in consultation with a physical activity professional (CSEP-Professional Fitness and Lifestyle Consultant). To assist in this, the following instructions are provided:

PAGE 1: • Sections A, B, C, and D should be completed by the participant BEFORE the examination by the physician. The bottom section is to be completed by the examining physician.

PAGES 2 & 3: • A checklist of medical conditions requiring special consideration and management.

PAGE 4: • Physical Activity & Lifestyle Advice for people who do not require specific instructions or prescribed exercise.
• Physical Activity Readiness Conveyance/Referral Form - an optional tear-off tab for the physician to convey clearance for physical activity participation, or to make a referral to a medically-supervised exercise program.

This section to be completed by the participant

A PERSONAL INFORMATION:
NAME
ADDRESS
TELEPHONE
BIRTHDATE ___ GENDER
MEDICAL No.

B PAR-Q: Please indicate the PAR-Q questions to which you answered YES
- Q 1 Heart condition
- Q 2 Chest pain during activity
- Q 3 Chest pain at rest
- Q 4 Loss of balance, dizziness
- Q 5 Bone or joint problem
- Q 6 Blood pressure or heart drugs
- Q 7 Other reason:

C RISK FACTORS FOR CARDIOVASCULAR DISEASE: Check all that apply
- Less than 30 minutes of moderate physical activity most days of the week.
- Currently smoker (tobacco smoking 1 or more times per week)
- High blood pressure reported by physician after repeated measurements.
- High cholesterol level reported by physician.
- Excessive accumulation of fat around waist.
- Family history of heart disease.

Please note: Many of these risk factors are modifiable. Please refer to page 4 and discuss with your physician.

D PHYSICAL ACTIVITY INTENTIONS:
What physical activity do you intend to do?

This section to be completed by the examining physician

Physical Exam: Ht ___ Wt ___ BP (i) / BP (ii) /

Conditions limiting physical activity:
- Cardiovascular
- Respiratory
- Other
- Musculoskeletal
- Abdominal

Tests required:
- ECG
- Blood
- Exercise Test
- Urinalysis
- X-Ray
- Other

Physical Activity Readiness Conveyance/Referral:
Based upon a current review of health status, I recommend:
- No physical activity
- Progressive physical activity
  - with avoidance of:
  - with inclusion of:
  - with Physical Therapy:
- Only a medically-supervised exercise program until further medical clearance
- Unrestricted physical activity — start slowly and build up gradually

Further Information:
- Attached
- To be forwarded
- Available on request

PARmed-X — PHYSICAL ACTIVITY READINESS MEDICAL EXAMINATION

Following is a checklist of medical conditions for which a degree of precaution and/or special advice should be considered for those who answered "YES" to one or more questions on the PAR-Q, and people over the age of 69. Conditions are grouped by system. Three categories of precautions are provided. Comments under Advice are general, since details and alternatives require clinical judgement in each individual instance.

	Absolute Contraindications	Relative Contraindications	Special Prescriptive Conditions	
	Permanent restriction or temporary restriction until condition is treated, stable, and/or past acute phase.	Highly variable. Value of exercise testing and/or program may exceed risk. Activity may be restricted. Desirable to maximize control of condition. Direct or indirect medical supervision of exercise program may be desirable.	Individualized prescriptive advice generally appropriate: • limitations imposed; and/or • special exercises prescribed. May require medical monitoring and/or initial supervision in exercise program.	**ADVICE**
Cardiovascular	aortic aneurysm (dissecting); aortic stenosis (severe); congestive heart failure; crescendo angina; myocardial infarction (acute); myocarditis (active or recent); pulmonary or systemic embolism—acute; thrombophlebitis; ventricular tachycardia and other dangerous dysrhythmias (e.g., multi-focal ventricular activity)	aortic stenosis (moderate); subaortic stenosis (severe); marked cardiac enlargement; supraventricular dysrhythmias (uncontrolled or high rate); ventricular ectopic activity (repetitive or frequent); ventricular aneurysm; hypertension—untreated or uncontrolled severe (systemic or pulmonary); hypertrophic cardiomyopathy; compensated congestive heart failure	aortic (or pulmonary) stenosis—mild angina pectoris and other manifestations of coronary insufficiency (e.g., post-acute infarct); cyanotic heart disease; shunts (intermittent or fixed); conduction disturbances — complete AV block — left BBB — Wolff-Parkinson-White syndrome; dysrhythmias—controlled; fixed rate pacemakers; intermittent claudication; hypertension: systolic 160-180; diastolic 105+	• clinical exercise test may be warranted in selected cases, for specific determination of functional capacity and limitations and precautions (if any). • slow progression of exercise to levels based on test performance and individual tolerance. • consider individual training program under medical supervision (indirect or direct). progressive exercise to tolerance; progressive exercise; care with medications (serum electrolytes; post-exercise syncope; etc.)
Infections	acute infectious disease (regardless of etiology)	subacute/chronic/recurrent infectious diseases (e.g., malaria, others)	chronic infections; HIV	variable as to condition
Metabolic		uncontrolled metabolic disorders (diabetes mellitus, thyrotoxicosis, myxedema)	renal, hepatic, & other metabolic insufficiency; obesity; single kidney	variable as to status; dietary moderation, and initial light exercises with slow progression (walking, swimming, cycling)
Pregnancy		complicated pregnancy (e.g., toxemia, hemorrhage, incompetent cervix, etc.)	advanced pregnancy (late 3rd trimester)	refer to the "PARmed-X for PREGNANCY"

References:

Arraix, G.A., Wigle, D.T., Mao, Y. (1992). Risk Assessment of Physical Activity and Physical Fitness in the Canada Health Survey Follow-Up Study. J. Clin. Epidemiol. 45.4 419-428.

Mottola, M., Wolfe, L.A. (1994). Active Living and Pregnancy. In: A. Quinney, L., Gauvin, T. Wall (eds.), Toward Active Living: Proceedings of the International Conference on Physical Activity, Fitness and Health. Champaign, IL: Human Kinetics.

PAR-Q Validation Report, British Columbia Ministry of Health. 1978.

Thomas, S., Reading, J., Shephard, R.J. (1992). Revision of the Physical Activity Readiness Questionnaire (PAR-Q). Can. J. Spt. Sci. 17.4 338-345.

The PAR-Q and PARmed-X were developed by the British Columbia Ministry of Health. They have been revised by an Expert Advisory Committee assembled by the Canadian Society for Exercise Physiology and the Fitness Program, Health Canada (1995).

You are encouraged to copy the PARmed-X, but only if you use the entire form

Disponible en français sous le titre «Évaluation médicale de l'aptitude à l'activité physique (X-AAP)»

	Special Prescriptive Conditions	ADVICE
Lung	chronic pulmonary disorders	special relaxation and breathing exercises
	obstructive lung disease	breath control during endurance exercises to tolerance; avoid polluted air
	asthma	
	exercise-induced bronchospasm	avoid hyperventilation during exercise; avoid extremely cold conditions; warm up adequately; utilize appropriate medication.
Musculoskeletal	low back conditions (pathological, functional)	avoid or minimize exercise that precipitates or exasperates e.g., forced extreme flexion, extension, and violent twisting; correct posture, proper back exercises
	arthritis—acute (infective, rheumatoid; gout)	treatment, plus judicious blend of rest, splinting and gentle movement
	arthritis—subacute	progressive increase of active exercise therapy
	arthritis—chronic (osteoarthritis and above conditions)	maintenance of mobility and strength; non-weightbearing exercises to minimize joint trauma (e.g., cycling, aquatic activity, etc.)
	orthopaedic	highly variable and individualized
	hernia	minimize straining and isometrics; strengthen abdominal muscles
CNS	convulsive disorder not completely controlled by medication	minimize or avoid exercise in hazardous environments and/or exercising alone (e.g., swimming, mountainclimbing, etc.)
	recent concussion	thorough examination if history of two concussions; review for discontinuation of contact sport if three concussions, depending on duration of unconsciousness, retrograde amnesia, persistent headaches, and other objective evidence of cerebral damage
Blood	anemia—severe (< 10 Gm/dl)	control preferred; exercise as tolerated
	electrolyte disturbances	
Medications	antianginal; antihypertensive; beta-blockers; diuretics; others; antiarrhythmic; anticonvulsant; digitalis preparations; ganglionic blockers	NOTE: consider underlying condition. Potential for: exertional syncope, electrolyte imbalance, bradycardia, dysrhythmias, impaired coordination and reaction time, heat intolerance. May alter resting and exercise ECG's and exercise test performance.
Other	post-exercise syncope	moderate program
	heat intolerance	prolong cool-down with light activities; avoid exercise in extreme heat
	temporary minor illness	postpone until recovered
	cancer	if potential metastases, test by cycle ergometry, consider non-weight bearing exercises; exercise at lower end of prescriptive range (40–65% of heart rate reserve), depending on condition and recent treatment (radiation, chemotherapy); monitor hemoglobin and lymphocyte counts; add dynamic lifting exercise to strengthen muscles, using machines rather than weights.

*Refer to special publications for elaboration as required.

The following companion forms are available by contacting the Canadian Society for Exercise Physiology (address below):

The Physical Activity Readiness Questionnaire (PAR-Q)—a questionnaire for people aged 15–69 to complete before becoming much more physically active.

The Physical Activity Readiness Medical Examination for Pregnancy (PARmed-X for PREGNANCY)—to be used by physicians with pregnant patients who wish to become more physically active.

To order multiple printed copies of the PARmed-X and/or any of the companion forms (for a nominal charge), please contact the:

Canadian Society for Exercise Physiology
185 Somerset St. West, Suite 202
Ottawa, Ontario CANADA K2P 0J2
Tel. (613) 234-3755 FAX. (613) 234-3565

Note to physical activity professionals...
It is a prudent practice to retain the completed Physical Activity Readiness Conveyance/Referral Form in the participant's file.

Physical Activity & Lifestyle Advice

We know that being physically active provides benefits for all of us. Physical inactivity is recognized by the Heart and Stroke Foundation of Canada as one of the four modifiable primary risk factors for coronary heart disease (along with high blood pressure, high blood cholesterol, and smoking). Physical inactivity has also been shown to reduce the incidence of hypertension, colon cancer, maturity onset diabetes mellitus, and osteoporosis. It can also reduce stress and anxiety, relieve depression, and improve self-esteem.

People are physically active for many reasons — play, work, competition, health, creativity, enjoying the outdoors, being with friends. There are also as many ways of being active as there are reasons. What we choose to do depends on our own abilities and desires. No matter what the reason or type of activity, physical activity can improve our well-being and quality of life. Well-being can also be enhanced by integrating physical activity with enjoyable healthy eating and positive self and body image. Together, all three equal VITALITY. So take a fresh approach to living. Check out the VITALITY tips below!

Active Living:
- make meaningful and satisfying physical activities a valued and integral part of daily living
- accumulate 30 minutes or more of moderate physical activity most days of the week
- choose from an endless range of opportunities to be active according to your own abilities and desires:
  • take the stairs instead of an elevator
  • get off the bus early and walk home
  • join friends in a sport activity
  • take the dog for a walk with the family
  • follow a fitness program

Healthy Eating:
- follow Canada's Food Guide to Healthy Eating
- enjoy a variety of foods
- emphasize cereals, breads, other grain products, vegetables and fruit
- choose lower-fat dairy products, leaner meats and foods prepared with little or no fat
- achieve and maintain a healthy body weight by enjoying regular physical activity and healthy eating
- limit salt, alcohol and caffeine
- don't give up foods you enjoy — aim for moderation and variety

Positive Self and Body Image:
- accept who you are and how you look
- remember, a healthy weight range is one that is realistic for your own body make-up (body fat levels should neither be too high nor too low)
- try a new challenge
- compliment yourself
- reflect positively on your abilities
- laugh a lot

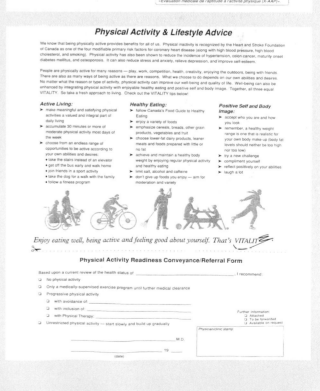

Enjoy eating well, being active and feeling good about yourself. That's VITALITY

Physical Activity Readiness Conveyance/Referral Form

Based upon a current review of the health status of ___, I recommend:
- No physical activity
- Only a medically-supervised exercise program until further medical clearance
- Progressive physical activity
  - with avoidance of:
  - with inclusion of:
  - with Physical Therapy:
- Unrestricted physical activity — start slowly and build up gradually

___ M.D.
(date) ___ 19 ___

Physician/clinic stamp:

Further Information:
- Attached
- To be forwarded
- Available on request

Physical Activity Readiness Medical Examination, Revised 2002. Canadian Society for Exercise Physiology. Ottawa, ON. Canada.

Dietary Reference Intakes: Macronutrients

Dietary Reference Intakes (DRIs): Recommended Intakes for Individuals, Macronutrients
Food and Nutrition Board, Institute of Medicine, National Academies

Life Stage Group	Total Water[a] (L/d)	Carbo-hydrate (g/d)	Total Fiber (g/d)	Fat (g/d)	Linoleic Acid (g/d)	α-Linolenic Acid (g/d)	Protein[b] (g/d)
Infants							
0–6 mo	0.7*	60*	ND	31*	4.4*	0.5*	9.1*
7–12 mo	0.8*	95*	ND	30*	4.6*	0.5*	**11.0**[c]
Children							
1–3 yr	1.3*	**130**	19*	ND	7*	0.7*	**13**
4–8 yr	1.7*	**130**	25*	ND	10*	0.9*	**19**
Males							
9–13 yr	2.4*	**130**	31*	ND	12*	1.2*	**34**
14–18 yr	3.3*	**130**	38*	ND	16*	1.6*	**52**
19–30 yr	3.7*	**130**	38*	ND	17*	1.6*	**56**
31–50 yr	3.7*	**130**	38*	ND	17*	1.6*	**56**
51–70 yr	3.7*	**130**	30*	ND	14*	1.6*	**56**
>70 yr	3.7*	**130**	30*	ND	14*	1.6*	**56**
Females							
9–13 yr	2.1*	**130**	26*	ND	10*	1.0*	**34**
14–18 yr	2.3*	**130**	26*	ND	11*	1.1*	**46**
19–30 yr	2.7*	**130**	25*	ND	12*	1.1*	**46**
31–50 yr	2.7*	**130**	25*	ND	12*	1.1*	**46**
51–70 yr	2.7*	**130**	21*	ND	11*	1.1*	**46**
>70 yr	2.7*	**130**	21*	ND	11*	1.1*	**46**
Pregnancy							
14–18 yr	3.0*	**175**	28*	ND	13*	1.4*	**71**
19–30 yr	3.0*	**175**	28*	ND	13*	1.4*	**71**
31–50 yr	3.0*	**175**	28*	ND	13*	1.4*	**71**
Lactation							
14–18 yr	3.8*	**210**	29*	ND	13*	1.3*	**71**
19–30 yr	3.8*	**210**	29*	ND	13*	1.3*	**71**
31–50 yr	3.8*	**210**	29*	ND	13*	1.3*	**71**

NOTE: This table presents Recommended Dietary Allowances (RDAs) in **bold** type and Adequate Intake (AIs) in ordinary type followed by an asterisk (*). RDAs and AIs may both be used as goals for individual intake. RDAs are set to meet the needs of almost all (97%–98%) individuals in a group. For healthy infants fed human milk, the AI is the mean intake. The AI for other life stage and gender groups is believed to cover the needs of all individuals in the group, but lack of data or uncertainty in the data prevent being able to specify with confidence the percentage of individuals covered by this intake.

[a]Total water includes all water contained in food, beverages, and drinking water.

[b]Based on 0.8 g/kg body weight for the reference body weight.

[c]Change from 13.5 in prepublication copy due to calculaton error.

Dietary Reference Intakes (DRIs): Additional Macronutrient Recommendations
Food and Nutrition Board, Institute of Medicine, National Academies

Macronutrient	Recommendation
Dietary cholesterol	As low as possible while consuming a nutritionally adequate diet
Trans fatty acids	As low as possible while consuming a nutritionally adequate diet
Saturated fatty acids	As low as possible while consuming a nutritionally adequate diet
Added sugars	Limit to no more than 25% of total energy

SOURCE: *Dietary Reference Intakes for Energy, Carbohydrate, Fiber, Fat, Fatty Acids, Cholesterol, Protein, and Amino Acids.*

Dietary Reference Intakes: Vitamins and Minerals

Dietary Reference Intakes (DRIs): Recommended Intakes for Individuals, Vitamins
Food and Nutrition Board, Institute of Medicine, National Academies

Life Stage Group	Vit A (μg/d)[a]	Vit C (mg/d)	Vit D (μg/d)[b,c]	Vit E (mg/d)[d]	Vit K (μg/d)	Thiamin (mg/d)
Infants						
0–6 mo	400*	40*	5*	4*	2.0*	0.2*
7–12 mo	500*	50*	5*	5*	2.5*	0.3*
Children						
1–3 yr	**300**	**15**	5*	**6**	30*	**0.5**
4–8 yr	**400**	**25**	5*	**7**	55*	**0.6**
Males						
9–13 yr	**600**	**45**	5*	**11**	60*	**0.9**
14–18 yr	**900**	**75**	5*	**15**	75*	**1.2**
19–30 yr	**900**	**90**	5*	**15**	120*	**1.2**
31–50 yr	**900**	**90**	5*	**15**	120*	**1.2**
51–70 yr	**900**	**90**	10*	**15**	120*	**1.2**
>70 yr	**900**	**90**	15*	**15**	120*	**1.2**
Females						
9–13 yr	**600**	**45**	5*	**11**	60*	**0.9**
14–18 yr	**700**	**65**	5*	**15**	75*	**1.0**
19–30 yr	**700**	**75**	5*	**15**	90*	**1.1**
31–50 yr	**700**	**75**	5*	**15**	90*	**1.1**
51–70 yr	**700**	**75**	10*	**15**	90*	**1.1**
>70 yr	**700**	**75**	15*	**15**	90*	**1.1**
Pregnancy						
14–18 yr	**750**	**80**	5*	**15**	75*	**1.4**
19–30 yr	**770**	**85**	5*	**15**	90*	**1.4**
31–50 yr	**770**	**85**	5*	**15**	90*	**1.4**
Lactation						
14–18 yr	**1,200**	**115**	5*	**19**	75*	**1.4**
19–30 yr	**1,300**	**120**	5*	**19**	90*	**1.4**
31–50 yr	**1,300**	**120**	5*	**19**	90*	**1.4**

NOTE: This table (taken from the DRI reports, see www.nap.edu) presents Recommended Dietary Allowances (RDAs) in **bold** type and Adequate Intakes (AIs) in ordinary type followed by an asterisk (*). RDAs and AIs may both be used as goals for individual intake. RDAs are set to meet the needs of almost all (97%–98%) individuals in a group. For healthy breastfed infants, the AI is the mean intake. The AI for other life stage and gender groups is believed to cover needs of all individuals in the group, but lack of data or uncertainty in the data prevent being able to specify with confidence the percentage of individuals covered by this intake.

[a] As retinol activity equivalents (RAEs). 1 RAE = 1 μg retinol, 12 μg β-carotene, 24 μg α-carotene, or 24 μg β-cryptoxanthin. The RAE for dietary provitamin A carotenoids is twofold greater than retinol equivalents (RE), whereas the RAE for preformed vitamin A is the same as RE.

[b] As cholecalciferol. 1 μg cholecalciferol = 40 IU vitamin D.

[c] In the absence of adequate exposure to sunlight.

[d] As α-tocopherol. α-Tocopherol includes RRR-α-tocopherol, the only form of α-tocopherol that occurs naturally in foods, and the 2R-stereoisomeric forms of α-tocopherol (RRR-, RSR-, RRS-, and RSS-α-tocopherol) that occur in fortified foods and supplements. It does not include the 2S-stereoisomeric forms of α-tocopherol (SRR-, SSR-, SRS-, and SSS-α-tocopherol), also found in fortified foods and supplements.

[e] As niacin equivalents (NE). 1 mg of niacin = 60 mg of tryptophan; 0–6 months = preformed niacin (not NE).

Riboflavin (mg/d)	Niacin (mg/d)[e]	Vit B_6 (mg/d)	Folate (μg/d)[f]	Vit B_{12} (μg/d)	Pantothenic Acid (mg/d)	Biotin (μg/d)	Choline (mg/d)[g]
0.3*	2*	0.1*	65*	0.4*	1.7*	5*	125*
0.4*	4*	0.3*	80*	0.5*	1.8*	6*	150*
0.5	6	0.5	150	0.9	2*	8*	200*
0.6	8	0.6	200	1.2	3*	12*	250*
0.9	12	1.0	300	1.8	4*	20*	375*
1.3	16	1.3	400	2.4	5*	25*	550*
1.3	16	1.3	400	2.4	5*	30*	550*
1.3	16	1.3	400	2.4	5*	30*	550*
1.3	16	1.7	400	2.4[i]	5*	30*	550*
1.3	16	1.7	400	2.4[i]	5*	30*	550*
0.9	12	1.0	300	1.8	4*	20*	375*
1.0	14	1.2	400	2.4	5*	25*	400*
1.1	14	1.3	400	2.4	5*	30*	425*
1.1	14	1.3	400	2.4	5*	30*	425*
1.1	14	1.5	400	2.4[h]	5*	30*	425*
1.1	14	1.5	400	2.4[h]	5*	30*	425*
1.4	18	1.9	600[j]	2.6	6*	30*	450*
1.4	18	1.9	600[j]	2.6	6*	30*	450*
1.4	18	1.9	600[j]	2.6	6*	30*	450*
1.6	17	2.0	500	2.8	7*	35*	550*
1.6	17	2.0	500	2.8	7*	35*	550*
1.6	17	2.0	500	2.8	7*	35*	550*

[f]As dietary folate equivalents (DFE). 1 DFE = 1 μg food folate = 0.6 μg of folic acid from fortified food or as a supplement consumed with food = 0.5 μg of a supplement taken on an empty stomach.

[g]Although AIs have been set for choline, there are few data to assess whether a dietary supply of choline is needed at all stages of the life cycle, and it may be that the choline requirement can be met by endogenous synthesis at some of these stages.

[h]Because 10% to 30% of older people may malabsorb food-bound B_{12}, it is advisable for those older than 50 years to meet their RDA mainly by consumng foods fortified with B_{12} or a supplement containing B_{12}.

[i]In view of evidence linking folate intake with neural tube defects in the fetus, it is recommended that all women capable of becoming pregnant consume 400 μg from supplements or fortified foods in addition to intake of food folate from a varied diet.

[j]It is assumed that women will continue consuming 400 μg from supplements or fortified food until their pregnancy is confirmed and they enter prenatal care, which ordinarily occurs after the end of the periconceptional period—the critical time for formation of the neural tube.

Reprinted with permission from (Dietary Reference intakes for Energy, Carbohydrates, Fiber, Fat, Fatty Acids, Cholesterol, Protein, and Amino Acids (Macronutrients)) © 2005 by the National Academy of Sciences, courtesy of the National Academies Press, Washington, D.C.

Dietary Reference Intakes (DRIs): Recommended Intakes for Individuals, Elements
Food and Nutrition Board, Institute of Medicine, National Academies

Life Stage Group	Calcium (mg/d)	Chromium (μg/d)	Copper (μg/d)	Fluoride (mg/d)	Iodine (μg/d)	Iron (mg/d)	Magnesium (mg/d)
Infants							
0–6 mo	210*	0.2*	200*	0.01*	110*	0.27*	30*
7–12 mo	270*	5.5*	220*	0.5*	130*	11	75*
Children							
1–3 yr	500*	11*	340	0.7*	90	7	80
4–8 yr	800*	15*	440	1*	90	10	130
Males							
9–13 yr	1,300*	25*	700	2*	120	8	240
14–18 yr	1,300*	35*	890	3*	150	11	410
19–30 yr	1,000*	35*	900	4*	150	8	400
31–50 yr	1,000*	35*	900	4*	150	8	420
51–70 yr	1,200*	30*	900	4*	150	8	420
>70 yr	1,200*	30*	900	4*	150	8	420
Females							
9–13 yr	1,300*	21*	700	2*	120	8	240
14–18 yr	1,300*	24*	890	3*	150	15	360
19–30 yr	1,000*	25*	900	3*	150	18	310
31–50 yr	1,000*	25*	900	3*	150	18	320
51–70 yr	1,200*	20*	900	3*	150	8	320
>70 yr	1,200*	20*	900	3*	150	8	320
Pregnancy							
14–18 yr	1,300*	29*	1,000	3*	220	27	400
19–30 yr	1,000*	30*	1,000	3*	220	27	350
31–50 yr	1,000*	30*	1,000	3*	220	27	360
Lactation							
14–18 yr	1,300*	44*	1,300	3*	290	10	360
19–30 yr	1,000*	45*	1,300	3*	290	9	310
31–50 yr	1,000*	45*	1,300	3*	290	9	320

NOTE: This table presents Recommended Dietary Allowances (RDAs) in **bold** type and Adequate Intakes (AIs) in ordinary type follwed by an asterisk (*). RDAs and AIs may both be used as goals for individual intake. RDAs are set to meet the needs of almost all (97%–98%) individuals in a group. For healthy breastfed infants, the AI is the mean intake. The AI for other life stage and gender groups is believed to cover needs of all individuals in the group, but lack of data or uncertainty in the data prevent being able to specify with confidence the percentage of individuals covered by this intake.

Sources: *Dietary Reference Intakes for Calcium, Phosphorous, Magnesium, Vitamin D, and Fluoride* (1997); *Dietary Reference Intakes for Thiamin, Riboflavin, Niacin, Vitamin B₆, Folate, Vitamin B₁₂, Pantothenic Acid, Biotin, and Choline* (1998); *Dietary Reference Intakes for Vitamin C, Vitamin E, Selenium, and Carotenoids* (2000); *Dietary Reference Intakes for Vitamin A, Vitamin K, Arsenic, Boron, Chromium, Copper, Iodine, Iron, Manganese, Molybdenum, Nickel, Silicon, Vanadium, and Zinc* (2001); and *Dietary Reference Intakes for Water, Potassium, Sodium, Chloride, and Sulfate* (2004). These reports may be accessed via http://www.nap.edu.

Manganese (mg/d)	Molybdenum (μg/d)	Phosphorus (mg/d)	Selenium (μg/d)	Zinc (mg/d)	Potassium (g/d)	Sodium (g/d)	Chloride (g/d)
0.003*	2*	100*	15*	2*	0.4*	0.12*	0.18*
0.6*	3*	275*	20*	3	0.7*	0.37*	0.57*
1.2*	17	460	20	3	3.0*	1.0*	1.5*
1.5*	22	500	30	5	3.8*	1.2*	1.9*
1.9*	34	1,250	40	8	4.5*	1.5*	2.3*
2.2*	43	1,250	55	11	4.7*	1.5*	2.3*
2.3*	45	700	55	11	4.7*	1.5*	2.3*
2.3	45	700	55	11	4.7*	1.5*	2.3*
2.3*	45	700	55	11	4.7*	1.3*	2.0*
2.3*	45	700	55	11	4.7*	1.2*	1.8*
1.6*	34	1,250	40	8	4.5*	1.5*	2.3*
1.6*	43	1,250	55	9	4.7*	1.5*	2.3*
1.8*	45	700	55	8	4.7*	1.5*	2.3*
1.8*	45	700	55	8	4.7*	1.5*	2.3*
1.8*	45	700	55	8	4.7*	1.3*	2.0*
1.8*	45	700	55	8	4.7*	1.2*	1.8*
2.0*	50	1,250	60	12	4.7*	1.5*	2.3*
2.0*	50	700	60	11	4.7*	1.5*	2.3*
2.0*	50	700	60	11	4.7*	1.5*	2.3*
2.6*	50	1,250	70	13	5.1*	1.5*	2.3*
2.6*	50	700	70	12	5.1*	1.5*	2.3*
2.6*	50	700	70	12	5.1*	1.5*	2.3*

Dietary Reference Intakes: Estimated Energy Requirements

Estimated Energy Requirements (EER) for Men and Women 30 Years of Age[a]
Food and Nutrition Board, Institute of Medicine, National Academies

Height (m [in])	PAL[b]	Weight for BMI[c] of 18.5 kg/m² (kg [lb])	Weight for BMI of 24.99 kg/m² (kg [lb])	EER, Men[d] (KCAL/DAY) BMI of 18.5 kg/m²	BMI of 24.99 kg/m²	EER, Women[d] (KCAL/DAY) BMI of 18.5 kg/m²	BMI of 24.99 kg/m²
1.50 (59)	Sedentary	41.6 (92)	56.2 (124)	1,848	2,080	1,625	1,762
	Low Active			2,009	2,267	1,803	1,956
	Active			2,215	2,506	2,025	2,198
	Very Active			2,554	2,898	2,291	2,489
1.65 (65)	Sedentary	50.4 (111)	68.0 (150)	2,068	2,349	1,816	1,982
	Low Active			2,254	2,566	2,016	2,202
	Active			2,490	2,842	2,267	2,477
	Very Active			2,880	3,296	2,567	2,807
1.80 (71)	Sedentary	59.9 (132)	81.0 (178)	2,301	2,635	2,015	2,211
	Low Active			2,513	2,884	2,239	2,459
	Active			2,782	3,200	2,519	2,769
	Very Active			3,225	3,720	2,855	3,141

[a]For each year below 30, add 7 kcal/day for women and 10 kcal/day for men. For each year above 30, subtract 7 kcal/day for women and 10 kcal/day for men.

[b]PAL = physical activity level.

[c]BMI = body mass index.

[d]Derived from the following regression equations based on doubly labeled water data:

Adult man: $EER = 662 - 9.53 \times age \ (yr) + PA \times (15.91 \times wt \ [kg] + 539.6 \times ht \ [ml])$

Adult woman: $EER = 354 - 6.91 \times age \ (yr) + PA \times (9.36 \times wt \ [kg] + 726 \times ht \ [ml])$

Where PA refers to coefficient for PAL

PAL = total energy expenditure ÷ basal energy expenditure

PA = 1.0 if PAL ≥ 1.0 < 1.4 (sedentary)

PA = 1.12 if PAL ≥ 1.4 < 1.6 (low active)

PA = 1.27 if PAL ≥ 1.6 < 1.9 (active)

PA = 1.45 if PAL ≥ 1.9 < 2.5 (very active)

Source: *Dietary Reference Intakes for Energy, Carbohydrate, Fiber, Fat, Fatty Acids, Cholesterol, Protein, and Amino Acids* (2002).

Percent Fat Estimate for Men: Sum of Triceps, Chest, and Subscapula Skinfolds

Sum of Skinfolds (mm)	Under 22	23–27	28–32	33–37	AGE TO LAST YEAR 38–42	43–47	48–52	53–57	Over 57
8–10	1.5	2.0	2.5	3.1	3.6	4.1	4.6	5.1	5.6
11–13	3.0	3.5	4.0	4.5	5.1	5.6	6.1	6.6	7.1
14–16	4.5	5.0	5.5	6.0	6.5	7.0	7.6	8.1	8.6
17–19	5.9	6.4	6.9	7.4	8.0	8.5	9.0	9.5	10.0
20–22	7.3	7.8	8.3	8.8	9.4	9.9	10.4	10.9	11.4
23–25	8.6	9.2	9.7	10.2	10.7	11.2	11.8	12.3	12.8
26–28	10.0	10.5	11.0	11.5	12.1	12.6	13.1	13.6	14.2
29–31	11.2	11.8	12.3	12.8	13.4	13.9	14.4	14.9	15.5
32–34	12.5	13.0	13.5	14.1	14.6	15.1	15.7	16.2	16.7
35–37	13.7	14.2	14.8	15.3	15.8	16.4	16.9	17.4	18.0
38–40	14.9	15.4	15.9	16.5	17.0	17.6	18.1	18.6	19.2
41–43	16.0	16.6	17.1	17.6	18.2	18.7	19.3	19.8	20.3
44–46	17.1	17.7	18.2	18.7	19.3	19.8	20.4	20.9	21.5
47–49	18.2	18.7	19.3	19.8	20.4	20.9	21.4	22.0	22.5
50–52	19.2	19.7	20.3	20.8	21.4	21.9	22.5	23.0	23.6
53–55	20.2	20.7	21.3	21.8	22.4	22.9	23.5	24.0	24.6
56–58	21.1	21.7	22.2	22.8	23.3	23.9	24.4	25.0	25.5
59–61	22.0	22.6	23.1	23.7	24.2	24.8	25.3	25.9	26.5
62–64	22.9	23.4	24.0	24.5	25.1	25.7	26.2	26.8	27.3
65–67	23.7	24.3	24.8	25.4	25.9	26.5	27.1	27.6	28.2
68–70	24.5	25.0	25.6	26.2	26.7	27.3	27.8	28.4	29.0
71–73	25.2	25.8	26.3	26.9	27.5	28.0	28.6	29.1	29.7
74–76	25.9	26.5	27.0	27.6	28.2	28.7	29.3	29.9	30.4
77–79	26.6	27.1	27.7	28.2	28.8	29.4	29.9	30.5	31.1
80–82	27.2	27.7	28.3	28.9	29.4	30.0	30.6	31.1	31.7
83–85	27.7	28.3	28.8	29.4	30.0	30.5	31.1	31.7	32.3
86–88	28.2	28.8	29.4	29.9	30.5	31.1	31.6	32.2	32.8
89–91	28.7	29.3	29.8	30.4	31.0	31.5	32.1	32.7	33.3
92–94	29.1	29.7	30.3	30.8	31.4	32.0	32.6	33.1	33.4
95–97	29.5	30.1	30.6	31.2	31.8	32.4	32.9	33.5	34.1
98–100	29.8	30.4	31.0	31.6	32.1	32.7	33.3	33.9	34.4
101–103	30.1	30.7	31.3	31.8	32.4	33.0	33.6	34.1	34.7
104–106	30.4	30.9	31.5	32.1	32.7	33.2	33.8	34.4	35.0
107–109	30.6	31.1	31.7	32.3	32.9	33.4	34.0	34.6	35.2
110–112	30.7	31.3	31.9	32.4	33.0	33.6	34.2	34.7	35.3
113–115	30.8	31.4	32.0	32.5	33.1	33.7	34.3	34.9	35.4
116–118	30.9	31.5	32.0	32.6	33.2	33.8	34.3	34.9	35.5

From A. S. Jackson and M. L. Pollock, "Practical Assessment of Body Composition" in *The Physician and Sportsmedicine*, 13(5):85, 1985. Copyright © 1985 McGraw-Hill Healthcare Group, Minneapolis, MN. Reprinted by permission.

Percent Fat Estimate for Women: Sum of Triceps, Abdomen, and Suprailium Skinfolds

Sum of Skinfolds (mm)	AGE TO LAST YEAR								
	18–22	23–27	28–32	33–37	38–42	43–47	48–52	53–57	Over 57
8–12	8.8	9.0	9.2	9.4	9.5	9.7	9.9	10.1	10.3
13–17	10.8	10.9	11.1	11.3	11.5	11.7	11.8	12.0	12.2
18–22	12.6	12.8	13.0	13.2	13.4	13.5	13.7	13.9	14.1
23–27	14.5	14.6	14.8	15.0	15.2	15.4	15.6	15.7	15.9
28–32	16.2	16.4	16.6	16.8	17.0	17.1	17.3	17.5	17.7
33–37	17.9	18.1	18.3	18.5	18.7	18.9	19.0	19.2	19.4
38–42	19.6	19.8	20.0	20.2	20.3	20.5	20.7	20.9	21.1
43–47	21.2	21.4	21.6	21.8	21.9	22.1	22.3	22.5	22.7
48–52	22.8	22.9	23.1	23.3	23.5	23.7	23.8	24.0	24.2
53–57	24.2	24.4	24.6	24.8	25.0	25.2	25.3	25.5	25.7
58–62	25.7	25.9	26.0	26.2	26.4	26.6	26.8	27.0	27.1
63–67	27.1	27.2	27.4	27.6	27.8	28.0	28.2	28.3	28.5
68–72	28.4	28.6	28.7	28.9	29.1	29.3	29.5	29.7	29.8
73–77	29.6	29.8	30.0	30.2	30.4	30.6	30.7	30.9	31.1
78–82	30.9	31.0	31.2	31.4	31.6	31.8	31.9	32.1	32.3
83–87	32.0	32.2	32.4	32.6	32.7	32.9	33.1	33.3	33.5
88–92	33.1	33.3	33.5	33.7	33.8	34.0	34.2	34.4	34.6
93–97	34.1	34.3	34.5	34.7	34.9	35.1	35.2	35.4	35.6
98–102	35.1	35.3	35.5	35.7	35.9	36.0	36.2	36.4	36.6
103–107	36.1	36.2	36.4	36.6	36.8	37.0	37.2	37.3	37.5
108–112	36.9	37.1	37.3	37.5	37.7	37.9	38.0	38.2	38.4
113–117	37.8	37.9	38.1	38.3	39.2	39.4	39.6	39.8	39.2
118–122	38.5	38.7	38.9	39.1	39.4	39.6	39.8	40.0	40.0
123–127	39.2	39.4	39.6	39.8	40.0	40.1	40.3	40.5	40.7
128–132	39.9	40.1	40.2	40.4	40.6	40.8	41.0	41.2	41.3
133–137	40.5	40.7	40.8	41.0	41.2	41.4	41.6	41.7	41.9
138–142	41.0	41.2	41.4	41.6	41.7	41.9	42.1	42.3	42.5
143–147	41.5	41.7	41.9	42.0	42.2	42.4	42.6	42.8	43.0
148–152	41.9	42.1	42.3	42.4	42.6	42.8	43.0	43.2	43.4
153–157	42.3	42.5	42.6	42.8	43.0	43.2	43.4	43.6	43.7
158–162	42.6	42.8	43.0	43.1	43.3	43.5	43.7	43.9	44.1
163–167	42.9	43.0	43.2	43.4	43.6	43.8	44.0	44.1	44.3
168–172	43.1	43.2	43.4	43.6	43.8	44.0	44.2	44.3	44.5
173–177	43.2	43.4	43.6	43.8	43.9	44.1	44.3	44.5	44.7
178–182	43.3	43.5	43.7	43.8	44.0	44.2	44.4	44.6	44.8

From A. S. Jackson and M. L. Pollock, "Practical Assessment of Body Composition" in *The Physician and Sportsmedicine*, 13(5):85, 1985. Copyright © 1985 McGraw-Hill Healthcare Group, Minneapolis, MN. Reprinted by permission.

Glossary

absolute $\dot{V}O_2$ the amount of oxygen consumed over a given time period; expressed as liters · min^{-1}.

acidosis an abnormal increase in blood hydrogen ion concentration (i.e., arterial pH below 7.35).

acids compounds capable of giving up hydrogen ions into solution.

acromegaly a condition caused by hypersecretion of growth hormone from the pituitary gland; characterized by enlargement of the extremities, such as the jaw, nose, and fingers.

actin a structural protein of muscle that works with myosin in permitting muscular contraction.

action potential the all-or-none electrical event in the neuron or muscle cell in which the polarity of the cell membrane is rapidly reversed and then reestablished.

adenosine diphosphate (ADP) a molecule that combines with inorganic phosphate to form ATP.

adenosine triphosphate (ATP) the high-energy phosphate compound synthesized and used by cells to release energy for cellular work.

adenylate cyclase enzyme found in cell membranes that catalyzes the conversion of ATP to cyclic AMP.

adequate intake (AI) recommendations for nutrient intake when insufficient information is available to set an RDA standard.

adrenal cortex the outer portion of the adrenal gland. Synthesizes and secretes corticosteroid hormones, such as cortisol, aldosterone, and androgens.

adrenaline *see* epinephrine.

adrenocorticotrophic hormone (ACTH) a hormone secreted by the anterior pituitary gland that stimulates the adrenal cortex.

aerobic in the presence of oxygen.

afferent fibers nerve fibers (sensory fibers) that carry neural information back to the central nervous system.

afferent neuron sensory neuron carrying information toward the central nervous system.

aldosterone a corticosteroid hormone involved in the regulation of electrolyte balance.

alkalosis an abnormal increase in blood concentration of OH^- ions, resulting in a rise in arterial pH above 7.45.

alpha receptors a subtype of adrenergic receptors located on cell membranes of selected tissues.

alveolar ventilation ($\dot{V}_A$) the volume of gas that reaches the alveolar region of the lung.

alveoli microscopic air sacs located in the lung where gas exchange occurs between respiratory gases and the blood.

amenorrhea the absence of menses.

anabolic steroid a prescription drug that has anabolic, or growth-stimulating, characteristics similar to that of the male androgen, testosterone.

anaerobic without oxygen.

anaerobic threshold a commonly used term meant to describe the level of oxygen consumption at which there is a rapid and systematic increase in blood lactate concentration. Also termed the *lactate threshold*.

anatomical dead space the total volume of the lung (i.e., conducting airways) that does not participate in gas exchange.

androgenic steroid a compound that has the qualities of an androgen; associated with masculine characteristics.

androgens male sex hormones. Synthesized in the testes and in limited amounts in the adrenal cortex. Steroids that have masculinizing effects.

angina pectoris chest pain due to a lack of blood flow (ischemia) to the myocardium.

angiotensin I and II these compounds are polypeptides formed from the cleavage of a protein (angiotensinogen) by the action of the enzyme renin produced by the kidneys, and converting enzyme in the lung, respectively.

anorexia nervosa an eating disorder characterized by rapid weight loss due to failure to consume adequate amounts of nutrients.

anterior hypothalamus the anterior portion of the hypothalamus. The hypothalamus is an area of the brain below the thalamus that regulates the autonomic nervous system and the pituitary gland.

anterior pituitary the anterior portion of the pituitary gland that secretes follicle-stimulating hormone, luteinizing hormone, adrenocorticotrophic hormone, thyroid-stimulating hormone, growth hormone, and prolactin.

antidiuretic hormone (ADH) hormone secreted by the posterior pituitary gland that promotes water retention by the kidney.

aortic bodies receptors located in the arch of the aorta that are capable of detecting changes in arterial PO_2.

apophyses sites of muscle-tendon insertion in bones.

arrhythmia abnormal electrical activity in the heart (e.g., a premature ventricular contraction).

arteries large vessels that carry arterialized blood away from the heart.

arterioles a small branch of an artery that communicates with a capillary network.

articular cartilage cartilage that covers the ends of bones in a synovial joint.

atherosclerosis a pathological condition in which fatty substances collect inside the lumen of arteries.

ATPase enzyme capable of breaking down ATP to $ADP + P_i + energy$.

ATP-PC system term used to describe the metabolic pathway involving muscle stores of ATP and the use of phosphocreatine to rephosphorylate ADP. This pathway is used at the onset of exercise and during short-term, high-intensity work.

atrioventricular node (AV node) a specialized mass of muscle tissue located in the interventricular septum of the heart; functions in the transmission of cardiac impulses from the atria to the ventricles.

autologous transfusion blood transfusion where the individual receives his or her own blood.

autonomic nervous system portion of the nervous system that controls the actions of visceral organs.

autoregulation mechanism by which an organ regulates blood flow to match the metabolic rate.

axon a nerve fiber that conducts a nerve impulse away from the neuron cell body.

basal metabolic rate (BMR) metabolic rate measured in supine position following a twelve-hour fast, and eight hours of sleep.

bases compounds that ionize in water to release hydroxyl ions (OH^-) or other ions that are capable of combining with hydrogen ions.

beta oxidation breakdown of free fatty acids to form acetyl-CoA.

beta receptor agonist (β-agonist) a molecule that is capable of binding to and activating a beta receptor.

beta receptors adrenergic receptors located on cell membranes. Combine mainly with epinephrine and, to some degree, with norepinephrine.

bioenergetics the chemical processes involved with the production of cellular ATP.

biological control systems a control system capable of maintaining homeostasis within a cell or organ system in a living creature.

blood boosting a term that applies to the increase of the blood's hemoglobin concentration by the infusion of additional red blood cells. Medically termed *induced erythrocythemia*.

blood doping *see* blood boosting.

blood packing *see* blood boosting.

Bohr effect the right shift of the oxyhemoglobin dissociation curve due to a decrease of blood pH. Results in a decreased affinity for oxygen.

bradycardia a resting heart rate less than sixty beats per minute.

brain stem portion of the brain that includes midbrain, pons, and medulla.

buffer a compound that resists pH change.

bulimia an eating disorder characterized by eating and forced regurgitation.

bulk flow mass movement of molecules from an area of high pressure to an area of lower pressure.

calcitonin hormone, released from the thyroid gland, that plays a minor role in calcium metabolism.

calmodulin part of second messenger system involving calcium that results in changes in the activity of intracellular enzymes.

capillaries microscopic blood vessels that connect arterioles and venules. Portion of vascular system where blood/tissue gas exchange occurs.

cardiac accelerator nerves part of the sympathetic nervous system that stimulates the SA node to increase heart rate.

cardiac output the amount of blood pumped by the heart per unit of time; equal to product of heart rate and stroke volume.

cardiovascular control center the area of the medulla that regulates the cardiovascular system.

carotid bodies chemoreceptors located in the internal carotid artery; respond to changes in arterial PO_2, PCO_2, and pH.

catecholamines organic compounds, including epinephrine, norepinephrine, and dopamine.

cell body the soma, or major portion of the body of a nerve cell. Contains the nucleus.

cell membrane the lipid-bilayer envelope that encloses cells. Called the *sarcolemma* in muscle cells.

cellular respiration process of oxygen consumption and carbon dioxide production in cells (i.e., bioenergetics).

central command the control of the cardiovascular or pulmonary system by cortical impulses.

central nervous system (CNS) portion of the nervous system that consists of the brain and spinal cord.

cerebellum portion of the brain that is concerned with fine coordination of skeletal muscles during movement.

cerebrum superior aspect of the brain that occupies the upper cranial cavity. Contains the motor cortex.

chemiosmotic hypothesis the mechanism to explain the aerobic formation of ATP in mitochondria.

cholesterol a twenty-seven-carbon lipid that can be synthesized in cells or consumed in the diet. Cholesterol serves as a precursor of steroid hormones, and plays a role in the development of atherosclerosis.

clo unit that describes the insulation quality of clothing.

concentric action occurs when a muscle is activated and shortens.

conduction transfer of heat from warmer to cooler objects that are in contact with each other. This term may also be used in association with the conveyance of neural impulses.

conduction disturbances refers to a slowing or blockage of the wave of depolarization in the heart, e.g., first-degree AV block, or bundle branch block.

conductivity capacity for conduction.

convection the transmission of heat from one object to another through the circulation of heated molecules.

Cori cycle the cycle of lactate-to-glucose between the muscle and liver.

coronary artery bypass graft surgery (CABGS) the replacement of a blocked coronary artery with another vessel to permit blood flow to the myocardium.

cortisol a glucocorticoid secreted by the adrenal cortex upon stimulation by ACTH.

coupled reactions the linking of energy-liberating chemical reactions to "drive" energy-requiring reactions.

critical power a specific submaximal power output that can be maintained without fatigue.

cromolyn sodium a drug used to stabilize the membranes of mast cells and prevent an asthma attack.

cycle ergometer a stationary exercise cycle that allows accurate measurement of work output.

cyclic AMP a substance produced from ATP through the action of adenylate cyclase that alters several chemical processes in the cell.

cytoplasm the contents of the cell surrounding the nucleus. Called *sarcoplasm* in muscle cells.

Daily Value a standard used in nutritional labeling.

deficiency a shortcoming of some essential nutrient.

degenerative diseases diseases not due to infection that result in a progressive decline in some bodily function.

delayed-onset muscle soreness (DOMS) muscle soreness that occurs twelve to twenty-four hours after an exercise bout.

dendrites portion of the nerve fiber that transmits action potentials toward a nerve cell body.

dental caries tooth decay; related to sugar content in foods.

deoxyhemoglobin hemoglobin not in combination with oxygen.

diabetes mellitus a condition characterized by high blood glucose levels due to inadequate insulin. Type I diabetics are insulin dependent, whereas Type II diabetics are resistant to insulin.

diabetic coma unconscious state induced by a lack of insulin.

diacylglycerol a molecule derived from a membrane-bound phospholipid, phosphatidylinositol, that activates protein kinase C, and alters cellular activity.

diaphragm the major respiratory muscle responsible for inspiration. Dome-shaped—separates the thoracic cavity from the abdominal cavity.

diastole period of filling of the heart between contractions (i.e., resting phase of the heart).

diastolic blood pressure arterial blood pressure during diastole.

Dietary Guidelines for Americans general statements related to food selection that are consistent with achieving and maintaining good health.

dietary reference intakes the framework for nutrient recommendations being made as a part of the revision of the 1989 RDA.

diffusion random movement of molecules from an area of high concentration to an area of low concentration.

direct calorimetry assessment of the body's metabolic rate by direct measurement of the amount of heat produced.

dose the amount of drug or exercise prescribed to have a certain effect (or response).

double-blind research design an experimental design in which the subjects and the principal investigator are not aware of the experimental treatment order.

double product the product of heart rate and systolic blood pressure; estimate of work of the heart.

dynamic refers to an isotonic muscle action.

dynamic stretching stretching that involves controlled movement.

dynamometer device used to measure force production (e.g., used in the measurement of muscular strength).

dysmenorrhea painful menstruation.

dyspnea shortness of breath or labored breathing. May be due to various types of lung or heart diseases.

eccentric action occurs when a muscle is activated and force is produced but the muscle lengthens.

ectomorphy category of somatotype that is rated for linearity of body form.

effect change in variable (e.g., $\dot{V}O_2$ max) due to a dose of exercise (e.g., 3 days per week, 40 min/day at 70% $\dot{V}O_2$ max).

effector organ or body part that responds to stimulation by an efferent neuron (e.g., skeletal muscle in a withdrawal reflex).

efferent fibers nerve fibers (motor fibers) that carry neural information from the central nervous system to the periphery.

efferent neuron conducts impulses from the CNS to the effector organ (e.g., motor neuron).

ejection fraction the proportion of end-diastolic volume that is ejected during a ventricular contraction.

electrocardiogram (ECG) a recording of the electrical changes that occur in the myocardium during the cardiac cycle.

electron transport chain a series of cytochromes in the mitochondria that are responsible for oxidative phosphorylation.

element a single chemical substance composed of only one type of atom (e.g., calcium or potassium).

endergonic reactions energy-requiring reactions.

endocrine gland a gland that produces and secretes its products directly into the blood or interstitial fluid (ductless glands).

endomorphy the somatotype category that is rated for roundness (fatness).

endomysium the inner layer of connective tissue surrounding a muscle fiber.

endorphin a neuropeptide produced by the pituitary gland having pain-suppressing activity.

end-plate potential (EPP) depolarization of a membrane region by a sodium influx.

energy of activation energy required to initiate a chemical reaction.

energy wasteful systems metabolic pathways in which the energy generated in one reaction is used up in another that leads back to the first, creating a futile cycle and requiring a higher resting metabolic rate.

enzymes proteins that lower the energy of activation and, therefore, catalyze chemical reactions. Enzymes regulate the rate of most metabolic pathways.

epidemiologic triad a model that shows connections between the environment, agent, and host that cause disease.

epidemiology the study of the distribution and determinants of health-related states or events in specified populations, and the application of this study to the control of health problems.

epilepsy a neurological disorder manifested by muscular seizures.

epimysium the outer layer of connective tissue surrounding muscle.

epinephrine a hormone synthesized by the adrenal medulla; also called *adrenaline*.

epiphyseal plate (growth plate) cartilaginous layer between the head and shaft of a long bone where growth takes place.

EPOC an acronym for "excess post-exercise oxygen consumption"; often referred to as the *oxygen debt*.

EPSP excitatory post-synaptic potential. A graded depolarization of a post-synaptic membrane by a neurotransmitter.

ergogenic aid a substance, appliance, or procedure (e.g., blood doping) that improves performance.

ergometer instrument for measuring work.

ergometry measurement of work output.

erythrocythemia an increase in the number of erythrocytes in the blood.

erythropoietin hormone that stimulates red blood cell production.

estrogens female sex hormones, including estradiol and estrone. Produced primarily in the ovary and also produced in the adrenal cortex.

evaporation the change of water from a liquid form to a vapor form. Results in the removal of heat.

exercise a subclass of physical activity.

exergonic reactions chemical reactions that release energy.

extensors muscles that extend a limb—that is, increase the angle at a joint.

FAD flavin adenine dinucleotide. Serves as an electron carrier in bioenergetics.

fasciculi a small bundle of muscle fibers.

fast-twitch fibers one of several types of muscle fibers found in skeletal muscle; also called Type II fibers; characterized as having low oxidative capacity but high glycolytic capacity.

ferritin the iron-carrying molecule used as an index of whole-body iron status.

field test a test of physical performance performed in the field (outside the laboratory).

flexors muscle groups that cause flexion of limbs—that is, decrease the angle at a joint.

follicle-stimulating hormone (FSH) a hormone secreted by the anterior pituitary gland that stimulates the development of an ovarian follicle in the female and the production of sperm in the male.

food records the practice of keeping dietary food records for determining nutrient intake.

free fatty acid (FFA) a type of fat that combines with glycerol to form triglycerides. Is used as an energy source.

G protein the link between the hormone-receptor interaction on the surface of the membrane and the subsequent events inside the cell.

gain refers to the amount of correction that a control system is capable of achieving.

General Adaptation Syndrome (GAS) a term defined by Selye in 1936 that describes the organism's response to chronic stress. In response to stress the organism has a three-stage response: (1) alarm reaction; (2) stage of resistance; and (3) readjustment to the stress, or exhaustion.

glucagon a hormone produced by the pancreas that increases blood glucose and free fatty acid levels.

glucocorticoids any one of a group of hormones produced by the adrenal cortex that influences carbohydrate, fat, and protein metabolism.

gluconeogenesis the synthesis of glucose from amino acids, lactate, glycerol, and other short carbon-chain molecules.

glucose a simple sugar that is transported via the blood and metabolized by tissues.

glucose polymer a complex sugar molecule that contains multiple simple sugar molecules linked together.

glycogen a glucose polymer synthesized in cells as a means of storing carbohydrate.

glycogenolysis the breakdown of glycogen into glucose.

glycolysis a metabolic pathway in the cytoplasm of the cell that results in the degradation of glucose into pyruvate or lactate.

Golgi tendon organ (GTOs) a tension receptor located in series with skeletal muscle.

graded exercise test *see* incremental exercise test.

gross efficiency a simple measure of exercise efficiency defined as the ratio of work performed to energy expended, expressed as a percent.

growth hormone hormone synthesized and secreted by the anterior pituitary that stimulates growth of the skeleton and soft tissues during the growing years. It is also involved

in the mobilization of the body's energy stores.

HDL cholesterol (high-density lipoprotein cholesterol) cholesterol that is transported in the blood via high-density proteins; related to low risk of heart disease.

hemoglobin a heme-containing protein in red blood cells that is responsible for transporting oxygen to tissues. Hemoglobin also serves as a weak buffer within red blood cells.

hemosiderin an insoluble form of iron stored in tissues.

high-density lipoproteins (HDL) proteins used to transport cholesterol in blood; high levels appear to offer some protection from atherosclerosis.

homeostasis the maintenance of a constant internal environment.

homeotherms animals that maintain a fairly constant internal temperature.

homologous transfusion a blood transfusion using blood of the same type but from another donor.

hormone a chemical substance that is synthesized and released by an endocrine gland and transported to a target organ via the blood.

hydrogen ion (H^+) a free hydrogen ion in solution that results in a decrease in pH of the solution.

hyperbaric chamber chamber where the absolute pressure is increased above atmospheric pressure.

hyperoxia oxygen concentration in an inspired gas that exceeds 21%.

hyperplasia an increase in the number of cells in a tissue.

hyperthermia an above-normal increase in body temperature.

hypertrophy an increase in cell size.

hypothalamic somatostatin hypothalamic hormone that inhibits growth hormone secretion; also secreted from the delta cells of the islets of Langerhans.

hypothalamus brain structure that integrates many physiological functions to maintain homeostasis; site of secretion of hormones released by the posterior pituitary; also releases hormones that control anterior pituitary secretions.

hypothermia a condition in which heat is lost from the body faster than it is produced.

hypoxia a relative lack of oxygen (e.g., at altitude).

immunotherapy procedure in which the body is exposed to specific substances to elicit an immune response in order to offer better protection upon subsequent exposure.

incremental exercise test an exercise test involving a progressive increase in work rate over time. Often graded exercise tests are used to determine the subject's $\dot{V}O_2$ max or lactate threshold. (Also called *graded exercise test.*)

indirect calorimetry estimation of heat or energy production on the basis of oxygen consumption, carbon dioxide production, and nitrogen excretion.

induced erythrocythemia causing an elevation of the red blood cell (hemoglobin) concentration by infusing blood; also called *blood doping* or *blood boosting.*

infectious diseases diseases due to the presence of pathogenic microorganisms in the body (e.g., viruses, bacteria, fungi, and protozoa).

inorganic relating to substances that do not contain carbon (C).

inorganic phosphate (P_i) a stimulator of cellular metabolism; split off, along with ADP, from ATP when energy is released; used with ADP to form ATP in the electron transport chain.

inositol triphosphate a molecule derived from a membrane-bound phospholipid, phosphatidylinositol, that causes calcium release from intracellular stores and alters cellular activity.

insulin hormone released from the beta cells of the islets of Langerhans in response to elevated blood glucose and amino acid concentrations; increases tissue uptake of both.

insulin-like growth factors groups of growth-stimulating peptides released from the liver and other tissues in response to growth hormone. Also called somatomedins.

insulin shock condition brought on by too much insulin, which causes an immediate hypoglycemia; symptoms include tremors, dizziness, and possibly convulsions.

integrating center the portion of a biological control system that processes the information from the receptors and issues an appropriate response relative to its set point.

intercalated discs portion of cardiac muscle cell where one cell connects to the next.

intermediate fibers muscle fiber type that generates high force at a moderately fast speed of contraction, but has a relatively large number of mitochondria (Type IIa).

ion a single atom or small molecule containing a net positive or negative charge due to an excess of either protons or electrons, respectively (e.g., Na$^+$, Cl$^-$).

IPSP   inhibitory post-synaptic potential that moves the post-synaptic membrane further from threshold.

irritability   a trait of certain tissues that enables them to respond to stimuli (e.g., nerve and muscle).

isocitrate dehydrogenase   rate-limiting enzyme in the Krebs cycle that is inhibited by ATP and stimulated by ADP and P$_i$.

isokinetic   action in which the rate of movement is constantly maintained through a specific range of motion even though maximal force is exerted.

isometric   action in which the muscle develops tension, but does not shorten; also called a *static contraction*. No movement occurs.

isotonic   contraction in which a muscle shortens against a constant load or tension, resulting in movement.

ketosis   acidosis of the blood caused by the production of ketone bodies (e.g., acetoacetic acid) when fatty acid mobilization is increased, as in uncontrolled diabetes.

kilocalorie (kcal)   a measure of energy expenditure equal to the heat needed to raise the temperature of 1 kg of water 1 degree Celsius; also equal to 1,000 calories and sometimes written as calorie rather than kilocalorie.

kilogram-meter   a unit of work in which 1 kg of force (1 kg mass accelerated at 1 G) is moved through a vertical distance of 1 meter; abbreviated as kg-m, kg · m, or kgm.

kinesthesia   a perception of movement obtained from information about the position and rate of movement of the joints.

Krebs cycle   metabolic pathway in the mitochondria in which energy is transferred from carbohydrates, fats, and amino acids to NAD for subsequent production of ATP in the electron transport chain.

lactate threshold   a point during a graded exercise test when the blood lactate concentration increases abruptly.

lactic acid   an end product of glucose metabolism in the glycolytic pathway; formed in conditions of inadequate oxygen and in muscle fibers with few mitochondria.

lateral sac   *see* terminal cisternae.

LDL cholesterol   form of low-density lipoprotein responsible for the transport of plasma cholesterol; high levels are indicative of a high risk of coronary heart disease.

lipase   an enzyme responsible for the breakdown of triglycerides to free fatty acids and glycerol.

lipolysis   the breakdown of triglycerides in adipose tissue to free fatty acids and glycerol for subsequent transport to tissues for metabolism.

lipoprotein   protein involved in the transport of cholesterol and triglycerides in the plasma.

low-density lipoproteins (LDL)   form of lipoprotein that transports a majority of the plasma cholesterol; *see* LDL cholesterol.

luteinizing hormone (LH)   also called "interstitial cell stimulating hormone"; a surge of LH stimulates ovulation in middle of menstrual cycle; LH stimulates testosterone production in men.

major minerals   dietary minerals including calcium, phosphorus, potassium, sulfur, sodium, chloride, and magnesium.

mast cell   connective tissue cell that releases histamine and other chemicals in response to certain stimuli (e.g., injury).

maximal oxygen uptake (V̇O$_2$ max)   greatest rate of oxygen uptake by the body measured during severe dynamic exercise, usually on a cycle ergometer or a treadmill; dependent on maximal cardiac output and the maximal arteriovenous oxygen difference.

mesomorphy   one component of a somatotype that characterizes the muscular form or lean body mass aspect of the human body.

MET   an expression of the rate of energy expenditure at rest; equal to approximately $3.5 \text{ ml} \cdot \text{kg}^{-1} \cdot \text{min}^{-1}$, or $1 \text{ kcal} \cdot \text{kg}^{-1} \cdot \text{hr}^{-1}$.

mineralocorticoids   steroid hormones released from the adrenal cortex that are responsible for Na$^+$ and K$^+$ regulation (e.g., aldosterone).

mitochondrion   the subcellular organelle responsible for the production of ATP with oxygen; contains the enzymes for the Krebs cycle, electron transport chain, and the fatty acid cycle.

mixed venous blood   a mixture of venous blood from both the upper and lower extremities; complete mixing occurs in the right ventricle.

molecular biology   branch of biochemistry involved with the study of gene structure and function.

motor cortex   portion of the cerebral cortex containing large motor neurons whose axons descend to lower brain centers and spinal cord; associated with the voluntary control of movement.

motor neurons   efferent neurons that conduct action potentials from the central nervous system to the muscles.

motor unit   a motor neuron and all the muscle fibers innervated by that single motor neuron; responds in an "all-or-none" manner to a stimulus.

muscle action   term used to describe muscle form development.

muscle spindle   a muscle stretch receptor oriented parallel to skeletal muscle fibers; the capsule portion is surrounded by afferent fibers, and intrafusal muscle fibers can alter the length of the capsule during muscle contraction and relaxation.

muscular strength   the maximal amount of force that can be generated by a muscle or muscle group.

myocardial infarction   death of a portion of heart tissue that no longer conducts electrical activity nor provides force to move blood.

myocardial ischemia   a condition in which the myocardium experiences an inadequate blood flow; sometimes accompanied by irregularities in the electrocardiogram (arrhythmias and ST-segment depression) and chest pain (angina pectoris).

myocardium   cardiac muscle; provides the force of contraction to eject blood; muscle type with many mitochondria that is dependent on a constant supply of oxygen.

myofibrils   the portion of the muscle containing the thick and thin contractile filaments; a series of sarcomeres where the repeating pattern of the contractile proteins gives the striated appearance to skeletal muscle.

myoglobin   protein in muscle that can bind oxygen and release it at low PO$_2$ values; aids in diffusion of oxygen from capillary to mitochondria.

myosin   contractile protein in the thick filament of a myofibril that contains the cross-bridge that can bind actin and split ATP to cause tension development.

NAD   coenzyme that transfers hydrogen and the energy associated with those hydrogens; in the Krebs cycle, NAD transfers energy from substrates to the electron transport chain.

negative feedback   describes the response from a control system that reduces the size of the stimulus, e.g., an elevated blood glucose concentration causes the secretion of insulin which, in turn, lowers the blood glucose concentration.

net efficiency the mathematical ratio of work output divided by the energy expended above rest.

neuroendocrinology study of the role of the nervous and endocrine systems in the automatic regulation of the internal environment.

neuromuscular junction synapse between axon terminal of a motor neuron and the motor end plate of a muscle's plasma membrane.

neuron nerve cell; composed of a cell body with dendrites (projections) that bring information to the cell body, and axons that take information away from the cell body to influence neurons, glands, or muscles.

nitroglycerin drug used to reduce chest pain (angina pectoris) due to lack of blood flow to the myocardium.

norepinephrine a hormone and neurotransmitter; released from postganglionic nerve endings and the adrenal medulla.

normocythemia a normal red blood cell concentration.

normoxia a normal PO_2.

nucleus membrane-bound organelle containing most of the cell's DNA.

nutrient density the degree to which foods contain selected nutrients, e.g., protein.

open-circuit spirometry indirect calorimetry procedure in which either inspired or expired ventilation is measured and oxygen consumption and carbon dioxide production are calculated.

organic describes substances that contain carbon.

osteoporosis a decrease in bone density due to a loss of cortical bone; common in older women and implicated in fractures; estrogen, exercise, and Ca^{++} therapy are used to correct the condition.

overload a principle of training describing the need to increase the load (intensity) of exercise to cause a further adaptation of a system.

oxidative phosphorylation mitochondrial process in which inorganic phosphate (P_i) is coupled to ADP as energy is transferred along the electron transport chain in which oxygen is the final electron acceptor.

oxygen debt the elevated post-exercise oxygen consumption (*see* EPOC); related to replacement of creatine phosphate, lactic acid resynthesis to glucose, and elevated body temperature, catecholamines, heart rate, breathing, etc.

oxygen deficit refers to the lag in oxygen uptake at the beginning of exercise.

oxyhemoglobin hemoglobin combined with oxygen; 1.34 ml of oxygen can combine with 1 g Hb.

pancreas gland containing both exocrine and endocrine portions; exocrine secretions include enzymes and bicarbonate to digest food in the small intestine; endocrine secretions include insulin, glucagon, and somatostatin, which are released into the blood.

parasympathetic nervous system portion of the autonomic nervous system that primarily releases acetylcholine from its postganglionic nerve endings.

partial pressure the fractional part of the barometric pressure due to the presence of a single gas, e.g., PO_2, PCO_2, and PN_2.

percent grade a measure of the elevation of the treadmill; calculated as the sine of the angle.

percutaneous transluminal coronary angioplasty (PTCA) a balloon-tipped catheter is inserted into a blocked coronary artery and plaque is pushed back to artery wall to open the blood vessel.

perimysium the connective tissue surrounding the fasciculus of skeletal muscle fibers.

peripheral nervous system (PNS) portion of the nervous system located outside the spinal cord and brain.

pH a measure of the acidity of a solution; calculated as the negative $\log_{10}$ of the $[H^+]$ in which 7 is neutral; values that are >7 are basic and <7 are acidic.

phosphocreatine a compound found in skeletal muscle and used to resynthesize ATP from ADP.

phosphodiesterase an enzyme that catalyzes the breakdown of cyclic AMP, moderating the effect of the hormonal stimulation of adenylate cyclase.

phosphofructokinase rate-limiting enzyme in glycolysis that is responsive to ADP, P_i, and ATP levels in the cytoplasm of the cell.

phospholipase C membrane-bound enzyme that hydrolyzes phosphatidylinositol into inositol triphosphate and diacylglycerol that, in turn, bring about changes in intracellular activity.

physical activity characterizes all types of human movement; associated with living, work, play, and exercise.

physical fitness a broad term describing healthful levels of cardio-vascular function, strength, and flexibility; fitness is specific to the activities performed.

pituitary gland a gland at the base of the hypothalamus of the brain having an anterior portion that produces and secretes numerous hormones that regulate other endocrine glands and a posterior portion that secretes hormones that are produced in the hypothalamus.

placebo an inert substance that is used in experimental studies, e.g., drug studies, to control for any subjective reaction to the substance being tested.

pleura a thin lining of cells that is attached to the inside of the chest wall and to the lung; the cells secrete a fluid that facilitates the movements of the lungs in the thoracic cavity.

posterior hypothalamus area of the brain responsible for regulation of the body's response to a decrease in temperature.

posterior pituitary gland portion of the pituitary gland secreting oxytocin and antidiuretic hormone (vasopressin) that are produced in the hypothalamus.

power a rate of work; work per unit time; $P = W/t$.

power test a test measuring the quantity of work accomplished in a time period; anaerobic power tests include the Margaria stair climb test and the Wingate test; aerobic power tests include the 1.5-mile run and cycle ergometer and treadmill tests in which power output and oxygen consumption are measured.

primary risk factor a sign (e.g., high blood pressure) or a behavior (e.g., cigarette smoking) that is directly related to the appearance of certain diseases independent of other risk factors.

progressive resistance exercise (PRE) a training program in which the muscles must work against a gradually increasing resistance; an implementation of the overload principle.

prolactin hormone secreted from the anterior pituitary that increases milk production from the breast.

proprioceptive neuromuscular facilitation technique of preceding a static stretch with an isometric contraction.

proprioceptors receptors that provide information about the position and movement of the body; includes muscle and joint receptors as well as the receptors in the semicircular canals of the inner ear.

protein kinase C part of second messenger system that is activated by diacylglycerol and results in the activation of proteins in the cell.

provitamin a precursor of a vitamin.

pulmonary circuit the portion of the cardiovascular system involved in the circulation of blood from the right ventricle to the lungs and back to the left atrium.

pulmonary respiration term that refers to ventilation (breathing) of the lung.

Quebec 10-second test a maximal effort 10-second cycle test designed to assess ultra short-term anaerobic power during cycling.

radiation process of energy exchange from the surface of one object to the surface of another that is dependent on a temperature gradient but does not require contact between the objects; an example is the transfer of heat from the sun to the earth.

receptor in the nervous system, a receptor is a specialized portion of an afferent neuron (or a special cell attached to an afferent neuron) that is sensitive to a form of energy in the environment; *receptor* is also a term that applies to unique proteins on the surface of cells that can bind specific hormones or neurotransmitters.

reciprocal inhibition when extensor muscles (agonists) are contracted, there is a reflex inhibition of the motor neurons to the flexor muscles (antagonists), and vice versa.

Recommended Dietary Allowances (RDA) standards of nutrition associated with good health for the majority of people. Standards exist for protein, vitamins, and minerals for children and adults.

relative $\dot{V}O_2$ oxygen uptake (consumption) expressed per unit body weight (e.g., ml · kg^{-1} · min^{-1}).

releasing hormone hypothalamic hormones released from neurons into the anterior pituitary that control the release of hormones from that gland.

renin enzyme secreted by special cells in the kidney that converts angiotensinogen to angiotensin I.

repetition the number of times an exercise is repeated within a single exercise "set."

residual volume (RV) volume of air in the lungs following a maximal expiration.

respiration external respiration is the exchange of oxygen and carbon dioxide between the lungs and the environment; internal respiration describes the use of oxygen by the cell (mitochondria).

respiratory compensation the buffering of excess H^+ in the blood by plasma bicarbonate (HCO_3^-), and the associated elevation in ventilation to exhale the resulting CO_2.

respiratory exchange ratio (R) the ratio of CO_2 production to O_2 consumption; indicative of substrate utilization during steady-state exercise in which a value of 1.0 represents 100% carbohydrate metabolism and 0.7 represents 100% fat metabolism.

resting membrane potential the voltage difference measured across a membrane that is related to the concentration of ions on each side of the membrane and the permeability of the membrane to those ions.

resting metabolic rate (RMR) metabolic rate measured in the supine position following a period of fasting (4–12 hours) and rest (4–8 hours).

rest interval the time period between bouts in an interval training program.

reversibility a principle of training that describes the temporary nature of a training effect; adaptations to training are lost when the training stops.

sarcolemma the cell (plasma) membrane surrounding a muscle fiber.

sarcomeres the repeating contractile unit in a myofibril bounded by Z-lines.

sarcoplasmic reticulum a membranous structure that surrounds the myofibrils of muscle cells; location of the terminal cisternae or lateral sacs that store the Ca^{++} needed for muscle contraction.

satellite cells undifferentiated cell found adjacent to skeletal muscle fibers. These cells can fuse with existing muscle fibers and contribute to muscle growth (hypertrophy). It may also be possible that these fibers can differentiate and form a new muscle fiber following muscle injury.

Schwann cell the cell that surrounds peripheral nerve fibers, forming the myelin sheath.

second messenger a molecule (cyclic AMP) or ion (Ca^{++}) that increases in a cell as a result of an interaction between a "first messenger" (e.g., hormone or neurotransmitter) and a receptor that alters cellular activity.

secondary risk factor a characteristic (age, gender, race, body fatness) or behavior that increases the risk of coronary heart disease when primary risk factors are present.

set a basic unit of a workout containing the number of times (repetitions) a specific exercise is done (e.g., do three sets of five repetitions with 100 pounds).

sex steroids a group of hormones, androgens and estrogens, secreted from the adrenal cortex and the gonads.

sham reinfusion an experimental treatment at the end of a blood doping experiment in which a needle is placed in a vein, but the subject does not receive a reinfusion of blood.

sham withdrawal an experimental treatment at the beginning of a blood doping experiment in which a needle is placed in a vein, but blood is not withdrawn.

sinoatrial node (SA node) specialized tissue located in the right atrium of the heart, that generates the electrical impulse to initiate the heartbeat. In a normal, healthy heart, the SA node is the heart's pacemaker.

SI units system used to provide international standardization of units of measure in science.

sliding filament model a theory of muscle contraction describing the sliding of the thin filaments (actin) past the thick filaments (myosin).

slow-twitch fibers muscle fiber type that contracts slowly and develops relatively low tension but displays great endurance to repeated stimulation; contains many mitochondria, capillaries, and myoglobin.

somatomedins groups of growth-stimulating peptides released from the liver and other tissues in response to growth hormone. Also called insulin-like growth factors.

somatostatin hormone produced in the hypothalamus that inhibits growth hormone release from the anterior pituitary gland; secreted from cells in the islet of Langerhans and causes a decrease in intestinal activity.

somatotype body-type (form) classification method used to characterize the degree to which an individual's frame is linear (ectomorphic), muscular (mesomorphic), and round (endomorphic); Sheldon's scale rates each component on 1–7 scale.

spatial summation the additive effect of numerous simultaneous inputs to different sites on a neuron to produce a change in the membrane potential.

specificity   a principle of training indicating that the adaptation of a tissue is dependent on the type of training undertaken; for example, muscles hypertrophy with heavy resistance training but show an increase in mitochondria number with endurance training.

spirometry   measurement of various lung volumes.

static stretching   stretching procedure in which a muscle is stretched and held in the stretched position for ten to thirty seconds; in contrast to dynamic stretching, which involves motion.

steady state   describes the tendency of a control system to achieve a balance between an environmental demand and the response of a physiological system to meet that demand to allow the tissue (body) to function over a period of time.

steroids   a class of lipids, derived from cholesterol, that includes the hormones testosterone, estrogen, cortisol, and aldosterone.

stroke volume   the amount of blood pumped by the ventricles in a single beat.

strong acids   an acid that completely ionizes when dissolved in water to generate H^+ and its anion.

strong bases   a base (alkaline substance) that completely ionizes when dissolved in water to generate OH^- and its cation.

ST segment depression   an electrocardiographic change reflecting an ischemia (inadequate blood flow) in the heart muscle; indicative of coronary heart disease.

summation   repeated stimulation of a muscle that leads to an increase in tension compared to a single twitch.

supercompensation   an increase in the muscle glycogen content above normal levels following an exercise-induced muscle glycogen depletion and an increase in carbohydrate intake.

sympathetic nervous system   portion of the autonomic nervous system that releases norepinephrine from its postganglionic nerve endings; epinephrine is released from the adrenal medulla.

sympathomimetic   substance that mimics the effects of epinephrine or norepinephrine, which are secreted from the sympathetic nervous systems.

synapses   junctions between nerve cells (neurons) where the electrical activity of one neuron influences the electrical activity of the other neuron.

systole   portion of the cardiac cycle in which the ventricles are contracting.

systolic blood pressure   the highest arterial pressure measured during a cardiac cycle.

tapering   the process athletes use to reduce their training load for several days prior to competition.

target heart rate (THR) range   the range of heart rates describing the optimum intensity of exercise consistent with making gains in maximal aerobic power; equal to 70%–85% HR max.

temporal summation   a change in the membrane potential produced by the addition of two or more inputs, occurring at different times (i.e., inputs are added together to produce a potential change that is greater than that caused by a single input).

terminal cisternae   portion of the sarcoplasmic reticulum near the transverse tubule containing the Ca^{++} that is released upon depolarization of the muscle; also called *lateral sac*.

testosterone   the steroid hormone produced in the testes; involved in growth and development of reproductive tissues, sperm, and secondary sex characteristics.

tetanus   highest tension developed by a muscle in response to a high frequency of stimulation.

theophylline   a drug used as a smooth muscle relaxant in the treatment of asthma.

thermogenesis   the generation of heat as a result of metabolic reactions.

thyroid gland   endocrine gland located in the neck that secretes triiodothyronine (T_3) and thyroxine (T_4), which increase the metabolic rate.

thyroid-stimulating hormone (TSH)   hormone released from the anterior pituitary gland; stimulates the thyroid gland to increase its secretion of thyroxine and triiodothyronine.

thyroxine   hormone secreted from the thyroid gland containing four iodine atoms (T_4); stimulates the metabolic rate and facilitates the actions of other hormones.

tidal volume   volume of air inhaled or exhaled in a single breath.

tonus   low level of muscle activity at rest.

total lung capacity (TLC)   the total volume of air the lung can contain; equal to the sum of the vital capacity and the residual volume.

toxicity   a condition resulting from a chronic ingestion of vitamins, especially fat-soluble vitamins, in quantities well above that needed for health.

trace elements   dietary minerals including iron, zinc, copper, iodine, manganese, selenium, chromium, molybdenum, cobalt, arsenic, nickel, fluoride, and vanadium.

transferrin   plasma protein that binds iron and is representative of the whole body iron store.

transverse tubule   an extension, invagination, of the muscle membrane that conducts the action potential into the muscle to depolarize the terminal cisternae, which contain the Ca^{++} needed for muscle contraction.

triiodothyronine   hormone secreted from the thyroid gland containing three iodine atoms (T_3); stimulates the metabolic rate and facilitates the actions of other hormones.

tropomyosin   protein covering the actin binding sites that prevents the myosin cross-bridge from touching actin.

troponin   protein, associated with actin and tropomyosin, that binds Ca^{++} and initiates the movement of tropomyosin on actin to allow the myosin cross-bridge to touch actin and initiate contraction.

twenty-four-hour recall   a technique of recording the type and amount of food (nutrients) consumed during a twenty-four-hour period.

twitch   the tension-generating response following the application of a single stimulus to muscle.

type I fibers   fibers that contain large numbers of oxidative enzymes and are highly fatigue resistant.

type IIa fibers   fibers that contain biochemical and fatigue characteristics that are between Type IIb and Type I fibers.

type IIb fibers   fibers that have a relatively small number of mitochondria, a limited capacity for aerobic metabolism, and are less resistant to fatigue than slow fibers.

underwater weighing   procedure to estimate body volume by the loss of weight in water; result is used to calculate body density and, from that, body fatness.

U.S. Dietary Goals   a series of nutritional goals to achieve better health for the American population: 58% carbohydrate; 30% fat (no more than 10% saturated fat); and 12% protein.

vagus nerve   a major parasympathetic nerve.

variable-resistance exercise   strength training in which the resistance varies throughout the range of motion.

veins   the blood vessels that accept blood from the venules and bring it back to the heart.

ventilation   the movement of air into or out of the lungs (e.g., pulmonary or alveolar ventilation); external respiration.

ventilatory threshold (Tvent)   the "breakpoint" at which pulmonary ventilation and carbon dioxide output begin to increase exponentially during an incremental exercise test.

venules   small blood vessels carrying capillary blood to veins.

vestibular apparatus   sensory organ, consisting of three semicircular canals, that provides needed information about body position to maintain balance.

vital capacity (VC)   the volume of air that can be moved into or out of the lungs in one breath; equal to the sum of the inspiratory and expiratory reserve volumes and the tidal volume.

web of causation   an epidemiologic model showing the complex interaction of risk factors associated with the development of chronic degenerative diseases.

whole-body density   a measure of the weight-to-volume ratio of the entire body; high values are associated with low body fatness.

Wingate test   anaerobic power test to evaluate maximal rate at which glycolysis can deliver ATP.

work   the product of a force and the distance through which that force moves ($W = F \times D$).

work interval   in interval training, the duration of the work phase of each work-to-rest interval.

Credits

Illustrations and Photos

CHAPTER 1

Figure 1.1A: Courtesy of Carnegie Institute of Washington, DC.
Figure 1.1B: Courtesy of Quinton Instrument Co.
Figures 1.2 and 1.3: Courtesy of W. B. Saunders Company.

CHAPTER 3

Figures 3.1 and 3.7: From Stuart Ira Fox, *Human Physiology*, 9th ed. New York: McGraw-Hill Companies, 2006.
Figure 3.2: From Rod R. Seeley, Trent D. Stephens, Philip Tate, *Anatomy and Physiology*, 6th ed., New York: McGraw-Hill, 2003.
Figures 3.3, 3.4, 3.6, 3.10, 3.11, and 3.16: From Stuart Ira Fox, *Human Physiology*, 5th ed. Copyright © 1996 Times Mirror Higher Education Group, Inc., Dubuque, IA. All Rights Reserved. Reprinted by permission.
Figures 3.5 and 3.22: From Stuart Ira Fox, *Human Physiology*, 7th ed., New York: McGraw-Hill, 2002.
Figures 3.12 and 3.17: From *Biochemistry* by C. K. Mathews and K. E. van Holde. Copyright © 1990 by The Benjamin/Cummings Publishing Company. Reprinted with permission.
Figure 3.13: Redrawn from Stuart Ira Fox, *Human Physiology*, 9th ed. New York: McGraw-Hill Companies, 2006.
Figure 3.19: From Stuart Ira Fox, *Human Physiology*, 4th ed. Copyright © 1993 Times Mirror Higher Education Group, Inc., Dubuque, IA. All Rights Reserved. Reprinted by permission.
Figure 3.20: From E. Widmaier, H. Raff, and K. Strong. *Vander's Human Physiology*, 10th ed., New York: McGraw-Hill Companies, 2006.
Figure 3.24: From S. K. Powers and S. L. Dodd, *Total Fitness: Exercise, Nutrition, and Wellness*, 2nd ed., Copyright © 1999 Allyn & Bacon, Needham Heights, MA. Reprinted by permission.

CHAPTER 4

Figure 4.4: From S. Dodd, 1984, "Blood Lactate Disappearance at Various Intensities of Recovery Exercise" in *Journal of Applied Physiology*, 57:1462–1465. Copyright © 1984 American Physiological Society, Bethesda, MD. Used by permission.
Figure 4.11: From G. Brooks and J. Mercier, "Balance of Carbohydrate and Lipid Utilization During Exercise: The 'Crossover Concept'" in *Journal of Applied Physiology*, 76:2253–2261, 1994. Copyright © 1994 American Physiological Society. Reprinted by permission.
Figures 4.15 and 4.16: From E. Coyle, "Substrate Utilization During Exercise in Active People" in *American Journal of Clinical Nutrition*, 61 (Suppl): 9685–9795, 1995. Copyright © 1995 American Society for Clinical Nutrition, Inc., Bethesda, MD. Reprinted by permission.
Figure 4.17: From Stuart Ira Fox, *Human Physiology*, 5th ed. Copyright © 1996 Times Mirror Higher Education Group, Inc., Dubuque, IA. All rights reserved. Reprinted by permission.

CHAPTER 5

Figure 5.1: From A. J. Vander et al., *Human Physiology: The Mechanisms of Body Function*, 4th ed. Copyright © 1985 McGraw-Hill, Inc., New York. Reprinted with permission.
Figure 5.2: From Stuart Ira Fox, *Human Physiology*, 3rd ed. Copyright © 1990 Times Mirror Higher Education Group, Inc., Dubuque, IA. All rights reserved. Reprinted by permission.
Figure 5.5: From Kent M., Van de Graaff, and Stuart Ira Fox, *Concepts of Human Anatomy and Physiology*, 4th ed. Copyright © 1995 Times Mirror Higher Education Group, Inc., Dubuque, IA. All rights reserved. Reprinted with permission.
Figure 5.7: Data from V .A. Convertino, L. C. Keil, and J. E. Greenleaf 1983, "Plasma Volume, Renin and Vasopressin Responses to Graded Exercises After Training." American Physiological Association, Bethesda, MD: *Journal of Applied Physiology: Respiration Environment Exercise Physiology*, 54: 508–514.
Figure 5.8: Data from J. T. Maher, et al., 1975, "Aldersterone Dynamics During Graded Exercises at Sea-level and High Altitudes." American Physiological Society, Bethesda, MD: *Journal of Applied Physiology* 39:18–22.
Figure 5.12: Data from J. E. Turkowski, et al., 1978, "Ovarian Hormonal Responses to Exercise." American Physiological Society, Bethesda, MD: *Journal of Applied Physiology: Respiration Environment Exercise Physiology*, 44:109–114.
Figure 5.13: Reprinted with permission from B. Saltin and J. Karlsson, 1971, *Muscle Metabolism During Exercise*, pp. 289–299, edited by B. Pernow and B. Saltin. Copyright © 1971 Plenum Press, New York, NY.
Figure 5.14: From M. Kjaer, 1989, "Epinephrine and Some Other Hormonal Responses to Exercise in Man. With Special Reference to Physical Training" in *International Journal of Sports Medicine*, 10:2–15. Copyright © 1989 Georg Thieme Verlag, Stuttgart, Germany. Reprinted by permission.
Figure 5.15: From R. C. Harris, et al., "The Effect of Propranolol on Glycogen Metabolism During Exercise" in *Muscle Metabolism During Exercise*, B. Pernow & B. Saltin, Eds. Copyright © 1971 Plenum Publishing Corporation, New York. Reprinted by permission.
Figure 5.18: Data from C. T. M. Davies and J. D. Few, 1973, "Effects of Exercise on Adrenocortical Function," American Physiological Society, Bethesda, MD: *Journal of Applied Physiology*, 35:887–891.
Figure 5.20A: Data from J. Sutton and L. Lazarus, 1976, "Growth Hormone in Exercise: Comparison of Physiological and Pharmacological Stimuli." American Physiological Society, Bethesda, MD: *Journal of Applied Physiology*, 41:523–527.
Figure 5.20B: Data from J. C. Bunt, et al. 1986, "Sex and Training Differences in Human Growth Hormone Levels During Prolonged Exercise." American Physiological Society, Bethesda, MD: *Journal of Applied Physiology*, 61:1796–1801.
Figure 5.22: Data from Scott Powers, et al., 1982, "A Different Catecholamine Response during Prolonged Exercise and Passive Heating." American College of Sports Medicine, Indianapolis, IN: *Medicine and Science in Sports and Exercise*, 14:435–439.
Figure 5.23: From W. W. Winder, et al., 1978, "Time Course of Sympathadrenal Adaptation to Endurance Exercise Training in Man" in *Journal of Applied Physiology: Respiration Environment Exercise Physiology*, 45:370–377. Copyright © 1978 The American Physiological Society, Bethesda, MD. Reprinted with permission.

Figure 5.25A: Data from L. H. Harley, et al., 1972, "Multiple Hormonal Responses to Graded Exercise in Relation to Physical Training." American Physiological Society, Bethesda, MD: *Journal of Applied Physiology*, 33:602–606.

Figures 5.25B and 5.26: Data from F. Gyntelberg, et al., 1977, "Effect of Training on the Response of Plasma Glucagon to Exercise." American Physiological Society, Bethesda, MD: *Journal of Applied Physiology: Respiration Environment Exercise Physiology*, 43:302–305.

Figure 5.30A: From: J. Issekutz and H. Miller, "Plasma-free Fatty Acids During Exercise and the Effect of Lactic Acid." 1962, in *Proceedings of the Society for Experimental Biology and Medicine*, 110:237–239. Copyright © 1962 Society for Experimental Biology and Medicine, New York. Reprinted with permission.

CHAPTER 6

Figure 6.1A: From W. E. Prentice, *Get Fit, Stay Fit*, 3rd ed. Copyright © 2004 The McGraw-Hill Companies, Inc. Reprinted by permission.

Figures 6.1B and 6.1E: Courtesy of Monark Exercise AB, Sweden.

Figures 6.1C and 6.1D: Copyright © Comstock Images/Alamy.

Figures 6.4 and 6.7: MasterScreen CPX, courtesy of VIASYS Healthcare, Höchberg, Germany.

Figure 6.10: From J. Coast and H. G. Welch, 1985, "Linear Increase in Optimal Pedal Rate with Increased Power Output in Cycle Ergometry" in *European Journal of Applied Physiology*, 53:339–342. Copyright © Springer-Verlag, Heidelberg, Germany. Reprinted by permission.

Figure 6.11: From P. Hopkins and S. Powers, 1982, "Oxygen Uptake during Submaximal Running in Highly Trained Men and Women" in *American Corrective Therapy Journal*, 36:130–132 (Now *Clinical Kinesiology: Journal of the American Kinesiotherapy Association*) (formerly the American Corrective Therapy Association). Reprinted by permission.

CHAPTER 7

Figure 7.1: From E. Widmaier, H. Raff, and K. Strang, *Vander's Human Physiology*, 10th ed, New York: McGraw-Hill Companies, 2006.

Figures 7.3, 7.9, 7.10, and 7.17: From David Shier, et al., *Hole's Human Anatomy and Physiology*, 7th ed. Copyright © 1996 Times Mirror Higher Education Group, Inc., Dubuque, IA. All rights reserved. Reprinted with permission.

Figure 7.4: From John W. Hole, Jr., *Human Anatomy and Physiology*, 3rd ed., Copyright © 1984 Times Mirror Higher Education Group, Inc., Dubuque, IA. All rights reserved. Reprinted by permission.

Figures 7.5, 7.6, 7.7, and 7.8: From Stuart Ira Fox. *Human Physiology*, 9th ed, New York: McGraw-Hill Companies, 2006.

Figure 7.11: From A.J. Vander et al., *Human Physiology: The Mechanisms of Body Function*, 4th ed. Copyright © 1985 McGraw-Hill, Inc., New York. Reprinted by permission.

Figure 7.12: From John W. Hole, Jr., *Human Anatomy and Physiology*, 5th ed., Copyright © 1990 Times Mirror Higher Education Group, Inc., Dubuque, IA. All rights reserved. Reprinted by permission.

Figure 7.13: From Stuart Ira Fox, *Human Physiology*. Copyright © 1984 Times Mirror Higher Education Group, Inc., Dubuque, IA. All Rights Reserved. Reprinted with permission.

Figure 7.15: From Kent M. Van de Graaff and Stuart Ira Fox, *Concepts of Human Anatomy and Physiology*, 2nd ed. Copyright © 1989 Times Mirror Higher Education Group, Inc., Dubuque, IA. All rights reserved. Reprinted by permission.

CHAPTER 8

Figures 8.1, 8.2, and 8.4: From David Shier, et al., *Hole's Human Anatomy and Physiology*, 7th ed. Copyright © 1996 Times Mirror Higher Education Group, Inc., Dubuque, IA. All rights reserved. Reprinted with permission.

Figures 8.3 and 8.6: From Stuart Ira Fox, *Human Physiology*, 5th ed. Copyright © 1996 Times Mirror Higher Education Group, Inc., Dubuque, IA. All rights reserved. Reprinted with permission.

Figures 8.5, 8.21, and 8.22: From Rod R. Seeley, Trent D. Stephens, Philip Tate, *Anatomy and Physiology*, 6th ed., New York: McGraw-Hill, 2003.

Figures 8.7 and 8.9: From A. J. Vander et al., *Human Physiology: The Mechanisms of Body Function*, 4th ed. Copyright © 1985 McGraw-Hill, Inc., New York. Reprinted with permission.

Figure 8.11: From R. Bottinelli, et al., "Myofibrillar ATPase Activity During Isometric Contractions and Myosin Composition in Rat Single-skinned Muscle Fibers," 1994, in *Journal of Physiology (London)*, 481:633–675. Copyright © 1994 Physiological Society, London. Reprinted by permission.

Figure 8.14: From S. Fox. *Human Physiology*, 7th ed, New York: McGraw-Hill Companies, 2002.

Figure 8.17: From Stuart Ira Fox, *Human Physiology*, 2nd ed. Copyright © 1987 Times Mirror Higher Education Group, Inc., Dubuque, IA. All rights reserved. Reprinted with permission.

CHAPTER 9

Figure 9.1: From John W. Hole, Jr., *Human Anatomy and Physiology*, 5th ed., Copyright © 1995 Times Mirror Higher Education Group, Inc., Dubuque, IA. All rights reserved. Reprinted by permission.

Figures 9.2, 9.15, and 9.17: From E. Widmaier, H. Raff, and K. Strang, *Vander's Human Physiology*, 10th ed, New York: McGraw-Hill Companies, 2006.

Figure 9.7: From Stuart Ira Fox, *A Laboratory Guide to Human Physiology: Concepts and Clinical Applications*, 4th ed. Copyright © 1987 Times Mirror Higher Education Group, Inc., Dubuque, IA. All rights reserved. Reprinted with permission.

Figures 9.8 and 9.16: From David Shier, et al., *Hole's Human Anatomy and Physiology*, 7th ed. Copyright © 1996 Times Mirror Higher Education Group, Inc., Dubuque, IA. All rights reserved. Reprinted with permission.

Figures 9.9, 9.10, 9.18, 9.20, and 9.21: From Stuart Ira Fox, *Human Physiology*, 5th ed. Copyright © 1996 Times Mirror Higher Education Group, Inc., Dubuque, IA. All rights reserved. Reprinted with permission.

Figures 9.11 and 9.14: From Kent M. Van de Graaf and Stuart Ira Fox, *Concepts of Human Anatomy and Physiology*, 4th ed. Copyright © 1995 Times Mirror Higher Education Group, Inc., Dubuque, IA. All rights reserved. Reprinted by permission.

Figure 9.12: Reprinted by permission of the publisher from Averill: "Critical Decisions in Cardiac Emergencies." *Emergency Medicine*, 2(2):63–79. Copyright © 1979 by Excerpta Medica, Inc.

Figure 9.13: From Stuart Ira Fox. *Human Physiology*, 9th ed, New York: McGraw-Hill Companies, 2006.

Figure 9.19: From Stuart Ira Fox, *Human Physiology*, 4th ed. Copyright © 1993 Times Mirror Higher Education Group, Inc., Dubuque, IA. All rights reserved. Reprinted with permission.

Figure 9.22: Data from L. Rowell, 1993, "Human Cardiovascular Adjustments to Exercise and Thermal Stress." American Physiological Society, Bethesda, MD: *Physiological Reviews*, 74:911–915 and L. Rowell, 1986, *Human Circulation Regulation During Physical Stress*. New York, NY: Oxford University Press.

Figure 9.23: Data from L. Rowell, 1986, *Human Circulation: Regulation During Physical Stress*. New York, NY: Oxford University Press.

Figure 9.24: From P. Astrand and K. Rodahl, *Textbook of Work Physiology*, 3rd ed. Copyright © 1986 McGraw-Hill Inc., New York. Reprinted by permission of the authors.

Figure 9.25: Data from L. Rowell, 1974, "Human Cardiovascular Adjustments to Exercise and Thermal Stress." American Physiological Society, Bethesda, MD: *Physiological Reviews*, 54:75–159 and L. Rowell, *Human Circulation: Regulation During Physical Stress*, 1986, New York, NY: Oxford University Press.

Figure 9.26: Data from P. Astrand, et al., 1965, Intra-arterial Blood Pressure During Exercise with Different Muscle Groups." American Physiological Society, Bethesda, MD: *Journal of Applied Physiology*, 20:253–257.

Figure 9.27: Data from G. Brenglemann, 1983. "Circulatory Adjustments to Exercise and Heat Stress," Annual Reviews, Inc., Palo Alto, CA: *Annual Review of Physiology*, 45:191–212; E. Fox and D. Costill, 1972, "Estimated Cardiorespiratory Responses during Marathon Running," Heldref Publications, Washington, DC: *Archives of Environmental Health*, 24:315–324; and L. Rowell, 1974, "Human Cardiovascular Adjustments to Exercise and Thermal Stress." American Physiological Society, Bethesda, MD: *Physiological Reviews*, 54:75–159.

CHAPTER 10

Figures 10.1, 10.3, and 10.11: From E. Widmaier, H. Raff, and K. Strang, *Vander's Human Physiology*, 10th ed, New York: McGraw-Hill Companies, 2006.

Figures 10.2, 10.5, 10.6, and 10.7: From Kent M. Van de Graaff and Stuart Ira Fox, *Concepts of Human Anatomy and Physiology*, 4th ed. Copyright © 1995 Times Mirror Higher Education Group, Inc., Dubuque, IA. All rights reserved. Reprinted by permission.

Figures 10.4, 10.19, 10.20, 10.24, and 10.25: From Fox S. *Human Physiology*, 9th ed, New York: McGraw-Hill Companies, 2006.

Figure 10.8: Courtesy of Sensor-Medics Corporation.

Figure 10.9: From John W. Hole, Jr., *Human Anatomy and Physiology*, 5th ed., Copyright © 1995 Times Mirror Higher Education Group, Inc., Dubuque, IA. All rights reserved. Reprinted by permission.

Figures 10.15, 10.16, and 10.18: From Stuart Ira Fox, *Human Physiology*, 5th ed. Copyright © 1996 Times Mirror Higher Education Group, Inc., Dubuque, IA. All rights reserved. Reprinted with permission.

Figure 10.17: From Stuart Ira Fox, *Human Physiology*, 3rd ed. Copyright © 1990 Times Mirror Higher Education Group, Inc., Dubuque, IA. All rights reserved. Reprinted with permission.

Figure 10.21: Data from J. Dempsey and R. Fregosi, 1985, "Adaptability of the Pulmonary System to Changing Metabolic Requirements," Yorke Medical Group, New York, NY: *American Journal of Cardiology*, 55:59D-67D; J. Dempsey, et al., 1986, "Is the Lung Built for Exercise?" American College of Sports Medicine, Indianapolis, IN: *Medicine and Science in Sports and Exercise*, 18:143–155; and S. Powers, et al., 1985, "Caffeine Alters Ventilatory and Gas Exchange Kinetics during Exercise" American College of Sports Medicine, Indianapolis, IN: *Medicine and Science in Sports and Exercise*, 18:101–106.

Figure 10.22: Data from J. Dempsey, et al., 1986. "Is the Lung Built for Exercise?" American College of Sports Medicine, Indianapolis, IN: *Medicine and Science in Sports and Exercise*, 18:143–155; and S. Powers, et al., 1982, "Ventilatory and Metabolic Reactions to Heat Stress During Prolonged Exercise" International Federation of Sportive Medicine, Turin, Italy: *Journal of Sports Medicine and Physical Fitness*, 22:32–36.

Figure 10.23: Data from J. Dempsey, et al., 1982, "Limitation to Exercise Capacity and Endurance: Pulmonary System" University of Toronto, Ontario, Canada: *Canadian Journal of Applied Sports Sciences*, 7:4–13; and K. Wasserman, et al., 1973, "Anaerobic Threshold and Respiratory Gas Exchange during Exercise" American Physiological Society, Bethesda, MD, *Journal of Applied Physiology*, 35:236–243.

CHAPTER 11

Figure 11-4: Data from E. Hultman and K. Sahlin, 1980, "Acid-base Balance during Exercise," in R. Hutton and D. Miller, Eds. Franklin Institute Press, Philadelphia, PA: *Exercise and Sport Science Reviews*, 8:41–128; N. Jones, et al., 1977, "Effects of pH on Cardiorespiratory and Metabolic Responses to Exercise," American Physiological Society, Bethesda, MD, *Journal of Applied Physiology*, 43:969–964;

and A. Katz, et al., 1984, "Maximum Exercise Tolerance after Induced Alkalosis," Stuttgart, Germany: *International Journal of Sports Medicine*, 5:107–110.

Figure 11.5: Data from E. Hultman and K. Sahlin, 1986, "Acid-base Balance during Exercise," R. Hutton and D. Miller, Eds. Orlando, FL, Academic Press, Inc.: *Exercise and Sport Science Reviews*, 8:41–128.

CHAPTER 12

Figure 12.10: Data from G. Brengelmann, 1977, "Control of Sweating and Skin Flow During Exercise," E. Nadel, Ed. Academic Press, Inc., Orlando, FL: *Problems with Temperature Regulation During Exercise*, and S. Powers, et al., 1982, "Ventilatory and Metabolic Reactions to Heat Stress During Prolonged Exercise," International Federation of Sportive Medicine, Turin, Italy: *Journal of Sports Medicine and Physical Fitness*, 2:32–36.

CHAPTER 13

Figure 13.4: From. E. F. Coyle, et al., 1984, "Time Course of Loss of Adaptation after Stopping Prolonged Intense Endurance Training" in *Journal of Applied Physiology*, 57:1857–1864. Copyright © 1984 American Physiological Society, Bethesda, MD. Reprinted by permission.

Figure 13.5: From T. J. Terjung, "Muscle Adaptations to Aerobic Training" in *Sports Science Exchange*, Vol. 6, No. 6, 1993. Copyright © 1993 Gatorade Sports Science Institute, Barrington, IL. Reprinted with permission.

Figure 13.6: Data from S. Powers, et al., 1994, "Influence of Exercise and Fiber Type on Antioxidant Enzyme Activity in Rat Skeletal Muscle" American Physiological Society, Bethesda, MD: *American Journal of Physiology*, 266:R375-380.

Figure 13.12: Reprinted with permission from D.Neiman, "Exercise, Infection, and Immunity" in *International Journal of Sports Medicine* 75 (1994) S131-S141, Georg Thieme Verlag, Stuttgart, Germany.

Figure 13.16: From D. G. Sale, 1988, "Neural Adaptations to Resistance Training" in *Medicine and Science in Sports and Exercise*, 20:S135-S143. Copyright © 1988 American College of Sports Medicine, Indianapolis, IN. Reprinted by permission.

CHAPTER 14

Figure 14.1: Data from R. Farmer and D. Miller, 1991, *Lecture Notes on Epidemiology and Public Health Medicine*. Boston, MA: Blackwell Scientific Publications, pp. 107–111.

Figure 14.2: Data from R. A. Stallones, 1966, U.S. Government Printing Office, Washington, DC: *Public Health Monograph 76*; and I.H. R. Rockett, 1994, "Population and Health: An Introduction to Epidemiology" Population Reference Bureau, Washington, DC: *Population and Health: An Introduction to Epidemiology*, 49(3):1–48.

Figure 14.3: Source: U.S. Department of Health, Education and Welfare, 1979, *Healthy People: The Surgeon General's Report on Health Promotion and Disease Prevention*.

Figure 14.4: From C. J. Casperson, "Physical Activity Epidemiology: Concepts, Methods, and Applications to Exercise Science," edited by K. B. Pandolf in *Exercise and Sport Science Reviews*, 17:457, 1989. Copyright © 1989 Williams & Wilkins, Baltimore, MD. Reprinted by permission.

Figure 14.5: Data from N. M. Kaplan, 1989, "The Deadly Quartet." American Medical Association, Chicago, IL: *Archives of Internal Medicine*, 149:1514–1520; and A. P. Rocchini, 1991, "Insulin Resistance and Blood Pressure Regulation in Obese and Nonobese Subjects." American Heart Association, Dallas, TX: *Hypertension*, 17:837–842.

CHAPTER 15

Figure 15.2: Copyright © Canadian Society for Exercise Physiology.

Figure 15.3: From A. D. Martin, "ECG and Medications" in E. T. Howley and B. D. Franks, *Health/Fitness Instructor's Handbook*. Copyright © 1986 Human Kinetics Publishers, Inc., Champaign, IL. Used by permission.

Figures 15.5, 15.7, and 15.9: From E. T. Howley and B. D. Franks. *Health/Fitness Instructor's Handbook.* Copyright © 1986 Human Kinetics Publishers, Inc., Champaign, IL. Used by permission.

Figure 15.6: From the YMCA Fitness Testing and Assessment Manual. Copyright © 2000 YMCA of the USA. Reprinted by permission.

CHAPTER 16

Figure 16.1: Data from L. S. Goodman and A. Gilman, eds., 1975, *The Pharmacological Basis of Therapeutics.* New York: Macmillan Publishing Company.

Figure 16.2: From G. L. Jennings, G. Deakin, P. Komer, T. Meridith, B. Kingwell, and L. Nelson, 1991. "What Is the Dose-Response Relationship between Exercise Training and Blood Pressure?" in *Annals of Medicine*, 23:313–318, Royal Society of Medicine Press, Inc.

Figure 16.3: Data from R. R. Pate, et al., 1995, "Physical Activity and Public Health" in *Journal of the American Medical Association*, 273:402–407, Chicago, IL: American Medical Association.

Figure 16.4: Data from M. M. Dehn and C. B. Mullins, 1977, "Physiologic Effects and Importance of Exercise in Patients with Coronary Artery Disease," Group Medicine Publications, Inc., New York, NY: *Cardiovascular Medicine*, 2:365; and H. K. Hellerstein and B. A. Franklin, 1984. John Wiley & Sons, Inc., New York, NY: *Rehabilitation of the Coronary Patient*, 2nd ed.

CHAPTER 17

Figure 17.1: From M. Berger, et al., 1977, "Metabolic and Hormonal Effects of Muscular Exercise in Juvenile Type "Diabetics" in *Diabetologia*, 13:355–365. Copyright © 1977 Springer-Verlag, New York, NY. Reprinted by permission.

Figure 17.2: From E. R. Richter and H. Galbo, 1986, "Diabetes, Insulin and Exercise" in *Sports Medicine*, 3:275–288. Copyright © 1986 Adis Press, Langhorn, PA. Reprinted by permission.

CHAPTER 18

Figure 18.2: Adapted from M. L. Pollock and J. H. Wilmore, *Exercise in Health and Disease*, 2nd ed., 1990. Philadelphia, PA: W. B. Saunders.

Figure 18.3: From T. G. Lohman, "The Use of Skinfold to Estimate Body Fatness in Children and Youth" in *Journal of Health, Physical Education, Recreation and Dance*, 98:102, November-December 1987. Copyright © 1987 American Alliance for Health, Physical Recreation and Dance, Reston, VA. Reprinted by permission.

Figure 18.6: From E. Jequier, "Calorie Balance vs Nutrient Balance" in *Energy Metabolism: Tissue Determinants and Cellular Corollaries*, John M. Kinney and Hugh N. Tucker, Eds. Copyright © 1992 Raven Press. Reprinted by permission of Lippincott-Raven Publishers, a Wolters Kluwer Company, New York.

Figure 18.7: From A. Keys, et al., *The Biology of Human Starvation*, Vol. 1. Copyright © 1950 University of Minnesota Press, Minneapolis, MN. Reprinted by permission.

Figure 18.8: From L. O. Schulz and D. A. Scholler, "A Compilation of Total Energy Expenditures and Body Weights in Healthy Adults" in *American Journal of Clinical Nutrition*, 60:676–81, 1994. Copyright © 1994 American Society for Clinical Nutrition, Inc., Bethesda, MD. Reprinted by permission.

Figure 18.10: From J. Mayer, et al., "Exercise, Food Intake, and Body Weight in Normal Rats and Genetically Obese Mice" in *American Journal of Physiology*, 177:544–548. Copyright © 1954 American Physiological Society, Bethesda, MD. Used by permission.

CHAPTER 19

Figure 19.1: From P. Astrand and K. Rodahl, *Textbook of Work Physiology*, 2nd ed. Copyright © 1977 McGraw-Hill, Inc., New York, NY. Reprinted by permission.

Figure 19.2: From H. Gibson and R. H. T. Edwards, 1985, "Muscular Exercise and Fatigue" in *Sports Medicine*, 2:120–132. Copyright © 1985 Adis Press, Langhorn, PA. Reprinted by permission.

Figure 19.3: From D. G. Sale, "Influence of Exercise and Training in Motor Unit Activation" in Kent B. Pandolf, Ed., *Exercise and Sport Sciences Review*, Vol. 15. Copyright © 1987 McGraw-Hill, Inc., New York. Reprinted by permission.

CHAPTER 20

Figure 20.5: Reprinted with permission from B. Scott and J. Houmard, "Peak Running Velocity Is Highly Related to Distance Running Performance" in *International Journal of Sports Medicine*, 75 (1994) 504–507, Georg Thieme Verlag, Stuttgart, Germany.

Figure 20.9: From P. Astrand and K. Rodahl, *Textbook of Work Physiology*, 2nd ed. Copyright © 1977 McGraw-Hill, Inc., New York, NY. Reprinted by permission.

Figure 20.11: Photo courtesy of Biodex Medical Sytems, Inc.

Figure 20.12: Photo courtesy of Lafayette Instrument Company.

Figure 20.13: Photo courtesy of Biodex Medical Systems, Inc.

CHAPTER 21

Figure 21.2: From M. Ikai and T. Fukunaga, 1968, "Calculation of Muscle Strength per Unit of Cross Sectional Area of a Human Muscle by Means of Ultrasonic Measurement" in *Internationale Zeitschrift fuer Angewanted Physiologie*, 26:26–31. Copyright © 1968 Springer-Verlag, Heidelberg, Germany. Reprinted by permission.

Figure 21.3: From J. Wilmore, et al., 1974, "Alterations in Strength, Body Composition, and Anthrometric Measurements Consequent to a 10-Week Weight Training Program" in *Medicine and Science in Sports*, 6:133–139. Copyright © 1974 American College of Sports Medicine, Indianapolis, IN. Reprinted by permission.

CHAPTER 22

Figure 22.5: From Kent M. Van de Graaff, *Human Anatomy*, 4th ed. Copyright © 1995 Times Mirror Higher Education Group, Inc., Dubuque, IA. All rights reserved. Reprinted by permission.

CHAPTER 23

Figure 23.1: From J. Bergstrom, et al., 1967, "Diet, Muscle Glycogen and Physical Performance" in *Acta Physiologica Scandinavica* 71:140–150. Copyright © 1967 Scandinavian Physiological Society, Stockholm Sweden. Reprinted by permission of Blackwell Scientific Publications, Ltd., Oxford, England.

Figure 23.2: From W. M. Sherman, 1983, "Carbohydrates, Muscle Glycogen, and Muscle Glycogen Super Compensation" in *Ergogenic Aids in Sports*, pp. 3–26, edited by M. H. Williams. Copyright © 1983 Human Kinetics Publishers, Inc., Champaign, IL. Used with permission.

Figure 23.3: From John O. Halloszy, Ed., in *Exercise and Sport Science Reviews*, 19:982, 1991. Copyright © 1991 Williams & Wilkins, Baltimore, MD. Reprinted with permission.

Figure 23.5: Data from P. W. R. Lemon and J. P. Mullin, 1980, "Effect of Initial Muscle Group Glycogen Levels on Protein Catabolism During Exercise" American Physiological Society, Bethesda, MD: *American Journal of Applied Physiology*, 48:624–629.

Figure 23.6: From C. T. M. Davies, et al., 1982, "Glucose Inhibits CO2 Production from Leucine during Whole Body Exercise in Man" in *Journal of Physiology*, 332:40–41. Copyright © 1982 Cambridge University Press, Cambridge, England. Reprinted by permission.

Figure 23.7: From. E. F. Coyle and S. J. Montain, 1995, "Benefits of Fluid Replacement with Carbohydrate During Exercise," in *Medicine and Science in Sports and Exercise*, 24:S324-S330. Copyright © 1995 Williams & Wilkins Company, Baltimore, MD. Reprinted by permission.

Figure 23.8: From D. L. Costill and B. Saltin, 1974, "Factors Limiting Gastric Emptying during Rest and Exercise" in *Journal of Applied Physiology*, 37:679–683. Copyright © 1974 American Physiological Association, Bethesda, MD. Reprinted with permission.

Figure 23.9: From K. Davies, et al., 1982, "Muscle Mitochondrial Bioenergetics, Oxygen Supply, and Work Capacity during Dietary Iron Deficiency and Repletion" in *Journal of Applied Physiology*, 242:E418-E427. Copyright © 1982 American Physiological Association, Bethesda, MD. Used by permission.

Figure 23.10: Photo courtesy of W. H. Sheldon Trust.

Figure 23.11: From J. M. Tanner, et al., *The Physique of the Olympic Athlete*. Copyright © 1964 George Allen & Unwin Publishers, Ltd., London England. Reprinted by permission.

CHAPTER 24

Figure 24.1: From E. T. Howley, "Comparison of Performances in Short Races in the 1964 and 1968 Olympic Games," in G. A. Stull and T. K. Cureton, *Encyclopedia of Physical Education, Fitness and Sports: Training, Environment, Nutrition and Fitness.* Copyright © 1980 American Alliance for Health, Physical Education, Recreation and Dance, Reston, VA. Reprinted by permission.

Figure 24.2: Data from Grover et al., 1967, "Muscular Exercise in Young Men Native to 3,100 m Altitude," American Physiological Society, Bethesda, MD: *American Journal of Applied Physiology* 22:555–564.

Figure 24.3: Data from L. G. C. E. Pugh, 1964, "Muscular Exercise at Great Altitudes," American Physiological Society, Bethesda, MD: *Journal of Applied Physiology*, 19:431–440.

Figure 24.4: From J. B. West and P. D. Wagner, 1980, "Predicted Gas Exchange on the Summit of Mt. Everest" in *Respiration Physiology*, 42:1–16. Copyright © 1980 Elsevier Biomedical Press, Amsterdam, The Netherlands. Reprinted by permission.

Figure 24.5: From J. B. West, et al., 1983, "Barometric Pressures at Extreme Altitudes on Mt. Everest: Physiological Significance" in *Journal of Applied Physiology*, 54:1188–1194.

Copyright © 1983 American Physiological Society, Bethesda, MD. Reprinted by permission.

Figure 24.7: From D. K. Mathews, et al., 1969, "Physiological Responses during Exercise and Recovery in a Football Uniform" in *Journal of Applied Physiology*, 26: 611–615. Copyright © 1969 American Physiological Society, Bethesda, MD. Reprinted by permission.

Figure 24.9: Data from G. W. Molnar, 1946. American Medical Association, Chicago, IL: *Journal of the American Medical Association*, 131:1046–1050.

Figure 24.10: From A. C. Burton and O. G. Edholm, *Man in a Cold Environment.* Copyright © 1955 Edward Arnold Publishers. Reprinted by permission of Edward Arnold Publishers, Division of Hodder & Stoughton Ltd., London, England.

Figure 24.11: From P. B. Raven, et al., 1974, "Effect of Carbon Monoxide and Peroxacetyle Nitrate on Man's Maximal Aerobic Capacity" in *Journal of Applied Physiology*, 36:288–293. Copyright © 1974 American Physiological Society, Bethesda, MD. Reprinted by permission.

CHAPTER 25

Figure 25.1: Data from G. Ariel and W. Saville, 1972. "Anabolic Steroids: The Physiological Effects of Placebos," American College of Sports Medicine, Indianapolis, IN: *Medicine and Science in Sports and Exercise*, 4:124–126.

Figure 25.2: From H. W. Welch, "Effects of Hypoxia and Hyperpoxia on Human Performance" in Kent B. Pandolf, Ed., *Exercise and Sport Sciences Reviews*, vol. 15. Copyright © 1987 McGraw-Hill, Inc., New York. Reprinted by permission.

Figure 25.3: From N. Gledhill, 1982, "Blood Doping and Related Issues: A Brief Review" in *Medicine and Science in Sports and Exercise*, 14:183–189. Copyright © 1982 American College of Sports Medicine, Indianapolis, IN. Reprinted by permission.

Figure 25.6: From John D. Cantwell, "Cocaine and Cardiovascular Events," in *The Physician and Sports Medicine,*14 (11):77–82. Copyright © 1986 McGraw-Hill Healthcare, Minneapolis, MN. Reprinted with permission.

Index

Page numbers for boxes are indicated by b, figures, by f, and tables by t.

A

Abbott, Bud, 4b
acclimatization
  cold, 256–257
  heat, 252b, 253, 254–256, 255b, 256t
  heat injuries and, 510
  heat shock proteins, 255, 255b
  loss of, 256
acetylcholine, 75, 145f
  in autonomic nervous system, 136
  in excitation-contraction coupling, 150b
  in heart rate regulation, 129, 182
  in synaptic transmission, 128
acetylcholinesterase, 128, 136
acetyl-CoA, 40–41, 42b, 68
acid-base balance. See also pH
  buffer systems, 234–236
  during exercise, 230–238
  hydrogen ion production during exercise, 232–233
  kidneys and, 236–237
  muscle, exercise-induced disturbances in, 233b
  regulation during exercise, 234, 237–238
  respiratory influence, 236
  ventilation and, 217
acidosis, 214, 231, 232b, 339
acids
  defined, 231
  fixed, 232–233
  organic, 233
  strong, 231
  volatile, 232
acromegaly, 82b
ACSM. See American College of Sports Medicine (ACSM)
ACTH (adrenocorticotropic hormone), 79, 80f, 84, 85b, 90t
actin, 142
  fatigue and, 412
  in muscle contraction, 145
action potentials, 126, 126f
Activity Pyramid, 331, 333f
adenohypophysis, 79
adenosine diphosphate (ADP)
  in ATP formation, 33
  endurance training and, 271, 271f
adenosine monophosphate, cyclic. See cyclic AMP (cyclic

3', 5' -adenosine monophosphate)
adenosine triphosphate (ATP). See also ATP-PC system
  aerobic tally, 46
  balance sheet, 45b
  chemiosmotic hypothesis, 44f
  in energy production, 33–34, 34f
  in muscle contraction, 145, 147f, 148
  oxidative phosphorylation and, 43f
  structure of, 33, 33f
adenylate cyclase, 76
adequate intakes (AI), 362
ADH (antidiuretic hormone), 90t
adipocytes, 67
adipose tissue. See body fat
adolescents, sudden cardiac death in young athletes, 469b
ADP. See adenosine diphosphate (ADP)
adrenal cortex, 82, 83–85, 91t
adrenal gland, 82–85
adrenal medulla, 82–83, 91t
adrenocorticotropic hormone (ACTH), 79, 80f, 84, 85b, 90t
aerobic fitness, men's and women's classifications, 303t
aerobic metabolism, 33
  ATP production, 38–43, 45, 46t
  free radical formation and, 43b
aerobic performance
  ergogenic aids for, 524, 526–529
  factors limiting, 415–418, 415f
  intermediate-length, 416, 417f
  long-term, 417, 417f
  maximal aerobic power, 262–263, 424–425, 425f
  moderate-length, 415–416
  oxygen supplementation and, 524, 526–527
aerobic power, maximal, and altitude, 501–503, 502f
aerobic power training
  high-intensity continuous exercise, 446–447
  interval training, 445–446
  long, slow-distance exercise, 446
Aerobics Center Longitudinal Study, 292b
Aerobics (Cooper), 9
afferent fibers, 121
afterload, 185, 267

aging
  cardiac output and, 188
  gene therapy for muscle loss, 157–158, 158b
  skeletal muscle and, 157–158
  skinfold measures, 383
  strength training and, 278b
  thermoregulation and, 253–254
  weight gain and, 374
air displacement plethysmography, 379
air pollution
  carbon monoxide, 517–518, 517f
  ozone, 517
  particulate matter, 517
  physiological responses to, 516
  sulfur dioxide, 517
Air Quality Index (AQI), 518
airway resistance, 206–207
  nasal strips and performance, 226b
  in obstructive lung diseases, 207
alanine, 32, 33, 482, 483
alarm reaction, in general adaptation syndrome, 84
aldosterone, 91t
  secretion of, 83–84, 84f
Ali, Muhammad, 133b
alkalosis, 231, 232b
  buffer use and, 235b
all-or-none law, 126–127
alpha glycerol phosphate, 100
alpha motor neuron, 131
alpha receptors, 82
altitude
  adaptation to high altitude, 503–504
  aerobic performance, long-term, 501
  anaerobic performance, short-term, 500–501
  atmospheric pressure, 500
  cardiovascular function, 502–503
  jumping through thin air, 501b
  lactate and, 508b
  "live high, train low" strategy, 505b
  long races, performances in Olympic Games (1964 and 1968), 502t
  maximal aerobic power and altitude, 501–502, 502f
  mountain climbing, 506–509
  program planning concerns, 332

  respiratory function, 503
  short races, performances in Olympic Games (1964 and 1968), 501t
  training for competition, 504–505
alveolar cells, type II, and alveolus, 204, 204f
alveolar ducts, 202
alveolar ventilation, 207
alveoli, 201, 202, 203f, 204, 204f
ambient temperature pressure and saturated (ATPS), A–2
amenorrhea
  exercise and, 89, 464–465, 464f, 466, 467b
  protein ingestion and, 485
American Alliance for Health, Physical Education, Recreation, and Dance (AAHPERD), 6, 302, 383
American Association for Health, Physical Education, and Recreation (AAHPER), 6, 10
American Association of Cardiovascular and Pulmonary Rehabilitation, 10
American College of Obstetricians and Gynecologists, 353
American College of Sports Medicine (ACSM), 7b, 278, 511
  cardiorespiratory fitness recommendations, 300
  certification programs, 9b, 11
  children's training recommendations, 470
  coronary heart disease risk factors, 293b
  exercise recommendations, 321, 323–324, 324b, 326, 347
  strength and flexibility training recommendations, 332b
  weight loss and maintenance recommendations, 397b
American Diabetes Association, 342
American Dietetic Association (ADA), 369
American Heart Association, 7b, 321, 360
  dietary fat recommendations, 373
  salt intake recommendations, 365
American Physiological Society (APS), 10

amino acids
  essential, 32
  formation of, 32
  as fuel source, 33, 67–68
  as nutrition supplements, 525t
  oxidation during exercise, 483–484, 485f
amphetamines, 530
anabolic steroids, 86, 87b
anaerobic metabolism
  aerobic/anaerobic ATP production, interactions between, 48
  ATP production, 33–34, 36, 38
  in short-term, intense exercise, 57
anaerobic pathways, 33
anaerobic performance
  ergogenic aids for, 529–530
  factors limiting, 413, 414f, 415
  genetics and, 449b
  short-term, 415, 415f, 500–501
  ultra short-term, 413, 414f, 415
anaerobic power testing
  cycling power tests, 432–434
  determination of, 430–434
  jumping power tests, 431
  running power tests, 431–432, 434
  short-term, 433–434
  sports-specific tests, 434
  ultra short-term maximal power tests, 431–433
anaerobic threshold, 59
analog-to-digital converter, 112
anatomical dead space, 207
androgenic steroids, 86, 87b
androgens, 83
androstenedione, 87b, 525t
anemia, 365
aneroid sphygmomanometer, 306
angina pectoris, 193, 302, 306, 347, 348
angioplasty, 347
angiotensin I, 83
angiotensin II, 83, 84f
angiotensin-converting enzyme (ACE), 83, 347
anorexia nervosa, 384, 465, 465f
anterior hypothalamus, 247
anterior pituitary gland, 79, 80f, 90t
antidiuretic hormone (ADH), 79–81, 90t
antioxidants, 525t
aorta, baroreceptors in, 178
aortic aneurysms, 469b
aortic bodies, 220, 221f
aortic pressure, stroke volume and, 185
aortic semilunar valve, 170
apneustic area, brain stem, 220
appetite, exercise and, 394–396
Applied Body Composition Assessment (Stolarczyk), 376
applied science, 10
arginine, 525t
arm crank ergometer, 109f
arm crank ergometry, net efficiency, 116f
arm exercises
  cardiovascular response, 193–194, 193f

metabolic rate, rectal temperature and, 249f
Armstrong, Lance, 416
arrhythmias, 195b, 306, 348
arsenic, 364
arterial blood pH, 231, 232b, 237f
arterial blood pressure. see blood pressure
arteries, 170
arterioles, 170, 185, 187–188, 187f
arteriosclerosis, risk factors, 177
arteriovenous oxygen difference, in endurance training, 267–268
articular cartilage, 470
ascorbic acid (vitamin C), 366–367t
Asmussen, E., 5
asthma
  asthma attack, 343f
  causes of, 342–343
  drug therapy, 343
  exercise-induced, 206b, 343–345
  prevalence of, 342
  prevention/relief of, 343
  screening for, 344b
  training and, 472
Astrand, P. O., 309b
atherosclerosis, 179b, 291, 372
athletes. See also female athletes; male athletes
  conditioning for, 457–458, 457f
  dietary goals for, 484–485
  elite, typical muscle fiber composition in, 155t
  iron deficiency in, 489–490, 489t
  as machine, 418
  paraplegic, 425
  physiological testing and gains for, 422–423
  predicting future champions, 430b
  sudden cardiac death in young athletes, 469b
  training programs (see training)
athletics. See sports
Atkins Diet, 391
atmospheric pressure, 500
ATP. See adenosine triphosphate (ATP)
ATPase, 33, 33f, 148, 149, 162
ATP-PC system. See also adenosine triphosphate (ATP); phosphocreatine (PC)
  in ATP production, 34
  control of, 47
  in short-term, intense exercise, 57
  in training programs, 448
(ATPS) ambient temperature pressure and saturated, A–2
atrioventricular (AV) node, 179, 182
atrioventricular (AV) valve, 170, 174, 181
atrium, heart, 171
atrophy, 155–156, 157b
autologous transfusion, 528

automobile racing, head injuries from, 134b
autonomic nervous system, 136, 137f
autonomic neuropathy, 340
autoregulation, 191
axons, 122, 123f, 142f

B

balance training, for older adults, 350
Baldwin, Kenneth, 156b
Balke, Bruno, 9b
Balke Standard protocol, 311, 312
ballistic stretching, 456
barometric pressure, 210, 507
  correction for, A–3
Bar-Or, Oded, 471b
baroreceptor reflex, 305
baroreceptors
  blood pressure regulation, 18
  cardiovascular system and, 178, 195, 196, 196f
basal metabolic rate (BMR), 391–393
bases
  conjugate, 234
  defined, 231
  strong, 231
Basic Four Food Group Plan, 374–375
Bassett, David, Jr., 295b
Beamon, Bob, 501, 501b
bench step, 109–110, 109f
Bernard, Claude, 15
beta carotene, 364
beta cells, 20b
beta oxidation, 40, 42b, 272
beta receptors, 82
beta-adrenergic receptors, 93f
beta-blockers, exercise heart rate and, 183b
beta-endorphin, 85b
beta-lipotrophin, 85b
beta-receptor agonist (β_2-agonist), 343
bety-hydroxy-beta-methylbutyrate, 525t
bicarbonate
  in blood buffering, 237
  extracellular buffers, 235–236
  ions, 231
  work rate and blood concentrations changes in, 238f
bicuspid valve, 170
Bigland-Ritchie, Brenda, 4b
binge eating, 384, 465
Biodynamics Laboratory (University of Wisconsin), 9b
bioelectrical impedance analysis (BIA), 379
bioenergetics, 23–49
  aerobic ATP production, 38–43, 45
  aerobic ATP tally, 46
  anaerobic ATP production, 33–34, 36, 37f
  cell structure, 24
  control of, 46–48
  defined, 24
  efficiency of oxidative phosphorylation, 46
  energy transformation, 25, 27–31

fuels for exercise, 31–33
high-energy phosphates, 33
interaction between aerobic/anaerobic ATP production, 48
biological control systems, 16–21. See also homeostasis
  cellular, 16
  components, 17, 18f
  defined, 17
  disease and failure of, 20b
  in exercise, 17b
  gain in, 18
  nature of, 17–18
  negative feedback in, 18
biopsy, 152b
biotin, 364, 366–367t
black globe temperature, 511
Blair, Steven N., 292b
blood
  diagnostic values of enzymes in, 29t
  heat transport, 242
  measuring enzyme activity in, 29b
  mixed venous, 170
  physical characteristics of, 186
  viscosity, 186, 187
blood boosting, 528
blood buffers, 529–530
blood doping, 527–529
blood flow. See also cardiovascular system
  afterload and, 267
  coronary, 171–172
  endurance training and, 275, 275f
  exercise during heat, 253
  heat acclimatization, 254
  hemodynamics, 186–188
  local, regulation during exercise, 190–191
  to lung, 211–212
  muscle and systemic physiology links, 275–278
  prolonged exercise in hot environment, 253
  redistribution of, during exercise, 189–190
  regional, within lung, 212f
  relationships with pressure and resistance, 186–187
  splanchnic, exercise intensity and, 189, 189f
  through systemic circuit, 187f
  vascular resistance, sources of, 187–188
  venous return, 184–185, 184f
blood gases. See also carbon dioxide; oxygen
  analysis, 210
  diffusion of, 201, 210–211
  exchange of, 201, 204
  hemoglobin and oxygen transport, 213
  ventilation and, 207–208
blood glucose. See also glucose
  biochemical adaptations, 271–272
  exercise and, 74, 339, 339f
  Glycemic Index and, 372b
  homeostatic control of, 19, 19f, 20b, 93
  hormone regulation of, 95
  insulin resistance and, 294

blood packing, 528
blood pH, biochemical adaptations, 273
blood pressure, 300
  arterial, 176–178, 177b, 178f
  baroreceptors and, 18
  diabetes and, 340
  diastolic, 176
  dynamic constancy in, 16
  factors influencing, 177–178
  in hypertension, 346
  mean arterial, calculation of, 176–177
  measurement in graded exercise test, 305
  negative feedback mechanism and, 19f
  regulation of, 18–19, 178
  resistance and flow in, 186–187
  systolic, 176
  work rate and, 188f
blood proteins, 235
blood sugar, 31
blood transfusion, 528
blood-gas barrier, 204
Bloomfield, Susan, 351b
body composition, 376–384
  body fatness for health and fitness, 383–384
  exercise and, 396
  performance and, 492
body composition measures
  air displacement plethysmography, 379
  bioelectrical impedance analysis, 379
  body mass index, 377–378
  dual energy x-ray absorptiometry, 378
  height/weight tables, 377, 377t, 384
  isotope dilution, 378
  near infrared interactance, 378
  nuclear magnetic resonance, 378
  photon absorptiometry, 378
  potassium-40, 378
  radiography, 378
  skinfold thickness, 379, 382–383, 386, 397
  total body electrical conductivity, 379
  two-component system, 379, 380–384
  ultrasound, 378
  underwater weighing, 378, 380–382, 381f
  whole-body density, 380
body fat
  brown adipose tissue, 393
  energy expenditure and, 515–516
  fat cell size and number, 386, 386f
  free fatty acid mobilization, 100–101, 101f
  health status and fitness, 383–384
  as insulation, 513
  nonbasal energy expenditure, 394, 394f
  performance and, 492–495, 494f
  somatotype, 492

body mass index (BMI), 296b, 377–378, 386
  obesity and, 384, 385b
body temperature. See also skin temperature
  calculating increase in, during exercise, 247b
  core-to-shell gradients, 242
  in enzyme regulation, 30, 31f
  heart rate and, 183
  heat loss, 244–245
  homeostasis and, 16, 16f
  hyperthermia, 251b
  hypothalamus and, 243, 247–248
  measurement during exercise, 243
  prolonged exercise and, 194
  regulation of, 241–257
  shivering and, 243
  specific heat, 246
  thermal events during exercise, 249–250
  ventilatory response to exercise, 223
body temperature pressure saturated (BTPS), A–2, A–3
Bohr, Christian, 4
Bohr effect, 214
bone health, exercise and, 350, 351b, 352
bone mineral density (BMD), 351b
bone mineral disorders, female athlete and, 466, 467b
Borg scale, 328, 354
boron, 525t
Boston Marathon, 489b
boxing, head injuries from, 134b
Boyle's Law, A–2
bradycardia, 266
brain
  anatomy, 132, 133f
  cerebellum, 134
  cerebrum, 133–134
  exercise and, 137
  motor control functions of, 132–134
brain serotonin (5-hydroxytryptamine), 410
brain stem, 132
  anatomy, 133, 133f
  injuries and Parkinson's disease, 133b
  motor control and, 132
breathing. See ventilation
bronchial asthma, 345
bronchial tree, 201, 202, 203f
bronchioles, 202
bronchitis, 345
bronchodilators, 342
bronchospasm, 206b, 344
Brooks, George, 69b
brown adipose tissue, 393
Bruce protocol, 311
BTPS (body temperature pressure saturated), A–2, A–3
buffers
  acid-base systems, 234–236, 235t
  extracellular, 235–236, 237
  intracellular, 234
  sodium, performance and, 235b
bulimia nervosa, 384, 465–466, 466f

bulk flow, 204
Buskirk, Elsworth R., 8

C
cable tensiometer, 435, 435f
caffeine, 531–534, 532t, 533f
  caffeine-ephedrine mixtures, 534
  as ergogenic aid, 531–534
  in lipid mobilization, 533
  mechanisms of action, 531–533, 533f
  sources of, 532t
calcitonin, 81–82, 90t
calcium, 370–371t
  dietary, 350, 351b, 364–365
  excitation-contraction coupling and, 150b
  glucose transporters and, 99
  as major mineral, 24
  in muscle contraction, 147f, 148
  sarcoplasmic reticulum and, 48
  in second messenger mechanisms, 76, 78, 78f
calcium channel blockers, 347
calcium-calmodulin pathway, glycogen breakdown, 63f
calmodulin, 63b, 78
caloric intake
  basal metabolic rate and, 392
  occupations and, 395, 395f
  weight control and, 388, 389
  weight loss and, 394b
calorimeter, 111
calorimetry
  direct, 111–112
  indirect, 112
Canadian Home Fitness Test (CHFT), 302, 304, 305f
cancer, 290
  as leading cause of death, 291b
  obesity and, 384
Cannon, W. B., 82
Cannon, Walter, 15
capillaries, 170
carbohydrate drinks, 483b
carbohydrates
  biosynthesis of, 31
  diet and performance, 478–482
  dietary fiber, 368–369
  dietary goals, 360
  energy and, 31–32
  during exercise, 65–67
  exercise intensity and, 64
  forms of, 31–32
  metabolic pool and, 41f
  metabolism, 62t, 63–64, 64f
  oxidation of, 61
  sports drinks, 66b, 483b
  starches, 368
  storage sites, 68t
  sugars, 368
carbon, in body composition, 24
carbon dioxide. See also blood gases
  blood transport, 215–216, 216f
  calculation of production, A–1
  comparison of old and new technology in measurement of production, 5f

partial pressure of, 210f
  as volatile acid, 232
carbon monoxide, 517
carbonic acid
  in carbon dioxide blood transport, 216
  Henderson-Hasselbalch equation, 236
cardiac accelerator nerves, 182
cardiac contractility, 183, 266–267
cardiac cycle, 174–175
cardiac output, 170, 181–185
  distribution of, during rest and maximal exercise, 189–190, 190f
  in endurance athletes, 181t
  exercise and, 170, 188–191
  during incremental exercise, 192–193
  maximal, 188
  maximal oxygen uptake and, 264–265, 502–503
  mean arterial blood pressure and, 177–178
  prolonged exercise and, 194, 194f
  rest to exercise transition and recovery from exercise, 192, 192f
  stroke volume and, 181–182, 185f
  work rate and, 188f
cardiac rehabilitation
  ACSM programs, 347
  effects, 349
  exercise programs, 348–349
  exercise testing, 348
  population served by, 347–348
cardiomyopathy, 195b
cardiopulmonary system, function of, 170. See also cardiovascular system
cardiorespiratory fitness
  decision tree, 300f
  elderly and, 349
  exercise prescription for, 325–329
cardiorespiratory fitness testing, 299–316
  Canadian Home Fitness Test, 304, 305t
  field tests, 302–305
  graded exercise tests (see graded exercise tests)
  maximal oxygen uptake and, 308–310
  resting and exercise measures, 302
  screening, 300
  step tests, 314–316
  testing procedures, 300–302
  walk tests, 304
cardiorespiratory function (CRF), 300
cardiorespiratory system, primary purpose of, 170
cardiovascular control center, 182
cardiovascular disorders, 290. See also names of specific disorders
cardiovascular drift, 194

cardiovascular system
    altitude and, 502–503
    blood flow (see blood flow)
    cardiac cycle, 174–175
    cardiac output (see cardiac output)
    central command, 195, 196f
    fitness testing (see cardiorespiratory fitness testing)
    heart (see heart)
    organization of, 170–171
    pulmonary and systemic circuits, 171, 172f
    training for children and, 469
cardiovascular system and exercise
    arm versus leg exercise, 193–194
    cardioprotective benefits of exercise, 172, 174b, 175b
    circulatory responses, 169–196
    emotional influence, 192
    incremental exercise, 192–193
    intermittent exercise, 194
    oxygen delivery to muscle, 188–191
    prolonged exercise, 194
    recovery from, 192
    regulation of adjustments to exercise, 195–196, 195f, 196f
    rest to exercise transition, 192
carnitine, 524, 525t
carnitine transferase, 272
carotid artery, baroreceptors in, 178
carotid bodies, 220, 221, 221f, 237
carrier molecules, 36
catalyzed reaction, 28f
catecholamines
    amphetamines and, 530
    diabetes and, 339
    in heat production, 243
    secretion of, 82
    in substrate mobilization, 96f, 97
    ventilatory response to exercise, 223
cell body, 122
cell membrane, 24
cells
    chemical reactions, 24, 25, 25f, 26b, 27
    major organelles of, 25f
    protein synthesis in, 26f
    structure of, 24, 25f
cellular respiration, 201
cellular stress response, 19–20, 20f, 21b
cellular theory, repeated bout effect and, 454b
cellulose, 32
Centers for Disease Control and Prevention (CDC), 7b, 296b
    exercise recommendations, 323–324
central chemoreceptors, 220
central command
    in cardiovascular control, 195, 196f
    endurance training and, 277–278
central command theory, 195, 196

central fatigue, 409–410
central nervous system
    anatomy, 121
    fatigue and, 148b, 409–410
    fuel sources, 74
    hyperthermia, 253
    muscle chemoreceptors, 130
    muscle spindle and, 163–164
    proprioceptors, 129–130
    reflexes, 130–131
    relationship with peripheral nervous system, 121, 122f
cerebellum, 132, 133f, 134
cerebral cortex, 133
cerebrospinal fluid (CSF), 220
cerebrum, 132, 133–134, 133f
certification programs, 11
Charles's Law, A–2
chemiosmotic hypothesis, 42, 44f
chemoreceptors
    central, 220
    humoral, 220, 222
    muscle, 163
    peripheral, 220, 221f
chewing tobacco, 535
children
    asthma in, 344b
    cardiovascular fitness standards for, 304b
    exercise and, 471b
    fat cell size and number in, 386
    future champions among, 430b
    maximal oxygen uptake in, 309b
    maximal run tests, 302, 303
    obesity in, 296b, 376, 378, 386
    skinfold thickness estimates for body fat, 383, 383t
    sports conditioning for, 469–470
    sports-related injuries, 470
    sudden cardiac death in, 469b
    whole-body density, 380
chloride, 24, 364, 370–371t
chloride shift, 216, 216f
cholera, 289
cholesterol, 372
    coronary heart disease and, 293, 293f, 321
    low-density vs. high-density, 372
    obesity and, 376
    physiology of, 32
    type 2 diabetes and, 341
Christensen, E. H., 5
chromium, 364, 370–371t, 525t
chronic obstructive pulmonary disease (COPD)
    disability grading, 345–346, 346t
    exercise and, 207b, 345–346
    spirometry for, 208
    testing and training, 345–346
cilia, respiratory, 202
circulation. See blood flow
circulatory system. See cardiovascular system
citrate synthase, 270b
citric acid cycle, 38
Civil Aeromedical Research Institute, 9b
Clarkson, Priscilla M., 455b

Clean Air Act, 518
clenbuterol, 531b
Clinical Guidelines on the Identification, Evaluation, and Treatment of Overweight and Obesity in Adults, 384
clo units, 513
clothing
    for cold weather exercising, 345
    for heat acclimatization, 255b
    heat injuries and, 510
    as insulation, 513, 515, 515f
    for walking, 329
cobalt, 364
cocaine, 534, 534f
cognitive-set point model, 387
cold and exercise
    clothing for, 255b, 345, 513, 515, 515f
    cold acclimatization, 256–257
    energy production, 515–516
    environmental factors, 512–513, 515
    hypothermia, 512, 512f, 516
    insulating factors, 513
    program planning concerns, 332
    water, 513
    wind chill index, 513
cold stress, physiological responses to, 248, 248f
coma, diabetic, 339
concentric action, 159
concussion, 134b
conditioning
    for children, 469–470
    diabetes and, 472
conducting zone, respiratory, 202, 203f, 204
conduction, heat, 244
conduction disturbances, cardiac, 306
conductivity, neuronal, 122
conjugate base, 234
conjugate base acids, 35b
connective tissue theory, repeated bout effect and, 454b
constant-load exercise, thermal events, 249–250
consumers, exercise physiology and, 11
contraceptives, oral, 88
contractile proteins, exercise and, 26b
control systems of body. See biological control systems
convection, heat, 244, 249, 249f, 250f
cool-downs, 325, 444
Cooper, Ken, 9b
Cooper Institute for Aerobics Research, 8
Cooper's run test, 302
copper, 364, 370–371t
core temperature. See body temperature
Cori cycle, 68b
coronary artery bypass graft surgery (CABGS), 347, 348
coronary artery disease (CAD)
    cholesterol and, 32
    diabetes and, 340
coronary heart disease (CHD), 291–293

    atherosclerosis, 291, 372
    exercise tests for, 6
    exercise training and, 347
    hypertension and, 346
    obesity and, 384
    pharmacologic stress tests, 307b
    physical inactivity and, 291b, 292–293, 300, 321
    risk factors, 291, 293b, 293f, 300
    sudden cardiac death, 195b
coronary sinus, 171
corporate fitness programs, 6–7, 6f
corticosteroids, 343
corticotropic-releasing hormone (CRH), 84
cortisol, 84–85, 84f, 91t, 94–95, 94f
coupled reactions, 25–27
creatine
    for muscle soreness, 455b
    as nutritional supplement, 525t
    for performance, 524
    supplements and athletic performance, 35b, 526b
creatine kinase, 47
critical power, measurement of, 428, 428f
cromolyn sodium, 343
cross-bridges, 145, 147f, 148, 150b, 151, 160, 412
cross-country skiing, training programs and maximal oxygen uptake, 263
crossed-extensor reflex, 131
crossover point, 62, 62f
cross-sectional area (CSA), 281
cross-sectional training studies, 262
Cureton, Thomas K., Jr., 8
cycle ergometer, 58, 109f, 110, 195, 250f
    for graded exercise test protocols, 313–314
    for graded exercise testing, 309, 310f
    net efficiency, 115
cyclic AMP (cyclic 3', 5'-adenosine monophosphate), 63b, 76, 77f, 78
    adrenergic receptor types, 82–83, 83t
    caffeine and, 533, 533f
    formation of, 48
    in muscle-glycogen utilization, 92
cycling
    asthma and, 344
    energy expenditure, 112, 113
    in exercise program, 330
    oxygen uptake in, 114b
    power tests, 432–433
    training programs and maximal oxygen uptake, 263
cytochrome chain. See electron transport chain
cytoplasm, 24, 272

D

Daily Value (DV), 362
Dalton's law, 210
Deadly Quartet, 294

dead-space ventilation, 207
death, leading *versus* actual causes of, 291b
deficiency diseases, 364
degenerative diseases, 290
dehydration, 252, 471b
    hyponatremia and, 489b
    preventing, 253b
dehydroepiandrosterone (DHEA), 525t
dehydrogenases, 30
delayed-onset muscle soreness (DOMS), 453, 453f, 454b
Dempsey, Jerome, 225
dendrites, 122, 123f, 127
dental caries, 535
deoxyhemoglobin, 213
deoxyribonucleic acid (DNA), 24, 26f
depolarization, 126
depression, obesity and, 384
detraining, 268–269, 268f, 270f, 413
DHEA (dehydroepiandrosterone), 525t
diabetes
    blood glucose control, 339
    coexisting conditions, 340
    coma in, 339
    competitive training and, 470–472
    diabetes mellitus, 85
    differences in types of, 338t
    exercise and, 339–342
    insulin and, 338, 339, 339f
    ketosis (ketoacidosis), 232b, 339
    nutrition and, 342
    obesity and, 296b, 338, 341b, 376, 384
    prevalence, 338
    type 1 (insulin-dependent), 338, 338t, 339–340
    type 2 (insulin-resistant), 338, 338t, 341–342, 341b
diabetic coma, 339
diacylglycerol, 78
diaphragm, 202f, 204
diastole, 175f, 176f
diastolic blood pressure, 176, 193
diet. *See* nutrition
Dietary Approaches to Stop Hypertension (DASH), 365, 375, 376t
dietary fats
    as nutrients, 372–373
    polyunsaturated, 373
    saturated, 373
dietary fiber, 368–369, 372
Dietary Guidelines for Americans, 7b, 360, 362
    carbohydrate recommendations, 368
    fiber recommendations, 369, 372
    food selection recommendations, 374–375
    physical activity recommendations, 396, 397b
    sodium intake recommendations, 365
Dietary Reference Intake (DRI), 362
    estimated energy requirements, A–24

macronutrients, A–18
    viamins and minerals, A–20—A–23
diffusion, of gases, 210–211
Dill, David Bruce, 4, 5, 5b
direct calorimetry, 111–112
disaccharides, 31
diverticula, 369
DNA (deoxyribonucleic acid), 24, 26f, 76
dopamine, 133b
dose-response relationship
    baseline physical activity status, 324f
    in exercise, 321, 322
    patterns of, 323–324, 324f
    physical activity and health, 323–325, 323b
    strength training, 332b
double product, 193, 193t, 306, 347
double-blind research design, 523
Douglas, C. J., 4
down-regulation, hormonal, 76
drugs
    amphetamines, 530
    for asthma, 343
    for blood pressure control, 347
    caffeine, 531–534, 532t, 533f
    clenbuterol, 531b
    cocaine, 534, 534f
    dose-response relationship, 322
    as ergogenic aids, 530–535
    nicotine, 535, 535f
    sympathomimetic, 530
dry bulb temperature, 511
dual energy x-ray absorptiometry (DEXA), 378
duration of exercise, influence on metabolism, 57–61
dwarfism, 82b
dynamic exercise, 159
dynamic neuromuscular imbalance, 468
dynamic stretching, 456
dynamometer, 436, 436f, 437f
dyslipidemia, 294
dysmenorrhea, 465
dyspnea, 206b, 302, 345
dystole, 174

E
eating disorders, 384, 465–466, 465f, 466f, 467b
eccentric action, 159
ECG. *See* electrocardiography (ECG)
ectomorphy, 492, 493f, 494f
effect (response), 321, 322
effectors, 17, 18, 18f
efferent fibers, 121
eicosanoids, 480b
Eisenhower, Dwight D., 6
ejection fraction, 267
elderly and exercise, 349, 352
    benefits of exercise, 350, 351b, 352
    osteoporosis prevention, 350, 351b, 352
    strength training and, 350
    training effect, 352b
    walking, 329, 350

electrically braked cycle ergometer, 109f
electrocardiogram, 179, 180f, 306
electrocardiography (ECG)
    exercise and diagnostic use, 179b
    normal, at rest, 179f
electrolytes, water and, 486–488
electron transport chain, 364
    in ATP production, 41–43, 45
    control of, 48
    defined, 41
    oxidation-reduction and, 41–42
    pathways, 41, 42f
elements, 364
emotions, 192
emphysema, 345
end-diastolic volume (EDV), 184, 265, 266
    stroke volume and, 183, 183f, 184
    ventricular filling and, 189b
endergonic reactions, 25, 27f
endocardium, 171, 173f
endocrine glands, 74, 90–91t
endomorphy, 492, 493f, 494f
endomysium, 141, 142f
endorphins, 85b, 90t
end-plate potential (EPP), 143
endurance exercise, respiratory muscle and, 206b
endurance training
    aerobic (*see* aerobic power training)
    blood pH, 273, 273f
    cardiac contractility and, 266–267
    central control in and, 277–278, 277f
    end-diastolic volume and, 266
    fatigue and, 410
    free fatty acids utilization, 272, 273f
    homeostasis and, 269–275
    injuries from, 447
    maximal oxygen uptake, 262–263, 268f
    muscle fiber alterations, 155, 157f
    oxygen deficit, 271, 271f, 272f
    performance and, 269–275
    peripheral feedback in, 277, 277f
    strength training combined with, 281, 451
    stroke volume and, 181t, 189b
    ventilation and exercise, 218, 223b
energy
    bioenergetics (*see* bioenergetics)
    energy of activation, 28–29, 28f
    forms of, 25
    rest and requirements for, 53
energy drinks, 483b
energy expenditure. *See also* metabolic rate
    basal metabolic rate, 391–393
    body fatness and, 515–516

cycling and, 114b
    direct calorimetry, 111–112
    estimation of, 112–114
    measurement of, 111–112
    net costs in, 398–399. 398t, 399t
    physical activity and exercise, 394
    for selected activities, A–5—A–16
    thermogenesis and, 392, 393–394
    treadmill running, 114b
    treadmill walking, 113b
    walking *vs.* running, 113f
    weight control and, 388, 391–399
energy transformation, 25, 27–31
energy wasteful systems, 393
environment
    altitude (*see* altitude)
    cold (*see* cold and exercise)
    exercise and, 332–333
    heat (*see* heat and exercise)
enzymes. *See also* specific *enzyme names*
    classification of, 30
    defined, 28
    diagnostic values of, in blood, 29t
    examples of specific enzymes within classes of, 30t
    factors regulating, 30, 31f
    lock-and-key model of action of, 29f
    measuring activity of, in blood, 29b
    naming of, 30
    rate-limiting, in metabolic pathways, 47, 47f, 47t
    regulation of chemical reactions, 30
    substrates, 28
ephedrine, caffeine and, 534
epicardium, 171, 173f
epidemiologic triad, 289, 289f
epidemiology, 288–290
    defined, 289
    risk factors in, 290, 291f
    web of causation, 290, 290f, 292, 296
epiglottis, 202
epilepsy, training and, 472–473
epimerases, 30
epimysium, 141, 142f
epinephrine, 63b, 91t
    in carbohydrate metabolism, 63–64
    in cyclic AMP formation, 48
    exercise effects on, 96–97, 97f, 99f
    in glycogenolysis, 92
    in lipolysis, 64
    physiologic responses to, 83t
    prolonged exercise and, 58
    secretion of, 82
    stroke volume and, 185
epinephrine-cyclic AMP (cAMP) pathway, glycogen breakdown, 63f
epiphyseal plate, 470, 470f
EPOC (excess post-exercise oxygen consumption), 55–56, 57f

ergogenic aids, 522–537
  for aerobic performance, 524, 525t, 526–527
  for anaerobic performance, 529–530
  blood buffers, 235b
  blood doping, 528–529
  defined, 523
  drugs, 530–534
  nicotine, 535
  nutritional supplements, 524
  physical warm-up, 536–537
  research concerns, 523
ergometers
  arm crank, 109f
  bench step, 109, 109f
  cycle, 109f, 110
  defined, 109
  treadmill, 109f, 110
  types of, 109f
ergometry, defined, 109
erythrocytes, 213
erythrocythemia, 528
erythropoietin (EPO), 529
esophageal temperature, 243, 487f
esterases, 30
Estimated Average Requirement (EAR), 362
Estimated Energy Requirement (EER), 362
estradiol, 87, 88, 88f
estriol, 87
estrogens, 83, 91t
  female sex characteristics and, 87, 88f
  muscle soreness and, 455b
  for osteoporosis, 349, 351b
  secretion of, 87–89
estrone, 87
ethics, in physiological testing, 418, 422
ethnicity
  obesity and, 384
  skinfold measures, 383
European Union, 82b
evaporation, 244, 246b, 249, 249f, 250f
excitation-contraction coupling, 145, 147–149, 150–151b
excitatory post-synaptic potentials, 127 (EPSPs)
excitatory transmitters, 127
exercise. See also physical activity
  appetite and, 394–396
  arm versus leg, 193–194, 193f
  arterial-mixed venous oxygen content during, 189
  asthma and, 206b
  beta-blocking medications and, 183b
  blood flow redistribution during, 189–190
  brain health and, 137
  carbohydrate sources during, 65–67
  cardiac output changes during, 188–191
  cardioprotective effects of, 172, 174b, 175b
  chronic obstructive lung disease and, 207b
  circulatory responses to, 192–194
  constant work-rate, oxygen uptake kinetics, 55b

defined, 321
diabetics and, 339–342
duration (see duration of exercise)
dynamic, 159
economy (see exercise efficiency)
electrocardiography and, 179b
endorphins in, 85b
environment and, 332–333
estimation of fuel utilization during, 61–62
fat metabolism and, 65b
fuels for, 31–33
glycogen breakdown during, 63b
heat and (see heat and exercise)
heat balance during, 242–243
homeostasis in, 17b, 21, 261, 261f
hormones and (see hormones)
hydration during, 253b
hydrogen ion production during, 232–233
indoor, 332
intensity (see intensity of exercise)
intermittent, 194
isometric, 194
lactic acid removal after, 56b
local blood flow regulation during, 190–191
lungs adapting to, 224
muscle fiber alterations, 155, 157
physiology (see physiology of exercise)
during pregnancy, 352–354
prescription (see exercise prescription)
recovery from: metabolic responses, 54–57
regulation of cardiovascular adjustments to, 195–196, 195f, 196f
resistance to infection and, 274b
respiratory muscles and, 206b
for special populations, 337–354
static, 158
stroke volume during, 183
sudden cardiac death during, 195b
temperature measurement during, 243
ventilatory control (see ventilation)
weight maintenance and, 394–396, 394b
exercise efficiency
  calculation of, 115–117
  fiber type, 116
  movement, speed and, 116
  net efficiency, 115
  running economy, 117
  tests for, 429
  work rate and, 115–116
Exercise in Education and Medicine (McKenzie), 7
Exercise Management for Persons with Chronic Diseases and Disabilities (ACSM), 347

exercise metabolism, 52–69
  body fuel sources, 65–68
  energy requirements at rest, 53
  exercise duration and fuel selection, 63–68
  fat/carbohydrate interaction, 64–65
  fuel selection factors, 62–63
  fuel utilization, estimation of, 61–62
  glycogen storage and, 32
  incremental exercise, 58–59, 58f
  lactate threshold, 59–61
  prolonged exercise, 58, 58f
  recovery from exercise, 54–56
  rest-to-exercise transitions, 53–54
  short-term intense exercise, 57
exercise physiology
  application of, to sports, 35b
  data collection equipment, 3–4
  graduate study and research, 8–10
  history of, 3–7
  investigation of significant subject matter areas in, 1954 and 1994, 9t
  overview of, 2–11
  physical education training programs, 7–8
  professional societies and research journals, 10–11
  research journals, 10
  translation to consumer, 11
exercise prescription, 320–333
  achieving health-related outcomes, 324b
  Activity Pyramid, 331, 333f
  for cardiorespiratory fitness, 325–328
  dose-response, 322
  dose-response patterns, 323–324
  duration, 322, 326f
  environmental concerns, 332–333
  frequency, 322, 326f
  games and sports, 330–331
  guidelines for improving fitness, 325
  intensity, 322, 326f
  jogging, 329–330
  physical activity and health, 323–325
  progression in, 325
  screening in, 325
  sequence for physical activity, 329–331
  strength and flexibility training, 331
  for type 2 diabetics, 341
  walking, 329
  warm-up/cool-down/stretch, 325
exercise pressor reflex, 195
exercise science, 8, 26b
exercise-induced asthma (EIA), 343–345
exergonic reactions, 25, 27f
expiration, 204, 205f, 206, 208
extensors, 130f, 141
extracellular buffers, 235–236, 237

extrafusal fibers, 163
extraocular muscles, innervation ratio, 132

F

FAD. See flavine adenine dinucleotide (FAD)
fascicle, 141, 142f
fast-acting hormones, 96
fast-twitch (type IIx) muscle fibers
  alteration by exercise training, 155, 157f
  central fatigue and, 413
  characteristics, 152, 153–154, 153b
  classification, 60, 149
  exertion of force, 154b
fat-free mass (FFM), 392, 480b
fatigue
  calcium and, 148
  central nervous system and, 409–410
  cross-bridges in, 412
  energetics of contraction, 412–413
  factors contributing to, 148b
  free radicals and, 41, 411b
  glycogen depletion and, 64
  heat-related, 254b
  mechanical factors, 412
  neural factors, 411
  peripheral, 410
  respiratory, performance and, 206b, 224–225, 225b
  sites of, 409–413, 410f
fats, 74, 372–373. See also body fat
  dietary (see dietary fats)
  energy and, 32, 40
  exercise intensity and, 65b
  exercise intensity and metabolism, 64f, 65b
  metabolic pool and, 41f
  metabolism, 64f
  respiratory exchange ratio for, 61
  storage of, 32, 67, 68t
  types of, 32
fat-soluble vitamins, 364
fatty acids, 32, 40. See also free fatty acids
  converting to acetyl-CoA, 42b
feedback, negative, 18
female athletes. See also gender
  amenorrhea in, 466, 467b
  body fat values, 494t
  bone mineral disorders in, 466, 467b
  dysmenorrhea in, 465
  eating disorders and, 465–466, 465f, 466f, 467b
  exercise-induced hypoxemia, 218
  knee injury in, 466, 468
  maximal oxygen uptake values in, 263, 263t
  menstrual cycle and, 87–89, 88f
  menstrual disorders in, 464–465, 464f, 467b
  triad of health problems, 467b
fen-phen (fen-fluramine and phentermine), 388b
ferritin, 365

fetus, exercise and, 353, 466
fever, 248
fiber
  dietary, 368–369, 372
  efficiency and type of, 116
  functional, 369
  total, 369
fibrinolysis, 321
Fick equation, 189
Fick's law of diffusion, 210
field tests, 302–305
fight or flight, 82
fitness
  heat injuries and, 510
  training principles, 443–444
fitness programs, corporate, 6–7, 6f
FITNESSGRAM, 304b
Fitts, Robert H., 414b
5-hydroxytryptamine (serotonin), 410
fixed acids, 232–233
flavin adenine dinucleotide (FAD)
  in ATP production, 36
  FADH (reduced), 41
  in Krebs cycle, 40f
flexibility training, 331, 456
flexors, 130f, 141
fluid replacement. See water replacement
fluoride, 364, 370–371t
folic acid, 364, 366–367t
follicle-stimulating hormone (FSH), 79, 80f, 86, 90t
follicular phase, of menstrual cycle, 87, 88f
Food Guide Pyramid, 374
food labels, 362, 363f
Food Quotient (FQ), 390
food records, 375
football
  head injuries from, 134b
  heat injuries from, 251b, 252, 252b, 511
  running power tests for, 431–432, 432f
football players, core temperature measurement in, 243
forced convection, 244
forced expiratory volume (FEV1), 209, 209f
force-velocity/power-velocity relationships, in muscle fibers, 161–162, 162f
four-component model, in body composition analysis, 379
Framingham Heart Study, 291, 384, 388
Franklin, Barry A., 307b
Frank-Starling law, 189b
Frank-Starling mechanism, 266
free fatty acids, 74
  caffeine and, 532, 533, 533f
  cortisol and, 84
  exercise and, 98, 99f, 100–101
  fat metabolism and, 64
  as fuel source, 67
  insulin resistance and, 295
  lactic acid and mobilization of, 101f
  transport of, 272
  weight loss and, 396
free radicals
  formation of, 41, 43b

muscle fatigue and, 148b, 254b, 411b
free-weight testing of strength, 435–436
friction-braked cycle ergometer, 109f
frostbite, 256
fructose, 31
FSH (follicle-stimulating hormone), 79, 80f, 86, 90t
fuel selection
  factors governing, 62–63
  intensity of exercise and, 62–63
fuel sources, body, 65–68, 67f, 74
fuel utilization, estimation of, during exercise, 61–62
functional fiber, 369
functional syncytium, 172

G

G protein, 76
gain, 18
gallbladder disease, obesity and, 384
games, in exercise program, 330–331
gamma motor neurons, 163
gases
  blood (see blood gases)
  BTPS correction of volumes, A–3
  correction of volumes to reference conditions, A–2
  standardization of volumes, A–2
  STPD correction of volumes, A–2
gel electrophoresis, 152b
gender. See also female athletes; male athletes
  aerobic fitness classifications, 303t
  body fatness and performance, 383–384, 492–495
  cardiac output and, 188
  cold exposure and, 515–516
  injury risk factors, 447
  knee injury risk and, 466, 468
  maximal oxygen uptake and, 265, 349, 350b
  obesity and, 387
  running economy and, 117
  skinfold thickness, 382, 383
  strength training and, 451, 453f
  thermoregulation and, 253–254
  training principles, 443
gene therapy, for age-related muscle loss, 157–158, 158b
general adaptation syndrome (GAS), 84, 85b, 94
genes, 26b
genetics
  obesity and, 386, 387
  training principles, 444
  training program response, 449b
  transcription, 26b
gigantism, 82b
Gladden, Bruce, 55b
glucagon, 91t
  diabetes and, 339
  exercise and, 97–100, 97f, 98f

in lipolysis, 64
  secretion of, 86
glucocorticoids, 83, 351b
gluconeogenesis, 55, 84, 482, 483
glucose. See also blood glucose
  aerobic ATP tally from breakdown of one molecule of, 46t
  anaerobic metabolism, 37f
  breakdown of, 27f
  cortisol and, 84
  creatine and, 526b
  defined, 31
glucose polymers, 479
Glycemic Index, 372b
glycemic load, 372b
glycerol, 32, 64
glycogen, 74
  defined, 32
  depletion of, 64, 478, 481
  diet and muscle stores, 478–479, 479f
  estradiol and, 88
  heat and muscle fatigue, 253, 254b
  muscle utilization of, 92–93, 93f
  regulation of breakdown of, during exercise, 63b
  storage of, 32, 65
glycogenolysis, 32, 92, 93f
glycolysis, 33, 147f
  in ATP production, 34, 36, 36f, 37f, 38f
  fatigue and, 413
  process of, 34, 36, 36f
glyconeogenesis, 68b
Golgi tendon organs, 163, 164, 165f, 195, 277, 279
Golgi-type receptors, 129
gonadotropins, 80f, 90t
goosebumps (piloerection), 248
graded exercise tests, 300
  blood pressure measurement, 305–306
  for cardiovascular fitness, 58
  for chronic obstructive pulmonary disease, 345
  cycle ergometer, 313–314, 313f
  electrocardiography in, 306
  heart rate measurement, 305
  measurements, 305–307
  protocol selection, 311
  protocols, 311–316
  rating of perceived exertion, 306–307
  step test, 314–316, 315f, 316f
  stopping, in low-risk adults, 308t
  termination criteria, 307
  treadmill, 312–313, 312f
graphs, interpretation of, 15b
Grassi, Bruno, 55b
growth hormone (GH), 79, 80f, 90t, 94
  abuse by athletes, 82b
  action of, 79, 81f
  exercise and, 95–96, 96f
  performance and, 82b
growth hormone-releasing hormone (GHRH), 79
growth plate, 470, 470f
guanosine triphosphate (GTP), 40

Guidelines for Exercise Testing and Prescription (ACSM), 307, 321, 347
gymnastics, head injuries from, 134b

H

Haldane, J. S., 4
Haldane respiratory gas analyzer, 4, 5
Haldane transformation, A–1
Harvard Alumni Study, 292b
Harvard Fatigue Laboratory, 4–5, 4t, 8, 9, 10
head injuries, 134, 134b
Health Canada, 362
Health-Related Physical Fitness Test Manual, 6
Healthy People (1979), 290, 296
Healthy People 2000, 296
Healthy People 2010, 296, 296b, 300
heart. See also cardiovascular system
  anterior view of, 171f
  arrhythmias, 195b
  arterial pH and, 231
  cardiac output (see cardiac output)
  conduction system of, 178f
  electrical activity of, 178–181, 180f
  intercalated disks, 172
  interventricular septum, 170
  layers of, 173f
  myocardium, 171–172, 173f
  skeletal muscle fibers vs. cardiac muscle fibers, 172, 173f
  structure of, 170
  sympathetic stimulation of, on stroke volume, 185f
  valves, 170
heart attack. See myocardial infarction
heart disease. See coronary heart disease (CHD)
heart mechanoreceptors, 195, 196f
heart rate, 300
  altitude and, 502–503, 503f
  arrhythmias, 306, 348
  cardiac output and, 188
  in endurance athletes, 181t
  exercise intensity and, 15b
  fluid intake and, 487f
  heat injury and, 511
  measurement in graded exercise test, 305
  pregnancy and exercise, 354
  prolonged exercise, 194, 194f
  regulation of, 182–183
  rest to exercise transition and recovery from exercise, 192, 192f
  resting and exercise measures, 302
  submaximal, maximal oxygen uptake estimation, 309–310, 310f
  target heart rate range, 327–328, 328f
  training and, 264
  walk tests, 304
  work rate and, 188f
heart rate reserve, 328

heart rate reserve method, 327b
heat and exercise
  acclimatization, 252b, 253, 254–256, 255b, 256t
  balance and, 242–243
  body temperature calculation, 247b
  children and, 471b
  fatigue and, 416
  heat loss mechanisms, 243–244
  heat production mechanisms, 243–244, 244f
  heat storage in body during exercise, 245–247
  heat-related problems, 509t
  hot environment and performance, 252–253
  injury prevention, 251b
  muscle fatigue, 254b
  overview, 250–251
  program planning concerns, 332
  prolonged, 217–218
  summary of heat exchange during exercise, 246f
  sweat rates, 251–252, 251f
  thermal events in, 249–250
heat cramps, 509t
heat exhaustion, 509t
heat gain, body, 242, 242f
heat injuries
  environmental heat stress, 511–512
  factors affecting, 510, 510f
  fitness implications, 510–511
  hyperthermia, 509–510
  performance implications, 511
  prevention of, 251b
heat load, physiological response to, 248f
heat loss
  body, 242, 242f, 244–245, 248, 251b
  calculation of, 245, 246b
heat shock proteins, 21b, 174b, 255, 255b
heat stroke, 509t
heat syncope, 509t
Heath-Carter scale, somatotyping method, 492
Hebbert, Oliver E., 6f
height/weight tables, 377, 377t, 384
hematocrit, 186f
hemodynamics, 186–188, 187f. See also blood flow
hemoglobin. See also oxyhemoglobin dissociation curve
  altitude and, 507
  blood doping and, 528, 528f
  defined, 213
  extracellular buffers, 235
  loading and unloading, 213
  normal concentrations, 213
  oxygen transport and, 213
hemosiderin, 365
Henderson, L. J., 4
Henderson-Hasselbalch equation, 236
Henry's law, 211, 236
HERITAGE Family Study, 264b
high-density lipoproteins (HDLs), 293b, 323–325, 323b

high-energy bonds, 25
high-energy phosphates, 33
Hill, A. V., 3, 3b, 4b, 54
Hill, James, 397f
hippocampus, 134
hockey, head injuries from, 134b
Hogan, Michael, 55b, 449b
homeostasis
  blood glucose regulation, 19, 19f, 20b, 93
  blood pressure regulation, 18–19
  body temperature and, 16, 16f
  defined, 15
  endurance training and, 269–275
  in exercise, 21, 261, 261f
  hormones in, 84
  pH regulation and, 231, 232b
  pulmonary system and, 201
  steady state versus, 15–16
  stress response in, 19–20, 20f, 21b
  temperature, 242, 242f
homeotherms, 242
homologous transfusion, 528
Hooke, Robert, 24
hormone replacement therapy (HRT), 349
hormones. See also neuroendocrinology; specific hormone names
  blood concentration of, 75–76
  chemical structure, 74–75
  classes of, 74
  defined, 74
  DNA stimulation, 76
  endocrine, 90–91t
  excretion of, 75
  exercise and (see hormones and exercise)
  hormone-receptor interactions, 76, 78
  hormones, 75
  mechanisms of action, 76, 77f, 78f
  membrane transport, 76
  metabolism, 75
  parathyroid, 82
  permissive, 94
  plasma volume, 75–76
  regulation and action of, 78–89
  second messengers, 76, 78
  secretion of, 75, 75f
  slow-acting, 76, 94
  steroid (see steroid hormones)
  thyroid, 81
hormones and exercise, 73–101
  blood hormone concentration, 75–76
  blood-glucose homeostasis, 93
  muscle-glycogen utilization, 92–93, 92f, 93f
  neuroendocrinology, 74–76, 78
  substrate mobilization, control of, 92–100
horse racing, head injuries from, 134b
Horvath, Steven, 5
Human Body Composition (Roche, Heymsfield, and Lohman), 376

human rights, physiologic testing and, 418
humidity
  exercise-induced asthma and, 344
  fatigue and, 416
  heat injuries and, 510
  heat loss and, 244–245
  hot environment and, 244, 250–251, 332
  prolonged exercise and, 58, 58f, 217–218, 218f
humoral chemoreceptors, 220, 222
Huxley, T. H., 10
hydration, heat injuries and, 510
hydrogen, in body composition, 24
hydrogen ions, 231. See also acid–base balance
  production of, during exercise, 232–233
  sources of, due to metabolic processes, 234f
hydrogen shuttle, 38b, 41, 59, 59f
hydrolases, 30
hydrostatic (underwater) weighing, 378
hydroxylases, 30
hyperbaric chamber, 524, 526–527
hyperinsulinemia, 294
hyperoxia, 500, 524
hyperplasia, 155, 280–281, 448
hyperplastic obesity, 385, 386
hypertension, 177
  classification, 176
  DASH eating plan and, 375, 376b
  exercise for, 346–347
  insulin resistance and, 294
  obesity and, 376, 384
  type 2 diabetes and, 341
hyperthermia, 251, 251b, 252, 253. See also heat and exercise
hypertriglyceridemic waist, 384, 385b
hypertrophic cardiomyopathy, 469b
hypertrophic obesity, 386
hypertrophy
  clenbuterol and, 531b
  gender and, 452
  strength training and, 155, 280–281, 448
hypoglycemia, 74, 254b, 339, 340, 480, 481
hyponatremia, 489b
hypothalamic somatostatin, 79
hypothalamus, 79
  anatomy, 79, 80f
  body temperature regulation and, 243
  growth hormone control, 79, 81f
  osmoreceptors in, 80–81
  pituitary gland control, 79
  thermostat set point, 247–248
hypothermia, 256, 516
hypothyroid state, 94
hypoxemia, exercise-induced, 218, 224, 225b

hypoxia, 59, 99, 500, 503, 508b
hypoxic threshold, 221, 221f

I
ibuprofen, 455b
ice hockey, head injuries from, 134b
Illinois Research Laboratory, 8
immune system, 458b
immunotherapy, 343
impaired fasting glucose (IFG), 341b
impaired glucose tolerance (IGT), 341b
inactivity. See physical inactivity
inclinometer, 110
incremental exercise
  arterial blood pH, 237f
  blood gases and, 218, 219f
  cardiovascular effects, 192–193, 193t
  lactate threshold in, 59–60, 60–61
  muscle pH, 237f
incremental exercise tests, 58
Inderal, 348
indirect calorimetry, 112
indoor exercise, 332
induced erythrocythemia, 528
infection, exercise and resistance to, 274b
infectious diseases, 290
ingestible temperature sensors, 243
inhibitory neurons, Golgi tendon organs and, 164, 165f
injury risk, seizures and, 472
innervation ratio, 132
inorganic compounds, 24
inorganic phosphate (P_i), 33
inositol triphosphate, 78
in-season conditioning, 457, 457f
inspiration, 204, 205f
Institute for Aerobics Research, 304b
Institute of Environmental Stress, 5
Institute of Medicine
  dietary recommendations, 360, 368, 369b
  exercise recommendations, 397b
insulin, 91t
  blood glucose regulation, 19, 19f, 20b, 97
  diabetes and, 338, 339, 339f
  exercise and, 97–100, 97f, 98f
  lipolysis inhibition by, 64
  membrane transport and, 76
  secretion of, 75, 85–86
insulin resistance, 294, 295
insulin shock, 339
insulin-like growth factor I (IGF-I), 158b
insulin-like growth factors (IGFs), 79
integrating center, 17, 18, 18f
intensity of exercise
  cardiovascular effects, 175b, 194
  cortisol and, 94–95, 95f
  endorphins and, 85b
  fuel selection and, 62–63
  heart rate and, 15f

hormonal responses summary, 100f
lactic acid production and, 233
metabolism and, 57–61
mitochondrial adaptations, 270b
muscle fiber recruitment, 413, 413f
muscle fuel source, 65–67, 67f
muscle glycogen utilization, 92–93, 92f
pH change during, 238f
pulmonary system and performance limits, 224–225
respiratory muscle and, 206b
splanchnic blood flow and, 189, 189f
sports drinks, 66b
sweat rates and, 486
vasodilation and, 191
$\dot{V}O_2$ Reserve Method for prescribing, 327b
intercalated disks, 172
intercostal muscles, 204
intermediate (type IIa) muscle fibers, 153
intermittent exercise, cardiovascular response to, 194
internal environment, control of, 14–22
International Association for the Study of Obesity, 397b
International Obesity Task Force, 397b
International Olympic Committee (IOC), 82b, 531
International Union of Biochemistry classification, 30
interstitial cell stimulating hormone (ICSH), 86
interval training, 194, 445–446, 445t
interventricular septum, 170
intracellular buffers, 234
intracranial hemorrhage, 134b
intrafusal fibers, 163
intrapleural pressure, 202, 204
intraventricular pressure, changes in, and ECG, 181f
involuntary heat production, 243, 244f
iodide, 370–371t
iodine, 364
ions, defined, 231
IPSP, 129
iron, 364, 365, 370–371t
as major mineral, 24
repletion, 490f
iron deficiency, 489–490
stages of, 489t
irritability, neuronal, 122
islets of Langerhans, 85, 86
isocitrate dehydrogenase, 48
isokinetic, defined, 436
isokinetic assessment of strength, 436–437
isokinetic dynamometer, 436, 437f
isoleucine, 33
isomerases, 30
isometric actions, 158, 159f
isometric measurement of strength, 435

isometric (static) exercise, cardiovascular response to, 194
isotonic (dynamic) exercise, 159
isotonic measurement of strength, 435–436
isotope dilution, 378

J
jogging. See also running
in exercise program, 329–330
injuries and, 350
net caloric cost per mile, 398, 398t
program for, 331t
John Wanamaker store (former), tracks and courts on roof, 7f
Johnson, Ben, 87b
joint receptors, 130
joules, 108
journals, research, 10
jumping power tests, 431

K
Karvonen method for target heart rate determination, 328
Keino, Kipchoge, 501
Kennedy, John F., 6
Kenney, Larry, 252b
ketoacidosis, diabetic, 232b, 339
ketoacids, 232b
ketosis, 339, 339f
Keys, Ancel, 8
kidneys
acid-base balance, 236–237
blood pressure regulation, 178
diabetes and, 340
hormone metabolism/excretion, 75
kilocalorie (kcal), 111
kinases, 30
kinesthesia, 129
knee injury risk, in female athletes, 466, 468
knee-jerk reflex, 163
Korean War, 6
Korotkoff sound, 306
Koroto koff sands, 177b
Kraus, Hans, 6
Krebs, Hans, 38
Krebs cycle
in ATP production, 38–41, 40f, 41f
compounds, enzymes, and reactions involved in, 40f
control of, 48
function of, 38–41, 40f
intermediates, 64–65
vitamins in, 364
Krogh, August, 3, 4b, 5
Krogh, Marie, 3

L
laboratory assessment
athlete gain, 423
of physical performance, 422
Laboratory for Human Performance Research (Pennsylvania State University), 8
Laboratory for Physiological Hygiene, University of Minnesota, 8

lactate. See also lactic acid
altitude and, 508b
biochemical adaptations and removal of, 274–275
Cori cycle and, 68b
criterion for achieving maximal oxygen uptake, 309b
endurance training and, 273–275, 273f
as fuel source, 68
lactic acid versus, 35b
muscle fatigue and, 148b
lactate dehydrogenase (LDH), 36
endurance training and, 273, 273f
function of, 38f
isoenzymes, 59, 60
lactate shuttle, 68, 69b
lactate threshold, 59f
critical power and, 428
defined, 59
direct determination of, 427
in endurance performance testing, 429–430, 430f
explanation for, 59–61, 61f
performance evaluation and, 426–428, 426b, 427f
practical use of, 61
specificity and, 262
ventilatory alterations and, 427–428, 427f
lactic acid. See also lactate
exercise and production of, 233, 234
formation of, 34, 35b, 36, 38f
free fatty acids and, 101f
incremental exercise and, 59
lactate versus, 35b
muscle soreness and, 60b
pH balance and, 30
post-exercise removal of, 56b
production of, during exercise, 237
work rate and blood concentrations changes in, 238f
Lagrange, F., 8
larynx, 201
lateral sac (terminal cisternae), 142, 148
Leading Health Indicators, 296b
left ventricular hypertrophy, 176
leg exercises
cardiovascular response, 193–194, 193f
metabolic rate, rectal temperature and, 249f
training effect, 276
leucine, 33, 483, 484, 485f
leukotriene inhibitors, 343
Life, Heat, and Altitude (Dill), 4
ligases, 30
lipases, 64
lipids. See fats
lipolysis, 32, 64
lipoprotein, 372
Little League elbow, 470
liver, Cori cycle and, 68b
livery glycogenolysis, 65, 66
loading/unloading hemoglobin, 213
locomotion. See movement
locomotor muscles, 206b
long, slow-distance training (LSD), 446
longitudinal training studies, 262

long-term aerobic performance, 501
Loucks, Anne B., 89b
Loughborough Intermittent Shuttle Test, 432
low-density lipoproteins (LDLs), 372
low-fat, complex carbohydrate (LFCC) diet, 373b
low-intensity exercise, fat metabolism and, 65b
Luft, Ulrich, 9b
lungs
adaptation to exercise, 224
blood flow to, 211–212
function of, 201
gas exchange, 204
position of, 202f
regional blood flow within, 212f
respiratory zone, 202, 203f
volumes and capacities, 208–209, 208f, 209t
luteal phase, of menstrual cycle, 87, 88, 88f
luteinizing hormone (LH), 79, 80f, 87, 88f, 90t
lyases, 30
lysine, 484, 525t

M
macronutrients, Dietary Reference Intake (DRI), A–18
macrophages, 202
magnesium, 364
function of, 370–371t
as major mineral, 24
Major League Baseball (MLB), 87b
malanocyte-stimulating hormone (MSH), 79, 80f
male athletes. See also gender
body fat values, 494t
exercise-induced hypoxemia, 218
maximal oxygen uptake values in, 263, 263t
maltose, 31
manganese, 364, 370–371t
Margaria, Rudolpho, 5
mast cells, 342, 344
Maughan, Ronald J., 483b
maximal effect (efficacy), in dose-response relationship, 322
maximal oxygen uptake ($\dot{V}O_2$ max), 3b, 263, 263t
aging and, 188
altitude and, 502–503, 504
cardiac output and, 188, 189, 264–265
in cardiovascular fitness testing, 308–310
in children, 309b
concurrent strength/endurance training and, 281
critical power and, 428
defined, 3b, 424
detraining and, 268–269, 268f
in different populations, 265t
in distance running, 426b
double product and, 193t
in endurance training, 189b, 262–263, 268f

maximal oxygen uptake (*cont.*)
  energy expenditure and, 398, 399t
  estimation errors, 310b
  estimation from last work rate, 309
  estimation from submaximal HR response, 309–310
  estimation of, 311
  exercise and fat metabolism, 65b
  fatigue and, 413
  gender and, 349, 350b
  in incremental exercise, 58
  lactate criterion for achieving, 309b
  longitudinal data on changes in, 265t
  maximal run tests, 302–304
  in paraplegic athletes, 425
  in pregnancy, 353
  in sedentary individuals, 266b
  strength training and, 278–279
  training intensity and, 446, 446f
  values in healthy and diseased populations, 263t
  weight maintenance and, 396, 397
McArdle's syndrome, 64b
McKenzie, R. T., 7
mean arterial pressure (MAP)
  arm and leg exercises, 193f
  calculation, 176
  factors influencing, 177–178, 178f
  stroke volume and, 185
mean skin temperature, calculating, 243
measurement
  of energy expenditure, 111–112
  exercise efficiency calculation, 115–117
  units of, 107
  of work, power, and energy expenditure, 106–117
  of work and power, 109–111
mechanistic research, 17b
mechanoreceptors, 222
medications
  cardiorespiratory fitness screening and, 300
  dose-response relationship for, 321f
medulla oblongata, 195
membrane transport, of hormones, 76
men. *See* gender; male athletes
menstrual cycle
  anorexia nervosa and, 384
  exercise and disorders of, 464–465, 464f, 467b
  hormones and, 87–89, 88f
  training and, 465, 467b
mesomorphy, 492, 493f, 494f
messenger RNA (mRNA), 26b, 76
metabolic acids, 232b, 339, 339f
Metabolic Cardiovascular Syndrome (Syndrome X), 294–295, 296, 296b, 373b
metabolic cart, computerized, 115f

metabolic energy production, in cool environment, 249f
metabolic equivalent (MET), 113, 115, 311, 311t, 324, 327b, A–5
metabolic pool, 41f
metabolic rate. *See also* energy expenditure
  calorimetry for, 111–112
  cardiac output during exercise, 188
  heat injuries and, 510
metabolism. *See also* aerobic metabolism; anaerobic metabolism; exercise metabolism
  aerobic, 33
  defined, 24
metric system, 107
  common prefixes, 107t
Metropolitan Life Insurance Company, height/weight tables, 377, 377t, 384
Meyerhof, August, 4b
Meyerhof, Otto, 3, 3b
micrograms, hormone measurement, 75
mineralocorticoids, 83
minerals, 364–365, 368
  calcium, 364–365
  Dietary Reference Intake for, A–20—A–23
  iron, 365, 489–490
  major, 364
  sodium, 365, 368
  summary of, 370–371t
Minnesota Starvation Experiment, 392, 392f
mitochondria, 24
  ATP production in, 36, 38b, 41–43, 45
  chemiosmotic hypothesis and, 44f
  exercise intensity and, 270b
  free fatty acid transport and oxidation, 272
  muscle cell before/after training, 271f
  NADH shuttling during glycolysis, 269
mixed venous blood, 170, 211
molecular biology, 24, 26b
molybdenum, as trace element, 364, 370–371t
Monark friction-braked cycle, 110
monosaccharides, 31, 32
motor cortex, 134
motor cycle racing, head injuries from, 134b
motor end plate, 143
motor function
  control of, 135–136
  Parkinson's disease and, 133b
  somatic, 131–132
  spinal cord and, 134–135
motor neurons, 143
motor units, 131, 131f, 143, 160
mountain climbing, 506–508
movement
  speed and exercise efficiency, 116, 116f
  voluntary, 135f, 136
multiple sclerosis (MS), nervous system function and, 124b

muscle
  biochemical properties of, 149, 151
  chemoreceptors, 195, 196, 196f
  enlargement, 280–281
  expiration, 204, 206f
  force regulation in, 160, 160f, 161f
  free fatty acid transport, 272
  innervation ratio, 132
  inspiration, 204, 206f
  mechanoreceptors, 195, 196, 196f
  oxygen transport in, 215
  sarcoplasm, 142
  skeletal (*see* skeletal muscle)
  systemic physiology and, 275–278
muscle actions, 158
  speed of, and relaxation, 159–160
  summary of classifications of exercise and types of, 159t
muscle contraction
  energetics of, 412–413
  energy for, 145
  excitation-contraction coupling, 145, 147–149, 150–151b
  sliding filament model, 144–145, 146f
muscle fatigue. *See* fatigue
muscle fiber types, efficiency and, 116
muscle glycogen, storage, 65, 66
muscle pH, incremental exercise and, 237f
muscle pump, circulatory, 184
muscle soreness, 453, 454b, 455b
  exercise-induced, 454b, 455b
  lactic acid and, 60b
  protection against, 454b
muscle spindle, 163–164, 164f, 195
muscular strength, defined, 434
muscular strength evaluation, 434–437
  criteria for method selection, 434–435
  free-weight testing, 435–436
  isokinetic assessment, 436–437
  isometric measurement, 435
  specificity in, 434
  variable-resistance measurement, 437
musculoskeletal system, training in children, 469–470
mutases, 30
myelin, 123f
myelin sheath, 124b
myocardial infarction (MI), 172
  cardiac rehabilitation for, 348
  exercise protection against, 172, 174b, 175b
  waist girth and, 385b
myocardial ischemia, 179b, 306
myocarditis, 195b
myocardium, 171–172, 173f, 195b
myofibrils, 142, 142f

myoglobin, oxygen-hemoglobin dissociation curve and, 215, 215f
myosin
  cross-bridges, 145, 160
  fatigue and, 412
  in muscle contraction, 142, 142f, 145
  in skeletal muscle, 152b, 153b
MyPyramid Food Groups, 374, 375t

N

NAD (nicotinamide adenine dinucleotide), 36, 38f
NADH. *See* nicotinamide adenine dinucleotide, reduced (NADH)
Nagle, Francis J., 9b
nanograms, hormone measurement, 75
nasal cavity, 201, 202
nasal strips, 226b
National Academy of Sciences, Food and Nutrition Board, 362
National Athletic Trainers Association, 253b
National Collegiate Athletic Association, 468
National Exercise and Heart Disease protocol, 311
National Research Council, 365
National Strength and Conditioning Association, 10, 11
National Weather Service, 513
National Weight Control Registry (NWCR), 397b
near infrared interactance (NIR), 378
negative feedback, 18, 81–82, 86
nephropathy, 340
nervous system, 120–137
  anatomical divisions of, 121f
  autonomic, 136, 137f
  brain (*see* brain)
  central, 121
  control of motor functions, 135–136
  functions of, 121
  motor control functions of brain, 132–134
  multiple sclerosis and, 124b
  neurons (*see* neurons)
  organization of, 121–122, 124–129
  peripheral, 121
  sensory information and reflexes, 129–131
  somatic motor function and, 131–132
  spinal cord (*see* spinal cord)
  vestibular apparatus and equilibrium, 132
net cost, for walking, jogging, and running, 398t
net efficiency, 115
neural theory, repeated bout effect and, 454b
neuroendocrine response, 74
neuroendrinology, 74–76, 78
  blood hormone concentration, 75–76
  defined, 74
  hormone secretion, 75

hormone-receptor interaction, 76, 78
plasma volume, 75–76
transport protein, 75
neurohypophysis, 79
neuromuscular cleft, 143
neuromuscular junction, 143–144, 145f, 411
neurons, 121
    action potential, 126, 126f
    all-or-none law, 126–127
    conductivity, 122
    electrical activity in, 122, 124–129
    irritability, 122
    motor (see motor neurons)
    neurotransmitters, 127–129
    parts of, 123f
    postganglionic, 136
    preganglionic, 136
    resting membrane potential, 124–126
    structure of, 122
    synaptic transmission, 124f, 127–129
neurotransmitters, 127–129, 136, 137f
niacin, 366–367t
nickel, 364
nicotinamide adenine dinucleotide (NAD), 36, 38f
nicotinamide adenine dinucleotide, reduced (NADH)
    ATP production by, 36, 40
    in electron transport chain, 41
    in Krebs cycle, 40–41, 40f
    lactate formation and, 273
    transport into mitochondria, 36, 38b, 269
nicotine, 535, 535f
Nielsen, M., 5
nitric oxide, 191b
nitrogen
    in amino acid oxidation, 483–484
    atmospheric, 500
    in body composition, 24
    nitrogen balance during exercise, 482, 484f
    partial pressure of, 210
    whole-body nitrogen balance studies, 484
nitroglycerin, 348
Nobel Prize in Physiology or Medicine, 3, 4b
nodes of Ranvier, 123f
Noll Laboratory (Pennsylvania State University), 8
nonbiological control system, 17f
noncatalyzed reaction, 28f
nonprotein R, 62, 62f
nonresponders, 526b
nonshivering thermogenesis, 248, 256, 257, 393
nonsteroidal anti-inflammatory drugs (NSAIDs), 455b
norepinephrine, 75, 91t
    body heat production and, 248, 256, 393
    exercise effects on, 96–97, 97f, 99f
    heart rate regulation and, 182
    in lipolysis, 64
    physiologic responses to, 83t

secretion of, 82
stroke volume and, 185
normocythemia, 528
normoxia, 500
nose, 201
nuclear magnetic resonance (NMR), 378
nucleus, cell, 24, 76, 133
nutrients
    balance and weight control, 389–390
    carbohydrates, 363, 368–369
    classes of, 363–365, 368–369, 372–374
    density of, 374
    diet supplements (see nutritional supplements)
    fats, 363, 372–373
    minerals, 362, 363, 364–365, 370–371t
    in pregame meal, 491–492
    proteins, 362, 363, 373–374
    recommended range of, 478
    vitamins, 362, 363, 364, 366–367t
    water, 363–364
nutrition
    Basic Four Food Group, 374–375
    for bone health, 351b
    DASH eating plan, 375, 376t
    for diabetes, 342
    diet evaluation, 375
    dietary goals, U.S., 360–361
    Food Guide Pyramid, 374
    food labels, 362, 363f
    for hypertension, 347
    Institute of Medicine recommendations, 360, 361, 368, 369b
    objectives, 296
    standards, 362–363
    weight control and, 389, 390–391
nutrition and performance
    carbohydrate diets, 478–480
    carbohydrate intake, timing of, 480–482
    minerals, 489–490
    pregame meal, 491–492, 491t
    proteins, 482–485
    salt, 488
    vitamins, 490
    water and electrolytes, 486–488
    water replacement (see water replacement)
nutritional supplements
    in athletic performance, 524
    creatinine, 35b

O
obesity, 7b
    basal metabolic rate and, 392
    body fat distribution, 384–385
    causes of, 386
    childhood, 376, 386
    dietary supplements and, 388b
    diseases associated with, 376, 384
    ethnicity and, 384
    genetics and, 386, 387
    height/weight tables, 377, 377t, 384
    hyperplastic, 385

hypertension and, 294
    hypertrophic, 386
    increase in, 296b
    insulin resistance and, 294
    measures for assessment of, 377–378
    nonbasal energy expenditure, 394, 394f
    overweight vs. overfat, 378
    prevalence, 296b, 384
    set point theory of, 387–388, 387f, 388f
    social pressure against, 386
    tracking risks related to, 385b
    type 2 diabetes and, 341, 341f
    weight control and, 384–388
obesity index, 377
occupations, caloric intake and, 395, 395f
off-season conditioning, 457, 457f
one-repetition maximum (1-RM) method, 436
onset of blood lactate accumulation (OBLA), 59
open-circuit spirometry, 112, 112f
oral cancer, 535
oral cavity, 202
oral contraceptives, 88
organelles, 24, 25f
organic acids, 233
organic compounds, 24
Ornish Diet, 391
ornithine, 525t
osteoarthritis, obesity and, 384
osteoclasts, 351b
osteoporosis, 349
    calcium intake and, 350, 351b, 364–365
    in female athletes, 89, 466, 467b
Otis, Arthur B., 11
ovaries, 91t
overload, 261–262
overtraining
    fatigue and, 410
    immune system and, 458b
    symptoms of, 458f
overuse injuries, 447
overweight children, 296b
oxidases, 30
oxidation
    of amino acids, 483–484, 485f
    of carbohydrates, 61
    defined, 27
oxidation-reduction reactions, 27–31, 28f
oxidative capacity, of muscle, 149, 155
oxidative phosphorylation, 38, 147f
    in ATP production, 38, 43f
    defined, 38
    efficiency of, 46
    stages of, 39f
    thermogenesis and, 393
oxidizing agent, 27–28
oxidoreductases, 30
oxygen. See also blood gases
    in ATP production, 45
    blood transport of (see hemoglobin)
    in body composition, 24
    consumption (cost) (see oxygen uptake (V̇O2))

muscle transport of, 215
    partial pressure of, 210, 210f
    supplementation in exercise, 524, 526–527
oxygen debt
    defined, 54
    in gluconeogenesis, 55
oxygen deficit
    biochemical adaptations, 271
    defined, 53
    endurance training, 272f
    trained vs. untrained subjects, 53–54, 54f
oxygen uptake (V̇O2)
    calculation of, A–1
    in cycling, 114b
    in incremental exercise test, 58–59, 58f
    kinetics, at onset of constant work-rate exercise, 55b
    maximal (see maximal oxygen uptake (V̇O2 max))
    measurement of, 5f, 112–113, 115
    open circuit-spirometry, 112
    post-exercise, 55–56, 57f
    in prolonged exercise, 58, 58f
    in rest-to-exercise transitions, 53–54, 53f
    steady-state, 3b
    in treadmill running, 114b
    in treadmill walking, 113b
oxygenases, 30
oxyhemoglobin dissociation curve, 4, 213–215, 213f
oxytocin, 79, 90t
ozone, 517

P
P wave, ECG, 179, 180f
PACER (Progressive Aerobic Cardiovascular Endurance Run) test, 302, 303b
pacinian corpuscles, 129, 130
Paffenbarger, Ralph S., 292b
pancreas, 85–86, 91t
    beta cells, 20b
    glucagon secretion, 86
    hormone secretion, 85–86
    insulin release, control of, 85–86
    somatostatin secretion, 86
pantothenic acid, 364, 366–367t
paraplegic athletes, 425
parasympathetic division, of autonomic nervous system, 136
parasympathetic nervous system, heart rate and, 182
parasympathetic neurons, 75
parasympathetic tone, 182
parathyroid gland, 82, 90t
parathyroid hormone, 90t
parietal pleura, 201, 202f
Parkinson's disease, 133b
PAR_med-X, 300, A–17
PAR-Q (Physical Activity Readiness Questionnaire), 300, 301f, 304
partial pressure
    atmospheric gases, 500
    defined, 210
    of oxygen and carbon dioxide, 210f
    oxyhemoglobin dissociation curve and, 213, 213f

particulate matter, air-borne, 517
PC. *See* phosphocreatine
peak expiratory flow rate, 344b
peak running velocity, 426b
pectoralis minor muscle, 204
Pennsylvania State University, Noll Laboratory, 8
peptidases, 30
perceived exertion scales, rating of, 306–307, 306t
percent fat estimate
  for men: triceps, chest, and subscapula skinfolds, A–25
  for women: triceps, abdomen, and suprailium skinfolds, A–26
percent grade, treadmill, 110, 111f
percentage of maximal heart rate, 328
percutaneous transluminal coronary angioplasty (PTCA), 348
performance
  aerobic (*see* aerobic performance)
  anabolic steroids and, 87b
  anaerobic (*see* anaerobic performance)
  body fat and, 492–495
  creatine supplements and, 35b
  dehydration and, 253b
  endurance training and, 269–275
  factors affecting, 408–418, 409f
  fatigue and (*see* fatigue)
  in hot environment, 252–253
  laboratory assessment of, 421–437
  nutrition and (*see* nutrition and performance)
  nutritional supplements and, 524
  pulmonary system and, 224–225
  sodium buffer ingestion and, 235b
  training for (*see* training)
perimysium, 141, 142f
periodization, of strength training, 280b
peripheral chemoreceptors, 220, 221f
peripheral fatigue, 410–411
peripheral feedback, 277, 277f
peripheral nervous system (PNS), 121
  relationship with central nervous system, 121, 122f
  sections of, 121, 122f
peripheral neuropathy, 340
peripheral resistance, 266, 267
permissive hormones, 94
peroxidases, 30
personal record (PR), 500
pH. *See also* acid-base balance
  calculation of, 236
  defined, 231
  in enzyme reaction, 30, 31f
  intense exercise and, 238f
  normal values, 231, 231f

oxyhemoglobin dissociation curve and, 213–215, 214f
  scale, 231, 231f
  work rate and blood concentrations changes in, 238f
pharmacologic stress tests, 307b
pharynx, 201, 202
phosphagen system, 34
phosphatases, 30
phosphates
  high-energy, 33
  inorganic (P_i), 33
phosphocreatine (PC), 147f. *See also* ATP–PC system
  in ATP production, 33
  depletion in exercise, 35b
  as energy source, 526b
  in muscle contraction, 412
  performance and, 524
phosphodiesterase, 78, 343
phosphofructokinase (PFK), 47, 529
phospholipase C, 76, 78, 78f
phospholipids, 32, 372
phosphoric acid, 32
phosphorous, 364, 370–371t
phosphorylase, 47, 63b, 64b
phosphorylation, 34, 40, 43. *See also* oxidative phosphorylation
photon absorptiometry, 378
phrenic nerves, 204
physical activity. *See also* exercise
  bone health and, 351b
  defined, 321
  dose-response and health, 323–325, 323b
  energy expenditure and, 395–396, 395f
  favorable changes due to, 322
  objectives, 296
  sequence of, 329–331
  in weight control, 397b
Physical Activity and Health: A Report of the Surgeon General, 293, 321, 324b
Physical Activity Readiness Questionnaire (PAR-Q), 300, 301f, 304
physical fitness
  corporate interest in, 6–7, 6f
  defined, 321
  historical overview, 5–7
  public health concern, 6
physical inactivity, 395, 395f
  as disease risk factor, 291b, 292–293
  heart disease risk, 321
  maximal oxygen uptake and, 266b
  muscle atrophy due to, 155–156, 157b
  as risk factor, 300
  type 2 diabetes and, 341
physiological testing
  anaerobic power (*see* anaerobic power testing)
  approaches to, 422
  athlete gain by, 422–423
  benefits of, 422–423
  components, 423–424
  critical power measurement, 428, 428f
  distance running, estimating success in, 429–430, 430f

distance running, peak running velocity, 426b
  endurance performance tests, 426–428
  ethics of, 418, 422
  exercise economy, 429
  limitations of, 423
  maximal aerobic power, 424–425
  muscular strength (*see* muscular strength evaluation)
  power tests, 430–434
  predicting future champions, 430b
  reliability of, 423b
  specificity of, 424–425
  test protocols, 425
physiology, disease risk and, 294–295
Physiology of Bodily Exercise (Lagrange), 8
picograms, hormone measurement, 75
piloerection (goosebumps), 248
pituitary glands, 79
  anterior, 79
  hormones released by, 79–81, 80f
  posterior, 79
placebo, 523, 523f
plasma
  in blood, 186, 186f
  hormone concentration in, 75
  transport protein in, 75
plasma erythropoietin (EPO), 505b
plasma free fatty acids, 67
plasma glucose. *See* blood glucose
plasma membrane, 24
plasma volume, 75–76
  endurance training and, 266
  heat acclimatization, 254
platelets, 186, 186f
pleura, 201, 202, 202f
pneumotaxic area, brain stem, 220
pollution, air, 516–518
polysaccharides, 31
polyunsaturated fats, 373
pons, 220
population attributable risk, 293
Position Stand on the Prevention of Thermal Injuries During Distance Running (ACSM), 511
posterior hypothalamus, 247, 248
posterior pituitary gland, 79, 90t
posture, brain stem and, 133
potassium, 364, 370–371t
  blood levels and ventilation, 220–221, 221f
  electrical activity in neurons, 125
  as major mineral, 24
  ventilatory response to exercise, 223
potassium-40, 378
potency, in dose-response relationship, 322
power
  defined, 108
  measurement of, 109–111
power tests, defined, 431
pregame meals, 491–492, 491t

pregnancy
  exercise during, 352–354
  obesity and, 384
  training during, 466
preload, 183, 265
preseason conditioning, 457, 457f
President's Council on Physical Fitness, 6
President's Council on Physical Fitness and Sports, 6
President's Council on Youth Fitness, 6
pressure receptors. *See* baroreceptors
primary risk factors, 293b
progesterone, 87, 88f
progressive resistance exercise (PRE), 450
prolactin, 79, 80f, 90t
prolonged exercise
  carbohydrates and, 481f
  cardiovascular response, 194, 194f
  fuel selection and, 63–64, 64f
  in hot environment, 217–218, 252
  metabolic response, 58
  proteins as fuel source, 67–68
  respiratory muscle and, 206b
  shift from carbohydrate metabolism toward fat metabolism, 64f
Promoting Health/Preventing Disease: Objectives for the Nation, 296
propranolol, 92, 97, 348
proprioceptive neuromuscular facilitation (PNF), 456
proprioceptors, 129–130
prostaglandins
  in dysmenorrhea, 465
  muscle soreness and, 453
  in Zone diet, 480b
proteases, 68
protein kinase C, 78
protein synthesis
  in cell, 26f
  steps in, 26f
proteins
  biosynthesis, 32–33
  dietary goals for athletes, 484–485
  energy and, 32–33, 40–41
  as exercise fuel source, 67–68
  extracellular buffers, 235
  metabolic pool and, 41f
  as nutrients, 373–374
  as nutrition supplements, 525t
  requirements during exercise, 482–483, 485
  stress (*see* stress proteins)
  transport protein, 75
provitamins, 364
Public Health Service, 6
pulmonary circuit, 171
pulmonary circulation, 211, 211f
pulmonary diseases. *See* respiratory diseases
pulmonary respiration, 201
pulmonary semilunar valve, 170
pulmonary system
  conducting zone, 202, 203f, 204
  maximal exercise performance, 224–225

respiratory zone, 202, 203f, 204
pulmonary ventilation. *See* ventilation
pulmonary volume, 208–209, 209t
pulse pressure, 176
purging, 465
Purkinje fibers, 179
pyridoxine (vitamin B-6), 366–367t
pyrogens, 248
pyruvate, formation of, 38
pyruvate oxidase activity, 490
pyruvic acid, 34
    Krebs cycle intermediates and, 64–65
    lactic acid and, 36, 38b, 56b, 60

Q
QRS complex, ECG, 179–180, 180f, 181f
Q_{10} effect, 56
Quebec 10-second test, 432–433

R
radiation, 249, 249f, 250f
    heat loss and, 243
radiography, 378
rate-pressure product, 193
Rating of Perceived Exertion (RPE), 306–307, 306t, 481, 487f, 531
receptors, 18. *See also* chemoreceptors
    baroreceptors, 195, 196, 196f
    in biological control, 17, 18f
    hormone-receptor interaction, 76, 78
    mechanoreceptors, 195, 196f
    skeletal muscle, 163–164
    skin temperature, 247–248
reciprocal inhibition, 130
recombinant human GH (rhGH), 82b
Recommended Dietary Allowances (RDAs), 362
rectal temperature, 243, 249f
red blood cells (RBCs)
    hematocrit and, 186, 186f
    oxygen-hemoglobin dissociation curve and, 215f
    2, 3 diphosphoglyceric acid concentrations, 215
reducing agent, 27
reductases, 30
reduction, defined, 27
reference standards, gas volumes, A–2
reflexes, sensory information and, 129–131
registry assemblies, 43
Rehabilitation of the Coronary Patient (Wenger and Hellerstein), 347
rehydration. *See* water replacement
relative humidity (RH)
    evaporative heat loss, 244, 245
    temperature, vapor pressure and, 245, 245t
relative $\dot{V}O_2$, 117
relative weight (RW), 377, 384
releasing hormones, 79

renin, 83, 84f
repeated bout effect, 453, 453f, 454b
repetition, defined, 446
repetitions maximum (RM), 280b
repolarization, 126
reproductive disorders, 89b
research
    as career specialty, 10
    historical overview, 8–10
    journals, 10
    mechanistic, 17b
    placebo, 523, 523f
    research design, 262, 523–524, 523f
    subject selection, 523
Research Quarterly, 8
residual volume (RV), 208
resistance exercise, progressive, 450
resistance training. *See* strength training
Resource Manual for Guidelines for Exercise Testing and Prescription (ACSM), 347
respiration, defined, 201. *See also* ventilation
respiratory chain. *See* electron transport chain
respiratory compensation, 238
respiratory control center, 219, 220, 220f, 221–222
respiratory diseases. *See also* names of *specific disorders*
    exercise and infections, 263, 264b
respiratory exchange ratio (R), 61, 62t
respiratory pump, 184
respiratory quotient (RQ), 389, 390f
respiratory system, 200–226
    acid-base balance and, 236
    airway resistance, 206–207
    altitude and, 503
    breathing, mechanics of, 204–207
    bulk flow in, 204
    carbon dioxide transport in, 213–217
    cellular respiration, 201
    conducting zone, 202, 203f, 204
    diffusion of gases in, 210–211
    exercise and (*see* exercise)
    lungs (*see* lungs)
    major organs of, 202f
    muscles of, 205f, 206b
    oxygen transport in, 213–217
    pulmonary physiology symbols, 207
    pulmonary respiration, 201
    respiratory control center, 221–222, 222f
    structure of, 201–204
    ventilation, pulmonary (*see* ventilation)
respiratory zone, 202, 203f, 204
responders, 526b
rest, energy requirements at, 53
rest interval, 446
resting membrane potential, 124–126, 125f
resting metabolic rate (RMR), 391, 392, 393

rest-to-exercise transitions, 53–54
reticular formation, 133
retinopathy, diabetic, 340
reversibility principle, 262
Ribisl, Paul M., 385b
riboflavin (vitamin B-2), 364, 366–367t
risk factors, epidemiology and, 290
Ritchie, Murdoch, 4b
RNA, messenger (mRNA), 26b
Robinson, Sid, 5
Rowell, Loring, 10
RPE (rating of perceived exertion), 306–307, 306t, 328, 481, 487f, 531
rugby, head injuries from, 134b
runner's high, 85b
running
    altitude and, 505
    asthma and, 344
    cardiorespiratory fitness tests, 302–304
    distance running, estimating success in, 429–430, 430f
    economy in, 117, 117f, 429–430, 430f
    energy expenditure, 112–113, 113f
    hyponatremia and, 489b
    interval training distances, 445t
    maximal oxygen uptake and, 308, 426b
    net caloric cost per mile, 398, 398t
    peak running velocity and performance, 426b
    power tests, 431–432, 431f, 434
    training programs and maximal oxygen uptake, 263

S
salt. *See* sodium
sarcolemma, 141, 142, 142f, 411
sarcomeres, 142, 412
sarcopenia, 157
sarcoplasm, 24
sarcoplasmic reticulum, 48, 142, 142f, 144f, 148, 411
Sargent, Dudley, 6
satellite cells, 141
saturated fats, 373
saturation, 76
scalene muscles, 204
Schmit-Nielsen, Bodil, 3
Scholander, Peter F., 5
Schwann cells, 122, 123f
screening
    for asthma, 344b
    for cardiorespiratory fitness testing, 300
    in exercise prescription, 325
SCUBA diving, asthma and, 472
Sears, Barry, 480b
second messengers, 76, 78, 92
secondary ending, 163
secondary hypertension, 176
secondary risk factors, 293b
sedentary lifestyle. *See* physical inactivity
seizures, exercise and, 472
selenium, 364, 370–371t
Selye, Hans, 85b, 94

semilunar valves, 170
sensory neurons, muscle, 163
sensory receptors, 129
serotonin, fatigue and, 410
set, defined, 446
set point, in obesity, 387–388, 387f, 388f
sex steroids, 83
sham reinfusion of blood, 528
sham withdrawal of blood, 528
Sheldon, W. H., 492
shivering, 243, 248, 256, 257, 393, 513, 515, 516
shoes, 329, 340
shortness of breath. *See* dyspnea
short-term exercise
    altitude and anaerobic performance, 500–501
    intense, metabolic response, 57
SI (system international) units, 107
    for power, 108
    for quantifying human exercise, 107t
    terms and units for expression of, 108t
side effects, in dose-response relationship, 322
sinoatrial (SA) node, 178, 182
Siri equation, 382
skeletal muscle, 140–165
    acid-base disturbances in, 233b
    actions, 158–159
    age-related changes, 157–158
    atrophy, 155–157
    biochemical and contractile characteristics of, 149, 151–155
    blood flow to, during exercise, 190
    caffeine and, 531
    connective tissue surrounding, 142f
    contraction (*see* muscle contraction)
    Cori cycle and, 68b
    diaphragm, 204
    exercise-induced changes in, 155
    extensors, 141
    fiber types, 149
    flexors, 141
    force regulation, 160
    force-velocity/power-velocity relationships, 161–163
    functions of, 141
    gene therapy and muscle mass, 157–158, 158b
    insulin resistance and, 294
    lactate production, 69b
    length-tension relationships, 160, 161f
    microstructure, 143f
    muscle pump, 184
    neuromuscular junction, 143–144
    oxygen delivery to, 170
    receptors, 163–164
    space flight effects on, 156, 156b, 157b, 414b
    speed of action and relaxation, 159–160
    structure of, 141–143
    vasodilation and, 191

skeletal muscle fibers
  ATPase activity, 149, 151, 152, 152b, 154t
  cardiac muscle fibers *versus*, 172, 173t
  characteristics of fiber types, 152–154, 154t
  composition in athletes, 155t
  contractile properties, 151–152
  disease risk and fiber type, 295b
  efficiency of, 152
  endurance training, 157f
  exercise training and, 155
  fast fibers (*see* fast-twitch (type IIx) muscle fibers)
  force-velocity/power-velocity relationships, 161–162, 162f
  oxidative capacity, 149
  performance and fiber types, 154–155
  slow fibers (*see* slow-twitch (type I) muscle fibers)
  types of, 60, 152b
skin temperature, 242. *See also* body temperature
  heat loss and, 244–245
  measurement of, 243
  receptors, 247–248
skinfold thickness, in body composition analysis, 379, 380, 382–383, 386, 397
sleep, in cold environments, 257
sleep apnea, obesity and, 384
sliding filament model (muscle contraction), 144–145, 146f
slope, in dose-response relationship, 322
slow-acting hormones, 94
slow-twitch (type I) muscle fibers
  characteristics, 152–153
  classification, 149
  exercise alteration of, 155, 157f
  exercise intensity and, 60
  exertion of force, 154b
smokeless tobacco, 535
smoking, 347, 384, 535
Snow, John, 289
soccer, running tests for, 432
sodium, 364, 365, 368, 370–371t
  electrical activity in neurons, 125
  hypertension and intake of, 347
  as major mineral, 24
  salt replacement and exercise, 487–488
  in sweat, 488
sodium bicarbonate, 235b
sodium buffers, performance and, 235b
sodium citrate, 235b
sodium/potassium pump, 126, 126f
"Soft American, The" (Kennedy), 6
somatic motor function, 131–132
somatomedins, 79
somatostatin, 86
somatotype, 492–495, 493f, 494f
soreness. *See* muscle soreness

space flight, muscle adaptations in, 156, 156b, 157b, 414b
spatial summation, 127
special populations, exercise for, 337–354
specialization, in research, 10
specific heat, 246
specificity, in training, 262, 459
sperm production, 86, 86f
sphygmomanometer, 176, 177f
spinal cord, motor function and, 134–135
spirogram, 208f, 209f
spirometer, 208f, 209
spirometry, 112, 112f, 208
splanchnic blood flow, exercise intensity and, 189, 189f
sports. *See also* female athletes; male athletes
  acid-base disturbance risk and, 233t
  anaerobic/aerobic energy production, 49f
  energy systems for, 443t
  exercise physiology applied to, 35b
  in exercise program, 330–331
  head injuries in, 134, 134b
sports drinks
  carbohydrate, 66b, 483b
  for children, 471b
  for water replacement, 253b
Sports Illustrated, 6
sports medicine, 3
sports nutrition, 3
sports physiology, 3
ST segment depression, 306, 306f
stage of exhaustion, in general adaptation syndrome, 84
stage of resistance, in general adaptation syndrome, 84
StairMaster, 316
standard error (SE), 310b
Standard Metabolic Rate, 393
standard temperature pressure dry (STPD), A–2
starches, dietary, 32, 368
Starnes, Joe, 175b
starvation
  acidosis and, 232b
  basal metabolic rate and, 392f
static exercise, 158
static stretching, 456
steady state, 15
steady-state oxygen uptake, 3b
stenosis of aortic valve, 469b
stents, 348
step tests, 304, 314–316, 315f, 316f
sternocleidomastoids, 204
steroids, 32
  anabolic, 86, 87b
  androgenic, 86, 87b
  classification of, 83
  glucocorticoids, 83
  mechanism of action, 77f
  mineralocorticoids, 83
  secretion of, 82
  sex steroids, 83
  structure, 74–75
stimulus strength, force of contraction and, 160, 160f
STPD (standard temperature pressure dry), A–2

strength training
  age-related muscle mass and, 158b
  anabolic steroids in, 87b
  arm flexor strength of men and women, 452, 452f
  bone health and, 350
  in children, 470, 471b
  contractile proteins, exercise and, 26b
  for diabetics, 341
  endurance training combined with, 281, 451
  equipment, weight-training programs, 452t
  free weights *vs.* machines, 451
  gender and, 451, 453f
  muscle fiber alterations and, 155
  muscular enlargement, 280–281
  neural adaptations, 279–280
  nutritional supplements for, 524, 525t
  periodization of, 280b
  in physical fitness program, 331
  physiological mechanisms, 278–281, 448–449
  single sets *vs.* multiple sets, 332b, 450b
stress proteins
  in cellular homeostasis, 20, 21b
  exercise and, 174b, 175b
  in heat acclimatization, 255
stretch reflex, 163
stretching, 325, 456, 536
stroke
  obesity and, 384
  risks for, 177
stroke volume (SV)
  cardiac output during exercise and, 188
  defined, 181
  end diastolic volume, 183, 183f
  in endurance athletes, 181t, 189b
  endurance training and, 265–266
  increase in, 266f
  maximal oxygen uptake and, 264–265
  prolonged exercise, 194, 194f
  regulation of, 183–185, 183f
  rest to exercise transition and recovery from exercise, 192, 192f
  work rate and, 188f
strong acids, 231
strong bases, 231
substrate, enzyme, 28
substrate mobilization, hormonal control of, during exercise, 92–101
substrate-level phosphorylation, 40
succinate dehydrogenase, 269t
sucrose, 31
sudden cardiac death
  during exercise, 195b
  in young athletes, 469b
sugars, dietary, 368
sulfur, 364
sulfur dioxide, 517

sulfuric acid, 232
summation, 160, 161f
supercompensation, 479
surfactant, 204
Surgeon General's Report on Physical Activity and Health, 7b
sweat clothing, heat acclimatization and training in, 255b
sweating, 471b
  in football players, 252
  gender and, 253
  heat adaptation and, 249
  heat loss and, 244
  hypothalamus and, 248
  rates, during exercise, 251–252, 251f
  sodium content in sweat, 488
  sweat rate during exercise, 488
swimming
  asthma and, 344
  in exercise program, 330
  interval training distances, 445t
  during pregnancy, 466
  training programs and maximal oxygen uptake, 263
sympathetic division, of autonomic nervous system, 136
sympathetic nervous system
  in blood glucose regulation, 98, 99f
  heart rate and, 182
  insulin levels and, 294
sympathomimetic drugs, 530
synapses, 122, 127, 128f
synaptic cleft, 128
synaptic transmission, 124f, 127–129
Syndrome X (Metabolic Syndrome), 294–295, 296, 296b, 373b
systemic circulation, 211, 211f
systole, 174, 175f, 176f
systolic blood pressure, 176, 193

T

T wave, ECG, 180, 180f, 181f
"talk test," 353–354
tapering, 459
target heart rate (THR) range, 327–328, 328f
  direct method of estimation, 327
  environment and, 332
  indirect methods of estimation, 327
Taylor, Henry Longstreet, 8
temperature
  of body (*see* body temperature)
  enzymes and, 30, 31f
  heat injuries and, 510
  oxygen-hemoglobin dissociation curve, 214–215, 214f
  relative humidity, vapor pressure and, 245, 245t
temporal summation, 127
ten percent rule, in training, 447
tensiometers, 435, 435f
terminal cisternae (lateral sac), 142, 148
testes, 86, 91t
testosterone, 86, 86f, 87b, 91t
tetanic contractions, 160

tetanus, 161f
defined, 160
theophylline, 343
thermic effect of food, 393
thermistors, 243
thermocouples, 243
thermogenesis, 392, 393–394
nonshivering, 248, 256, 257, 393
thermoregulation, gender and age differences, 253–254
thiamin (vitamin B-1), 364, 366–367t
thigh muscle fiber types, succinate dehydrogenase and, 269t
thirst, 83–84, 84f
thorax, 204
three-component model, in body composition analysis, 379
thyroid gland, 81–82, 90t
thyroid hormones, 81, 94
thyroid-stimulating hormone (TSH), 79, 80f, 90t, 94
thyroxine (T$_4$), 90t, 94
function of, 81
in heat production, 243, 248
transport protein and, 75
tidal volume, 207
Tipton, C. M., 9
Tolerable Upper Intake Level (UL), 362, 364
tonic seizures, 472
total body electrical conductivity (TOBEC), 379
total body water (TBW), 378
total fiber, 369
total lung capacity (TLC), 208
total vascular resistance, mean arterial blood pressure and, 177
toxicity, vitamins, 364
trace elements, 364
trachea, 201, 202, 203f
training
for aerobic power (see aerobic power training)
age and, 278b
for anaerobic power improvement, 447–448
asthma and, 472
ATP-PC system improvement, 448
children and cardiopulmonary system, 469
chronic obstructive pulmonary disease and, 345–346
common mistakes of, 458–459
for competition at altitude, 504–505
components of, 444
diabetes and, 470–472
for endurance (see endurance training)
epilepsy and, 472–473
for flexibility, 456
glycolytic system improvement, 448
injuries from, 447
lung adaptations, 224
maximal oxygen uptake and, 264–265
menstruation and, 465, 467b

metabolism (see exercise metabolism)
for muscular strength (see strength training)
musculoskeletal system in children and, 469–470
overload principle, 261–262, 442–443
for performance, 441–459
physiology of, 260–281
during pregnancy, 466
principles of, 261–262, 442–444
research designs, 262
reversibility principle, 262, 442–443
specificity principle, 262, 442–443, 459
in sweat clothing in cool conditions, 255b
ten percent rule, 447
year-round conditioning, 457–458, 457f
training effect
endurance training and, 275–277, 276f
exercise in elderly, 352b
transaminases, 30
transcarboxylases, 30
transcription, genetic, 26b
transferases, 30
transferrin, 365
transfusion, blood, 528
transport protein, 75
transverse tubules, 142, 144f, 148, 411
treadmill, 109f
calculation of work performed, 110
electrocardiogram exercises, 179b
graded exercise test protocols, 312–313, 312f
net efficiency, 115
percent grade for, 110, 111f
protocols, 311t
tricuspid valve, 170
triglycerides, 32, 40, 372
metabolism, 67
triiodothyronine (T$_3$), 81, 90t, 94
tropomyosin, 147, 147f, 148
troponin, in muscle contraction, 147, 147f, 148
TSH (thyroid-stimulating hormone), 79, 80f, 90t, 94
tubule, kidney, 236
twenty-four-hour recall method, 375
twins, training programs, 263
twitch, 159, 159t
two-component model, in body composition analysis, 379, 380–384
tympanic temperature, 243
Type I muscle fibers. See slow-twitch (type I) muscle fibers
Type IIa muscle fibers, 153–154
Type IIb muscle fibers, 152, 153b
Type IIx muscle fibers. See fast-twitch (type IIx) muscle fibers

U

ultrasound, 378
undertraining, 458

underwater weighing, 380–382, 381f
United States Air Force, 9b
universal energy donor, ATP as, 33
upper respiratory tract infections (URTI), exercise and, 274b
up-regulation, hormonal, 76
U.S. Department of Agriculture, 360, 369b, 374
U.S. Department of Health and Human Services, 296
U.S. dietary goals, 361

V

vagus nerve, 182
valine, 33
Van Slyke blood-gas analyzer, 5
vanadium, 364, 525t
vapor, temperature, relative humidity and, 245, 245t
vapor pressure, 244
variability, in dose-response relationship, 322
variable, defined, 15b
variable-resistance exercise, 448
variable-resistance isokinetic dynamometer, 436
variable-resistance measurement of strength, 437
Varieties of Human Physique, The (Sheldon), 492
vasoconstriction, 190
vasodilation, 191, 191b
vasopressin, 79, 90t
veins, 170
velocity-force/velocity-power relationships, 161–162, 162f
venoconstriction, 184
ventilation. *See also* respiratory system
acid-base balance and, 217
altitude and, 503, 503f
alveolar, 207
control of, 219–224
defined, 201
hypoxic threshold, 221, 221f
mechanics of, 204, 206–207
potassium blood levels and, 220–221, 221f
pulmonary, defined, 207
pulmonary physiology symbols, 207
ventilation-perfusion ratio, 212–213, 212f
ventilation and exercise
blood-gas responses, 217–218
endurance training, 223b
exercise-induced asthma, 344
heavy exercise, 222
incremental exercise, 218, 219f
inspiration, 204
prolonged exercise in hot environment, 217–218
regulation at rest, 219–220
rest-to-work transitions, 217
submaximal exercise, 222
ventilation-perfusion ratio (V/Q), 212–213, 212f
ventilatory and blood-gas responses to exercise, 217–218

ventilation threshold (Tvent), 218
ventilatory threshold (Tvent), 427, 427f
ventricles, heart, 211
venules, 170
vestibular apparatus, 132, 132f
Vibrio cholerae, 289
visceral pleura, 201, 202f
vital capacity (VC), 208, 209f
vitamin A, 364, 366–367t, 525t
vitamin B-1 (thiamin), 364, 366–367t
vitamin B-2 (riboflavin), 364, 366–367t
vitamin B-6 (pyridoxine), 364, 366–367t
vitamin B-12, 364, 366–367t
vitamin C (ascorbic acid), 364, 366–367t, 525t
vitamin D, 366–367t
vitamin E, 366–367t, 525t
vitamin K, 366–367t
vitamins
deficiency diseases, 364
Dietary Reference Intake for, A–20–A–23
fat-soluble, 364
functions and food sources, 366–367t
immune function and, 274b
precursor forms, 364
supplemental, for athletes, 490
water-soluble, 364
Vmax, 151, 152, 152b, 154t
$\dot{V}O_2$ max. *See* maximal oxygen uptake ($\dot{V}O_2$ max)
$\dot{V}O_2$ Reserve ($\dot{V}O_2$ R) method for prescribing exercise intensity, 327b
volatile acids, 232
voluntary heat production, 243, 244
voluntary movement, 135f, 136
vomiting, self-induced, 465

W

walk tests, 304, 308, 313
walking
asthma and, 344
energy expenditure, 112–113, 113f
in exercise program, 329, 350
net caloric cost per mile, 398, 398t
program for, 330t
war, physical fitness and, 6
warm-ups
benefits of, 536
in exercise prescription, 325
in training session, 444
water
cold water injuries, 513
cooling and, 245
doubly labeled, 391
electrolytes and, 486–488
loss during exercise, 486
as nutrient, 363–364
in respiratory exchange ratio, 61
shipwrecked individuals and temperature of, 513, 515f
total body water, 378
weight fluctuation, 364

water replacement
  in children, 471b
  before exercise, 486
  during exercise, 252, 253b, 488f
  loss during exercise, 486–488
  sports drinks for, 253b
water vapor pressure, 515, A–2
  correction for, A–3
  heat injuries and, 510
water-soluble vitamins, 364
web of causation, 290, 290f, 292, 296
weight control
  basal metabolic rate, 391
  caloric intake in, 388, 389, 394, 395f
  diabetes and, 341b
  diet and, 390–391
  diet vs. exercise, 394b
  dietary supplements, 388b
  drugs for, 388b

energy expenditure and, 388, 391–399
fat balance and, 389–390
fat cells and, 386, 386f
nutrient balance in, 389–390
obesity and (see obesity)
overfeeding, 393
physical activity in, 397b
thyroid and, 81
walking for, 329
water weight, 364
weight loss vs. weight maintenance, 396–399
weight gain, aging and, 374
weight training. See strength training
Weight Watchers, 391
Wet Bulb GlobeTemperature (WBGT), 512
wheezing, 342
white blood cells (WBCs), hematocrit and, 186, 186f
whole-body density, 380
Willett, Walter, 374

wind, heat injury and, 510
wind chill index, 513, 514t
Wing, Rena, 397b
Wingate test, 433, 433t
women. See female athletes; gender
Woods, Joseph J., 4b
work
  defined, 107
  energy expenditure, measurement of, 111–112
  measurement of, 109–111
  treadmill exercise output, 110
  units of measurement, 107–108, 107f, 108f, 108t
work interval, 446
work rate, 108, 188f, 309, 311, 313
  energy expenditure, 116f
  exercise efficiency and, 115–116, 116f
work time to exhaustion, muscle glycogen concentration and, 478, 478f

workout, 444
World Anti-Doping Agency Web site, 87b
World War I, 6
World War II, 6
wrestling, head injuries from, 134b

Y

year-round conditioning, 457
YMCA (Young Mens' Christian Association), submaximal graded exercise test protocols, 313, 314, 314f
Youth Fitness Test, 6

Z

Z line, sliding filament model and, 144
zinc, 24, 364, 370–371t
Zone Diet, 391, 480b